Developmental-
Behavioral
Pediatrics

Developmental-Behavioral Pediatrics

3rd EDITION

Melvin D. Levine, M.D.

Professor of Pediatrics
Director, The Clinical Center for the
    Study of Development and Learning
University of North Carolina Medical School
Chapel Hill, North Carolina
Cochairman of the Board, All Kinds of Minds,
    A Non-Profit Institute Dedicated
    to the Understanding of Differences
    in Learning

William B. Carey, M.D.

Director of Behavioral Pediatrics
Division of General Pediatrics
Children's Hospital of Philadelphia
University of Pennsylvania School of Medicine
Philadelphia, Pennsylvania

Allen C. Crocker, M.D.

Program Director, Institute for Community Inclusion
Children's Hospital
Harvard Medical School
Boston, Massachusetts

W.B. SAUNDERS COMPANY
A Division of Harcourt Brace & Company
Philadelphia • London • Toronto • Montreal • Sydney • Tokyo

W.B. SAUNDERS COMPANY
A Division of Harcourt Brace & Company

The Curtis Center
Independence Square West
Philadelphia, Pennsylvania 19106

Library of Congress Cataloging-in-Publication Data

Developmental-behavioral pediatrics / [edited by] Melvin D. Levine, William B. Carey, Allen C. Crocker.—3rd ed.

p.   cm.

Includes bibliographical references and index.

ISBN 0–7216–7154–3

1. Pediatrics.   2. Pediatrics—Psychological aspects.   3. Child development.   4. Child psychology.   I. Levine, Melvin D.   II. Carey, William B.   III. Crocker, Allen C. [DNLM: 1. Child Development   2. Child Behavior.   3. Child Behavior Disorders.   4. Developmental Disabilities.   WS 105 D48912 1999]

RJ47.D48 1999   618.92'8—dc21

DNLM/DLC   98–12901

DEVELOPMENTAL-BEHAVIORAL PEDIATRICS   ISBN 0–7216–7154–3

Printed in the United States of America.

Last digit is the print number: 9   8   7   6   5   4   3   2   1

Contributors

George L. Askew, M.D. Assistant Professor of Pediatrics and Public Health, Boston University School of Medicine/School of Public Health; Medical Director, Pediatric Inpatient Service, Boston Medical Center, Boston, Massachusetts.
The Neighborhood: Poverty, Affluence, Geographic Mobility, and Violence

Marilyn Augustyn, M.D. Assistant Professor of Pediatrics, Boston University School of Medicine, Department of Pediatrics, Division of Developmental and Behavioral Pediatrics, and Boston Medical Center, Boston, Massachusetts.
Infancy and Toddler Years

Stephen A. Back, M.D. Instructor in Neurology, Harvard Medical School; Children's Hospital, Boston, Massachusetts.
Cerebral Palsy

Marion Taylor Baer, M.S., Ph.D. Professor of Clinical Pediatrics, University of Southern California School of Medicine; Adjunct Associate Professor, Department of Community Health Sciences, University of California, Los Angeles, School of Public Health; Associate Director and Nutrition Director, Center for Child Development and Developmental Disabilities, University of Southern California/Children's Hospital, Los Angeles, California.
Effects of Nutrition on Development and Behavior

Martin Baren, M.D. Clinical Professor of Pediatrics, University of California at Irvine Medical School, Irvine, California.
Pediatric Psychopharmacology

William Beardslee, M.D. Gardner Monks Professor of Psychiatry, Harvard Medical School; Chairman, Department of Psychiatry, Children's Hospital, Boston, Massachusetts.
Psychotherapy With Children

Myron L. Belfer, M.D., M.P.A. Professor of Psychiatry in the Department of Social Medicine, Harvard Medical School; Senior Associate in Psychiatry, Children's Hospital, Boston, Massachusetts.
Body Image: Development and Distortion

Rosemarie Bigsby, Sc.D. Clinical Assistant Professor of Pediatrics, Brown University School of Medicine, Providence; Coordinator of NICU Services for Infant Development Unit, Women and Infants Hospital, Providence, Rhode Island.
Stresses and Interventions in the Neonatal Intensive Care Unit

Boris Birmaher, M.D. Associate Professor of Psychiatry, University of Pittsburgh School of Medicine; Director, Child and Adolescent Bipolar Services, and Medical Director, Services for Teens at Risk (STAR), Western Psychiatric Institute and Clinic, Pittsburgh, Pennsylvania.
Major Psychiatric Disorders in Childhood and Adolescence

James A. Blackman, M.D., M.P.H. Professor of Pediatrics, University of Virginia School of Medicine; Director of Research, Kluge Children's Rehabilitation Center, Charlottesville, Virginia.
Developmental Screening: Infants, Toddlers, and Preschoolers

Nathan J. Blum, M.D. Assistant Professor of Pediatrics, University of Pennsylvania School of Medicine; Medical Director, Behavioral Pediatrics Clinic, Children's Seashore House, Philadelphia, Pennsylvania.
Repetitive Behaviors

W. Thomas Boyce, M.D. Professor of Epidemiology and Child Development, School of Public Health and Institute of Human Development, University of California, Berkeley; Head, Division of Health and Medical Sciences, University of California, Berkeley, Berkeley, California.
Critical Life Events: Sibling Births, Separations, and Deaths in the Family

M. Patricia Boyle, Ph.D. Instructor in Psychology, Harvard Medical School; Associate in Psychology, Department of Psychiatry, Children's Hospital, Boston, Massachusetts.
Evolving Parenthood: A Developmental Perspective

David Brent, M.D. Professor of Child Psychiatry, Pediatrics, and Epidemiology, University of Pittsburgh School of Medicine; Chief, Division of Child and Adolescent Psychiatry, and Director, Services for Teens at Risk (STAR), Western Psychiatric Institute and Clinic, Pittsburgh, Pennsylvania.
Major Psychiatric Disorders in Childhood and Adolescence

Christine M. Burns, Ed.M., M.B.A. Clinical Assistant Professor of Pediatrics, School of Medicine and Dentistry, University of Rochester, Rochester, New York.
Visual Impairment and Blindness

Bettye M. Caldwell, Ph.D. Professor, Department of Pediatrics, University of Arkansas for Medical Sciences, Little Rock, Arkansas.
Child Care

John Campo, M.D. Assistant Professor of Psychiatry and Pediatrics, University of Pittsburgh School of Medicine, Western Psychiatric Institute and Clinic; Director, Behavioral Science Division, Children's Hospital of Pittsburgh, Pittsburgh, Pennsylvania.
Major Psychiatric Disorders in Childhood and Adolescence

William B. Carey, M.D. Director of Behavioral Pediatrics, Division of General Pediatrics, Children's Hospital of Philadelphia, University of Pennsylvania School of Medicine, Philadelphia, Pennsylvania.
Acute Minor Illness; "Colic": Prolonged or Excessive Crying in Young Infants; Pediatric Assessment of Behavioral Adjustment and Behavioral Style; Comprehensive Formulation of Assessment; The Right to Be Different

Patrick H. Casey, M.D. Harvey and Bernice Jones Professor of Developmental Pediatrics, Department of Pediatrics, University of Arkansas for Medical Sciences; Director, Center for Applied Research and Evaluation and Director, Division of Developmental-Behavioral Pediatrics, Arkansas Children's Hospital, Little Rock, Arkansas.

Failure to Thrive

William J. Cashore, M.D., FAAP. Professor of Pediatrics, Brown University School of Medicine; Associate Chief of Pediatrics, Women and Infants Hospital, Providence, Rhode Island.

Stresses and Interventions in the Neonatal Intensive Care Unit

Suzanne B. Cassidy, M.D. Professor of Genetics and Pediatrics, Case Western Reserve University School of Medicine; Clinical Director for Center for Human Genetics, University Hospitals of Cleveland, Cleveland, Ohio.

Congenital Anomalies

Donna Madden Chadwick, M.T.-B.C., L.M.H.C., M.S., CCC-SLP. Faculty, Music Department, Emmanuel College, Boston; Director, Music Therapy Clinical Services, Westford, Massachusetts.

The Arts Therapies

Stella Chess, M.D. Professor of Child Psychiatry, New York University Medical Center, New York, New York.

The Development of Behavioral Individuality

Ken L. Cheyne, M.D. Associate Director of Pediatric Education, Adolescent Medicine, Blank Children's Hospital, Des Moines, Iowa.

The Emergency Department Management of Behavioral Crises

Walter P. Christian, Ph.D. Instructor in Psychology, Harvard Medical School; Adjunct Clinical Professor of Psychiatry, Boston University School of Medicine; Clinical Assistant Professor, Department of Counseling, Psychology, Rehabilitation, and Special Education, Northeastern University, Boston; Clinical Affiliate in Psychology, McLean Hospital, Belmont; Professional Staff, Developmental Evaluation Center, Children's Hospital, Boston, Massachusetts.

Legal Issues

Elin R. Cohen, M.D. Fellow in Developmental and Behavioral Pediatrics, Yale University School of Medicine, New Haven, Connecticut.

Brothers and Sisters

William I. Cohen, M.D. Associate Professor of Pediatrics and Psychiatry, University of Pittsburgh School of Medicine; Developmental/Behavioral Pediatrician and Director, Down Syndrome Center of Western Pennsylvania, Children's Hospital of Pittsburgh, Pittsburgh, Pennsylvania.

Down Syndrome: Care of the Child and Family

William Lord Coleman, M.A., M.D. Associate Professor of Pediatrics, Center for Development and Learning, Department of Pediatrics, University of North Carolina School of Medicine, Chapel Hill; Assistant Consulting Professor of Pediatrics, Duke University Medical Center, Durham, North Carolina.

Adolescent Development and Behavior: Implications for the Primary Care Physician; The Interview

Eve R. Colson, M.D. Assistant Professor of Pediatrics, Tufts University School of Medicine, Boston; Staff Pediatrician, Baystate Medical Center, Springfield, Massachusetts.

The Gifted Child

George D. Comerci, M.D. Professor of Pediatrics, University of Arizona College of Medicine, Department of Pediatrics, and Arizona Health Sciences Center, Tucson, Arizona.

Disordered Eating Behaviors: Anorexia Nervosa, Bulimia Nervosa, Cyclic Vomiting Syndrome, and Rumination Disorder

David L. Coulter, M.D. Associate Professor of Pediatrics and Neurology, Boston University School of Medicine; Director of Pediatric Neurology, Boston Medical Center, Boston, Massachusetts.

Central Nervous System Disorders

Susan E. Craig, Ph.D. Director of Training, AGH Associates, Inc., Hampton, New Hampshire.

Special Education Services for Children With Disabilities

Allen C. Crocker, M.D. Program Director, Institute for Community Inclusion, Children's Hospital, Harvard Medical School, Boston, Massachusetts.

Human Immunodeficiency Virus Infection in Children; Mental Retardation; The Child With Multiple Disabilities; The Right to Be Different

Timothy Culbert, M.D. Assistant Professor of Clinical Pediatrics, University of Minnesota Medical School, Department of Pediatrics, Minneapolis; Developmental/Behavioral Pediatrician, Alexander Center for Child Development and Behavior of the Park Nicollet Clinic, HealthSystem Minnesota, Bloomington, Minnesota.

Pediatric Self-Regulation

Philip W. Davidson, Ph.D. Professor of Pediatrics, School of Medicine and Dentistry, University of Rochester, Rochester, New York.

Visual Impairment and Blindness

Elisabeth M. Dykens, Ph.D. Assistant Professor, Psychiatry, Division of Child Psychiatry, Neuropsychiatric Institute, University of California, Los Angeles, Los Angeles, California.

Genes, Behavior, and Development

Ann R. Ernst, Ph.D. Pediatric Psychologist, Medical Associates Clinic, Dubuque, Iowa.

The Emergency Department Management of Behavioral Crises

Camille T. Fine, Ph.D. Pediatric Neuropsychologist, The Pinellas County Schools, St. Petersburg, Florida.

Neuropsychological Assessment of Children

Carol A. Ford, M.D. Assistant Professor of Pediatrics and Medicine and Director, Adolescent Medicine Program, University of North Carolina School of Medicine, Chapel Hill, North Carolina.

Adolescent Development and Behavior: Implications for the Primary Care Physician

Brian W. C. Forsyth, M.B., Ch.B. Associate Professor of Pediatrics and Child Study Center; Attending Pediatrician, Yale–New Haven Hospital, New Haven, Connecticut.

Early Health Crises and Vulnerable Children

Deborah A. Frank, M.D. Associate Professor of Pediatrics and Assistant Professor of Public Health, Boston University School of Medicine, Department of Pediat-

rics, Division of Developmental and Behavioral Pediatrics, Boston Medical Center, Boston, Massachusetts.
Infancy and Toddler Years

Carolyn H. Frazer, M.D. Instructor, Harvard Medical School; Assistant in Medicine, Children's Hospital, Boston, Massachusetts.
Recurrent Pains

Stuart Goldman, M.D. Assistant Professor of Psychiatry, Harvard Medical School; Senior Associate in Psychiatry, Children's Hospital, Boston, Massachusetts.
Psychotherapy With Children

Lauren Heim Goldstein, Ph.D. MacArthur Foundation Research Fellow, Institute of Human Development, University of California, Berkeley, Berkeley, California.
Critical Life Events: Sibling Births, Separations, and Deaths in the Family

Peter A. Gorski, M.D., M.P.A. Assistant Professor of Pediatrics, Harvard Medical School; Executive Director, Massachusetts Caring for Children Foundation; Director of Professional Education, The Brazelton Institute, Boston Children's Hospital, Boston, Massachusetts.
Pregnancy, Birth, and the First Days of Life

Robert M. Greenstein, M.D. Professor of Pediatrics and Director, Division of Human Genetics, Department of Pediatrics, University of Connecticut Health Center, Farmington, Connecticut.
Genes, Behavior, and Development

Linda Sayler Gudas, Ph.D. Instructor in Psychology, Harvard Medical School; Assistant in Psychiatry, Department of Psychology, Children's Hospital, Boston, Massachusetts.
Life-Threatening and Terminal Illness

Randi Jenssen Hagerman, M.D. Professor of Pediatrics, Department of Pediatrics, and Section Head of Developmental and Behavioral Pediatrics, University of Colorado Health Sciences Center; Co-Director of the Child Development Unit, The Children's Hospital, Denver, Colorado.
Chromosomal Disorders

Lawrence D. Hammer, M.D. Associate Professor, Department of Pediatrics, Stanford University School of Medicine, Stanford; Medical Director, Ambulatory Care Services, Lucile Packard Children's Hospital, Palo Alto, California.
Child and Adolescent Obesity

Marjorie S. Hardy, Ph.D. Assistant Professor, Department of Psychology, Muhlenberg College, Allentown, Pennsylvania.
The Emergency Department Management of Behavioral Crises

Sara Harkness, Ph.D., M.P.H. Professor, School of Family Studies, University of Connecticut, Storrs, Connecticut.
Culture and Ethnicity

Anne Bradford Harris, M.P.H., M.S., R.D. Nutrition Training Director, University of Southern California University Affiliated Program, Children's Hospital, Los Angeles, California.
Effects of Nutrition on Development and Behavior

Kathleen Hebbeler, Ph.D. Program Manager, SRI International, Menlo Park, California.
Early Intervention Services

Fred Henretig, M.D. Professor of Pediatrics, University of Pennsylvania School of Medicine; Director, Section of Clinical Toxicology, Division of Emergency Medicine, Children's Hospital of Philadelphia, Philadelphia, Pennsylvania.
Toxins

Stephen R. Hooper, Ph.D. Associate Professor, Department of Psychiatry; Psychology Section Head, Center for Development and Learning; Director, Child and Adolescent Neuropsychology, University of North Carolina School of Medicine, Chapel Hill, North Carolina.
Neuropsychological Assessment of Children

Roseanne B. Howard-Teplansky, M.P.H., R.D. Visiting Professor of Nutrition, Simmons College, Boston, Massachusetts.
Effects of Nutrition on Development and Behavior

Louanne Hudgins, M.D. Associate Professor, Department of Pediatrics, Division of Genetics and Congenital Defects, University of Washington School of Medicine; Director, Clinical Genetic Services, Children's Hospital and Regional Medical Center, Seattle, Washington.
Congenital Anomalies

Olson Huff, M.D. Associate Clinical Professor of Pediatrics, University of North Carolina School of Medicine, Chapel Hill; Medical Director of Pediatrics, Mission St. Joseph Hospital; Developmental Pediatrician, Olson Huff Center for Child Development, Thoms Rehabilitation Hospital, Asheville, North Carolina.
Developmental Assessment of the School-Aged Child

Carol Nagy Jacklin, Ph.D. Emerita Professor of Psychology, University of Southern California, Los Angeles, California.
Effects of Gender on Behavior and Development

Kathleen Bradley Kapsalis, M.M.H.S. Adjunct Faculty, Falmouth Institute for Quality Systems Management, Falmouth; Clinical Adjunct Professor, Northeastern University, Boston, Massachusetts; Founding Member, Substance Abuse Task Force; National Brain Injury Foundation, Washington, D.C.
Legal Issues

Constance H. Keefer, M.D. Instructor in Pediatrics, Harvard Medical School; Director of Newborn Nurseries, Brigham and Women's Hospital, Boston, Massachusetts.
Culture and Ethnicity

Desmond P. Kelly, M.D. Medical Director, Developmental Pediatrics, The Children's Hospital, Greenville Hospital System, Greenville; GHS Associate Professor of Pediatrics, University of South Carolina School of Medicine, Columbia, South Carolina.
Hearing Impairment; Disorders of Speech and Language

William Kessen, Ph.D. Eugene Higgins Professor of Psychology, Emeritus, and Professor of Pediatrics, Emeritus, Yale University School of Medicine, New Haven, Connecticut.
The Development of Behavior

John R. Knight, M.D. Instructor in Pediatrics, Harvard Medical School; Assistant in Medicine, Children's Hospital, Boston, Massachusetts.
Substance Use, Abuse, and Dependence

Gerald P. Koocher, Ph.D. Associate Professor,

Harvard Medical School; Chief Psychologist, Children's Hospital, Boston, Massachusetts.
Life-Threatening and Terminal Illness

Ernest F. Krug III, M.Div., M.D. Clinical Associate Professor, Department of Pediatrics, Wayne State University, Detroit; Director, Center for Human Development, and Chief, Division of Developmental-Behavioral Pediatrics, William Beaumont Hospital, Royal Oak, Michigan.
The Preschool Years

Karen Levine, Ph.D. Instructor, Harvard Medical School, Boston; Clinical Director, Autism Services, North Shore Arc, Danvers, Massachusetts.
Psychological Testing

Melvin D. Levine, M.D. Professor of Pediatrics, Director, The Clinical Center for the Study of Development and Learning, University of North Carolina Medical School, Chapel Hill, North Carolina; Cochairman of the Board, All Kinds of Minds, A Non-Profit Institute Dedicated to the Understanding of Differences in Learning.
Middle Childhood; Attention and Dysfunctions of Attention; Neurodevelopmental Variation and Dysfunction Among School-Aged Children; Social Ability and Inability; Comprehensive Formulation of Assessment; The Right to Be Different

Ronald L. Lindsay, M.D. Clinical Assistant Professor of Pediatrics, The Ohio State University College of Medicine and Public Health; Medical Director, Nisonger Center UAP, The Ohio State University, Columbus, Ohio.
Alternative Therapies

Iris F. Litt, M.D. Professor of Pediatrics, Stanford University School of Medicine; Director, Division of Adolescent Medicine, Lucile Packard Children's Hospital at Stanford, Stanford, California.
Development of Sexuality and Its Problems

Stephen Ludwig, M.D. Professor of Pediatrics and Associate Chair, Department of Pediatrics, University of Pennsylvania School of Medicine; Associate Physician-in-Chief for Education, John H. and Hortense Cassell Jensen Endowed Chair, The Children's Hospital of Philadelphia, Philadelphia, Pennsylvania.
Family Function and Dysfunction

John A. Martin, Ph.D. Clinical Psychologist, Private Practice; Director of Research, Council on Spiritual Practices, San Francisco, California.
Development of Sexuality and Its Problems

Lizbeth J. Martin, Ph.D. Assistant Professor, College of Notre Dame, Belmont, California.
Effects of Gender on Behavior and Development

Karen C. Mikus, M.Ed., Ph.D. Instructor, University of Michigan School of Social Work, Ann Arbor; Director, Early Childhood Program, Center for Human Development, William Beaumont Hospital, Royal Oak/ Berkley, Michigan.
The Preschool Years

Michael E. K. Moffatt, M.D., M.Sc., FRCP(C). Professor and Head, Department of Pediatrics and Child Health, University of Manitoba; Head of Pediatrics, Health Sciences Centre, Winnipeg, Manitoba, Canada.
Enuresis

Richard P. Nelson, M.D. Professor of Pediatrics and Executive Associate Dean, The University of Iowa College of Medicine, Iowa City, Iowa.
Mental Retardation; The Child With Multiple Disabilities

Steven L. Nickman, M.D. Clinical Assistant in Psychiatry, Harvard Medical School; Assistant in Psychiatry, Massachusetts General Hospital, Boston, Massachusetts.
Adoption and Foster Family Care

Howard J. Osofsky, M.D., Ph.D. Professor and Head, Department of Psychiatry, Louisiana State University School of Medicine, New Orleans, Louisiana.
Developmental Implications of Violence in Youth

Joy D. Osofsky, Ph.D. Professor of Pediatrics and Psychiatry, Louisiana State University School of Medicine, New Orleans, Louisiana.
Developmental Implications of Violence in Youth

Judith S. Palfrey, M.D. T. Berry Brazelton Professor, Harvard Medical School, Harvard School of Public Health; Chief, Division of General Pediatrics, Children's Hospital, Boston, Massachusetts.
Legislation for the Education of Children With Disabilities

David A. Pangburn, M.D. Clinical Preceptor, Harvard Medical School, Boston; Pediatrician, Alewife Brook Community Pediatrics, Arlington, Massachusetts.
Referral Processes

John M. Parrish, Ph.D. Associate Professor of Psychology in Pediatrics and Associate Professor of Child Psychology in Psychiatry, University of Pennsylvania School of Medicine; Head, Section of Pediatric Psychology, and Clinical Director, Biobehavioral Rehabilitation Service Line, Children's Seashore House of The Children's Hospital of Philadelphia, Philadelphia, Pennsylvania.
Child Behavior Management

Ellen C. Perrin, M.D., M.A. Professor of Pediatrics, University of Massachusetts School of Medicine, Worcester, Massachusetts.
Hospitalization, Surgery, and Medical Procedures

James M. Perrin, M.D. Associate Professor of Pediatrics, Harvard Medical School; Director, Division of General Pediatrics, Massachusetts General Hospital, Boston, Massachusetts.
Chronic Illness

Marie Kanne Poulsen, Ph.D. Professor of Clinical Pediatrics, University of Southern California School of Medicine; Psychology Director, USC University Affiliated Program, Children's Hospital, Los Angeles, California.
Effects of Nutrition on Development and Behavior

Harris Rabinovich, M.D. Associate Professor of Psychiatry, Jefferson Medical College, Division of Child and Adult Psychiatry, Philadelphia, Pennsylvania.
Major Psychiatric Disorders in Childhood and Adolescence

Leonard A. Rappaport, M.S., M.D. Associate Professor of Pediatrics, Harvard Medical School; Associate Chief, Division of General Pediatrics, Children's Hospital, Boston, Massachusetts.
Recurrent Pains

Martha S. Reed, M.Ed. Educational Specialist and Faculty Consultant, All Kinds of Minds Institute, Chapel Hill, North Carolina.
Educational Assessment

Sally M. Reis, Ph.D. Professor, Educational Psychology, University of Connecticut; Principal Investigator, National Research Center on the Gifted and Talented, Storrs, Connecticut.
The Gifted Child

Thomas N. Robinson, M.P.H., M.D. Assistant Professor, Department of Pediatrics, Stanford University School of Medicine, Stanford, California.
Child and Adolescent Obesity

Randal Rockney, M.D. Associate Professor, Pediatrics and Family Medicine, Brown University School of Medicine; Pediatrician, Hasbro Children's Hospital, Providence, Rhode Island.
Encopresis

John S. Rodman, M.D., M.P.H. Director of Quality Management Physician Services, Sarasota Memorial Hospital, Sarasota, Florida.
Legislation for the Education of Children With Disabilities

Anthony Rostain, M.D., M.S. Associate Professor of Psychiatry and Pediatrics, University of Pennsylvania School of Medicine; Attending Physician and Director, Medical Student Education in Psychiatry, The Children's Hospital of Philadelphia, Philadelphia, Pennsylvania.
Family Function and Dysfunction

Mark Ruggiero, M.D. Assistant Professor, Developmental and Behavioral Pediatrics, Oregon Health Sciences University; Developmental and Behavioral Pediatrician, Shriners Hospital for Children, Portland, Oregon.
Maladaptation to School

Janine I. Sally, M.S. Manager, Kidnetics, The Children's Hospital, Greenville Hospital System, Greenville, South Carolina.
Disorders of Speech and Language

Adrian D. Sandler, M.D. Clinical Associate Professor, Department of Pediatrics, University of North Carolina School of Medicine, Chapel Hill; Medical Director, Olson Huff Center for Child Development, Thoms Rehabilitation Hospital, Asheville, North Carolina.
Developmental Assessment of the School-Aged Child

John Sargent, M.D. Director, Education and Research, Menninger Clinic, Topeka, Kansas.
Variations in Family Composition

Neil L. Schechter, M.D. Professor of Pediatrics and Head, Division of Developmental and Behavioral Pediatrics, University of Connecticut School of Medicine, Farmington; Director, Section of Developmental and Behavioral Pediatrics, St. Francis Hospital and Medical Center, Hartford, Connecticut.
The Gifted Child

Barton D. Schmitt, M.D. Professor of Pediatrics, University of Colorado School of Medicine; Director, General Pediatrics Consultative Services, The Children's Hospital, Denver, Colorado.
Pediatric Counseling

David J. Schonfeld, M.D. Associate Professor of Pediatrics and Child Study, Yale University School of Medicine, New Haven, Connecticut.
Brothers and Sisters

Henry L. Shapiro, M.D. Assistant Professor of Pediatrics, University of South Florida College of Medicine, Tampa; Medical Director, Developmental-Behavioral Pediatrics, All Children's Hospital, St. Petersburg, Florida.
Electronic Media; Sleep Disorders

S. Norman Sherry, B.S., M.D. Clinical Assistant Professor in Pediatrics, Harvard Medical School; Consultant in Child Psychiatry, Massachusetts General Hospital;

Associate in Medicine (Pediatrics), Boston Children's Hospital, Boston, Massachusetts.
Adoption and Foster Family Care

Donna Spiker, Ph.D. Senior Research Associate, Department of Psychiatry and Behavioral Sciences, Stanford University, Stanford; Senior Research Associate, SRI International, Menlo Park, California.
Early Intervention Services

Martin T. Stein, M.D. Professor of Pediatrics, University of California, San Diego, San Diego, California.
Common Issues in Feeding

Max Sugar, M.D. Clinical Professor of Psychiatry at Louisiana State University School of Medicine, and Tulane University School of Medicine; Staff Psychiatrist, Veterans Affairs Medical Center, New Orleans, Louisiana.
Disasters

Charles M. Super, Ph.D. Professor and Dean, School of Family Studies, University of Connecticut, Storrs, Connecticut.
Culture and Ethnicity

Dale Sussman, M.D. Clinical Assistant Professor, Developmental-Behavioral Pediatrics, University of North Carolina Center for Development and Learning, Chapel Hill, North Carolina.
Pediatric Self-Regulation

Carl W. Swartz, Ph.D. Clinical Assistant Professor, Department of Psychological Studies, School of Education, and Research Scientist, Center for Development and Learning, University of North Carolina, Chapel Hill, North Carolina.
Schools as Milieux

Ludwik S. Szymanski, M.D. Associate Professor of Clinical Psychiatry, Harvard Medical School; Director of Psychiatry (Emeritus), Institute for Community Inclusion, Children's Hospital, Boston, Massachusetts.
Emotional Problems in Children With Serious Developmental Disabilities

Helen Tager-Flusberg, Ph.D. Professor of Psychology, University of Massachusetts, Boston; Senior Scientist, Eunice Kennedy Shriver Center, Waltham, Massachusetts.
Intelligence: Concepts, Theories, and Controversies

Stuart W. Teplin, M.D. Associate Professor of Pediatrics, Clinical Center for the Study of Development and Learning, University of North Carolina School of Medicine, Chapel Hill, North Carolina.
Autism and Related Disorders

Alexander Thomas, M.D. Professor of Psychiatry, New York University Medical Center, New York, New York.
The Development of Behavioral Individuality

Ute Thyen, M.D. Medizinische Universität zu Lübeck, Klinik für Pädiatrie, Lübeck, Germany.
Chronic Illness

Michael G. Tramontana, Ph.D. Associate Professor, Vanderbilt University Medical School, Department of Psychiatry, Nashville, Tennessee.
Neuropsychological Assessment of Children

David K. Urion, M.D. Assistant Professor of Neurology, Harvard Medical School, Boston, Massachusetts; Member of the Faculty, Harvard Graduate School of Education, Cambridge, Massachusetts; Director, Learning Disabilities/Behavioral Neurology Program, Department of Neurology, Children's Hospital, Boston, Massachusetts.

Diagnostic Studies of the Central Nervous System

Betty R. Vohr, M.D., FAAP. Professor of Pediatrics, Brown University School of Medicine; Director of Neonatal Follow-up, Women and Infants Hospital, Providence, Rhode Island.

Stresses and Interventions in the Neonatal Intensive Care Unit

Judith S. Wallerstein, Ph.D. Senior Lecturer Emerita, School of Social Welfare, University of California, Berkeley, Berkeley; Founder and Past Executive Director, Judith Wallerstein Center for the Family in Transition, Corte Madera, California.

Separation, Divorce, and Remarriage

Lynn Mowbray Wegner, M.D. Clinical Assistant Professor, Department of Pediatrics, University of North Carolina School of Medicine, Chapel Hill, North Carolina.

Gross Motor Dysfunction: Its Evaluation and Management

Paul H. Wise, M.D. Associate Professor of Pediatrics, Boston University School of Medicine/School of Public Health; Director of Social and Health Policy Research, Department of Pediatrics, Boston Medical Center, Boston, Massachusetts.

The Neighborhood: Poverty, Affluence, Geographic Mobility, and Violence

W. S. Yancy, M.D. Clinical Professor of Pediatrics and Associate Clinical Professor of Psychiatry, Duke University Medical Center, Durham, North Carolina.

Aggressive Behavior and Delinquency

Barry S. Zuckerman, M.D. Professor and Chair, Department of Pediatrics, Boston University School of Medicine and Boston Medical Center, Boston, Massachusetts.

Infancy and Toddler Years

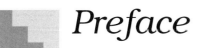

Preface

On the Need to Put the Right Thing to its Root

*A tree's leaves may be ever so good,
So may its bark, so may its wood;
But unless you put the right thing to its root
It never will show much flower or fruit.*

*But I may be one who does not care
Ever to have tree bloom or bear.
Leaves for smooth and bark for rough,
Leaves and bark may be true enough.*

*Some giant trees have bloom so small
They might as well have none at all.
Late in life I have come on fern.
Now lichens are due to have their turn.*

Excerpted from "Leaves Compared with Flowers"
by Robert Frost, *A Mountain Interval* (1936)

The third edition of *Developmental-Behavioral Pediatrics* comes at a time in history when the professional discipline the book represents is receiving increasing acknowledgment as a major participant in the celebration of childhood. We have become serious innovators and integrators, collaborating with others to overcome the obstacles that threaten the effectiveness and life experience of young people. The discipline has seized its unique opportunity, its ability to contribute to specialized clinical wisdom aimed at dealing with significant morbidity at the same time that it exerts an impact on the everyday practice of pediatrics and family medicine.

Thus, this comprehensive volume maintains its dual mission as a definitive reference work for subspecialists in developmental-behavioral pediatrics and as a guide to generalists who seek to foster optimal behavioral adjustment and development in all children. The current edition has added abundant vignettes that exemplify the challenges faced by all clinicians in this field. There is, as well, a strong emphasis on practical management suggestions, graphic illustrations, and thoughtful clinical description. Some new chapters have been added. These include coverage of behavioral emergencies, motor coordination weaknesses, and unpopular children. There is an expanded section on psychopharmacology and many totally rewritten

and updated chapters by authors who are new to *Developmental-Behavioral Pediatrics*.

As with earlier editions, there is a serious attempt to "preserve the hyphen," to demonstrate and apply the inseparability of development and behavior. The message is at least implicit throughout this volume: behavior affects development and development is dependent upon and productive of behavior. This text also strongly advocates a decidedly multifaceted approach to the understanding and management of children who elicit developmental-behavioral concerns, stressing repeatedly that no single discipline or approach holds all the answers for an individual child or adolescent. This text advocates a constant blending of knowledge from multiple sources.

Most importantly, *Developmental-Behavioral Pediatrics* resonates with the philosophy and dual themes in the Robert Frost poem represented at the beginning of this preface. First, we need to think profoundly about how we are nurturing the formative phase of a life, indeed "how you put the right thing to its root." Second, we must commit ourselves to support of human individuality. We vigorously reject implications that there is only one acceptable set of criteria for childhood competency, the misguided notion that, one way or another, all must satisfy identical requirements and meet preordained standards of excellence. To the contrary, as Frost so effectively reminds us, nature yields multiple forms of positive outcome. Not only is there beauty in a tree's blossoms (which may be disappointing), but also some trees may boast of attractive bark or leaves rather than the more obvious and conventionally appealing blooms. We are reminded of the need to discover and uncover nature's abundant durable and insidiously appealing products:

*Late in life I have come on fern.
Now lichens are due to have their turn.*

All of us who support childhood need to appreciate and honor the diverse patterns of function and style with which children continue to educate us all regarding nature and the human condition. The third edition of *Developmental-Behavioral Pediatrics* seeks to inform this redemptive process.

MELVIN D. LEVINE
WILLIAM B. CAREY
ALLEN C. CROCKER

Contents

PART IV

Effects of Medical Illness   321

PART V

Outcomes During Childhood   357

PART I

Patterns of Variation Over Time

1   *The Development of Behavior*

William Kessen

Developmental study through much of the last century has been dominated by the opinions and observations of Piaget.

Vygotsky's work has given new spirit and justification to the researchers of the effects of culture and of social-cognitive change in children.

For friends of children, tension between the belief in internal forces and the belief in external determination has been especially painful over the last 40 years.

This book is a careful and systematic characterization of the current need in pediatrics to take into account the social and behavioral aspects of human development that have often been underappreciated by clinicians and scholars alike.

The curious mixture of stability and variety in human development—the texture of change and continuity—has fascinated parents and scholars at least since Aristotle. In a sense, this book is a contemporary statement of that fascination. One part of the continuing mystery has been psychological and psychosocial (misleadingly but conventionally called *behavioral*) development: that is, the course of changes over time in perception, learning, thinking, language, and personality. The vast domain of behavioral development has been worked over intensely for the last century, chiefly by biologists, pediatricians, and psychologists. Of necessity, any single-chapter survey of the domain today will be incomplete and selective. There is an endeavor here to explore four aspects of the study of behavioral development. These include (1) a brief historical statement of the several lines of thought and work, descending almost entirely from Darwin, that have organized the developmental study of behavior over the last 100 years or so; (2) an exposition of the core prejudicial or conceptual issues that have defined—and divided—the field; (3) a summary statement of five theoretical positions that have been influential in the study of child development; and (4) the primary methods used in the major empirical fields of developmental study.

A Brief History of Developmental Study, 1850–1990

Unlike babies, fields of study do not have rules for establishing birth dates; however, if a conventional opening date for the systematic study of human behavioral development is required, the best time is early in 1877 when Charles Darwin published his observations on his first child's first months, "A Biographical Sketch of an Infant," in *Mind*. And, whether or not a specific birthday for developmental studies is accepted, there can be no doubt that Darwin's observations about human change—especially in *The Descent of Man* (1871)—both forecast and began the flood of theoretical and empirical studies about child development that bridge Darwin's time to ours. In fact, a look at Darwin's intellectual lineage will form a sound introduction to contemporary research in psychological and psychosocial development; one of several possible genealogies is shown in Figure 1–1.

The first line of descent in the Darwinian pedigree called on the analogy between the development of children and the development of species (represented most famously in Haeckel's cry, "Ontogeny recapitulates phylogeny" [Haeckel, 1874]). The *child-animal analogy* has since appeared in many guises; ludicrous to us now is the turn-of-the-century assignment of children to fish stages, ape stages, and the like (Chamberlain, 1901; Romanes, 1889). The founder of American child psychology, Hall (1923), was not as extravagant in his claims for the parallel between species and person, but his confessed "intoxication" with evolutionism marked the early years of child study in the United States. Far more sophisticated applications of the child-animal analogy derived from the work of von Uexküll (1909), who understood better than any of his contemporaries the social context of animal behavior, and Tinbergen (1951), from whom productive speculations were derived about the nature of the attachment between parent and child. In the last years of the 20th century, the child-animal analogy appeared with new virulence in the work of Wilson (1978), who enlarged it to form an account of human social behavior.

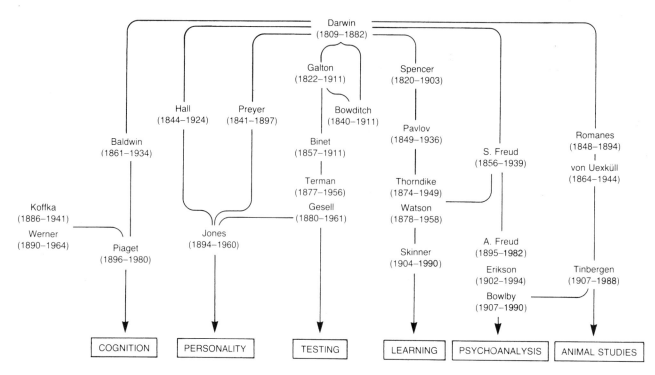

Figure 1–1. Pedigree for the study of human behavioral development.

Less productive of empiric work but richly influential in theory has been the allied analogy between embryologic development and postnatal behavioral development. Laid out explicitly by Gesell (1928, 1945) in his well-regarded opera, the embryologic image of all human change returned to child development with the revival of the work of Piaget. In more focused form, Waddington's (1957) notion of "canalization" offered developmentalists a possible escape from the vise formed by nature opposing nurture.

Never far from the child-animal association was the line of influence labeled "Learning" in Figure 1–1. Even before Darwin's major work, Hippolyte Taine and Herbert Spencer had suggested the powerful idea that human behavior was selected by the action of the environment. Pavlov (1927) and Watson (1928), with one model of learning, and Thorndike (1932), with another, provided the learning-theoretical fuel that was to keep American child psychology running for many years. The simplicity of the learning vision was its major strength—development could be understood as the action of rewards and punishments on behavioral atoms—and it was left to Skinner (1961) to forge the most relentless and powerful version of the argument for development as learning.

Darwin's concern with variation also led steadily from his cousin Francis Galton's (1889) early studies of the inheritance of talent to the still flourishing field of individual testing. Galton's central purpose was to demonstrate the genetic superiority of the English ruling classes, but the possibility of systematically measuring individual variation had educational implications as well. Binet and Simon (1905–1911) in France and, somewhat later, Gesell (1928) and Terman (1916) in the United States set in motion a line of research on and application of the testing of intelligence, aptitude, achievement, and personality that

has probably produced a larger literature than any other segment of developmental study over the last century. It is telling that Galton's invention, "intelligence," should return to the center of theoretical debate in the late 20th century, exactly in the terms he first used—an argument about the priority of nature over nurture. Two less dramatic consequences of the interest in individual variation have persisted in scholarly attention—the close study of physical growth and the assessment of the developmental status of newborn and young infants.

In the 1970s, the ancient commitment to intelligence as a simple, single marker—usually the IQ score—underwent serious critical and empiric revision. Led by the work of Sternberg (1977, 1980), developmentalists formed theories and measures of social intelligence and the ability to solve practical problems; weakened, perhaps forever, was the notion that we could provide *one* number to represent the complexities of human intelligence (see Chapter 70).

It is difficult to imagine Galton and Freud (1905, 1949) maintaining a conversation much beyond initial stiff greetings, and it is a measure of the enormous power of the Darwinian vision that they are intellectual joint heirs. Freud's biologism, his commitment to development, and his emphasis on conflict are part of the heritage he shared with and derived from Darwin. We will say more about psychoanalysis later on, but Freud's place in the genealogy—uneasily between the animal folk and the students of cognition—is secure. In the second half of the 20th century, Freud's flag has been carried by his daughter Anna (1966), the only true descendant in the pedigree, by the deviationists Erikson (1950) and Bowlby (1969, 1973, 1980), and by a host of engaged scholars (see, for example, Lidz and Lidz, 1989).

Developmental study through much of the last century has been dominated by the opinions and observations of Piaget (1937, 1947), who brought together the strands of European interest in the philosophy of human thought and the evolutionary models of phylogenetic and ontogenetic development. Drawing on the work of the brilliant and neglected American Baldwin (1906–1911), Piaget built a unique form of the evolutionist argument. Still, his persistent use of physiologic analogies, his insistence on the construction of new thought from the interaction of organism and world, and his certainty that a small set of orderly rules could encompass the explanation of human development set him surely in the line of intellectual march we have been sketching.

As might be expected, some parts of the developmental story do not easily fit into the structure of the family tree. The most important aberrant group consists of those researchers who studied the development of human individuality across more or less wide stretches of age. Allied to the sturdy Darwinian Preyer (a physiologist who wrote two volumes [1881] on his observations of babies and commentary thereon), the so-called baby biographers were succeeded in the 1930s by industrious investigators at several centers (Berkeley, Fels, Denver, and Harvard, among others) devoted to collecting as much information as could be found about the changes over time in the lives of samples of American children. Their new empiricism left little room for the play of theory.

Because they fit even less neatly, some significant chapters of the developmental story cannot properly be drawn from our Darwinian display. The Gestalt movement, which contributed three important theorists concerned with children—Koffka (1924), Lewin (1935), and Werner (1948)—drew its strength from continental sources in philosophy and physiology. Similarly, the interest in human thought and language that engaged American philosophers such as William James and Charles Pierce did not draw heavily on evolutionist dogma.

The most notable theorist to escape the heritage of Darwin was Vygotsky (1896–1934), a Russian student of language and literature, a devoted Marxist theorist, and a keen commentator on art and art history. He attracted passing attention in the United States with the translation of his *Thought and Language* (1962), but Piaget so fully occupied the attention of the new cognizers that Vygotsky remained in the background until Piaget's death and intellectual recession. After 1980, it seemed as though Vygotsky would become the central intellectual force of developmental psychology. His work from the 1930s was translated into English and it was remarked on with a zeal that had not been seen since the revival of Piaget in the 1960s. Vygotsky's work has given new spirit and justification to the researchers of the effects of culture and of social-cognitive change in children (Rogoff, 1984; Wertsch, 1985). But the American use of the Russian's ideas has been largely in support of independent theorizing and empiric research about cultural psychology. The work on the values and theories of childhood held in different human cultures has been led by Shweder (1991) and by Cole (1996); the work does not fit into any of the classic categories of developmental study, and its perturbation may require a shift in how children are studied.

Weaving through the story of these scholars and their relation to one another is the more important story of the critical issues that have defined and divided the field of developmental study. In keeping with the convictions about the complexity and variety of the human mind, one finds that people and issues do not always smoothly dovetail. The closer one gets to children, the less secure become the historical and conceptual simplifications.

Persistent Conceptual Issues in Developmental Study

A neat antithesis—nature versus nurture or whole child versus separated functions—is often misleading, chiefly because the wisest theorists and scholars in a field of study find adroit and innovative ways to evade it. Nonetheless, in this truncated staking out of the territory, a discussion of several dimensions of disagreement among developmentalists will create a conceptual space in which theorists and research studies can be located. Recognizing that serious workers rarely occupy either end of the dichotomies, the following contrasts are used to present the most persistent conceptual issues in development study.

LAWS OF DEVELOPMENT *OR* UNDERSTANDING INDIVIDUAL VARIETY

Folk knowledge as well as somewhat sturdier empiric evidence suggests that people favor either a search for the simple general rules governing a domain of study or an exploration of the domain's marvelous intricacy. For the developmentalist, this contrast can be represented in the difference between an interest in *the child* and an interest in *this child*. In the larger definition, the contrast is between those of us who consider development a characteristic of the species and those who consider it a characteristic of a particular individual child. Many disputes in developmental study have persisted because the contestants were arguing at cross purposes; to put the point in statistical terms, the phenomenon of special interest for the "individualist" constitutes experimental error for the "law seeker." Cronbach (1957) has presented an elegant analysis of how, over the years, this difference in attitude has produced striking variations in research method and analysis as well as in theoretical stance.

The group of developmental researchers least ambivalent in their attitude toward the law-and-variety dimension are the experimental psychologists concerned with perception, learning, and cognition. When a study was made of infants' responses to voice-onset time (the acoustic parameter that permits adults to tell the difference between the sounds *b* and *p*, for example), the baby subjects certainly did not all behave in the same way. As a matter of fact, some of them would not play in the experiment at all. But the empiric question posed—"Do infants perceive voice-onset time in the manner of adults?"—required the researchers to treat the resulting creative individuality as noise in the observations. A great number of studies of children, particularly in the years from 1950 to 1970, fell near the law end of the law-and-variety dimension. Of course, the law-seeking developmentalists know as well as anyone else that children are not alike. But their research problems are chosen and their data-analysis procedures are devised under the guidance of an overarching search for general principles.

But the devotion of the law-seeker can be more subtly revealed. When Darwin described the behavior of his son Doddy or when Preyer described, in a much longer account, the behavior of his son Axel, their parental pride may have been aroused by the uniqueness of their offspring, but their scientific interest was in Doddy and Axel as particular children representing general human characteristics. To the degree that the children were different from other children they were false witnesses to developmental laws. Later, Piaget (1936, 1937, 1945), on the basis of his observations of his three children, elaborated a theory of infancy—a statement that can also stand as a general theory of human development. His strategies were the same as Darwin's. Both believed that beneath the surface variations of style and pace and personality, one can see in operation—if one has cut nature at the joints—general, unexceptionable principles of human development.

Galton, both because of his interest in variety and because of his lifelong fascination with statistics, carried the law-variety debate a long way forward by describing individual variation as being distributed about some central tendency of the group. The central tendency—the middle place in the array of variation—stood as the description of the species, while the scatter around the center—shorter people, dumber people, stronger people—was understood as departures from the middle. Binet had no fondness for the statistical simplicities of Galton; ironically, when the Binet "tests" had been laundered by Terman and Gesell, most human variation came to be seen as statistical deviation from "the norm."

The Galtonian interpretation of variety remains the most powerful idea used nowadays in attempts to resolve the tension of our first dichotomy; the laws of species development can be described by placing the person in the appropriate position within the general distribution of values obtained from many observations. In their reach to understand variation among infants, Gesell and his successors (Griffiths [1954] and Brazelton [1973], to name only two) follow in the same tradition. A closer look at Gesell's writings suggests that however much he wanted to fulfill his clinical obligation to describe individuality accurately, the heart of his scientific task was the statement of universal laws of human development.

Who, then, speaks for the special character of each of us? We will not consider here the sentimentalists who are satisfied to declare the wonder of human uniqueness and who would attack all systematic attempts to understand it. Three strategies of research and theory remain: First is the *trait theory*, whose proponents postulate a spectrum or—if the metaphor will survive—several intersecting spectra of personal characteristics. We are each of us defined by the assembly of several, or many, basic human qualities. As a waggish statistician has noticed, one needs only eight traits at about 15 different levels of intensity to designate uniquely every human being in the world. The task for the trait theorists, thus far unresolved, has been to detect the correct eight traits. The second strategy, sup-

ported by even less certain supportive research, is the *personal history theory*, whose advocates propose that human uniqueness depends on variations in our personal histories and circumstances (Mischel, 1968), those subtle and sometimes not-so-subtle turns in our lives that determine our present position. We will meet this idea later; it represents so inchoate a strategy of explanation of human variation that we can only note its recent re-emergence. Then, of course, there is the *interactionist strategy*, which would, sensibly enough, account for human variation by adducing a version of trait theory to work in harness with a version of personal history theory. The proposal is so balanced and so plausible that it can be faulted only by the absence of any significant empiric demonstration of its accuracy.

As we noted at the outset, the dichotomy of development defined by species and development defined by person is rationally based and thus artificial. Its appeal—with the possible exception of dissent concerning internal and external causation (see later)—is that it is the dimension of theoretical stance most useful for determining what students of children believe about the primary tasks of developmental study. The range of emphasis on either *individual* or *species* has been awesome; even putting aside the recognitions of artists such as Wordsworth and Salinger, informative developmental analysis stretches from Piaget's account of Jacqueline's patterns of grasping to the thousand-subject study of prematurity by The Infant Health and Development Program (1990).

NORMAL *OR* EXCEPTIONAL

Floating through the foregoing discussion has been an unstated distinction between those of us most concerned with empiric research and those most concerned with caring for sick and needy children. Even before the relation between research and practice can be clarified, however, there is the linking issue of whether one's primary interest is in the normal or usual or "garden variety" child or, by contrast, in the exceptional or unusual or deviant child. In fact, the two issues can scarcely be separated. Everyone is aware of the correlation between research interest and normal behavior on the one hand and clinical interest and the exceptional child on the other. Of course, significant empiric work on exceptional children has been carried out (the rich research literature on mental retardation stands as a measure), but, by and large, the center of scientific developmental study has been on the normal or typical paths of development. Only psychoanalysis, among the major visions of development, includes a systematic theory of deviance.

Not surprisingly, several important consequences have derived from the long-standing difference between studying the abnormal and studying the normal and its correlated distinction between empiric research and clinical practice. The most obvious consequence—which we will meet again in different forms—is that different research methods, different avenues of publication, and different networks of colleagues have been established for the two strategies of study. Thus it is not the case that some people were interested in normal behavior whereas others were interested in deviant behavior and all shared a common set of theories, methods, and colleagues. Rather, two cultures of study emerged, each with its own sense of scientific value and professional standing. Over the years, it has become increasingly difficult to establish a group for sharing problems in which members of the two cultures could bring their best skills to bear jointly on a research issue. The need for productive interaction is now critical to the lives of children; although a glimmering of such an exchange has recently appeared in the disparate fields of cognitive-behavior therapy, behavioral medicine, and the study of at-risk infants, we are still far from the cooperation that is called for.

A less often noted consequence of the separation of cultures between the normalists and the abnormalists has been the common but by no means universal tendency for developmental deviation—whatever its character—to be seen as a function of personality differences. Reasons for this curious outcome are not hard to find. Empiric scientists (particularly those whose workspace is the laboratory) who study memory and problem solving rarely become interested in memory disturbances or eccentric problem solving. Laboratory students of simple learning rarely become concerned with educational problems in the classroom. Therefore, when a child at home or in school is judged to need attention on the basis of unusual behavior, the professional person most likely to be called in is someone trained in one of the several schools of trait or personality variation rather than an expert on the mental structure underlying the disturbance. Again, however, particularly in the recent application of behavioral and biobehavioral procedures, there are signs of a broader definition of the sources of developmental deviation. Especially in the last decade, scholars have turned attention toward everyday behavior in our culture (Rogoff, 1984) and toward the child's life in other cultures (Cole, 1985). Thereby the definition of *normal* has been made richer, and *development* can be seen as a matter of *context* rather than of unfolding. It is one of the consequences of thoughtful observations of children in varying cultural settings (see the discussion in the preceding section of this chapter) that the hard-edged distinction between *normal* and *abnormal* becomes uncongenial to good sense.

In our survey of the disciplinary space that contains developmental study, however, we can detect a significant defining characteristic of investigators in the relative emphasis given to the normal or to the deviant.

INNER FORCES *OR* EXTERNAL DETERMINATION

The war (no weaker word will do) between those scholars who see human development and behavior as directed by internal organizing forces (Nature) and those who see development and behavior as determined by personal history and experience (Nurture) has been going on for thousands of years. Despite valiant attempts at compromise— "all behavior is 100% genetic and 100% environmental," "development occurs in the interaction of nature and nurture," "biology sets limits from within which personal experience selects"—there is little sign of a truce. Even the people who are reasonable on the issue (and all of us *believe* that we are) are "reasonable" on one side or the

other. The debate that took its first formal statement from the 5th century BC reached a new frenzy of polemic rhetoric in 20th century America. No one has ever matched the soaring promise of the behaviorist Watson:

> Give me a dozen healthy infants, well formed, and my own specified world to bring them up in and I'll guarantee you to take any one at random and train him to become any type of specialist I might select—doctor, lawyer, artist, merchant, chief and, yes, even beggarman and thief, regardless of his talents, penchants, tendencies, abilities, vocations, and race of his ancestors (1925).

And, in continuation of the everlasting debate, Watson was answered in his own time and has been answered repeatedly in ours:

> It is doubtful whether the basic temperamental qualities of infants can be measurably altered by environmental influence. Training and hygiene may exert [a] very palpable and important influence on the organization of the personality without necessarily altering the underlying nature or habitus (Gesell, 1928).
>
> The positions of genes having indirect effects on the most complex forms of behavior will soon be mapped on the human chromosomes. These genes are unlikely to prescribe particular patterns of behavior. . . . The behavioral genes more probably influence the ranges of the form and intensity of emotional responses, the thresholds of arousals, the readiness to learn certain stimuli as opposed to others . . . (Wilson, 1978).

When a disagreement persists for so long and with such vehemence among intellectuals who are committed to the steady use of mind and method to solve problems rationally, one has to suspect (1) that the problem has been wrongly stated, (2) that there is not yet sufficient research information, or (3) that the conflict is fired by ethical and political beliefs outside the usual canons of science. In this case, all three conditions obtain.

For friends of children, tension between the belief in internal forces and the belief in external determination has been especially painful over the last 40 years of this century. Reforms of the 1960s, best exemplified by the enactment of the Head Start program, were based on a commitment made by the political establishment and supported by academic developmentalists that there was great space in the lives of children for the impact of environmental intervention. After a few tentative years, the balance shifted sharply with the renewed debate over the genetic basis of intelligence. Since 1970, both the national policy and the scientific establishment have been divided and ill at ease about the chances that society could be transformed by manipulating changes in the lives of the children of deprived and dispossessed members of our culture.

Two advances in terms of the antique division between Nature and Nurture are worth noting; both address the issue of our common ignorance. First, theoretical models for elucidating the action of genes have become enriched in their complexity and thereby have become more ambiguous with regard to their ultimate effect on behavior and research methods; both in biochemical embryology and in behavioral genetics, the biological models are now more ingenious and more revealing of the variety of human development. If the study of behavioral development follows its traditional imitation of biological advances, the complications of genetic theory will be mirrored in new complexities of behavioral explanation. And there has been a significant shift in the confidence of theorists about the certainties of evolutionary progress (Gould and Lewontin, 1979; Kessen, 1990). In brief, no longer can the developmentalist leave productive change to the inevitable working out of Darwin's rules.

The second advance has been slower in coming but is no less important for our ideas about development. During the recent period of prodigious change in our understanding of genetic mechanisms, there has been no corresponding advance in our ability to talk about and research the remarkable variety of environments in which children find themselves. In brief, we have not had theories of environment with power comparable to that of our theories of gene action. This imbalance is slowly being redressed, chiefly in the recognition that earlier conceptions of the environment were too narrowly drawn; fewer developmental psychologists nowadays are committed to a view of the environment as an assembly of atomistic stimuli, and fewer still believe that the child's social surroundings are fully captured by describing characteristics of a mother. Recent work in several cultures has shown anew that the child's world comprises cultural values, economic constraints, and networks of adult interaction that defy simplistic analysis. If environmental theory over the next years advances at half the pace that gene theory advanced between 1960 and 1990, our conceptions of child development will be radically transformed.

Despite the visible improvement in our comprehension of the relation between genetic influence and environmental influences on human development, the acrimony of the Nature-Nurture debate will not be significantly reduced as long as the conflict is tied to our varying visions of the just society.

DEVELOPMENTAL CHANGE: SUDDEN *OR* SLOW

It is a long descent from the tortuous and politically vital tensions of the Nature-Nurture debate to the academic feuds over whether development is continuous or proceeds in sudden spurts, usually called "stages." But, for reasons rooted in philosophic traditions since Aristotle, developmentalists have been testy concerning their colleagues' position on whether development leaps or slinks (Brainerd, 1978).

At the grosser level of theory, the issue of *stage* divides the positions of Freud and Piaget, dependent as they both are on radical and relatively sudden transformations in mental structure, from the positions of the learning theorists and most of the cognitive developmentalists, who prefer to see changes in the child as gradual and continuous. However, the disagreement goes deeper than a theorist's epistemologic prejudice; it reveals a sharp distinction in the meaning of developmental change.

For stage theorists, particularly Piaget (and it is his theory that has provoked the most intense debates), to say that the child has entered a new stage of cognitive development is to say that a fundamental change has taken place in the way the child understands and uses the environment. In a useful analogy to computer software, a new

stage requires an entirely new program. Although psychoanalytic theorists have not fussed about stages as often as the Piagetian folk have, it is plausible to see the transformation from one psychosexual stage to another as representing a saltatory shift in the way impulses and prohibitions are organized.

The other side of the argument derives from the traditions of 19th century biology and physics. Nature does not proceed by leaps. Rather, if we have secure control of the underlying reasons for change—the relevant variables—we could display a family of smoothly changing functions. In the most extreme statement of the position, age itself is only a parameter in forming the most elegant mathematical statement of a continuous function.

Controversy over the rate and nature of developmental change cooled somewhat in the 1970s, but a scholar's opinion on the stage issue remains a revealing way of finding out his or her position in the larger developmental domain.

WHOLE CHILD *OR* REDUCED CHILD

Advances in knowledge seem inevitably linked to increasingly refined and necessarily narrower analysis. Thus the marvelous intricacy of a newborn is compressed into a bilirubin level; the attractive, troubled second-grader becomes a case of learning disability; and the particularity and social complexity of the adolescent are screened into a heroin addict. The tendency to see only parts of the child—the "organ systems" of our special interest—is surely not confined to the laboratory developmentalist. Dramatic examples of simplification can be advanced by looking in the laboratory—the assessment of reaction times as a measure of problem solving or the use of adrenalin levels to measure anxiety—but the clinician seems just about as likely as the bench scientist to reduce the fullness of a child to the comprehensible, smaller package of a diagnosis.

We must analyze, then, in order to understand. Is there a defensible scholarly and humane alternative to that ancient strategy, a way of reassembling the child to make a whole recognizable being?

With cyclic regularity and in all the developmental sciences, a new look at the *whole child* has been called for. Whether in child psychology or in pediatrics, there is a recurrent professional declaration that the child is not just a laboratory report or an aptitude test score, that a new try must be made to broaden our vision of the growing infant and child. The book you are now reading in fact is a careful and systematic characterization of the currently perceived need in pediatrics to take into account the social and behavioral aspects of human development that have often been underappreciated by clinicians and scholars alike. Unhappily for our joint attempt here, as for the whole-child argument more generally conceived, developmental workers have been notoriously deficient in their ability to devise theories of reconstruction, ways of sewing back the pieces of the child that were cut apart to study their weave and structure more closely.

The human and scientific problem is compounded by the apparent fact that the dichotomy between advocacy of the whole child and advocacy of the reduced child is not a division among schools or philosophies; rather, it is a division that occurs chiefly *within* concerned developmentalists. That is, each of us, as scholar-researcher, is necessarily committed to one form or another of the strategies of methodical analysis; each of us, as a student of the larger issues of development (not to speak of our roles as parents and citizens), wants to get back to the child entire. Unlike the earlier contrasting views on conceptual issues, which tend to divide groups, the search for the whole child divides each developmentalist. The solution to this dilemma, at least for the foreseeable future, is to recognize that the reconstruction of the whole child will not soon become part of the scientific enterprise as it is usually defined; rather, the cyclic call for a broader vision must be seen as a philosophic and ethical caution to the analytic scientist in us: Do the best science you can, but remember that you are working on a tiny fragment of the entire mosaic and, above all, do not claim that your fragment is the whole. The sometimes lyrical calls for attention to the whole child threaten the integrity of the scientific process in ways both subtle and obvious.

EMOTION *OR* COGNITION

Developmentalists differ on many specific questions about content of the field and about what critical problems deserve close study. In our examination of the general topography of developmental study we cannot pause to describe all the diverging paths; however, one among them has been so enduring and so divisive that it reaches the status of an epistemologic separation. The dividing question has been: Shall we conceive of behavioral development as turning centrally around emotion (or motivation) or as based on cognition (or thought)?

In the United States, the early years of child study did not elaborate the dichotomy between feeling and knowledge. G. Stanley Hall's vision of the child was so aggregative and far-reaching that he was able (in his questionnaire studies of development) to range from the investigation of children's fears to studies of language to inquiries about the nature of dolls. However, the general psychology of the time was heavily biased toward the study of thought and language and perception and consciousness with almost no place left for the systematic study of the conative, or emotional, side of the human experience.

The standard emphasis was severely disturbed when Freud visited the United States in 1909, and it is convenient to date from that event the slow but steady growth of interest among developmentalists in the emotional life of the child. The Freudian image, or at least the American version of this image, had a couple of surprising effects. One, directly influencing Watson, led to the laboratory study of infantile emotion and the postulation of primitive stages of rage, fear, and love. The second and far more extended effect was the introduction of the notion of *drive* or *motivation* into the powerful emerging field of learning studies. From the early 1920s until Dollard and Miller's statement of the intersection between psychoanalysis and learning theory (1950), the mainstream of American psychology (and its deposits in developmental study) saw the energetic and emotional side of the child's experience chiefly as a matter of primary and learned "drives" (hunger, comfort, desire for learned rewards such as praise, and

the like). But the psychoanalytic emphasis on the emotional life of children did not modify the field overnight; rather, the study of emotion seeped into American developmental study and came to the surface most often in studies of personality variation and in the great longitudinal studies of the 1930s and 1940s.

The domination of American developmental studies by learning theory—motivation and all—and by students of personality development received a toppling challenge with the reappearance of the work of Piaget in the United States. Although Piaget had been anticipated by Baldwin and had a mild youthful success among American psychologists between 1925 and 1930, his impact on the larger pattern of developmental study was felt with decisive force in the years between 1950 and 1975. Piaget presented a rich and persuasive vision of the child (as we shall see in the next section) that was organized around the idea that development was primarily cognitive; human change was a matter of the child's epistemologic development, the child's increasingly rational theory of the way the world worked. The Piagetian revolution was supported by the concurrent and vigorous increase in American interest in computer models of human mental structures and by the renewed empiric study of thought and language. For 15 years, American developmental psychology and allied fields were devoted to an examination and extension of Piaget's image of the child as thoughtful or on the way to being thoughtful.

Since Mandler's provoking books on emotion (1975, 1984), there has been a revival of interest in untangling the knots of early emotional expression in children. The groundwork for renewed study was established by Bowlby's (1969) and by Ainsworth's (1979) observations of *attachment* in the first year of life. From their beginnings, a research industry has been built, a network that has infiltrated common American speech and has become an interest and a concern of parents and developmentalists alike.

SUMMARY

We have proposed six rough dimensions along which to locate the predispositions and attitudes of developmental scholars in the late 20th century. The dimensions are neither linear nor orthogonal, but they will serve to set some boundaries on the conversations among serious researchers of children in our time. The fully sensible reader would, we suppose, choose to take a middling position on all the seesaws, claiming the sixfold fulcrum. However balanced such a solution seems, the message of the foregoing paragraphs is that no one can maintain that calm neutrality; we will be able to understand the major developmental theories about to be discussed if we understand first that all of us bring to these theories several biasing commitments that are rendered intellectually unhurtful only by being made visible.

Five Images of Development

Perhaps the first discriminating characteristic of all major theories of development is that they are social entities as well as conceptual ones. Put in the baldest terms, developmental theories are separated not only by their methods, applications, and core theoretical ideas; they are, as noted earlier, separated as professional associations. Theories are collections of people who agree on the main terms of the child's nature and who gather together—at conventions, in departments, and through journals—to debate their residual minor disagreements. Such chasmic separation of different points of view has two consequences: (1) the members of each group are protected, to some degree, from doubt about their convictions because they are surrounded by other convinced people, and (2) more sadly, exigent problems arising from the lives of children can rarely be addressed from several sides because the group definition—the theoretical purity—must be protected against leakage. No more will be said here about the cult character of developmental theory; the formation of the social clusters of developmental science has been insufficiently studied by historians and demographers of academic disciplines.

Setting the social meaning of theories aside, there are a number of other dimensions along which we can compare different systematic ways of seeing children. For each of the five theoretical attitudes discussed in the following pages, we select a prototypical theory and then present four summary statements about each position: (1) a word about the history of the theory; (2) the major theoretical ideas tied to the position (specifically, the structural unit of development and the major mechanism of change); (3) the theory's favored methods and favored empiric problem; and (4) some implications of the theory for the people, professionals or parents, who care for children.

DEVELOPMENT AS MATURATION

> The body grows; behavior grows. The infant is a growing action system. He comes by his mind in the same way that he comes by his body, through the processes of development. As the nervous system undergoes growth differentiations, the forms of behavior also differentiate (Gesell and Amatruda, 1947).

History. The idea that the child becomes more sensible and more competent in much the same way that he or she becomes taller and stronger is surely the most ancient folk theory of development. A million-year-old phylogenetic heritage has laid down regularities of mind just as it has laid down regularities of tibial elongation. Unexamined commitment to the maturationalist attitude was behind Darwin's willingness to present his son Doddy as a model of mankind; internal forces of growth required the unfolding of predictable patterns of behavior.

Gesell remains the smartest and best informed champion of the conviction that development is maturation. He collected miles of film about babies and wrote numerous books to demonstrate the thesis that human behavior is as lawful in its changes with age as any other aspect of human physiology. Moreover, Gesell formulated a series of principles—the principles of developmental direction, reciprocal interweaving, functional asymmetry, and self-regulating fluctuation—that were meant to carry the maturational theory of grandmother onto a scientific plane. Not insensitive to the variety of human growth, Gesell suggested that many differences among children could best be

understood as early, perhaps genetic, biases of temperament, but he knew that children were different from one another, and he spent a good part of his career devising procedures to describe the differences in precise ways.

Structure and Change. For Gesell, the structural unit of development, that is, what develops, is behavior. Although the maturationalists are persuaded that there are biological structures underlying all visible changes in the actions of children, it is one of the ironies of history that Gesell shared with his intellectual enemy, Watson, the commitment to the notion that what had to be explained in development were changes over age in observable acts. Like less thoughtful maturationalists, Gesell saw age as the primary mechanism of change. Of course, age was a countable marker for more fundamental biological processes, but the central variable in human development is, for maturational theorists, level of maturity.

Method and Problem. In the hands of the baby-biographers, natural observation was the primary method for finding out about developmental change. Gesell and other later scholars constrained the range of observations and looked at babies and children either in controlled environmental situations or more specifically through the use of standard tests.

Gesell was particularly concerned that his observations be made in as rigorous and reliable a way as possible; he introduced the use of film as a method of data collection, and he organized his observations into what came to be known as developmental scales, a layering of test performance that would indicate each child's relation to the expected performance for children of that age. A number of developmental tests (especially aimed at infants) have been proposed since Gesell's early observations; most widely used since the 1970s has been the Brazelton Infant Assessment Scale, a test that combines many earlier devices.

Implications. For parents, the maturationalist position is quietly reassuring. The child will develop at his or her individual pace according to the program that inheres in biological makeup; the task of the parents is to provide the care and sustenance that good gardeners provide for their plants. And, in the popular literature of the maturationalist school, specific measures are given so that parents and professional practitioners may determine whether the baby is on the expected maturational course or how far (in weeks or months or years) the child departs from the predicted species pattern (Gesell and Ilg, 1943, 1946).

DEVELOPMENT AS LEARNING

History. Opposite maturation on the theoretical seesaw has been the equally ancient and equally exaggerated notion that human development could be understood by an examination of the individual child's personal history, environment, and social interactions. The idea of development as learning was forcefully stated in the late 17th century by Locke; it was refined in the work of the associationistic British philosophers; and it reached its apogean claims by the mid-20th century in the proposals of the American psychologists Watson and Skinner and their students. As maturationalist theory depends on evolutionist ideas of regularity and species differentiation, so learning theory depends on evolutionist ideas about selection. In the course of each individual life, particular ways of behaving and thinking are chosen by the exigencies of environmental variation (in most readings, by rewards and punishments) to shape the character and personality of each child. In the statement by Watson that appeared earlier in this chapter, we find the most arrogant presentation of the learning position.

Structure and Change. What changes during development? The answer from the learning theorists has been remarkably consistent—"the responses of the child." Because Watson and Skinner reflect an epistemologic as well as a developmental position, it has been an integral part of learning theories of development to see the "structural unit" (a term none of them would use!) of change as the aggregation of learned responses of more or less generality that are acquired over a lifetime. The only data that can be admitted into the scientific canon are those that can be seen and described by several objective observers. Subdermal processes such as images or thoughts or ideas or dreams need not be called on to understand the development of the child.

Proposals about the mechanisms of change in children have been relatively straightforward as well. The most general answer is environmental contingencies, those varied ways in which the inanimate and social environments respond to the behavior of the child. Conditioning in the Pavlovian manner has been called on as a specific mechanism of change, and subtle conceptions of stimulus differentiation and response generalization have been used in explaining behavioral change, but the most persistent theoretical mechanism used by learning theories of development to comprehend variation in behavior has been reinforcement, a notion that in earlier folk theories was encompassed by the ideas of reward and punishment.

Less radical learning theorists than Watson and Skinner—such as Dollard and Miller, earlier on, and Bandura, more recently—have proposed less adamant versions of the learning model; however, throughout, the emphasis has remained on simplicity of behavior description and elegance of explanatory paradigms.

Method and Problem. The method of choice for the student of children's learning has been the laboratory experiment; literally thousands of studies have been performed in which infants and children were seen in a carefully monitored setting where tight controls were maintained over environmental change, where the child's responses were measured with care and precision, and where experimental effects could be unambiguously assigned to some variation of circumstances designed by the experimenter. It is somewhat more difficult to specify the prototypical problem of the learning theorists. To be sure, studies of simple learning have predominated (for example, left-right choices guided by reward or the tendency of a child to aggress as a function of the behavior of a valued adult), but a great diversity of phenomena has been brought under the explanatory umbrella of learning theory. The discriminating marks of the learning approach have been explanatory simplicity, close definition of the experimental procedures, and an unyielding insistence on the efficacy of definable environmental contingencies.

Implications. The messages for practice of the learning ideology are mixed. On one hand is the almost boundless optimism of a theory that maintains that if you control the environmental contingencies, you control all development. Like Archimedes, with sufficient leverage, parents and practitioners can move the developmental world. On the other hand, there is the more hidden message of assigned responsibility; if the child does not grow well and fruitfully, then one or another of the caretakers was inadequate or ill-informed. The underside of an Archimedean theory of human development is that failure of normal development must be assigned, not to some recessed and unobservable physiologic or genetic source, but rather to the adult manipulators of the environmental rewards and punishments.

Since the 1890s at least, one form or another of the "learning" vision has dominated American culture. Its optimism, its assignment of personal responsibility, and its theoretic simplicity have been the critical signs of American behavioral science in the 20th century.

DEVELOPMENT AS RESOLUTION OF CONFLICT

History. The proposition that life and mind are results of conflict—the resolution of antitheses—is as old as philosophy itself, and the idea of development as the resolution of conflict had a lively effluence in the speculations of a number of 19th century scholars. Perhaps a derivative of that tradition, perhaps another expression of Darwin's implied phylogenetic struggle, Freud, in the first years of the 20th century, stated a textured and elaborate theory of the human mind that, first, leaned heavily on a conflict theory of change and, second, irreversibly transformed our conceptions of children. The working out of the implications for child development of the general theory of psychoanalysis was left largely to Freud's disciples and to his vaguely ambivalent intellectual successors. However conveyed, the psychoanalytic image of children has become (in curiously naturalized forms) almost unconsciously part of the American folk theory of children.

Structure and Change. Freud's proposals about the nature of the human mind and, by implication, of human development were the most intricate and conceptually demanding of any psychological theory prior to the arrival of the chip-based computer. Therefore, the easy simplicities of Gesell and Skinner are barred to us. Nonetheless, it is not a distortion of Freud's vision to see the primary structural unit of development as the child's theory of impulse and prohibition and the primary mechanism of change as the resolution of personal conflict. In the expression of the operation of his major theoretical ideas, Freud depended as well on a maturational premise about developmental changes in sensitive areas of the body. His unique attempt to reconcile the demands of physiology and the demands of society made Freud's image of the child the most pervasive and influential theory of the 20th century.

Largely because of neuroanatomical development, the child's focus of pleasure-seeking interest was held by Freud to move from sucking to defecation to stimulation of genitals over the first years of life. Such a progression poses parallel problems in social development—the ambivalent and continually significant relation with the child's mother, the conflict that arises from the demands of adults for the child to exercise personal control, and the far more complicated prohibitions on the expression of unlimited sensual gratification. Freud emphasized a critical conflict between the child's impulse and the requirements of his parents (standing in for the larger society) for graded limitation of pleasure. Some stable resolution of the resulting conflicts was established in most children by age 6 or so and, healthy or unhealthy, the resolution marked the rest of their lives.

Freud explored all the forbidden areas of conventional child development in his time—dreams, wishes, terrors, craziness, and defensive maneuvers—and he presented to a shocked and disbelieving world a version of the child that was discrepant from all the contemporaneous standard stories of innocent peaceful youth. In spite of the grim and pessimistic tone of Freud's speculations, American interpreters were able (thanks to the wildly optimistic temper of our society when Freud was worrying his theory through) to see the psychoanalytic vision as a liberating and uplifting message: children had only to be allowed to indulge in their impulsive, sensuous urges in order to become healthy and fully formed. Someday the story of a marvelous irony will be told: while Freud's ideas were being shredded into a form acceptable to the American temper, that is, total freedom and a slack rein on childish urges, Watson was simultaneously advocating and persuading parents to accept rigidly controlled procedures for childrearing, devoid of pacifiers, late toilet training, or masturbation. Here we find yet another demonstration of the capacity of the American temper to find support for individualism, self-control, and progressivism no matter what the intentions of the theorist.

Freud's emphasis on the importance of conflict in development brought to general child development theory a sensitivity to human motivation and intention. Also, observers became concerned about the pathology of children; the almost unbroken commitment of American psychology to the rational and the ordinary was severely tested by Freud's delving into the hidden and the strange in childish behavior.

Method and Problem. Despite Freud's dream of a physiologic psychology and despite his early training in laboratory science, psychoanalysis evolved a method of test and proof that was and still is eccentric to the usual canons of empiric science. The critical problem for psychoanalytic child psychology is the child's attempt to reconcile the demands of impulse, danger, and social restriction. Elaborate mental structures are erected to monitor and control the child's interpretation of what is felt in desire and what is required by the parental surround. To plumb the mysteries of this set of interpretations, the primary method of study for Freud came to be the therapeutic encounter between child and analyst. Early on, the difficulties of applying the required therapeutic style to children led to a substitution of speculation and natural observation as ways to the child's mind. It is a measure of the complexities and difficulties of the psychoanalytic research mode that, almost a century after Freud's observations on Little Hans, there exists no established and defensible empiric literature on the early psychodynamic lives of children.

Implications. Because of the general seepage of psychoanalytic ideas into the American culture alluded to earlier, it is not easy to specify the major implications of psychoanalytic child psychology for the lives of practitioners and parents. Without doubt, Freud taught us that the child, like the adult, is a far more conflicted, troubled, and vulnerable being than other theories had maintained. He also drove our attention to the importance for the child of early social encounters, particularly those encounters having to do with the continuing struggle between the push of ancient urges on one side and the controlling modifications of civilization on the other. Finally, by elaborating a theory of pathologic variation, of alternative endings to the struggle, Freud presented conventional developmental study with the task of understanding why some of the variations in human growth were frightening and beyond ordinary experience.

DEVELOPMENT AS COGNITIVE CHANGE

History. The line of 19th century philosophy that led from Schopenhauer to Nietzsche to Freud was contrasted by a line that ran from Kant to Piaget. Barely touched by questions of human drives and urges, the cognitive line had as its main intention understanding the ways in which human beings came to know—that is, how we are able to use the regularities of mind and the regularities of personal history to build the traditional epistemologic notions of time, space, object, and cause. Although American developmental scholars were concerned with problems of human knowledge early in the 20th century—found in particular in the brilliant work of Baldwin—questions about the development of memory, thought, and inference were off-base for the usual American student of children until the revival of interest in the work of Piaget in the 1950s. For the three ensuing decades, the cognitive vision of children dominated academic child study; thousands of studies were published that extended, refuted, modified, or commented on the work of the great Genevan theorist. And even when enthusiasm for Piaget's ideas began to fade, an even older tradition of American interest in cognitive issues—now clothed in the language of information processing and artificial intelligence—appeared in new strength.

Structure and Change. Like psychoanalytic theory, Piaget's cognitive theory saw the child's growth, in the largest view, as a series of quantal changes—from the hand and eye construction of the world (sensorimotor) to a primitively theoretical way of dealing with intellectual problems in an immediately relevant here-and-now fashion (concrete operations) to a fully abstract understanding of the structure of the world (logical operations). Each state in the child's developing comprehension of his or her universe was a newly organized theory of the world and self; the core structural unit of development for Piaget was the scheme, an integrated theory, correct or not by adult standards, that permitted the child to receive information from the world, make sense of it, and predict the future. Development is the increase in scope and elegance of the child's schemes, the growth of intellectual sophistication. What is sometimes difficult for adults—even professionally trained adults—to comprehend is Piaget's recognition that the child's world view differs from ours. The child's theory of the world is not an incomplete adult view; rather, it is a different theoretical organization of presented evidence.

As a mechanism for change, Piaget proposed an analogy with two biological processes of adaptation *assimilation* and *accommodation*. In a parallel with ingestion and growth, the process of cognitive change is seen as a taking in of information from the world and making it useful for the child's present mental structures (e.g., a wooden block may stand for a cat in play) balanced against a changing of mental structures in order to adapt to the requirements of the environment (e.g., the child modifies the gestural repertory to conform with the practices of the parents). Piaget saw human development as truly constructive, depending neither on maturation nor on learning for its working out. Rather, on each problem the child encounters in the world, a theory is brought to bear (at whatever level of generality and elegance). If confirmed, the theory is strengthened; if not, the child will adapt, or attempt to adapt, to the new demands of the environment. Thus, through the processes of assimilation and accommodation the child becomes more effectively adapted to the surrounding world, both inanimate and social.

Following on the work of Piaget and the much older work of the psychology of adult thought, there has been in the late 20th century a sudden growth of interest in understanding the child's thinking as a system of information coding, storage, organization, and retrieval. Backed up by the technology of digital computing and often using the computer as a powerful metaphor, the newer developmental psychology of thought has concentrated its attention on memory, language studies, and problem solving.

As noted earlier, the mark of the 1980s was the American rediscovery of Vygotsky. His work addressed many of the problems Piaget had seen, but Vygotsky gave to the child far more interest in and far more dependence on the social environment. Cognitive change is the consequence of an exchange between a knowing adult and the child in a domain Vygotsky called the *zone of proximal development*. Here—in that part of the child's mind that educators have called "optimal lead"—the presentation of problems by the adult brings the child to a higher and higher level of development. Vygotsky's ideas share the commitment to progress and perfectibility that has characterized all developmentalists, save Freud alone. Only in the last years of the century has that central commitment come under new and critical examination (Kessen, 1990; Morss, 1990).

Method and Problem. The study of cognitive change has drawn on just about every method in the developmentalist's kitbag. Piaget presented his seminal account of the first 3 years of intellectual life as commentaries on observations he made on his own three children. In his work with older children, Piaget used a method of conversational inquiry with children in which he probed, gently and sympathetically, their reasons for believing in their theories of physics or chemistry or morality. Finally, both Piaget and his imitators have used the laboratory experiment extensively to test particular propositions about the variables that influence cognitive change. Through all the variation in method, the core problem for students of the development of thought has been the child's conception of the world, the ways in which evidence from the world is organized and used to understand how things (and people) work. Thus, the emphasis for Piaget and other cognizers shifted from behavior as the focus of attention to mental structures as the focus of attention. The similarity to Freud's strategies is clear, but there should be no confusion about the fact that Freud and Piaget were in pursuit of far different domains of mental structure.

Implications. The images of the thinking child that Piaget and Vygotsky brought so dramatically to the attention of developmental scholars have been widely influential in shaping the character of academic research and, to a lesser degree, in the design of school curricula and teaching procedures. In contrast, the view of the child as a largely cognitive being has had relatively little direct impact on the behavior of parents and clinical practitioners concerned with children. If there is an effect to be detected, it is from the general cultural diffusion of the conviction that intelligence and academic competence are the major markers of successful modern life.

Over the last four decades of the 20th century, there has been a persistent interest in the development of human language. The work has been various, from the early work of Piaget to the pattern-setting writings of Chomsky to the integrative work of Nelson (1996). The study of language as a special arena of cognitive development continues apace, with the usual selection of defining academic arguments and professional fighting over turf.

DEVELOPMENT AS CULTURAL (ECOLOGICAL) ADAPTATION

History. The scholarly interest in variation that sprouted from Darwin's proposals and produced systematic studies of the development of children also produced the anthropologic interest in variation from one cultural group to another. A number of early explorations of cultural variation had as part of their agenda the demonstration of the superiority of Western European forms; however, over the years, the emphasis on deficiency of cultures has been supplanted in anthropologic studies by an emphasis on understanding how cultures come to vary, without assignment of evaluative labels (Jahoda, 1980; Geertz, 1973).

Strange to say, after an initial flurry of attention, for many years American students of children did not draw on cultural variation in patterns of development to amplify their understanding of children. The search for uniformity, the desire for simple descriptions of growth and development, was uncongenial to attempts to account for the nonuniform and the unusual. Then a bubble of interest in the 1950s was followed by an explosion of research on cultural variation in the development of children. Moreover, the focus of study was no longer the exotic ranges of isolated and nonliterate groups alone, but also the subdivisions of American society itself—for example, ethnic variation and social class variation in the rearing of children.

Structure and Change. The revived enthusiasm for the comparative study of human development has not brought in its train a well–worked-out theory of structure and a statement of mechanisms for change. However, commentaries on cultural variation tend to lean toward a cognitive interpretation of the child's initiation into the peculiarities of his or her culture. Ritual, social patterns, power structures, caretaking arrangements, theories of the inanimate world—all are seen as problems posed for the child's solution. Becoming a member of a particular society is in large measure a matter of adapting to the theories of action and intention that adult members of the culture share. Therefore, the child in middle class white American culture can be understood as differing from the peasant child in a Chinese commune primarily in terms of the varying theories of social structure and the natural order. From such a point of view, developmentalists are only beginning to formulate systematic theories of cultural differences in child development.

Method and Problem. The problem of cultural, or ecological, developmental study is easy enough to state superficially—the examination of the nature and sources of variation in the mind of the child from one culture to another—but, just as in the case of theory, investigators have only preliminary and borrowed ways of addressing the problem. What is required is a meeting of anthropologic sensitivities and historical knowledge with the rigors and care of empiric research in psychology. Signs of such a meeting can now be detected (Cole and Scribner, 1974; Cole, 1985; Shweder, 1991).

Implications. Just as early anthropologists sought the better and the worse in cultural patterns, so early developmentalists interested in cultural variation in child development sought to define the ways in which one pattern of child care or education was preferable to another. An evaluative stance about variation was notably present in the first attempts by social scientists to understand variation within American culture—the differences between poor African American and poor white families, for instance. Happily, derogatory evaluation has usually given way to the recognition that in childrearing, as in other aspects of cultural variety, different does not mean deficient. It is too early to say how the new appreciation among academic scholars of cultural variety will affect the lives of American parents and their children.

The five theoretical positions just presented are a selection and an abstraction of a vast range of attitudes and beliefs that have been expressed concerning the lives of children over the last century. All are attempts to encompass the richness—or the jumble—of children's variety and, in a way, to provide systematic answers to the core conceptual questions with which we began the chapter.

REFERENCES

Ainsworth M. Infant-mother attachment. Psychol 34:932–937, 1979.

Baldwin JM: Thought and Things: Genetic Logic. 3 vols. New York, The Macmillan Co, 1906–1911.

Binet A, Simon T: The Development of Intelligence in Children. (Translation of papers in L'Année Psychologique, 1905–1911.) Baltimore, Williams & Wilkins, 1916.

Bowlby J: Attachment and Loss. New York, Basic Books, 1969, 1973, and 1980.

Brainerd CJ, et al: The stage question in cognitive-developmental theory. Behav Brain Sci 2:173, 1978.

Brazelton TB: Neonatal Behavioral Assessment Scale. Philadelphia, J.B. Lippincott, 1973.

Chamberlain AF: The Child: A Study in the Evolution of Man. London, Walter Scott, 1901.

Cole M: Cultural Psychology. Cambridge, MA, Harvard University Press, 1996.

Cole M: Society, mind, and development. *In* Kessel F, Siegel AW (eds): The Child and Other Cultural Inventions. New York, Praeger, 1985.

Cole M, Scribner S: Culture and Thought. New York, John Wiley & Sons, 1974.

Cronbach, LJ: The two disciplines of scientific psychology. Am Psychol 12:671, 1957.

Darwin CR: A biographical sketch of an infant. Mind 2:286, 1877.

Darwin CR: The Descent of Man; and Selection in Relation to Sex. New York, Appleton, 1871.

Dollard J, Miller NE: Personality and Psychotherapy. New York, McGraw-Hill Book Co, 1950.

Erikson EH: Childhood and Society. New York, WW Norton, 1950.

Freud A: Normality and Pathology in Childhood. London, Hogarth Press, 1966.

Freud S: An Outline of Psychoanalysis. New York, WW Norton, 1949.

Freud S: Three contributions to the theory of sex (German edition, 1905). *In* Brill AA (ed): Basic Writings of Sigmund Freud. New York, Modern Library, 1938.

Galton F: Natural Inheritance. New York, The Macmillan Co, 1889.

Geertz C: The Interpretation of Cultures. New York, Harper & Row, 1973.

Gesell A: The Embryology of Behavior. The Beginnings of the Human Mind. New York, Harper Brothers, 1945.

Gesell A: Infancy and Human Growth. New York, The Macmillan Co, 1928.

Gesell A, Amatruda CS: Developmental Diagnosis: Normal and Abnormal Child Development. 2nd ed. New York, Hoeber, 1947.

Gesell A, Ilg FL: The Child from Five to Ten. New York, Harper Brothers, 1946.

Gesell A, Ilg FL: Infant and Child in the Culture of Today: The Guidance of Development. New York, Harper Brothers, 1943.

Gould SJ, Lewontin RC: The spandrels of San Marco and the panglossian paradigm: a critique of the adaptationist programme. Proc R Soc Lond (Biol) 205:581–598, 1979.

Griffiths R: The Ability of Babies: A Study in Mental Measurement. New York, McGraw-Hill Book Co, 1954.

Haeckel E: Anthropogenie oder Entwicklungs-Geschichte des Menschens. Leipzig, Engelmann, 1874.

Hall GS: Life and Confessions of a Psychologist. New York, Appleton, 1923.

The Infant Health and Development Program: Enhancing the outcomes of low birthweight, premature infants: a multisite randomized trial. JAMA, 1990.

Jahoda G: Theoretical and systematic approaches in cross-cultural psychology. *In* Triandis HC, Lambert WW (eds): Handbook of Cross-Cultural Psychology: Perspectives. Boston, Allyn and Bacon, 1980, pp 69–141.

Kessen W: The Rise and Fall of Development. Worcester, MA, Clark University Press, 1990.

Koffka K: The Growth of the Mind. London, Kegan Paul, 1924.

Lewin K: A Dynamic Theory of Personality. New York, McGraw-Hill Book Co, 1935.

Lidz T, Lidz R: Oedipus in the Stone Age: A Psychoanalytic Study of Masculinization in New Guinea. Madison, CT, International Universities Press, 1989.

Mandler G: Mind and Body. New York, WW Norton, 1984.

Mandler G: Mind and Emotion. New York, John Wiley & Sons, 1975.

Mischel W: Personality and Assessment. New York, John Wiley & Sons, 1968.

Morss J: The Biologising of Childhood. Hillsdale, NJ, Lawrence Erlbaum Associates, 1990.

Nelson K: Language in Cognitive Development. Cambridge, Cambridge University Press, 1996.

Pavlov IR: Conditioned Reflexes. London, Oxford University Press, 1927.

Piaget J: The Construction of Reality in the Child (French edition, 1937). New York, Basic Books, 1954.

Piaget J: The Origins of Intelligence in Children (French edition, 1936). New York, International University Press, 1952.

Piaget J: Play, Dreams, and Imitation in Childhood (French edition, 1945). New York, WW Norton, 1951.

Piaget J: The Psychology of Intelligence (French edition, 1947). London, Routledge & Kegan Paul, 1950.

Preyer WT: The Mind of the Child (German edition, 1881). New York, Appleton, 1888–1889.

Rogoff B, Lave J: Everyday Cognition. Cambridge, MA, Harvard University Press, 1984.

Romanes GJ: Mental Evolution in Man. Origins of Human Faculty. New York, Appleton, 1889.

Shweder R: Thinking Through Cultures. Cambridge, MA, Harvard University Press, 1991.

Skinner BF: Cumulative Record (enlarged edition). New York, Appleton-Century-Crofts, 1961.

Sternberg RJ: Intelligence, Information Processing, and Ontological Reasoning. Hillsdale, NJ, Lawrence Erlbaum Associates, 1977.

Sternberg RJ: Natural, unnatural, and supernatural concepts. Cognitive Psych 14:1–16, 1980.

Terman LJ: The Measurement of Intelligence. Boston, Houghton-Mifflin, 1916.

Thorndike EL: The Fundamentals of Learning. New York, Teachers College, 1932.

Tinbergen N: The Study of Instinct. Oxford, Clarendon Press, 1951.

von Uexküll JJ: Umwelt and Innerwelt der Tiere. Berlin, Springer-Verlag, 1909.

Vygotsky LS: Mind in Society: The Development of Higher Psychological Processes. *In* Cole M, et al (ed). Cambridge, MA, Harvard University Press, 1978.

Vygotsky LS: Thought and Language. Translated and edited by Hanfman E and Vakar G. Cambridge, MA, MIT Press, 1962.

Waddington CH: The Strategy of the Genes. London, Allen & Unwin, 1957.

Watson JB: Psychological Care of Infant and Child. New York, WW Norton, 1928.

Watson JB: Behaviorism. New York, The Macmillan Co, 1925.

Werner H: Comparative Psychology of Mental Development. New York, Follett Publishing Co, 1948.

Wertsch JV: Vygotsky and the Social Formation of Mind. Cambridge, MA, Harvard University Press, 1985.

Wilson EO: On Human Nature. Cambridge, MA, Harvard University Press, 1978.

2 Pregnancy, Birth, and the First Days of Life

Peter A. Gorski

 With this chapter begins the story of the growing child and his or her interactions with the multitude of biological and psychosocial factors influencing development and behavior during pregnancy, delivery, and the newborn period. Some of the factors and influences are transient and others more enduring. The limited surveillance role of the pediatrician during pregnancy shifts in the newborn period to one of major importance. In addition to strengthening the doctor-patient relationship and the traditional child care issues (e.g., supporting breast-feeding), clinical opportunities then include building parental skills, helping parents understand newborn behavior, promoting parent-infant synchrony, and dealing with distorted perceptions.

Pregnancy—Parental Transitions and Pediatric Surveillance

Fetal life marks the emergence and initial growth of the infant organism as well as the infant-parent relationship. As the fetus grows in size, draws increasingly from the mother's supply systems, initiates autonomous activity and discrete reactivity, and ultimately demands to begin extrauterine life, so too does the developing pregnancy give shape to a growing sense of emotional connection, relationship, upheaval, and commitment in the expectant parents. Although stressful biological or psychological conditions can overwhelm and disturb this natural process of somatopsychic development of the child and of the child's primary caregiving relationships, childbearing offers every parent the chance to start over, to make a profound contribution to others and, ultimately, to feel human.

The work of pregnancy involves at least five psychological domains and social circumstances. All contribute to perinatal outcome and to the parents' will and capacity to support long-term health and development. Pediatricians who meet with expectant parents can use the five subject areas to quickly engage with them in discovering their stage of preparedness and use of support. The five areas are (1) attachments and commitments, past and future; (2) forming a mental representation of the fetal infant; (3) social and professional support—past history; (4) history of loss; (5) parents' sense of security.

ATTACHMENTS AND COMMITMENTS, PAST AND FUTURE

Pregnancy causes expectant parents to reconsider and renegotiate relationships to each other, to older children, to family of origin (parents and siblings), to career, and to friends, community, and culture. Existing ties and commitments necessarily open, although they do not necessarily loosen. Indeed, new insights and attachments may strengthen relationships with individual and institutional sources of support. The history and current nature of the relationship between expectant parents and their own parents become central for expectant parents and for helping professionals to understand the sources of support and conflict that will likely influence the interactive relationship with the fetus and newborn.

FORMING A MENTAL REPRESENTATION OF THE FETAL INFANT

Expectant mothers and fathers begin early in pregnancy to identify increasingly specific behavioral characteristics, temperamental attributes, and intentionality in their baby. Prenatal ultrasound augments the process that is biologically triggered by the perception of fetal movement, activity states, and motor reactivity to intrauterine and environmental sensory stimuli. The direction and shape of such mental representations, or personifications, are influenced equally by fetal behavior patterns and by parents' self-concept, self-esteem, temperamental world view, physical condition, mood, sense of hope, doubts, dreams, and fears. Especially during the last trimester, the health professional has a unique opportunity to elicit powerful personal insights from parents and to jointly interpret and anticipate caregiving possibilities or consequences.

SOCIAL AND PROFESSIONAL SUPPORT—PAST HISTORY

Expectant parents' use of and need for social and professional support reflect their past history of dependence, interdependence, connectedness, isolation, or alienation. Here there is a chance to gather insight into the way to structure professional interventions after the infant's birth. Questions concerning this issue can also stimulate the expectant parents to consider and plan their future child care support needs.

HISTORY OF LOSS

The parents' history of personal loss can take many forms. Each can affect a person's sense of vulnerability about life in general and about human attachments in particular. The physical as well as emotional stretching and unknown consequences of pregnancy heighten expectant parents' sensitivity to potential (as well as universally inevitable) loss. In addition to physical losses, there is symbolic loss of a person's imagined, hoped for, or idealized infant, giving a rich menu to sample with parents that can help identify, distinguish, and organize important influences and interferences upon parents' developing perceptions and interactions with their infant. Examples of past losses include death of a family member (especially if the death occurred just before or during the pregnancy or if the pregnancy or delivery coincides with an anniversary associated with the birth or death of that family member), marital separation or divorce, previous pregnancy losses, onset of disease or disability (loss of a person's good health), and departure from a dear relative, friend, community, or job.

PARENTS' SENSE OF SECURITY

Parents' sense of security is a crucial contemporary subject for concern. Beyond the timeless developmental challenge for people to acquire a basic sense of trust in themselves and others that they will be cared for, many parents, and half of all women, have suffered some form of violent threat or action against them. Family or domestic violence, as well as impersonal violations by strangers, endanger the safety of adults and children alike. Beyond any real ongoing threat, perceived danger can paralyze a new parent's trust and modeling of intimate relationships. Health professionals who inquire about the expectant parent's sense of safety can organize protection that might enable the parent to communicate the hope of unconditional love to her newborn infant.

Pediatric Prenatal Interview—Format and Questions

Pediatricians who start their relationship with families during the poignant developmental transition of pregnancy gain distinct advantage toward supporting later stages of healthy development and facing physical, behavioral, or emotional crises as they arise. The 20- to 30-minute prenatal interview (Table 2–1) should be scheduled after the 30th week of gestation. The father should always be invited to attend. If the interview is conducted by a pediatric primary care provider, the visit with expectant parents can introduce them to the staff, philosophy, and policies of the practice. The following guidelines offer a structured approach to obtaining medical and personal histories to identify expectant parents' psychological stages and issues. Equally important, such questions are intended to further stimulate parents' own mental process of creating and individuating their infant. The suggested sets of questions direct the health care professional's attention to the five clinically applied conceptual domains previously discussed. Complementary guidelines for conducting pediatric prena-

Table 2–1 • Topics to Cover in a Pediatric Prenatal Interview

I. Attachment history
   A. Family relationships—nuclear and extended
   B. Parents' own parenting histories
   C. Work history and plans
   D. Relationship issues with existing children
II. Mental representation of fetus
   A. Expectations regarding gender and personality
   B. Fetal activity patterns
   C. Parental concerns related to pregnancy complications
   D. Plans for feeding infant
III. Social support
   A. Help from family or nonfamily child care
   B. Friendships with other expectant families or families of newborns
   C. Description of pediatric practice
IV. Experience with loss
   A. Previous pregnancies
   B. Family members
   C. Moves from community
   D. Employment changes
V. Safety/security
   A. Physical safety
   B. Emotional security
   C. Recommendation of confidential resources

tal interviews have been published by the American Academy of Pediatrics (American Academy of Pediatrics, 1996).

The interview should be opened with welcomes, congratulations, and general questions such as "How are you feeling?", "When are you due?", and "How has the pregnancy gone so far?". Answers to these questions may lead the health care provider to further explore any of the five aforementioned psychological domains. The question "How difficult was it to get pregnant?" may lead to asking whether the parents had planned to have a baby and from there to a conversation about how pregnancy will affect their current activities and plans.

ATTACHMENTS AND COMMITMENTS, PAST AND FUTURE

The health care worker should ask the expectant parents where they live and how they each occupy their time. Are they planning any changes around the birth of the new baby? How much time away will mother and father take from commitments outside of parenting? Where do their families live? How close are they to family members, physically and emotionally? How did their own parents rear them? What roles did parents and children play in their family of origin? If they have other children, ask the parents to describe them and their relationships.

These questions should spark insights by, as well as issues for, the expectant parents regarding possible changes in the direction, intensity, and commitment of their relationship to specific persons and pursuits.

FORMING A MENTAL REPRESENTATION OF THE FETAL INFANT

The following sample questions are designed to open conversation toward parents' identification with their baby: Do you know whether you're having a girl or a boy? How do you feel about that? Which gender would you prefer? Tell me about your baby. How active is the baby? Do you feel any patterns of fetal activity and rest? How do these correlate with your own activity and rest cycles? When you dream about your baby, what thoughts, hopes, and anxieties come to mind? What were you like as a child? How would you describe yourself and your partner now? What is your worst fear about your baby's health or personality? How are you planning to feed your infant? How did you make that choice?

Emotional valence might be alternately directed positively, negatively, or ambivalently. The health care professional's interest, sympathy, effort to understand, and support of the full range of possibilities help secure a therapeutic alliance and a safe base for discussing future conflicts.

SOCIAL AND PROFESSIONAL SUPPORT—PAST HISTORY

Questions to ascertain the expectant parents' social and professional support needs include the following: Who will help you care for your baby at home? What kind of support do you imagine you will want? What are your thoughts about sharing child care responsibilities with other family members or hired substitutes in your home or at a day care center? Will your family's help be welcome with or without some reservations?

The expectant parents should be counseled on the health care provider's professional availability, schedule of planned office visits, and procedures for accessing staff during day and night hours. The expectant parents' reaction should be noted. For example, are the scheduled visits too frequent or not sufficiently often? The health care provider should inquire about the parents' access to transportation and communication (telephone). Have they met and formed an enduring connection with other expectant parents?

This discussion should help the health care provider to consider individual needs and benefits to specific community-based resources during the initial adjustment to parenting (e.g., nurse home visitation, community parent drop-in center, professional counseling, child care resource network, lactation consultant, and more frequent pediatric office and telephone contact).

HISTORY OF LOSS

When opportune during the interview, the health care provider should express sympathy for expressed losses and sensitively inquire further into the timing, emotional significance, and resolution or active influence of particular experiences with personal loss. Examples, if relevant, include asking the following: How old were you when he or she died? How do you feel now that you are pregnant and expecting to become a mother yourself? How much do you miss your mother at this time? What month did that happen? How much do you still miss living in that community? What is it about those times that you miss most? Who helps you or to whom do you turn when these strong feelings arise? Tell me about your previous attempts to have a baby. How does that experience affect your sense

of your baby's fragility or vulnerability? When do you think you will be able to trust that the baby will survive? How will you know when to stop worrying whether that might happen to this baby?

The health care provider should be able to follow a parent's invitation to learn better how to care for them, how the past influences the present and the future, and how, when, and why they may feel most comfortable with specific offers of professional support.

PARENTS' SENSE OF SECURITY

After a rapport is established with the expectant parent or parents, they should be asked directly how safe they feel. If the health care provider suspects vulnerability in one parent, a confidential conversation about personal safety should be arranged with that parent. At that time, such parents should be asked specifically whether they have ever been hit or threatened. Do they feel that they and their baby will be protected from harm where they live? How careful does the parent have to be about what is said to the other parent, partner, family member, boss, or other threatening person? The person may opt to speak with someone outside the family about this concern. The health care provider can offer names and telephone numbers at any time that the parent feels ready and able to use such help.

Gestational Influences on Newborn Behavior

Newborn behavior develops over the course of gestation under the influence of genetics as well as exposure to maternal metabolic and psychological states and placental circulation. The developing brain and nervous system are constantly exposed and responsive to various conditions, substances, and stimuli within the fetal-placental circulation and from the external environment. Among the known fetal environmental influences on newborn behavior and development, the most studied include maternal metabolic imbalance, in utero drug exposure, hypoxic-ischemic encephalopathy, and maternal stress and depression.

METABOLIC INFLUENCES

Studies of the effects on newborn behavior of antepartum maternal metabolism have focused on gestational and pregestational diabetes as an exemplary model. Whereas influence on long-term neurodevelopmental outcome is inconclusive, direct effects on the behavioral organization of newborn infants are measurable (Rizzo et al, 1990). Compared with infants matched for gestational age, birth weight, perinatal complications, socioeconomic status, and ethnicity but whose mothers were under better glucose regulation, study infants demonstrated poorer physiological control, more immature motor processes, and weaker interactive capacities. Important questions remain to be answered concerning whether these neurobehavioral deficits mark teratogenic influences that challenge behavioral processes throughout development or whether these differences are transient effects dependent upon active exposure to maternal fuels. Nonetheless, clinicians must recognize and respond to the potential for initial parental difficulty in understanding the behavioral cues of these newborns.

SUBSTANCE EXPOSURE

The developing brain and nervous system are constantly exposed and responsive to various conditions, substances, and stimuli from the external environment. Consequently, perinatal medical risks and intrauterine exposure to chemicals used by or prescribed to women during pregnancy and birthing contribute to newborn behavioral capacities and characteristics. There has been long-standing concern as to the behavioral effects of narcotic drugs on the developing fetus. Heroin-addicted newborns are at high risk for sleep disturbances (with abnormal electroencephalograms), growth retardation, central nervous system (CNS) irritability associated with narcotic withdrawal, sudden infant death syndrome, and behavioral disorganization of state and alerting and motor processes (Strauss et al, 1975). Similar findings have been reported for infants prenatally exposed to numerous other narcotic and nonnarcotic drugs. Poor-quality prenatal care, poor maternal nutrition, and unstable home environment compound, or even exceed, the developmental risks associated with maternal drug addiction.

The potential neurodevelopmental and behavioral effects of cocaine on the human infant are of serious concern, ranging from perinatal cerebral infarction to intrauterine growth retardation, abnormal sleep and feeding patterns, irritability, and tremulousness (Chiriboga et al, 1993). More recently, studies have found that cocaine may have less direct neurobehavioral teratogenicity than the associated or synergistic influences of an impoverished, depressed, polydrug caregiving environment (Brooks-Gunn, McCarton, and Hawley, 1994).

Other substances that cross the placental circulation may contribute to neonatal behavioral disturbances and later developmental dysfunction. These include, among others, alcohol, caffeine, and compounds in cigarette smoke (Emory et al, 1988; Johnson et al, 1996; MacArthur and Knox, 1988). It is often impossible to discriminate the extent to which drugs directly cause long-term CNS damage, whether drugs act primarily to contribute to hypoxic-ischemic conditions, or whether they serve as a proxy for a suboptimal social environment.

OBSTETRIC AND NEONATAL INTERVENTION EFFECTS

Compounds that create regional depression of sensory pathways in the mother during labor may cross placental circulation and cause CNS depression in the newborn. However, studies that carefully control for the effects of parity and length of labor indicate that when minimum quantities needed to achieve anesthesia are applied in tightly controlled dosage, behavioral signs of neurologic depression are minimal and short-lived. This finding has been replicated across studies that tested the effects of a variety of drugs and routes of administration (Sepkoski et al, 1992). Current clinical concern, however, centers on the possibly disorganizing effect of obstetric medication on newborn sucking and feeding.

Neonatal medical procedures may themselves affect newborn behavior during the first days or weeks of life. For example, research on the disorganizing effects of phototherapy cautions about the prudent use of this therapeutic intervention in cases of mild to moderate nonhemolytic hyperbilirubinemia (Ju and Lin, 1991). Newborn circumcision has also received empiric scrutiny with respect to pain sensation and effectiveness of anesthesia (Anand and Hickey, 1987).

MATERNAL EMOTIONAL STRESS DURING PREGNANCY AND CHILDBIRTH

There is a burgeoning field of research examining the impact of emotional stress and support during pregnancy and childbirth on newborn behavior, parental mood, infant-parent relationship, and infant health and development. In studies using primates, sustained stress during pregnancy has been associated with impaired newborn neurobehavior, specifically immature motor abilities, impaired equilibrium reactions, and vestibular functioning as well as shorter episodes of looking and visual attention (Schneider and Coe, 1993). In addition, increased incidence of low birth weight has been found to be associated with mothers who report stress or clinical depression during pregnancy. Several causal mechanisms could explain the newborn neurobehavioral effects of emotional stress during pregnancy. Recurrent maternal sympathetic activation can alter placental blood flow and create transient fetal hypoxia. The flood of stress-induced corticoids chronically engages the pituitary-adrenal axis. In fetal monkeys given dexamethasone for 3 days at midgestation (Moyer et al, 1977), the size of the newborn's hippocampus is diminished. An alternative explanatory model suggests that infant behavior may become modified by stress-induced increases in tryptophan production with consequent increases in serotonin in the fetal cortex (Gennaro and Fehder, 1996). Even though definitive understanding of causality awaits further research, intervention programs offering childbirth education and social-emotional support to expectant women have successfully reduced the numbers of low–birth weight and small for gestational age infants born to this population (Edwards et al, 1994).

Emotional support for expectant women during labor and delivery itself can have positive influence on pregnancy outcome. Whether provided by trained professional obstetric staff or midwife or lay companions, also known as doulas, social support during labor has been found to be associated with improved physical outcomes for women and newborns, more positive childbirth experiences for laboring women, more physiologically stable and behaviorally organized infants, and more satisfying breast-feeding interactions (Zhang et al, 1996).

In studies of support during labor conducted in both Guatemala and the United States, researchers found impressive positive effects. Compared with a control group of women who were passively observed during labor, those who received continuous support from a doula had significantly reduced rates of cesarean section and forceps deliveries. In addition, the experimental group used dramatically less epidural anesthesia as well as less oxytocin to enhance labor; they had shorter duration of labor, briefer stay in the hospital for newborn infants, and less maternal fever (Kennell et al, 1991). Simply changing the physical setting of childbirth in the hospital does not, by itself, improve perinatal outcome. Obstetric programs that integrate emotional care with the medical support of labor and delivery contribute to healthier starts for infants and mothers, and, in the process, reduce health care costs.

Neurologic Basis and Clinical Importance of Newborn Behavior

ONTOGENY OF BEHAVIORAL SYSTEMS

Health professionals and parents anticipate the thrill of greeting a wide-awake newborn infant at birth (Fig. 2–1). Often, infants remain alert, calm, and physiologically stable for the first 1 to 4 hours following medically uncomplicated delivery. Over the next 24 to 36 hours, newborn behavior is less predictable with respect to alerting, feeding, sleeping, and crying. Behavioral self-regulation with increasingly predictable patterns of activity, rest, and attention begin to emerge by the 3rd day of life. Contemporary pressures for early hospital discharge of postpartum mothers and infants seriously challenges the opportunity for professionals to support parental understanding of and comfort with the influence of newborn behavioral organization on the emerging social relationship and emotional attachment.

These fundamental characteristics of newborn behavior reflect CNS maturation as well as innate individual differences of neurobehavioral functioning. The following discussion describes the neurologic basis of the most commonly observed newborn behavioral capacities.

Intrinsic Activity Cycles: Earliest Organization of Behavior

Much research has concentrated on the search for a basic cycle of human movement, rest, and alerting that might describe a fundamental characteristic of behavioral organization and underlying brain activity that exists from early fetal life. Robertson (1987) has documented the existence of spontaneous motility cycles in human newborns across all behavioral states of sleep and wakefulness. This cyclic variation in spontaneous movement every 1 to 10 minutes is observed in utero in human fetuses during the second half of gestation and perhaps earlier. These patterns of human cyclic motility are weaker and less regular during less organized behavioral states of active sleep and may be influenced by alterations in the metabolic environment of the fetus and newborn. Most importantly, the finding of remarkable stability of these cycles of spontaneous movement from midgestation through the first 10 weeks of post-term life adds evidence for a dramatic shift in brain organization and behavioral self-regulation, not at the time of birth at 40 weeks, but after 50 postconceptual weeks. Previous studies of electrophysiologic organization of the CNS, structural maturation of the cerebral cortex, and behavioral development of infant crying and sleep patterns indicate relative CNS immaturity during the first 2 to 4 months post-term with respect to fundamental organization of cortical activity as well as of higher perceptual and cognitive processes (Parmelee, 1977). Therefore, despite substantial environmental and physiologic changes that accompany birth, the human fetus and newborn share basic continuities of behavior and responsiveness.

Behavioral States

In general, healthy full-term infants display a regular series of distinct states over a period of time. These were first described and systematized by Wolff (1966). A number of other classification schemes have been published. For example, Brazelton has proposed a system with the following six states: (1) quiet sleep, (2) active sleep, (3) drowsiness, (4) alert inactivity, (5) active awake, and (6) crying. Each state can be distinguished on the basis of a number of distinct clusters of behavior (Table 2–2).

The study of behavioral states in infants has attracted wide interest as an indicator of the functional integrity of the CNS during the fetal, neonatal, and infant periods of development. Maturational changes in sleep-wake cycles have been studied, and neonatal state periodicities have been correlated with later neurodevelopmental, especially mental, outcome. These investigations have found that earlier maturation of electrophysiologic and behavioral patterns of quiet sleep in the newborn period predict higher performance on cognitive tests at preschool and school age (Whitney and Thoman, 1993).

Sleeping and waking states in infants reflect the competency of the CNS as well as modulate the infant's interactions with the external environment. A number of studies

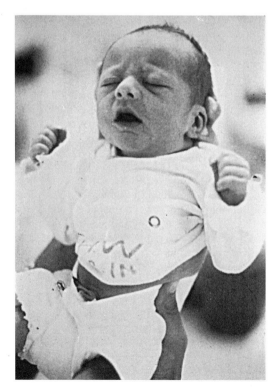

Figure 2–1. The remarkable newborn.

Table 2–2 • Neonatal State Classification Scale

State	Characteristics
Quiet sleep	Breathing is regular and eyes are closed; spontaneous activity is confined to startles and jerky movements at regular intervals. Responses to external stimuli are partially inhibited, and any response is likely to be delayed. There are no eye movements, and state changes are less likely after stimuli or startles than in other states.
Active sleep	Breathing patterns are irregular and infant makes sucking movements; eyes are closed but rapid eye movements can be detected underneath the closed lids. Infants also have some low-level and irregular motor activity. Startles occur in response to external stimuli and can produce a change of state.
Drowsiness	While the newborn is semidozing, eyes may be open or closed; eyelids often flutter; activity level is variable and interspersed with mild startles. Drowsy newborns are responsive to sensory stimuli but with some delay, and state change frequently follows stimulation.
Alert inactivity	Infant has a bright alert look, with attention focused on sources of auditory or visual stimuli; motor activity is inhibited while attending to stimuli.
Active awake	Eyes are open and there is considerable motor activity, thrusting movements of extremities, and occasional startles set off by activity. Infant is reactive to external stimulation with an increase in startles or motor activity. Discrete responses are difficult to distinguish because of the generally high activity level.
Crying	There is intense irritability in the form of sustained crying and jerky limb movement. This state is difficult to break through with stimulation.

Adapted from Brazelton TB: Neonatal Behavioral Assessment Scale, 2nd ed. London, Heinemann, 1984.

have documented the influence that an infant's state has on his or her response to stimulation; the response may differ depending on whether the infant is in a sleep, drowsy, or alert state (Berg and Berg, 1979). For example, a visual stimulus that captures the attention of a quietly awake infant does not elicit a response from a more aroused, crying infant. This arousal distinction applies not only between states but also within a particular state. A newborn infant displays a different pattern of responsiveness at the beginning of an alert period compared with the end of the period. This difference is analogous to the daytime pattern of adults who commonly go through periods of higher and lower arousal while awake. This pattern, called the basic rest-activity cycle, is distinct from the sleep-wake cycle and is theoretically related to the cyclic activity of the autonomic nervous system (ANS). The ANS mediates the infant's responsivity to the external environment and is responsible for regulating a number of homeostatic functions.

The infant cry state is itself attracting interest in the effort to develop predictive measures of CNS functioning based on newborn behavior. Successful prediction of developmental outcome from neonatal cry analyses corroborates a relation between the characteristics of the infant's cry and the functional integrity of the infant's nervous system (Lester, 1987).

Maturational Differences Between Full-Term and Preterm Infants

Neonatal behavioral and psychophysiologic measures of state organization are among the most frequently applied methods in neonatal behavioral research. These techniques highlight maturational differences, for example, between preterm and term infants that could affect their responses to caregiving and treatment practices (Table 2–3). Research findings suggest that the underlying difference in CNS organization between premature and full-term infants lies in an unevenness in the development of premature infants. Aspects of greater CNS maturity (more alertness and less sleep) coexist with characteristics of less CNS maturity

(more nonalert waking activity and more frequent sleep-wake transitions). Most distinctively, then, premature infants exhibit irregular state development as compared with full-term infants, rather than either increased maturity or immaturity. These early neurobehavioral differences between infants of different gestational ages could reflect significant changes in brain organization that may continue throughout childhood development. Current long-term follow-up studies of preterm infants tend to find that the mental development and neurologic status of medically uncompromised preterm infants at school age does not differ from that of full-term infants, yet these same children are more likely to show visual-motor and spatial difficulties, with associated school underachievement (Hack et al, 1994). Infants who experience severe perinatal medical complications, such as bronchopulmonary dysplasia or severe intracranial hemorrhage, are more vulnerable to continued long-term neurodevelopmental disabilities (Brazy et al, 1991; Vohr et al, 1991) (see Chapter 26).

Sensory-Perceptual Functions

Infant behavior is premised upon sensory processes that serve as avenues of communication between the infant and the world. Sensory systems undergo rapid changes during the last trimester of pregnancy and the first several months after birth.

There appears to be an orderly sequence in the functional development of the sensory systems of human infants. This sequence unfolds starting with the cutaneous

Table 2–3 • Behavioral Differences Between Full-Term and Preterm Newborns

1. Preterm infants have disorganized patterns of sleep-wake activity
2. Preterm infants have less coordination of behavior with physiology (e.g., activity states and cardiorespiratory control)
3. Extremely premature infants show less behavioral response to stimulation but more exaggerated physiologic reactivity.

(somesthetic or tactile) system in the 3rd month of gestation, through vestibular, auditory (becoming functional between the 25th and 27th weeks of gestation), and visual (maturing 3–6 months after term) (Gottlieb, 1971). The visual system, the one that is usually dominant in everyday interactions with the environment, is the last system to start functioning during gestation and the least well-developed at birth. Still, the healthy full-term newborn can fixate visually with a variety of stimuli, exhibiting differential attention to inanimate versus animate stimuli.

The development of the sensory nervous system also informs clinicians about the effects of some common medical practices on newborns. For example, because somatosensory structure and function is in place by midgestation, pain fibers are responsive in all newborn infants, including preterm infants. Using regional anesthesia during newborn circumcision reduces behavioral and physiologic reactivity to that painful medical procedure (Anand and Hickey, 1987).

INDIVIDUAL DIFFERENCES IN NEWBORN BEHAVIOR

The preceding discussion highlighted aspects of behavioral and neurobiologic development that are common to all human infants. Differences in development were noted to be caused by idiosyncrasies of gestational age at birth or other medical risk factors. How, then, can the range and stability of differences in the behavior of infants born at the same gestation with similar medical courses be accounted for? The pattern of behavioral and psychophysiologic responses to animate and inanimate stimuli that characterize children (beyond early infancy) and adults is often referred to as temperament. Temperament describes the style without supplying the explanation of individual patterns of behavior.

Researchers tend to agree that temperamental dimensions reflect behavioral styles rather than discrete behavioral acts, have biological underpinnings, and enjoy continuity of expression relative to other aspects of behavior. Newborn infants born at identical gestational ages and sharing common biological conditions often exhibit distinct patterns of behavior. Although not always stable from day to day, individual behavioral differences among newborn infants can be observed, particularly with respect to sensitivity to stimulation, state range and regulation, intensity of reactions, alerting, and ability to modulate motor activity. Disagreements exist about the extent to which a newborn infant's behavior represents the analogues of later temperament. Scientists wrestle with questions concerning the stability of individual temperament over time, the influence of varied social contexts, and the nature of its inheritance (see Chapter 8). Formal neonatal behavioral examination helps parents and professional caregivers to systematically identify and portray the nature of interaction that each infant brings into the caregiving world.

Caregivers and children bring their individual behavioral patterns into the relationship that they create with each other. Similarities or differences can produce understanding and comfort or confusion and conflict. Whether stable or changed over time, individual behavioral characteristics influence the ease, harmony, and pleasure between the child and the environment at each stage of development. In return, the child continuously learns to find those environments and relationships that best support his or her needs and style. These lessons begin immediately through the new relationship between newborn infant and parent. The neonatal period serves to launch parents' perceptions and infants' expectations in the direction of contented anticipation of the future or toward frustration and learned helplessness (Table 2–4) (Seligman, 1975; Sroufe, 1986).

Newborn Behavioral Assessment

Brazelton elaborated on earlier assessments of newborn behavior to complement and potentially enrich basic neurologic assessment of motor tone and reflexes. Framed within the matrix of observing and manipulating changes in states of arousal of newborns, the Neonatal Behavioral Assessment Scale (NBAS) (Nugent and Brazelton, 1995) follows the infant through sleep, drowsiness, bright and active alertness, and crying while the examiner interacts with the newborn infant. The examination elicits 20 neurologic reflex behaviors. It also scores 26 behavioral responses to unique stimuli as well as common caregiving routines such as cuddling, consoling, and visual and auditory stimulation.

A most important concept of the NBAS lies in assessing the infant's capacities to initiate support from the environment, modulate or terminate his or her response to excess outside stimulation, and rely on self for coping with a rewarding or distressing situation. Reflecting the range of behavioral capacities of the normal newborn, the behavioral items assess the infant's ability to (1) organize states of consciousness, (2) habituate reactions to disturbing events, (3) attend to and process simple and complex environmental stimuli, (4) control motor tone and activity while attending to these stimuli, and (5) perform integrated motor acts for self-defense and social interaction.

The NBAS is designed and validated to elicit the behavioral capacities of full-term infants, from birth to 2 months of age. Although attempts have been made to apply this tool to premature infants, results are not wholly satisfying or meaningful because the neurologic organization of these infants is qualitatively different. As a result, responses to stimuli are often uninterpretable using the scoring system of the full-term scale.

Als and colleagues (1994) have developed a complex set of assessment techniques packaged to evaluate quality of behavioral organization at various ages in the preterm and high-risk full-term newborn. The Assessment of Preterm Infant Behavior (APIB) and its related clinical observation method called the Newborn Individualized Developmental Care and Assessment Program (NIDCAP) is an

---

Table 2–4 • Summary of Influences on Newborn Behavior

Metabolic (e.g., glucose metabolism)
Pharmacologic (e.g., nicotine, alcohol, drugs)
Iatrogenic (e.g., medications and interventions)
Psychological (e.g., maternal stress)
Maturational (e.g., gestational age)
Individual differences in neurophysiologic reactivity

extension of the NBAS that provides a comprehensive description of the range of behavioral functions in the less mature infant. APIB scores indicate functional maturity as well as the infant's degree of fragility and ability to tolerate sensory activity during caregiving and handling. From this information, an individualized developmental care plan can be generated. Preliminary research results of clinical trials using the NIDCAP demonstrate positive hope toward stabilizing infants' initial physiologic fragility, improving developmental outcome following premature birth, and lowering cost of neonatal hospitalization.

The aforementioned instruments for assessing the behavioral competencies and individuality of full-term and biologically at-risk newborns are complicated to learn and apply. They are primarily useful as research instruments. An abstracted form of the NBAS is being studied to be useful as a clinical guide for practitioners to engage parents in assessing the behavior of newborns and young infants.

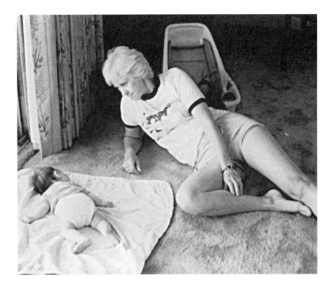

Figure 2–2. Beginnings of mother-infant synchrony.

Clinical Opportunities in the Newborn Period

BUILDING PARENT SKILLS AND PARENT-PHYSICIAN RELATIONS

Powerful circumstances combine during the perinatal period to heighten the pediatrician's opportunities to effectively support healthy infant development (Table 2–5). As discussed earlier in this chapter, the birth family is exceptionally exposed with respect to their emotional anticipation and uncertainty. The newborn infant comes remarkably equipped to communicate interests and needs through physiologic and behavioral signal systems. Capitalizing on the parents' open availability and the infant's compelling responsivity, the pediatrician's visits during the newborn hospitalization can cement a lasting relationship built on trust, honesty, and optimism. By examining newborns together with the parents at the mother's bedside, the pediatrician can demonstrate the range of the newborn's physical and behavioral competencies and individual behavioral reactions. As the baby moves from sleep to increasingly wakeful, active, and even irritable states, the physician can observe the parents' personal responses to each behavior. Not only are newborn infants hard to resist, parents can hardly resist projecting intentionality about the infant's movements, sounds, and sleep-wake states (Fig. 2–2). The observant physician can make use of such affect, whether positive or not, for diagnostic and therapeutic advantage. The baby is a most effective psychotherapeutic agent in

the hands of an attentive pediatric professional who uses the newborn assessment to engage the family's love and attention for their child. The adroit clinician sweetens the emotional juices that flow so opportunely as newborns and parents begin to bond the glue that cements the initial valence of their lifelong relationship (Kennell et al, 1991).

UNDERSTANDING ATYPICAL INFANT BEHAVIOR

Even though birth is almost always a magnificent celebration of life, occasionally perinatal circumstances for the infant or mother are distressing or even life threatening. This chapter has already discussed the disorganizing or disabling effects on newborn behavior often associated with prematurity and gestational insult or stress. Another group of infants born at risk for atypical patterns of behavioral development are infants born small for gestational age. Whether preterm or full-term, these infants are susceptible to a particular set of challenging behaviors. These infants, who are born less than the 10th percentile by ponderal index (weight in grams divided by the cube of length in centimeters), are unusually likely to exhibit the effects of extremely low sensory thresholds (Als et al, 1976). Their nervous systems have difficulty organizing adaptive responses to more than one or two concurrent sources of stimulation from the ambient sensory environment. These infants have certain clinical concerns, including frequent gaze aversion from face-to-face interaction, disjointed movement patterns, frequent startles and tremors, mottling or wild fluctuations of skin color (including acrocyanosis), and, rarely, dyspnea or apnea (see Chapter 26).

Follow-up studies find this population of infants to be at higher risk for failure to thrive, behavioral disturbances, particularly of self-regulation (e.g., colic and inattention), and activity, as well as child abuse and neglect. Early diagnosis through newborn behavioral assessment and attention to parental frustration can direct effective therapeutic strategies for diminishing sensory overload and provid-

Table 2–5 • Clinical Opportunities in the Newborn Period

Integrate behavior into the physical examination.
Assess and support infant self-regulation and parent-infant synchrony.
Help parents to understand and nurture infants with atypical behavioral patterns or responses.
Help families deal with distorted perceptions.
Promote breast-feeding.
Build parent-physician relationship.

ing external organization until the infant can develop higher sensory limits and consistent behavioral self-regulation.

DEALING WITH DISTORTED PERCEPTIONS

Even when no medical risks occur, the fragile faith of parents of newborns can be wounded by seemingly minor or even tangential disappointments, tensions, or misfortunes. All too easily, then, parents may transfer the real vulnerability of the moment or of another person into the mental representation of the newborn baby. These infants' normal behavioral signals may get misinterpreted by anxious or depressed parents who imagine that their child is physically vulnerable. Overprotecting or overindulging the child from infancy onward, distressed parents often fail to guide these infants toward healthy social autonomy. A classic syndrome, known as the vulnerable child syndrome, can develop (Gorski, 1988; Green and Solnit, 1964). These children often have prolonged separation anxiety well beyond early childhood; prolonged infantile, often aggressive, behaviors; sleep and feeding problems; psychosomatic disorders; or school underachievement months or years after the signal event that triggered the parents' malaise. Over time, the young child internalizes the caregivers' insecurities into his or her own self-concept, avoiding the risks that all children must take in order to stretch beyond what is comfortable to develop new abilities and relationships. Pediatricians, through their early and frequent encounters with families of newborns, can identify and sympathetically help shift the family's perception of their child from vulnerable to adaptive and strong (see Chapter 33).

PROMOTING BREAST-FEEDING

Increasingly, American women are choosing to breast-feed their newborn infants. By 1995, 60% of newborns were breast-fed, a 20% increase over the previous 5 years. However, less than half of the original number continued to be fed mother's milk 6 months after birth, despite accumulating empiric evidence that human milk is nutritionally superior to synthetically prepared formula and significantly reduces the risk of many common illnesses, including diarrheal diseases, lower respiratory infections, otitis media, bacteremia, meningitis, and allergies (Lawrence, 1994). Furthermore, new studies support the health benefits of human milk for hospitalized preterm infants. The composition of milk expressed from postpartum women changes over time and over the course of each feeding. In particular, protein and lipid content of human milk adapts to the needs and capacities of the infant's intestinal and immunologic systems at each stage of development.

Efforts to guide and support successful initiation of breast-feeding are extremely challenged by the current practice of discharging healthy newborn infants and mothers from the hospital 1 to 2 days following birth. Few women have begun lactating confidently by then. Many return home without help for child care or social support. While lobbying hospitals for postpartum stays to be determined by the needs of individual families, health providers should also augment the traditional pediatric care of the newborn with early office and home visits as necessary.

Social Significance of Newborn Behavior

This chapter reviewed evidence for the newborn infant's competence to perceive, respond to, and communicate with its environment. Newborn infants help adults succeed as caregivers by being readable, predictable, and responsive. No longer can professionals allow parents to feel totally responsible for all of their infant's behavior. The newborn, once thought to be a "blank slate to be written upon by his environment, his world a blooming, buzzing confusion" (James, 1890), has come to be respected as a social partner who can effectively engage and, to some extent, guide caregivers to support his or her growth and development.

Not all infants are born after a full intrauterine gestation and without CNS pathology or behavioral dysfunction. Premature and other high-risk newborns, born with disorganized signaling systems, challenge their caregivers to understand their behavior and support their physiologic and psychological development. Similarly, families stressed by untoward pregnancy outcome, social isolation, insecure spousal relationship, a history of child abuse or neglect, or emotional depression may not be able to cope with a behaviorally disorganized, or even an alert, self-regulated infant. Early intervention, through the physician-patient relationship and other community-based family resources that provide emotional support and developmental counseling for parents of high-risk newborns at home and in the hospital, can help prevent negative outcomes and foster positive infant growth and family relationships (Olds, Henderson, and Kitzman, 1994; Rauh et al, 1990). Health professionals have a distinct opportunity to note the psychological condition of the parents in addition to the medical status and behavior of the newborn. By offering attention and support to the family as well as to the newborn, caregivers can contribute most effectively to the quality of infant health and development.

Moreover, as trusted members of communities, pediatric health care professionals can influence public deliberation and policy to ensure that infants and families are valued and supported as they take their first steps toward preserving a just, caring, and peaceful world. Only then will newborn infants ultimately grow able and willing to cultivate their biological endowment and relational experience in order to inspire themselves and their society.

REFERENCES

Als H, Lawhon G, Duffy FH, et al: Individualized developmental care for the very low birth weight preterm infant. Medical and neurofunctional effects. JAMA 272:853–858, 1994.

Als H, Tronick EZ, Adamson L, Brazelton TB: The behavior of the full-term but underweight newborn infant. Develop Med Child Neurol 18:590–602, 1976.

American Academy of Pediatrics: Committee on Psychosocial Aspects of Child and Family Health. The Prenatal Visit. Pediatrics 97:141–142, 1996.

Anand KJS, Hickey PR: Pain and its effects in the human neonate and fetus. N Engl J Med 317:1321–1329, 1987.

Berg WK, Berg KM: Psychophysiologic development in infancy: state, sensory function, and attention. *In* Osofsky JD (ed): Handbook of Infant Development. New York, John Wiley, 1979, pp 283–343.

Brazy JE, Eckerman CO, Oehler JM, et al: Nursery neurobiologic risk score: important factors in predicting outcome in very low birth weight infants. J Pediatr 118:783–792, 1991.

Brooks-Gunn J, McCarton C, Hawley T: Effects of in utero drug exposure on children's development. Arch Pediatr Adolesc Med 148:33–39, 1994.

Chiriboga CA, Bateman DA, Brust JC, Hauser WA: Neurologic findings in neonates with intrauterine cocaine exposure. Pediatr Neurol 9:115–119, 1993.

Edwards CH, Cole OJ, Oyemade US, et al: Maternal stress and pregnancy outcomes in a prenatal clinic population. J Nutr 124(6 Suppl):1006S–1021S, 1994.

Emory EK, Konopka S, Hronsky S, et al: Salivary caffeine and neonatal behavior: assay modification and functional significance. Psychopharmacology 94:64–68, 1988.

Gennaro S, Fehder WP: Stress, immune function and relationship to pregnancy outcome. Nurs Clin North Am 31:293–303, 1996.

Gorski PA: Fostering family development following preterm hospitalization. In Ballard RA (ed): Pediatric Care of the ICN Graduate. Philadelphia, WB Saunders, 1988, pp 27–32.

Gottlieb G: Ontogenesis of sensory function in birds and mammals. In Tobach E, Aronson LR, Shaw E (eds): The Biopsychology of Development. New York, Academic Press, 1971, pp 67–126.

Green M, Solnit A: Reactions to the threatened loss of a child: a vulnerable child syndrome. Pediatrics 34:58–66, 1964.

Hack M, Taylor G, Klein N, et al: School-age outcomes in children with birth weights under 750 g. N Engl J Med 331:753–759, 1994.

James W: The Principles of Psychology. New York, Henry Holt, 1891.

Johnson VP, Swayze VW, Sato Y, Andreasen NC: Fetal alcohol syndrome: craniofacial and central nervous system manifestations. Am J Med Genet 61:329–339, 1996.

Ju SH, Lin CH: The effect of moderate non-hemolytic jaundice and phototherapy on newborn behavior. Acta Paediatr Sin 32:31–41, 1991.

Kennell J, Klaus M, McGrath S, et al: Continuous emotional support during labor in a US hospital. JAMA 265:2197–2201, 1991.

Lawrence PB: Breast milk: best source of nutrition for term and preterm infants. Pediatr Clin North Am 41:925–941, 1994.

Lester BM: Developmental outcome prediction from acoustic cry analysis in term and preterm infants. Pediatrics 80:529–534, 1987.

MacArthur C, Knox EG: Smoking in pregnancy: effects of stopping at different stages. Br J Obstet Gynaecol 95:551–555, 1988.

Moyer JA, Herrenkohl LR, Jacobowitz DM: Effects of stress during pregnancy on catecholamines in discrete brain regions. Brain Res 121:385–393, 1977.

Nugent JK, Brazelton TB: Neonatal Behavioral Assessment Scale, 3rd ed. London, Mac Keith Press, 1995.

Olds DL, Henderson CR, Kitzman H: Does prenatal and infancy nurse home visitation have enduring effects on qualities of parental caregiving and child health at 25 to 50 months of life? Pediatrics 93:89–98, 1994.

Parmelee AH Jr: Remarks on receiving the C. Anderson Aldrich Award. Pediatrics 59:389–395, 1977.

Rauh VA, Nurcombe B, Achenbach T, Howell C: The mother-infant transaction program. The content and implications of an intervention for the mothers of low-birthweight infants. Clin Perinatol 17:31–45, 1990.

Rizzo T, Freinkel N, Metzger BE, et al: Correlations between antepartum maternal metabolism and newborn behavior. Am J Obstet Gynecol 163:1458–1464, 1990.

Robertson SS: Human cyclic motility: fetal-newborn continuities and newborn state differences. Dev Psychobiol 20:425–442, 1987.

Schneider ML, Coe CL: Repeated social stress during pregnancy impairs neuromotor development of the primate infant. J Dev Behav Pediatr 14:81–87, 1993.

Seligman MR: Helplessness: on development, depression, and death. San Francisco, WH Freeman, 1975.

Sepkoski CM, Lester BM, Ostheimer GW, Brazelton TB: The effects of maternal epidural anesthesia on neonatal behavior during the first month. Dev Med Child Neurol 34:1072–1080, 1992.

Sroufe A: Attachment and the construction of relationships. In Hartup WW, Rubin Z (eds): Relationships and Development. Hillsdale, NJ, Erlbaum, 1986, pp 51–71.

Strauss ME, Lessen-Firestine JK, Starr RH, et al: Behavior of narcotic-addicted newborns. Child Dev 46:887–893, 1975.

Vohr BR, Coll CG, Lobato D, et al: Neurodevelopmental and medical status of low-birthweight survivors of bronchopulmonary dysplasia at 10 to 12 years of age. Dev Med Child Neurol 33:690–697, 1991.

Whitney MP, Thoman EB: Early sleep patterns of premature infants are differentially related to later developmental disabilities. J Dev Behav Pediatr 14:71–80, 1993.

Wolff PH: The causes, controls, and organization of behavior in the neonate. Psychol Issues 5:1–105, 1966.

Zhang J, Bernasko JW, Leybovich E, et al: Continuous labor support from labor attendant for primiparous women: a meta-analysis. Obstet Gynecol 88:739–744, 1996.

3 Infancy and Toddler Years

Barry S. Zuckerman • Deborah A. Frank •
Marilyn Augustyn

 The description of the first 2 years of life stresses the importance for development and behavior of the transactions between the innate capabilities and traits of the child and the influences of the environment. The common clinical developmental-behavioral issues occurring in this period are considered from that point of view. The discussion is subdivided into the norms and problems observed in the principal areas: social-emotional; neuromaturation; cognition, play, and language; and nutrition and growth.

No single theory of behavior and development provides a practical framework for dealing with the diverse developmental issues that arise in the everyday practice of pediatrics. Development is a complex process that continues throughout the life cycle. Various explanatory models have been postulated by members of different disciplines. We propose a transactional model that incorporates data and theory from several fields: neurology, developmental psychology, child psychiatry, and pediatrics. Although it is not all-inclusive, this model facilitates informed developmental surveillance of children's behavior and development from birth to age 2 years.

At birth, a child's biological endowment includes (1) limbs, a central nervous system, organs, and sensory systems (intact or impaired) and (2) capacities for organizing experiences and interacting with the environment. As outlined in Chapters 1 and 8, the transactional model of development assumes that infants and caretakers together determine the child's developmental and behavioral outcome. This differs from other models in which *either* the child *or* the caretaking environment can unilaterally determine outcome. This approach is supported by emerging research on early brain development showing that caretaking, which may involve the infant's vision, hearing, smell, food, and taste, actually influences the number of synaptic connections; specifically, enriched environments increase synaptic connections in animals by 25% (Comery, Shah, and Greenough, 1995). At the other extreme, significant stress or trauma experiences result in central nervous system neurochemical alterations that may shape behavior and development (Perry et al, 1995). To promote or assess a child's development, contributions from "nature" and "nurture" need to be identified and understood. This approach to promotion and surveillance of development and behavior has three goals: (1) to nurture the child's primary attachment and promote development (internal security and self-control), (2) to decrease parent-child conflicts and increase the parents' understanding of and empathy for the child, and (3) to identify remediable disabilities and problems. This chapter discusses the multiple developmental processes that take place during the first 2 years of life across all the classic "streams of development": social

and emotional development, sensory and motor maturation, cognitive development, language acquisition, and physical growth. For each developmental process, possible normal variations and indications for clinical concern are described.

Social-Emotional Development

Sequential social-emotional and interactive patterns are based on how infants form relationships and interact with their caregivers. The process by which parents support a child's attempts at self-regulation can be understood as mutual regulation. Mutual regulation typically refers to the process by which infants thrive through the support and responsive interactions provided by their caregivers. This sequence is described in Table 3–1.

In addition, three theoretical constructs—attachment, separation, and autonomy/mastery—provide a framework for additional understanding of social and emotional development on a clinical level.

ATTACHMENT

Attachment describes the discriminating, enduring, and specific affective bond that develops over time between children and caregivers. Although infant behaviors that create and maintain this bond vary from one developmental stage to the next, their goal—to maintain the child's internal security—remains constant. Attachment is bidirectional: primary caregiver to infant and infant to primary caregiver, although these can be mutually exclusive. For example, a caregiver may have a strong attachment to a child but not be optimally responsive to that particular child's needs, and thus the child may feel ambiguously attached to the caregiver.

The process of attachment begins in utero. With quickening, parents begin to perceive the fetus as a separate individual and enter into an intense relationship with the imagined child to be (see Chapter 2). After birth, parents modify the expectations, hopes, and fears that evolved during the pregnancy as they become acquainted with the

Table 3–1 • Socioemotional Development of Infants and Children: Themes and Behaviors

Age	Developmental Goals	Clinical Observations
3 months	Can be calm/recovers from crying with comforting Able to be alert/looks at speaker when talked to	Attends visual/auditory stimulus for ≥3 seconds Remains calm/focused for ≥2 minutes
5 months	Displays positive affect toward primary caregiver Displays full range of emotions	Responds to social overtures (smiles, makes happy vocalization) Can display negative affect (frowns, makes angry arm/leg movements)
9 months	Makes purposeful two-way interactions	Makes intentional gestures such as pointing for a desired object or holding up arms to be picked up
13 months	Forms chains of communicative interaction ("circles"), that is, multiple verbal exchanges with "openings" and "closings"	Makes verbal exchanges with caregiver. For example child says "milk," parent brings bottle, child smiles and laughs appreciatively, and parent smiles (2 "circles").
18 months	Elaborates interactions that convey complex emotions	Imitates behavior and uses it to convey emotional theme. For example, child may rock and feed a doll.
24 months	Creates mental representations that can be used symbolically	Simple pretend play patterns of at least one idea, for example, "playing house"

Adapted from Greenspan SJ: Monitoring social and emotional development of young children. *In* Parker S, Zuckerman B (eds): Behavioral and Developmental Pediatrics. Boston, Little, Brown, 1995, p 35.

real baby. The process occurs for both mothers and fathers as illustrated in Figure 3–1.

Mothers who are emotionally available, sensitive, perceptive, and effective at meeting the needs of their child are likely to have securely attached infants. However, the child also makes a substantial contribution. For example, an alert infant who reacts readily to parents' faces and responds promptly to consoling maneuvers enhances parents' positive feelings and a sense of competence in the parents. Conversely, a drowsy, relatively hypotonic infant who provides less satisfying feedback may disappoint parents who anticipate the usual emotional satisfaction from their infant. Interventions in early infancy to increase sensitive responsiveness in mothers resulted in more securely attached infants at 12 months of age (van den Boom, 1994). Likewise, maternal unresponsiveness to infant behavior can be associated with 12-month-old infants' not wanting to interact with their mothers following a brief separation (Crockenberg, 1981). From these and other studies, lack of predictable or timely caretaker response appears to be a mechanism that prevents secure attachment from developing.

The process of parent-child attachment is not instantaneous. Most families require several months before they feel they know their infant. During this initial attachment period, parents strive to understand their infant's needs. Through trial and error, they gradually learn effective responses to the infant's need for food, rest, or social interaction. Parents begin to demonstrate an intuitive understanding of how to enhance their child's social responsiveness. For example, in face to face interactions, parents exaggerate their facial expressions and slow their vocalizations in response to the infant's limited ability to process social information. Eyebrows go up, mouths open wide, and conversation consists of "aahs" and "oohs." In response to such maneuvers, the neonate's eyelids widen, the pupils

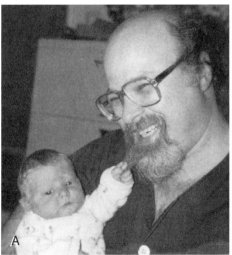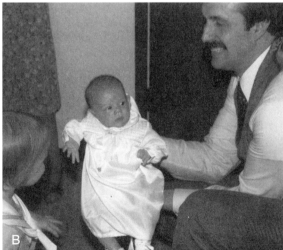

Figure 3–1. Two involved fathers.

dilate, and mouths become rounded. These signs of social interest occur long before the development of responsive smiling at 6 to 8 weeks of age. The newborn has all the necessary neurologic pathways to perform the seven universal facial expressions (happiness, sadness, surprise, interest, disgust, fear, and anger). Newborns are able to produce these expressions although they are much more readily identifiable at 2 to 3 months of age (Field et al, 1984).

By 3 months of age, the child and parents achieve social synchrony manifested by reciprocal vocal and affective exchanges. Parental displays of pleasure are followed by a build-up of smiling, cooing, and movement in the infant. When the excitement peaks, the infant transiently disengages to reorganize for another cycle of excitement. Infants also initiate these pleasurable exchanges. Occurrence of this mutually satisfying synchrony signals the end of the early adjustment period. Affect regulation and sharing by the infant is enabled by empathic responsiveness of the parent, and this synchrony may be the earliest precursor to the development of values (Sameroff and Emde, 1989), perhaps as expressed in the golden rule: "Do unto others as you would have them do unto you."

The next important step in the attachment process is the development of a clear preference for primary caretakers. By 3 to 5 months of age, a baby stops crying more readily for familiar caretakers than for strangers. Babies smile sooner and more brightly for their parents, and this clear behavioral preference enhances the parents' formation of positive emotional ties to their infant. At about the same time, infants look to their primary caregiver for signals (smile, comfort, fear) on how to respond to new experiences; this is referred to as *social referencing*. For example, during this period when a pediatrician enters the examination room, the infant looks to the mother to see if it is "all right" to allow this stranger to approach. If the mother smiles comfortably, the infant is more likely to remain calm. However, if the mother herself is upset about the possible pain the child will experience with immunizations, for example, the child is more likely to cry. The classic experiment for social referencing is mother-staged comfort or fear related to an infant's propensity to crawl over or avoid a visual cliff.

As recall memory for absent objects emerges between 7 and 9 months of age, the infant's preference for primary caretakers produces the well-recognized phenomena of *separation protest* and *stranger anxiety*. Separation protest is a 9-month-old infant's reaction of distress when the primary caretaker leaves as opposed to stranger anxiety, which also begins at about 9 months, in which the infant is distressed upon encountering a stranger. Attachment involves close proximity and provides a secure base that allows infants to explore their world. Initially attachment figures provide a sense of security by their physical proximity. Later in the 1st year, the infant internalizes this relationship with attachment figures, thus developing an internal model of security. By 18 months of age, infants have the ability to hold an image of the attachment figure continuously in their mind (memory) when they are not physically present, which helps comfort them in times of stress. For example, a scene commonly observed at child care drop-off is the child who walks around somewhat

aimlessly repeating "Mommy, mommy, mommy." The child is working to maintain the image of the mother and therefore security by repeating her name when she leaves (see Cognition, Play, and Language). There are two behavioral hallmarks of a secure attachment relationship in the first 2 years of life: *security* and *exploration* (Sroufe, 1979). This internalized working model of attachment can be seen in infants' behavior as they use their parents for security and progressive exploration of the world.

The creation of a secure relationship of attachment requires consistent availability of adults who are affectionate and responsive to the child's physical and emotional needs. Children given the opportunity to develop such a relationship possess a foundation on which to build positive relationships with peers and unrelated adults. Such a child is also associated at a later age with more effective coping with stress and better performance at school (Sroufe, 1988; Waters, Wippman, and Sroufe, 1979). The possibility of forming these relationships with more than one caring adult has been tested in studies of both adoptive families and communal living situations. Most adoptive mothers and their infants develop warm and secure attachment relationships (Singer et al, 1985). Similarly, in the kibbutz, children form attachment relationships of similar quality with two different nonfamilial caregivers (Sagi et al, 1995).

The research method commonly used to describe infant attachment is called the "strange situation" (Ainsworth and Bell, 1970). The purpose of the paradigm is to assess the quality of the infants' attachment to mother and to evaluate the infant's capacities for coping with stress. The theory is that the separation of the child from an attachment figure should activate the child's attachment system, and the infant's distress response to strangers is one indication of attachment to the primary caretaker. Attachment could then be studied during the reunion by assessing the child's proximity to the primary caretaker and the ease of being soothed and returning to play. The actual procedure consists of eight episodes in a prearranged sequence during which the infant is with the mother, with a stranger, separated from the mother, and reunited with the stranger and then the mother. The entire episode is videotaped and takes about 25 minutes. Attachment theory suggests that infants who are securely attached are able to use their caretaker to quickly soothe themselves and return to play (secure attachment [B]). Avoidantly attached infants demonstrate no overt response to the return of their caretakers and continue to play as if their caretakers did not return or leave (anxious/avoidant [A]). Anxiously attached infants turn to their mothers but are not easily soothed and do not return to play (anxious/resistant [C]). A disorganized attached infant demonstrates chaotic and/or self-destructive behavior, with the child first approaching and then backing away from the parent (disorganized/disoriented [D]). Although primary care providers do not use the full research paradigm in their clinical practice, this model and classification system may be useful as a reference when observing separations and reunions in the office.

The importance of forming a secure attachment between infant and parent has achieved prominence in the past several decades, particularly as the presence of surrogate child care has increased. A possible confounder to this attachment relationship classification system is the role of temperament and "goodness of fit." Temperament, or the "how of behavior," may make the initial adjustment to a separation harder; that is, "difficult" children may do better with a familiar situation, "easy" children may not display any problems, and "slow to warm up" children may initially exhibit problems and then be fine. An infant's temperament may not "fit" with parental expectations initially, and the attachment process may be prolonged or require adjustments on the part of both the infant and the caretaker (see Chapter 8 regarding temperament).

Putting Theory Into Practice

The transactional model provides a context for examining variability in the attachment process as a function of both the infant's behavior and the parents' responses to that behavior. The clinician can facilitate the evolution of secure relationships of attachment by being available to counsel caretakers during periods of difficulty. Although some infants appear intrinsically more difficult to nurture than others, parental handling from the earliest months of life appears to be a major determinant of the quality of the attachment relationship (Spieker and Booth, 1988). Inconsistent, inappropriate, or punitive responses to a child's physical or emotional needs may threaten the development of secure parent-child attachment. Parents burdened by illness, psychiatric impairment, drug abuse, or other crises may find it particularly difficult to respond warmly and consistently to the infant's frequent demands. Infants and toddlers who have experienced chronically inconsistent nurturing may appear uninterested in exploring the surrounding world, even in the caretaker's presence. Some of these children appear unusually clingy without the presence of obvious stress. Others appear actively angry and distrustful of their primary caretakers, ignoring or resisting caretakers' efforts to comfort them after brief separations or other stress (Sroufe, 1979).

An even more serious disturbance of the attachment process should be suspected when youngsters between the ages of 9 months and 2 years fail to demonstrate a behavioral preference for familiar caretakers in response to stress. Lack of discriminate attachment behaviors toward familiar caretakers can be an ominous sign, requiring the clinician to search for developmental delay in the child, serious family dysfunction, neglect, or abuse (Gaensbauer and Sands, 1979). Long separation from parents and disorganized patterns of multiple caretaking—conditions that occur in many prolonged hospitalizations—can also produce indiscriminate attachment behaviors. When a child exhibits indiscriminate, avoidant, or resistant attachment behaviors, the clinician should encourage caretakers' availability, warmth, and responsiveness whether the child is at home, in child care, or in the hospital. Hospital and child care personnel should provide the child with one or two nurses or teachers who are assigned consistently to augment parents' efforts to restore the child's sense of internal security. If the child's avoidant, resistant, or indiscriminate attachment behaviors persist, mental health referral for the family is indicated.

SEPARATION

Negotiation of separation, both psychological and physical, poses a continuous challenge to parent and child. In psychiatric theory, best outlined by Mahler and associates (1975), separation refers to the internal processes by which the child evolves a satisfying identity as an individual distinct from the parents. Depending on the psychological context, actual physical separations can enhance or impede the child's ability to develop a comfortable individuality. During infancy, as the reliable physical availability to responsive caretakers encourages the infant's efforts toward independence, a complementary process of acceptance of the child's internal separation must take place within the parents. Some parents readily accept an infant's total dependence but have difficulty tolerating a toddler's striving for an independent identity.

Putting Theory Into Practice: Bedtime, Child Care, and Hospitalization

The child's and parents' responses to everyday experiences of physical separation, such as bedtime, child care, parental travel, or hospitalization of parent or child, can vary widely. In assessing the developmental progress of the child's internal process of separation, the clinician should anticipate that both parents and child will show mixed feelings about separations. Appropriate management of a physical separation depends on its duration and context as well as on the developmental readiness of both parents and child. A brief observation of an unstructured interaction between a parent and infant in the primary care provider's office can provide valuable clinical data from which to gauge the child's social-emotional development. Observation of caregiving patterns include the caretaker's ability to comfort the infant, to find an appropriate level of stimulation to interest and engage the infant pleasurably, and to read and respond to the infant's emotional signals. If any of the clinical observations or behavioral responses are suboptimal, then hypersensitivity or hyposensitivity to environmental stimulation should be considered (Greenspan, 1996).

Brief, predictable physical separations from the parents facilitate successful psychological separation for young children. The first such separation occurs when the infant is put to bed alone at night. The next occurs the first time parents leave their new infant with a relative or baby-sitter. Most parents are uncomfortable with these first separations. When parents express apparently disproportionate anxiety about their child's well-being during routine separations, they are often expressing ambivalence about the child's evolution of independence. Explicit discussion of the parents' feelings about internal and external separations can be more effective than reassurance about the ostensible concern. For example, the clinician might suggest that it is not easy for parents to be away from their babies, rather than say, "Crying doesn't make children sick."

Initial difficulties with separation subside only to become acute again when, at 7 to 9 months of age, children begin to show *separation protest* (crying when the caretaker leaves their presence). As described in subsequent sections, clinicians can help parents recognize that the separation protest that results from normal cognitive phenomena will diminish as the child learns from multiple brief separations and reunions that parents reliably return.

As the psychological process of separation proceeds,

the child develops the ability to form relationships with caretakers other than the parents. Parents can facilitate the formation of these new relationships by their physical availability to the child as the relationship is first formed. A new baby-sitter should be introduced with the mother present for at least 1 day. When the child begins attending a new child care center, a parent should stay at the center with the child for the first 5 to 7 days, leaving for successively longer periods each day. Parents should expect that the child will initially protest their departure. The child's distress diminishes as familiarity with the new caretakers increases and experience teaches that the parent's return is assured.

Overwhelming stress, such as physical illness and the painful experiences entailed in hospitalization, exceeds any infant's capacity to tolerate physical separation from his or her parents. When the child is tired or ill or has recently sustained a prolonged separation from caretakers, the physical presence of the parent paradoxically supports the process of internal separation by preventing the child from becoming overwhelmed by internal or external stress. The clinician should recommend that a parent or other familiar caretaker remain with a young child during hospitalization (see Chapter 32).

Because the separation process is mutual, clinicians should be alert to parental issues that can unintentionally sabotage the child's establishment of a separate identity. This process is particularly in jeopardy when the parents perceive the child as unusually "vulnerable" because of past illness or other factors that make a child special (e.g., only boy, only girl, last child). A recent loss in the parents' lives, such as a death or divorce, can also threaten the separation process.

When parents regard their child as uniquely susceptible to harm or illness, they can become overprotective, which involves the parents' difficulty in supporting age-appropriate, socioculturally concordant separation and individuation in the child. This leads to the *vulnerable child syndrome*, which involves separation difficulties, insufficient setting of limits, somatic concerns, and overuse of the health care system (Thomasgard and Metz, 1995). A clinician who encourages parents to discuss their real or imagined losses and their ambivalence about separation can help to liberate both parent and child. The process of internal separation does not end in infancy for either parent or child but must be negotiated repeatedly throughout the life cycle (see Chapter 33).

AUTONOMY AND MASTERY

The infant's intrinsic need for autonomy and mastery drives developmental progress from the earliest weeks of life. *Autonomy* refers to the achievement of behavioral independence. *Mastery* describes the child's quest for ever-increasing competence. These complementary processes require that caretakers and infants continually renegotiate control of the infant's bodily functions and social interactions.

Self-consoling behavior marks the beginning of autonomy. From the earliest days after birth, a crying infant tries to bring the hand to the mouth. Once the hand is inserted, the infant begins to suck and stops crying. Several studies have demonstrated that sucking facilitates the infant's ability to regulate his or her level of arousal. For example, Brazelton (1962) found that during the first 3 months of life, infants who engage in frequent hand-sucking cry less than other infants. Studies show sucking on sucrose may further reduce a reaction to a painful stimulus, possibly through a neurally mediated pathway (Bucher, 1995).

As the infant matures, the repertoire for self-consolation expands to include rhythmic behaviors such as body rocking (20% of all children) and head banging or rolling (6% of all children); these behaviors usually begin between 6 and 10 months of age. In the 2nd year of life, toddlers use favored possessions such as blankets (transitional objects) and repetitive rituals (e.g., saying goodnight to stuffed animals in a fixed order) to cope autonomously with bedtime and other stressful situations (see Chapter 45).

The infant's drive to master the environment serves as an important motivating force in itself, independent of the need for food, warmth, sleep, and social approval. This intense striving for competence and independence can lead to struggles with caretakers over feeding, sleep, toileting, and exploration. For instance, many 9-month-old children are so intent on practicing new fine motor skills that they will insist on feeding themselves with their fingers, refusing to allow parents to feed them. Like the legendary mountaineer George Leish Mallory, an 18-month-old child will repetitively scale a forbidden sofa "because it's there."

Putting Theory to Practice: Thumb-Sucking, Tantrums, and Toilet Training

As the transactional model predicts, the child's struggles for autonomy and mastery produce varying degrees of discord depending on the temperamental style of the child and the attitudes of the caretakers. For example, temperamentally persistent youngsters delight parents by working at a new task until they have mastered it. However, such persistent children may also infuriate parents by refusing to abandon unsafe explorations of the kitchen stove.

Parental concerns about thumb-sucking, temper tantrums, and toilet training provide three common clinical examples of autonomy issues. *Sucking*, the first organized behavior under the infant's control, is used both to obtain nutrition and to achieve self-regulation (by sucking on a pacifier, a hand, or nothing). Parents unaware of the self-regulatory function of nonnutritive sucking, which occurs in between 23% and 46% of children ages 1 to 4 years, may interpret it as a sign of hunger and inadvertently overfeed the infant (Friman, 1990). With increasing age, nonnutritive sucking on fingers or pacifiers decreases, becoming a selective coping response to fatigue, illness, or distress.

If parents ignore this harmless self-regulating behavior, most children spontaneously relinquish it between the ages of 4 and 5 years as other strategies for coping develop. However, if parents try to discourage finger sucking through criticism or restraint, a positive coping mechanism becomes an occasion for a negative struggle over who controls the child's body. To assert their autonomy, children then stubbornly persist in thumb-sucking longer than they would otherwise. Clinicians can help parents perceive the positive functions of nonnutritive sucking and alleviate unnecessary anxiety about orthodontic problems or digital deformity, which arise only if thumb-sucking persists and is extensive past the age at which permanent teeth erupt (Friman and Schmitt, 1989).

Tantrums, common in the 2nd year of life, arise from the child's efforts to exercise mastery and autonomy. Clinicians and caretakers can better devise appropriate management if they understand the developmental issues that give rise to tantrums. For example, some tantrums result from the child's frustration at failing to master a task. Distracting the child and permitting success in a more manageable activity can be a helpful maneuver to alleviate this type of tantrum. Most toddlers respond with tantrums as parents impose limits that restrict their autonomy. Parental response to such tantrums should encourage self-control and limitation of the child's frustration by paying attention to temperamental characteristics. Ignoring is an effective way to avoid reinforcing tantrums, although young children may need to be held so that they can regain control. Older children should be left alone in a safe place until they have calmed themselves. In using a "time out" procedure, parents should not attempt to inflict a fixed number of minutes of isolation. The goal should be to help the child develop self-regulation. As soon as the tantrum subsides, isolation should end and the child should receive praise for the quieter state.

An appropriate balance between necessary limits and support for independence requires frequent renegotiation as the child's level of development changes. In general, successful limits are firm, consistent, explicit, and selective. Children thrive on routine and structure. Setting limits should include praise for desired behavior ("time in") as well as disapproval for or removal from an undesired behavior. Parents of toddlers often need help in choosing which issues are worth a battle. Breaking the child's will should never become an end in itself. Constant tantrum behavior indicates that both family and child have lost control. Such families may benefit from mental health referral. (See Chapter 78 for further suggestions on behavioral management.)

Toilet training proceeds optimally when parents appreciate the child's need for autonomy and mastery. Anticipatory guidance around toilet training should begin toward the end of the 1st year because many parents plan to initiate toilet training after the child's 1st birthday. If toilet training is begun on an arbitrary schedule, before the child has shown an interest in mastery of this skill, unnecessary tension can be created between parent and child. Between the ages of 2 and 3 years, most children spontaneously begin to imitate the toileting behavior of siblings and parents. At first, youngsters may just want to sit on the toilet without producing urine or stool. Parents should permit the child to pace the process as they would the learning of any other new skill (such as riding a tricycle). The drive for autonomous control of body functions and the desire to master socially approved tasks enable children to train themselves within a few days when they choose the time. Toilet training need not be a charged issue. By respecting the child's autonomy and pride in mastery, parents can make toilet training an occasion for growth rather than conflict.

Neuromaturation in Infancy

Maturing sensory and motor abilities progressively refine the quality of information available to the growing infant. To learn about the social and inanimate world, the baby must actively coordinate the three systems that result in (1) regulation of state (i.e., level of arousal), (2) reception and processing of sensory stimuli, and (3) voluntary control of fine and gross motor movements. Neuromaturation of these regulatory systems in conjunction with mutual regulation with the caretaker forms the basis of social and emotional development as discussed earlier in this chapter and in Table 3–1.

STATE CONTROL

The newborn's level of arousal creates six organized clusters of behaviors called *states*. There are two sleep states (quiet and active); a drowsy state; an alert, responsive state; a fussy state; and a state characterized by vigorous crying (see Chapter 2). These six states provide the neurophysiologic foundation for the infant's motor and sensory responses. For example, muscle tone appears hypertonic in crying infants and hypotonic in sleeping ones. During sleep, infants gradually decrease responses to repetitive loud noises or bright lights. The same stimuli presented to infants in drowsy or alert states can increase their alertness and activity (Nugent, 1985).

Most learning occurs when the baby is alert but not moving, because newborns cannot use their large muscles and attend simultaneously. As the baby becomes active and fussy, orienting behavior toward sights and sounds ceases. Periods of quiet alertness are fleeting in the early weeks of life. The ability of some awake, fussy newborns to interact with caretakers may be improved by swaddling, which inhibits movement and facilitates a quiet, alert state.

During the first 3 months of life, neurophysiologic changes (doubling of quiet sleep and diminishing latency of the visual evoked potential) and neuroanatomic changes (rapid myelinization and increased dendritic branching) progressively permit the infant to regulate arousal. This improved regulation of arousal produces increased sustained alertness, decreased crying, and longer periods of sleep (Table 3–2).

Table 3–2 • State Changes in Early Infancy

	Behavior (hours/day)			
Age	*Longest Awake Period*	*Crying*	*Longest Sleep Period*	*Total Sleep*
2 weeks old	2.61	1.75	4.41	16.25
6 weeks old	NA	2.75	NA	NA
12 weeks old	3.41	1.00	7.67	15.11
16 weeks old	3.56	NA	8.48	14.87

NA = not available

Data from Parmelee AH Jr., Weiner W, Schultz H: Infant sleep patterns: from birth to 16 weeks of age. Pediatrics 65:576, 1974, and Brazelton TB: Crying in infancy. Pediatrics 29:579, 1962.

Putting Theory Into Practice: Colic and Sleep

The infant's first social responses consist of attaining or maintaining an alert state in response to caretaking maneuvers. The crying baby who quiets when picked up or the drowsy one who suddenly becomes wide-eyed and attentive at the sound of mother's voice delights caretakers.

There are wide individual variations in the infant's control of state, responsiveness to environmental input, and sleep-wake patterns. Some babies spontaneously rouse from active sleep into quiet alertness. Others move directly from sleep to crying, becoming alert only after being consoled. Once roused, many infants independently inhibit their movements in order to attend to an interesting sound or sight. However, some youngsters cannot sustain an alert, receptive state unless assisted by an adult who swaddles them or gently restrains their hands. These inattentive infants can be frustrating to caretakers. The clinician can suggest various methods to help such infants maintain alertness and can also alleviate parents' distress by pointing out that the baby's inattentiveness reflects immaturity and will improve with time.

Like the inattentive infant, the colicky infant suffers from a disorder of state control that improves with maturation (Zuckerman, 1981) (see Chapter 37). *Colic*, or "paroxysmal fussiness," tends to occur in infants with low sensory thresholds. Parents who try to soothe the inexplicably crying infant may inadvertently overstimulate the baby further and prolong the crying bout. Recent studies have examined various "treatment interventions" from supplemental carrying to increased parental responsiveness (Parkin, Schwartz, and Manuel, 1993; St. James-Roberts et al, 1995) as well as a potential relationship between maternal behavior and early infant temperament (Parker and Barrett, 1992). In opposition to standard pediatric advice to "be responsive," supplemental carrying does not reduce crying and fussing behavior further in *infants who have colic as compared to infants who do not have colic;* this resistance to carrying may indicate an important difference in state regulation and control in infants with colic (Barr et al, 1991).

Clinical supervision of *sleep disorders* requires an understanding of the normal variability in children's sleep patterns. Newborns typically sleep 16½ hours per day, including naps; by the 6th month of life, the amount of sleep declines to approximately 14½ hours. One- and two-year-old children sleep approximately 13 hours a day including naps, and 3-year-old children have 12 hours of sleep per day (Ferber, 1985). A longitudinal study of 104 infants aged 1 to 12 months found that 71% of the children "settled" (slept from midnight to 5 AM) by the 3rd month, 83% settled by the 6th month, and 10% never completely settled during the 1st year (Moore and Ucko, 1957).

Duration of sleep depends both on the maturation of the child's central nervous system and on parental handling. The clinician can help parents devise strategies that can gradually mold the infant's innate biological rhythms into more socially convenient patterns. By 9 months of age (and particularly during the 2nd year), children are motivated to control their bodies and the environment. Letting go of daytime exploration and excitement is difficult, leading to resistance to sleep as an issue of autonomy and self-regulation. By 9 months, waking at night is normal although many infants can then return to sleep themselves (*self-regulation*); other infants need their parents to provide the sleep onset association (e.g., holding, sucking) to return to sleep (*mutual regulation*). Infants who return to sleep without calling for parental attention are generally regarded as sleeping through the night.

Some new parents require help with distinguishing active sleep from wakefulness. Active sleep occurs every 50 to 60 minutes during a sleep cycle. If parents rush to check or feed the infant at every rustle or moan made during active sleep, the development of sustained sleep is delayed. The clinician who suspects this to be the case can advise parents to wait until their infant seems fully awake before picking him or her up (see Chapter 44).

SENSORY ABILITIES

Sensory abilities in the infant mature rapidly during the 1st year of life. Although immature, the infant's innate visual capacities are preset to select socially relevant stimuli. The newborn's visual field is relatively narrow, and only objects at the fixed focal distance of 19 cm (approximately 12 inches) are perceived clearly. Infants ignore visual stimuli that are too close or too distant (Cohen, DeLoach, and Strauss, 1979). Thus, the mother's face is seen more clearly by the newborn than are his or her own hands. By 2 to 3 months of age, visual accommodation matures. The baby then discovers hands and other near objects. Between 6 months and 1 year of age, the infant achieves visual acuity and a visual field functionally similar to an adult's, although measured visual acuity does not approach adult values until the preschool years (Cohen, DeLoach, and Strauss, 1979).

Very young infants modify their behavior in response to information gathered by smell and taste. By 7 days of age, infants reliably discriminate between their own mother's breast pads and those of other nursing mothers (MacFarlane, 1975). Infants vary their sucking patterns in response to the taste of breast milk, formula, and salty or sweet liquid. The flavor aspects of food eaten by mothers are transmitted through their milk to their infants. For example, the infant feeds longer and sucks more overall when the milk is flavored with garlic (Mennella and Beauchamp, 1991). Infants suck less on an unsweetened liquid, such as breast milk, after they have tasted a sweet solution (Lipsitt, 1979). Newborns can differentiate varying degrees of sweetness and different kinds of sugars (Desor, Maller, and Turner, 1977).

Putting Theory Into Practice: Low Sensory Threshold and Sensory Deficit

Parents subliminally monitor their infant's responses to sensory input and then modulate that input to enhance the infant's responsiveness. A mother, for example, moves her head slowly back and forth until the infant's expression signals that her face is now in focus. When the baby is startled by the father's deep voice, the father switches to falsetto, also known as "parentese" (caretaker speech).

Although caretakers usually make these adjustments automatically, clinicians may need to provide explicit guidance for families whose infants are unusually hypersensitive or unresponsive. Some premature or small for dates infants have low sensory thresholds. Sounds and sights that are attractive to most infants are aversive to these hypersensitive babies. For example, even though most infants prefer to track a moving face that is making sounds, a hypersensitive infant may avert his or her gaze, vomit, or startle when confronted with this simultaneous visual and auditory stimulation. Clinicians can assist parents in sustaining social interaction with these infants by suggesting that stimulation be offered to only one of the baby's senses at a time. Extraneous stimuli, such as bright lights and loud radios, should be decreased.

Healthy infants should turn to voices and track faces with their eyes. Parents are exquisitely sensitive to their infant's responses. When parents express concern that their infant does not seem to hear or see, that infant should be formally assessed. No child is too young for audiologic testing. In 1994, the Joint Committee on Infant Hearing and Testing of the National Institutes of Health recommended universal newborn screening (see Chapter 57).

MOTOR DEVELOPMENT

Fine Motor Development

It is in large part through motor acts that the very young child develops and expresses perception, emotion, and cognition. Between 2 and 3 months of age, decline of the asymmetric tonic neck reflex and expansion of accommodative abilities permit infants to look at their hands and touch one hand with the other. By furnishing simultaneous information to the senses of vision and touch, this mutual hand grasp provides a foundation for later visual motor skills. During the 3rd month of life, as the world of close proximity comes into focus, infants begin swiping at objects with loosely fisted hands. At this stage, infants swipe with one hand only at objects in front of one shoulder or the other. By 6 months of age, they reach persistently toward objects in the midline, at first with both hands and then with one.

Between 3 and 6 months of age, the coordination of grasping and reaching gradually comes under visual guidance and voluntary control. During early reaching efforts, grasping may occur, but only after the hand has contacted the object. After 6 months of age, infants begin to shape their hands for grasping in the horizontal or vertical plane of the desired object immediately before touching it. By 9 months of age, shaping of the hand occurs before the object is reached. One-year-old children orient the hand in the appropriate plane when starting to reach for an object (Twitchell, 1965).

Once the infant can reliably obtain an object, clumsy whole-hand grasping becomes progressively refined. At 4 months of age, the child holds an object between fingers and palm; at 5 months of age, the thumb becomes involved. By 7 months of age, thumb and fingers can grasp and retain an object without resting on the palm at all. At this time, the child uses a raking motion between the thumb and several fingers to scoop up small objects. By 9 months of age, the child manipulates small objects with a neat pincer grasp, using thumb and forefinger perpendicular to the surface. Every nook and cranny is then accessible to the child's exploration. During the 2nd year of life, toddlers develop a palmar grasp and wrist supination that permits them to use tools such as spoons and pencils.

Gross Motor Development

Three processes enable the infant to attain upright posture and the ability to move the limbs across the midline of the body: (1) balance of flexor and extensor tone, (2) decline of obligatory primary reflexes, and (3) evolution of protective and equilibrium responses.

First, the infant's muscle tone progresses from the neonatal state of predominant flexion to a balance in the tone of flexor and extensor muscles. As this balance develops, the flexed newborn posture gradually unfolds until by 6 months of age babies can extend their legs so far that they can put their toes in their mouths.

Second, the decline of obligatory primary reflexes (such as the Moro or asymmetric tonic neck reflex) permits the infant more flexible movement. A 1-month-old child cannot look to one side or the other without assuming the fencing posture of the asymmetric tonic neck reflex. Until this reflex disappears, the child's arm position is determined by the head's orientation. As this reflex disappears, the infant develops the ability to bring his or her hands toward the midline.

Third, in order to sit and walk, the child must establish equilibrium and protective responses. These responses are the automatic changes in trunk and extremity positions that the baby uses to balance and keep from falling. The familiar parachute response of 9-month-old children who extend arms or legs to catch themselves when dropped toward the ground is an example of such protective reactions. Table 3–3 summarizes the age ranges for acquisition of selected milestones in motor development.

The age range for normal development of gross motor skills is wide (see Table 3–3). Parents and clinicians should not focus on any rigid timetable of discrete motor milestones but should appreciate the ongoing process. In general, infants learn to maintain new positions weeks to months before they can attain them voluntarily. For example, many infants at 6 months of age sit briefly unsupported

Table 3–3 • Age Range in Acquisition of Skills

Skill	Range* (months)
Fixates on disappearance of ball	4–5
Uses whole hand to grasp rod	3–6
Sits alone while playing with toy	3–6
Uses partial thumb opposition to grasp pellet ("pincer grasp")	7–9
Supports weight momentarily	6–8
Grasps pencil at farthest end	8–12
Walks alone with good coordination	10–16
Runs with coordination	14–25
Uses eye-hand coordination in tossing ring	29–42

*Fifth to ninety-fifth percentile

Adapted from Bayley N: Manual for the Bayley Scales of Infant Development, 2nd ed. Copyright © 1993 by The Psychological Corporation. Adapted and used by permission. All rights reserved.

if placed in that position, but they cannot get themselves into a sitting position until 8 months of age. Coordinated motion from a new posture takes even longer to develop. Most children cannot walk independently until 4 to 5 months after they have learned to pull themselves up to a standing position.

Putting Theory Into Practice: Gross and Fine Motor Development

The developmental route to walking varies with the child's tone and temperament. Mildly hypotonic (loose-limbed) youngsters sit at the usual age but are late in rolling from back to front or walking. These hypotonic infants scoot or hitch on their buttocks rather than crawl. By 3 years of age, these mildly hypotonic youngsters have developed a normal gait. Temperamentally inactive children or those who adapt slowly may not attempt independent walking until long after they are neurologically able to do so. Conversely, very active babies start taking steps as soon as they can stand. During the 2nd year of life, these active infants rarely walk if they can run.

Parents are often relieved to know that, within the wide range of normal variation, there is no correlation between intelligence and the age at which gross motor skills are acquired. No single motor skill can be used as an indicator of neurologic integrity or dysfunction. In general, the clinician should investigate when delayed milestones are associated with global delays, opisthotonic posturing, persistent fisting of the hands, consistent disuse of a limb or side of the body, obligatory and prolonged infantile reflexes, or failure to develop a neat pincer grasp by the 1st birthday. The early diagnosis of cerebral palsy and other motor disabilities is described in Chapter 59.

Cognition, Play, and Language

COGNITION

The developmental theories of Jean Piaget, as outlined by Ginsberg and Opper (1979), provide the most useful clinical framework for understanding infant cognitive growth. These theories of cognitive development describe learning as a process of adaptation. Piaget believed that infants are active initiators and not passive recipients in learning; infants are aware of their environment and begin to modify their behavior in response to environmental demands. Infants can take in (assimilate) information and use it to revise existing mental structures, structures that have evolved from primitive reflex responses and were created in response to interactions with the environment. The infant can create new structures/schemas or change existing ones to accommodate new information that does not conform to existing schemas.

Piaget organizes cognitive development during the sensorimotor period (birth to 2 years of age) into six stages. Each stage represents a temporary equilibrium between the infant's skills and the challenges of the environment. A toy that is too familiar no longer engages the toddler, who prefers the greater challenges posed by the contents of the kitchen cupboard. Conversely, a completely insoluble

problem (such as the use of a crayon presented to a 9-month-old child) does not hold the infant's interest. Cognitive development requires opportunities for exploration and manipulation that are neither too easy nor too hard. Piaget believed that infants and young toddlers are multisensory and active in this learning process; infants use their whole bodies and minds to explore the world and the people in it.

Object Permanence

The newborn behaves as though the world consists of shifting images that cease to exist when they are no longer perceived. "Out of sight, out of mind" is a literal description of the infant's world during the first stage of sensorimotor development (stage I). Gradually, stable mental images of absent objects and people develop. By 2 months of age, a baby continues to look expectantly at a person's empty hand after an object has been dropped from sight (stage II). Between 4 and 8 months of age, the infant can locate a partly hidden object and visually track objects through a vertical trajectory. If a baby sees someone hide an object, however, he or she will not search for it (stage III). Between 9 and 12 months of age, infants can find an object that they see hidden (stage IV). At this age, however, infants cannot retrieve an object that is moved in plain view from one hiding place to another. By 18 months of age, babies reliably find objects after multiple changes of position as long as those changes are observed, but they cannot deduce the whereabouts of an object if they do not see it being moved (stage V). Finally, by age 2 years, the toddler has sufficient symbolic abilities to infer the position of a hidden object from other cues without actually observing it being moved to that position (stage VI). People and things then reliably exist for the child as stable entities whether or not they are perceptually present. Behaviors characteristic of each stage of the child's understanding of object permanence are outlined in Table 3–4.

Causality

Piaget observed an orderly sequence of changes in the child's understanding of causal relationships over the first 2 years of life. First, the infant learns to recreate satisfying bodily sensations by maneuvers such as thumb-sucking (primary circular reaction). At about 3 months of age, the child begins to use causal behaviors to recreate accidentally discovered, interesting effects (secondary circular reaction). For example, babies at this age may repeatedly kick a mattress once they have discovered by chance that this behavior sets in motion a mobile above the bed. The infant's understanding of cause and effect gradually leads to increasingly specific behavior patterns aimed at particular environmental effects. During the 2nd year of life, the infant becomes more of an experimenter, intent on causing novel events rather than reinstituting familiar ones (tertiary circular reactions). At the same time, the child begins to comprehend that apparently unrelated behaviors can be combined to create a desired effect. For example, by age 2 years, a child can spontaneously wind up a toy to make it move.

Table 3-4 • Cognition, Play, and Language

Piagetian Stage	Age	Object Permanence	Causality	Play	Receptive Language	Expressive Language
I	Birth to 1 month	Shifting images	Generalization of reflexes		Turns to voice	Range of cries (hunger, pain)
II	1–4 months	Stares at spot from which object disappeared (looks at hand after yarn drops)	Primary circular reactions (thumb-sucking)		Searches for speaker with eyes	Cooing Vocal contagion
III	4–8 months	Visually follows dropped object through vertical trajectory (tracks dropped yarn to floor)	Secondary circular reactions recreates accidentally discovered environmental effects (e.g., kicks mattress to shake mobile)	Same behavioral repertoire for all objects (bangs, shakes, puts in mouth, drops)	Responds to own name and to tones of voice	Babbling Four distinct syllables
IV	9–12 months	Finds an object after watching it being hidden	Coordination of secondary circular reactions	Visual-motor inspection of objects Peek-a-boo	Listens selectively to familiar words Responds to "no" and other verbal requests	First real word "Jargoning" Symbolic gestures (shakes head "no")
V	12–18 months	Recovers hidden object after multiple visible changes of position	Tertiary circular reactions (deliberately varies behavior to create novel effects)	Awareness of social function of objects Symbolic play centered on own body (drinks from toy cup)	Can bring familiar object from another room Points to parts of body	Many single words—uses words to express needs Acquires 10 words by 18 months
VI	18 months to 2 years	Recovers hidden object after invisible changes in position	Spontaneously uses nondirect causal mechanisms (uses key to move wind-up toy)	Symbolic play directed toward doll (gives doll a drink)	Follows series of two or three commands Points to picture when named	Telegraphic two-word sentence

Infant Recognition, Memory, and Habituation of Attention

Research shows that an infant's capacity for memory is predictive of later cognitive functioning. Low to moderate correlations have been found between an infant's preference for novel visual stimuli and IQ at age 3 years and vocabulary up to age 7 years (Fagan, 1982). The research paradigm often used to assess infant memory consists of the presentation of a stimulus and subsequent observation of whether the infant spends more time attending to a novel rather than a familiar stimulus (Bornstein and Sigman, 1986). Preference for novelty is thought to represent a better memory and an attraction for exploring new stimuli, which leads to developmental progression and learning.

PLAY

"Play is a window through which we come to understand the child from both inside and outside" (Sheridan, Foley, and Radlinski, 1995). Peek-a-boo signals the emergence of object permanence. An elaborate detour to retrieve a ball rolled under the couch shows that the child understands invisible displacements. The repetitive dropping of food from the high chair completes many tertiary circular reactions in a child's learning process, as long as someone is there to pick up the food and close the circle.

The infant's handling of objects also reflects his or her progressive understanding of the world. At 5 to 6 months of age, an infant can reliably reach and grasp attractive objects. At this stage, the baby subjects all toys to the same behavioral repertoire, regardless of their particular properties. A toy car, a bell, or a spoon all are mouthed, shaken, banged, and dropped. By 9 months of age, the baby systematically manipulates the object to inspect it with eyes and hands in all orientations, thus demonstrating the cognitive ability to process information simultaneously instead of sequentially.

By the 1st birthday, the baby demonstrates understanding of the socially assigned function of objects. A toy car is pushed on its wheels; a bell is rung. Next, early representational play, which reflects stable concept of objects, appears. At first such *symbolic play* centers on the child's own body as the youngster "drinks" from a toy cup or puts a toy telephone to his or her ear. Between 17 and 24 months of age, the child's thought and play become less egocentric; for example, the doll is offered a drink. When the child becomes facile in the use of symbols (between 24 and 30 months of age), truly imaginative play begins. In such play, the child uses one object to represent another (such as putting bits of paper on a plate to symbolize food). Table 3–4 outlines the concurrent development of object permanence, causality, and play.

Putting Theory Into Practice: Separation Protest, Stranger Awareness, and Cognitive Assessment

Each cognitive transformation alters the infant's social behavior. Although babies as young as 2 to 3 months of age can recognize their parents, they have no recall memory—that is, no internal symbolic representation of their parents—until they attain stage IV object permanence (the stage at which they search for a completely hidden object). The child's recall memory for parents evolves before memory for inanimate objects (Bell, 1970). The child's experience of "missing" the parent after separation results from the discrepancy between the recalled image of the parent and the parent's absence from the child's perceptual field. For the 4-month-old child, the parent does not exist when not seen. The 10-month-old child knows that parents still exist when they are not there, but the child of this age cannot imagine where they might be. The child may vigorously protest separation and anxiously track parents even into the bathroom. Not until the child attains stage V object permanence (at 15 to 18 months of age) can he or she predict the position of an object from a series of displacements. Once this cognitive capacity emerges, the child has the ability to infer parents' whereabouts in their absence, and separation protest diminishes.

Infants learn primarily from exploration and play. It is through these activities that the infant experiences the world, comes to know it, and predicts it. According to Piaget, infants learn by *assimilation* (applying existing skills/responses to events/experiences) and *accommodation* (changing behavior to fit new experiences). When observing the child for cognitive skills, exploratory skills (mouthing, shaking, tracking) as well as insightful strategies (imitation, modeling) are sought.

The ability to deal simultaneously with several pieces of information develops at the same time that the child achieves stage IV object permanence. Stranger awareness results, because the child can then actively compare unfamiliar people to familiar people. The 4-month-old child smiles at any smiling adult. The 7- to 9-month-old child glances warily from parent to stranger to parent and then howls. The child health professional can reduce parents' bewilderment at separation protest and stranger anxiety by explaining that these behaviors are positive signs of normal cognitive development rather than results of inexplicable emotional disturbance. It is often difficult to sort out cognitive function from the child's overall developmental function (including communication and motor function) in the first 2 years of life. Several screening tests use developmental milestones such as object permanence (playing peek-a-boo, following a dropped object) as a means of assessing cognition and learning.

LANGUAGE

Like other developmental phenomena, the infant's acquisition of language follows a predictable sequence. However, the rate and quality of the infant's progression through linguistic development can be more sensitive to caretaking practices than other sensorimotor skills. Infants communicate actively from birth. Lacking words, infants communicate through numerous sensory channels with four major purposes to their communication efforts: (1) to regulate another person's behavior, (2) to attract or maintain another person's attention for social interaction, (3) to draw joint attention to objects and events, and (4) to experience the inherent pleasure of communicating.

Infants can acquire reciprocal language only through

interaction with responsive sources. Television and radio have negligible effects on language learning in infants.

Parents and infants begin to construct the basis for later language acquisition long before the baby can understand or produce a single word. Through games and caretaking rituals during the 1st year, children learn to take turns communicating. With vocalization and nonverbal cues, caretakers and infants learn to direct each other's attention to interesting environmental events, to signal needs and feelings, and to interpret each other's intentions. During the 2nd year of life, the child begins to extend the rules of communication learned in action to the use of spoken words.

The production of meaningful speech is the result of cognitive, oral-motor, and social processes. By 1 month of age, the infant has a range of cries that parents associate with, for example, hunger or pain. Between 1 and 3 months of age, the infant develops a range of nondistress vocalizations, onomatopoetically described as "cooing." When the caretaker imitates the baby, the infant's production of sound is prolonged. The caretaker's contingent responses to these early vocalizations shape the infant's vocalization into conversation-like patterns. Adult speech both elicits and reinforces infant speech (Bloom, 1977).

By 3 to 4 months of age, infants can produce babbling repetition of all vowel sounds and some consonants. At least two distinct syllables are produced. As babbling matures, the infant starts to produce repetitive two-syllable combinations, such as mama and dada, even though, at this time, these combinations have no symbolic reference.

The emergence of actual words, or sounds used as symbols, depends on the infant's attainment of rudimentary object permanence. Before a person or object can be named, it must have a stable existence in the infant's mind. The first true words usually refer to parents and other family members, because the concept of object permanence occurs for people before inanimate objects. Between 10 and 15 months of age, infants speak their first real words. During this time, infants also begin to use symbolic gestures, such as shaking the head to indicate no. "Jargoning," long utterances that sound like statements or questions but contain no real words, also occurs initially around the 1st birthday.

Receptive language ability precedes expressive ability during the toddler years. When asked to do so, children can point to pictures or objects before they can name them. Most 1-year-old infants can respond to simple commands, such as "bye-bye" or "no-no," and most 18-month-old children can point to one or two body parts.

During the 2nd and 3rd years of life, expressive vocabulary expands exponentially. Infants have acquired a mean of 10 words by age 18 months and about 1000 words by age 3 years. At the same time, the child begins to construct two-word telegraphic sentences, first to comment on his or her own needs ("more cookie") and then to comment on events in the immediate environment ("mommy go"). By conversing with children and expanding statements ("mommy's going out"), caretakers help children to become generally competent speakers of their native language by the age of 5 years.

Literacy may also begin during infancy (McLane and McNamee, 1991). Through exposure to books, infants gradually become increasingly aware of the importance of written language. Just as with spoken language, infants use their keen powers of observation and their desire to imitate activity to learn about books and written language long before they can read and write. Sharing books with children can stimulate their interest as early as 6 months of age, when infants may merely pat the faces in a picture book. In addition to enhancing language development, book sharing enhances parent-child relationships by establishing joint attention. Because literacy is a critical determinant of eventual child outcome, the surveillance of "early literacy milestones" can be clinically useful (Table 3–5).

Putting Theory Into Practice: Language

During physical examinations, clinicians can provide a model for talking to even the youngest infant. In addition, clinicians should help parents differentiate between immaturity and pathologic conditions in children's language abilities. Pronunciation should not be a focus of concern for children younger than 2 years of age. At this age, children frequently make sound substitutions and omit final consonants. Parents should provide a model but not demand correct speech. Clinicians must distinguish difficulties with speech (sound production) from difficulties with language (use of symbols). Ability to use symbols can be easily observed in children's play. Isolated speech difficulties from either anatomic or neurologic abnormalities may be seen in children with normal symbolic skills. Such children often have difficulty with other oral motor behaviors, such as eating or blowing kisses, or with other fine motor skills. They are not necessarily cognitively or emotionally impaired. If half a child's speech output is unintelligible by age 3 years, referral to a speech pathologist and audiologist for evaluation is appropriate.

True delay in acquisition of language constitutes a

Table 3–5 • Developmental Milestones of Early Literacy

Age	Motor	Cognitive/Language	Interaction
6–12 months	Reaches for book Puts book to mouth	Looks at pictures Vocalizes, pats picture	Face-to-face gaze Parent follows baby's cues for "more" and "stop"
12–18 months	Holds book with help Turns several pages at a time	Points at pictures with one finger Labels pictures with same sound	May bring book to read Child becomes upset if parent does not let child "control" reading
18–36 months	Turns one page at a time Carries book around house	Names familiar pictures Attention highly variable Demands story over and over	Parent asks "what's happening?" questions Parent shows pleasure when child supplies word

serious developmental dysfunction. An 18-month-old child who uses no single words other than mama or dada, a 24-month-old child without multiple real words, or a 30-month-old child without two-word phrases should undergo evaluation. Language delays of this magnitude do not result from spoiling or laziness, as parents sometimes suggest (e.g., "He never has to ask for anything"). When evaluating a child with delayed expressive language, the clinician should assess receptive language abilities and search for evidence of global developmental delay, impaired hearing, autism, or an extremely deprived environment. It is extremely important that a formal hearing assessment be performed sooner rather than later. Full evaluation and treatment of language impairments are described in Chapter 63.

Nutrition and Growth

Caretakers must provide infants with nutrients that will sustain the rapid growth of body and brain, which is greater during the first 2 years of life than at any other time after birth.

An infant's own feeding behavior also affects the intake of adequate nutrition. At birth, an infant has a rooting reflex the helps in locating the nipple. An extrusion reflex pushes out solids to prevent ingestion of inappropriate foods. The infant's small, elongated mouth, combined with forward and backward movements of the tongue, squeeze the nipple so that milk is suckled.

Extrusion and rooting reflexes disappear after 4 months of age. By 3 months of age, as the mouth enlarges, neuromaturation of the cheek and tongue allows the infant to become progressively efficient at true sucking, which incorporates negative pressure to obtain milk from the nipple. By 6 to 8 months of age, infants begin chewing motions and are able to close their lips over the rim of a cup and drink. By 9 to 12 months of age, the development of the pincer grasp permits the child to eat finger foods. During the 2nd year of life, infants acquire the ability to use a spoon and hold a cup or bottle efficiently. Parental concerns about messiness, decreased appetite, and selective tastes emerge at this time (see also Chapter 40).

Infant nutrition affects both concurrent and future growth patterns. Both overfeeding and underfeeding can jeopardize the infant's later well-being. During this period of rapid growth, the brain is uniquely vulnerable to nutritional insult. Seventy percent of adult brain weight is attained by 2 years of age.

Although growth of the brain is the most critical organic achievement of infancy, most adult attention focuses on the rapid growth of the baby's body. Birth weight should double by 5 months of age, triple by 1 year of age, and quadruple by 2 years of age. Length at birth increases 50% in the 1st year of life and doubles by age 4 years.

The rate of growth and consequent caloric requirement per unit of body weight decline gradually over the first 2 years of life. As caloric needs change during maturation, so does the infant's capacity to ingest and digest an increasing variety of foods.

Putting Theory Into Practice: Growth Deficits

Newborn boys are larger than their female counterparts at birth, and they continue to grow at a faster rate during the first 3 to 6 months of life. After the first 6 months of life, there are no sex differences in infant growth rate. A decreased rate of weight gain in underprivileged children during the first 2 years of life should be investigated, because it usually reflects inadequate nutrition or complicating illness, not immutable genetic potential (Smith, 1977).

The rate of increase in the length of the child during the first 2 years of life is variable. Two thirds of normal infants cross percentile measurements (Smith, 1977). An infant's genotype for height is expressed by 2 years of age. Children's height can be evaluated, by means of standard charts, as a function of midparental height.

Premature infants and infants who are small for gestational age have distinct growth patterns. A statistically significant difference in growth percentiles is found unless correction for prematurity is done for head circumference until 18 months of postnatal age, weight until 24 months of postnatal age, and length until 40 months of postnatal age (Brandt, 1978). Small for gestational age infants show less predictable growth patterns, depending on the timing, severity, and cause of their intrauterine failure to grow; those who show growth acceleration in the first 6 months of life have the best prognosis for later outcome.

Neuromaturation, cognitive and social development, and temperament all influence feeding during infancy. Lethargic infants are difficult to feed. Management should focus on maintaining alertness. A hyperresponsive extrusion reflex (tongue-thrusting), dyskinetic tongue movements, or both result in difficult and prolonged feeding. These responses warrant further evaluation because they are often associated with dysfunction of the central nervous system.

Anticipatory guidance at the 6- and 9-month checkups should address potential feeding conflicts. Children's need for autonomy may result in their refusing food from parents. In this case, parents can present finger foods to facilitate independent feeding. Parents should also be warned that most children at this age explore by banging and dropping. Most parents do not mind when infants repetitively drop toys but may become annoyed when food is dropped. Parents can be told that this behavior is not intentionally provocative but reflects the child's need to practice new cognitive and motor abilities.

Some feeding problems need to be seen in the context of development and temperament, because newly acquired skills can present difficulties. For example, parents should anticipate that new gross motor abilities will make eating less interesting to most toddlers. The clinician can help parents by pointing out the contribution of the child's temperament to feeding behavior. For example, a child with a high activity level may have difficulty sitting long enough to complete a meal. Similarly, children who are distractible and nonpersistent are also unlikely to finish a meal. Children with a withdrawal response are often unwilling to try unfamiliar foods. Toddlers who adapt slowly may have a selective diet because they do not readily learn to like new foods. The clinician can work with parents to devise specific strategies for dealing with such feeding problems.

Conclusion

An understanding of infant and toddler development and behavior provides a framework for child care during the first 2 years of life. This knowledge can be applied to a transactional model for child development, which stresses the contributions of both child and caretaker to developmental outcome. Usually, the child health professional is the only professional involved with families of young children, and he or she may thus be able to promote maximal child development and prevent unnecessary parental concerns or parent-child conflicts that can contribute to later behavior disturbances. When growth deficits, developmental delays, sensory deficits, or serious behavioral problems already exist, the clinician can minimize their long-term impact by early identification and appropriate management and referral as well as by providing ongoing support to the family.

REFERENCES

Ainsworth MDS, Bell SM: Attachment, exploration and separation: illustrated by one year olds in a strange situation. Child Dev 41:49, 1970.

Barr RG, McMullen SJ, Spiess H, et al: Carrying as colic "therapy": a randomized controlled trial. Pediatrics 87:623, 1991.

Bell SM: The development of the concept of object as related to infant-mother attachment. Child Dev 41:291, 1971.

Bloom K: Patterning of infant vocal behavior. J Child Psychol 23:367, 1977.

Bornstein MH, Sigman MD: Continuity in mental development from infancy. Child Dev 57:251, 1986.

Brandt J: Growth dynamic of low birthweight infants with emphasis on the perinatal period. *In* Falkner F, Tanner J (eds): Human Growth: Postnatal Growth. New York, Plenum Press, 1978.

Brazelton TB: Crying in infancy. Pediatrics 29:579, 1962.

Bucher H, Moser T, von Siebenthal, et al: Sucrose reduces pain reaction to heel lancing in preterm infants: a placebo controlled, randomized and masked study. Pediatr Res 38:332, 1995.

Cohen LB, DeLoach S, Strauss MS: Infant visual perception. *In* Osofsky JD (ed): Handbook of Infant Development. New York, John Wiley & Sons, 1979.

Comery TA, Shah R, Greenough WT: Differential rearing alters spine density. Neurobiol Learn Mem 63:217, 1995.

Crockenberg S: Infant irritability, mother responsiveness, and social support influences on the security of infant-mother attachment. Child Dev 52:857, 1981.

DeSor JA, Maller O, Turner RE: Preference for sweet in humans: infant children and adults. *In* Weiftenbh JM (ed): The Genesis of Sweet Preference. Washington, DC, US Government Printing Office, 1977.

Fagan JF: New evidence for the prediction of intelligence from infancy. Infant Mental Health J 3:219, 1982.

Ferber R: Solving Your Child's Sleep Problems. New York, Simon & Schuster, 1985.

Field T, Greenberg R, Woodson R, et al: Facial expressions during Brazelton neonatal assessments. Infant Mental Health J 5:61, 1984.

Friman P: Concurrent habits. Am J Dis Child 144:1316, 1990.

Friman P, Schmitt BD. Thumb-sucking: pediatrician's guidelines. Clin Pediatr 28:438, 1989.

Gaensbauer T, Sands K: Distorted affective communications in abused, neglected infants and their potential impact on caretakers. J Acad Child Psychiatry 18:236, 1979.

Ginsberg H, Opper S: Piaget's Theory of Intellectual Development. Englewood Cliffs, NJ, Prentice-Hall, 1979.

Greenspan SJ: Assessing the emotional and social functioning of infants and young children. *In* Meisels SJ, Fenichel E (eds): New Visions for the Developmental Assessment of Infants and Young Children, Zero to Three, Arlington, VA, 1996, p 231.

Lipsitt LP: The newborn as informant. *In* Kearsley RB, Sigel IE (eds): Infants at Risk. Assessment of Cognitive Functioning. Hillsdale, NJ, Lawrence Erlbaum Associates, 1979.

MacFarlane JA: Olfaction in the development of social preferences in the human neonate. *In* Parent-Infant Interactions. CIBA Foundation Symposium 33. New York, Elsevier, 1975, p 103.

Mahler M, Pine F, Bergman A: The Psychological Birth of the Human Infant. New York, Basic Books, 1975.

McLane JB, McNamee GD: Early Literacy. Cambridge, MA, Harvard University Press, 1991.

Mennella JA, Beauchamp GK: Maternal diet alters the sensory qualities of human milk and the nursling's behavior. Pediatrics 88:737, 1991.

Moore T, Ucko C: Night waking in early infancy: Part I. Arch Dis Child 32:333, 1957.

Nugent JK: Using the NBAS With Infants and Their Families. White Plains, NY, March of Dimes, 1985.

Parker S, Barrett DE: Maternal type A behavior during pregnancy, neonatal crying, and early infant temperament: do type A women have type A babies? Pediatrics 89:474, 1992.

Parkin PP, Schwartz CJ, Manuel BA: Randomized controlled trial of three interventions in the management of persistent crying of infancy. Pediatrics 92:197, 1993.

Parmelee AH Jr., Weiner W, Schultz H: Infant sleep patterns: from birth to 16 weeks of age. Pediatrics 65:576, 1974.

Perry B, Pollard R, Blakley TL, et al: Childhood trauma, the neurobiology of adaptation, and "use dependent" development of the brain: how "states" become "traits." Infant Mental Health J 16:271, 1995.

Sagi A, van Ijzendoorn MH, Aviezer O, et al: Attachments in a Multiple-Caregiver and Multiple Infant Environment: The Case of the Israeli Kibbutzim. Monograph of the SRCD, Chicago, University of Chicago Press, 1995, pp 71–91.

Sameroff A, Emde R: Relationship Disturbances in Early Childhood: A Developmental Approach. New York, Basic Books, 1989, p 223.

Sheridan MK, Foley GM, Radlinski SH: Using the Supportive Play Model: Individualized Intervention in Early Childhood Practice. New York, Teachers College Press, 1995.

Singer LM, Brodzinsky DM, Ramsay D, et al: Mother-infant attachment in adoptive families. Child Dev 56:1543, 1985.

Smith DW: Growth and Its Disorders. Philadelphia, WB Saunders, 1977.

Spieker SJ, Booth CL: Maternal antecedents of attachment quality. *In* Belsky J, Nezworski T (eds): Clinical Implications of Attachment. New York, Erlbaum, 1988, p 95.

Sroufe LA: The role of infant-caregiver attachment in development. *In* Belsky J, Nezworski T (eds): Clinical Implications of Attachment. New York, Erlbaum, 1988, p 18.

Sroufe LA: The coherence of individual development: early care, attachment, and subsequent developmental issues. Am Psychol 34:834, 1979.

St. James-Roberts I, Hurry J, Bowyer J, et al: Supplementary carrying compared with advice to increase responsive parenting as interventions to prevent persistent infant cying. Pediatrics 95:381, 1995.

Thomasgard M, Metz WP: The vulnerable child syndrome revisited. J Devel Behav Pediatr 16:47, 1995.

Twitchell T: The automatic grasping responses of infants. Neuropsychologia 3:247, 1965.

Van der Boom: The influence of temperament and mothering on attachment and exploration: an experimental manipulation of sensitive responsiveness among lower class mothers with irritable infants. Child Develop 65:1457, 1994.

Waters E, Wippman J, Sroufe LA: Attachment, positive affect and competence in the peer group: two studies in construct validation. Child Dev 50:821, 1979.

Zuckerman B: Crying and colic. *In* Gabel S (ed): Behavioral Problems in Childhood. New York, Grune & Stratton, 1981, p 257.

4 The Preschool Years

Ernest F. Krug III • Karen C. Mikus

 Multiple environmental and intrinsic forces congregate within the minds of preschool children. The unfolding patterns of behavior, skill mastery, and discovery are harbingers of performance to come. In the years leading up to formal schooling, children begin to reveal their unique profiles of strength, weakness, and ecological variation. This chapter offers a matrix of critical dimensions along which development begins to interact meaningfully with early educational experience.

The preschool years, extending from approximately 18 months to 5 years of age, are an exciting period of transition from a time of limited language ability and primarily sensory-motor engagement with the surrounding environment to mastery of communication, a high degree of motor control, significant competence in self-regulation, expanding cognitive capacities, and a heightened ability to empathize with others (Table 4–1). The accomplishments of the period are mediated by continual transactions between the child and the child's environment. Theories emphasizing the primacy of genetic expression of individual capabilities or of environmental influence on a passive organism have generally been rejected in favor of a concept that recognizes that the child and the environment modulate each other through interactions that influence behavioral outcome in a variety of subtle and more overt ways.

Understanding the normal development of the preschooler is important, not only because it enables proper recognition of abnormal development but also because it provides the basis for appreciating normal developmental variation. The development of the child is a complex process in which the relative contributions of biological and environmental variables are influenced by multiple factors. Central nervous system damage or chromosomal abnormalities may, for example, exert considerable biological influence. An abusive home environment may exert a strongly negative effect. The child, particularly the preschooler, is amazingly resilient, in part because of the plasticity of the nervous system at this age and in part because the striving for competence and control is so strong. Comprehending the preschooler's behavior requires a multifactorial approach and sensitivity to the particular developmental tasks of this period.

As the pediatrician seeks to determine whether a preschooler's development is normal or abnormal, it is useful to take a functional perspective that analyzes the child's adaptive accommodations to internal and external forces. A delay in the achievement of a particular milestone may have no significance. On the other hand, failure to progress in the achievement of increasing competence and independence indicates a more significant problem. The pattern of achievement may vary considerably among different children because of the large number of variables involved, but it is critical to detect as early as possible those barriers to full development that may have lasting negative effects unless removed or modified through appropriate intervention.

Foundations of Neurodevelopmental Competence

A critical factor in any child's development is the biological substrate that defines his or her capacities for motor and language accomplishments, behavioral self-regulation, and cognitive awareness. Temperament is also largely biologically determined and influences developmental outcome in significant ways because of its effect on how the child is perceived by others. Stella Chess and Alexander Thomas, through their New York Longitudinal Study (see Chapter 8), have provided practitioners with invaluable insight into the effect of temperament on the course of development (Chess and Thomas, 1986; Thomas and Chess, 1977). Two-year-old children are typically difficult, but the "difficult" child with a feisty temperament and a poor "fit" with parents and caretakers encounters additional challenges.

Underlying what is manifest behaviorally are patterns of neuronal proliferation and migration, the elaboration of interneuronal connections, and the expression of neurotransmitters. Myelination improves the rate and efficiency of neuronal communication. A variety of insults or damage to these processes clearly affects brain function, although outcome cannot be predicted accurately using presently available laboratory measures. Such predictions may never be possible because of the complexity of the human mind and the vast number of variables that affect outcome. Even so, the following discussion examines the major streams of development in the preschool child, also taking into account the tremendous range of expression along these lines.

MOTOR DEVELOPMENT

The preschool child normally grows about 3 to 5 pounds and 2½ to 3 inches per year. Approximately half the child's adult height is attained by 2½ years of age. Appetite often

Table 4–1 • Developmental Milestones in Preschoolers

Milestone	Typical Age at Presentation	Age at Which Absence of Milestone Is Abnormal*
Gross motor		
Jumping and clearing ground	24 months	30 months
Doing a broad jump of 18 inches	36 months	48 months
Alternating feet downstairs	36 months	48 months
Balancing on one foot for 2 seconds	36 months	48 months
Hopping on one foot	42 months	60 months
Fine motor		
Stacking five 1-inch cubes	20 months	27 months
Stacking seven 1-inch cubes	24 months	36 months
Copying a circle	36 months	48 months
Holding pencil with mature grasp	36 months	48 months
Copying a cross	40 months	60 months
Language		
Combining two ideas (e.g., "Mommy, go!")	18 months	24 months
Naming one picture in a book	18 months	27 months
Following a two-step command	18 months	27 months
Using three- to four-word sentences	24 months	36 months
Using pronouns (I, you) appropriately	24 months	30 months
Identifying two colors	36 months	42 months
Naming the use of common objects	30 months	36 months
Speaking in a way understandable to a stranger	36 months	48 months
Social-adaptive		
Independent feeding with spoon and fork	24 months	36 months
Independent dressing without tying shoes	36 months	48 months
Independent toileting	36 months	48 months
Cognition		
Searching for lost object in several places other than place object was last seen	18 months	24 months
Playing with toys in functional way (e.g., pushing a toy car around)	18 months	24 months
Reenacting familiar activities	18 months	30 months
Being able to imitate actions later	18 months	30 months
Using one object to stand for another object in play (a block for a telephone)	18 months	30 months
Using imaginary objects in play	36 months	48 months
Role playing several familiar people	36 months	48 months
Drawing face of a person with crude features	36 months	48 months
Planning out a story and assigning roles to self and others	48 months	60 months
Social-emotional		
Demonstrating shared attention: "Do you see what I see?"	18 months	30 months
Showing strong sense of self: using "No," "Mine"	18 months	36 months
Playing side by side with a single peer	24 months	36 months
Separating from parent without crying	36 months	48 months
Labeling feelings in self	36 months	48 months
Taking turns and sharing	36 months	48 months
Playing group games with simple rules	48 months	60 months

*The significance of an absent milestone must be assessed in the context of the child's complete physical and neurologic examination. Furthermore, the absence of a particular milestone may be "abnormal" earlier than indicated in the table in the context of a child's other accomplishments.

Data from Bayley Scales of Infant Development–II (N Bayley: Bayley Scales of Infant Development, 2nd ed. San Antonio, The Psychological Corporation, 1993); Denver II (Frankenburg WK, Dodds J, Archer P, et al: Denver II. Denver, Denver Developmental Materials, 1990; Frankenburg WK, Dodds J, Archer P, et al: The Denver II: A major revision and restandardization of the Denver Developmental Screening Test. Pediatrics 89:91, 1992); Developmental Rainbow: Early Childhood Development Profiles (Mahoney G, Mahoney F: Developmental Rainbow: Early Childhood Development Profiles. Tallmadge, OH, Family Child Learning Center, 1996); Early Language Milestone Scale (Coplan J: Early Language Milestone Scale, 1983. Modern Education Corp., P.O. Box 721, Tulsa, OK, 74101); The Revised Developmental Screening Inventory–1980 (Developmental Evaluation Materials, P.O. Box 27391, Houston, TX, 77277); Transdisciplinary Play-Based Assessment (Linder T: Transdisciplinary Play-Based Assessment. Baltimore, Paul II Brookes, 1990).

Valid screening for developmental delays should be done using a carefully developed or normed instrument/reference such as one of the preceding.

decreases and activity level increases, with the development of a leaner appearance. In conjunction with this physical growth, the motor competence of the child increases. Motor performance can be assessed in terms of movement, posture, and tone. High or low levels of tone typically reflect some degree of central nervous system dysfunction. Infants who display low levels of tone of a benign nature generally show at least low-normal, if not normal, tone by the preschool years.

- By 2 years of age the awkward toddler gait gives way to a normal, fluid gait, although normal variations in tone have an impact on this phenomenon.
- By age 2 years, the typical child runs well.
- By age 2½ years, the child stands on one foot briefly and climbs stairs (bringing the feet together on each step).
- By age 3 years, the average child alternates feet climbing stairs, rides a tricycle, and does a broad jump.

- By age 3½ years, the child throws a ball accurately at a target and hops on one foot.
- By age 4 years, the child is proficient at hopping.
- By age 5 years, the child skips and can swing himself or herself on a swing.

Throughout this period, the quality of movement is refined, although some normal preschoolers appear clumsy because of weak balance or proprioception, and some demonstrate the motor overflow characteristic of a neuromaturational lag. Constitutional and environmental factors also play a role in the broad range of motor expression exhibited in the preschool period. For example, in a family in which many members have strong athletic skills or in which the parents enjoy taking their preschool son or daughter outdoors to develop motor skills, earlier demonstration of motor competence may be seen.

Fine motor control progresses from a neat pincer grasp by age 1 year to the ability to oppose the thumb to each finger sequentially by age 5 years and to hold a pencil with a tripod grasp. In most cases, the child with excellent gross motor skills also develops very good fine motor controls, although there are clumsy children whose fine motor skills are proficient and athletes who are dysgraphic. Temperament factors (e.g., attention and activity level) can significantly affect performance. Even so, the 2-year-old child is expected to stack six blocks and imitate a vertical stroke. The 3-year-old child can usually copy a circle, use scissors, and stack 10 blocks. The average 4-year-old child can imitate drawing a square and can draw a person with at least three parts. Most 5-year-old children can print their first names, build a six-block staircase, and copy an open square with a circle at one corner. Many normal children, particularly boys, have early difficulty with form copying tasks, and this may or may not predict later difficulty in this area.

COGNITIVE DEVELOPMENT

Basically, preschoolers are busy scientists as they actively explore their environment and gain knowledge of the world, themselves, and other people. They seek to understand and to construct a model of the world: What is this made of? How does it work? If I do this, then what happens? Through observation and hands-on experimentation, they acquire cause and effect understanding and become increasingly adept at problem solving.

A major accomplishment of the preschool years is the development and consolidation of the ability to use symbols and mental representations. That is, children learn to use one object to stand for another object and internal mental images to carry people, other living creatures, objects, events, routines, and places within their own minds without the concrete stimuli being visibly present. This cognitive capacity opens the door for deferred imitation; language development; pretend play; understanding the use of pictures, drawings, and models; the ability to use numbers to represent quantity and letters to represent sounds; comprehension of reality-fantasy distinctions; and the development of humor. The 18- to 24-month-old child can engage in rudimentary forms of mental representation as evidenced by early language and simple pretend play.

A 5-year-old child can develop elaborate scripts, direct others regarding their roles in play scenarios, and even weave the others' ideas into various story lines. One of the most sophisticated constructions devised by preschoolers is a *theory of mind*. By age 3 years, children realize that other people have internal mental states, and they think about needs and emotions in others as possibly being different from their own. They seem to understand that mental states can and do influence behavior. By age 4 or 5 years, youngsters can think about internal states such as desires and beliefs (Flavell, Miller, and Miller, 1993). Elder preschoolers develop understandings about what is going on in the minds of other people, have an awareness of false beliefs, and more reliably and stably differentiate between appearance and reality. However, it often seems that the child's perceptions remain a stronger influence on behavior than does reality.

The development of the theory of mind reflects increasingly complex comprehension and manipulation of internal mental representations. It is the same cognitive phenomenon that helps young children learn to take the role of the other. The perspective-taking capabilities of young children are more developed than once was assumed; that is, preschoolers are not quite as egocentric as they were once thought to be (Flavell, Miller, and Miller, 1993). However, seeing a situation from another person's point of view is an achievement even for some adults and one that remains fragile and tenuous for young children. Even though the concrete, perceptual aspects of the "data" often dominate young children's thinking, they can also think abstractly at times and can make inferences and deductions about unobservable mental stimuli and relationships. Furthermore, children's attention spans lengthen as they age from 1½ to 5 years, and their abilities to categorize, analyze, and synthesize information become stronger and more efficient.

One aspect of cognitive development is the child's progress in handling anxiety. When the child perceives something that is discrepant from his or her present understanding of the world, this causes arousal. Initially, the child may become excited, but this gives way to uncertainty if the experience cannot be resolved in some way. Uncertainty turns into anxiety if the discrepancy between experience and cognitive comprehension persists (Kagan, 1984). At approximately 2 years of age, the child recognizes peers as a separate force, and this peer anxiety must be resolved. As the child's conceptualization and representational abilities increase, poorly understood forces, both within and without, become personified in "the dark," "monsters," and "bad people." Every anxiety contains an element of real or potential threat, but the cognitive task is to name that threat and thereby gain some control over the fear that it generates (Fig. 4–1).

LANGUAGE DEVELOPMENT

Of all the streams of development, language proficiency most closely mirrors intellectual competency. Furthermore, it is deviance in language development that is the most frequent developmental complaint brought to the pediatrician in the preschool years. The progression in language proficiency during the first 5 years of life is exponential.

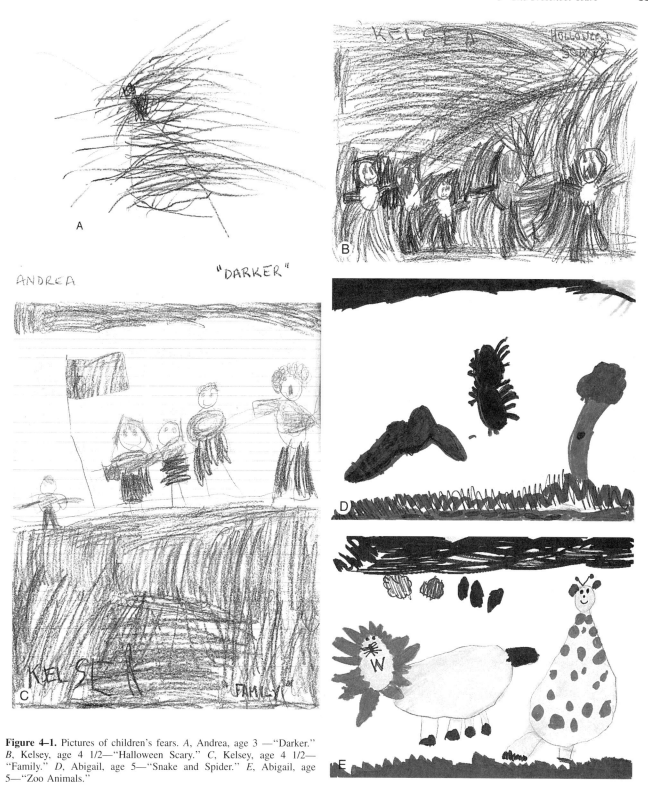

Figure 4–1. Pictures of children's fears. *A,* Andrea, age 3 —"Darker." *B,* Kelsey, age 4 1/2—"Halloween Scary." *C,* Kelsey, age 4 1/2—"Family." *D,* Abigail, age 5—"Snake and Spider." *E,* Abigail, age 5—"Zoo Animals."

At age 1 year, the child understands simple requests but has very little verbal expressive ability, with a typical vocabulary of two to four words. By age 5 years, a child can define familiar words, argue, tell stories, comment on future events, and lie (Fletcher, 1987). At the end of the preschool period, a typically developing child often has a vocabulary of close to 10,000 words.

Assessing the language development of the preschool child is best accomplished by examining separately four major components of language: phonology, semantics, syntax, and pragmatics. Phonology comprises the science of sounds and specifically the range of sounds that actually occur in language. Semantics addresses the meaning of words and larger components of language. Syntax relates to the structure or grammatical use of language. Pragmatics is the study of the social use of language, that is, communication in a social context.

With respect to phonology, it is common for children to demonstrate numerous articulation immaturities at age 2 years (e.g., "Tum heah!" for "Come here!"). Some sounds are altered (e.g., "tee" for "see"), multiple sounds are reduced (e.g., "play" becomes "pay"), and final consonants are often dropped. By age 3½ years, the child has usually achieved normal pronunciation, although immaturities are often still present. A child's inability to make steady progress in the maturation of sound production is cause for concern, and referral to a speech-language pathologist may prevent abnormal phonologic patterns from becoming ingrained. Phonologic impairments beyond age 4 years are also highly correlated with later evidence of developmental dyslexia.

As preschool children's verbal abilities develop, they understand more sophisticated language and demonstrate increasing ability to encode relevant meaning in conversational situations. This phenomenon usually parallels the increasing grammatical complexity of the child's utterances. Syntactic sequences such as "more juice" in the 18-month-old child give way to the incorporation of verbs ("want more juice") by age 2 years and the use of pronouns by age 2½ years ("I want more juice"). Mean length of utterance steadily increases, and by age 4 years the child is formulating complex sentences. As syntactic competencies develop, dysfluency (stuttering) is relatively common and usually resolves spontaneously. Persistence of dysfluency for several months, despite parents' efforts to give close attention to the child when he or she is talking without criticizing her stuttering, should raise suspicion of a chronic problem that requires intervention.

The development of conversational speech is usually evident by 3 years of age. Between the ages of 3 and 5 years, children become elaborate story-tellers, depending on the temperament of the particular child. The first indication of normal pragmatics is the child's use of pointing by age 14 months to communicate shared attention. By age 2 years, the child reflects the development of inner language through the problem-solving nature of play. It is common for children with language delays to have behavioral problems in the early preschool period because they lack the ability to solve problems in social situations and they "act out" their frustrations.

There is a wide range of normal in preschool language development, and it is likely that there is more than one acceptable route to language proficiency (Shonkoff, 1992). Deciding whether a particular child's language is abnormal or normal depends on a variety of variables: the child's ability to imitate sounds accurately (at age-appropriate levels), to demonstrate communicative intent, to solve problems initially using symbolic play at age 2 years and progressing to simple verbal analysis by age 5 years, to steadily build a meaningful vocabulary, and to engage in the give and take of normal conversation by age 3 years.

EMOTIONAL AND SOCIAL DEVELOPMENT

Three phenomena are especially significant during the preschool years for a child's emotional and social development: regulation, reciprocity, and representation. The beginning of all three are (usually) developed in the 1st year of life, but capacities in each must be expanded substantially in order for the 5-year-old child to have a smooth and productive year in kindergarten.

During the preschool years, a child must learn to regulate his or her impulses, affect, and behavior. In interaction with others, for example, the child must learn not to bite or hit others and not to grab or fling toys even when the discharge of such impulses might have a measure of sensory or motor satisfaction. The young child must work hard to manage his or her emotions. Understanding, for instance, that it is "OK" to feel angry but "*not* OK" to strike out or call names is a major accomplishment in regulation of emotion and action. Most children achieve these milestones to some extent by the age of 4 to 5 years, although relapses in impulse control and regulation still occur.

The ability to participate in back-and-forth exchanges with others begins in infancy and occupies children in their preschool years. At first, a child's partners are mainly adults (parents, relatives, caregivers) and siblings. Gradually, children are expected to be able to participate in give-and-take sequences with peers. Learning to share, take turns, and incorporate other children's ideas into their play falls within this category, as does the ability to recognize another's point of view. Children's play with peers changes from a side-by-side format to a more cooperative, interactive, and elaborated format. The child who is not able to participate in complex social imaginative play with fellow kindergartners is likely to be left out or, worse, rejected and avoided (Chapter 54).

The ability to create and understand internal mental representations (see Cognitive Development) enables children to convey their ideas and desires through spoken language, to make and play with friends, to appreciate other people's points of view, to demonstrate empathy and compassion, and to learn preliminary negotiation skills for settling conflicts with peers. These are important social skills that children need to successfully navigate the world outside of their family. These skills also make family life more manageable and enjoyable.

A solid concept of self and positive feelings about oneself as well as a sense of personal efficacy are essential to the development of a competent child. Greenspan suggests that children usually develop a complex sense of self by the age of 18 months (Greenspan, 1996; Greenspan and Greenspan, 1989). From 18 to 30 months, children are able to deal with *emotional ideas*; that is, they work on expression of their feelings and feeling-related ideas through words and in pretend play. *Emotional thinking* characterizes youngsters from 30 to 48 months in Greenspan's typology; during this period, children are able to comprehend and work with increasingly complex intentions, wishes, and emotions in themselves and others. Having a theory of mind and more sophisticated communication skills (abilities in the developmental domains of cognition and language) support a child's emotional and social development.

Preschoolers experience and wrestle with many intense emotions, including anger, anxiety, shame, excitement, pleasure, frustration, sadness, and joy. Children frequently confront and try to resolve significant emotional issues having to do with trust, autonomy-dependency, closeness with and separation from loved ones, and assertiveness and initiative, to name a few (Erikson, 1968; Greenspan, 1996). They often become overwhelmed by their strong feelings, and they have much to learn about expressing feelings in ways that do not alienate others and get themselves into trouble. Before language is well established (and even afterward), tantrums may be a child's most available vehicle for expression and discharge of painful or exasperated responses. Throughout the preschool years, many children tend to express their feelings first in behavior; this highlights the importance of looking for the function and communicative intent that underlie surface actions.

Temperament is particularly salient with regard to children's social and emotional development (Chapter 8). The child's temperamental style influences his or her experience and management of emotions and the emotional tasks of early childhood. A particularly intense youngster may react in extreme and dramatic ways when frustrated or confronted with a separation or a conflict. A less active and expressive child may appear to be untroubled when, in fact, she is also anxious. Parental understanding of temperament and ways to help children navigate rough emotional and social waters are particularly important if this period of growth and development is to have a positive influence.

Moral and Spiritual Development

The primary "moral" tasks of the preschool period are learning self-control and learning to share. There has been much debate about how parents can best facilitate this process, and most parents are concerned about how they can produce a "good child." Discipline issues take on great import. Parents ask questions about spanking and are concerned about being manipulated. One conclusion appears incontestable: the nature and quality of the parents' love for the child affects the child's ability to love others. Discipline is an important vehicle by which the parents teach the child certain behavioral standards and values, and it reflects the quality of the parents' love. This, in turn, is affected by the parents' upbringing and by the parents' personalities and temperament.

Robert Coles (1997) has described the preschool child as a *moral listener.* Beyond simply experiencing reality, the preschooler reflects on the behavior of parents and significant others through symbolic play and other representations. If parental love conveys shared respect, the child is more likely to respect others. If discipline is harsh or arbitrary, or if it is lacking altogether, the child does not experience that mutuality which is a key enabler of moral development. Throughout this process the child tries to make sense of discrepancies between what the parents say and do and between what he or she sees on television or in society and what happens at home. Preschoolers pick up on consistent themes and try to maximize positive feedback from parents, but they do test limits, use "unacceptable" behavior to gain attention, and re-enact situations that they perceive to be discrepant from their present moral understanding.

The young preschool child is often egocentric. According to Selma Fraiberg (1959), the young preschooler attributes great power to his or her own thoughts. Children believe the world is there for their benefit, but everything does not go their way. There are battles over independence, although there is also anxiety every time a battle with the parent appears to have been won. By age 3 years, the child is usually interested in rules and becomes increasingly insistent that rules be followed. A sense of guilt evolves as the child becomes sensitive to behaviors that hurt or disappoint significant others. Parental and societal values begin to have a clear impact on the child's values. The maturing preschool child's play often demonstrates the careful attention paid to the parents' behavior, at times much to the parents' embarrassment. In addition, children who manifest a sense of basic trust in their environment have the foundation for developing a concept of God by age 4 or 5 years. However, they tend to rely on their parents and their parents' religious institution to be mediators of God for them. Hence, parental inconsistencies in this realm may influence the child's understanding of meaning in life and may create confusion about moral standards. Furthermore, preschoolers think in concrete terms about God, heaven, and other religious concepts, and this both results from and creates certain specific expectations about life and death.

Gradually, egocentrism, to the degree that it exists in any particular child, gives way to a sense of obligation toward others. The preschooler moves from a preoccupation with control and independence to a sense of self, which enables productive participation in the world of peers and the shifting of some attachment to the peer group. The child wants increasingly to please loved ones, and this concern evolves into what Freud called a superego. Initially, the child requires an external presence (e.g., the parent) to implement behavioral controls. This gives way to the child's use of language to mediate behavior (e.g., saying "No hit, no hit!" while the child is hitting somebody). Finally, the child internalizes these language and moral constructs, and they are incorporated into the conscience.

The child develops a concept of self and of the world that is informed by the parents' style of discipline, the predictability of the environment, and the degree to which the child feels respected as a person. If the child experiences too much guilt and shame, he or she may feel ineffectual as a moral agent; if the child experiences no guilt or shame, he or she may develop little sense of obligation toward and concern for the rights and feelings of others. Another important phenomenon is the development of an understanding of intentionality. Three-year-old children can distinguish intentional acts from mistakes or accidents but tend to assign blame on the basis of the visible outcome. Four- and five-year-old children are more likely to assign punishment based on the perpetrator's intention. Most children by age 4 or 5 years, moreover, demonstrate the intent to care about the health and well-being of peers, teachers, and parents.

INTERACTION OF THE STREAMS AND THE CAREGIVING CONTEXT

The foregoing analysis of the separate streams of development is useful, but children are whole packages, not developmental territories exclusive of one another. Representational play is the primary means by which children construct reality for themselves to make it meaningful at each level of their understanding. If the child's motor skills predominate as a strength, motor play may be the preferential way in which the child "expresses" anxiety and experiences autonomy. If language skills are particularly strong, the child's problem solving may be more verbal. If a particular area is weak, efforts should be made to assist the child with compensatory strategies. For example, the clumsy child can be introduced to swimming or horseback riding to nurture the self-esteem that comes from using one's body competently.

The caregiving context plays an important role in the development of the young child. In addition to meeting the child's basic needs, caregivers need to be emotionally and physically available to preschoolers in predictable and supportive ways. Characteristics of caregivers that promote neurodevelopmental competence in children include warmth, responsiveness, sensitivity, flexibility, and the ability to be empathic. Being able to read and understand a child's cues and the meaning of a child's sometimes difficult behaviors helps parents and other caregivers provide the emotional and behavioral sustenance that a child needs to flourish. The caregiving context also encourages normal development by ensuring opportunities for play and exploration while providing a stable, secure base where the child can refuel. A delicate balance between adult-imposed structure and child-directed choice must also be achieved. An atmosphere of trust and respect encourages children to believe in themselves yet be responsive to others. It is important for parents to be aware of the detrimental patterns from their own childhood so that these are not repeated in the next generation. A high-quality caregiving context does not mean that parents have to be perfect in the provision of flawless care; rather, the concept of solidly "good-enough" parenting and nurturance can be a useful goal to pursue (Winnicott, 1986).

Providing such a caregiving environment is no small task. Parenting is extremely challenging especially in the contemporary fast-paced, highly stressful world. Many parents do not have sufficient concrete resources, and limited social and emotional support for parenting further complicates the rigorous jobs of father and mother. Pediatricians have a unique opportunity to provide support and information that can enhance the effectiveness of the caregiving context (Table 4–2).

THREATS TO NEURODEVELOPMENTAL COMPETENCE

There is much evidence to suggest that neurodevelopment is a string of discontinuities, rather than a steady unidirectional progression (Thatcher et al, 1996). In other words, development consists of progress in a particular realm followed by consolidation, which, in turn, creates a readiness to address a new challenge. A weakness at one point in the early life of a child may become a relative strength later on. The preschooler's goal is to build a sense of competence in understanding and in exerting some control over the world. Every success adds to the child's confidence; every failure potentially weakens it. The consolida-

Table 4–2 • Developmental Tasks of Preschoolers

Child	How Parents Can Help
Consolidation of basic trust in self and significant others	Be dependable, consistent, responsive, and respectful.
Achievement of mental representation of people, events, routines, places	Engage child in conversation about people and past events; encourage pretend play; read books together.
Achievement of gross motor competency	Encourage exploration and activities that challenge motor skills.
Development of fine motor skills	Provide opportunities to play with clay, water, blocks, building materials, and art supplies.
Achievement of cooperation and positive peer interaction	Provide peer experiences that help child develop negotiation skills.
Achievement of adequate task persistence and attentional capacity	Provide experiences that challenge attentional skills and restrict experiences that do not (e.g., television).
Achievement of impulse control and other self-regulatory skills	Help the child learn to calm self; use "time out."
Achievement of self-care and toileting independence	Reinforce independence in the child; do not shame.
Development of close, reciprocal relationships with family figures	Take time to listen to the child, be sensitive to the child's feelings, and play on the child's terms. Consciously avoid using child's love to meet one's own needs.
Achievement of conversational skills	Talk in back-and-forth way with the child; provide exposure to normal language models through play groups with peers.

tion phase may be long or short and varies in length in part because of the internal and external factors that can affect the youngster's capacity to solve problems. For example, a severe illness may cause behavioral regression as a response to feeling threatened or overwhelmed. A mood disorder (e.g., depression) can paralyze cognitive effort. Extremes of temperament can elicit hostility in the environment, for example, in the case of the child with negative mood who is poorly adaptable, unpredictable, and intense. Neurologic dysfunction of various degrees may significantly reduce a child's capacity for self-regulation, resulting in irritability, poor sleep, and frequent tantrums.

External threats may have less impact on the resilient preschooler than his or her own fantasy life, but they create the context for the child's fears. Probably the most prevalent is family dysfunction and divorce. One out of every two marriages in the United States ends in divorce, and this can cause significant disruption in the child's life, depending on the custody arrangements and the degree of animosity between the parents. Most preschoolers seem to adapt well, but they do act out through their behavior the consequences of parental inconsistency, anger, and threats. Dreams about being abandoned or left are an example.

A more subtle threat is the effect of the media, particularly television. Many preschoolers spend large blocks of their waking time in front of television. Values are conveyed in a multisensory format, and it is common for preschool boys, in particular, to imitate the violent behavior they see portrayed. In addition, this passive inter active mode of learning may become habitual, and active learning experiences through play may increasingly be abandoned, unless parents insist on limiting television viewing time and encourage opportunities for exploration and creative play.

Poverty, violence, and fragile (or nonexistent) community supports do have an effect on neurodevelopment. (The impacts of socioeconomic deprivation are discussed in Chapter 17.) There are significant differences with regard to that impact among families in the same neighborhood, mediated by a family's degree of hope, internal resilience, and strength of connection to a social network that supports and builds up its members. Issues related to nutrition, basic health, and adequate housing, as well as the presence and availability of one or two parents, may also be influential. Early intervention programs (e.g., The Brookline Early Education Project and the High/Scope Perry Preschool Project) have demonstrated clear, positive effects in the short term for modifying negative socioeconomic influences. Long-term benefits have been demonstrated, but not consistently (Bryant and Maxwell, 1997). This argues for the crucial importance of the child's environment for sustaining and encouraging active learning and the curiosity that grows out of early enrichment opportunities.

UNDERSTANDING THE PRESCHOOL CHILD

It may be nearly impossible for the pediatrician to understand the preschooler's behavior (Table 4–3) in the context of a 10-minute office visit. Some children cry and some are stoic but avoid eye contact. Some converse and appear older than their years. In most cases, however, preschoolers preferentially represent their feelings through art or play, rather than through language. Furthermore, preschoolers' concept of reality is based on their own perceptions rather than on empiric reasoning. In other words, preschoolers draw conclusions about the world based on what makes sense to them, not by simultaneously testing hypotheses. Moreover, the preschooler can be rigid in insisting that things be done a certain way.

Parents want their preschool children to eat independently whatever is put in front of them and to use the toilet appropriately. Many children are ready to do these things by the age of 2 years, but, for many, age 3 years is more realistic, and some push the boundary to age 3½ years. What factors explain these differences? In addition to the varieties of developmental and temperamental variables, the parents' demands upon the child, family and cultural values, and the "fit" between the child and his or her environment affect the child's openness to external demands, expectations about what can be accomplished, and his or her sense of accomplishment.

The issue of where and how much the child sleeps illustrates the complexity of understanding preschool behavior. There are wide differences of opinion among parents. Some parents think that a "family bed" reduces anxiety for the child; others are adamant that such a practice is unhealthy and prolongs dependency. Some parents initiate independent sleeping in a separate room soon after birth; others keep the infant in the parents' room until a later transition to a separate room. Children vary considerably as well. Some want all lights out and the door to the room closed; some want a night-light. Some children sleep in a bed, some on the floor, and some in the bedroom doorway. In any event, bedtime is a time when the day's events are reviewed and children bring closure to the day. It seems to help if the child at least falls asleep in the same location where he or she may awaken during the night. A bedtime ritual can be extremely helpful to provide consistent structure regarding location for sleep, review of the day, and, through the vehicle of a story, rehearsal of any situation that causes anxiety. Here, as in other circumstances, the child's behavior is interwoven with the parent's, and change is transactional.

For example, a young girl may be very sensitive to textures, poorly adaptable to changes, and clingy because of unresolved separation anxiety. If her mother finds it difficult to set limits and needs (rather than likes) affection from the child, then the youngster may have picky eating habits, be resistant to toilet training, and be insistent on sleeping with her parents. Changes in either side of this equation might result in a different outcome. A less anxious child would be more willing to accept new challenges. A less needy parent would conceivably be more free to coax the child into new experiences and to tolerate short bursts of anxiety and frustration.

Particularly in this age range, a person must look behind the child's behavior to comprehend it. "Lying" and "stealing" are examples. Preschool children do not usually lie because of an intent to fabricate and deceive. They simply relate a story that conforms to their understanding or longing without concern for the verity of the elements of the story. If confronted about a specific behavior, preschoolers respond without regard for the principle of truth, because they do not begin to comprehend abstract principles until the end of the preschool period, and then only in a contextual sense. In other words, the "truth" has to do with what the child believes or wishes to be true in a particular situation. Similarly, the concept of stealing is meaningful for persons having a sense of ownership and an understanding of the boundary between self and others. This sense develops in the preschool period, but the young child may impulsively take things without asking, learning, however, that this results in a negative parental response. Positive reinforcement of desired behavior and consistent parental modeling of truthful behavior, as well as respect for others, play an important role in the child's behavioral development and facilitate the evolution of socially acceptable behavior.

The preschooler's art and play behavior are valuable, if not essential, windows into understanding the child's world. The problem solving that occurs through play and the symbolic representation of art reflect those discrepancies in the child's experience, which the child attempts to resolve (Fig. 4–2). Fear of impulses, fear of the unexpected, fear of pain or loss of bodily integrity, and fear of abandonment, among other feelings, must be dealt with before establishing a foundation of ego strength and the confi-

Table 4–3 • Normal Variations in Preschool Development

Vignette: Serena

Serena is a bright young girl whose verbal capabilities are strong and far outstrip her motor skills, which are immature, although not abnormal. She is shy with a slow-to-warm-up temperament. Although her parents wish Serena were a bit more outgoing and adaptable, they seem to work well with her need for predictability. So far, her developmental progress has been "on-time" enough that no additional intervention has been warranted and recommendations for gross motor play and child management strategies have been sufficient.

Serena at 18 months
  Motor: Learned to walk 2 months ago and is still unsteady; crawls up stairs and resorts to crawling when she could walk.
  Language: Says many single words; uses more two-word combinations every day.
  Cognitive: Feeds baby doll with bottle and then covers and kisses doll; moves trucks along and has two cars chase each other.
  Social/emotional: Protests any separation from mother very strongly and persistently; follows mother from room to room.
  Moral/spiritual: Generally does what she is told and does not challenge authority.

Serena at 3 years
  Motor: Climbs stairs slowly with care, holding on to railing and placing her feet together on each step; pushes herself on her tricycle, rather than pedaling.
  Language: Speaks in full and complex sentences; has a large vocabulary; converses with mother about past events.
  Cognitive: Loves to pretend; does not need realistic props; sequences several ideas/actions in her stories.
  Social/emotional: Slow to warm up in nursery school; does not like to go to other children's homes to play unless mom goes along.
  Moral/spiritual: Articulates household rules; complains to mother when peers break rules.

Serena at 5 years
  Motor: Not interested in riding a two wheeler; not yet skipping; just beginning to figure out how to "pump" on a swing.
  Language: Can tell complicated stories; uses language to negotiate and solve problems; interested in reading and writing.
  Cognitive: Imaginative play is varied, elaborate, and rich in content; can tell peers what their roles are in her stories.
  Social/emotional: Shy, quiet; has one good friend in neighborhood; watches others a long time before she joins in.
  Moral/spiritual: Wants to do what is right and checks with mother. Talks about God as a kind father.

Vignette: Michelle

Michelle is active with definite strengths in the motor arena. In contrast, her verbal skills are developing more slowly. She has a very intense temperament (some might call her a child with a "difficult temperament"). She often reacts strongly and persistently to frustrations. Her difficulties with verbal expression in conjunction with her temperamental style frequently result in tantrums and some aggression. Michelle's outbursts distress her mother, who is more mild-mannered and prefers to avoid confrontations. Play-based home activities that stimulate and promote language development have been the primary intervention.

Michelle at 18 months
  Motor: Has been walking since 10 months old; runs with fair balance; climbs out of her crib easily.
  Language: Has eight single words and no two-word combinations.
  Cognitive: Explores actively; is curious; is fascinated with machines and vehicles; takes toys apart; sits only briefly to have a picture book read to her.
  Social/emotional: Sometimes bites a sibling or a peer; gets overstimulated easily and then has a hard time settling down; has difficulty falling asleep without parent present.
  Moral/spiritual: Says "No, no" as she climbs up onto tipsy antique rocking chair that is always off-limits.

Michelle at 3 years
  Motor: Always on the go; kicks soccer ball with accuracy; alternates feet on stairs, up and down.
  Language: Speaks in very short sentences, often in phrases; does ask questions; vocabulary grows slowly and steadily.
  Cognitive: Likes cause and effect toys; builds elaborate block structures; counts Matchbox cars and knows different makes of cars.
  Social/emotional: Has intense tantrums with crying and screaming; has slow recovery from distress.
  Moral/spiritual: Screams at peers who do not follow rules she establishes for games, but manipulates rules to suit her own needs.

Michelle at 5 years
  Motor: Rides two-wheeler without training wheels; climbs deftly.
  Language: Uses full sentences; vocabulary continues to grow; some mild word retrieval difficulties.
  Social/emotional: Easily frustrated; has some friends but can be impatient with others' pace.
  Moral/spiritual: Manipulative and domineering; asks questions about hell.

---

dence necessary to separate from parents and meet new challenges. In a similar fashion, the preschooler's play and art often reflect the child's hope for how the world should be. Different roles can be explored through play, and positive pictures of reality can be created to convey the child's hopes.

KEY INDICATORS OF DYSFUNCTION

A number of behavioral issues are associated specifically with the preschool period. Parents often come to the pediatrician with concerns about difficulty managing their child's behavior, and power struggles may erupt around feeding, bedtime and sleeping, toilet training, and behavior in public—areas where the child recognizes that he or she has some degree of control. It is well known that preschoolers normally do not eat all that is put before them at the table, yet eating disorders in this period are uncommon, and the children usually follow their growth curves with predicted regularity. Excessive pickiness about what the child eats may reflect either sensitivity to certain food products (e.g., avoidance of milk in the presence of a lactose intolerance) or a need for predictability and control that is outside the norm. It is unlikely that a metabolic disorder would manifest at this late time, but this should be considered if the clinical findings suggest such a possibility.

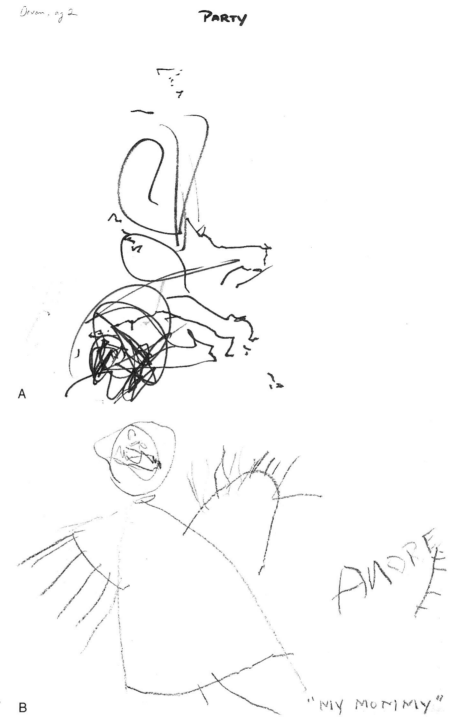

Figure 4–2. Children's drawings. *A*, Devon, age 2. *B*, Andrea, age 3.

In the United States, attempts to toilet train children are generally deferred until age 2 years, and many children show no interest until age 3 years. Parents are frequently upset when their youngster runs behind the couch to squat and produce a stool in the diaper, knowing that the child could just as easily go to the potty chair. But the child goes through a period of testing sphincter control and experimenting with autonomy. The busy parent may find it difficult to be consistent. Furthermore, the attention that the parents give this task in terms of their emotional re-

sponse may prolong the process. As in all other areas of discipline, consistency—as difficult as that is for all parents to achieve—and positive reinforcement—in contrast to negative contingencies—produce the most permanent gains and avoid emotional sequelae.

Of all the circumstances in which parents feel most inclined to spank their preschooler, misbehavior in the mall must rank very high. No parent likes to be embarrassed in a public place, particularly when a hasty exit is impossible. Making the child stop the unwanted behavior quickly and experiencing some relief of parental frustration are usually achieved with a spanking. How much is actually taught through spanking is hotly debated by experts, but certainly one message given is that aggression toward another person can get results. Children usually resent such attacks and may even feel that the punishment cancels the crime, allowing the unwanted behavior to be repeated on some other occasion (Fraiberg, 1959). Simply removing the child from the situation, with a brief, age-appropriate explanation, is probably the best course of action (see Wolraich et al, 1998).

Beyond these rather common behavioral issues are certain behavioral symptoms that indicate dysfunction. *Hyperactivity* may be a temperament variable, but it may also reflect neurologic dysfunction, anxiety, depression, or bipolar disorder. The child whose activity appears driven, particularly when associated with excessive tantrums or sleep disturbance, requires a more careful look. Conflicts over bedtime and its location are not uncommon among preschoolers, but *sleep disturbance* (see Chapter 44) in the form of frequent nightmares or night awakening may signal anxiety and require intervention. Evidence of *generalized anxiety* in situations tolerated by most children, which the child cannot diminish through play or with basic reassurance from the parent, also warrants referral. *Poor social relatedness/responsiveness* is another worrisome symptom, although some children may be normally shy. Shyness, however, is preferentially displayed outside the home and with strangers. At age 2 years, *inability to communicate needs* to others and *abnormalities of movement, posture, or tone* warrant referral for evaluation, even if the child appeared normal at 18 months. *Aggressive behavior* is seen more commonly in boys and is often influenced by television, but the parents' inability to modify this behavior indicates the presence of a true dysfunction. Finally, persistent *parent-child conflict* demonstrates a need for intervention to create productive communication and avoid negative patterns that can persist into later years.

RESILIENCY

There is no single factor that protects children from risk or that places them at risk. There is an interplay of multiple factors, and it is more likely the effects of accumulated neurodevelopmental deficits that produce risks and of accumulated neurodevelopmental assets that provide protection. These factors exist within the child, within the caregiving environment, and within the larger sociocultural context.

Within the child, temperament, intelligence, and sociability interweave to produce important protective capacities. There is the capacity to elicit attention and warmth from others, the capacity to be affectionate and responsive to others, the capacity to delay gratification, and the capacity to solve problems by entertaining at least two (or more) solutions. Temperament characteristics of particular value for resiliency are the youngster's adaptability to changes (i.e., smooth transitions to new settings), high energy and persistence (in contrast to high activity and low persistence), and a desire to investigate—and master—new situations (approach). A sense of personal autonomy coupled with a basic hopefulness about the future round out the

resilient child's profile (Seifer and Sameroff, 1987; Werner, 1990).

As has been emphasized throughout this discussion, the child interacts continually with a caregiving environment that either promotes resilient qualities in the child or gives little or no nurturance to such qualities. It is clear that secure attachment between child and parent as well as emotional availability of the primary caregiver are critical in this regard. Thomas and Chess (1977) noted that the ability of a parent to perceive positively and value his or her child's difficult temperament usually meant that such a child, even if at high risk for a behavior disorder, would not develop one. The environment thus has a redemptive role by instilling faith in the child's abilities and by establishing a sense of meaning and rootedness for the child's existence. This does not happen without some effort on the parent's part and is less likely to happen if the parent lacks a strong sense of self or is emotionally unavailable. The parent needs to understand, through training or experience, when to allow the child to make decisions, when to reduce frustration and provide comfort, and how to give the child increasing levels of responsibility. For example, the parent should resist the temptation to dress the 3-year-old child if she, like most children that age, is capable of dressing herself with supervision. Similarly, socialization for girls and boys should be individualized and should encourage appropriate risk taking, acceptance of limits, and awareness of others' needs through structure and emotional support. Furthermore, the structure provided should be authoritative without being permissive or authoritarian. In other words, the parent acts from a position of knowledge (learned or natural), rather than from a position of either power or avoidance.

There is also responsibility that the larger society shares to support the development of resiliency in children. Public policy must be perceived by children and families to value children. The larger society must elicit and nurture the protective factors discussed previously because it is the dynamic interaction of these factors (Seifer and Sameroff, 1987) that makes resiliency more or less prevalent in a society. Parental leave policies, funding for high-quality day care, a commitment to strengthening families, support for adoption programs, programs to reduce violence, funding for programs that provide positive socialization experiences, and universal health care for children are examples of policies that demonstrate a commitment to children by society. The values demonstrated by the commitments and actions of society influence the priorities and actions of the employers of the parents and of parents themselves. Optimally, the values espoused by churches, synagogues, mosques, and other religious entities are not a prophetic cry in the wilderness but rather a reinforcement of values shared by the larger society, which promote civility, caring, and respect for all persons—particularly their special, individual differences.

PROMOTING NEURODEVELOPMENTAL COMPETENCE

Enabling preschool children to grow into emotionally healthy individuals who reach their potentials is the hope of all parents. It should also be the commitment of the society that provides the political and economic environment in which they live. The primary medical care provider has an important role to play as well.

The preschool years are a wonderful time for the pediatrician to build a special relationship with the child, conveying respect and concern about the youngster's feelings. Carefully explaining what is going to be done and seeking the child's assent to procedures is a part of that respect. There are times when procedures must be done even if the child objects, but ideally, these are uncommon occurrences.

The pediatrician should also seek to develop a parent-professional partnership that establishes the physician as the parents' consultant, to understand the parents' values, and to provide advice and counsel that is congruent with those values. The ability of the parent and child to relate well to each other and the treatment of conditions that damage or impede growth and development are the physician's focus, rather than family values with which the physician disagrees. If the physician does not understand a family's values, he or she should try to listen and learn.

In that context, the physician makes anticipatory guidance a major priority. The physician helps the parents understand their child's behavior and prepares them for the peculiar challenges of each developmental period. Reassuring a parent not to become preoccupied with the child's feeding and elimination can forestall potentially harmful conflicts. By exploring the child's magical thinking and fears, the physician enables the parent to be a more effective support and comfort for the child. Interpreting the child's temperament can take some of the mystery out of parent-child conflict. Providing guidance in the area of behavioral management gives parents valuable tools to deal effectively with their child's behaviors; bolstered by such anticipatory guidance and forethought, parents need not react to those behaviors with embarrassment or anger (Brazelton, 1992).

Developmental surveillance is central to this process, because the physician must understand the patient's developmental strengths and weaknesses in order to be an informed advocate. When the physician detects significant delays or dysfunction, referrals to community resources for complete diagnosis and early intervention can prevent or modify abnormal developmental patterns. A goal of early intervention is to expand the child's behavioral repertoire with potential for improvement in outcome. Understanding the strengths and limitations of local resources—medical, school, and other—enables the physician to guide parents appropriately.

Parents inevitably raise the question of whether to enroll their child in preschool and other enrichment activities. Some think that preschool is a necessary preparation for kindergarten, although there is little evidence to support this. Preschool should be viewed as an opportunity for socialization and confidence building, not academic preparation. Creative abilities should be fostered in contrast to rote learning. Parents should visit preschools under their consideration to identify the one with the happiest atmosphere and the most nurturing personnel. First and foremost, the child's needs should govern program selection. Furthermore, parents wishing to keep the child at home should be reassured that this places the child at no disadvantage (apart from children with special needs who warrant specialized intervention services). Indeed, for some preschoolers, not being able to meet the behavioral expectations of a preschool teacher may impart early feelings of inadequacy with which the child is ill-equipped to deal.

The preschool years are a time of extremely fertile mental development. Introduction of music instruction (with the music being taught as a "second language") or a foreign language during this period seems to produce lasting impressions that facilitate later learning in those areas. It is possible to teach 3- and 4-year-old children to read and spell, but this rote learning is not active problem solving, nor does it have much relevance for the preschool child. Rather, the encouragement of age-appropriate conceptual development and the development of alternative forms of personal expression can produce long-lasting and fruitful results. The physician's task is to prevent or treat disease, advocate for the child's individual differences, and provide sensitive and informed guidance to the parents, so that the benefit of neurodevelopmental assets is maximized and the impact of neurodevelopmental deficits is minimized.

REFERENCES

Bayley N: Bayley Scales of Infant Development, 2nd ed. San Antonio, TX, The Psychological Corporation, 1993.

Brazelton TB: Touchpoints. Reading, MA, Addison-Wesley, 1992.

Bryant D, Maxwell K: The effectiveness of early intervention for disadvantaged children. *In* Guralnick MJ (ed): The Effectiveness of Early Intervention. Baltimore, Paul H Brookes, 1997.

Chess S, Thomas A: Temperament in Clinical Practice. New York, Guilford Press, 1986.

Coles R: The Moral Intelligence of Children. New York, Random House, 1997.

Coplan J: Early Language Milestone Scale, 1983. Modern Education Corp., PO Box 721, Tulsa, OK 74101.

Erikson EH: Identity: Youth and Crisis. New York, WW Norton, 1968.

Flavell JH, Miller PH, Miller SA: Cognitive Development, 3rd ed. Englewood Cliffs, NJ, Prentice-Hall, 1993.

Fletcher P: Aspects of language development in the preschool years. *In* Yule W, Rutter M (eds): Language Development and Disorders. London, Mac Keith Press, 1987.

Fraiberg S: The Magic Years. New York, Charles Scribner's Sons, 1959.

Frankenburg WK, Dodds J, Archer P, et al: Denver II. Denver, Denver Developmental Materials, 1990.

Frankenburg WK, Dodds J, Archer P, et al: The Denver II: A major revision and restandarization of the Denver Developmental Screening Test. Pediatrics 89:91, 1992.

Greenspan SI: Assessing the emotional and social functioning of infants and young children. *In* Meisels SJ, Fenichel E (eds): New Visions for the Developmental Assessment of Infants and Young Children. Washington, DC, Zero to Three, 1996.

Greenspan SI, Greenspan NT: The Essential Partnership. New York, Penguin Books, 1989.

Kagan J: The Nature of the Child. New York, Basic Books, 1984.

Knobloch H, Stevens F, Malone AF: Manual of Developmental Diagnosis. Hagerstown, MD, Harper and Row, 1980.

Mahoney G, Mahoney F: Developmental Rainbow: Early Childhood Development Profiles. Tallmadge, OH, Family Child Learning Center, 1996.

Seifer R, Sameroff AJ: Multiple determinants of risk and invulnerability. *In* Anthony EF and Cohler BJ (eds): The Invulnerable Child. New York, Guilford Press, 1987.

Shonkoff JP: Preschool. *In* Levine MD, Cary WB, Crocker AC (eds): Developmental-Behavioral Pediatrics, 2nd ed. Philadelphia, WB Saunders, 1992.

Thatcher RW, Lyon GR, Rumsey J, Krasnegor N: Developmental Neuroimaging. San Diego, Academic Press, 1996.

Thomas A, Chess S: Temperament and Development. New York, Brunner/Mazel, 1977.

Werner EE: Protective factors and individual resilience. *In* Meisels S, Shonkoff J (eds): Handbook of Early Childhood Intervention. Cambridge, MA, Cambridge University Press, 1990.

Winnicott DW: The Maturational Processes and the Facilitating Environment: Studies in the Theory of Emotional Development. New York, International Universities Press, 1986.

Wolraich ML, et al: AAP Policy Statement: Guidance for Effective Discipline. Pediatrics 101:723, 1998.

Suggested Readings

Ausubel DP, Sullivan EV, Ives SW: Theory and Problems of Child Development, 3rd ed. New York, Grune & Stratton, 1980.

Bjorklünd DFB: Children's Thinking: Developmental Function and Individual Differences, 2nd ed. Pacific Grove, CA, Brooks/Cole Publishing, 1995.

Coles R: The Spiritual Life of Children. Boston, Houghton Mifflin, 1990.

Linder T: Transdisciplinary Play-Based Assessment. Baltimore, Paul H Brookes, 1990.

5 *Middle Childhood*

Melvin D. Levine

 The years of middle childhood may well fall between the cracks, as society commits to early education and contends actively with the social, cultural, educational, and behavioral issues posed by adolescents. Yet the functions and dysfunctions of children in middle childhood represent revealing tentative outcomes of early childhood influences. At the same time, one can see the emergence of potent risk factors transacting with forces of resiliency to promote or deter readiness for adolescence. In this chapter, the missions of middle childhood are delineated. There follows a detailed discussion of the ways in which physicians can become active allies in their accomplishment.

Childhood's middle years are not a latent era. They are characterized by activation and change and are a time of earnest searching, of goal-directed exploration and problem solving, and of increasingly sophisticated decision making. This is a period for preparation and rehearsal. It also is an era of debuts and refined performances and of trials and errors. Further, it leads to a critical moment called "readiness for adolescence."

Diverse challenges and constraints entice and imperil the school-aged child. To begin with, this chapter explores some of the principal missions that await youngsters entering this age span. It then surveys some developmental acquisitions that facilitate the pursuit of these missions. Finally, there is consideration of the health professional and the ways in which such an adult relates, forms alliances, and collaborates in the missions of middle childhood.

Developmental Missions

Children in this age group, motivated by sociocultural and endogenous forces, undertake unspoken missions in their quest for growth and fulfillment. Ongoing self-assessment and feedback either reinforce or inhibit the missions, which may be elucidated and classified according to various schemas. In the following section, 12 such missions are described briefly as a way of offering insights into the life scenario of this age group.

MISSION ONE: TO SUSTAIN SELF-ESTEEM

Feeling good about oneself is a prime requisite for mental health. For the school-aged child, daily life brings forth exposures and experiences that have the potential for strengthening, maintaining, or reducing self-esteem (Brooks, 1992).

To explain the quest for self-esteem, certain generalizations can be helpful. Many factors influence a child's feelings of worth. In this age group, these include feedback (i.e., either praise or criticism) from peers, reinforcement from respected adults, a record of success or mastery, an accommodation with social standards, a sense of having met endogenous or personal needs, confidence in the ability to recover from anxiety, a feeling of being in control, and optimism regarding future challenges or stresses. Self-esteem also entails having identifiable "islands of compe-

tence," areas of performance or potential performance that represent true assets (Brooks, 1992).

Influences on self-esteem are multiple and diffuse. Patterns of nurturance, early life experiences, successes and failures, and innate abilities may interact with an internal system of self-assessment to produce either feelings of worthiness or predominantly negative sentiments and reduced self-esteem.

Self-esteem is not a fixed or absolute attribute. As children progress through their school years, their feelings about themselves are likely to fluctuate from day to day and even hour to hour. Although a general level can be described, it is normal for the developing school-aged child to engage in a cyclic process of questioning and reconstructing feelings about self-worth (Stipek and MacIver, 1989). Occasional crises or influential encounters may necessitate drastic re-evaluations. Often such momentary turmoil is not evident to adults.

It should be emphasized that it is healthy for school-aged children to struggle somewhat with issues of self-esteem. It is appropriate that they explore different techniques and measures to sustain self-esteem, to test and to prove for themselves their own merit.

It is important to recognize that self-esteem is not always a generalized entity. A child may show uneven self-esteem across areas, for example displaying low academic self-esteem but good social and athletic self-esteem. When there are no areas of intact self-esteem, middle childhood becomes a time of growing emotional vulnerability.

51

MISSION TWO: TO FIND SOCIAL ACCEPTANCE

The school years are a time of coming out—a challenge to the child to "make it" beyond the protective shroud of his or her family. Primarily, the mission entails a quest for social acceptance and admission into one's peer group (see Chapter 54). For most school-aged children, this is a matter of utmost concern, and it commonly becomes a strong preoccupation. For some youngsters peer acceptance is gained with ease, whereas for others it exacts inordinate effort and the expenditure of great energy and anxiety. On the list of a child's priorities, popularity is likely to rank near the top. It is not unusual in this age group to observe the sacrifice of autonomy and free will for the cause of social success.

The acquisition of social skills is described later in this chapter. Children are variably prepared to confront the testy challenges set up by peer groups. School becomes a critical arena, a site with little or no privacy, in which one interacts and makes comparisons between oneself and one's peers. When faced with the choice of pleasing the teacher or appealing to a peer group, many school-aged children feel constrained to select the latter.

As children grow older, their social effectiveness is measured by their status among peers in general and by the richness of their close relationships. A child's social status may be influenced by many factors, such as physical appearance, the presence or absence of acceptable mannerisms, patterns of behavior, competence in specific performance areas (especially gross motor function and sports), personality, somatic maturation, and the child's own repertoire of social skills. Some children who are lacking in one or more of these areas develop a most recalcitrant condition, namely, a bad reputation.

It is possible for a child to receive too much gratification from his or her social standing. This phenomenon of "too much too soon" may eclipse other priorities for the child. For example, a youngster may underachieve academically as a result of excessive peer adulation.

MISSION THREE: TO RECONCILE INDIVIDUALITY WITH CONFORMITY

The school-aged child becomes increasingly aware of his or her unique preferences, strengths, and styles. These then find expression in a range of social contexts. The growing child faces enormous pressures to conform both to adult expectations and to the stringent standards of taste and performance mandated by peers. A child's unique characteristics or interests may differ from those of the peer group, sometimes engendering ostracism and isolation. For most children there is a process of transaction that allows them to modify but not totally sacrifice natural inclinations to yield authentic but socially acceptable patterns of behavior and taste. Eccentricity in this age group is rare. Many cultural-social forces and traditions coerce children toward conformity and uniformity.

A child who likes to collect insects while most others in the neighborhood opt for sports, one who prefers to stay indoors and read rather than pleasing parents and peers by being outside on a beautiful day, a child who disdains the "cool" vernacular used by peers, a youngster who does not wish to accept contemporary dress codes and fashions—all such children may have to struggle to sustain these individual preferences. For most, a conflict between individuality and the pressure to conform may not be as dramatic; nevertheless, the need to reconcile innate preferences with exogenously conditioned expectations is a constant tension, one that may lead to confusion over a child's authentic needs and tastes. The impact of this process increases during this age span. Children of late elementary and junior high age are particularly susceptible to such coercion. In fact, the subculture between ages 11 and 14 may resemble the harshest of totalitarian governments, the despot being the peer group. These young citizens may sacrifice freedom of speech, follow a stiff behavioral code, act in accordance with preset standards (e.g., "coolness," "macho"), and adorn themselves in uniforms that adhere meticulously to current modes.

MISSION FOUR: TO DISCOVER AND EMULATE ROLE MODELS

Children in this age group often seek out and try out prototypes. Various attributes and interests may be borrowed from peers, older children, and adults. In a sense, the school-aged child embarks on an expedition, studying those he or she esteems, sometimes exaggerating their virtues or fantasizing about them and commonly adapting or attempting to incorporate their qualities. Models may include a parent, an older sibling, other children, a television star, a well-known athlete, a teacher, or a physician.

The process of modeling and identification is a helpful one, and it is universal. At times parents may feel that a child is emulating an inappropriate prototype or is excessive or even obsessive about it. Sometimes entire communities of children extract attributes from the same model—perhaps a television personality or musical sensation. Commercial enterprises may, in fact, exploit the propensity by issuing T-shirts and other paraphernalia that can induce and energize imitation and adulation.

Role models within a family are particularly influential. To some extent, all children identify with mothers or fathers. One parent may be a particularly compelling influence. It is not unusual for a child to try on attributes of a favorite and close grandparent, aunt, or uncle. Modeling can influence academic achievement. Children who have never seen their parents read a book or write a letter may experience more trouble in acquiring academic skills than those who have witnessed these practices throughout early childhood. The drive to imitate is an important part of modeling. In a sense, the school-aged child often rehearses or tries out an assortment of practices and modes of behavior observed in the adults he or she respects. Some imaginary play and even athletic efforts of children are based on this desire to assume the identity and functions of adult role models, to move in and, in a sense, become that model. A strong sense of fulfillment is bestowed on a child who watches his favorite football star on television and hours later finds himself on the playing field going through the identical motions and perhaps fantasizing that he is that very star.

MISSION FIVE: TO EXAMINE VALUES

Emergence from the security of home and entry into an outside world entail a series of cognitive and behavioral adjustments for the school-aged child. One of these involves the reconciliation of disparate values. Expectations at home may contrast with those at school. A child's personal and family beliefs may be diametrically opposed to those of a neighborhood friend and his or her parents. Standards of discipline may differ from those of friends and from friend to friend, and economic values may be sharply contrasting. For the school-aged child encountering such discrepancies, there is a constant reawakening and sometimes a chain of disconcerting realizations.

Before entering kindergarten, the child assumes that the values assimilated at home are absolute and universal. Social exposures in school and the neighborhood begin to introduce relativism, or the notion that standards are dependent on contexts and backgrounds. Monetary values depend in part on how much money you have. Religious beliefs are founded both on one's creed and on the extent to which it is observed by a family. These awakenings may lead to a child to question personal norms; it is not unusual for the seeds of rebellion to be sown as an older school-aged child comes to recognize not only that there exist other possibilities, but also that at least some may be superior to those of his or her own family. The child who begins the early school years assuming that the way things are done at home is universally acceptable soon discovers that there may be more than one set of criteria; ultimately, in preadolescence, she or he recognizes that at least some of the cherished values at home may be abnormal, arbitrary, or inappropriate. This may even lead to periodic bouts of intense cynicism.

MISSION SIX: TO "MAKE IT" IN A FAMILY

Although "breaking away" from earlier dependence on the family is an important accomplishment of the school years, home remains a critical arena for development throughout this period. Children need to feel as successful at home as they are in their other performance arenas. In this age group, youngsters return home each day like warriors back from the plains of battle. They would like to feel and be perceived as triumphant. They would like to get credit at home for what they have achieved afield. In this age group, youngsters have a profound appetite for well-earned positive feedback from family members. They desperately need to overhear their parents boasting about them. When parental admiration fails to be communicated regularly, either because such reinforcement is unavailable or because there is actual success deprivation and failure in the world beyond the domicile, some of the impetus for healthy development may be lost.

The need to "measure up" at home is a compelling one. Probably the most convenient and most accessible gauges for such measurement are siblings. Brothers and sisters form an influential part of a child's environment, and the standards they set must be taken seriously. They serve as models and competitors, as playmates and adversaries, as gratifiers and humiliators. Therefore, sibling rivalry is an expected phenomenon. Intense competition,

conflict, and resentment may be intermittent or constant between siblings during school years. Indulgence in such intense crossfire may actually serve as useful training and practice in the art of social conflict resolution. At an appropriate level, sibling rivalry may also facilitate a child's social education. Parents may need help in their efforts to contain but not suppress such transactions and to ensure that no one child is overly oppressed by this developmentally normal warfare.

Being able to "make it" with parents is critical. School-aged children need to know not only that they are loved by their elders but also that they are respected. There may be a constant drive to impress parents, to solicit their approval, to meet or surpass their expectations.

In addition to seeking respect from a family, a child seeks to acquire respect for his or her family. Pride in one's family is a critical component of pride in one's self. Children who are ashamed of their families (of one or more family members) are apt to question their own self-worth.

MISSION SEVEN: TO EXPLORE AUTONOMY AND ITS LIMITS

It is not unusual for the school-aged child to experiment with the constraints imposed upon him or her by the adult world. A child may simultaneously take comfort in the regulations promulgated at home and in school while deriving satisfaction from violating them. In particular, older school-aged children may commit relatively benign social taboos (such as using vulgar language, lying, and stealing insignificant objects). In moderation, these experiments may represent normal testing behaviors during the school years. Various manifestations of defiance may also be within normal limits. Parents may be concerned about minor infractions, about a child's tendency to exaggerate or make up stories, or about his or her unwillingness to accept discipline or assume responsibility. In fact, it can be hard for parents to draw the line between a normal testing of limits and truly difficult behavior.

As school-aged children progress toward early adolescence, their drive for autonomy intensifies. There may be internal conflict between an intense desire for greater freedom, on the one hand, and lingering feelings of dependency, on the other. In later elementary school, this precarious balance or slight imbalance engenders seemingly contradictory scenarios. A child may want to stay out and play later but be equally desirous of having his parents available when he returns. It should be emphasized that when children seek autonomy, not only are they experimenting with the constraints imposed by parents and society, they are also—perhaps more importantly—testing themselves. There may be an unconscious rehearsal process, an attempt to discover whether they can survive without the help of adults, an effort to find out what it will be like to be grown up. Cigarette smoking, use of adult language, membership in cliques, and increasing adventures after dark may all represent auditions for the biggest show—adult autonomy.

MISSION EIGHT: TO ACQUIRE KNOWLEDGE AND SKILL

To observe oneself becoming increasingly competent and masterful is a reinforcing experience for a school-aged child. Children in this age group need to feel that they are growing more able, that they are mastering skills. School is of course the principal arena for this effort; however, skill and knowledge acquisition are not confined to the classroom. Children in this age group also learn from one another, from their parents, and from a wide range of avocational and recreational exposures. There is greatly expanded knowledge of how things work. As is discussed later in this chapter, there is a growing ability to generalize, to understand processes, to think in abstract terms. Knowledge of the universe expands. Children also strive for physical mastery. For the school-aged child, the process of learning may be a constant source of gratification and reward, or it may erode self-esteem. School performance thus plays a critical role in development. A youngster in a classroom is aware of the accomplishments of the peer group. Maladaptive strategies may be appropriated to save face and to avoid the feeling of not "measuring up" intellectually, socially, or motorically. The school-aged child is armed with very little tolerance for failure. When knowledge and skill are not accruing rapidly enough, giving up may seem better than facing the humiliation of having tried and failed.

Beginning at about age 7, children are preoccupied with whether they are "smart." Derogatory terms such as "retard" unfortunately are quite common and reflect a concern for at least a modicum of intellectual prowess. Many children would rather be regarded as "bad" than as "dumb." They would prefer to get into trouble for not completing an assignment in school than to endure the humiliation of bad grades and pages streaked with a teacher's critical red marks.

MISSION NINE: TO LIVE WITHIN ONE'S BODY

An important component of the development of the school-aged child is the progressive realization of the extent to which one is entrapped in a body. Various anatomic and physiologic advantages and constraints become an important part of experience. The school-aged child is a student of bodies—his or her own, those of peers, and those of adults—but may feel uncomfortable talking about personal somatic concerns. Becoming reconciled with one's own body is a critical and ongoing developmental challenge. Much experimentation occurs during these years, as children set out to investigate bodily functions and limitations. A child self-evaluates to determine whether his or her physical appearance, body build, and coordination compare favorably with those of his peers. Sporting events can be one mechanism for this, because they permit the child to explore a variety of corporal performance frontiers. This is but one of many physical challenges. The school-aged child must also learn to deal with pain and discomfort (see Chapter 36) and to tolerate illness.

Acquisition of secondary sexual characteristics becomes an increasing interest as children approach early adolescence, and it is not unusual for youngsters throughout this age group to become curious about the bodies of other children. A common occurrence, one that frequently alarms parents, is when two or more youngsters unclothe (to varying degrees) and "play doctor." Experiments and explorations such as this allow youngsters to pursue one of their major interests, namely, bodily similarities and differences. In a sense, they are acquiring norms. They also experiment with their own bodies. Various forms of masturbation, for example, may be developmental learning experiences. It is only when they become obsessive or extreme or when adults overreact to such activities that they become clinically problematic. It is probably fortunate that most children who undertake bodily investigations never get caught. For those who are surprised in the act, it is most helpful to provide reassurance of normalcy and to alleviate needless anguish or guilt.

It is not unusual for school-aged children to believe that their bodies are not right, that one or more anatomic parts are of the wrong size or shape, that something does not work right, that the soma is defective in some manner. Usually they do not discuss such concerns with parents. With encouragement, they may be willing to confide in a physician. It can be helpful for a school-aged child to learn of the universality of this phenomenon. Youngsters in this age range may not be aware of the wide normal variation in bodies with respect to looks and functions or of how common it is to worry about one's body.

School-aged children express somatic concerns in a variety of manners. Some conceal the blemishes about which they are most concerned. Extreme modesty about undressing may be evident. Other youngsters may refrain from activities that expose self-perceived shortcomings of anatomy or body performance. A child with nocturnal enuresis may refrain from sleeping at a friend's house (see Chapter 42). A youngster who is obese may decline an invitation to go swimming. Certain children may conveniently forget their gym suits when they are likely to be humiliated over their poor gross motor function on the playing fields. It is a common phenomenon in many communities for children to be required to take a shower in physical education classes beginning at about age 12 or 13. Word may spread throughout town, and youngsters may fret for months over the prospects of this threatening exposure. It is important to reassure children about both the uniqueness and the sameness of their bodies while at the same time respecting their privacy and allowing them to appropriate protective strategies.

MISSION TEN: TO DEAL WITH FEARS

A young child approaches the school years with a bevy of fears, many of which were established considerably earlier in life. There is of course wide variation among youngsters in terms of the targets of their apprehension. In early elementary school, fears of the dark, concerns about monsters and ghosts, idiosyncratic phobias, squeamishness about certain animals (such as snakes, mice, and spiders), and preoccupations with death and injury are typical. Particularly common are fears involving food intake. A child may like peas and enjoy mashed potatoes but become quite anxious when the two come in contact with each other. Some children fear lumps in oatmeal, while others are reluctant to swallow pills, firmly believing somehow that they are likely to choke on them.

No 6- or 7-year-old is entirely liberated from such fears. An important mission during school years is the attempt to explore and modify, minimize, and perhaps entirely eliminate targeted fears. Children may do so by becoming increasingly educated about the foci of their concern. Intellectualization and knowledge can be used to overcome anxiety. Through education and experience, a youngster may come to realize and confirm that ghosts do not exist. Usually this requires more than parental reassurance; somehow a child must arrive at a state of readiness to accept and assimilate such an accommodation.

School-aged children are likely to employ many mechanisms to deal with fears. They may explore these through play. A child with an inordinate fear of injury may actually enjoy playing imaginary dangerous games. Some youngsters with concerns about monsters take great pleasure in reading or observing horror stories on television. Others compensate by showing a great deal of bravery and "macho," trying somehow to acquire equanimity by pretending to be tough. There is a sense that one can become fear-free by acting fearless.

Fear of the future (anticipatory anxiety) is common in school-aged children. They may be apprehensive about what comes next, about future challenges, about environmental disasters, or about the possibility of failure and humiliation. Life transitions may be particularly difficult. A fear of future losses (of relatives, of friends, of possessions) also may be prevalent.

MISSION ELEVEN: TO DEAL WITH APPETITES AND DRIVES

Learning how to obtain satisfaction is an important mission for school-aged children. As the school-aged child experiences appetites and desires, there is a drive toward fulfillment and satisfaction. As is discussed in Chapter 52, some youngsters with attention deficits suffer because of their insatiability. They appear to be in a steady state of hunger. As school-aged children mature, they become increasingly sophisticated at identifying and finding ways to satisfy or curb appetites. Multiple hungers come forth, including desires for specific foods, sexual drives, quests for praise and success, want of material things, searches for pleasure, and the wish for the attention of others. Each of these is represented to varying degrees at various times in the development of school-aged children. Any one or more may become excessive (even obsessive).

An important mission thus involves finding the tools to limit and control such appetites and drives. The means of doing so may be painful yet in the long run more rewarding than total capitulation to desire. Included are such processes as compromising with others when there is a conflict over desires, sharing, settling for fulfillment in less than anticipated dosages, delaying gratification, and accepting substitutes or replacements. The process of maturing for the school-aged child entails, in part, the acquisition and assimilation of these means of control. When this does not occur, children become increasingly frustrated and anxious. There is enormous variation with regard to the capacity to satisfy or extinguish "burning desires."

MISSION TWELVE: TO REFINE SELF-AWARENESS

The age-old admonition "Know thyself" characterizes another mission. Throughout elementary school a youngster is acquiring increasing insight into himself or herself. Formal education is one source of such knowledge, while studying of peers and their attributes is also informative. Observations and feedback regarding one's own performance and limitations further shape the child's sense of identity. Finally, a process of introspection is applied to this effort. The school-aged child progressively develops a sense of what he or she is "good at" and what he or she is "bad at." There is a growing capacity to articulate and confess specific strengths and weaknesses. Children between ages of 6 and 8 are more apt to deny deficits or to refuse to think or talk about them. By age 12, youngsters are more prepared to reckon with these, although commonly they will still be reluctant to discuss the ways in which they might be different from peers.

The first 11 missions described in this section play roles in shaping a child's identity. As school-aged children accumulate experience, they become increasingly perceptive about themselves. They observe their own patterns of behavior, ways of reacting, and targets of fear and confidence. They integrate these as they climb toward higher levels of self-awareness. In doing so, they are liable to pass through brief or prolonged periods of confusion. Parents may report occasional outpourings of despair. Children may use a variety of indirect means to discover more about themselves, such as making provocative comments such as "Nobody likes me" or "I'm not good at anything." The responses to these experimental self-effacing statements can be important in helping children see themselves as others see them. As children grow older they learn more about themselves by talking about other youngsters. In gossiping with friends or being "catty" about someone else, children, in reality, may be analyzing themselves. Some older elementary school children become very interested in reading biographies. They become close to a particular friend and like to engage in intimate discussions partly as a means of increasing self-awareness. By finding someone to whom they can confess, someone whom they feel they can trust, they may be able to define their own identity simply by describing it.

As children grow in their self-awareness, several issues become increasingly important: To what extent is the child willing and able to accept the way he or she is? How realistic are the youngster's self-perceptions? How prepared does the child feel to meet the challenges of adolescence and adulthood? Those who live with and help children in this age group need to be sensitive to the child's own sense of identity. To the degree that school children develop an authentic or viable version of who and what they are, they are likely to find fulfillment and gratification during adolescence.

Developmental Acquisitions

Success in the school years is facilitated through the acquisition of new abilities, strategies, and insights that become the means for discovery and accomplishment, the implements for carrying out the aforementioned missions. Psychologists, developmentalists, and other students of childhood have advanced various conceptual models relevant to development in this age group. The reader is referred to the classic works of Freud (1965), Erikson (1959), Piaget (1968), and Gesell and Ilg (1946) (see also Chapter 1). Many possible schemes can be suggested to account for change over the school years. In the present section, a framework has been constructed to be particularly relevant to developmental pediatrics and to the understanding of variation and deviation in this age group. Some basic developmental acquisitions are described:

Attention, persistence, and goal-directedness
Orientation and perception
Storage and retrieval
Interpretation and generalization
Expression and production
Social reception and interaction
Protective resiliency and strategy formation
Other acquisitions

The following sections elaborate upon each of these eight areas of developmental acquisition.

ATTENTION, PERSISTENCE, AND GOAL-DIRECTEDNESS

During middle childhood, children acquire increasing control over attention. The specific attention controls are described in some detail in Chapter 52. These controls undergo considerable strengthening between the years of 6 and 13. Children become increasingly selective in their concentration and in the allocation of mental effort. There is far less randomness of focus and output with a much higher level of goal-directed activity and highly selective attention.

In particular, the processing controls gain greatly in their effectiveness. A child's ability to detect saliency amid less relevant detail represents a major accomplishment of middle childhood development. A first-grader struggles to focus on the teacher instead of looking out the window, while a 7th-grade child can look at a chapter in a social studies book and decide what is most likely to be asked on tomorrow's quiz.

Children in this age group also become more adept at activating their minds, relating new facts or ideas to prior knowledge or experience. They become increasingly able to process information in sufficient depth and to concentrate for appropriate durations of time.

A number of acquired traits contribute to the strengthening of selective attention and the lengthening of task persistence in this age group. Important is the child's growing ability to delay gratification and function effectively without immediate rewards or instant excitation. A toddler or preschool youngster commonly demands a swift and pleasurable "payoff" for any actions taken. His goals generally are of short range. Desires and felt needs call for instantaneous satisfaction. Delayed consequences and events in the distant future have far less motivating power for preschool children. As youngsters enter the school years, the very foundations of education emphasize the concept of preparation (a form of delay). Children become increasingly receptive to the notion of "getting ready" for later life. Enormous pressure is brought to bear, coercing them to look ahead, to sacrifice immediate pleasure for

something better later on. Even the Boy Scout troop leader keeps reiterating his faithful motto, "Be Prepared"!

Most school-aged children encounter little difficulty in sustaining delays of gratification. Initially, they are apt to harbor weak satisfaction control or insatiability. As they proceed through the elementary school years, successful youngsters increasingly realize the rewards of work and sacrifice. Earlier hedonistic inclinations are tempered as they come to recognize that completing homework, delivering newspapers, performing family chores, or enduring dull sermons in a place of worship may portend later and greater benefits than those attained through instant gratification. By being able to postpone their reinforcement, children become increasingly able to persist at tasks, to find their way through immediately unrewarding detail, and to engage in activities whose short-term motivational content is minimal. These capacities clearly are strengthened when there is likelihood that children can reap some immediate profits along the way; those whose efforts consistently meet with failure may have little reason to invest persistence and patience.

Linked to the enhancement of the attention controls is the child's improved function as a planner, one who grows steadily in the capacity to preview potential actions and their likely outcomes before undertaking them. Children learn to predict social and personal consequences. Increasingly, they are able to inhibit counterproductive impulses or first responses, such as those that are apt to lead to inevitable punishment or ridicule. Competent school children become increasingly proficient at "editing" the many possibilities for action that present themselves. Some plans are facilitated, whereas others are aborted or modified. Multiple factors are integrated as part of this process. Language is often used to control impulses, to think through alternatives before taking an action. Cultural standards, moral values, and social skills play a role. Selective inhibition of impulses and the development of reflective behaviors also have a profound impact on learning and school performance (see Chapter 52).

Another conditioner of persistent attention is the child's capacity to stave off fatigue, to remain aroused and alert during prolonged purposeful activity or concentration. This too is a progressive acquisition during school years.

ORIENTATION AND PERCEPTION

School-aged children continue the exploratory work of earlier life and become increasingly knowledgeable about their environment. There is a continuing stabilization of orientation, one that enables the children to perceive themselves relevant to various ordinate points in daily life. Three principal forms of orientation can be cited: body awareness, appreciation of spatial attributes, and awareness of time relationships. In their daily activities and in the process of learning, school-aged children gain sophistication in these three dimensions.

School-aged children's perception of their own bodies evolves steadily. During late preschool and early elementary years, they become increasingly proficient at naming body parts. Fantasies about the purposes of various anatomic components give way to knowledge and demystification, while children become adept at managing their bodies independently. They are able to respond appropriately to bodily needs and become more autonomous in managing discomfort and other inconveniences incurred by the soma. As they progress through school years, children take increasing pride in their appearance. They may agonize over blemishes, unwanted protuberances, conspicuous dimensions, and the like.

Sense of body position and gross motor function improve, so that children can acquire feelings of mastery over physical space. This is a requisite for effective participation in sports and also for artistic, writing, and craft skills. By age 7, most children are able to discriminate left from right. They then perform increasingly complex operations regarding left-right distinctions, including the ability to identify right and left parts on other people or objects facing them, a sign of enhanced sophistication with regard to body awareness and "outer space."

Spatial perception is another area of development in this age group. It entails the capacity to perceive physical relationships beyond one's own body. The child's interpretation of visual, haptic (i.e., touch), proprioceptive, and kinesthetic data becomes increasingly strengthened. Children are able to perceive more complex and more detailed configurations in the spatial environment. Standardized tests requiring them to copy geometric forms or match complicated designs demonstrate a growing ability to attend simultaneously to multiple aspects of a pattern and to see their interrelationships. Thus, a preschool child may be able to interpret and copy only a simple right triangle, while a 9-year-old can perceive and utilize a triangle that is at a 45-degree angle on the page and has a second triangle embedded within it. A 12-year-old can add to this array the attributes of three-dimensionality. Such progressively sophisticated spatial orientation and perception is important in learning to read and write.

Subtle discriminations in the visual symbol system are facilitated as the child's spatial orientation and perceptual abilities improve. As school-aged children grow older, in fact, actual perceptions and visual analyses become increasingly less important insofar as they are able to interpret incoming data with more reliance on memory, language, and conceptualization. Thus, a word may be decoded not exclusively by its spatial attributes but more by the overall semantic context and its nearly instant recognition through visual memory and attached verbal associations.

Orientation in time and the capacity to assimilate and make good use of temporal relationships are critical themes of development in this age group. Closely linked is the ability to understand and store sequences of information when the serial order of their components is critical to their meaning. Arranging words in the correct order to form a grammatically acceptable sentence, remembering the sequence of letters in a word, processing three- and four-step instructions, and completing long-division problems are examples of these sequential operations. As is discussed in Chapter 53, children with dysfunctions of temporal-sequential ordering often experience academic lags. Time and sequential awareness also contribute to a child's organizational abilities. The school years are characterized by an increasing ability to retain, retrieve, and deploy sequences. Between ages 6 and 13, a youngster is able to

engage in activities that depend on increasingly complex sequences. A 5-year-old may be able to follow only a three-step instruction, whereas at age 12 he masters six- or seven step directions. The ability to tell time, to learn the days of the week and months of the year, and to master time-related vocabulary (e.g., before and after, now and later, yesterday and tomorrow) may be markers of this aspect of development.

STORAGE AND RETRIEVAL

During the school years, the facility for storage and easy retrieval of information undergoes steady expansion. The capacity to preserve and then find previously encountered data is critical for learning, for the interpretation of new experience, and for the acquisition of skills.

In the early grades there is a predominant stress on paired association memory, involving the coupling in memory of two items (such as a sound and an alphabetic symbol or a quantity and a number symbol). This form of memory function becomes increasingly effective and automatic during elementary school. In the middle grades of elementary school, there is an increasing call for rapid and precise retrieval from memory. For children to succeed, facts and skills must be recalled with virtual no cueing and with increasing speed (progressive automaticity), another capacity that grows through the course of middle childhood.

As children move on toward their middle school years, they develop increasing capacity in active working memory. This is a form of memory that entails the maintenance of certain facts or processes in memory while they are being developed or applied. This form of memory is critical for success in mathematics but also plays a role in areas such as reading and written output (Ramsdell and Levy, 1996).

Many trends during the school years produce a generalized enhancement of memory. A growing proportion of stored fact and routine becomes easy to recall quickly. This progressive automatization is a prime facilitator of learning and productivity. A 5- or 6-year-old child may struggle to recall the "blueprints" for constructing certain letters. As she or he progresses through the school years, visual retrieval of symbolic configurations becomes increasingly efficient, unconscious, and rapid. Such facilitated memory enables the child to concentrate on more sophisticated ideas and processes rather than on the mechanics of letter formation. Progressive automatization, the expanding mass of skill and knowledge that can be drawn upon effortlessly, is a most accelerated aspect of memory growth in this age group.

Another important trend with regard to memory is the emergence of a series of strategies for retaining new information. Youngsters acquire a repertoire of "tricks" needed to store relevant data more effectively. These include mnemonics, the ability to associate newly presented information with previous experience, and the use of highly specific memory-strengthening techniques. Students also become increasingly effective at putting new knowledge in pre-existing categories. Such systematic categorization greatly facilitates the speed and accuracy of recall from long-term memory (see Chapter 53).

INTERPRETATION AND GENERALIZATION

The rapid growth of language and cognitive ability in the school-aged child has been studied and written about extensively. The preadolescent child displays competence in thought processes and in comprehension that dramatically surpasses that of the prekindergarten youngster. Greater facility with language and the ability to understand phenomena on an increasingly abstract level characterize these revolutionary processes.

Perhaps the most widely accepted conceptual model of cognitive development in this age group stems from the work of Piaget. The Swiss epistemologist thought of the school years as representing a period in which children master so-called concrete operations (Piaget and Inhelder, 1968). The phenomenon is illustrated vividly in what may be the most well-known experiment in developmental psychology. Piaget and his collaborator, Inhelder, presented children with two identical beakers, each of which contained the same quantity of liquid, such as water. Each child was asked whether both containers possessed the same amount of water. Necessary adjustments were made until children agreed that this was the case. Subsequently, with the child watching, the investigator poured the liquid from one beaker into a third receptacle, one that was taller and thinner than either of the other containers. Not surprisingly, the water rose to a higher level in the taller and thinner beaker. The children were then asked, "Does this (i.e., the tall, thin) beaker contain as much water as the other (i.e., the initial) beaker, does it contain more water, or does it contain less?" The researchers were interested in finding out whether children would understand that the amount of liquid is "conserved" regardless of the apparent change of height of the liquid in the taller and thinner beaker. They wanted to determine whether children could "conserve continuous quantities." This would provide some evidence that they were able to transcend their own direct sensory observations and appeal to a higher order of logic or reasoning.

In this experiment, 4-year-old children commonly believed that the total amount of water had changed. They attended to only one component of what they saw, justifying their responses by saying such things as "I know there is more; it's higher" or "The glass is bigger, so there is more." Such responses were not changed, even when the experimenter pointed out that no liquid had been added or taken away. Children aged 5 or 6 years tended to give intermediate responses. Often they were not sure. Some were able to conserve the liquid when a difference in appearance was only slight but had more difficulty when it was great. Sometimes they could foresee what would happen (i.e., "When you pour the water, it will stay the same"), but they actually answered incorrectly when confronted with the dramatic visual difference. In other words, they were not yet prepared to overrule sensory data with logical thought.

Beginning at about age 7 or 8, genuine conservation was detectable. Children were absolutely sure that the amount of liquid had not changed. Three basic concepts were used to justify their answers, and these were characterized as "compensation," "identity," and "reversal."

Children invoking compensation noted that although the liquid was higher, the container was thinner and one made up for the other. Those citing identity pointed out that there could be no difference, since nothing was added or taken away; while those invoking reversal asserted that if one pours the liquid back into the original container, one can prove that the same amount was there all along. As youngsters gain in sophistication they become less exclusively reliant on concrete or sensory data. A child may state, "You know, I really didn't need to look when you were pouring, since I knew you were just pouring. I knew that just by pouring you can't change the amount of water."

It was Piaget's conviction that subjects in the middle childhood years made extensive use of these concepts of compensation, reversibility, and identity to make sense of a multitude of phenomena that went beyond continuous quantities (such as the water in the experiment). Included were discontinuous quantities (such as the conservation of length, area, solid substance, and number). As noted, Piaget characterized this phase of development as concrete operations. By operations he meant those mental activities (i.e., efforts carried out in one's head) through which a youngster derives a more lucid understanding of time, space, number, amount, and other conceptual areas. They are "concrete" because they are applied to the physical entities of everyday life, substances such as pecan pie, blocks, and money. It is not until adolescence, during a stage Piaget referred to as "formal operations," that these processes are applied on a more abstract level to symbols, words, and numbers in addition to observable objects (see Chapter 6).

Thus it can be seen that the cognitive development of the school-aged child entails the increasing ability to draw inferences, build on previous experience, and see relationships between newly acquired data and data encountered previously. Toward the end of middle childhood, youngsters become increasingly adept at interpreting analogies and metaphors. Their inferential powers grow, and they are able to detect irony, paradox, ambiguity, double-entendre, and hidden meanings. Further development of these functions, however, awaits the adolescent years.

Closely linked to a child's conceptual development is increasing sophistication in the understanding of language. In the earliest grades, children are honing their phonologic awareness, their reception of the basic sounds in their language. Such awareness is essential for the acquisition of early reading and spelling skills. At the same time, words and sentences become important tools—methods of characterizing relationships, rules, and generalizations. As noted earlier, language skills reinforce memory and attention. Thus they facilitate the mission of skill and knowledge acquisition. Language is also critical for social development (see Chapter 54).

By age 5, most children have acquired a large vocabulary and have mastered the basic grammar and syntax of their language. At the same time that their vocabulary continues its growth in size, children in this age group acquire a rich semantic network. That is, they become increasingly adept at linking words to each other, at recognizing how words in their vocabulary relate meaningfully to each other. As a result, the words that children know accrete greater meaning during middle childhood.

There is also significant progress at the sentence level

of language. Between age 5 and the onset of adolescence, children add a relatively small number of syntactic formations that were lacking in kindergarten (Smith, Goodman, and Meredith, 1970). They become increasingly adept at using and understanding embedded clauses. Carol Chomsky (1969) and others provide interesting examples of this aspect of development. She cites the child's ability to interpret sentences such as, "The monkey promises the dog to jump off." In this kind of sentence a complement verb (i.e., "to jump") occurs, and the challenge is to assign the correct subject (i.e., which will jump, the monkey or the dog?). At age 5, a child will select the noun phrase that is closest in the sentence to the complement verb. Therefore, most early elementary school students respond that it is the dog that will jump off. The capacity to deal with exceptions to this rule for certain verbs (such as "promises") is not developed until close to age 10. As children develop in middle childhood, their abilities to interpret and formulate language at the sentence level represent sensitive indicators of their overall language abilities.

Other language acquisitions are also relevant. The child becomes sensitive to figurative language, to metaphor and simile. During the school years, children are more discerning of figures of speech that equate two elements from different realms of experience (Winner, Rosenstiel, and Gardner, 1976). In one study, early elementary school students were asked to interpret the sentence "My friend John is a real tiger." Most believed that John really was a tiger. By about age 8, youngsters surmised that this sentence was really nonsense, and they attempted to alter it to make sense. For example, some tried to change the sentence into a story, stating, "John is friendly with a tiger." It was not until age 10 or 11 that the metaphoric interpretation of this sentence was possible. To accomplish this, the children had to be sensitive to multiple meanings and the ways in which various classes of words can interrelate. School-aged children become progressively skilled at penetrating beyond literal meanings, proceeding toward flexibility and even creativity of interpretation.

EXPRESSION AND PRODUCTION

Development of the school-aged child is conditioned to some extent by exogenous expectations and challenges dispatched from the adult world. An example of this is the transition from a predominantly decoding experience in the early elementary grades to the expectation for high-efficiency encoding (Levine, Oberklaid, and Meltzer, 1981). Youngsters in kindergarten and first grade need to learn to recognize and interpret various symbols and operations. Although they may be required to perform some writing, to "show and tell," and to solve some arithmetic problems, the volume and complexity of these outputs are relatively low. At ages 6 to 8, children are mastering the alphabet and the number system. They are learning to recognize words and to associate these with sounds and meanings. Beginning around fourth grade, there is a fairly rapid shift, and they are expected to become increasingly productive, to synthesize and express ideas of their own, to write more lengthy assignments, to take tests under timed conditions, to complete long-term projects, and to solve multistep mathematics problems. All these

activities have in common their emphasis on output, on efficient productivity, on encoding more than decoding, and on expressive skills more than receptive ones.

Fortunately, school-aged children grow in their productivity. There are many reasons for this. As attention and concentration improve, more sustained and more focused effort is feasible. Enhanced abilities in the language and motor areas (see later) further facilitate output, as do the growing abilities to integrate data from multiple sources, to retrieve stored information rapidly and with relatively little conscious effort, and to tap functions of memory and cognition simultaneously. The school-aged child becomes increasingly efficient and organized. Thus most youngsters are able to satisfy demands for effective output.

A child's verbal expressive ability undergoes a metamorphosis that parallels in many ways the acquisition of receptive language skills described in the previous section. Fluency and word finding improve markedly. The size of the child's active vocabulary grows exponentially under the influence of an educational setting and a stimulating home environment. The child has available increasing options for the use of language as he or she becomes adept for the first time at figurative speech. The latter does not become highly developed until late in adolescence (and often beyond). The school-aged child grows in the awareness of the uses of language. For example, words and phrases can be mobilized to win friends and influence people. During school years, the child begins to acquire the skills to employ writing as an alternative language mode. Those who have not as yet mastered oral speech may encounter particular difficulties with fluent written expression. As mentioned earlier, during the school years the child improves in his or her ability to use language to reinforce memory, to think, to imagine, and to create. Language also can be used to help a child gain social acceptance.

School-aged children become increasingly able to exploit language to initiate, modify, and sustain relationships with peers and adults. Subtle regulations of voice tone, word usage, and even rhythm can connote social nuances that lubricate relationships. This facility is known as verbal pragmatic skill (see Chapter 54). The growing awareness of this aspect of communication aids in the socialization of the school-aged child.

Gross motor skills represent another conduit for output. Physical mastery over space is a valued aspiration for many school children. Maturation and changes in body size facilitate the process. Growing muscle strength adds to physical efficacy. During school years, youngsters become increasingly able to interpret incoming information from their eyes and from proprioceptive-kinesthetic fibers in muscles and joints. These data can be used to program effective motor activities. They become better able to organize complex motor operations, to master and retrieve multistep motor processes and sequential motor patterns. Complicated athletic pursuits become possible. School-aged children become better able to plan a motor activity, to inhibit extraneous muscle function, and to become motor-efficient. Young children show an abundance of associated movements (such as synkinesias), that is, muscle activities not relevant to the task at hand. By age 7 or 8 these tend to disappear, and increasing motor efficiency is noted.

Availability of motor memory increases. School-aged children are able to store and retrieve rapidly the blueprints for various forms of motor output, such as particular athletic skills or dance steps. Children differ markedly in their capacity to store and retrieve these motor plans.

Most likely there is a close relationship between gross motor function and confidence and self-esteem (Cratty, 1979). A child who is well coordinated, one who succeeds in sports and other motor enterprises, is likely to be bolstered in fulfilling the mission of sustaining self-esteem. Motor success can also help youngsters gain social acceptance and come to terms with their own bodies. Children who are delayed or deficient in gross motor abilities may encounter ostracism by peers.

Much of what has been stated regarding gross motor output is applicable to the area of fine motor function. During the school years, youngsters become increasingly adept at planning, coordinating, monitoring, and remembering a range of activities requiring effective finger manipulation. Arts and crafts and the act of writing depend heavily upon the ability to take in data from visual and proprioceptive-kinesthetic pathways and then program appropriate fine motor responses. Increases in skill in eye-hand coordination, in the rate of fine motor output, and in overall precision become important developmental acquisitions for school-aged children.

It is essential that a school-aged child feel effective in one or more of the output conduits just delineated. Strengths in one may compensate for weaknesses in another. If all four of these outputs are blocked or are chronically deficient, the mission to sustain self-esteem is likely to be abortive.

SOCIAL RECEPTION AND INTERACTION

It was pointed out earlier that the quest for social acceptance is an important mission of the school years. A youngster emerges from the protective custody of the home into a social milieu dominated by peers. A wide range of developmental acquisitions during this period facilitates socialization (Flavell and Ross, 1981). Social perceptual and conceptual skills develop under the influence of culture and experience. They are bolstered by innate sensitivities or instincts and further conditioned by ongoing feedback. Through successful social encounters, a child gains in other missions also. Socialization helps a child select and conform to models. It is a way of both studying and assimilating values or cultural influences and learning. Interactions with other children help youngsters increase their self-awareness as they "study" the attributes and behaviors of others with whom they are intimate. Peers become allies in the exploration of autonomy and its limits. They collaborate in the satisfaction of appetites and drives. They serve as sources of comparisons that even help a child understand, appreciate, or criticize his or her own body. Finally, through peer interaction, youngsters come to understand their individuality and to strike a balance between uniqueness and conformity.

In acquiring social cognition, a youngster grows aware of the dynamics of relationships. Late elementary school students talk about making friends. They are interested in what it means to be popular, becoming preoccupied in many cases with physical appearance (such as looks and clothing) and likely to offer highly stereotyped discourses on "taste." Although the early elementary school student is likely to interact on a less self-conscious level, with little planning or forethought, for the older child social relationships constitute a matter of interest. From the study of socialization, the child begins to refine his basic social skills. In particular, he learns to sublimate immediate desires in the interest of long-term relationships. He learns to share with others, to praise someone else, to balance competition with cooperation, to say and do things that are likely to please a friend, and to inhibit actions and words that could be damaging to relationships.

PROTECTIVE RESILIENCY AND STRATEGY FORMATION

Children hate to feel hurt. In this regard, of course, they are not different from infants or adults. During school years, they amass an arsenal of defensive material to fortify themselves against the threat of humiliation, physical harm, frustration, fear, and failure. They learn to cope and to apply strategies to prevent such injuries. They develop a resiliency that enables them to recover promptly after setbacks. They acquire some immunity from prolonged feelings of despair and find protection through coping, which enables them to succeed at the following life tasks:

Managing Success and Failure. An important developmental acquisition is a repertoire of tactics for dealing with failure and, analogously, a method of handling success. Too much of either may be problematic. A variety of different styles are appropriated. Children may practice denial. After a defeat, they may pretend that they won or that "It wasn't important." Rationalization may be incorporated into such a style.

As children pass through elementary school, they sense a need not to become complacent or "cocky" about their successes. They may show a tendency to tone these down, to apply modesty, or to proclaim in a self-deprecatory manner, for example, "I wasn't that good today," or "It was too easy." This serves as a good social strategy, and, at the same time, it shields the child from some deleterious effects of excessive gratification.

Saving Face. Children develop face-saving techniques to insulate themselves from humiliation. A youngster who strikes out every time he is at bat in baseball may proclaim that he is not really trying or, alternatively, he may clown at home plate. Another way of coping with potential or actual humiliation is avoidance—strategies to evade intolerable situations. He may conveniently forget his gym suit when the class is playing baseball or may feign illness on the day of a science examination. A girl may deny that she is concerned about her weight or physical appearance in general, as a way of concealing concern over her inability to "keep up" in the quest for physical attractiveness. Most youngsters acquire a battery of face-saving skills during the elementary school years. Various styles and strategies are apt to be tried. It is important for the adult world to acknowledge and recognize these but not to try to discourage face-saving techniques without, at least, suggesting better ones.

Managing Frustration, Disappointment, and Loss. Losses and disappointments are not unusual at any stage of life. The preschool child may have a difficult time coping with such occurrences. Temper tantrums, violent outbursts, and prolonged tearfulness may be characteristic of the "terrible twos." Although sadness and grief are common and appropriate, children need mechanisms for recovery within a reasonable amount of time. There is wide variation in the extent to which this occurs, and a range of acceptable devices may be appropriated.

Some children deal with frustration and loss through denial and rationalization: "I didn't really like that bicycle anyway," or "I don't care if I failed that test. They can't really do anything to me." At other times and in other cases, youngsters can displace or dislodge a source of frustration. They can gain resiliency by seeking alternative routes after a disappointment.

Accommodating Discomfort. The capacity to deal with pain and discomfort becomes increasingly strengthened during the school years. Pain tolerance develops in some unique ways (see Chapter 36). Closely linked to this aspect of coping is the process of delaying gratification, referred to earlier in the context of task persistence. Youngsters may be better able to endure boredom, drudgery, and inconvenience, knowing that there is a "light at the end of the tunnel." They increasingly postpone gratification and recognize that immediate discomfort may lead to greater pleasure later on. A clearer picture of the need to sacrifice some comfort in the present as a way of enhancing future pleasure becomes evident during this period. The ability to keep future gains in sight may make current pain or boredom easier to tolerate.

Dealing With Feelings. The school child becomes increasingly adept at talking about and coping with personal feelings. Many styles are encountered as one surveys how youngsters experience and react to their models. Most become more skilled in expressing feelings, in trying to control those that appear to be wasteful and self-destructive, and in modifying inappropriate emotions. The range of coping mechanisms includes "letting it all out," denial, and displacement.

Channeling Appetites. During the school years, the child must cope with a whole range of emerging appetites that demand satisfaction. One example is burgeoning sexual awareness, in which various forms of sublimation are appropriate. The older school-aged child may struggle to reach a balance between repression of desires and their outward, judicious expression. In this effort, children may need to use adults as resources. Considerable guilt can be associated with appetites, and to some extent this is normal. Growth of sexual awareness and various methods of coping with it are elaborated in Chapter 48. In addition, appetites for food, attention, and pleasure in general also need to be dealt with. Once again, youngsters appropriate a range of coping styles to pursue, contain, deny, and channel their cravings.

Designing and Implementing Strategies. Some youngsters are master strategists and rational problem-solvers—skills likely to be of great value for coping with a wide range of setbacks and potentially troublesome challenges. Other children are less adept at masterminding. Strategy formation pervades social and cognitive realms. In acquiring skill and knowledge, some children are particularly talented at developing good learning techniques, being able to bypass intrinsic weaknesses and apply their strengths effectively.

OTHER ACQUISITIONS

Although particular school-aged acquisitions have been singled out for elaboration in this chapter, one could cite many others that facilitate the pursuit of childhood missions. Several are particularly worthy of mention.

The moral development of school children represents one important theme. School-aged children show a progression in this area. Much of the work in this field (some of it controversial) was originally carried out by Kohlberg. He elaborated six stages of "moral reasoning" (Kohlberg, 1963) that corresponded with the stages of cognitive development depicted by Piaget and his coworkers.

During the earliest stage, moral choices are made to avoid punishment, to acknowledge power, and to "stay out of trouble." At a second stage, doing the right thing entails doing what basically satisfies personal needs and desires, although there may also be some elements of reciprocity and fair play. The latter tend to be pragmatic (i.e., "If you help me, I'll help you"). With the third stage of moral development, the child tries to be a "good" boy or girl, striving to make choices that will conform to what the majority of people want. An action becomes acceptable if it is well intended. In the fourth stage, there is said to be a "law and order" fixation. The child develops a rather inflexible attitude toward authority, laws, and the stabilization of society. The child does her duty; motives become irrelevant. At stage five, she begins to base her actions on her conscience. Correct acts are defined in terms of general individual rights and criteria agreed upon by everyone in society. Also, at this stage, values become somewhat more relative—the law can be changed if it violates principles. Circumstances sometimes justify breaking the law. In the sixth stage, actions are based on personal ethical principles that have been arrived at over time. These are based on universal notions of justice, fair play, equality, and respect. Although as children progress through the various stages of moral development they may not necessarily agree on their moral decision making, there is a tendency for them to base their choices on thought processes or standards appropriate for their stage of development.

Another developmental acquisition concerns the growth of a sense of humor. One can learn a great deal by studying the ways in which children joke and interpret the humor of others, and much research has been done in this area (Wolfenstein, 1954). Cultural, cognitive, and affective issues have an impact on this particular acquisition. Certain characteristic patterns are evident. For example, during the early elementary years, children are said to be interested in issues of competence, becoming particularly fascinated with riddles and games concerning "morons." They are attracted to stories about people who do something "dumb."

In early elementary school, children are able to memorize jokes for the first time. They are preoccupied with "getting them right." As they progress toward late elementary school, they are able to appreciate increasingly subtle humor. In particular, the element of irony becomes accessible. Children can use humor to work through painful issues, as joke telling becomes another medium of experimentation and exploration. Troublesome themes may be incorporated in joking in a relatively nonthreatening manner as a way of demystifying them for the child. This is seen particularly in the older elementary school youngster's preoccupation with "dirty jokes," which may be employed as a means of discovery. It is not unusual, for example, for a 10-year-old youngster to tell such jokes without really understanding them. Audience reaction can be used as a form of education and confirmation. Joke telling and humor responsiveness can aid in a number of school-aged missions. Their social applications, their usefulness for acquiring knowledge, and their deployment as strategies to save face and overcome frustration may be invaluable, especially to youngsters adept in their use.

A closely related developmental acquisition concerns the increasing sophistication and application of play (Erikson, 1977). Children can use their play for a variety of purposes. Playing can help with coping. According to Erikson, "The child's play is the infantile form of the human ability to deal with experience by creating model situations and to master reality by experiment and planning." Play obviously has other purposes. It can help a child to build skills—in the motor area, in visual-spatial orientation, in rule compliance, and in language. Play can be used as a medium to explore consequences of actions. Imaginary play affords an opportunity to alter outcomes and plots and is also a way of testing fate without experiencing true pain or risk.

School-aged children ultimately lose their inclination or option to participate in imaginary games. As they progress in elementary school, such activities are perceived as "babyish." More time is spent in competitive recreation and in activities that enhance skill, focus interest, and build knowledge. To some extent, this progression is culturally determined. Some youngsters may not wish to give up imaginary play but are forced to do so because this activity is perceived as inappropriate after a certain age.

During school years another developmental acquisition involves changing notions about gender identity. This too is highly conditioned by culture and by the expectations of peers and adults. As a result, there can be considerable variation in its evolution. This vital component of development in the school child is covered in Chapter 9.

Finally, many school-aged children are acquiring individuality, a unique sense of personal identity. Often this process of individuation is facilitated through the pursuit of personal affinities. The latter are strong areas of interest (perhaps even passion) that the child discovers and pursues over time. These domains of personal preference and the quest for expertise within them can do much to sustain the self-esteem and overall motivation of a growing child.

The various developmental acquisitions and the approximate time course of their appearances are summarized in Table 5–1.

The Health Care Professional and the School-Aged Child

Health care professionals, like other adults who play a role in the lives of school-aged children, can have a profound influence on the outcomes of the various missions of this period. The next two sections explore some issues and procedures relevant to what might be termed the "developmental-behavioral health maintenance" of the school-aged child.

ON ORCHESTRATING A VISIT

When there is sufficient time, a health visit for a school-aged child can be rewarding. A well-child examination or

Table 5–1 • Developmental Acquisitions During Middle Childhood

Area of Developmental Acquisition	Age (years)		
	5 to 7	*8 to 10*	*11 to 13*
Attention, persistence, and goal directedness	Steady improvement in processing controls, especially saliency determination and satisfaction control; also heightened ability to allocate, sustain mental energy		Marked enhancement of production controls, reflective behaviors
Orientation and perception	Growth in body awareness, left-right, basic sequences	Handling of greater spatial detail and complexity, including three-dimensionality; mastery of complex sequential verbal and nonverbal inputs	
Storage and retrieval	Gains in paired associative learning	Increasing ease of storage and retrieval in long-term memory; growing capacity and use of active working memory; progressive automatization of skills and knowledge	
Interpretation and generalization	Concrete thinking; growing phonology and word learning	Conservation; complex sentence comprehension growth	Formal operations, greater understanding of symbolic, abstract language
Expression and production	Steady progression toward greater verbal fluency, gross motor, fine motor, and graphomotor proficiency; steady improvement in the allocation and maintenance of goal-directed mental effort		
Social reception and interaction	Egocentricity; home-based values	Friends as collaborators; rapid growth in social cognition	Heavy dependence on friendships; increasing influence by peer group
Resiliency and strategy formation	Steady growth in coping skills, in the mastery of strategic approaches to problem solving, growing ability to recover from stress, frustration, and setbacks		
Other acquisitions	Progressive trends toward increasingly sophisticated moral reasoning, play dominated by rules and the need for skills acquisition, the cultivation and deepening of affinities, and greater sophistication of humor		

a specific consultation can become an important event in his or her development. Parents can also find such an encounter informative, reassuring, and influential. The flow of events during a visit can facilitate the process.

Whenever possible (and at least occasionally), both parents should accompany the child. Each child should come for a separate visit (i.e., without siblings), because this approach communicates a highly individualized focused interest in that child as a person.

Often it is helpful for the physician to begin a visit alone with one or both parents. Several key questions can be framed to elicit issues regarding the developmental missions of this age group. Open-ended questions can be asked. Relevant domestic stress, or other environmental factors, or recent critical events in the life of the family should be sought. Usually the parent's feelings about the child and about the job they are doing can be inferred from the comments. By spending time alone with parents, one is in a better position to evoke concerns or "hidden agendas" that may not emerge when the youngster is present.

If they are seeing the physician for a specific complaint, some important matters can be explored: Why are they coming in now? What are their real concerns? What is it they are most worried about? Are there any "skeletons in the closet"? A child may be brought to the pediatrician because he or she seems to be "hyperactive." The physician may wonder why they are coming in now—at the age of 9—when the child has had problems like this all along. With some inquiry, it may turn out that a neighbor's child, now a teenager, had a similar problem and was recently indicted for car theft and possession of drugs. The association between that child and their own may haunt the parents. It is important for the pediatrician to be aware of this real but perhaps concealed concern.

The physician can also use this time alone with the parents to get a sense of how they perceive the visit, what they expect the outcome to be, and what they think they need. To pursue the previous example, parents who bring in a child who is thought to be "hyperactive" may expect that some blood tests will be done and that their child will be given a special diet. In other instances, they may want a referral to a mental health professional, some assistance in formulating an individualized educational plan at school, or advice on day-to-day management. Some parents want and expect an electroencephalogram, while others just crave support and a trusting relationship with the physician. Still others approach the physician to gather influence as they request services in school. Identifying these expectations can be very helpful for the physician.

After meeting with parents, the physician should spend time alone with the child. Pediatricians accustomed to dealing with preschoolers and infants may not feel inclined to be alone with children. On the other hand, this is an important part of the developmental health maintenance of the school-aged child. The physician needs to construct a positive "one-to-one," trusting relationship with the child, whether the visit is for a specific problem or for an annual physical examination. Time spent talking with the youngster and forming an alliance can be profitable (see the next section).

For any child over age 6, the child and parents should be given the option of a physical examination without parents in the room. Many school-aged children never get undressed in front of their parents. They are likely to be more self-conscious before a mother or father than they are to be barely clothed before their physician. Often they are more embarrassed about being embarrassed than they are embarrassed.

The physical examination can be a rich source of information and an excellent medium for education and counseling. The physician should carry on a dialogue during the physical assessment, reassuring the youngster about any somatic concerns. Sometimes the physician may need to be aggressive in eliciting these. For example, if a child is obese, one may want to comment on this and state that many children who are overweight are concerned about their appearance. When eliciting potential somatic concerns, it is important for the physician to universalize or generalize the problem, pointing out that many other youngsters face the same anxieties, since children of this age group seem to fear that their problems are unique. The obese 11-year-old boy may be self-conscious because he believes that his genitalia are too small. In reality, they are embedded in a prepubic fat pad. It might be important to reveal this to the youngster, while stating that many overweight boys harbor this concern but that they are all very normal. Frequently a youngster is too embarrassed or threatened by such a problem to bring it up himself, so that the physician may need to take the initiative. When dealing with potentially humiliating somatic issues, the physician must, of course, promise the youngster complete confidentiality.

After some discussion and a physical examination, the physician should reconvene the entire group—parents and child. It would be inappropriate to see the parents alone at this time. If the physician closes the door and excludes a child following a physical examination, it is likely that the youngster will fantasize about this. "What is he telling them? Does he think I'm a 'mental case'? Did he find out that I have cancer? How come he has to tell them alone after he promised he would not tell them anything I said?" Meeting alone with the parents following a physical examination could thus be perceived as a betrayal and may disrupt the physician-child alliance. Instead, it is appropriate for all to meet together. If for some reason the physician needs to speak to the parents alone, this should be done by telephone or on a subsequent visit. In an atmosphere of openness, the physician can share his or her feelings, offer guidance, and jointly plan for the future. The child can also use this forum to reassure himself that the physician has not failed to honor the pledge of confidentiality. Forging this kind of relationship among the physician, the patient, and the family during middle childhood can be extremely important later during the adolescent years.

COLLABORATING WITH PARENTS

The pediatric role in counseling, advice-giving, anticipatory guidance, and parent education is a familiar one (see Chapter 76). Traditionally, these activities tend to be better informed and more vigorous with regard to younger children rather than to those of school age. Some pediatricians may feel more comfortable counseling parents about an infant feeding problem than they do advising about how to manage a rivalry between 10- and 12-year-old siblings. Notwithstanding, the demand for advice on school-aged issues is intense and may often remain unfulfilled (Shonkoff et al, 1979; Levine, 1982). Certain aspects of developmental education and management are particularly relevant and therefore form the core of pediatric developmental health maintenance.

Elucidating the Missions and Attainments. It is difficult to separate the responsibilities of the health care professional from those of a health and developmental educator. The physician plays an important role in acquainting parents with the missions and developmental events of this age group, particularly when parents do not seem to understand some of the struggles of their own children.

Asking the Age-Relevant Questions. In providing primary care for school-aged children, it is helpful to inquire about the most relevant areas of function. Certain performance arenas become particularly germane. One wants to gain a sense of how the child is functioning at home, in the neighborhood, and at school. Specific inquiries may yield information about the success or failure of the child's developmental missions.

Anticipating Next Steps. A physician can be helpful by sensitizing parents to the "coming attractions" of development. Simultaneously, one can assess and encourage preparedness. For example, the physician might mention to a parent that the youngster is reaching an age of increasing sexual awareness and may inquire about anticipated methods of sex education. An older school-aged child may be showing early signs of experimenting with autonomy, and parents may need to be clued in about the need to develop ways of handling the child's intensifying yearning for independence. Anticipatory guidance can be offered regarding a wide range of normal events, such as entering school, going away to summer camp, dealing with peer abuse, socializing with the opposite sex, and developing good study habits.

Collaborating to Induce Mastery. The physician can help parents induce success in their children. An important question to ask about school-aged children during a well-child visit concerns their level of success: "When was the last time he had a real triumph?" or "What are the activities or endeavors that bring her consistent rewards and praise?" In this age group, success deprivation, a feeling of not being masterful at anything, is devastating. True success (in one or more areas) is like a developmental vitamin; without it serious complications are likely to set in. The physician can help parents to recognize the importance of helping a child taste success.

Praising, Idolizing, and Criticizing. Parents may need to be helped to achieve a good balance between praise and criticism, between boasting and condemnation, between adulation and approbation. Sometimes it is helpful for a physician to suggest that a child's parent keep some sort of mental ledger to sustain these balances. If one is spending too much time criticizing and nit-picking, a conscious effort may be called for to provide positive reinforcement for the youngster. Parents may need to "catch him doing something right."

Differentiating Between Extreme Normality and Deviance. The health care professional can be an important source of information with regard to the appropriateness of various problems and occurrences in the lives of school-aged children. It is common for parents to want to know what is normal. One set of parents may report that their 10-year-old son has stolen money from them. Another may lament that their 9-year-old seems to lie around too much, or that a 12-year-old daughter is too concerned about her appearance. Still another may have discovered their 12-year-old masturbating. Some may fret because their daughter came home intoxicated or stayed out too late and may have taken drugs.

During middle childhood, parents may be haunted by fears of the kind of adolescent their youngster will become. The parents of a 6-year-old may call their physician and anxiously relate the fact that they caught their son or daughter undressed and playing doctor with the little girl or boy next door. There may be an underlying concern that he or she is becoming a "sex fiend" or is somehow making an abnormal psychosexual adjustment. Even greater panic may ensue when such activities transpire between children of the same sex. The physician will find himself in the position of having to look at the whole child. Is the reported event or concern an isolated finding in an otherwise well-adjusted child? Is it extreme or chronic or recurrent? Or is this a single or "experimental" event? What are the parents' concerns? What are their worst fantasies about this problem? How realistic are they?

Sometimes parental reaction to perceived abnormal behavior can be most damaging to a child. The physician can help temper parents' responses, while remaining vigilant for early signs of seriously troubled behavior. Reassurance can be helpful, although there also is some danger in overreliance on the old adage, "He'll outgrow it." Physicians have a natural sense of normal variation in behavior and development. The primary care doctor sees a vast number of normal children. It can be redemptive for parents to learn that a particular struggle they perceive as unique is also occurring in many other families.

Helping to Prioritize. Sometimes parents overwhelm their children, expecting too much too soon. They may be trying to superimpose rigid adult values on the often fluid and amorphous configurations of the school-aged child's life. In such cases, the physician can help parents prioritize and decide what is really important. An older elementary school child, for example, may be heavily preoccupied with outside interests (such as sports, dance, or music). Life is further encumbered with academic concerns, coercive social pressures from peers, and anxieties about incipient puberty. If, amid all this disquietude, the youngster must come home each day to parents who "hassle" over the cleanliness of a bedroom, dirt under fingernails, a C minus on the last report card, coming home late last Saturday night, and the low caliber of chosen friends, life can become increasingly confused and frustrating.

Parents may have to recognize that they cannot have everything their way. They must determine what is most important to them. This may necessitate ignoring dirt lodged under fingernails or allowing a child to continue to live in the substandard conditions of a condemned bedroom. They may need help to decide that developing better study habits and coming home on time at night are the most important things to them, and that they will overlook more trivial infractions. The physician can play an important role by encouraging parents to think through their priorities rather than insisting on perfection or compliance in all areas.

Helping to Cope. Sometimes parents primarily need advice about how to handle their own reactions rather than the actions of the child. They themselves need to evolve a coping style, a way of managing the frustration of cohabiting with a school-aged child (or children). They need to program a time for themselves. They may seek advice about how to channel their own anger, despair, frustration, or disagreements about child rearing. It may have been easier for them to raise infants than school-aged children, and the physician may need to assist parents to identify and perhaps modify their own coping strategies when they are very angry at their youngster, when they feel like hurting him, or when things seem out of control. There may be a need to rework these strategies and to support parents.

Listening and Reinforcing. The physician can be a trusted and valuable "sounding board." At times it is appropriate merely to lend an ear, since parents may need to talk about their children and the way they manage them. At other times, they may want to boast about a child or about the success of their own rearing techniques. The physician can do a great deal to offer parents positive reinforcement. By listening and supporting, the health care professional can also alleviate guilt and anxiety. Whenever possible, the physician should help parents feel good about themselves and the job they are doing to develop confidence in their own values, judgments, and practices. Parenting can become increasingly effective to the extent that it is so perceived by competent and confident parents. The physician should always seek, find, and point out to the caretakers areas in which they have shown good practice and judgment.

Managing Crises. All families have their quota of crises and critical life events. A trusted physician, one who has established a good alliance with parents and their children, can be an invaluable ally during critical times of decision making. A parent may approach a physician for advice about how to handle the child when there is an impending separation or divorce, how to present a terminal illness or death, or how to prepare a youngster for hospitalization or surgery. Through experience, training, and reading appropriate material, health care professionals can become skilled at educating parents about the proper management of commonly occurring life crises in the school-aged child. In particular, with this age group, mothers and fathers may need help in learning to be honest and open, to find the right words, to share family problems with children, and to balance their candor with warmth and reassurance. They may need help in recognizing that it is difficult and potentially dangerous to deceive, conceal, or deny problems with youngsters of this age group. School children have extraordinary insights of their own and can actually help parents meet a crisis or solve a problem in some cases.

Acknowledging and Accepting Individuality. Parents must sometimes be reminded that no two children are alike. It is important that they define the unique attributes and needs of their individual progeny and perceive a separate profile of strengths and weaknesses for each. They may need help in allowing a child to expand his or her assets, to express a unique style, to engage in or to avoid activities according to unique inclinations. There is potential for conflict between a parent's expectations and a child's individuality. A parent may be determined to have a child become an outstanding athlete, although that youngster's gross motor abilities are limited and he displays potential for musical or artistic talent. A young girl may be inclined toward computers rather than ballet lessons. The physician can help parents celebrate the individuality of the child and pursue rearing strategies consistent with this. Parents can be encouraged not to force square pegs into round holes. At times, they need to be encouraged not to try too hard to mold offspring after their own images or to model them after some immutable preconceived ideals.

COLLABORATING WITH THE SCHOOL-AGED CHILD

As noted earlier in this section, the physician has a unique opportunity to form a strong supportive alliance with a school-aged child. To some extent this depends on establishing the routine practice of spending time alone with children in this age group. Whether a youngster is being seen in consultation for a specific problem or being followed for routine medical care, a one-to-one interaction can be highly gratifying and informative for the child.

Privacy and Confidentiality. The child in the early elementary school grades may find it relatively easy to relate to an adult authority figure such as a physician. The youngster may anticipate visits eagerly and enjoy sharing experiences and thoughts with the clinician. As children progress through the elementary school years, they may become more wary and, at times, even suspicious of the doctor-patient relationship. They may come to view the visit to a physician as an intrusion on their privacy. The doctor may be perceived as an agent for the parents rather than a confidant and ally of the child. For this reason, it is especially important to reassure an older school-aged child regarding confidentiality. Sometimes it is even appropriate to state initially in front of the parents that everyone should understand that the child and the doctor may want to keep a few secrets about very personal things. The youngster may seek periodic reassurance regarding this. The physician can say something like "I want to keep you as my patient and have you trust me. If I tell anyone else what you have said to me, I'm afraid you won't want to come back here anymore. I'm going to be very careful not to let that happen."

To what extent should a physician invade a child's traditionally private life? Should one ask personal questions? Or, alternatively, should inquiries be open-ended (such as, "Are there any matters I can help you with?")? The physician should individualize her or his approach to these issues. Certain youngsters who appear to be harboring problems or about whom there are concerns may benefit from a more "invasive" approach. Direct questions should be asked in an effort to uncover underlying concerns, particularly if there are problems within the family, if the child is in difficulty at home or in school, of if one has the clinical impression that the youngster is anxious about his health, development, or other matters. By spending some time alone with the parents prior to seeing the youngster, one sometimes may use parents' perceptions to formulate leading questions to ask the child. In "invading" various private domains of a school-aged child, care must be taken in the manner in which questions are asked.

How to Ask. Visiting a physician includes many constraints, not the least of which are limitations of time. This may necessitate a direct approach, without an opportunity to "break the ice." Nevertheless, every attempt should be made to avoid embarrassing the youngster or making him or her feel too different or "singled out." As suggested earlier, one way to avoid pitfalls is to state questions in such a way that they highlight the universality of issues. For example, if one suspects that a child may be concerned about not growing fast enough, one might initiate the discussion in the following manner: "So many kids who come in here at your age seem to have questions about the way they're growing. Some of them think they're growing too fast, and others are worried that they're not growing fast enough! There are so many different normal ways to grow at your age that almost everyone wonders if he is okay or not. Do you ever have any thoughts about this?" By generalizing issues to all children in that age group, some of the possible pathologic implications are removed, making it easier for the child to express concerns that might not otherwise be discussed with any adults.

Sometimes a physician may not suspect that a child has any problems at all. Open-ended questions could therefore conceivably uncover unsuspected anxieties. First, the physician should obtain a sense of how the usual developmental missions are progressing for the child. Questions can be framed in a nonthreatening manner to pursue areas of socialization, academic success, self-esteem, family life, and so on. Concrete questions are more likely to yield results. For example, if one wants to derive a sense of how a child is doing with peers, one may want to depict a particular scenario: For most school-aged children, critical sites of social interaction include the bus stop, the bus, the corridors at school, the gymnasium, the cafeteria, and the playground. One might ask specifically about one or more of these. "How are things on the playground at your school? Is there a lot of fighting and arguing? Do kids ever call each other names? What do you usually do on the playground? Are there certain kids you spend most of your time with? Have you ever gotten called any names on the playground?"

In this way one progresses from a general discussion of the anthropology of a playground to a more specific inquiry about the youngster's own status therein. The physician can use certain common occurrences as a way of signaling to the child that she understands what things are really like. By choosing questions appropriately, the physician can demonstrate to the child that she sympathizes with him and takes seriously the issues that are confronted in daily life. Some youngsters may be reluctant to mention concerns they have because they feel that these are not viewed as legitimate by the adult world. The following are examples of some good "lead-ins":

"I bet your sister really makes you mad sometimes."

"A lot of kids think that their parents hassle them too much. Have you ever had this problem?"

"I bet there are some teachers at school that really make you mad. Do you find this sometimes?"

The physical examination, as noted earlier in this section, can be a good source of information about a child's body image. The physician can use this experience to elicit concerns or feelings about growth, about physical attractiveness, and about feelings and anxieties over somatic vulnerability of one sort or another.

Sometimes a physical examination can be a good way to facilitate dialogue with a school-aged child. During a direct interview, the youngster may indulge only in monosyllables and remain relatively unresponsive. However, after a physical examination, the child may "open up" and become more responsive. Somehow the laying on of the hands may help build rapport and trust. Therefore, in many cases it may be better to postpone discussion of how things are going until after the physical examination has been completed. In some cases, a youngster may be worried about the check-up and may feel much more relaxed once it has been completed.

How to Listen. Despite time constraints, the physician should become a listener. Many important insights are likely to come forth. School-aged children should feel comfortable using a physician as a confidant. The latter in turn may respond by taking concerns seriously and by revealing a sincere interest in the child's enterprises and accomplishments. Children should be encouraged to gather trophies, report cards, or artwork to show their doctor. The physician can become an influential and valued participant-observer in the development of a school-aged child. The youngster can look forward eagerly to periodic visits, in part to have a chance to boast and to harvest praise. Children with problems may feel more comfortable confiding in a physician who has also shared their triumphs.

A physician can also spend time watching and listening as the child interacts with parents. At the end of a visit, when all participants are called together for feedback or discussion, one may gather some notion of the quality of communication between the child and parents as well as the style of communication between the two parents, if both are present.

How to Advise and Educate. The school-aged child may solicit advice from a pediatrician. The physician should not minimize or try to render trivial the concerns that a youngster expresses and should try to achieve a balance between reassurance and overreaction. A sympathetic response is important, even when the child's anxieties really are unfounded. The physician must resist the temptation to moralize, preach, or devalue an articulated concern. Whenever possible, the child should be given an opportunity to suggest solutions of his or her own. When the physician wishes to offer advice, presenting several choices will make the child feel like more of a collaborator. It also conveys respect for the youngster by implying that he or she has the ability to make important decisions.

Availability and Accessibility. The physician should communicate to a school-aged child awareness of and interest in the various missions of the child's age group. Children might want the freedom to telephone the physician. They should have the sense that the doctor is available for advice and education. The child should know that, in a confidential and private way, the physician can serve as a source of normative feedback, since so many youngsters are concerned with whether they are normal. Parents, too, should feel comfortable asking for advice and presenting concerns about their school-aged child's development. They may seek help from the physician as a diagnostician, educator, advisor, and advocate. When well informed and conscientiously fulfilled, these roles can strengthen the formative developmental acquisitions of the school-age years. Along with parents, other family members, and other professionals in the community, the physician can co-conspire actively in the processes through which the missions pursued become missions accomplished.

REFERENCES

Brooks R: The Self Esteem Teacher. Circle Pines, MN, American Guidance Service, 1992.

Chomsky C: The Acquisition of Syntax in Children from Five to Ten. Cambridge, MA, MIT Press, 1969.

Cratty BJ: Perceptual and Motor Development in Infants and Children. Englewood Cliffs, NJ, Prentice-Hall, 1979.

Erikson EH: Toys and Reasons. New York, WW Norton, 1977.

Erikson EH: Identity and the Life Cycle. New York, International Universities Press, 1959.

Flavell JH, Ross L (eds): Social Cognitive Development. Cambridge, Cambridge University Press, 1981.

Freud S: New Introductory Lessons on Psychoanalysis. New York, WW Norton, 1965.

Gesell A, Ilg F: The Child from Five to Ten. New York, Harper and Brothers, 1946.

Kohlberg L: Development of children's orientation towards a moral order. I. Sequence in the development of moral thought. Vita Humana, 6:11, 1963.

Levine MD: The school child with school problems: an analysis of physician participation. Except Child 48:296, 1982.

Levine MD, Oberklaid F, Meltzer L: Developmental output failure—a study of low productivity in school aged children. Pediatrics 67:18, 1981.

Piaget J: Quantification, conservation, and nativism. Science 162:976, 1968.

Piaget J, Inhelder B: The Psychology of the Child. New York, Basic Books, 1968.

Ransdell S, Levy CM: Working memory constraints on writing quality and fluency. *In* Levy CM, Ransdell S (eds): The Science of Writing. Hillsdale, NJ, Lawrence Erlbaum, 1996.

Riesman D, Glazer N, Denney R: The Lonely Crowd. New Haven, Yale University Press, 1950.

Shonkoff J, Dworkin P, Leviton A, Levine MD: Primary care approaches to developmental disabilities. Pediatrics 64:506, 1979.

Smith EB, Goodman KS, Meredith R: Language and Thinking in the Elementary School. New York, Holt, Rinehart, and Winston, 1970, pp. 9–29.

Stipek K, MacIver D: Developmental change in children's assessment of intellectual competence. Child Dev 60:521, 1989.

Winner E, Rosenstiel A, Gardner H: The development of metaphorical understanding. Dev Psychol 12:289, 1976.

Wolfenstein M: Children's Humor. Glencoe, IL, Free Press, 1954.

6 Adolescent Development and Behavior: Implications for the Primary Care Physician

Carol A. Ford • William Lord Coleman

 Adolescent patients demand unique skills from their pediatricians and family physicians. Those caring for teenagers need to be sensitive to the rapid changes that occur at the junctions between their bodies and their minds. In this chapter, the authors provide the kinds of background information that can facilitate sensitive communication so desperately needed for the optimal health care and nurturing of the rapidly growing minds and bodies of those in this vulnerable age group.

Physician: "What's new?"

Adolescent patient: "Not much . . . just trying to figure out who I am."

Introduction

Adolescence, the unique developmental period between childhood and adulthood, is generally associated with the second decade of life and is characterized by tremendous biological, cognitive, psychosocial, and sexual change. All adolescents experience a variety of opportunities for health-promoting and health-risking behaviors as they traverse the pathway to adulthood and answer the question "Who am I?" Whereas most children reach adulthood with few difficulties, others engage in behaviors that can lead to significant health problems or outcomes that dramatically influence the trajectory their life will take.

To monitor adolescent behaviors that have an impact on mortality, morbidity, and social problems among youth and adults, the Centers for Disease Control and Prevention has developed the Youth Risk Behavior Surveillance System. This biennial survey of a nationally representative sample of high school students assesses behaviors that contribute to unintentional and intentional injuries, substance use, behaviors related to unintended pregnancy and sexually transmitted diseases (STDs), unhealthy dietary behaviors, and physical inactivity (Centers for Disease Control and Prevention, 1996). Substantial numbers of adolescents are at increased risk of motor vehicle crashes, other unintentional injuries, suicide, and homicide, which together account for 72% of all deaths among youth and young adults 5 to 24 years of age (Table 6–1). For example, on a monthly basis, 50% of high school students drink alcohol; 12% of female and 19% of male students drive a motor vehicle after drinking alcohol. On a yearly basis, 21% of female and 14% of male high school students make a suicide plan; 12% of female and 6% of male students report making at least one suicide attempt. One fifth of all high school students (8% of female and 31% of male) report carrying a gun, knife, or club at least once a month. Each year, 3% of female and 6% of male high school students experience an injury from a physical fight serious enough to require medical treatment (Centers for Disease Control and Prevention, 1996).

Most adolescents become sexually active during adolescence. By 12th grade, 66% of students report having a history of sexual intercourse, and 50% are sexually active (defined as having sexual intercourse within the preceding 3 months). Substantial numbers of sexually active adolescents report behaviors, such as having multiple sexual partners and inconsistent condom use, that place them at increased risk of acquiring sexually transmitted infections and experiencing unintended pregnancy. By high school graduation, 1 of 10 students has either been pregnant or fathered a pregnancy (Centers for Disease Control and Prevention, 1996).

Health care professionals are well positioned to assist children and their families through the adolescent years by promoting healthy adolescent development, helping adolescents choose behaviors that enhance rather than risk health, and addressing specific health needs (Millstein, Petersen, and Nightingale, 1993). Most adolescents visit a physician at least once a year, and among adolescents 10 to 18 years of age, 58% of all office visits are to primary care physicians (Ozer et al, 1997). Adolescents and their parents view physicians as credible sources of information and want clinicians to address issues unique to adolescent development (Fisher, 1992; Malus et al, 1987; Rawitscher, Saitz, and Friedman, 1995; Schuster et al, 1996). In contrast to most community and school-based health education programs, patient-physician conversations provide the opportunity for highly individualized counseling. For some adolescents, a physician visit may be the only opportunity to discuss sensitive health issues openly with a responsible, knowledgeable, trusted adult in a private and confidential setting.

Several organizations, including the American Medi-

Table 6–1 • Behaviors Reported by High School Students on the 1995 United States Youth Risk Behavior Surveillance Survey

Behavior	Female Students %	Male Students %	Total %
Rode with a driver who had been drinking ≥1 times within preceding 30 days	37.8 (±4.3)*	39.5 (±4.4)	38.8 (±3.9)
Drove after drinking alcohol ≥1 times within the preceding 30 days	11.9 (±3.7)	18.5 (±3.2)	15.4 (±3.2)
Carried a weapon (e.g., a gun, knife, or club) on ≥1 of preceding 30 days	8.3 (±1.4)	31.1 (±2.0)	20.0 (±1.3)
Injured in a physical fight seriously enough for medical treatment ≥1 times during past 12 months	2.5 (±0.9)	5.7 (±1.0)	4.2 (±0.6)
Made a suicide plan during past 12 months	21.3 (±1.7)	14.4 (±1.7)	17.7 (±1.5)
Attempted suicide ≥1 times during past 12 months	11.9 (±1.8)	5.6 (±1.1)	8.7 (±0.9)
Smoked cigarettes on ≥1 of the preceding 30 days	34.4 (±3.1)	35.4 (±2.4)	34.8 (±2.2)
Drank alcohol on ≥1 of the preceding 30 days	49.9 (±3.5)	53.2 (±2.6)	51.6 (±2.3)
Used marijuana ≥1 times during the preceding 30 days	22.0 (±2.8)	28.4 (±2.1)	25.3 (±2.0)
Ever used illegal steroids	2.4 (±0.6)	4.9 (±0.8)	3.7 (±0.6)
Ever sniffed glue, breathed the contents of aerosol spray cans, or inhaled any paint sprays to get high	18.4 (±2.5)	22.1 (±2.3)	20.3 (±2.1)
Ever had sexual intercourse	52.1 (±5.0)	54.0 (±4.6)	53.1 (±4.5)
Had four or more sex partners during lifetime	14.4 (±3.3)	20.9 (±2.6)	17.8 (±2.5)
Among sexually active students, used condom at last intercourse	48.6 (±4.8)	60.5 (±4.3)	54.4 (±3.4)
Ever been pregnant or fathered a pregnancy	8.0 (±2.0)	5.9 (±1.0)	6.9 (±1.2)

* Numbers in parentheses indicate 95% confidence interval.
Adapted from Centers for Disease Control and Prevention: CDC Surveillance Summaries, September 27, 1996. MMWR 45(No. SS-4), 1996.

cal Association, Maternal and Child Health Bureau, US Preventive Task Force, and the American Academy of Pediatrics, have published guidelines to help clinicians provide adolescent health care (American Academy of Pediatrics, 1997; Elster and Kuznets, 1994; Green, 1994; US Prevention Task Force, 1996). These guidelines encourage primary care clinicians to begin discussing adolescent development and behaviors associated with potential risks of negative health outcomes with all patients during late childhood or early adolescence. Physicians who are reluctant to discuss sensitive health topics with patients by early adolescence should be aware of information available about age of initiation of behaviors associated with potential negative health outcomes. High school students reported that before the age of 13 years, 25% smoked a whole cigarette, 8% tried marijuana, 32% drank alcohol (other than a few sips), and 9% experienced sexual intercourse (Centers for Disease Control and Prevention, 1996).

The American Medical Association (1996) has designed Guidelines for Adolescent Preventive Services (GAPS) specifically to help health professionals provide comprehensive screening and preventive services to adolescents between the ages of 11 and 21 years in primary care settings (Levenberg and Elster, 1995). As shown in Figure 6–1, these guidelines encourage yearly visits that include screening for abnormal eating patterns, change in or poor school performance, substance use (tobacco, alcohol, and other drug use), sexual activity, depression, and risk for suicide. GAPS also suggests yearly health guidance for adolescents regarding normal development, nutrition and exercise, injury prevention, sexual behaviors, and substance use. Anticipatory guidance for parents is recommended on a periodic basis.

Thus, the responsibility of all primary care physicians who see adolescent patients includes assessment of development, screening for behaviors associated with potential negative health outcomes, and provision of prevention and risk-reduction counseling. An understanding of normal adolescent development assists clinicians in preparing for these tasks.

Adolescent Development

CULTURAL CONTEXT

> When a girl has her first menstrual period the whole camp celebrates with the wild elima festival, in which the girl, and some of her chosen girl friends, are the center of all attention, living together in a special elima house. Male youths sit outside the elima house and wait for the girls to come out, usually in the afternoon, for the elima singing. They sing in antiphony, the girls leading, the boys responding. Boys come from neighboring territories all around, for this is a time of courtship (Turnbull, 1983).

An individual's experience of adolescence is dramatically shaped by cultural context (Friedman, 1989). As illustrated in the foregoing passage, biological maturation occurs within the context of socioculturally defined expectations. Young Mbuti pygmy girls experience menarche, or first menses, very differently from girls in the United States (Turnbull, 1983).

Even within the United States, an individual's experience of the transition from childhood to adulthood is influenced by a variety of environmental factors. For example, many adolescents are encouraged to extend education beyond high school in preference to early marriage and employment; others are implicitly or explicitly expected to finish schooling by 18 years of age. Variation in the economic status of youths' homes and communities have a profound influence on available opportunities. Shifts in family configuration, schools, and peer culture may all have an impact on children's negotiation of adolescence (Feldman and Elliott, 1990). Thus, it is important to assess

Age of adolescent

Procedure	Early				Middle			Late			
	11	12	13	14	15	16	17	18	19	20	21
Health guidance											
Parenting*		●———●				●———●					
Development	■	■	■	■	■	■	■	■	■	■	■
Diet & physical activity	■	■	■	■	■	■	■	■	■	■	■
Healthy lifestyles**	■	■	■	■	■	■	■	■	■	■	■
Injury prevention	■	■	■	■	■	■	■	■	■	■	■
Screening history											
Eating disorders	■	■	■	■	■	■	■	■	■	■	■
Sexual activity***	■	■	■	■	■	■	■	■	■	■	■
Alcohol & other drug use	■	■	■	■	■	■	■	■	■	■	■
Tobacco use	■	■	■	■	■	■	■	■	■	■	■
Abuse	■	■	■	■	■	■	■	■	■	■	■
School performance	■	■	■	■	■	■	■	■	■	■	■
Depression	■	■	■	■	■	■	■	■	■	■	■
Risk for suicide	■	■	■	■	■	■	■	■	■	■	■
Physical assessment											
Blood pressure	■	■	■	■	■	■	■	■	■	■	■
BMI	■	■	■	■	■	■	■	■	■	■	■
Comprehensive exam	———	●	———		———	●	———	———	●	———	
Tests											
Cholesterol	———	1			———	1		———	1		
TB	———	2			———	2		———	2		
GC, Chlamydia, Syphilis & HPV	———	3			———	3		———	3		
HIV	———	4			———	4		———	4		
Pap smear	———	5			———	5		———	5		
Immunizations											
MMR	■										
Td	■				———	○	———				
Hep B	■				———	6	———	———	6	———	
Hep A	———	7	———		———	7	———	———	7	———	
Varicella	———	8	———		———	8	———	———	8	———	

Figure 6–1. The American Medical Association's Guidelines for Adolescent Preventive Services (GAPS). (From American Medical Association: Guidelines for Adolescent Preventive Services, 3rd ed. Chicago, American Medical Association Department of Adolescent Health, 1996.)

1. *Screening test performed once if family history is positive for early cardiovascular disease or hyperlipidemia.*
2. *Screen if positive for exposure to active TB or lives/works in high-risk situation, eg, homeless shelter, health care facility.*
3. *Screen at least annually if sexually active.*
4. *Screen if high-risk for infection.*
5. *Screen annually if sexually active or if 18 years or older.*
6. *Vaccinate if high risk for hepatitis B infection.*
7. *Vaccinate if at risk for hepatitis A infection.*
8. *Vaccinate if no reliable history of chicken pox.*
* *A parent health guidance visit is recommended during early and middle adolescence.*
** *Includes counseling regarding sexual behavior and avoidance of tobacco, alcohol, and other drug use.*
*** *Includes history of unintended pregnancy and STD.*
○ *Do not give if administered in last five years.*

adolescent development and behaviors within the context of environmental and cultural factors.

BIOLOGICAL DEVELOPMENT

Whereas the term *adolescence* refers to the general developmental changes that occur between childhood and adulthood, the term *puberty* refers specifically to biological changes. Even though changes in the reproductive system are most associated with puberty, virtually all body tissues are affected. Skeletal growth during puberty accounts for nearly 25% of final adult height. Skull bones increase approximately 15% in thickness, the forehead becomes more prominent as the underlying brow ridges and sinuses develop, and the jaw grows forward. Predictable gender-specific changes in mean body fat and lean body mass occur. Lymphoid tissue decreases by approximately 50% between the ages of 12 and 20 years. The heart doubles in weight, but the heart rate, which has been decreasing during childhood, stabilizes. Systolic blood pressure increases in boys and plateaus in girls. Red blood cell mass, blood volume, and hematocrit increase in boys while remaining relatively constant in girls. Lung size increases, vital capac-

ity increases, and respiratory rates decrease. Although the brain and spinal cord have reached nearly final adult mass by early puberty, there is a slow evolution of electroencephalographic changes during puberty from predominately low-frequency waves to the alpha rhythm characteristic of adulthood (Slap, 1986; Tanner, 1978).

Dramatic changes in the reproductive system and the development of secondary sexual characteristics are unique characteristics of puberty. The sequence of changing events is similar, although not exactly the same, for most individuals. For girls, the onset of puberty begins between 8 and 13 years of age (Tanner, 1978), although recent evidence suggests that in the United States, pubertal changes are beginning at earlier ages, especially among African American girls (Herman-Giddens et al, 1997). The first sign of puberty is usually the appearance of breast buds (thelarche), characterized by elevation of the breast and papilla as a small mound with slight enlargement of the areolar area. Pubarche, the onset of the growth of pubic hair, is less often the first sign of puberty. Girls typically experience a height spurt during early puberty or midpuberty, which is followed by first menses (menarche) during midpuberty to late puberty. In the United States, the mean age of menarche among white girls is 12.9 years (SD = 1.2) and among African American girls is 12.2 years (SD = 1.21) (Herman-Giddens, 1997). Early menstrual cycles are often anovulatory and may be irregular until the reproductive system reaches full maturity (Tanner, 1978).

In boys, the normal range of onset of puberty is between 9.5 and 13.5 years of age, with the first sign usually being enlargement of the testes. Early pubertal events include the growth of pubic hair and coarsening and reddening of the scrotal skin. Midpubertal events include lengthening of the penis and occurrence of ejaculation (spermarche). The height spurt and facial hair growth occur relatively late in the sequence of pubertal events. There is a typical sequence of facial hair growth, with hair first developing on the upper lip, then on the upper cheeks and the midline below the lip, and finally on the cheeks and lower chin. Another relatively late pubertal event is lengthening of the vocal cords, which causes a lowering of the tone of the voice. Gynecomastia occurs in more than 60% of adolescent boys during early puberty to midpuberty; this resolves in 70% of boys within 1 year and in 90% of boys within 2 years (Slap, 1986; Tanner, 1978).

COGNITIVE DEVELOPMENT AND LEARNING

Cognition is the process of accumulating and organizing information about the world and using it to solve problems and modify behavior. Cognitive development involves the interplay of neuropsychological maturation, environmental stimulation, environmental responsiveness, and constant internal cognitive reorganization. Cognitive development accelerates rapidly as the adolescent enters middle school, finishes high school, and then continues on to college, vocational school, the military, or the job market.

The young adolescent enters the cognitive phase of formal operations, which continues to develop through middle and late adolescence (Inhelder and Piaget, 1968). This phase is characterized by cognitive flexibility, complex reasoning, and the forming and testing of hypotheses. The level of cognitive maturity proceeds from simple to complex, from concrete to abstract and symbolic, and from self-centered to other-centered; it affects the adolescent's understanding and perception of the world and how decisions are made. The adolescent begins to grasp political, moral, social, and philosophical concepts such as liberty, justice, democracy, totalitarianism, capitalism, free market, irony, and faith. Other cognitive abilities include the use of analogies, inductive and deductive reasoning, and higher-order cognition such as inferential thinking. To be effective, the adolescent must develop metacognition, which is the cognitive ability to think about thinking, the ability to critique the process of thinking and problem solving, and to analyze performance. An adolescent may use this skill to reflect on any particular function, for example, attention (meta-attention) or language (metalanguage). An athlete or dancer who uses mental imagery and videotapes to improve performance is using metacognition and metamotor techniques.

Furthermore, a variety of other higher-order functions develop in the adolescent: (1) memory skills (e.g., rapid, simultaneous retrieval, active working memory, and cumulative memory), (2) language skills (e.g., grasp of sophisticated semantics and syntax, and sustained and active listening), (3) analytical thinking (e.g., critical reasoning), (4) organizational skills (e.g., effective note-taking, efficient study skills, time management, and test preparation), and (5) increasingly sophisticated writing skills.

Learning is often restricted to the adolescent's areas of cognitive strengths or affinities or to professional or vocational interests. Learning is most productive in times of high motivation and low anxiety. Stress often inhibits the ability to plan, produce, predict, or think in futuristic terms. On the other hand, cognitive development is partially dependent on experiences, even stressful experiences. For example, an adolescent with chronic illness may be unusually knowledgeable and understanding about disease processes, physiology, impending death, and finality. For a more detailed description of cognition and learning, see Chapter 53.

PSYCHOSOCIAL DEVELOPMENT

Current theories of adolescent psychosocial development have historical roots in general theories of human development. G. Stanley Hall (1844–1924) was the first to advance a psychology specific to adolescence, although many others have developed theories of adolescence since (Muuss, 1988). Erikson (1963) conceptualized human psychosocial development as a process of successfully resolving a series of predictable developmental conflicts or "crises" that occur during eight stages within the life span; the fourth through sixth stages occur or have their onset during adolescence.

In Erikson's model, the fourth developmental stage, industry versus inferiority, begins when the child enters school. The task of this stage is to achieve a sense of industry and avoid the emergence of feelings of inferiority. During this stage, the child is learning to win recognition by producing things and achieving outside of the home. Learning occurs through experience and manipulation, not just explanation. Basic motor skills are mastered and applied to tasks that yield a sense of accomplishment, while the pleasure of becoming part of a productive situation gradually surpasses the pleasure of play. However, the individual needs adequate skills to join or contribute to the situation or group; without these prerequisites, the individual experiences a sense of inferiority and withdraws into the family and develops social isolation. Resolution by early adolescence is important so that teenagers feel competent and are able to meet the intensifying demands to be "industrious" while simultaneously facing the next crisis.

Erikson's fifth stage, the identity versus confusion stage, emerges in early and middle adolescence when childhood experiences have been consolidated and the teenager must establish a sense of personal identity. During this stage, adolescents experience the need for autonomy, individuation, privacy, and separation from family. Adolescents are increasingly influenced by social values and customs outside the family, and they become less dependent on their families. Relationships with peers help adolescents develop their roles and establish a clear identity. Adolescents may become preoccupied with social, religious, and political issues, often having idealized views. Selecting and "trying on" a variety of roles and occupations while wondering about others' perceptions and judgments is an important activity during this stage. The adolescent's developmental task is to answer questions such as "Who am I as a physical being?" and "Who am I as a vocational being?"

Sexual identity is an integral part of an adolescent's sense of self. Sexual development occurs within the context of biological maturation, cultural expectations, and psychosocial development. Gender identity and sexual orientation (heterosexual, homosexual, or bisexual) are consolidated during adolescence, and exploration, experimentation, and questioning are normal. Adolescents, to varying degrees, engage in sexual fantasies and sexual activity. The adolescent's developmental tasks include answering the question "Who am I as a sexual being?"

Erikson's sixth stage, the intimacy versus isolation stage, occurs in late adolescence. The older adolescent, with a newly established personal identity, wants to fuse this identity with another and develop a sense and state of intimacy. Empathy, an essential quality in forming meaningful relationships, develops. Adolescents experience the need and capacity to commit to a relationship, whether sexual, intellectual, or social. Close relationships with friends, fellow students, teachers, or other adult figures become very important and permit glimpses of the true self. Separation from the family is almost complete, but undercurrents of dependency may still exist and are especially evident in times of stress or self-doubt, which are often associated with unresolved issues and unmet goals. To fail in the tasks of this stage is to experience isolation. Such failure may be accompanied by wishes for the destruction of those who threaten the adolescent or the adolescent's relationships, or by prejudice against those who are different or threatening.

According to Erikson's theory, healthy adolescence is the culmination of the successful resolutions of the conflicts or crises described in these three stages and the consolidation of individual identity. The adequacy of resolving prior crises strongly influences the outcome of the next crisis. Persisting conflicts or unresolved crises interfere with further development and contribute to possible psychopathology (Erikson, 1963).

INDIVIDUAL VARIATION

The sequence of events that occur during biological, cognitive, and psychosocial development is much less variable than the age at which these events occur and the speed with which maturation occurs. Figure 6–2 shows six normal adolescents and illustrates the enormous variability in timing of biological development. All three boys are 14.75 years of age, and all three girls are 12.75 years of age. The boy and girl on the left are just experiencing the first signs of puberty, whereas the boy and girl on the right are in the late stages of biological maturation (Tanner, 1978). These differences are explained by the normal variation in the timing of onset of puberty and because some adolescents pass rapidly and some pass slowly through puberty. For example, the average length of time for completion of the biological events of puberty for girls is 4 years, with a range of 1.5 to 8 years; the mean duration of puberty for boys is 3 years, with a range of 2 to 5 years (Slap, 1986).

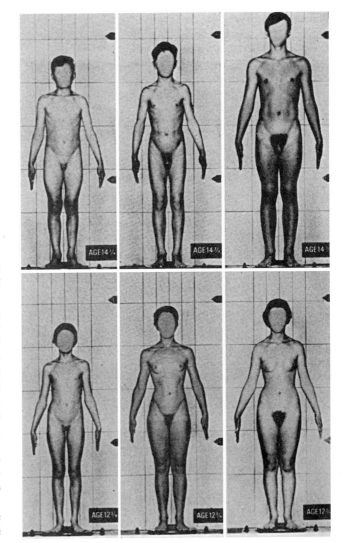

Figure 6–2. Normal variation in timing of pubertal development. (From Tanner J: Foetus into Man: Physical Growth from Conception to Maturity. Cambridge, MA, Harvard University Press, 1978.)

There is also wide variation in the cognitive transitions of adolescence. The sequence of cognitive development is characterized by the evolution from concrete-operational to formal-operational thinking (Inhelder, 1968), but not all adolescents begin this change at the same time, nor do they achieve it at the same rate or to the same level. The timing and pace vary within each individual and are not always predictable and smooth; for example, the cognitive processes of a 13-year-old child may develop rapidly for 2 years, then level off for a year, seemingly not to progress before they take off again to an even higher order of cognition. Similarly, psychosocial development varies greatly in its onset, timing, quality, and outcome. The process by which adolescents strive for a feeling of competence and productiveness, a sense of self-identity, and mature relationships varies enormously.

Importantly, maturation in one domain of development may not be synchronous with maturation in other domains. For example, level of biological maturity does not necessarily reflect level of cognitive maturity or psychosocial development. Adolescents who are physically mature are not necessarily abstract thinkers, and this needs to be taken into consideration when communicating with adolescent patients. In addition, asynchronicity of development may put adolescents at risk of behaviors with negative health outcomes. For example, adolescents who experience early biological maturation develop a mature physical appearance while in early adolescence; this may provide entry into older peer groups who are engaging in health-risking behaviors during a time when young adolescents may be less likely to have the cognitive and emotional maturity required to make responsible decisions about their behaviors in this situation (Crockett and Petersen, 1993).

Implications for Provision of Primary Adolescent Health Care

It is of fundamental importance that physicians consider developmental issues when providing primary health care to adolescent patients. The structure and dynamics of the patient-physician relationship undergo a tremendous transition between childhood and adulthood. With each patient, the clinician is faced with the challenge of assessing the level of maturation across multiple developmental realms, with wide variation possible within each developmental domain. In contrast to screening for potential health problems in younger children, screening for potential health problems in an adolescent population requires asking about sometimes exquisitely sensitive personal behaviors in a developmentally appropriate manner. Finally, all management strategies should take into consideration the individual patient's stage of development.

TRANSITION IN PATIENT-PHYSICIAN RELATIONSHIP

Structure of Clinical Visit

The structure of health care visits should change before or during early adolescence so that all adolescent patients spend at least part of each visit privately with their physicians (American Academy of Pediatrics, 1997; Elster and Kuznets, 1994). This routine change in procedure gives patients and their parents the message that physicians recognize adolescents' increasing desire for privacy and increasing independence from parents, and that adolescents may have issues that they are reluctant to discuss with their parents. Most parents support this arrangement when it is explained (1) as a routine strategy to teach adolescents to take increasing responsibility for their own health, (2) as a way for adolescents to develop a relationship with another responsible, caring, trusted adult who is available to help with problems that may develop during adolescence, and (3) that parents will be immediately notified of life-threatening problems.

Although the primary focus of visits should be the adolescent patient, the importance of involvement of parents should not be overlooked. Physicians should inquire about parental concerns and seek validation of information obtained from the adolescent patient when appropriate. In addition, physicians have an opportunity to offer parents guidance specific to their son's or daughter's developmental stage and behaviors (Steinberg and Levine, 1990). Common areas of concern include communication, conflict resolution, setting of appropriate limits, helping adolescents to resist peer pressure, and finding ways to be a responsive parent.

Patient-Physician Communication

There is transition in patient-physician communication as children become adolescents and then young adults. In contrast to the patient-physician communication of early childhood, when physicians spend most of their time communicating with patients' parents, during adolescence, physicians spend an increasing amount of time directly communicating with the patients themselves. Most adolescents appreciate the opportunity to talk to an adult who is a good listener, respectful, nonjudgmental, interested, and caring. Creating a supportive environment in which adolescents feel comfortable talking with a physician increases the chances of effective prevention and risk-reduction counseling. Special issues related to interviewing adolescent patients are described in Chapter 66.

Confidentiality and Informed Consent

Adolescent patients are sensitive to the issue of privacy in clinic settings. Even when adolescents have the opportunity to talk with physicians in a private setting, they may be concerned about the confidentiality of the information they disclose. Physicians who discuss confidentiality with adolescent patients increase the likelihood of open communication about sensitive health topics related to sexuality, substance use, and mental health issues (Ford et al, 1997).

Multiple legal and ethical issues influence physicians' abilities to assure adolescents of confidentiality (English, 1990; English et al, 1995; Hillard et al, 1997), and professional organizations have developed policy statements to guide physicians regarding this complex issue (Gans, 1993). In general, these policies recommend that physicians be aware of state laws regarding confidential health services for adolescents, support adolescents' access to confidential health services, and explain confidentiality policies (including the conditions requiring the limitations of confidentiality such as suspected physical or sexual abuse, suicidal or homicidal intent, and, in some states, injuries resulting from violence such as gunshot and stab wounds) to all adolescent patients and their parents.

ASSESSMENT OF ADOLESCENT DEVELOPMENT AND BEHAVIORS

A physician evaluating an adolescent patient during a routine comprehensive primary care visit is continually assessing development. A physician collects information to answer questions such as "Where is this patient in terms of biological, cognitive, and psychosocial development?" "Is this patient engaging in behaviors with the potential of negative health outcomes?" "Is this patient experiencing significant emotional difficulties?" and "What are this patient's strengths?" Observation of adolescent-parent interactions, questions asked by the patient and parent, information shared by the patient or parent, information collected during a comprehensive psychosocial history performed alone with the patient, and physical examination collectively provide the information needed to assess development within all realms. Furthermore, all adolescents should be directly asked about behaviors that have been associated with major causes of adolescent morbidity and mortality.

Several strategies have been developed to assist physicians organize a comprehensive adolescent developmental and behavioral assessment (American Academy of Pediatrics, 1997; Goldenring and Cohen, 1988; Green, 1994; Levenberg and Elster, 1995; US Prevention Task Force, 1996). Many physicians prefer performing all assessments during a face-to-face interview with the adolescent patient in a private and confidential setting, particularly when discussing sensitive information. One strategy to organize this assessment is based on the acronym HEADSS (Table 6–2) (Goldenring and Cohen, 1988). This acronym stands for *Home, Education/employment*, peer group *Activities, Drugs, Sexuality*, and *Suicide*. This organizational strategy guides the clinician from least to most sensitive topics and provides the opportunity for in-depth questioning when potential problem areas are identified. Physicians who are reluctant to initiate direct questioning regarding sensitive personal behaviors may first ask about the behaviors of peers. An adolescent patient's description of peer behaviors gives clinicians an impression of the types of decisions the patient is facing, an opportunity to hear what the patient thinks about peer behaviors, and an opportunity to ask about the patient's personal behaviors via a less direct route of inquiry.

An alternative method of collecting information to assess adolescent development and behavior is by use of questionnaires developed to screen for important psychosocial and behavioral issues in a time-efficient manner. The American Medical Association has recently developed patient and parent questionnaires as part of its implementation package for GAPS. Patients and parents complete questionnaires before seeing the clinician, providing a mechanism

for clinicians to quickly recognize topics that need further exploration during the actual interview (Levenberg and Elster, 1995). Examples of GAPS "trigger questions" are listed in Table 6–3 (American Medical Association, 1996). If questionnaires are used to obtain information, it is important to offer adolescent patients an additional opportunity to communicate directly with a physician in a private and confidential setting. This is particularly important when patients have completed the questionnaire in a nonprivate setting (particularly in the presence of a parent), changed responses, or left selected portions of the questionnaire blank. All information related to sexuality, substance use, and mental health (particularly suicide) should be reviewed with the teenager in a face-to-face confidential interview.

When a potential problem is identified by screening questions on a questionnaire or by direct communication, further information should be gathered to clarify whether there is a problem and, if so, the extent of the problem. Prioritization, with input from the patient and parent, determines which problems need to be further evaluated and managed acutely and which problems can be further assessed during a later visit.

MANAGEMENT ISSUES

Developmental Context

All management plans should take into account the individual patient's level of maturation to increase the chance of promoting healthy development and creating successful management plans (Table 6–4). For example, adolescence is a period of natural curiosity, and physicians are provided with a rich opportunity to convey information on an array of health-related topics. Concerns about physical development or attractiveness can provide impetus for discussion of puberty, exercise, nutrition, and sexuality. As adolescents develop increasing autonomy, choices about behaviors that influence health can be introduced within the context of personal choice and control. The physician's role in helping

Table 6–2 • The HEADSS Psychosocial Interview for Adolescents

Topic	Questions
Home	Who lives with patient? What are relationships like at home? Recent moves? Ever run away? New people in home environment?
Education/employment	Any change in school/grade performance? Favorite and worst subjects? Any years repeated/classes failed? Future goals? Any current or past employment? Number of schools in past 4 years?
Activities	What do you do for fun with peers? Where and when? What activities do you do with family? Sports or regular exercise? Church attendance, clubs, projects, hobbies? How much TV and favorite shows? Favorite music? Do you have a car? Wear seat belts? History of arrests or crime?
Drugs	Tobacco, alcohol, or drugs used by peers? By patient? By family members? Amounts, frequency, patterns of use, car use when intoxicated? Source? How paid for?
Sexuality	Orientation? Degree and types of sexual experiences and acts? Number of partners? Masturbation (normalize)? History of pregnancy/abortion (or partner pregnancy/abortion)? Sexually transmitted infections? Sexually transmitted disease knowledge and prevention? Contraception? Frequency of use? Condoms? Comfort with sexual activity, enjoyment/pleasure obtained? History of sexual/physical abuse?
Suicide	Sleep disorders? Appetite/eating behavior change? Feelings of "boredom," hopelessness, helplessness? Emotional outbursts and highly impulsive behavior? History of withdrawal, isolation? History of past suicide attempts, depression, counseling in patient? In family? In peers? History of drug, alcohol abuse, acting-out, crime? Recent change in school performance? Recurrent serious "accidents"? Suicidal ideation? Significant current or past losses? Preoccupation with death (clothing, music, media, art)?

Adapted from Goldenring J, Cohen E: Getting into adolescent heads. Contemp Pediatr 5:75–90, 1988.

Table 6–3 • Selected Items From American Medical Association Guidelines
for Adolescent Preventive Services (GAPS) Questionnaires

Topic	Question
Eating/weight	Are you satisfied with your eating habits?
School	Are your grades this year worse than your grades the year before?
Friends/family	Do you have at least one friend who you really like and feel you can talk to?
Weapons/violence	Have you been in a *physical fight* during the past 3 months?
Tobacco	Do you ever smoke cigarettes or use snuff or chew tobacco?
Alcohol	In the past month, did you get drunk or very high on beer, wine, wine coolers, or other alcohol?
Development	Do you have any concerns or questions about the size or shape of your body, or your physical appearance?
	Are you physically and emotionally attracted to people of your own sex?
	Have you ever had sexual intercourse?
	Do you and your partner *always* use condoms when you have sex?
Emotion	In general, are you happy with the way things are going for you these days?
	Ever *seriously* thought about killing yourself, made a plan to kill yourself, or actually tried to kill yourself?
Self	What do you like best about yourself?
	If you could, what would you change about your life or yourself?

Adapted from American Medical Association: Guidelines for Adolescent Preventive Services (GAPS) Initial Adolescent Preventive Services Visit Form. Chicago, American Medical Association Department of Adolescent Health, copyright 1996.

adolescents choose responsible and health-promoting behaviors includes ensuring that adolescents are well-informed about possible consequences of various behaviors, improving their decision-making skills by providing practice in considering alternative perspectives, enhancing self-confidence, and teaching peer resistance skills to reduce adolescents' susceptibility to antisocial peer influence. In addition, physicians can assist parents and adolescents to recognize ways to reduce opportunities for behaviors that have negative consequences (Crockett and Petersen, 1993).

It is particularly important to consider cognitive development when giving instructions and explanations to adolescents. In general, younger adolescents require more concrete approaches, whereas older adolescents may benefit from more abstract, symbolic approaches. However, all patients are less likely to exercise their capacity for abstract, formal reasoning when unfamiliar or sensitive topics are being addressed, which makes it important to be clear, explicit, and concrete when discussing issues such as substance use or sexuality (Crockett and Petersen, 1993). As-

Table 6–4 • Implications of Adolescent Development on Health Promotion

Domain	Implications for Health Promotion
Biological	Concerns about physical development can provide impetus for instruction regarding health-related topics (e.g., puberty, sexuality, nutrition).
	Pubertal development is associated with increased sexual motivation.
	Mature appearance may provide entry into older peer groups.
Cognitive	In general, younger adolescents require more concrete approaches, whereas older adolescents benefit from more abstract, symbolic approaches.
	Training in decision making can be effective; a key aspect for adolescents is learning to consider alternatives. Experiential components such as role playing may be helpful, especially for emotionally charged issues.
	Adolescents become better able to comprehend health risks, reflect on their behavior, and consider long-term consequences.
Self and identity	Opportunities to feel competent and successful support self-esteem and self-worth.
	Self-understanding is fostered when adolescents learn to express personal points of view while keeping an open mind to alternative perspectives.
	Adult mentors can promote identity development by providing guidance and support, serving as role models and challenging young people to consider new options and to do their best.
Autonomy	Adolescents should be given opportunities to exercise their autonomy while minimizing risks of negative consequences.
	Health should be introduced in the context of personal choice and control, something for which the adolescent has personal responsibility.
Family	Parents can be key players by setting standards for behavior, instilling values, and providing emotional support.
	Efforts toward strengthening parent-adolescent relationships and facilitating authoritative parenting are important.
	When good relationships with parents are not possible, links with other adults for support and mentoring are important.
Peers	Peer relationships are important. Loneliness and peer rejection should be targeted for intervention. Social skills training may improve adolescents' peer relationships.
	The potential contribution of peers to development of health-risking behaviors needs to be confronted. Increasing self-confidence and teaching social skills can decrease adolescents' susceptibility to peer pressure. Another strategy is to link adolescents to peers with prosocial values.
	Older peers can encourage health behaviors by serving as positive role models and promoting pro-health norms in peer groups.

Adapted from Crockett L, Petersen A: Adolescent development: health risks and opportunities for health promotion. *In* Millstein S, Petersen A, Nightingale E (eds): Promoting the Health of Adolescents: New Directions for the Twenty-First Century. New York, Oxford University Press, 1993, pp 13–37. Copyright © 1994 by Oxford University Press, Inc. Used by permission of Oxford University Press, Inc.

sessing whether adolescent patients have understood important messages is a practical way of checking to be sure that effective communication has occurred. For example, when instructing a patient on the use of oral contraceptive pills, the physician may ask "So if you start your period next Wednesday, when will you take the first pill?" and "What will you do if you have any questions or problems?"

General Management Strategies by Level of Risk

Upon completion of an assessment, physicians have an impression of the types of decisions that an adolescent is facing regarding initiation of a variety of behaviors and of behaviors that an adolescent patient is already engaging in that may have health-compromising consequences. It is useful to conceptualize an adolescent patient's "level of risk" of potential negative health outcomes when developing management strategies.

Low Risk

Many adolescent patients are "on track" in all developmental realms and at low risk of negative health outcomes from their behaviors. Management strategies for these patients include communicating the physician's assessment that things are going well developmentally, acknowledging awareness of the potential stresses of adolescence, positively reinforcing choices and behaviors that promote healthy development, and discussing common issues that are salient to patients at that developmental stage. Because intervention programs to influence adolescent behaviors may be most effective when adolescents are enrolled before initiation of behaviors associated with risk (Kirby et al, 1994), anticipatory guidance with low-risk patients is important. Adolescents may appreciate discussions of a range of topics, including counseling about issues such as "how to say 'no'" (Ford, 1996; Malus et al, 1987; Rawitscher, Saitz, and Friedman, 1995; Schuster et al, 1996). Finally, because adolescence can be a time of rapid changes, physicians should clearly convey the message that they are available to help with issues that may emerge in the future.

For example, a physician who determines that an adolescent has not used drugs and is not currently at risk of trying drugs may comment, "I think it's great you have decided to stay away from trying cigarettes, alcohol, or other drugs. That's a very intelligent and courageous choice. I'm really proud of you! I also want you to know that I understand how tempting it can be for teens to try them, and so I still plan to ask you this again on our next visit. If things change, I hope you'll trust me enough to talk about it. My only concern is your health." (Knight, 1997).

Moderate Risk

Along a continuum, patients who are at moderate risk include (1) adolescents who are engaging in behaviors with moderate risks of negative health outcomes but are otherwise generally on track developmentally and (2) those who are not yet engaging in potential health-compromising behaviors but are at increased risk of initiating these behav-

iors because of problems within one or more developmental domains (e.g., adolescents having school problems) or because of situational factors (e.g., family dysfunction or immediate peer group engaging in problem behaviors). General management strategies for these patients include clearly communicating that there are issues of concern; addressing health needs; providing individualized counseling; arranging further assessment of problem areas if indicated; identifying and engaging school, community, or mental health resources if appropriate; and arranging regular follow-up.

When adolescents are participating in behaviors that have the potential for negative health outcomes, it is particularly important that physicians not miss the opportunity to provide individualized risk-reduction counseling. This may be the only opportunity for some adolescent patients to discuss their particular situation with a responsible, trusted adult in a private and confidential setting. Counseling strategies should be appropriate to the adolescent patient's willingness to address worrisome behaviors. Initially, the physician should identify with the patient a clearly defined problem behavior (Hofmann, 1990; Knight, 1997). If a patient does not perceive the behavior as problematic, a useful strategy can be to provide pertinent facts to help the patient see connections between behaviors and negative outcomes (e.g., "I believe that your asthma is being negatively affected by your smoking of marijuana, and this may be one reason you're not playing basketball anymore") (Knight, 1997). If a patient agrees that the behavior is problematic but is not willing to change the behavior, a physician can try to increase the motivation to change. Useful strategies include acknowledging that ambivalence about changing behavior is normal and encouraging the patient to identify the pros and cons of continuing the behavior. For example, a physician who is attempting to motivate a patient to change his or her alcohol use may ask "What do you like about using alcohol?" followed by "Now tell me the down side of your alcohol use." Prompting the patient with suggestive questions such as "Do you think your decline in grades could be related to your alcohol use?" assists the patient in creating a complete list of pros and cons. The physician can then ask the patient to summarize the pros and cons of continuing a problematic behavior, while supporting the statements favoring change (Knight, 1997).

When patients are willing to change a problem behavior, a realistic and specific strategy must be developed with a concrete plan for implementation. For example, if a patient is choosing to abstain from alcohol use, it may be helpful to plan ways the patient can avoid situations in which alcohol is being used by peers or adults, to plan how the patient will refuse an alcoholic drink if it is offered, and to plan ways to obtain safe transportation if alcohol is consumed. Follow-up visits should include specific assessment of the success or failure of the implemented plan, with modifications as appropriate. If problem behaviors escalate or continue despite a series of office visits, referral is indicated.

High Risk

Patients who are at high risk include adolescents who are engaging in behaviors with significant risks of negative health outcomes (e.g., having frequent unprotected sexual intercourse; regularly driving while intoxicated) and adolescents engaging in multiple risky behaviors. Adolescents who are participating in behaviors associated with high risks of negative outcomes may be developmentally "off track," have significant underlying psychological issues (e.g., depression), have a history of past or present abuse, or be living in chaotic environments or dysfunctional home situations. If present, these underlying issues must be identified; successful management of underlying issues is usually associated with a clear reduction in problem behaviors.

General management strategies for adolescents at high risk of negative health outcomes from their behaviors include addressing the patient's acute health needs (e.g., provision of STD screening, condoms, and contraception if the adolescent engages in unprotected sexual intercourse); providing specific and thorough risk-reduction counseling; addressing existing underlying global issues, if present; and arranging frequent follow-up visits. Evaluation and management of patients in this category may involve mental health professionals, school professionals, and professionals associated with community resources.

Protective Factors

It is important to recognize personal and environmental factors that increase a patient's chance of successfully navigating adolescence. Many adolescents experience a smooth transition from childhood to adulthood despite considerable obstacles. Recent research shows that protective factors decrease the likelihood of adolescents' engaging in problem behaviors and play an important role in the developmental course of adolescent problem behavior (Compas, Hinden, and Gerhardt, 1995; Jessor et al, 1995; Resnick, Harris, and Blum, 1993; Resnick et al, 1997). Thus, an important component of any management plan is the identification of factors in the child, family, and community that may provide protection from unhealthy development and behaviors.

Physicians can assist patients and their families in identifying and nurturing adolescent patients' strengths. Nurturing strengths may involve improving a young person's competence in traditionally approved areas such as academics as well as improving competence outside of academics. This is especially important for less academically inclined students and may include nurturing strengths in areas such as the arts, athletics, hobbies, technical skills, or community service. Opportunities for adolescents to feel competent and successful promote the development of self-esteem, feelings of self-worth, and self-confidence. Adolescents who have self-confidence are more likely to resist peer pressure to engage in risky behaviors (Crockett and Petersen, 1993).

In addition to identifying an adolescent's strengths, it is helpful to identify protective factors related to family and community. Parents play a critical role in setting standards for behavior, instilling values, and providing emotional support. Physicians can encourage efforts toward strengthening parent-adolescent relationships and facilitating authoritative parenting styles. Links to other responsible, trusted adults for support and mentoring are also important, especially when good relationships with parents

are not possible (Crockett and Petersen, 1993). A sense of "family connectedness" is a powerful protective factor and is not necessarily dependent upon family composition. Family connectedness refers to an adolescent's sense of belonging and closeness to family, with the core being an adolescent's experience of being connected with at least one caring, competent adult in a loving, nurturing relationship (Resnick, Harris, and Blum, 1993; Resnick et al, 1997).

Adolescents who feel a positive orientation to school and who feel connected to school are less likely to engage in problem behaviors (Jessor et al, 1995; Resnick, Harris, and Blum, 1993; Resnick et al, 1997). This does not always correspond with high academic performance, which emphasizes the importance of schools in promoting a sense of belonging among students with all levels of academic proficiency. Physicians should encourage activities that increase patients' feelings of connectedness to school as a strategy to promote healthy development.

Conclusion

Adolescence is a period of dramatic biological, cognitive, psychosocial, and sexual development. Physicians have the opportunity to promote healthy adolescent development and encourage behaviors that enhance health. Physicians foster optimal development and healthy behavior by (1) maintaining a biopsychosocial perspective of the adolescent, (2) constructing a comprehensive profile of each aspect of the adolescent's development and behavior, (3) assessing relevant risk and protective factors, (4) addressing the adolescent's specific health care needs, and (5) providing appropriate prevention and risk-reduction counseling.

ACKNOWLEDGMENTS

The authors would like to express sincere appreciation to Margaret R. Morris, MD, for her helpful review of this manuscript.

REFERENCES

American Academy of Pediatrics: Guidelines for Health Supervision III. Elk Grove Village, IL, American Academy of Pediatrics, 1997.
American Medical Association: Guidelines for Adolescent Preventive Services (GAPS) Initial Adolescent Preventive Services Visit Form. Chicago, American Medical Association Department of Adolescent Health, 1996.
American Medical Association: Guidelines for Adolescent Preventive Services, 3rd ed. Chicago, American Medical Association Department of Adolescent Health, 1996.
Centers for Disease Control and Prevention: CDC Surveillance Summaries, September 27, 1996. MMWR 45(No. SS-4), 1996.
Compas B, Hinden B, Gerhardt C: Adolescent development: pathways and processes of risk and resilience. Annu Rev Psychol 46:265–293, 1995.
Crockett L, Petersen A: Adolescent development: health risks and opportunities for health promotion. *In* Millstein S, Petersen A, Nightingale E (eds): Promoting the Health of Adolescents: New Directions for the Twenty-First Century. New York, Oxford University Press, 1993, pp 13–37.
Elster A, Kuznets N: AMA Guidelines for Adolescent Preventive Services (GAPS): Recommendations and Rationale. Baltimore, Williams & Wilkins, 1994.
English A: Treating adolescents: legal and ethical considerations. *In* Farrow J (ed): The Medical Clinics of North America. Philadelphia, WB Saunders, 1990, pp 1097–1112.

English A, Matthews M, Extravour K, et al: State Minor Consent Statutes: A Summary. Cincinnati, OH, Center for Continuing Education in Adolescent Health, 1995.

Erikson E: Childhood and Society. New York, Norton Publishing, 1963.

Feldman S, Elliott G (eds): At the Threshold: The Developing Adolescent. Cambridge, MA, Harvard University Press, 1990.

Fisher M: Parents' views of adolescent health issues. Pediatrics 90:335–341, 1992.

Ford C, Millstein S, Eyre S, et al: Anticipatory guidance regarding sex: views of virginal female adolescents. J Adolesc Health 19:179–183, 1996.

Ford C, Millstein S, Halpern-Felsher B, et al: Influence of physician confidentiality and assurances on adolescents' willingness to disclose information and seek future health care: a randomized controlled trial. JAMA 278(12):1029–1034, 1997.

Friedman H: The health of adolescents: beliefs and behaviour. Soc Sci Med 29(3):309–315, 1989.

Gans J: Policy Compendium on Confidential Health Services for Adolescents. Chicago, American Medical Association, 1993.

Goldenring J, Cohen E: Getting into adolescent heads. Contemp Pediatr 5:75–90, 1988.

Green M: Bright Futures: Guidelines for Health Supervision of Infants, Children, and Adolescents. Arlington, VA, National Center for Education in Maternal and Child Health, 1994.

Herman-Giddens M, Slora E, Wasserman R, et al: Secondary sexual characteristics and menses in young girls seen in office practice: a study from the Pediatric Research in Office Settings Network. Pediatrics 99(4):505–512, 1997.

Hillard P, Coupey S, Goldfarb A, et al: Preserving confidentiality in adolescent gynecology. Contemp Pediatr 14(6):70–92, 1997.

Hofmann A: Clinical Assessment and Management of Health Risk Behaviors in Adolescents. Adolescent Medicine: State of the Art Reviews. Philadelphia, Hanley & Belfus, 1990, pp 33–44.

Inhelder B, Piaget J: The Growth of Logical Thinking from Childhood to Adolescence. New York, Basic Books, 1968.

Jessor R, Van Den Bos J, Vanderryn J, et al: Protective factors in adolescent problem behavior: moderator effects and developmental change. Developmental Psychology 31(6):923–933, 1995.

Kirby D, Short L, Collins J, et al: School-based programs to reduce sexual risk behaviors: a review of effectiveness. Public Health Rep 109(3):339–360, 1994.

Knight J: Adolescent substance use: screening, assessment, and intervention. Contemp Pediatr 14(4):45–72, 1997.

Levenberg P, Elster A: Guidelines for Adolescent Preventive Services (GAPS): Clinical Evaluation and Management Handbook. Chicago, American Medical Association, Department of Adolescent Health, 1995.

Malus M, LaChance P, Lamy L, et al: Priorities in adolescent health care: the teenager's viewpoint. J Fam Pract 25(2):159–162, 1987.

Millstein S, Petersen A, Nightingale E: Promoting the Health of Adolescents: New Directions for the Twenty-First Century. New York, Oxford University Press, 1993.

Muuss RE: Theories of Adolescence, 5th ed. New York, McGraw-Hill, Inc., 1988.

Ozer E, Brindis C, Millstein S, et al: America's Adolescents: Are They Healthy? San Francisco, University of California, National Adolescent Health Information Center, 1997.

Rawitscher L, Saitz R, Friedman L: Adolescents' preferences regarding human immunodeficiency virus (HIV)-related physician counseling and HIV testing. Pediatrics 96:52–58, 1995.

Resnick M, Harris L, Blum RW: The impact of caring and connectedness on adolescent health and well-being. J Paediatr Child Health 29(suppl 1):S3–S9, 1993.

Resnick M, Bearman P, Blum RW, et al: Protecting adolescents from harm: findings from the national longitudinal study on adolescent health. JAMA 278(10):823–832, 1997.

Schuster M, Bell R, Petersen L, et al: Communication between adolescents and physicians about sexual behavior and risk prevention. Arch Pediatr Adolesc Med 150:906–913, 1996.

Slap G: Normal physiological and psychosocial growth in the adolescent. J Adolesc Health Care 7(65):13S–23S, 1986.

Steinberg L, Levine A: You and Your Adolescent: A Parent's Guide for Ages 10–20, 1st ed. New York, Harper Collins, 1990.

Tanner J: Foetus into Man: Physical Growth from Conception to Maturity. Cambridge, MA, Harvard University Press, 1978.

Turnbull C: The Mbuti Pygmies: Change and Adaptation. New York, Holt, Rinehart & Winston, 1983.

US Prevention Task Force: Guide to Clinical Preventive Services, 2nd ed. Baltimore, Williams & Wilkins, 1996.

7 *Evolving Parenthood: A Developmental Perspective*

M. Patricia Boyle

 As Dr. Boyle eloquently demonstrates in this chapter, it is not only children who transport themselves across developmental destinations. Parents too develop. Parenthood becomes shaped by experiences with parenting. The challenges presented by an individual child may alter the parenting practices of a parent. It is the reciprocity of parent and child interactions that is a constant influence on both parties. This chapter depicts evolving parenthood in such a way that its implications for physicians are most plentiful.

Pediatrician-Family Relationship

As with most physicians in practice, the pediatrician's role and identity have evolved from that of the family doctor. Although major changes have inevitably occurred, certain critical components remain. Modern-day pediatricians do not deliver the babies for whom they give care, are rarely required to make house calls, and to an increasing degree must deal with the complexities of managed health care; yet these specialists, perhaps more than any other, still have an opportunity to develop and maintain a strong, meaningful, and rewarding relationship with a stable population of families. Moreover, many physicians find this opportunity for long-term commitment to be among the most compelling features of pediatric medicine.

Similarly, there is no greater potential for patient attachment than that experienced by parents toward the physician who cares for their children. Changing patterns of childrearing and geographic distance from extended family members are among the societal shifts that have heightened parental needs and diminished support. In response, some parental perspectives and expectations of the pediatrician's role have undergone further change. The impact of recent sociocultural effects and the pressure many parents feel to be well-informed about and responsive to the latest thoughts and theories proposed by pediatric professionals have contributed to making the pediatrician a most important childrearing adjunct, often perceived as a trusted family friend.

Pediatricians know that the demands of a contemporary practice are multidimensional. Along with the child's physical health and well-being, many other aspects of growth and development have properly become areas for their concern. As both the study and understanding of behavioral pediatrics have advanced, the value of a phenomenologic approach to the child within the family has been widely recognized. Pediatricians, together with other child health specialists, now focus more attention on the contextual factors of childrearing. There is a growing ap-

preciation for how rich this subject is when considered within the framework of a life-span perspective. Among the developmental theorists who argue this position, Hetherington and Baltes (1988) maintain, "There is no complete account of child development unless we understand its aftermath and contributions to later life."

Adult Development

Subscribing to a life cycle principle of adult development is of particular value to the pediatrician because it offers a theoretical paradigm for improving counseling skills and other interventional techniques. Perceiving parents as engaged in identifiable developmental issues of their own can increase the pediatrician's empathic response and lead to a stronger bond between physician and parent. It can also contribute to clarifying diagnoses and enlisting parental cooperation.

Over the years many theorists have promulgated the concept of an adult life cycle (Erikson, 1950; Levinson, 1978, 1996; Lidz, 1976; Vaillant, 1977). In his discussion of the "eight ages of man," Erikson posited a theory of development extending from birth to old age. In his book *The Seasons of a Man's Life,* Levinson (1978) elaborated specific stages in adult development, each of which occurs in an orderly progression and has its own developmental tasks. Like Erikson, Levinson proposes a lifelong sequence that is fixed yet interdependent. Problems or issues unresolved in earlier stages of childhood or adulthood can significantly hamper the resolution of an ongoing period.

Even though Levinson (1978) initially studied the lives of adult men, he concluded, at that time, that ". . . everyone lives through the same developmental periods in adulthood, just as in childhood, though people go through them in radically different ways." In his more recently published *The Seasons of a Woman's Life,* he confirms his earlier view: "There is, in short, a single human life cycle through which all lives evolve, with myriad variations related to gender, class, race, culture, historical epoch, specific circumstances and genetics" (Levinson, 1996).

Some elaboration of the concepts of adult development is essential to any consideration of parent-child relationships and the adult-parent role. A major finding of Levinson's evolution of life structure is that of an orderly sequence consisting of alternating stable "structure-building" periods and transitional "structure-changing" periods in the lives of adults. The meaning of these principles is provided by Levinson (1978):

> The developmental tasks are crucial to the evolution of the periods. The specific character of a period derives from the nature of its tasks. A period begins when its major tasks become predominant in a man's life. A period ends when its tasks lose their primacy and new tasks emerge to initiate a new period. The orderly progression of periods stems from the recurrent change in tasks. The most fundamental tasks of a stable period are to make firm choices, rebuild the life structure and enhance one's life within it. Those of a transitional period are to question and reappraise the existing structure, to search for new possibilities in self and world and to modify the present structure enough so that a new one is formed.

Parenting in a Changing Society

Because this chapter examines the changing and complex demands of the parenting role within the course of "normal" adulthood, it is critical to recognize that parents, who are subject to adult imperatives, are also faced with unavoidable developmental tasks throughout their lives. In becoming adults they must eventually leave the ordered safety of school and the sanctuary of home as they negotiate separation, achieve self-support, and enter into a stable, intimate relationship. In meeting the changing and complex demands of the parenting role, husbands and wives must strive to evolve as individuals in their own right and to secure a deep and lasting relationship with each other. Most adults encounter stressful life experiences that affect and can significantly alter all family members. Unemployment, physical or mental illness, accident, or sudden death can challenge family stability and cause serious developmental disruption from which it is difficult to recover.

In addition to these unpredictable and nonnormative events, family development is inevitably influenced by the changing sociohistoric context in which the family lives. There are increasing rates of maternal employment, participation in infant and child day care, separation and divorce, and teenaged and other single parenting, as well as extended life expectancy. Other societal shifts of concern include the abortion controversy, the rapid increase in substance abuse and rate of violent crimes, the threatening presence of acquired immunodeficiency syndrome, and the growing number of homeless families.

In view of such vulnerability, there is a far greater need within society to maintain some idealized view of its social patterns and structures as real and certain. In the same way that belief in idealistic goals and methods of parenting has evolved, people are inclined to assume the existence of a model family unit. However, the image of a nuclear family, composed of two natural parents living in the home with one or more children born of that union, is, of course, less and less reflective of society. An increasing number of children are being raised by single parents, many of whom are teenaged mothers, and an increasing number of children live in restructured families with siblings who were born to one of their parents in another marriage. With the increasing rate of divorce and remarriage, unconventional parenting styles seem to represent changing social patterns more realistically.

There are countless parental permutations, yet there is a commonality of basic parental issues that extends across the widest experiential gaps. Certain components of "conventional" childrearing continue to provide the most familiar and meaningful structure for organizing concepts about the interrelatedness of parenting and adult development. However, recognition of the inescapable and potentially debilitating impact of both nonnormative events and social historical change to which all families are subject cannot be overlooked. Individual and collective responses to disruption and disturbance are determined by many factors: (1) the style, philosophy, and emotional resource of each parent, (2) the level and stability of their individual adult development, and (3) the availability of adult support from within the marriage, from their respective families, from friends, and from appropriate professionals, among whom the pediatrician may be the key figure.

Transitions of Parenthood

The pediatrician may feel ill-prepared to counsel parents (and perhaps extended family members) in matters that are grave and seemingly insoluble. Having the ability to understand the myriad parental responses to ever-changing life events and how these responses can affect childrearing behavior is often of inestimable value. To achieve some sense of how useful such knowledge can be, Levinson's conception of adult development relative to becoming and being a parent is examined. The primary focus of attention is on how the transition to and transitions within ordinary parenthood are made, how the ease and success of transitions are facilitated, and, finally, in what ways being a parent contributes to the critical development of the adult. A summary of Levinson's adult stages with corresponding developmental tasks is presented in Table 7–1.

Any exploration of parental development within a life span perspective focuses on the initial phase of this critical life event. Goldberg (1988), in her description of how intricate this transitional process is, advised, "The transition to parenthood may be the most universally occurring adult developmental transition, with psychological, sociocultural, and biological components, all of which interact and influence one another." Adaptation to parenthood can create a state of disequilibrium in the new mother and father, both as individuals and in their relationship to each other. The following discussion focuses on the ongoing and ever-increasing complexity of the parenting process throughout the lives of the family.

This chapter explores the developmental odyssey of the child, from infancy through adolescence, and the parent-child relationships as they evolve during the parents' life stage transformations. Five childhood stages of development are elucidated: infancy, toddlerhood, preschool-age, school-age, and adolescence. Problem situations familiar to

Table 7–1 • Stages and Tasks of Adult Development
Relative to Becoming and Being a Parent

Early adult transition (17 to 22 years)	Begin moving out of preadult world. Make preliminary step into adult world.
Early adulthood (22 to 45 years)	
Entering the adult world (22 to 28 years)	Explore possibilities for adult living and keep options open. Create a stable structure for life.
Age 30 transition (28 to 33 years)	Work out flaws of first adult life structure. Create basis for more satisfactory structure.
Settling down stage (33 to 40 years)	Establish place in society. Acquire seniority, "becoming one's own [person]."
Midlife transition (40 to 45 years)	This is a time of questioning. Seek expressions for neglected parts of self.
Middle adulthood (45 to 60 years)	Great variability in satisfaction and well-being. Occurrence of at least moderate crisis followed, for many, by stable period.

Adapted from Levinson D: The Seasons of a Man's Life. New York, Alfred Knopf, 1978. Copyright 1978 by Daniel J. Levinson.

many pediatricians are presented, as are situations reflecting the dramatic impact of current social and political upheaval on children and their families.

TIMING OF THE FIRST PREGNANCY

There is general agreement among developmental theorists that it makes a great difference when, in the evolution of a developmental period, parenthood begins. According to Goldberg (1988), "Certainly, becoming a parent for the first time at age 20 is qualitatively different from becoming a parent at age 35." The timing of a first birth in the adult's life cycle critically affects not only the development of the marriage but also the evolution of the self. An optimal time, therefore, for a first pregnancy is toward the end of a successfully negotiated developmental period. Many couples attend seriously to the timing of the initial phase of establishing a family—the one irreversible step in the life of the individual that, perhaps more than any other, precipitates assumption of the adult role.

According to Erikson (1964), "Parenthood is, for most, the first, and for many, the prime generative encounter . . . ." In his essay "Human Strength and the Cycle of Generations," Erikson further states, "The love of young adulthood is, above all, a *chosen,* an *active* love . . . the problem is one of transferring the experience of being cared for in a parental setting, in which one happened to grow up, to a new, an adult affiliation which is actively chosen and cultivated as mutual concern" (Erikson, 1964). In his writing, Erikson (1950) advanced the concept of "generativity," which he defined as "concern in establishing and guiding the next generation," a concern of far greater complexity than biological reproduction alone because "the mere act of having, or even wanting children, however, does not 'achieve' generativity." Less well

known but of significant value are the works of LeMasters (1968) and Rossi (1974). One of the first to posit parenthood as a developmental crisis, LeMasters (1968) believed that parenthood and not marriage denotes the final transition to adult responsibility: "The arrival of the first child forces young married couples to take the last painful step into the adult world." Interested in the effect of parenthood on adults and on parental development, Rossi (1974) examined the social aspects of the transition to parenthood, focusing on the parent more than the child. She, too, believed that the first pregnancy, rather than marriage, is the major point of transition.

Although the timing of the first pregnancy is of great significance, the decision to have a baby is not always well considered. Some babies are conceived after much careful thought, some after very little thought, and an increasingly large number after no thought at all. The most carefully arranged pregnancies are those of the nonconventional older husbands and wives who have accorded priority to business or professional careers and postponed parenting until they are well into the later "settling-down period" (age 32 to 40 years), or even right after entering the "midlife transition" (age 40 to 45 years) described by Levinson. Many younger couples briefly defer having a first child while they resolve concerns related to housing, finance, or advanced educational goals. Other young married adults manifest a willingness or, perhaps, an ambivalence related to becoming parents by the degree of casualness or inefficiency with which they attend to contraception. Finally, there is a growing population of young and very young girls who, having become pregnant, decide to keep their babies with or without outside support from either the baby's father or their own family.

THE PEDIATRICIAN AS CONSULTANT

The need for anticipatory guidance for minor and more complex parenting situations is derived from a society in which heightened tensions and uncertainty occur within the context of a diminishing sense of community. Many couples, expecting their first child, seek out resources with which they are familiar as a means of acquiring a sense of support. After securing obstetric care and enrolling in a childbirth program, they often contact a pediatrician to arrange a prenatal visit. Many behavioral pediatricians and family practitioners appreciate this opportunity to become acquainted with prospective parents while they are free of the anxiety and confusion of the postpartum period. At this time, they can answer questions and allay fear. They may also recognize an early need for intervention and prepare the way for its implementation.

Prospective Parents

With careful interviewing, it is often possible to ascertain the individual level of maturity of each spouse, to identify vulnerability, and to begin to develop an alliance. The ages of the parents suggest at what point they might be in the developmental scheme of their lives. Expressing interest in early familial experiences can be of value, because it often uncovers myths and legends from one or the other's nuclear family: "My mother was in labor for 48 hours before I was born" or "Both our mothers adored homemaking; they say they cannot understand how our generation thinks." Such remarks, offering important clues to underlying concerns, might have been made by a seemingly untroubled couple during a first meeting with their new pediatrician. The following is an example of how a prenatal visit can provide the pediatrician with an understanding of prospective parents.

EXAMPLE

Asked "to tell something about themselves," the 29-year-old husband readily recounts his recent graduation from a prestigious law school and subsequent recruitment by a well-known firm in which his prospects for a future partnership seem excellent. With slightly more reserve, but no less confidence, his 27-year-old wife presents her educational and career credentials, describing how happy and successful she is in her position with a consulting firm. In a spontaneous, rather abashed tone, she says that although they hadn't exactly planned this "interruption," they were simply thrilled with the idea of having a baby. Almost in unison, they spoke of maternity leave and benefits and expressed the hope that the pediatrician would be able to help them to "think about" arranging appropriate child care, because they had no immediate family nearby.

Becoming a little more expansive, the wife emphasized how very busy their lives were, noting that they should be looking for a new apartment because their lease would expire within the month. Shifting abruptly to the subject of breast-feeding, she shrugged unexpectedly, saying, "Oh well, I'll probably decide to wean 'it' before I return to work." In response to the pediatrician's query as to when that might be, the couple again seemed to speak together, "Not for at least 10 weeks." Although continuing to discuss various aspects of child care in a calm, controlled voice, the wife had increased difficulty in remaining focused and there was evidence to suggest underlying and perhaps acute feelings of distress. Unable to follow or interrupt her narrative, the pediatrician was soon disconcerted. She decided to postpone further questioning and to request instead a second prenatal interview in 2 weeks. After some negotiation, an appointment was arranged.

As she later reviewed her notes, the pediatrician perceived both husband and wife to be developmentally stable as they approached the "age 30 transition" of Levinson's (1978) schema. Comfortably established in their careers, they had betrayed no evidence of marital disharmony. She could not, however, dismiss her own uneasiness about their approach to home relocation and child care investigation, as well as the presence of unidentifiable tension between them; nor could references to the baby as "it" and an "interruption" be ignored.

Clarification was provided sooner than expected. An early morning telephone call from the young attorney began with a query regarding confidentiality. Not waiting for a response, he asked whether the physician had noticed that his wife was upset. He added that she felt a great deal of conflict and was unhappy about the upcoming birth. She loved her job, had applied and been accepted in a master's of business administration program, and had even in the

beginning mentioned terminating the pregnancy. The baby's future grandparents express continued concern at the thought of day care. While dismissing such comments angrily, his wife referred to them daily, saying she would never be the "slave to her family" that her mother had been. The husband, sounding increasingly anxious and upset, asked the pediatrician for advice and help.

Indicating her willingness to help, the pediatrician reminded herself not to overdo reassurance at this time and to make comments and recommendations slowly and with caution. As she contemplated the seriousness of the situation, she recalled a recent study on the transition to parenthood, which indicated that psychological variables associated with postpartum depression included low motivation for pregnancy and a low level of psychological health, particularly among first-time mothers (Grossman et al, 1980). Aware, too, of the studies indicating the widely ranging ill effects of maternal depression on infant development (Tronick and Field, 1986), she knew that some support would be needed in the forthcoming weeks. The nature and extent of the intervention would require careful interviewing and consideration. The pediatrician knew of a well-established intervention program that included a prenatal "dual-career couples' group" and excellent individual or marriage counselors.

A greater source of disquietude for the pediatrician was an earlier consultation with an unmarried adolescent girl and her parents as they struggled with their feelings about the daughter's decision to keep her baby.

Failure to anticipate the impact of a child on one's life is seen most clearly in this group of adolescent girls trying to be mothers. There is little doubt that a pregnant teenager of 16 years is at great risk (Osofsky, Osofsky, and Diamond, 1988). Not having fully negotiated adolescence, she has yet to begin the transition to early adulthood. She must, in a sense, attempt to "skip" several developmental stages to achieve a maturity beyond her years and experience. The pediatrician perceives the need to provide immediate support and assistance during this period of initial stress. Recommending and conferring with an obstetrician is an obvious objective, as is preparing the family for a referral to a mental health professional experienced with young, unmarried prospective mothers. Exploring and resolving feelings is a task for all those involved, as is making practical decisions and arrangements. Planning for and learning about pregnancy, childbirth, and child care are left for the young patient to explore with a counselor, as are matters relating to the father of the baby. These and other sensitive issues are not broached by the pediatrician who recognizes the complexity of the family's needs. Yet, the foregoing situation exemplifies the timely and effective ways in which a physician, committed to providing comprehensive pediatric care, can serve in a most critical role before a baby is born.

BEFORE AND AFTER THE BABY ARRIVES

With the arrival of the first child, some of the life changes parents experience are immediately apparent, although the degree to which their lives will be modified by the child's power to transform and transcend all other aspects of their development may be blissfully obscured. Until recently, the initial impact of pregnancy and delivery was felt directly by the mother and, by way of her response, indirectly by the father. The trend toward fathers' participating more in preparing for childbirth has contributed to their feeling less isolated and excluded from the early birthing process. Yet, the intimate awareness of the child's growing within her provides the mother with a head start in adjusting to the idea of her baby as a real person. Having gradually detached herself somewhat from daily concerns to "plan for the baby," she pursues a state of psychological preparedness directed toward providing nurturance and fostering reciprocity.

Without the physical sensations and discomforts of pregnancy as well as being deprived of the positive emotional and psychological experiences, the father may feel some exclusion and experience psychological upset. Concerns about a wife's negotiation of pregnancy and delivery, financial stress created by the expanding family and, perhaps, loss of a wife's income, or the need to work out child care arrangements are among the issues with which the father is faced. Deprived of the physical closeness of his wife as the pregnancy progresses, he may begin to perceive the infant as divisive and to dread its arrival. The prospect of future loss as his wife attends to their dependent infant can create increasing tensions for him. The father may be caught in the dilemma of wanting the child to be born immediately and not wanting the child at all. The birth of the child can stress parents and threaten their closeness almost as readily as it can enhance their relationship.

During the early neonatal period, the responsibilities can seem inordinate. Anxieties that result from lack of experience, the tedium and demands of providing constant care, the exhaustion that comes from sleep deprivation, worry about feeding problems, and a cranky or colicky infant can make this a time for which, in retrospect, parents have only a blurred recollection. Unable to create a comfortable environment or soothe an infant, some mothers can lose a sense of confidence and adequacy. Fathers who share caretaking responsibilities often feel similar frustration. Others, deeply invested in their work and left somewhat on their own, can become driven. Feeling deprived and abandoned, some fathers become angry and demanding, contributing further to the stress within the family. Any unusual crisis from outside, from work or extended family, adds further to the upset feelings parents experience. Even under the most optimal circumstances, the neonatal period may seem to be more one of survival than of transition. Although with the birth of subsequent children, the parents have the added concern of sibling adjustment and rivalry, they are increasingly expert and sanguine. Self-assured and purposeful parents are the most accomplished and successful throughout the parenting years. This experience is frequently achieved through hard-won struggles and often at some expense to the first-born child.

Because all first-born children are recognized to be at some risk, pediatricians should be alert to the significance of problems in the first child's neonatal period. Frequent or anxious telephone calls and emergency department or office visits may indicate the presence of a real problem such as postpartum depression or other serious parent-child disruption. The capability of each individual to accept and fill the parental role depends to some degree on his or her own experience and maturity. The young mother or father whose early childhood was one of emotional deprivation and neglect requires generous increments of nurturing and support. In addition, either parent may require some professional help.

Because the baby's beginning emotional security rests on the parents' ability to understand and meet the earliest nonverbal needs, the mother and father must be readily available and committed. It is critical that the baby's emotional support be secured at this time. The developmental task of the first stage of life is to achieve a sense of mutuality and reliability—the attainment of basic trust, as Erikson (1950) defined it, wherein the meeting of one's needs by the first caretakers is the primary condition from which evolves trust in one's self and trustworthiness in others. Not all parents and babies begin their relationships under optimal circumstances, regardless of the positive, even eager, attitudes parents may have. Some babies are born with physiologic sensitivities and some with difficult or uneven temperaments, and some may simply not live up to parental expectation. There are parents who respond well to placid, smiling, sleepy babies and parents who like their babies active, alert, and more wakeful. Pediatricians benefit from understanding that early difficulties rarely arise from a conscious decision on the part of parents and that an effective response to distressed and troubled parents is to accept and support them and to avoid becoming impatient and making critical judgments.

EXAMPLE

A pediatrician received a telephone call from a parent who sounded hysterical, saying that the baby had not slept in 2 days. The pediatrician recalled having been prepared for such signs of family tension. These new parents, after several miscarriages, had finally resigned themselves to childlessness. Then, joyously accepting the "surprise baby," they seemed, at first, to make a conflict-free adjustment. Listening to the sleep problem, the pediatrician schedules an office visit with both parents. Before the visit, he reviews the family history. The 30-year-old father had recently started his own business, and the loss of the wife's income had created additional financial worry, with both parents struggling with the question of whether she should return to work.

Because of their inexperience and recent entry into a transitional period in their own development, the couple manifest normal, predictable stress. By providing them with ample time to describe the baby's irregular sleep patterns and making some suggestions about management, the pediatrician confirms his interest and support. Encouraging the couple to discuss how things are going may or may not elicit a detailed commentary about their current woes. Whether the pediatrician is offered an opportunity to address the problems directly may not be as critical as the concern and availability implicit in his response. An alliance of this nature can create a sense of comfort and support for a husband and wife that proves meaningful to their development as parents.

THE POSTNATAL PERIOD

Having survived the neonatal period, many parents' experience of the remainder of their child's infancy is calm and pleasurable. They tend, under ordinary circumstances, to begin reinvesting some of their energies in earlier interests and considerations. A husband who has been feeling distracted and fragmented becomes more stimulated and productive in his work and more actively involved in projects related to the home. With the lessening of the baby's demands on her time and body, a wife rediscovers herself as a separate person and as a wife. Perhaps either or both of the new parents felt at times during the procreative period that they had regressed and were infantile, but they become more fully aware of how far they have advanced in establishing themselves as mature adults. Having been separated by the demands and anxieties of producing and providing care to a newborn, they may enjoy reunion, gaining new happiness in each other.

PARENTING AND ONE'S OWN CHILDHOOD

Despite the lessening of stress and adaptation to parenthood, problems can still occur. As Fraiberg, Edelson, and Shapiro (1975) said, there are ghosts in every nursery. The ghosts to which they refer are the unresolved conflicts from a parent's own past that may "... break through the magic circle in an unguarded moment, and a parent and his child may find themselves re-enacting a moment from another time with another set of characters." There is some pain and irresolution in every person's childhood; it is one reason why people not only forget details but are sometimes unable to recall entire periods from their early lives. The application of this defensive process is known clinically as *repression*. According to Fraiberg and colleagues, it is a form of repression, together with the mechanism of isolation, that children most commonly use to bury painful feelings. Both repression and isolation are unconscious activities that serve to banish anxiety and other painful processes from the child's consciousness. Fraiberg and colleagues' theory holds that parents who have blocked the early sensations of pain associated with certain childhood experiences tend to be more closely identified with the aggressive adult who inflicted the pain and to repeat with their children the unpleasant and even cruel behaviors they experienced. An extreme example is the father who, having been beaten by his father, physically abuses his child.

Pediatricians often encounter and are puzzled by this phenomenon operating in a much milder form. For example, an irate father attributes consciously malevolent motivation to his smiling, adorable 20-month-old toddler by saying, "As soon as my wife and I sit down to dinner, we hear her screaming in her crib; she is always trying to keep us apart" or "She wakes us up night after night, demanding to sleep in our bed." Although it is relatively simple to recognize and understand such statements as representing distortion, it is difficult to help a parent realize how inaccurate or inappropriate the perception is. The parent's account, while seemingly simple and straightforward to the pediatrician, may be related to an experience or area so personal, sensitive, and painful that interpretation is the least felicitous approach. Forcing awareness is seldom, if ever, productive; it often jeopardizes an alliance and should be avoided. When the disruption is mild, the pediatrician can begin by offering behavioral management techniques

that often smooth the way for improved interaction. If the problem appears intractable or seems to escalate, the pediatrician can consult a mental health professional or suggest that a direct consultation be arranged by the parents. In the foregoing example, the pediatrician knows that such a recommendation is indicated. The 50-year-old husband with two grown children by a previous marriage had agreed to father "one and only one" child with his second, young wife. Marrying this time for companionship and attention, his capacity for childrearing is more limited than even he had anticipated.

Another situation with which pediatricians are most familiar often arises when a preschooler continues to struggle to assert himself or herself. A parent for whom the development of autonomy was thwarted and for whom the maternal relationship is one of long-standing tension and conflict is particularly vulnerable to a child's emerging strong-mindedness. With increasing conviction, the parent describes the interaction as a battlefield, failing to recognize, perhaps, his or her own overriding need to be victorious. Because the establishment of a continuing sense of self and a beginning sense of self-control is the developmental goal of this stage, a young child feels the need to achieve autonomy at any cost. Therefore, even though setting limits is of critical importance, the child's psychological health can be preserved when a graceful way of yielding is offered.

Parents report skirmishes around all the early basic functions: eating, sleeping, and toileting. It often appears that the negative interaction begins to develop a life of its own. Unable to withdraw from the battle, the parent and child may become far too entrenched and, perhaps, too gratified to yield. If the child's negativism becomes generalized, as it often tends to do, interrupting such circular patterning is a difficult process. The pediatrician must rely on tact, the strength of the alliances with the parents and the child, and knowledge of innovative child management techniques. Avoiding any reference to the possibility that a parent's own underlying conflict may be causal (of which the parent is likely to be unaware), the pediatrician supports parental efforts to reverse direction. This pediatric problem exemplifies the "the sooner the better" principle; left too long it may require outside intervention such as enrollment in a special play group or nursery school or a referral for counseling, or both. Often, a pediatrician can be truly effective by encouraging the parent's recollection of similar childhood frustration, thereby creating an empathic climate for the child. When not successful in these efforts, the pediatrician should be prompt in recommending further intervention. A cautionary note for the pediatrician is a reminder that his or her own life stage and experiences can create misperceptions that affect understanding, responsiveness, and the ability to counsel wisely.

PARENTING AND ONE'S OWN DEVELOPMENT

It should not be inferred that negative displacement by a parent always produces opposing behavior in the child or that the pattern becomes automatically circular. Furthermore, such projective identification by a parent can occur at any time in the child's development with varying intensity and outcome. Because this projective identification is affected directly by the interrelatedness of a parent's and a child's respective life cycle states, it may be moderated or heightened accordingly. As the last child to leave her family, a young mother who continues to struggle with her own separation issues may have far more difficulty when her child first boards the school bus than does a woman in her middle 30s for whom the same landmark represents freedom to take courses or return to work. A father 40 years of age who has successfully established himself in the business world, thereby "becoming one's own man" (Levinson, 1978), may have less need to prove himself through his child's academic or athletic achievement than does perhaps a 44-year-old father who is not satisfied with his own progression on the corporate ladder.

Family physicians and pediatricians might feel dismayed by much of the foregoing discussion if it seems to suggest that they must be all things to all parents. It is not likely, however, that they would react with surprise or unfamiliarity to the interactional patterns and problems discussed so far. Although perhaps not systematically attentive to such occurrences in daily practice, physicians recognize that the complexity of parent-child interaction is a major determinant in the quality of pediatric care they are able to provide.

Because it is the mother who most often serves as principal caretaker, rule maker, and disciplinarian, it is she with whom the infant, toddler, or preschooler naturally has the greatest opportunity to begin to resolve the critical issues of attachment, individuation, and separation and to acquire autonomy, independence, and a sense of competence. With the increase in maternal employment and shared child care, however, many children negotiate and resolve issues with either parent—whoever is there at the time or with whom the issue and the temperamental match provide an impetus. Yet during the earlier stages of a child's development, pediatricians hear much more about mother-child conflict and have far less opportunity to meet with fathers, unless such a meeting is specifically arranged.

In many families, fathers at this stage of their own development and at this stage of the development of their family are preoccupied with being productive, proving themselves, and attaining gratification from work. They seek to settle themselves in a stable position vocationally, yet are open to discovering other options for making the best possible decisions and advancements. Many men feel a sense of comfort when they enter manager-level positions; for others, a move upward is accompanied by a renewed sense of urgency. Some fathers in the "age 30 transition" described by Levinson (1978) find themselves moving smoothly along an "occupational path" and feeling freer to enjoy their school-aged children when they are old enough to express ideas or to understand and share interests. They fail to realize the degree to which they themselves are more available and the positive effects that result from that availability.

It may be that societal demands create added stress for some fathers who are expected to share child care responsibilities and be actively involved in the daily happenings of their offspring. In many households, involvement of the fathers often occurs more naturally and greatly enhances father-child relationships.

An early positive experience in his family of origin inspires a father to nurture and support his own family readily and well. A harsh and depriving childhood produces resolve on the part of some fathers to prevent their children from having a similar experience. A father whose parents structured and stimulated him toward academic achievement, athletic excellence, and a strong sense of self creates similar childrearing conditions naturally. Another father who believes ignorance or disinterest on the part of his parents led to his school failure and inadequate vocational training is determined to provide his children with "every opportunity." Parental motivation is derived from many sources. It varies according to the child's developmental stage, the parents' developmental tasks, and conditions (familial, political, and economic). Having aspirations and expectations for one's children is natural and universal. Many parents, aware of their child-directed goals, accurately perceive their motivation and seek to foster their children's optimal growth in a reasonable fashion.

Less consciously and with too little restraint, some parents are engaged with their children in striving and maneuvering related to their own unmet needs from earlier periods of development. There is generally a further lack of awareness that the pursuit of certain qualities or accomplishments for the child reflects the parents' wish to undo or assuage old hurts, humiliations, and feelings of inadequacy. In some such situations, the essence and true potential of a child are obscured because of the endless adjusting and readjusting of a parental "template." The degree of success achieved by a parent in this pursuit varies widely, depending on many factors: the natural endowment of the child, the cooperation or interference of the other parent, the available resources and other environmental conditions, the strength of the parent's determination, and the intensity of the need to succeed.

A bright preschooler can be taught to read and memorize many facts. A sturdy kindergarten youngster can begin skating lessons at 5 years of age and go on to be playing hockey by 7 years of age. Cello lessons or French tutoring for a talented second-grader may be within the child's level of ability and energy to manage. Yet a mother who plans to have her offspring begin school as a reader can suffer and create suffering for her intellectually average child when they both experience frustration and failure. Some children are poorly coordinated and learn to skate only after long hours of practice at an age when they are sufficiently physically mature and personally motivated to do so. Musical ability and language facility are not inherent in all children. When they are lacking, some modest expertise depends on the child's effort and investment.

A child's entrance into school precipitates the emergence of overdetermined aspirations in many families hitherto uninvolved in "pushing" their children. Although it is fairly commonplace for children to enter day care as infants and toddlers, entry into kindergarten symbolizes a formal coming of age for many children and their parents. It represents the opening phase of a complicated process whereby children and their parents are measured by an independent agency for many years to come. Beginning to acquire learning skills, entering competitive sports, getting along with children of the same age, and behaving well in the classroom are perceived by many parents as the start of serious business. Setting inordinately high standards and responding harshly to mediocrity or failure is extreme but not uncommon parental behavior. Consider the very successful businessman who, as a school-aged boy, received a whipping from his father when he failed to achieve "all As." Having repressed his early humiliation and anger, he expresses gratitude for the parental guidance that motivated him. While not physically punitive with his seventh-grader, he "psychologically whips" him with coldness and rejection.

It is difficult for many parents to discover the right motivational approach—that is, being interested, supportive, and helpful while avoiding overinvestment, nagging, anger, and control. It is even more difficult to attain such an attitude when an unmotivated child refuses to study, demonstrates a learning disability, or has trouble socializing. Pediatricians who have ongoing relationships with schools—public, private, and special schools—can often intervene effectively in the process of having children evaluated and referred for remediation and counseling. In addition, advocating for their child patients is a proper role for pediatricians, helping parents understand the child's perspective as they also provide the child with support and understanding.

The effects of sex-typing, documented by Kagan (1964), continue to have an impact on children both at home and at school. Many mothers, fathers, and teachers maintain a double standard for their children, expecting girls to be quiet, alert, and compliant while allowing their male counterparts to be at least slightly noisy, distracted, and obstreperous. But what happens when the parents of a 13-year-old daughter press her to be assertive, competitive, and academically superior? In many typical classroom settings, she may be destined to be somewhat at odds with her teachers and peers. In this example, the girl strides forward, seemingly unaware or unconcerned with the "different" way in which she is perceived. Closely identified with parental values and intellectually talented, she is determined to excel. Her parents, on the other hand, discouraged and disappointed by their own career achievement and with each other, rarely show pleasure in or approval of their daughter; her successes only heighten their expectations and demands.

The parents in this example, fully cognizant of their goals for their only child, are convinced that they are directing her wisely. Having come from modest familial and educational backgrounds themselves, theirs is a narrow, rigid perspective. Moreover, accustomed to their daughter's complete cooperation, they have never considered the possibility of her having a developmental disruption. It is, therefore, not remarkable that they fail to attend to some changes in her eating habits or to note that she has lost 10 pounds. It is noted, however, by her pediatrician in a routine check-up. Both her pediatrician and the parents become alarmed. As physical causes are ruled out, psychological questions are raised. While the young high school student denies dieting and the presence of a problem, anorexia nervosa is finally diagnosed. The pediatrician decides to meet with his young patient to counsel her as well as recommending a psychological evaluation. She reluctantly agrees; she and her parents subsequently accept a referral for family therapy. Diagnosed and treated at an early stage, the physical symptoms of the anorexic condition abate fairly soon. The underlying conflicts, reflective of the daughter's adolescent turmoil, respond somewhat slowly to individual and family therapy. Clearly, the necessary significant alterations and shifts in the family structure are difficult to attain.

There are many problems that arise as parents and children confront and are confronted by the crisis of adolescence. Reminiscent of the very early attempts of the toddler to separate and establish autonomy and independence, normal adolescence differs in that it is so often experienced as a developmental upheaval. Many more parents seek support and guidance at this stage of parenthood than at any other. As the children change in size and contour, they reveal new interests and longings. Eschewing parental advice and assistance, they seem to immerse themselves in the values and standards of the peer group. With a qualitative change in the way they are able to hypothesize and think conceptually, the cognitive stage of "formal operations," identified and described by Inhelder and Piaget (1950), can lead to adolescents' overvaluing their cognitive solutions. They often seem to have all the answers and adhere with tenacity to a single point of view.

Parents, well able to describe adolescent behavior, are at a loss as to how it should be managed. They consult the family pediatrician and are supported by his or her interest and understanding. Acknowledging their own negative feelings of anger and disappointment, parents are helped to see that the adolescent, struggling with ambivalence about growing up, uses conflict and disruption as a means of moving away and achieving independence. The parents are encouraged to continue to set limits and enforce rules. Advised of the need to provide continued caring, investment, and protection for their adolescents, who, in turn, seem to reject, defy, and disown them, parents often feel tempted or goaded to abdicate their responsibility. It is important at this time to remind parents that it is critical that they remain stable, even stolid, in the face of such unpleasant and turbulent interaction.

A far more challenging task for the pediatrician is to help parents become aware of those aspects of the conflict to which they are contributing. This awareness is often relatively inaccessible because it approaches areas of vulnerability that parents are unwilling and unprepared to address. Taking refuge in their feelings of anger and disappointment with the child's behavior is a poignantly successful way to avoid the true issues. In fact, the more actively parents struggle, the more energy they unknowingly invest in maintaining a state of conflict so they may be spared the sadness and pain they have to experience about the child's growing up and eventually leaving home. For parents, being needed and needing are closely related, as are separating and being separated from. Trying to prevent children from making the same mistakes they made, keeping them secure and safe, and monitoring their motives and whereabouts are necessary activities with which parents protect themselves from a deeper and more searing sense of loss. Asking a parent to affirm and encourage the child's wish for independence may be unconsciously experienced as being asked to participate in the amputation of one's own limb.

PARENTING AND LIFE EVENTS

As painful and full of conflict as the experiences that parents have with a child's adolescence may be, they are heightened further by other circumstances and conditions. Adolescent turmoil occurs coincidentally with the time when parents reach a critical period in their own lives. Recognition of the many aspects of "midlife transition" (Levinson, 1978, 1996) has illuminated the stresses that arise for a parent who is also parenting an adolescent child. Levinson times the midlife transition in the adult as taking place between the ages of 40 and 45 years. Both he and Jacques (1965) addressed themselves to this period of the middle years. Jacques, the first theorist to posit the concept of "midlife crisis," differs from Levinson in the age span of the transition, which he identifies as beginning in the late 30s and continuing for several years. Like Levinson, he sees the core of the crisis to be experiencing one's own mortality. Levinson, moreover, is rigorous in his view that although a modest decline in functioning may occur with some frequency, it is not developmentally normal. Rapoport and colleagues (1980) hypothesize a different time determinant for the "midlife phase," fixed not by chronology but by the period between the first child's and the last child's reaching adolescence.

Regardless of the exact age at which it occurs, all parents reach a time when they begin to realize their mortality and a time when their children reach young adulthood. In addition, the parents' position often becomes a midgenerational one wherein the mortality they must first confront is that of *their* parents. There is a time when they must perceive and accept their parents' decline and assume responsibility for their care. It is critical to recognize how rapidly the patterns shift at this juncture. Adjusting to and accepting the psychological loss of aging parents represents a final yielding of dependency, with the sad and reluctant knowledge that one's parents are ill or growing old and that a time will come when they are no longer there. Caught between the loss of support from their parents and the beginning of the loss of their adolescent children, parents may be unable to find solace in their relationship with each other. Although they are often financially more secure than at any other time in their lives, parents are faced with new responsibilities and demands at a period in which they had anticipated a respite. Many marriages reflect the stresses of this period of transition and are vulnerable to disruption as well. For women, recent changes in occupational role patterns have created a new philosophy and new opportunities that may relieve some of the familial tension of this period. Conversely, in some marriages, the entry of a wife into an interesting and engaging job may create added dissatisfaction for the husband.

There are endless variations in the human life cycle drama of adults sharing their lives with the lives of their aging parents and their growing children. Stage settings and scene changes are often beyond the control of the members of the cast. On one hand, many parents achieve career success, acquire status, gain community respect, and grow in wisdom and perspective. On the other hand, there are those who lose jobs, fail to meet self-actualizing goals, suffer ill health, and experience marital disruption and dissolution. Given the trials and tensions of negotiating the many stages of human development, the degrees of success achieved by so many parents is impressive and reassuring. With the many shifts and changes that occur during parenthood, mothers and fathers often encounter disappointments. These disappointments are, however, offset by the many satisfactions and rewards children bring to their lives. As the children grow older, they cease to be a major responsibility but continue as a source of interest, affection, and caring. Parents look forward to their children's assuming adult status and to their establishing homes and families of their own. The arrival of grandchildren confirms the parents' lives and closes the circle of creativity to which they have made a lasting contribution.

REFERENCES

Erikson E: Insight and Responsibility. New York, WW Norton, 1964.

Erikson E: Childhood and Society. New York, WW Norton, 1950.

Fraiberg S, Edelson E, Shapiro V: Ghosts in the nursery: a psychoanalytic approach to the problems of impaired infant-mother relationship. J Am Acad Child Adolesc Psychiatry 14:387–421, 1975.

Goldberg WA: Introduction. Perspectives on the transition to parenthood. *In* Michaels GY, Goldberg WA (eds): The Transition to Parenthood. Cambridge, Cambridge University Press, 1988.

Grossman FK, Eichler LS, Winikoff LS, et al: Pregnancy, Birth and Parenthood. San Francisco, Jossey-Bass, 1980.

Hetherington EM, Baltes PB: Child psychology and life-span development. *In* Hetherington EM, Lerner RM, Perlmutter M (eds): Child Development in Life-Span Perspectives. Hillsdale, NJ, Lawrence Erlbaum, 1988, p 19.

Inhelder B, Piaget J: The Growth of Logical Thinking From Childhood to Adolescence. New York, Basic Books, 1950.

Jacques E: Death and the mid-life crisis. Int J Psychoanal 46:203, 1965.

Kagan J: Acquisition and significance of sex-typing and sex-role identity. *In* Hoffman LW, Hoffman ML (eds): Review of Child Development Research. New York, Russell Sage, 1964.

LeMasters EE: Parenthood as crisis. *In* Sussman H (ed): Sourcebook on Marriage and the Family. Boston, Houghton Mifflin, 1968.

Levinson D: The Seasons of a Woman's Life. New York, Alfred Knopf, 1996.

Levinson D: The Seasons of a Man's Life. New York, Alfred Knopf, 1978.

Lidz T: The Person. New York, Basic Books, 1976.

Osofsky JD, Osofsky HJ, Diamond MO: The transition to parenthood: special tasks and risk factors for adolescent parents. *In* Michaels GY, Goldberg WA (eds): The Transition to Parenthood. Cambridge, Cambridge University Press, 1988.

Rapoport R, Rapoport N, Shelitz Z: Fathers, Mothers and Society. New York, Random House, 1980.

Rossi A: Transition to parenthood. *In* Greenblatt C (ed): The Marriage Game. New York, Random House, 1974.

Tronick EZ, Field T: Maternal Depression and Infant Disturbance. Child Development Series, No 34. San Francisco, Jossey-Bass, 1986.

Vaillant G: Adaptations to Life. Boston, Little, Brown, 1977.

8 The Development of Behavioral Individuality

Stella Chess • Alexander Thomas

 Children's temperaments are the predominantly congenital, increasingly stable patterns of behavioral style, the characteristic ways they experience and react to their environments. When the child's temperament makes a "poor fit" with the particular environment, conflict and stress develop, and a reactive clinical problem is likely in development, social behavior, school performance, or physical health. Pediatricians need to recognize the temperament patterns of their patients and help parents understand, tolerate, and accommodate them. Care must be taken not to ignore or trivialize, nor to create a pathologic origin for them or try to change them.

Interactional (Transactional) Model

The interactional or transactional model has become accepted in the biology, developmental psychology, and psychiatry fields. In this view, behavioral as well as biological attributes must be considered in their reciprocal relationship to other characteristics of the organism at all times, as must their interaction with environmental opportunities, demands, and expectations. Consequences of this "interactional" process can modify or change selective features of behavior, and the new behavior can, in turn, alter recurring or new environmental influences. New environmental features can emerge independently or can result from organism-environmental interactional processes. The same process can modify or change abilities, motives, behavioral style, or psychodynamic defenses. Development is a fluid dynamic process that can reinforce, modify, or change specific psychological patterns at all age periods.

This interactional concept was emphasized in longitudinal studies from their inception in the mid-1950s and has become a dominant position. A number of important theoretical and practical implications are cited briefly in this chapter. (See Chess and Thomas, 1996b, for a more detailed exposition.)

Early life experience, although important, is not decisive for later development. Psychological development is characterized by both continuity and change, and in any individual case, a linear one-to-one prediction from early to later life is unreliable. Development continues through all age periods. No single pathogenic factor can be labeled as the sole cause of disturbed psychological development. All possible factors and their interactions must be considered in the analysis of the ontogenesis and evolution of an individual's behavior disorder. Such an approach avoids what Mischel (1977) describes as "the shortcomings of all simplistic theories that view behavior as the exclusive result of any narrow set of determinants."

In analyzing the nature of the organism-environment interactional process, the concept of "goodness of fit" and the related ideas of consonance and dissonance are very useful. "Goodness of fit" results when the properties of the environment and its expectations and demands are in accord with the organism's own capacities, motivations, and style of behavior. When this *consonance* between organism and environment is present, optimal development in a progressive direction is possible. "Poorness of fit" involves discrepancies and *dissonances* between environmental opportunities and demands and the capacities and characteristics of the organism so that distorted development and maladaptive functioning occur. Consonance is never an abstraction but is always "goodness of fit" in terms of the values and demands of a given culture or socioeconomic group (Fig. 8–1).

"Goodness of fit" does not imply a lack of stress and conflict. These are inevitable concomitants of the developmental process, in which new expectations and demands for change and progressively higher levels of functioning occur continuously as the child grows older. When in keeping with the child's developmental potential and capacity for mastery, stress and conflict can have constructive consequences. The issue involved in disturbed behavioral functioning is rather one of *excessive* stress resulting from "poorness of fit" between environmental expectation and demands and the capacity of the child at a particular level of development.

The "goodness of fit" concept is a formulation that facilitates the application of the interactional conceptual model to specific counseling, early intervention, and treatment situations. The formulation structures a strategy of intervention that includes an assessment of the individual's motivations, abilities, and temperament; his or her behavioral patterns and their consequences; and the expectations, demands, and limitations of the environment. The specific potential or actual dissonance between individual and environment can then be proportioned. For example, if consultation is requested for a girl who stands passively at the periphery of a group and assessment reveals a temperamental pattern of one who is "slow to warm up," attention can

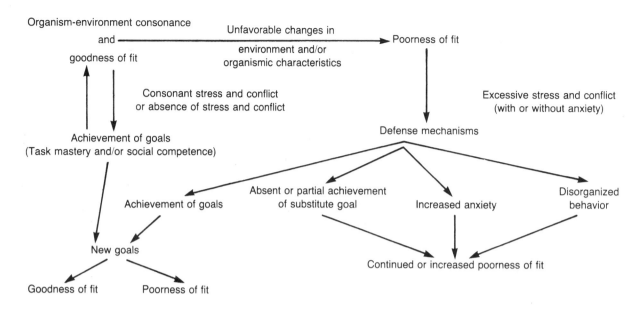

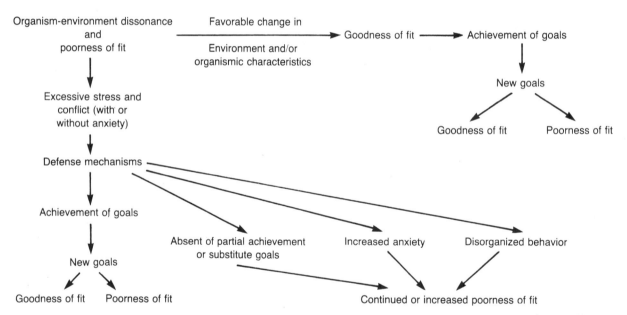

Figure 8–1. The "goodness of fit" model and the roles of stress, conflict, and development are shown. All kinds of permutations and combinations are possible in the course of any one child's development. Goodness or poorness of fit is rarely global. At any age period for any individual, certain environmental demands and expectations may be consonant with his or her capacities and coping mechanisms, whereas others may be dissonant. These consonances and dissonances may even shift with succeeding age periods.

be focused on whether the parents and teachers are making a demand for quick, active group involvement. If a boy disrupts his class with bizarre behavior, the assessment may show a severe reading difficulty, with defensive avoidance behavior. If a disabled youngster has difficulties in mastering complex demands and expectations in adolescence, preventive intervention can ensure continued "goodness of fit." (See Chapter 75 concerning diagnostic formulation.)

Temperament

Pediatricians and experienced nurses know that even newborns exhibit marked individual differences in behavior. Some of these characteristics appear to persist and to influence the response of the baby to handling by the parents and also the response to new situations.

For psychiatrists and psychologists, however, the

concept of the infant as a tabula rasa led them increasingly to ignore individual differences in the infant during the 1950s. Developmental level was an acknowledged factor in structuring the child's reactions to the environment. Initially, "developmental level" referred to general laws of responsiveness and time sequences in which universals in personality organization were achieved but not to the issue of uniqueness of functioning. By the 1950s, some theoreticians and researchers, such as Freud, Gesell, and Shirley, had noted significant individual differences in infants' behavior, and studies had described these differences in specific, discrete areas of functioning (Thomas and Chess, 1977). However, no long-term investigations had been reported that defined these differences systematically and comprehensively or studied the relationship between these findings in early life and the later course of healthy and deviant psychological development.

In 1956, we began the New York Longitudinal Study (NYLS) to identify, categorize, and rate individual differences in children and to explore their significance for the developmental process. We have followed up the behavioral development of 133 subjects from early infancy to early adult life, using a variety of data-gathering and analytical procedures. Several other longitudinal studies of special populations were added to supplement the NYLS data. Our methods and findings are detailed in the following references: Thomas and Chess, 1977; Chess and Thomas, 1996b.

Temperament may best be viewed as a general term referring to the *how* of behavior. It differs from ability, which is concerned with the *what* and *how well* of behaving, and from motivation, which accounts for *why* a person does what he or she does. Temperament, by contrast, concerns the style or the *way* in which an individual behaves. Two children may dress or ride a bicycle with equal skill and have the same motives. Two adolescents may display similar intellectual interests, and their academic goals may coincide. Two adults may show equal expertise and similar devotion to their jobs. Yet these children, adolescents, or adults may differ significantly with regard to the quickness with which they approach a new physical environment, social situation, or task; the intensity and character of their mood expression; and the effort required by others to distract them when they are absorbed in an activity.

Like any other characteristic of the organism—whether it is height, weight, intellectual competence, or perceptual skills—temperament is influenced by environmental factors in its expression and even in its nature as development proceeds.

In the 1970s, Buss and Plomin (1975) and Torgersen and Kringlen (1978) presented the first twin studies that indicated a partial genetic basis for temperament. In 1987, Jerome Kagan and coworkers found a number of biological variables such as heart rate and variability, and cortisol salivary levels that correlated with behavioral inhibition in children. Since then, there has been an explosion of research exploring the correlates of temperament with brain structure (Steinmetz, 1994), the hypothalamic-pituitary-adrenocortical systems (HTP) (Gunnar, 1994), and other physiologic correlates (Calkins and Fox, 1994). These studies are an impressive indication that temperament has a biological source. They also point to the interplay of biol-

ogy and environment to shape the expression of temperament through the life span.

Underlying genetic and physiologic features do not nullify the presence of both continuity and change in temperament over time. Stability and change in response to both environmental influences and genetically determined hormonal influences are features of maturation and development (McCall, 1986; McDevitt, 1986).

Temperamental Characteristics

Nine categories describing temperament were established by an inductive content analysis from the first group of infant behavioral records in the NYLS, which were obtained through parental interviews:

1. *Activity level*, which is the motor component in functioning and the diurnal proportion of active and inactive periods. Mobility during bathing, eating, playing, dressing, the sleep-wake cycle, reaching, crawling, and walking are used in scoring this category.
2. *Rhythmicity (regularity)*, which is the predictability or unpredictability in time of function. It is related to the sleep-wake cycle, hunger, feeding pattern, and elimination schedule.
3. *Approach or withdrawal*, which is the nature of the initial response to a new stimulus, be it a new food, a new toy, or a new person. Approach responses are positive, displayed by mood expression or motor activity. Withdrawal reactions are negative, displayed by mood expression or motor activity.
4. *Adaptability*, which pertains to responses to new or altered situations. One is not concerned with the nature of the initial response but with the ease with which it is modified in a desired direction.
5. *Threshold of responsiveness*, which is the intensity level of stimulation necessary to evoke a discernible response, regardless of the specific form that the response may take. It is displayed in reactions to sensory stimuli, environmental objects, and social contacts.
6. *Intensity of reaction*, which is the energy level of response, regardless of its quality or direction.
7. *Quality of mood*, which is the amount of pleasant, joyful, and friendly behavior, as contrasted with unpleasant, crying, and unfriendly behavior.
8. *Distractibility*, which is the effectiveness of extraneous environmental stimuli in interfering with or in altering the direction of the ongoing behavior.
9. *Attention span and persistence*. Attention span concerns the length of time a particular activity is pursued by the child. Persistence refers to the continuation of an activity in the presence of obstacles.

Temperamental Constellations

Three functional temperamental constellations have been defined by combined qualitative and factor analyses. The first group includes regularity, positive approach responses to new stimuli, high adaptability to change, and a mild or moderately intense mood that is preponderantly positive. Children with these characteristics adapt to regular schedules, take easily to most new foods, smile at strangers, adapt readily to school, and accept most frustration and new rules with little fuss. This group composed about 40% of our NYLS sample. These children are called "easy."

Children at the opposite end of the temperamental spectrum demonstrate irregularity in biological functions, negative withdrawal responses to new stimuli, nonadaptability or slow adaptability to change, and intense mood expressions that are frequently negative. These children characteristically display irregular sleep and hunger patterns, slow acceptance of new foods, prolonged adjustment periods, and relatively frequent and loud periods of crying. Laughter is also loud. Frustration produces tantrums. This is the "difficult child," as mothers and pediatricians can attest. This group composed about 10% of our NYLS sample.

The third noteworthy temperamental constellation combines negative responses of mild intensity to new stimuli with slow adaptability after repeated contact. These youngsters are characterized by mild intensity of reactions, whether positive or negative. If given the opportunity to reexperience each new situation gradually and without pressure, these children finally show quiet and positive interest and involvement. These children who are "slow to warm up" made up about 15% of our NYLS sample.

As can be seen from the preceding percentages, not all children fit into one of these three temperamental groups. Varying and different combinations of temperamental traits are manifested by individual children, and there is a wide range in degree of manifestation. A few children are extremely easy or difficult with all new situations and demands; others show only some of these characteristics, and relatively mildly. Some children warm up slowly in any new situation; others warm up quickly in a few situations.

The various temperamental constellations represent variations within normal limits, and an extreme rating score may be seen in a sample of children for any specific temperamental attribute. Such amodal ratings are not a criterion of a psychopathologic condition but indicate the wide range of normal behavioral styles.

Each of the nine categories of temperament has been identified in each child at different age periods in all our longitudinal samples. These temperamental characteristics have also been identified in other centers in the United States and abroad. It is clear, therefore, that these behavioral traits are ubiquitous among children and can be categorized systematically. Our NYLS subjects have been rated on these same nine categories in adolescence and early adult life.

Several parental questionnaires for rating temperament at various age periods in childhood, as well as self-rating questionnaires that can be used for both adolescents and young adults, have been developed. The childhood questionnaires developed by William Carey and coworkers have been used especially widely in a large number of studies and clinical settings in the United States and abroad (see Chapter 67).

Some workers have suggested modifications in our scheme of categorization of temperament, whereas others present alternative models.

Impulsivity is a term frequently used to describe the rate at which a child translates thoughts or feelings into action, whether rapidly with little hesitation or more slowly after some deliberation. Little agreement has been achieved, however, as to where impulsivity comes from and what it consists of. Some regard it as a dimension of temperament and others do not. The *Diagnostic and Statistical Manual of Mental Disorders IV* defines it as "impatience, difficulty in delaying responses, blurting out answers before questions have been completed, difficulty awaiting one's turn, and frequently interrupting or intruding on others to the point of causing difficulties in social, academic, or occupational settings." It appears likely that although impulsivity probably has strong temperamental components, it is more an aspect of the child's behavioral adjustment with equally important environmental contributions. The temperamental factors may be activity, approach, and distractibility, but it seems probable that the establishment of impulse control lies as much or more in the degree to which caregivers teach children to restrain themselves.

Temperament and Behavioral Disorders

Studies carried out in our research unit and by other investigators using our formulations of temperament have indicated its significant role in normal and deviant psychological development. These findings are summarized in the following discussion (Thomas and Chess, 1980; Chess and Thomas, 1996a, 1996b). Children with the "difficult child" pattern are most vulnerable to the development of behavioral problems in early and middle childhood. Their intense negative withdrawal reactions to new situations and slow adaptability, together with their biological irregularity, make the demands of early socialization especially stressful. In the NYLS, 70% of children in this group experienced clinical behavioral disorders (a mild reactive behavioral disorder in most cases) before 10 years of age. With parental counseling and other therapeutic measures, the great majority recovered or improved markedly by adolescence.

Children with physical disabilities or mild mental retardation in the difficult child group are at even greater risk for the development of behavioral problems and are vulnerable to psychiatric disorders if they have a parent with mental illness. Infants with colic are also more likely to show a low sensory threshold or the difficult child pattern (Carey, 1972).

However, behavioral disorders can develop in children with any temperamental pattern if demands for change and adaptation are in dissonance with the particular child's capacities and therefore are excessively stressful. Thus, excessive stress results in the distractible child when he or she is expected to concentrate without interruption for long periods, in the persistent child if absorption in an activity is prematurely and abruptly terminated, and in the high-activity child if all possibilities for movement are restricted. Teachers may underestimate the intelligence of the child who warms up slowly or the low-activity child, with unfavorable consequences for the learning situation.

Temperament is not always a significant factor in the development of a behavioral disorder. This is also true of motivation, ability, or specific environmental influences. In any specific instance, the pattern of interaction of factors responsible for disturbed function cannot be assumed a priori, inasmuch as it may vary qualitatively from case to case.

Importance of Temperament to the Pediatrician

The pediatrician's role with regard to the child's temperamental individuality is multiple and includes advice on child care practices, routine examinations and procedures, management of minor problems, evaluation of the acutely ill child, management of the chronically ill child or child with disability, and preventive counseling (Table 8–1) (Carey and McDevitt, 1989, 1995).

In carrying out these activities, it is necessary for the pediatrician to be able to assess the child's temperamental characteristics in a minimum amount of time. This can be accomplished through the information that the pediatrician obtains from the parents and from observations of the child in ongoing care and management. We have been impressed by the ability of pediatricians to rate a child's temperamental qualities once they are familiar with the categories and the behavioral criteria for these ratings. Furthermore, the pediatric examination—whether in the office, in the clinic, or at home—provides an opportunity to observe the child's behavior in multiple situations. More systematic data on temperament can be obtained quickly by asking the mother to fill out the Carey questionnaire for the appropriate age period (see Chapter 67). Finally, the pediatrician can include questions on temperament as part of the clinical history (Thomas and Chess, 1977).

Table 8–1 • Issues and Situations in Which Consideration of Temperament May Be Significant for the Clinician

Reassurance of parents that the child's deviation from a culturally desirable norm does not mean a pathologic condition in child or bad parenting; especially true with difficult child or one who is slow to warm up

Child care advice specified in terms of child's temperament, such as approach to weaning and toilet training

Evaluation of severity of actual physical illness by estimating deviation of child's behavior from usual temperament; also, temperament can affect reaction to illness

Evaluation and management of specific symptoms such as colic, night awakening, or "hyperactivity" as partially influenced by temperament

Child's adaptation to beginning nursery school or day care center as influenced by reactions to new situation and speed of adaptation; especially relevant in a difficult child or one who is slow to warm up

Ease or difficulty of child's establishing peer relationships

School functioning—optimal style of classwork and homework schedule in relation to degree of persistence and distractibility

In behavior disorders, identification of influence of temperament and the specific pattern of "poorness of fit"

Special influences of temperament in the physically disabled child and the child with mental retardation

ADVICE ON CHILD CARE

Knowing the infant's temperamental characteristics can be useful to the pediatrician and the parents in developing an optimal approach to early child care. For the inexperienced mother who has been bombarded with pat formulations warning her that every move or expression can affect her infant's future mental health, any difficulty or problem in her infant's management can appear ominous. Fussing at night, avoiding new foods, crying at strangers, resisting toilet training, or ignoring safety rules may all be interpreted by mothers as proof of bad mothering. The pediatrician can evaluate the issue, identify the aspects of the child's temperament that are relevant, and advise the mother appropriately. By contrast, simply brushing aside the mother's concern with responses such as "Do not worry, everything will be all right" or "Be patient, your baby will outgrow this" will most often have limited and temporary value. More useful for the difficult child or the child who warms up slowly is outlining ways of gradual exposure to new events in advance of the finite situation.

ROUTINE EXAMINATIONS AND PROCEDURES

An infant's response to new people and procedures is strongly influenced by his or her temperamental characteristics. When the infant is brought to the pediatrician's office initially or at irregular intervals, he or she is confronted with a strange place, a number of unfamiliar persons, and unusual sounds and is then subjected to a physical examination and immunizations that are restraining, discomforting, and sometimes painful. Depending on his or her temperament, the child may fuss quietly and briefly, squirm a bit, and then be immediately cheerful once the procedures are completed. Conversely, the child may howl loudly from the moment he or she enters the pediatrician's office, struggle violently during the physical examination and inoculation, take up to several hours to calm down, and respond even more intensely at the next visit. The child with a low activity level sits quietly in the waiting room, whereas the youngster with a high activity level fidgets, jumps around, tries to poke into drawers and closets, and becomes a nuisance if he or she has to wait a long time to see the pediatrician.

The pediatrician who evaluates the temperament of his or her patient is in a good position to minimize the distress of each child's office visit. With the easy child, no special management approach is necessary. The child who warms up slowly should be given time to get used to the waiting room before proceeding to the physical examination. The highly active child should be examined quickly; if a wait is inevitable, toys and space to move around in are desirable for both the child and the waiting room. Even though the difficult child is given a period to warm up, he or she may still respond to the examination with loud and long protests. The pain or discomfort of any office procedure should be minimized for all patients, and especially for the child with a low sensory threshold.

MANAGEMENT OF MINOR PROBLEMS

Minor problems in a young child brought to the pediatrician's attention are in many cases significantly related to temperamental issues (Carey, 1972). Frequent night waking, as reported by Carey (1974), is more likely to occur in an infant with a low sensory threshold. He suggests two possible explanations: (1) the greater responsiveness to daytime stimulation makes the infant with a low sensory threshold more arousable at night or (2) these infants are more responsive to internal and external stimuli at night as well. Carey recommends reducing environmental stimulation before bedtime and, if necessary, during the night.

The prolonged loud crying spells of the infant with colic present a difficult and disturbing management problem to parents. Our impression that this is related to the difficult child's temperament is confirmed by Carey's work, which also suggests a relationship to a low sensory threshold. The pediatrician can provide much-needed reassurance and support to the parents in such cases, in addition to any other specific therapeutic measures he or she uses (see Chapter 37 concerning colic).

Sleep problems can develop in easy children after a minor acute illness. Although the child slept well through the night previously, he or she frequently awakens crying when ill. Parental care usually involves picking up the child each time while soothing and alleviating his or her discomfort. Following recovery from the illness, the child, having adapted to the timing of events, continues to awaken crying each night. The parents interpret this as a sign of anxiety. If there is no other evidence of anxiety, evaluation shows that night awakening undoubtedly reflects the quick adaptability of the child to the nighttime pattern of the illness. One might safely predict that the nocturnal crying will quickly disappear if the child is no longer picked up (see Chapter 44).

The response of a child to the irritation of a skin rash can be significantly influenced by temperamental traits. The child who reacts intensely may cry loudly and complain vigorously even if treatment is proceeding effectively. The child with a low sensory threshold may need special measures to reduce the sensory irritation from the rash.

The preceding instances illustrate—but by no means exhaust—the many ways in which the child's temperament influences the response to physical symptoms and the management of minor ailments. Every pediatrician can document this relationship extensively from his or her own clinical experience.

Recently there has arisen a trend to identify at-risk temperamental qualities as pathologic. All temperamental qualities are, by definition, normal behavior. When management difficulties arise, it is because caretakers fail to foster the positive. Assigning a label of pathology is a "blame the child" tactic. High activity level, while inconvenient in a small living space or on a long car ride, does not qualify the child for the diagnosis of attention deficit disorder with hyperactivity. Permitting opportunities for constructive motor outlet is more appropriate than giving medication. The "difficult child" cluster is not a pathologic entity. An extreme example of this trend to identify some temperamental qualities as having pathologic origin can be found in the discussion by Greenspan (1995) of five "challenging" types of children: (1) highly sensitive, (2) self-absorbed, (3) defiant, (4) inattentive, and (5) active/aggressive. These five types are described as disturbed personality patterns with pathologic symptoms interdig-

itated throughout with temperamental characteristics. For example, the "active/aggressive child" (Greenspan, 1995) is clearly described as being a highly active and an "angry, aggressive, frustrated" child.

EVALUATION OF THE ACUTELY ILL CHILD

A major professional responsibility of the pediatrician is to evaluate the gravity of symptoms in an acutely ill child. Is the sudden high fever the first sign of a serious illness or a minor infection? Is lethargy an indication of severe toxicity or a reaction to the discomfort and malaise of a more benign condition? Are acute restlessness and thrashing ominous signs or intense reactions to pain? These judgments depend primarily on careful diagnostic clinical evaluation. There are many occasions, however, in which knowledge of the child's temperamental characteristics can be helpful in making judgments. All other things being equal (which often they are not), if the child's behavior when acutely ill is qualitatively different from his or her usual temperamental style, it is a more serious indication than if the behavior is similar but exaggerated. Mothers are aware of this issue pragmatically when they report that the acutely ill child "is not behaving as usual."

The high-activity, high-intensity child who is restless, thrashes around vigorously, and complains loudly when ill is exhibiting a quantitative exaggeration of the usual temperamental traits. The same behavior in a low-activity, low-intensity child represents a qualitative change from the normal temperament. By and large, the qualitative change is more likely to reflect a more severe acute physical change than is the simple quantitative exaggeration of the child's usual temperament. The same considerations apply in reverse; that is, listlessness in a child who is normally very active is more ominous than is an increase in activity. The complaint of intense pain in a child with a high sensory threshold is likely to have substantial significance, whereas the same complaint in a child with a low sensory threshold may be significant or merely reflect a relatively minor irritation.

Although these and similar temperamental phenomena are not the decisive issues in the evaluation of an acutely ill child, their consideration is often valuable to doctors and nurses in making diagnostic judgments.

The preceding considerations are complicated, however, by the phenomenon some mothers have reported that their child's behavioral pattern when ill is different in a typical way. The child seems to express one kind of temperament when healthy and another when acutely ill. The "good patient" behavior during illness of a difficult child may be an expression of extreme discomfort, in contrast to the vigor of negative mood expression at other times. Here, too, both doctor and parent must be alert to the significance of the acutely ill youngster's behavior.

MANAGEMENT OF THE CHRONICALLY ILL OR DISABLED CHILD

In the management of the more chronically ill or physically disabled child, temperamental issues are frequently of major importance. The ease with which a child can follow a regimen of restricted physical activity, accepting stringent demands of prolonged bedrest, is strongly influenced by temperamental characteristics. Children who exhibit low activity and highly adaptive children find such regimens easier to tolerate than those who are highly active or slowly adaptive. The child who is persistent and has a long attention span can be content once engaged in a sedentary activity. Conversely, the necessity to terminate a physically exhausting activity for a persistent youngster can be difficult. The child who is easily distracted is much more easily diverted from an undesirable activity, but it may be difficult to keep him or her interested in any lengthy sedentary occupation. When hospitalization is required, the need to adapt to a host of new people and situations can be especially stressful to the difficult child or the child who warms up slowly.

It is important for the physician, together with the parents and nurses, to formulate schedules and routines for the physically restricted child that will be most consonant with the youngster's temperament. This ensures the maximum cooperation of the child and the best accomplishment of necessary management procedures. It also minimizes the danger that the stress imposed by the illness or disability will precipitate a reactive behavioral disorder.

The child's temperament is not a crucial or even important factor in every pediatric consultation and treatment. The importance of temperament can be considerable in certain pediatric practice situations, moderate or modest in others, and negligible in still others. However, it is only when the potential influence of temperament is appreciated that its actual significance can be evaluated in any specific situation with an individual child.

PREVENTIVE COUNSELING

As discussed previously, all temperamental qualities are normal and each has a potential, in an environment that provides a poor fit, to lead to the development of behavioral problems. Similarly, each temperamental quality in an environment with a good fit usually leads to harmonious interaction. For example, both short attention span and high distractibility are assets in infant caregiving. It is easy to distract the infant's attention with a toy until the task is complete. These same qualities—short attention span and high distractibility—are frequent causes of difficulty in the school-aged child who fails to complete a chore or homework because attention has run out or interest is easily diverted by peripheral stimuli. By accepting both the reality of the child's temperament and the necessity for task completion, a good fit can be attained by permitting the child who is easily distracted to take frequent breaks, provided that they are offered without rancor and with consistency, and by redirecting attention when it has wandered. Both the caregiver who thinks that the child is being deliberately oppositional and creates an adversarial atmosphere and the caregiver who opts for personal harmony by dropping a demand potentiate problems. In the first instance, confrontation and enmity are needlessly created; in the second instance, the child is deprived of social and task learning and fails to be introduced to styles of functioning that would permit development of a personal style of task orientation. In another example, high or swift adaptability

is, in the short run, usually a temperamental quality that makes parenting easy. However, a highly adaptive school-aged child, enchanted with all the extracurricular activities, signs up for more than he or she can manage. Parents, anticipating such reactions, should be ready to mandate a ceiling. In the opposite instance, the slowly adaptive child needs to be given stepwise opportunities to experience new foods, people, places, and activities—under duress if needed. Having become familiar with the new experience and having been helped by parents, who by this time are aware of the child's long-term preferences, the slowly adapting child can move from participant-observer to full participant.

Scenarios of this sort can be provided for each extreme of each temperamental quality, with variations depending on the developmental stage and the opportunities and demands of each (Table 8–2).

Social Competence and Task Mastery—the Goals of Behavioral Development

A fundamental characteristic of all living organisms is that their functioning is goal directed. The student of biology must ask the question "What for?" This question reflects human-centered teleology and is forbidden to the nonbiological scientist, who is allowed to ask only "How?"—a question the biologist must also ask.

The psychoanalytic movement ushered in a search for goals and motives of human behavior. At the historical period in which Freud developed his instinct theories, only animal models of instincts, drive state satisfaction, and drive state frustration were available. These concepts have been found to be increasingly inadequate for both human developmental theory and animal behavior studies, leading many psychoanalysts to propose modifications of libido theory. However, no consensus has yet been achieved in the psychoanalytical movement for a revision of its traditional formulations of the goals of behavior in light of current research findings (Thomas and Chess, 1980).

In contrast, behaviorism avoided the issue of human goals by focusing on the stimulus-response paradigm, as typified by the conditioned reflex, with the judgment that goals and motives are hidden in the mind's scientifically unknowable "black box." Those behaviorists who have incorporated intrapsychic factors into their conceptual framework have moved to the social learning field but have not developed a systematic theoretical model for considering the goals of behavior developmentally.

An alternative approach is possible, based on the weight of recent research involving infants. The goals of human behavior, starting at birth, can be conceptualized as social competence and task mastery. Both are highly developed in the human being, with his or her unique capacity for learning. Both proceed developmentally as the individual's capacities mature, as learning takes place, and as the environment makes successive new demands and presents new opportunities. Both proceed by a constant reciprocal interaction. Task mastery facilitates social relationships, and increased social competence promotes the

Table 8–2 • Suggestions for Management of Variations in Temperament

Child's Temperamental Qualities	Management Approaches
Activity level	
High	Provide periodic opportunities for constructive high-speed activities.
	Demand motor quietness in socially appropriate places, but arrange that it be needed for short periods only.
Low	Allow sufficient time for tasks so that child need not be rushed or scolded for slow pace.
	Do not denigrate slowness or allow quicker sibling to take over task.
	Compliment quality of completed task if genuine effort has been made.
Rhythmicity	
Irregular	In early infancy, accommodate (eating, sleep).
	By toddler stage and older, accept lack of hunger, sleepiness, but impose social rules (next food at snack time, must be in own room if cannot sleep but allowed to play by self).
	Impose regular wakening time for school.
Regular	In early infancy, accommodate.
	If irregularity is imposed by outside circumstances, make provision for actual regularity (bring food, diaper, pajamas, and so on).
	At older ages, warn child of impending disruption of usual regular schedule; commiserate.
Approach-withdrawal	
Withdrawal	Be alert to the possibility that the activity refused by the child may actually bring pleasure; parent should be guided by awareness of child's interests. If this is the case, insist on a time-limited trial.
Approach	If suitable, express pleasure and interest.
	Be alert that child's first positive response may be short-lived; if so, make it a learning experience ("we must remember," not "I told you so").
Adaptability	
Slow	For mandated (as school) or desirable (as social exposures) activities, provide advance multiple opportunities of brief, graduated exposure.
	Do not force child into a "sink or swim" introduction to a shaky situation.
Quick	For the most part, quick adaptability is an asset; enjoy.
	Be alert to child's selection of concepts and people for adaptation; find alternatives to adaptation to socially undesirable people or antisocial mores.
Threshold of responsiveness	
Low	Avoid exciting stimuli immediately before and during sleep time for infants and toddlers.
	Provide nonirritating surroundings; avoid high decibels, tight or itchy clothing, using degree of child's threshold as guide.
	Encourage positive aspects, as empathy with people's feelings, reasonable preferences.
High	Compensate child who misses cues by drilling in safety rules, social formulas—at developmental level.
Intensity of reactions	
High	Do not respond with counterintensity; wait out child's blast but consider the content.
	Make judgment according to actual reasonableness and state it with quiet persistence, whether denying or accepting child's demand.
	Do not assume that child's high intensity equals deep desire—it may be a trivial matter.
	Do not give in to "buy" peace.
Low	Be alert to possibility that child's deep and valid interest may be expressed mildly.
	Take complaints of pain very seriously; investigate.

capacity to master the environment. Most activities, such as play, school functioning, sex, and athletics, contain both social and task features.

A number of developmental psychologists have emphasized the central role of social competence and task mastery for goal-directed functioning. Bruner, for example, says that "the forms of early competence can be divided into those which regulate interaction with other members of the species and those involved in mastery over objects, tools, and spatially and temporally ordered sequences of events. Obviously, the two cannot be fully separated, as can be seen in the importance of imitation and modeling in the mastery of 'thing skills'" (Bruner, 1973).

Within the research in child development, the past few decades have presented a number of studies of the mechanisms by which the infant achieves self-awareness and self-mastery. Self-esteem, self-control, social intelligence, self-awareness of motivation, and self-awareness of temperament have all been areas of scrutiny. These have been cogently summarized in an excellent review article by Susan Harter (1983). Common to a wide range of theoretical backgrounds have been such formulations as modeling upon the behavior of caretakers, motivation for approval, and self-instruction to attain control over desired behaviors. The changing developmental capacities are constant background to such studies.

Recent research has provided an impressive body of data on the capacities of the neonate and very young infant. The newborn can recognize visual patterns and show preferential attention to complexity, movement, three-dimensional objects, and representations of the human face. Sound can be localized at birth, and there are data suggesting a spatially relevant and functional relationship between vision and hearing. The neonate also shows a wide range of capacities with regard to neurobehavioral organization, including orienting responses, habituation reactions, and correlation between intensity of auditory stimulation and direction of eye movements. Learning, as demonstrated in the formulation of conditioned reflexes, starts actively at birth. Learning by imitation has been demonstrated in

Table 8–2 • Suggestions for Management of Variations in Temperament *Continued*

Child's Temperamental Qualities	Management Approaches
Quality of mood	
Negative	Do not feel guilty; it is not your fault.
	In making judgments, be aware of child's style of expressing positive involvement, e.g., persistence.
	Be alert to child's genuine distress, which may be camouflaged by a general negative mood.
Positive	Appreciate your good fortune.
	Be alert to possibility that child may overvalue people and situations because of general positive mood.
	Teach (at developmental level) social, moral, and safety safeguards as a protection against undeserved positive judgments.
Distractibility	
High	Aim is to compensate, not to change.
	Do not denigrate, but redirect child's wandering attention without rancor.
	Help child set up reminders to return to task; act as a colleague.
	Give high praise for final accomplishment, if it is of reasonable quality.
Low	If child continues task, seemingly ignoring another demand, insist but do not accuse of disobedience, as child really did not hear or notice.
Attention span and persistence	
Low	Quality and completion are the goals, not style of functioning.
	Plan brief periods of task involvement (take into account both developmental stage and temperamental style).
	Rule: It is child's responsibility to return to task (after reminder) after each planned break, until completion; monitor nevertheless.
High	Give advance warning when task must be interrupted.
	Teach child to estimate time required; do not permit starting a lengthy task if time is brief, unless child accepts the reality of need to stop short of completion.
Easy child	Enjoy each other.
	Be alert to child's insufficiently vigorous expression of pain or social discomfort; investigate mild complaints.
Difficult child	Anticipate child's negative mood and withdrawal response to new demands and situations; respond quietly and permit child's initial retreat.
	Make plans to expose child gradually to these new circumstances in order to create familiarity.
	Because loud complaints may be given by child to both major and minor fears and injuries, investigate all before determining appropriate action.
	Wait out tantrums, then quietly inquire about the problem.
	Do not "buy" peace by giving in to child's loud excessive demands; yet, if the complaint is valid, do not ignore it because of the child's excessive commotion.
Child who is slow to warm up	Provide advance familiarity with elements of coming events.
	Refrain from hurrying child into unfamiliar situations; be satisfied with child's being a participant-observer initially.
	Seek out legitimate occasions for praise.

See also Carey and Jablow, 1997; Chess and Thomas, 1986; and Turecki and Tonner, 1989.

the 1st week of life. The newborn is capable of active social communication—the most basic element of social exchange. Manipulative-exploratory behavior of increasing complexity in the first few weeks of life has been described by a number of investigators.

Thus, the neonate and young infant are biologically equipped for the pursuit of two basic adaptive goals—the development of social relations (social competence) and the acquisition of skills (task mastery). Achievement of these goals sequentially with increasing levels of complexity and maturation is a source of satisfaction and gratification and a crucial factor in the progressive development of a positive self-concept.

Whether it is walking, weaning, self-feeding, toilet training, self-dressing, or acquring language, the normal child is highly motivated at the appropriate developmental level to engage in these task and carry them through to completion. It is true that many humans carry out the process of mastery through stress and tension, whether it is the infant learning to walk and to drink from a cup or the adult artist or scientist struggling with a painting or laboratory experiment. To view such stress as undesirable and, if inevitable, regrettable is to misinterpret profoundly the dynamics of healthy psychological development. It is only when demands are made for a level and quality of performance that are excessive and inappropriate for the individual that the stress and tension can have unfavorable consequences. If the demands are not excessive and the stress is resolved by mastery, the effects are positive. Unfavorable consequences can result not only from excessive demands but also from misguided efforts by parents to "protect" their child from stress and tension.

Adaptive and Coping Styles

In responding to the demands and expectations of parents, teachers, and peers and in the pursuit of social competence and task mastery, the child's ideal coping strategy is direct engagement with successful outcome. Even partial coping brings a sense of mastery of a new demand or expectation. For example, a boy who is clumsy because of delayed neuromuscular development may not be able to meet the expectations of his peer group as a ball player. However, he may stay with the group despite their initial criticisms and teasings, practice assiduously on his own with a parent or older sibling, improve gradually, and gain the respect of his peers as they begin to appreciate his determined efforts and improvement. Successful achievement also enhances self-esteem and the child's confidence that successful direct struggle is possible even when the stress is substantial.

However, if the new demand is highly excessive for the child, direct mastery is not possible unless the level of expectation is modified to bring it within the scope of the individual's capacities. If the level of expectation is not modified, the excessive stress and impossibility of direct mastery can cause the child to resort to one defensive strategy or another. This can happen for many reasons: dysphasia, dyslexia, temperament-environment dissonance, academic demands that are beyond an individual's intellectual abilities, overwhelming environmental stress, or severe distortions of brain functioning. On many occasions, and for various reasons, an individual can have the capacity to cope directly and effectively with the new demand yet fail to do so, turning instead to some defensive strategy. Certain past experiences may have created a conditioned response that any stress is dangerous, or the demand may be presented by parent, teacher, or employer in an ambiguous or confusing form. As another example, the kind of effort required to master the demand can appear, rightly or wrongly, to alienate the individual from his or her peer group.

Defensive strategies, or defense mechanisms as they are usually called, can be defined operationally as behavioral strategies that attempt to cope with demands or conflicts that the individual cannot or will not master directly. This definition does not assume, as Freud did, that defense mechanisms are necessarily unconscious, nor does it assume any a priori theoretical formulations of the causes of stress and conflict. Thus, although derived originally from psychoanalytical theory and practice, the concept of defense mechanism as defined here can be used in the analysis of behavioral dynamics independent of the psychoanalytical framework.

Specific defense mechanisms can also be defined operationally and identified by simple inference from empiric data, again without commitment to any one theoretical scheme. *Suppression-repression* represents the attempt to extinguish feelings or ideas; *denial* is the posture that the stressful environmental demands are really insignificant and need not be confronted; *avoidance* exemplifies the detachment from the stressful situation; *reaction formation* signifies the attempt to cope by transforming the motivation into its opposite; *rationalization* represents ascribing a socially acceptable motive to behavior that has other motivations; *displacement* denotes the involvement with a less meaningful but less stressful object or situation than the one at issue; *projection* means ascribing motives, feelings, or ideas to others that are really one's own; and *fantasy* expresses the retreat into intrapsychic thoughts and feelings as a substitute for confronting external reality. *Sublimation*, or avoidance through a socially desirable activity, and *humor* are generally more constructive defense strategies. *Delusional thinking*, the reconstruction of reality to eliminate stress and threat, usually occurs in severe mental illness. Fantasy and humor are not always defensive ma-

neuvers; they can even be prominent features of healthy and creative functioning.

The use of defense mechanisms is by no means always undesirable. An individual can at one time or another be faced with excessively stressful demands or conflicts that cannot be mastered directly. This can evoke the temporary use of a defensive strategy, which then gives the person the opportunity to resolve the stress positively. In these situations, it would appear that the use of the defense mechanism is necessary to organize the strengths and capacities needed for successful mastery. For example, an adolescent boy who warms up slowly may experience a typically uncomfortable shy response when joining a new peer group. He may rationalize his initial peripheral and outwardly detached involvement to the group by making various excuses (he is worried about a friend who is ill, he has a sprained ankle, or he has to get home early) and gain the time necessary to make a gradual positive adaptation. A young girl may be aware that the severe and frequent arguments between her parents threaten to break up her home and family. She may deal with the potential anxiety this creates by denying the seriousness of the situation and displacing her anxiety by worrying over a pet dog's well-being. Although the denial and displacement are unrealistic, they enable her to pursue her own life activities without crippling anxiety.

At times, the price paid for the achievement of psychological equilibrium through a defensive strategy is so high that it must be challenged at all costs. Thus, a child with a school phobia may avoid the anxiety of attending school by elaborating various somatic symptoms. If not attending school, the child may be completely comfortable with active pursuit of friendships and other activities, but he or she may be incapable of returning to school without severe acute anxiety. In such a case, this pattern of adaptation has so many serious consequences that it must be treated as an emergency.

Finally, there are instances in which a defense mechanism, no matter how strongly and decisively it is used, fails to achieve or sustain a state of psychological equilibrium. The resulting disequilibrium can find expression in a panic state, acute dissociative state, severe depression, or behavioral disorganization (see Chapter 64).

Defense mechanisms vary tremendously in their influence on the developmental course of different individuals. These mechanisms can have little or no importance, can be of transient significance at one time or another, or can be intermittent or constitute a continuous and highly important factor. In this regard, they are similar to other factors that influence the course of development—temperament, intellectual level, specific abilities or defects, parental practices and attitudes, other family influences, special events, and the social environment—all of which vary greatly in their impact on different individuals (see Chapter 75 regarding comprehensive diagnostic formulation).

REFERENCES

Bruner J. Organization of early skilled action. Child Dev 41:1, 1973.
Buss AH, Plomin R: A Temperament Theory of Personality. New York, John Wiley & Sons, 1975.
Calkins SD, Fox N: Individual differences in the biological aspects of

temperament. *In* Bates J, Wachs TD (eds): Temperament: Individual Differences at the Interface of Biology and Behavior. Washington, DC, American Psychological Association, 1994.

Carey WB: The Difficult Child. Pediatr Rev 8:39, 1986.

Carey WB: Night waking and temperament in infancy. J Pediatr 84:756, 1974.

Carey WB: Clinical applications of infant temperament measurements. J Pediatr 81:823, 1972.

Carey WB, Jablow M: Understanding Your Child's Temperament. New York, Macmillan, 1997.

Carey WB, McDevitt SC: Coping With Children's Temperament. New York, Basic Books, 1995.

Carey WB, McDevitt SC: Clinical and Educational Applications of Temperament Research. Amsterdam, The Netherlands, Swets & Zeitlinger, 1989.

Chess S, Thomas A: Know Your Child. Northvale, NJ, Jason Aronson, 1996a.

Chess S, Thomas A: Temperament Theory and Practice. New York, Brunner/Mazel, 1996b.

Chess S, Thomas A: Temperament in Clinical Practice. New York, Guilford Press, 1986.

Greenspan S: The Challenging Child. Reading, MA, Addison-Wesley, 1995.

Gunnar MR: Psychoendocrine studies of temperament and stress in early childhood. *In* Bates J, Wachs TD (eds): Temperament: Individual Differences at the Interface of Biology and Behavior. Washington, DC, American Psychological Association, 1994.

Harter S: Developmental Perspectives on the Self-System. *In* Mussen PH (ed): Handbook of Child Psychology. New York, John Wiley & Sons, 1983, pp 275–355.

Kagan J, Reznick JS, Snidman N: The physiology and psychology of behavioral inhibition in children. Child Dev 58:1459, 1987.

McCall RB: Issues of stability and continuity in temperament research. *In* Plomin R, Dunn J (eds): The Study of Temperament: Changes, Continuities, and Challenges. Hillsdale, NJ, Lawrence Earlbaum, 1986.

McDevitt S: Continuity and discontinuity of temperament. *In* Plomin R, Dunn J (eds): The Study of Temperament. Changes, Continuities, and Challenges. Hillsdale, NJ, Lawrence Earlbaum, 1986.

Mischel W: On the future of personality measurement. Am Psychol 32:246, 1977.

Steinmetz JE: Brain substrates of emotion and temperament. *In* Bates J, Wachs TD (eds): Temperament: Individual Differences at the Interface of Biology and Behavior. Washington, DC, American Psychological Association, 1994.

Thomas A, Chess S: Temperament and Development. New York, Brunner/Mazel, 1977.

Thomas A, Chess S: Dynamics of Psychological Development. New York, Brunner/Mazel, 1980.

Torgersen AM, Kringlen E: Genetic aspects of temperamental differences in infants. J Am Acad Child Psychiatry 17:433, 1978.

Turecki S, Tonner L: The Difficult Child, 2nd ed. New York, Bantam Books, 1989.

BOOKS FOR PARENTS

Carey WB, Jablow M: Understanding Your Child's Temperament. New York, Macmillan, 1997.

Chess S, Thomas A: Know Your Child. Northvale, NJ, Jason Aronson, 1996.

Kurcinka MS: Raising Your Spirited Child. New York, HarperCollins, 1991.

Turecki S, Tonner L: The Difficult Child, 2nd ed. New York, Bantam Books, 1989.

9 Effects of Gender on Behavior and Development

Carol Nagy Jacklin • Lizbeth J. Martin

 Popular opinions have been and continue to be confident in describing extensive inborn differences in development and behavior between male and female children. Such genetic variations do exist, but scientific study has revealed that they are few and small. Much of the behavior diversity related to gender differences appears to be the result of socialization influences.

Much emphasis is placed on possible differences between girls and boys, even though there are many other kinds of distinctions to be made among children. People rarely wonder, for example, whether blue-eyed children differ from brown-eyed children in temperament or intellectual abilities, but people do care whether the sexes differ in these and many other psychological attributes. The relative contribution that biology plays in the development of sex differences is also of interest. This chapter first considers the ways that girls and boys are similar and different, no matter what the cause, in the context of (1) the neonatal period, (2) temperamental and emotional measures, and (3) intellectual abilities. Second, this chapter discusses research in the area of socialization of gender by parents, teachers, and peers.

It has become increasingly common to describe the developmental process from a biopsychosocial framework. Although there are few truly sexually dimorphic behaviors in humans, any behavior that is differentiated by sex raises the question of its cause. Both biology and psychology describe behavior. The origin of a specific behavior, let alone a cluster and pattern of behaviors, as seen in gender identity, for example, can be viewed only from an interactional model.

Neonatal Period

BIRTH PROCESSES THAT ARE SEX DIFFERENTIATED

Conception results in more male zygotes than female zygotes. Conservative judgments of this primary sex ratio estimate 120 male zygotes conceived for every 100 female zygotes. Fetal and neonatal deaths are more common among male than among female zygotes, thus reducing the sex ratio at birth. The birth process itself is somewhat different for the average boy compared with the average girl, with the mean length of labor being about an hour longer for male infants than for female infants. Although there is evidence that the length of labor is related to a child's subsequent development, in most studies, long labor is confounded by a greater use of perinatal medication so that the effect of either the length of labor or drugs alone is difficult to determine (Jacklin, 1989). (See Chapter 26 on perinatal stresses.)

In an article that chronicles greater male vulnerability from conception to early death, Gualtieri and Hicks (1985) hypothesize an immunoreactive theory of selective male affliction. They suggest that there is "something about the male fetus that evokes an inhospitable uterine environment." Simply stated, they believe that because the male fetus is genetically different from the mother, the mother's body is stimulated to produce a kind of antibody against the male fetus (but not against the female fetus, which is genetically similar to her). They believe these antibodies lead either directly or indirectly to fetal damage. This manuscript has caused considerable controversy. (Twenty-five peer commentaries are published with the article.)

The male vulnerability may be related to higher levels of learning, attention, and retardation problems. These developmental and behavioral deviations are discussed in Chapters 52, 53, and 56. (See also Chapter 6 concerning normal changes in adolescence.)

SEX STEROID HORMONES AT BIRTH

Considerable research is underway to study the course of some of the sex steroid hormones during development. These hormones are somewhat different in male and female neonates. Testosterone concentrations are higher in boys, whereas levels of other hormones (androstenedione, estrone, estradiol, and progesterone) are not differentiated between the sexes.

There is considerable overlap in the male and female frequency distributions of testosterone, the one hormone that has been shown to be at different levels in the two sexes. This overlap in the distributions among male and female humans contrasts with the differentiation of sex hormones in the neonatal nonhuman primate. Sex differences in sex steroid hormones are much larger at birth in nonhuman subjects. Progesterone levels, which do not differ in human neonates, are twice as high in newborn female rhesus monkeys as in males. Similarly, estradiol levels in umbilical cord plasma are twice as high in newborn female rhesus monkeys as in males, but there are no sex differences for this hormone in human neonates. The sex difference for testosterone in humans is much smaller than in rhesus monkeys, with the male to female ratio of testosterone in the umbilical plasma of rhesus monkeys being about 2:1.

Because of the discrepancy in the magnitude of sex differences between human and nonhuman hormone concentrations, simple generalizations about sex differentiation in animals should be applied to humans only with great caution.

BEHAVIOR AT BIRTH

At birth, boys and girls seem alike. Nonetheless, investigators have carried out numerous tests to detect behavioral differences. In a landmark study, Bell and colleagues (1971) performed approximately 60 different behavioral assessments on neonates in the first 4 days of life; of these assessments, 12 revealed stable characteristics (i.e., scores correlated significantly from day to day for individual infants during the first 4 days of life). Of these 12 assessments, two involved sex differences, with prone head raising involving the clearest sex difference and tactile threshold involving a sex difference in breast-fed infants but not in bottle-fed infants. More recent studies have failed to find the sex differences in tactile sensitivity. The results of many such studies are summarized in Table 9–1 (Maccoby and Jacklin, 1974).

Brain Development

The only confirmed sexual dimorphism in the human brain present at birth is the small difference in brain weight. Other differences between male and female brains seen in later life have not been confirmed to exist at birth. During the first 10 years of development, the sex difference in brain and body size becomes larger. The sex differences in body size and adult brain weight represent the largest nongenital differences between the sexes, and brain weight may simply be another body size difference. Even here, the overlap of the distributions of male and female data is substantial, and the overlap of distributions only increases for all other variables (Breedlove, 1994).

HORMONAL REGULATION

It has long been believed that the sexually dimorphic nucleus of the preoptic area (SDN-POA) of the hypothalamus in humans is permanently differentiated during a critical period in prenatal life by steroid hormone regulation. It has become clear that the influence of fetal androgen on neural tissue is not necessarily immutable but, rather, responds in a plastic fashion not only to pubertal hormonal events but also to environmentally triggered hormone regulation. It is possible to appreciate the tremendous influence of the prenatal hormonal milieu on sexual neural dimorphism without discarding effects of socialization processes (Pilgrim and Hutchison, 1994). The two, rather than being mutually exclusive, are mutually interactive. The nature-nurture controversy has evolved into the concept of biological and social interaction.

CEREBRAL HEMISPHERE ASYMMETRY

Young girls who suffer left hemisphere brain damage are more likely to show better recovery of language function than boys, suggesting greater female ability to transfer language function to the right hemisphere of the brain. Later in life, women's brains have been found to display less rigid lateralization of function in relation to men's brains, such that female stroke patients tend to recover function better than their male counterparts (Breedlove, 1994; Kandel et al, 1995).

Female fetuses exposed to diethylstilbestrol (DES) show a more malelike lateralization of brain function, and greater numbers of these females declare themselves to be homosexual or bisexual relative to the non–DES-exposed female population (Breedlove, 1994).

Temperament and Emotions in Childhood

Emotional states are believed to be stable temperamental characteristics. Most of the work measuring emotional stability in young children has measured irritability, sometimes as a naturally occurring state. For example, Moss and Robson (1970) measured crying or fussiness when there was no discernible stimulation. Others have measured fussiness as a reaction to a wide range of unpleasant stimulations from mild to somewhat harsh. Although Moss did find boys crying more than girls, when hours asleep were equated in his sample, the sex difference disappeared. Other studies do not tend to find sex differences in crying or irritability. How "difficult" a child is labeled is related in part to his or her irritability. Sex differences are not found in numbers of "difficult" children reported.

Timidity is commonly believed to be more intense, more frequent, or elicited upon weaker stimulation in girls than in boys. Although many studies using both observational measures and parent reports do not find differences by sex, when differences are found, girls are reported to show more timidity. Related work on behavioral inhibition in children finds large individual differences but no average difference between girls and boys.

Activity level includes a variety of behaviors and, as is often true in development, the specific behaviors that form the basis of a behavioral cluster change with age. Research in this area is mixed with respect to sex differences. Although it is commonly believed that boys are

Table 9–1 • Sex Differences and Similarities in Behavior at Birth

Characteristic	Sex Differences	Comments
Tactile sensitivity	None	
Prone head raising	Boys higher	Differences so small studies must be aggregated to find significance
Activity level	None	

more active than girls, most studies do not find differences in the first 3 years of life. When differences are found, however, boys are likely to be more active than girls.

Situational factors may play a role in the inconsistency of findings. At least three situational factors relate to activity level: the size of the space in which activity level is measured, the presence or lack of rough-and-tumble play, and the size of the group of peers with whom the child is interacting. Boys tend to play in larger groups, and larger groups tend to be more active. Imitation of organized sports seems to be a factor for boys even in these early years. If children are tested in small spaces, sex differences are unlikely, but when children are observed in large play yards, differences are more likely to emerge, because there are greater opportunities for rough play, an activity that is more common among boys.

An additional factor may be how activity is organized. Boys are more frequently diagnosed as "hyperactive" than are girls (Safer and Allen, 1976), but when actual activity is measured, "hyperactive" children do not move from place to place more than normal children do. However, they do show more restless, squirmy movements when staying in one place and lack of purpose when moving from place to place. Thus, sex differences in activity level may prove to be differences in kind of activity rather than in amount; however, this issue is not yet settled.

Aggression refers to a cluster of actions and motives that are not necessarily related to one another. Included in all forms of aggression is a desire to dominate and control. Aggression may therefore include assertiveness, vigor, and antisocial behavior. There is some evidence that the level of aggression is higher in boys than in girls, but again these are small average differences (Maccoby and Jacklin, 1980).

Sex differences and similarities in temperament and emotions are summarized in Table 9–2.

Measurement of Intellectual Abilities

DECLINES IN GENDER DIFFERENCES IN INTELLECTUAL ABILITIES OVER TIME

Earlier reviews of studies comparing male and female performance on intellectual tasks found sex differences in verbal behavior, but current research does not. In their comparison of verbal ability scores of girls and boys, Hyde and Linn (1988) found that the differences between the

sexes had been reduced across the past decades. They conclude that these changes are a result of efforts to make test items in verbal ability areas gender neutral.

Similar decreases in gender differences over the past 2 decades have been shown in a variety of other intellectual abilities in high school and college students. Using meta-analysis (a statistical technique for estimating the size of effects and comparing large numbers of studies), Rosenthal and Rubin (1982) concluded that they could not pinpoint a cause for this change. In addition, when reviewing meta-analyses of studies investigating a wide variety of psychological sex differences, Hyde and Plant (1995) reported that ". . . there are more effect sizes in the close-to-zero range for gender differences than for other areas of psychological research."

In summary, tests of intellectual abilities have differentiated girls and boys less and less over recent decades. The only exception to this trend is at the highest end of the mathematics ability continuum, in which the ratio of boys outscoring girls has remained constant over the years. There is evidence that mathematical test items are less gender neutral than are the verbal items.

THE MATHEMATICS CONTROVERSY

In the early 1980s, Benbow and Stanley (1980) published a series of articles that caused a stir in both the media and academia. They described the scores on a standardized test of mathematic ability for a large population of bright boys and girls. In every study, the boys scored higher than the girls. What was particularly important about these results was that the authors speculated about the biological causes of their findings. These speculations were exaggerated in media accounts, and they became the overriding message of the studies.

Seemingly, Benbow and Stanley's studies supported the popular myth about gender differences in mathematic ability. However, Benbow and Stanley only speculated about biological causes for their results; they had no biological data. Furthermore, many aspects of their studies were criticized in professional journals. For example, the results were reported as ratios of girls to boys at the highest scores, an analysis that exaggerates the actual group differences in scores. The Benbow and Stanley studies also failed to take into account the children's differential mathematics-related experiences, assuming that enrollment in equal numbers of mathematics classes would equate for this factor (Eccles and Jacobs, 1986).

During the time that the Benbow and Stanley studies were published and the associated media blitz occurred, Eccles and colleagues were collecting data for a large-scale study of mathematics course taking and achievement by seventh through ninth graders. Thus, these researchers had a unique opportunity to record how the media's presentation of a scientific study affects the attitudes of people directly concerned with the subject matter of the study (Eccles and Jacobs, 1986).

The conclusions of the larger, primary study were that mathematics anxiety, gender-stereotyped beliefs of parents, and the perceived value of mathematics to the student account for the major portion of sex differences in mathematic achievement. In addition, Eccles and colleagues

Table 9–2 • Sex Differences and Similarities in Temperamental and Emotional Characteristics

Characteristic	Sex Differences	Comments
Irritability	Negligible	
"Difficulty"	None	
Level of timidity	Girls higher	Small differences
Behavioral inhibition	None	
Level of activity	Boys higher	Small differences only in gross motor activities
Level of aggression	Boys higher	Small differences

found that students' attitudes about mathematics are most strongly related to their mothers' beliefs concerning the difficulty of mathematics for their children. Mothers' beliefs were also important in that they directly and strongly influenced their children's anxiety over mathematics. Similar results have also been reported for younger children. (The influence of teachers in mathematics achievement is discussed later.)

The related research on the effects of the popular reports of the Benbow and Stanley results compared the attitudes of parents who were aware of the Benbow and Stanley work as reported in the media ("misinformed" parents). Briefly, Eccles and Jacobs (1986) found that uninformed mothers believed that the mathematic ability of their sons and daughters was equivalent, whereas misinformed mothers of girls thought that mathematics was more difficult for their children than did mothers of boys. Thus, the media campaign had a direct effect on the same attitudes of parents that have a direct effect on their children's taking mathematics courses and their subsequent achievement. Clearly, the effects were deleterious to girls. As mothers came to believe that mathematics were much more difficult for girls than for boys, their daughters became less likely to take additional mathematics courses. Teachers and parents, by and large, do not know the power of expectations in mathematics learning. This is a symptom of a larger problem. Current findings in psychology are not prominent in the education of teachers. Nationally organized parents groups (e.g., the Parent Teacher Association) could bring this kind of information to parents. Professionals such as pediatricians, interacting with parents and children, could bring such information to parents.

Recently, Benbow and Lubinski (1993) reported finding hemispheric activation differences by sex and intellectual precocity as measured by electroencephalogram. They stated that "mathematical talent seems to have biological co-variates" (Benbow and Lubinski, 1993), but no direct biological connection to any of the sex differences has been proven.

Socialization of Gender

The process whereby children grow into adults is of central interest to developmental psychologists and pediatricians. Questions about how and how much parents can influence their children's attitudes and behaviors have been an important part of developmental psychology since some of the earliest studies. This discussion considers the role of parents and teachers in this process as well as the role of socialization by association.

Most of this research has been carried out in middle class white American populations, and more cross-subcultural data are needed before these findings can be generalized.

PARENTS' EXPECTATIONS AND BELIEFS BEFORE THEY GAIN EXPERIENCE WITH THEIR CHILDREN

In terms of behavior, boys and girls are similar at birth. The one difference that has been established, muscle strength, is a difference of which parents are probably not aware. How parents do see their children at birth has been investigated. When asked to rate their children, parents describe many more sex differences than researchers have been able to document.

In one study (Rubin, Provenzano, and Luria, 1974), parents described their newborn infants in sex-stereotyped ways. Although the infants did not differ appreciably in height or weight, for example, parents rated their girl infants as small and their boy infants as big. Mothers had held and looked at their infants before filling out the rating scales, whereas fathers were only able to see their infants through the window of the nursery before they produced their ratings. Fathers gave more strongly stereotyped ratings than did mothers. Perhaps stereotyping is most likely when little information is available.

Consistent with this view, stereotyping by parents appears to be less evident for older infants. A modified version of Rubin's checklist was given to parents of two cohorts in the Stanford Longitudinal Study. One group of parents had children 6 months old, and the other had children 33 months old. At both ages, only minimal sex differences were noted in the responses to checklist items.

DIFFERENTIAL SOCIALIZATION BY PARENTS

As discussed earlier, parents describe their newborn infants in sex-stereotyped ways but they are less likely to do so after they have had some experience with their children. But, how do they behave toward their sons and daughters?

Studying the interaction between a parent and a child is complex. It is difficult to determine which individual is determining the nature of the interaction. Is a child treated in a certain way because of stereotyped views that a parent has about that child or because the child is acting in a way that elicits a particular behavior from the parent? For many years, parent-child interactions were assumed to consist of encounters in which parents trained and influenced their children. The evidence given for this influence was the correlation between parent and child behaviors. Given only correlational evidence, it is not clear who is "shaping" or influencing whom.

Even with the difficulties involved in dyadic research, if evidence is examined for differential treatment by parents of boys and girls in the first 3 or 4 years of life, boys and girls are seen to be treated similarly. For example, in areas such as warmth, nurturing, acceptance, restrictiveness, allowing dependency, and allowing aggression, very young boys and girls do not seem to be treated differently by their parents (Maccoby and Jacklin, 1974). Boys do seem to receive more physical punishment. This may be a case in which boys and girls are eliciting different behavior from parents because of different initial behavior (Maccoby and Jacklin, 1980).

In most areas of parent-child interaction there appears to be little difference in the first few years of life in the way boys and girls are socialized, although there is an exception. In the area of sex-role stereotyped play, differential socialization can be documented. Fathers offer more sex-appropriate toys to sons and daughters as early as 1 year of age and react negatively to sex-inappropriate toy play as early as 3 years of age. Rough-and-tumble play and high arousal play are more likely to be initiated by fathers toward their sons than toward their daughters.

As children age, some areas of differential socialization can be seen. Parents are more likely to know where their girls are after school or on the weekend. Daughters receive more of what has been called "chaperonage" than do sons. Knowing where the child is or allowing the child to roam may be partly a function of the task that a child is asked to do in the household. Girls are more likely to be assigned household chores and child care. Why girls are so often given these tasks is an interesting question. Task assignment, particularly child care, does have an effect on a child's behavior. In the relatively few cases in which this task is assigned to boys, it seems to increase their nurturing abilities and decrease their aggression outside the child care situation (see Socialization by Association).

TEACHERS' DIFFERENTIAL SOCIALIZATION IN PRESCHOOL

Recent research in tracing differential socialization of boys and girls in the schools is promising and is described here for two age groups. Data pertaining to the preschool child are discussed first, followed in a later section by a discussion about the school-aged child.

In the preschool class, the positive reinforcement that boys and girls receive is dependent on different circumstances. Girls are more likely to receive positive reinforcement from their teachers when they stand close to the teachers. For boys, receiving positive reinforcement from the teachers is unrelated to their distance from their teachers. When teachers change their reinforcement pattern, girls adjust their distance from the teacher, so it can be concluded that the different reinforcement pattern by the teachers is at least partially responsible for the girls' greater closeness. Where the child stands with respect to the teacher is also an important determinant of what activities the child engages in, being that the preschool teacher tends to be involved in the areas of fine motor skill activities (e.g., stringing beads, playing with clay). If teachers move to other activity areas, the girls follow them. The girls' play experience is thus shaped by the contingencies involved in the teacher's close presence. Play experience with different types of toys has been shown to correlate with the child's tested cognitive ability (Connor and Serbin, 1978).

We do not wish to exaggerate the teacher's role in generating sex differences. Peer influences (discussed previously) are no doubt important. Teachers do not appear to respond differentially to aggression in the two sexes, for example. Boys may be reprimanded more often for fighting, because this occurs more often among boys, but the teacher's response is similar regardless of the sex of the child.

TEACHERS' DIFFERENTIAL SOCIALIZATION IN THE PRIMARY AND SECONDARY CLASSROOMS

Boys receive somewhat more praise in class than do girls, and recent research has confirmed this finding. Perhaps more importantly, a different pattern of feedback is given to boys than to girls. Girls tend to receive negative feedback for the content of their academic work, whereas boys receive most of their negative feedback for aspects of their work that do not involve its content, such as lack of neatness or not trying hard enough. These feedback patterns lead boys and girls to different attributions about the reasons for their own poor performance when they do fail; boys tend to believe the problem is lack of effort, whereas girls more often believe they failed because of lack of ability. These self-attributions relate, in turn, to how hard a child persists at a task after he or she experiences failure. Girls give up more easily after academic failure, but if the feedback contingencies are experimentally changed, "learned helplessness" can be reversed.

Researchers have also documented differential treatment of boys and girls by mathematics teachers. For example, mathematics teachers provide more feedback to boys. Perhaps even more importantly, boys are more likely to get feedback when they get an answer wrong. Teachers sustain the interaction with boys when boys give a partially correct, incorrect, or no response answer, but the same is not true for girls. Teachers are also more likely to initiate verbal contact with male students than with female students. Most of the research in this area has been limited to frequency counts of teacher behavior in direct instruction. One study also documented differential behavior by mathematics teachers in less formal contacts in the classroom—70% of all encouragement in academic abilities and pursuits by the teachers was directed toward boys. Although active discouragement was rare, female students received 90% of the discouraging comments from teachers. These findings come from a variety of schools and involve teachers of both sexes and all ages. In sum, boys and girls do receive differential treatment in the classroom.

DEVELOPMENT OF GENDER IDENTITY

Prenatal Hormonal Influences

When attempting to identify a biological marker of behavioral differences between the sexes, a readily accessible variable is that of steroid hormone levels. Androgen insensitivity, the essential lack of androgen receptor function in an XY male human, illustrates hormonal effects on the development of gender identity. Genetic male infants who through mutation are insensitive to androgen during fetal development are born with external female genitalia; they are raised as female and are not identified as genetically male until a medical workup is done to explain the lack of menses (Breedlove, 1994). These individuals continue life as female, have normal feminine gender identity, and are sexually attracted to men.

Androgen-insensitive male children appear to show the same cognitive sex differences identified among their normal sisters, that is, a propensity toward higher verbal than spatial skills as measured by the WISC (Wechsler Intelligence Scale for Children) (Breedlove, 1994). As stated earlier, this propensity exists but is shrinking. Is this a result of receptor malfunction, socialization from birth, or both?

Girls suffering from congenital adrenal hyperplasia are prenatally androgenized. Is their behavior masculinized by hormones or differences in parental treatment?

People in society behave differentially toward boys and girls. Social reactions are triggered by the biological appearance of the infant, which is, in turn, directed by genetic blueprint. Hence, separation of social and biological influences becomes moot.

Cognitive and Environmental Influences

By 2 years of age, children begin to display sex-typed preferences (for same-sex playmates, toys, games, and clothes). In general, sex-typed preferences increase through middle childhood in tandem with increasing cognitive ability. Exposure to the larger world might be expected to *decrease* sex-typed choices and play preferences because of wider experience. On the contrary, as children grow through middle childhood, male and female play environments become increasingly different (Martin, 1993). There is a snowballing effect of these sex-typed gender preferences. As the sexes choose same-sex playmates and sex-typed play activities, their social microenvironments become increasingly different and, consequently, their social experiences diverge. Sex-typing becomes a developmental self-fulfilling prophecy.

Children of 2 or 3 years of age are able to correctly gender-label photographs of male and female children as well as adults. They also correctly identify their own gender. It is not until several years later, however, that most children acquire gender constancy, the concept that gender is a permanent characteristic. Own-sex favoritism is found in children as young as 2 to 3 years of age and increases until puberty, another example of differential social and cognitive experiences among the sexes during development (Serbin, Powlishta, and Gulko, 1993).

Figure 9–1 (Serbin, Powlishta, and Gulko, 1993) shows the complexity of forces at work in the development of sex-typing. Figure 9–1 is a schema displaying the interaction between cognitive and social variables affecting the development of sex differences in behavior. This bidirectional interaction is further complicated by the biology of the individual, not shown on the figure. Although the number of variables involved is daunting, the biopsychoso-cial analysis of gender differences in behavior is necessary to gain an understanding of the complete process.

Effects of Hormones at Puberty

No studies have been able to disentangle the effects of pubertal hormones on adolescent behavior from society's expectations for opposite-sex peer interactions in adolescence. For additional information on development of sex-typed behavior in adolescence, see Eccles and coworkers (1996) and Chapter 48.

SOCIALIZATION BY ASSOCIATION

Additional research on the socialization of gender is being done outside of the field of developmental psychology by psychological anthropologists. In a landmark study, Whiting and Edwards (1988) reanalyzed the historical six-culture sample by gender and have added five new cultures. This research adds an important cross-cultural perspective to issues surrounding the socialization of gender.

Eleven cultures have been analyzed for differences by sex in dyadic interactions of adults with children and children with children of different ages. The authors concluded that "we are the company we keep," that is, the individuals with whom a person interacts, whether they are infants, peers, or older individuals, elicit particular behaviors from the person. If an individual spends his or her time with an infant, the infant seems to bring forth nurturing responses. If that individual spends enough time with infants, he or she becomes a nurturer. For example, in many cultures, young girls are given child care responsibilities, whereas young boys are not (Whiting and Edwards, 1988). As a function of those responsibilities, girls are more likely to become nurturers. When boys are given child care responsibilities, however, they become more nurturing.

Choices about assigning company may entail choices about shaping personality. Gender roles and the division of labor may play a strong role in causing gender differences. There is considerable evidence that interacting with infants and children brings forth nurturing characteristics. Cur-

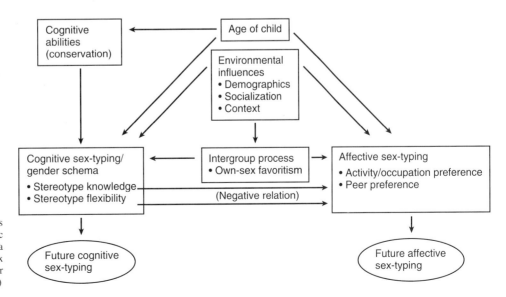

Figure 9–1. The sex-typing process in middle childhood—a schematic model. (From Serbin LA, Powlishta KK, Gulko J: The development of sex typing in middle childhood. Monogr Soc Res Child Dev 58[2]:61, 1993.)

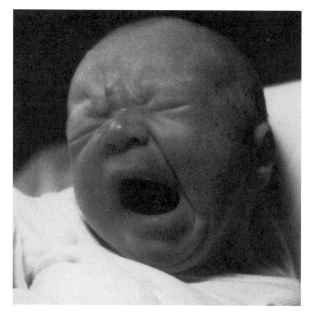

Figure 9–2. What's all this fuss about gender? (Photo by H. Belluci)

rently, women and girls do most of this care, whereas men and boys may even be discouraged from doing it. Should nurturing be encouraged in only one sex? Nurturing may be an antidote for violence. It may be even more important to encourage nurturing qualities in boys than in girls, given the slightly higher average levels of male aggressive behavior.

Conclusion

The most important point about explaining sex differences is that there is very little to explain. Many aspects of human functioning are not particularly dimorphic with respect to sex (Fig. 9–2). Recent publications concentrate not on whether a sex difference exists but on how large a difference really exists. These analyses are sobering if the social implications of the work are considered. It is completely impossible to predict an individual's personality or abilities on the basis of his or her sex. Large numbers of both sexes score at the high and low ends of distributions of birth measures, temperament measures, and intellectual ability tests. Certainly, large numbers of girls and boys are at the high end of distributions for all cognitive tests—enough to fill society's need for persons of exceptional skill. This has important implications both for the individual and for the nation's collective ability to function well.

Researchers often take biological measures (e.g., steroid hormones) and try to predict specific behavioral outcomes as a result of those measures. This is a confusion of research *measures* with behavioral *influences* (Breedlove, 1994). The fault lies in the belief that hormonal *measures* are purely biological when, in fact, they are subject to simultaneous psychological and social influences upon the developing organism.

Parents can play an important role by encouraging their children according to their capabilities and not according to their sex. Teachers can be more aware of their reward systems, which often limit rather than encourage children. Pediatricians are in a unique position to be myth-breakers. They can help parents and teachers to understand that adult expectations can limit or empower children. In regard to psychological functions, attention should be focused on the individual and not on his or her sex. Our goal should be that each child be allowed to fully develop her or his potential.

REFERENCES

Bell RQ, Weller GM, Waldrop MF: Newborn and preschooler: organization of behavior and relations between periods. Monogr Soc Res Child Dev 36:1, 1971.

Benbow CP, Lubinski D: Psychological profiles of the mathematically talented: some sex differences and evidence supporting their biological bases. *In* The Origins and Development of High Ability. Chichester, England, John Wiley & Sons, 1993.

Benbow CP, Stanley IC: Sex differences in mathematics ability: fact or artifact? Science 210:1262, 1980.

Breedlove SM: Sexual differentiation of the human nervous system. Annu Rev Psychol 45:389, 1994.

Connor IM, Serbin LA: Behaviorally-based masculine and feminine activity preference scales for preschoolers: correlates with other classroom behaviors and cognitive tests. Child Dev 8:1411, 1978.

Eccles JS, Flanagan C, Lord S, et al: Schools, families, and early adolescents: what are we doing wrong and what can we do instead? J Dev Behav Pediatr 17:267–276, 1996.

Eccles JS, Jacobs JF: Social forces shape math attitudes and performance. Sign 11:367 1986.

Gualtieri T, Hicks RE: An immunoreactive theory of selective male affliction. Behav Brain Sci 8:427, 1985.

Hyde JS, Linn MC: Are there sex differences in verbal abilities? A meta-analysis. Psychol Bull 104(1):53, 1988.

Hyde JS, Plant EA: Magnitude of psychological sex differences: another side to the story. Am Psychol 50(3):159, 1995.

Jacklin CN: Female and male: issues of gender. Am Psychol 44(2):127, 1989.

Kandel ER, Schwartz JH, Jessell TM, eds: Essentials of Neural Science and Behavior. Norwalk, CT, Appleton & Lange, 1995.

Maccoby EE, Jacklin CN: Sex differences in aggression: a rejoinder and reprise. Child Dev 51:563, 1980.

Maccoby EE, Jacklin CN: The Psychology of Sex Differences. Stanford, CA, Stanford University Press, 1974.

Martin CL: Theories of sex typing: moving toward multiple perspectives. Monogr Soc Res Child Dev 58(2), 1993.

Moss H, Robson K: The relation between the amount of time infants spend at various states and the development of visual behavior. Child Dev 41:509, 1970.

Pilgrim C, Hutchison JB: Developmental regulation of sex differences in the brain: can the role of gonadal steroids be redefined? Neuroscience 60(4):843, 1994.

Rosenthal R, Rubin DB: Further meta-analytic procedures for assessing cognitive gender differences. J Educat Psychol 74:708, 1982.

Rubin JS, Provenzano FJ, Luria Z: The eye of the beholder: parents' views on sex of newborns. Am J Orthopsychiatry 5:353, 1974.

Safer DJ, Allen RP: Hyperactive Children. Baltimore, University Park Press, 1976.

Serbin LA, Powlishta KK, Gulko, J: The development of sex typing in middle childhood. Monogr Soc Res Child Dev 58(2), 1993.

Whiting BB, Edwards CP: Children of Different Worlds: The Formation of Social Behavior. Cambridge, MA, Harvard University Press, 1988.

PART II
Milieux and Circumstances

10 *Culture and Ethnicity*

Sara Harkness • Constance H. Keefer •
Charles M. Super

This chapter about the impact of the child's environment on development and behavior deals with the general culture milieu. The child's "developmental niche" consists not only of the psychological characteristics of his or her immediate caregivers but also of the physical and social settings and prevailing customs of child care. Cultures differ in many ways that bear on childrearing, such as the amount of individuality or privacy encouraged. These variations affect the generation, reporting, and management of behavior problems. The authors offer suggestions on culturally sensitive assessment and interventions.

Pediatricians, like other people who serve children and their families, must increasingly deal with sociocultural differences in the context of their practice. This chapter addresses culture and ethnicity as the most general and pervasive aspect of children's environments. From this perspective, there are three challenges for pediatricians: (1) to develop a broader knowledge base about cross-cultural variation in childrearing and child development, (2) to integrate this knowledge with developmental perspectives and use of standard developmental-behavioral assessment tools to make more informed clinical assessments, and (3) to develop a culturally sensitive attitude in interaction with all patients, including those from the same cultural background as the pediatrician. This chapter first reviews the concepts of culture and ethnicity, presenting a framework for the pediatrician to use in learning about the cultural organization of child life. Also discussed are major dimensions of cross-cultural variation in children's environments and related differences in development, the role of the pediatrician in evaluating individual clinical cases in cultural context, and advocacy issues in culturally sensitive general and developmental-behavioral pediatrics.

Culture, Ethnicity, and Children's Environments

Culture and *ethnicity* are closely linked terms as used by scholars, educators, and clinicians across several fields. Anthropologists use the term culture to mean the way of life of a people, including both the external, socially constructed environments for living (e.g., political systems or housing patterns) and the internalized rules, expectations, and values that guide communication, thinking, and behavior (LeVine, 1973). The idea of culture as being "in

people's heads" has gained attention recently in cognitive approaches to culture (Holland and Quinn, 1987; Schwartz, White, and Lutz, 1992), and this approach seems particularly relevant to the pediatrician who learns about patients' lives mainly through conversation. Central to both external and internal concepts of culture is the idea of *systematicity*. The "culture" of a people is not a random collection of customs, beliefs, and values, but rather an organized and meaningful system, even though it may (and probably does) contain internal contradictions. Parents play a crucial role as mediators and creators of culture (Harkness and Super, 1995).

Ethnicity refers to membership in a culturally defined group, usually in the context of a larger dominant society as is the case with immigrant groups or "minorities." The internal cognitive and emotional dimensions are also sometimes considered under the rubric of ethnicity. Giordano (1973) states

> Ethnicity from a clinical point of view is more than distinctiveness defined by race, religion, national origin, or geography. It involves conscious and unconscious processes that fulfill the deep psychological need for security, identity, and a sense of historical continuity. It is transmitted in an emotional language within the family and is reinforced by similar units in the community.

Ethnic categories often include several groups of varied cultural or national origin, which may differ in important ways, as is the case with both Hispanic and Asian peoples. Growing familiarity with these differences has led to a finer appreciation of the distinctive needs of particular ethnic groups in the clinical setting (McGoldrick, Pearce, and Giordano, 1982). On the other hand, it is also becoming clear that many themes transcend cultural boundaries and that these themes relate systematically to shared aspects of social and family organization as well as to tradition. Thus, consideration of cultural and ethnic issues in pediatrics need not imply building an endlessly elaborated compendium of knowledge. Rather, what is needed is an understanding of the basic dimensions of cultural difference as they operate in families, in combination with knowledge of specific aspects of the backgrounds of particular children and their families.

THE DEVELOPMENTAL NICHE

A useful framework for learning about children's lives from a cultural perspective is the developmental niche (Harkness and Super 1994; Super and Harkness 1997). In this approach, one takes the perspective of the child, looking outward to the environment as it is shaped by features of the larger sociocultural setting. Three groups of factors can be seen to operate: (1) Physical and social settings of everyday life, (2) customs of child care, and (3) the psychology of the caretakers. The three components of the developmental niche operate together as a system, and they interact with features of the larger culture (e.g., customary child care practices are strongly influenced by parents' work patterns). From the pediatric perspective, an important aspect of the developmental niche of any particular child is the adaptability of the niche to the child's temperament and developmental status.

Physical and Social Settings of Everyday Life

Children's environments are organized first in terms of where, with whom, and in what activities they usually spend their days. Is the infant at home alone with mother or in day care for 9 hours each day? Does the 6-year-old girl spend afternoons with a group of neighborhood children at the playground, does she stay home watching television with her brother, or does she help out at the family-run convenience store? What is the learning environment offered in each of these settings with regard to parental involvement, cognitive stimulation, development of interpersonal skills (e.g., cooperation), and the acquisition of social roles? What are the differential patterns of risk with respect to accidental injury, physical abuse, and exposure to pathogens?

Customs of Child Care

Customs of child care involve the caretakers' repertoire of normative strategies for childrearing. Insofar as these are part of shared cultural patterns, they are comfortable and familiar methods that do not call for careful analysis or justification—they seem "natural" and obvious to parents. Is it customary to breast-feed beyond 1 year? Do toddlers normally sleep in the same bed with their parents? Is reading a story naturally part of the bedtime routine? Do parents customarily help with homework in the evening? What are the traditional methods of discipline?

Psychology of the Caretakers

Parental theories about their children's behavior and development are influenced by the larger environments that they and their children occupy, and they are important in making decisions about children's settings of daily life (Harkness and Super, 1996). Although parental theories are often not explicit or developed into a coherent and internally consistent set of beliefs, they underlie customs of child care. When parents confront choices, however, the culturally influenced assumptions that give meaning to the available options may be talked about more explicitly. Should each child have his or her own room? Should young children be encouraged to help out at home—and if so, should they be paid? How should one prepare an older sibling for the birth of a new baby?

Cross-Cultural Variation in Children's Environments and Development

Studies of children and families around the world have shown that American middle class culture is unusual compared to the environments for children derived from many other traditions (DeGenova, 1997; Greenfield and Cocking, 1994; Whiting and Edwards, 1988), including European societies. The following contrasts suggest some of the major dimensions that are relevant for the pediatrician's understanding of the child's culturally structured developmental niche and its implications for behavior and development. These group differences are normal variations built around universal age-related changes (Kagan, 1982).

LOW SOCIAL DENSITY VERSUS HIGH SOCIAL DENSITY

American middle class homes are, by comparison with most other societies, rather sparsely populated: the child may thus spend much time at home with only one caretaker and perhaps a sibling. In contrast, children in many other societies and in some American ethnic groups (e.g., Hispanic Americans) are likely to live in households with more members or where other people are more likely to be around as frequent visitors. This may be true even in societies in which the small nuclear family is the most typical household form. For example, children in some European countries (including Holland, Spain, Italy, and Poland) have more frequent contact with the extended family than do most American children.

In societies in which the nuclear family is closely embedded in the extended family, such as in India and Africa, child care is more likely to be shared and the influence of the mother is seen as less uniquely powerful. The mother may function as an "executive," as is typical in sub-Saharan African groups in which baby-sitting is delegated to older siblings. Related to these variations in settings and customs of child care is an absence of concern about "attachment" in folk theories of child development. The mother does not worry about the effects on the child's development of having her child taken care of by someone else, especially a relative. Empiric research supports this robust view of development. Kermoian and Leiderman (1986), for example, found that Gusii infants in rural Kenya routinely developed secure attachments to both mother and sibling caretaker. Shared child care in the home in US families may also show similar patterns of secure multiple attachments.

PRIVACY VERSUS SHARING

A second dimension of variation is the extent to which the organization of the living space promotes physical separateness and individual ownership of objects in contrast to shared space and few if any individual possessions. In many cultures, the lives of family members are not parceled into different, private spaces and consciously distinct schedules. For example, rural African babies and young children sleep in close proximity to their mothers, and fathers sleep separately; in Japan children sleep on mats next to their parents. In settings such as these, it is not possible to maintain separate regular schedules for different members of the family. Children's sleeping and eating must fit around the activities of other, older members of the family. Likewise, mothers may be more prepared to respond in an ad hoc fashion to the baby's or child's need for food or a nap. Parental ideas about childrearing in these settings do not emphasize the importance of regularity in the baby's or child's daily routines.

There are well-documented differences in development associated with this cultural variation. Among Puerto Rican families living in high-density households in New York City, for example, individual variation in the diurnal regularity of biological functioning (eating, sleeping, elimination) was of little importance and was not related to the manifestation of behavior problems during the preschool years; among a middle class Jewish sample (Chess and Thomas, 1984), however, battles over bedtime and other family routines were far more common and were significantly related to adjustment at age 5 years.

INDIVIDUAL ACHIEVEMENT VERSUS GROUP RESPONSIBILITY

Closely related to the contrast between privacy and sharing is the relative emphasis that different cultural groups place on individual achievement as opposed to the development of a sense of responsibility within the group. American middle class culture places great emphasis on individual achievement, and parents are encouraged to provide children with as much "stimulation" as possible in order to develop their potential talents to the fullest. In some societies and in some groups within US society, however, responsibility is more valued; children may be assigned more household chores at an early age, including the care of younger siblings and tasks that are vital to the family's economic well-being (Fig. 10–1). Children in the rural Kenyan community that we studied, for example, spent half of their time at home in work activities by the age of 6 years. In this setting, parents defined "intelligence" as the ability to do what needed to be done around the homestead *without being asked*. By cross-cultural standards, American middle class children do few household chores, and "intelligence" is defined more in terms of school-related skills.

One effect of this difference in orientation is in children's early language and cognitive development. Studies of young children in non-Western cultures in Africa and the Pacific region, as well as in African American families, have documented many differences in how young children are talked to and how they learn to talk. Although children in all cultures become competent users of their own languages, there are wide differences in the kinds of language-related skills that are learned; for example, arguing effectively according to cultural rules, relating the story of one's day to the assembled family at dinner, or expressing verbally the nuances of one's inner emotional experience. In developmental testing situations, these differences can appear as wide disparities in children's performance on tasks such as retelling a story to an adult tester, with American middle class children scoring much higher than children from different cultures. On the other hand, cross-cultural comparisons of children's development of responsible behavior at home show the opposite contrast:

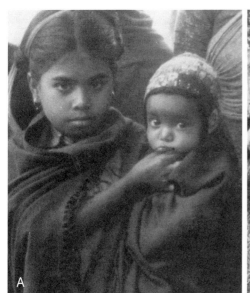
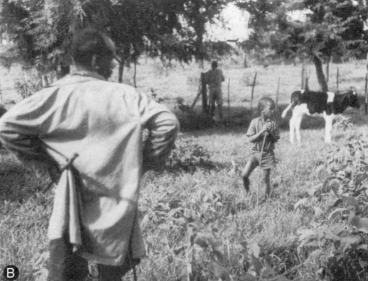

Figure 10–1. Varying responsibilities of children. *A,* In Bangladesh, an older sister carries a baby to keep him safe and contented. *B,* In Kipsigis, Kenya, a father and son keep an eye on the family herd of cows.

children in African societies, for example, routinely take on responsibilities for child care, cooking, housekeeping, and animal care that would be thought beyond their developmental capacities in urbanized Western societies.

INDEPENDENCE VERSUS INTERDEPENDENCE

Another related dimension of variation concerns the way cultures emphasize training for independence as opposed to interdependence (Fig. 10–2). In American middle class culture, the achievement of independence is seen as such a fundamental aspect of normal development that both parents and professionals tend to interpret many behaviors in this framework. The toddler who does not want to be constrained in a car seat is seen as showing a need for independence, just as the uncooperative teenage boy is showing ambivalence about giving up his dependence. Independence is a personal quality that is perceived as essential for success in adult life, not surprisingly in that American young people leave their parents' homes at a very early age when viewed from either historical or cross-cultural perspectives. Furthermore, independent children may be able to cope more easily with the absence of parents who work outside the home. In contrast, interdependence is valued in many other cultures in which parents expect to live in close proximity to at least some of their children for the rest of their lives.

Although these differences in training do produce variation in children's competence in specific skills such as tying one's own shoes and saying good-bye to one's parents without showing distress, many of the same behaviors can be achieved in the service of different cultural goals. Children in rural Kenya learn to walk several miles to the store to do an errand for their mother by about age 6, but, in this case, the "independent" behavior develops in the service of interdependent family relations. Furthermore,

different contexts may be used to emphasize different kinds of behavior. For example, although Japanese patterns of child care at home emphasize dependence on the mother, young Japanese children are customarily sent to nursery school to learn to "get along in a group."

HIERARCHY VERSUS EQUALITY

The modern American middle class family is not only small and individually oriented, it is also egalitarian. In contrast, in societies in which the extended family is important, there is a hierarchy of authority that includes not only parents in relation to dependent children but also adults of different ages, genders, and relationships. In traditional communities of north India, for example, the young married woman is subservient to her husband, but both may be subject to his parents. This difference is expressed in many different domains, but a particularly important one is discipline. In societies characterized by authoritarian relationships within the family, discipline tends to be harsher, and the parent (especially the father) may be emotionally more distant. This pattern is also apt to apply to relationships between the father and mother.

INDIVIDUALISM VERSUS COLLECTIVISM

In recent years, a number of researchers have suggested that the aforementioned differences can be conceptualized as belonging to a general cultural orientation toward either individualism or collectivism (Greenfield and Cocking, 1994; Kagitcibasi, 1997) and that the social development of children must be understood as a process of learning the appropriate orientation through both explicit and implicit communications. As summarized by Killen and Wainryb (in press):

> Cultures with an individualistic orientation are said to value the person as detached from relationships and from the

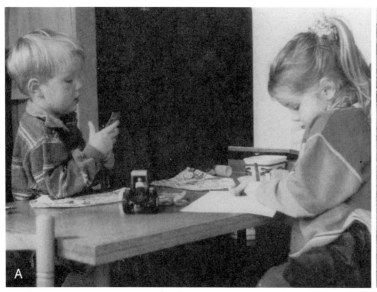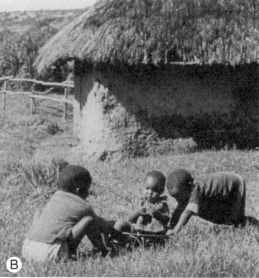

Figure 10–2. Differing styles of sibling play. *A,* In Holland, a sister and brother do artwork together at their own table in the family room. *B,* In Kipsigis, Kenya, two older siblings play with baby sister, pulling her in a cooking pot like a sleigh. The older children are responsible for their little sister while the mother is busy nearby.

community, as independent from the social order, and as motivated to attain personal goals. By contrast, collectivistic cultures value the individual in relation to others and by his or her roles and interdependent duties within the social system.

Further research within this conceptual framework has led to the recognition that even in collectivistic cultures, there is room for individual choice and development, and even the most individualistic societies need to promote a collectivistic orientation to maintain some sense of the social group. Nevertheless, the individualism-collectivism contrast has proved useful for understanding how a variety of different dimensions of cultural difference may relate to each other.

Cultural Considerations in the Clinical Assessment of Developmental-Behavioral Issues

CLINICAL ILLUSTRATIONS

Cultural differences such as those previously described manifest themselves not only in normal development but also in developmental and behavioral problems that parents and others bring to the clinical setting. The following section describes and comments on three clinical cases in which cultural knowledge was needed for the assessment and management of developmental-behavioral issues.

EXAMPLE 1: PORTUGUESE-AMERICAN TODDLER WITH EATING AND SLEEPING PROBLEMS

Mr. and Mrs. Gomes brought their son John, 20 months, to the developmental-behavioral clinic because of his refusal of food, inadequate weight gain, and poor sleeping patterns. Mrs. Gomes (and her mother), dreading every meal and ending each one in tears, had taken to feeding John all day long, following him around with food and a spoon as he played. In addition, they had begun giving him high-calorie, milk-based supplements at bedtime. John was not, and never had been, allowed to feed himself. He looked thin, pale, and weak to his mother and grandmother, and that image was reinforced by neighbors and relatives. Mrs. Gomes was vulnerable to their many comments on his size, accepting them as confirmation of her inadequacy as a mother and allowing her guilt to soar. She was certain that John was anorexic, especially after hearing on the Oprah Winfrey Show that infants could have the disorder.

The feeding problem had been identified early. As a newborn John had difficulty latching on to the breast, a pattern that Mrs. Gomes saw as rejection of food and, very quickly, as her failure. She stopped breast-feeding and initiated feeding solids before 3 months of age. Sleep emerged as a problem abruptly, within a week of the Gomes' moving from the maternal grandparents' home to their own place when John was 9 months of age. Although initially they tried to let him cry out his repeated wakenings in his own room, soon he was sleeping with them. They had lived with Mrs. Gomes' parents since

John's birth, and although he was extremely attached to his grandfather, the Gomes had not realized he would notice the change. In fact, they had not anticipated any of their reactions to the separation until their first visit to the grandparents', about 2 weeks after the move, when John and all four adults burst into tears.

Developmental screening of John showed normal to superior performance in motor, language, cognitive, and social areas, but he would not leave his parents, despite his interest in going to the playroom with the psychologist. He showed great pleasure in play and initiated many contacts with the psychologist, but only a few with his father and none with his mother.

A few points in the Gomes' family histories proved to be most useful in understanding and untangling the problem. Mrs. Gomes' sister had been diagnosed with anorexia as a child, and Mrs. Gomes vividly remembered scenes of her mother fighting, unsuccessfully, to get food into her. Mr. Gomes and his mother, who was apparently obese, had fought with each other over his poor eating as a child, and as an adult he had been significantly overweight.

By reflecting with Mr. and Mrs. Gomes, the clinical team uncovered cultural and generational implications of these histories in the parents' current difficulties with John. Among their Portuguese family and community, a baby should look fat in order to be seen as healthy and normal, and a mother would interpret any comment about her baby's size as a reflection of her success as a good Portuguese mother. The team acknowledged the family's transgenerational feeding and eating problems as history that was clouding the parents' current views of John and themselves, but that the history need not repeat itself. Having clarified those implications, the team proposed parental behavioral changes based on developmental principles. The changes were acceptable to Mr. and Mrs. Gomes, even though previously they had not been obvious. Specifically, the team talked about the emergence of autonomy in the child's 2nd year of life as well as the high degree of awareness that even young infants have for important people around them. The team focused only on the feeding issues because the sleep difficulties were thought to be secondary to the feeding interactions. The parents were asked to stop their involvement in John's eating and allow him total control over his intake, despite the messes and despite their fear of losing him to starvation. The team also suggested that the parents discontinue the bedtime supplements. The parents were asked to keep a record of what John ate each day.

On the return visit 2 weeks later, Mr. and Mrs. Gomes reported dramatic change in John's eating. He was entirely self-feeding, consuming amounts that were more than adequate for the comfort of his mother and grandmother. Even more striking was Mrs. Gomes' description of a day with John. For the first time, he would approach her with toys for positive interaction and for the first time, she enjoyed being with him. She told the pediatrician that she had not realized she *could* play with him, having no recollection of her parents playing with her. John still insisted on sleeping with his parents, but they showed resolve in their need to be together in bed without him and he was wakening less often, probably because of the decrease in bedtime feedings. John's behavior in the clinic supported the team's optimistic appraisal of the situation. He was as pleased as before with the play, but this time he went several times to his mother's knee to show her a toy or for a cuddle, before he approached his father for the same. The parents already had plans for dealing with the sleep problem, asking only for the pediatrician's approval and fine-tuning.

This case illustrates a common kind of behavioral-developmental issue for parents of toddlers in ethnic groups including not only Portuguese but also Hispanic, Italian, and some Asian (notably Indian) populations. In these cultures, mothers feed infants and young children up to a much later age than is considered appropriate in US middle class families. In these cultures also, feeding is often considered *the* core function and defining feature of motherhood. A baby's difficulties with breast-feeding or a toddler's refusal of food is thus interpreted as more generally a rejection of the mother herself. For children with certain temperamental dispositions or for other reasons, however, such feeding practices can lead to conflicts such as that which the Gomes family experienced. It seems likely that the other eating disorders reportedly suffered in earlier generations of the family may have developed along similar lines. The clinical response to the Gomes' case, although based on developmental principles, also substituted an American middle class cultural model of development as involving increasing autonomy and separation as an alternative to the parents' previous cultural model based on interdependence. That the parents could accept this different view so readily may be because the idea of autonomy was presented in relation to only one (admittedly problem) domain and because it was in the service of achieving the parents' primary cultural goal of getting the child to eat more.

EXAMPLE 2: ANGLO-AMERICAN INFANT WITH BEHAVIORAL AND SLEEPING PROBLEMS

At the time that Mr. and Mrs. Pearce brought 6-month-old David to the behavioral-developmental clinic, they were desperate for relief from his constant and demanding irritability and his highly irregular sleep schedule, including nighttime sleep periods of, at most, 1½ hours. The problem had begun at birth, with his parents responding to his every cry, which they heard as signaling hunger. In response, they had continually increased his feedings, which amounted to an almost unbelievable 48 ounces of milk per day in addition to a small amount of solids. David had had a few longer stretches of nighttime sleep in the past 2 months when the parents let him cry after wakening, but they said, "He still needs us to put him to sleep" for naps, bedtime, and after wakening at night.

Mr. Pearce was very supportive of and concerned about his wife, finding her in tears at the end of his working day. No one was getting enough sleep and he felt their lives were drifting apart. These difficulties had seriously challenged their confidence in themselves as parents. Mrs. Pearce had been given up to foster care by her mother at the age of 6 years. She had very fond memories of her foster mother, but the early break with her own mother and the death of her foster mother several years

before David's birth had contributed to her vulnerability to self-doubts as a parent, thus increasing her need to respond to his every cry.

The clinical team's assessment of David showed that his development was normal in cognitive, language, and fine and gross motor development. His temperament was not extreme on most dimensions, although his diurnal schedule as reported by his parents was irregular. It was difficult for the team to imagine him as irritable all day long. An attempt at napping during the clinic revealed behavior typical of David's difficulty falling asleep. He repeatedly raised his head from the mattress, turning it from side to side, bobbing up and down and whimpering. The team also observed, however, that his mother constantly intervened, patting his head with every bob.

Both parents accepted the team's observation of their overintervention with David in this brief episode in the clinic and as they described it at home. They seemed relieved to learn about the concept of overprotection that might be "no favor to the child," as Mr. Pearce later put it. They also quickly saw that their reading of most of David's cries as hunger or a need for attention, and their consequently rapid responses, had actually prevented him from developing his own skills in state regulation even though he seemed by temperament to have the capacity to do so. Based on this understanding, the parents accepted the team's recommendations to reduce his intake of formula and increase solid food, to let him cry for short periods during the day if they had to attend to a task, and to keep a diary of his daily schedule.

Within a week, Mrs. Pearce reported in a telephone call that she had limited David's formula intake and that he was eating much more solid food. Along with these changes in eating, she commented that David seemed happier during the day and was even able to nap without "help" from his parents. On a return visit 2 weeks later, the positive ripple effects of the change in feeding were apparent in other areas of his behavior, such as David's requiring much less parental intervention for going to sleep and sustaining longer periods of nighttime sleep. Mrs. Pearce herself saw that she had overstimulated David in general—with radio playing, lights, mobiles, and a toy-filled bedroom, as well as with her own attentiveness. She was thankful for the permission to pull back, and, in doing so, she continued to discover on her own how to tolerate his cry, how his behavior at night affected his daytime behavior, and how she and her husband could modulate their interventions, entertainment, and activities with David.

This case, like the first one, illustrates the interaction between individual family history and cultural beliefs and practices in the development of a behavioral problem. As a foster child who had suffered twice the loss of her mother, Mrs. Pearce was anxious not to fail her own child. Her attentiveness, however, was also an exaggeration of the standard mainstream American cultural model of responsive parenting. In the parental advice literature, in the media, and through informal networks, American parents constantly receive the message that what infants and children most need is individual attention and "stimulation." Rarely is a concern for *over*stimulation communicated to parents. In contrast to this cultural approach, comparative research on American and Dutch families has shown that Dutch parents are very concerned with maintaining a regular and restful schedule for infants and young children, with the apparent result that Dutch babies sleep significantly more and, when awake, are quieter and less active (Super et al, 1996). In David's case, it seems that what the parents needed most was authoritative advice to counter what they had derived from a combination of personal experience and cultural images of good parenting, advice that demonstrated that being a good parent might be achieved through different routes.

EXAMPLE 3: CONTROL OF FEMALE ADOLESCENT SEXUAL BEHAVIOR IN A HAITIAN FAMILY

Dr. McHale, a Euro-American pediatrician, first met the Bernard family when they brought their children for an introductory visit. The Bernards had emigrated from Haiti several years earlier and had three children, of whom the oldest was 16-year-old Jacqueline. Both parents were present for the initial visit, but Mr. Bernard asked and answered most questions for the children and for his wife. The pediatrician's questions regarding school, sports, and social activities drew short answers from the children and some intrafamily glances as the father described the close supervision of the children that either he or his wife or his brother and sister-in-law provided. The children's out-of-school social activities were limited to extended family and church.

Almost a year later, Jacqueline was brought to the clinic by her father. Mr. Bernard wanted an examination to determine whether his daughter had engaged in sexual intercourse. He was angrily convinced that she had and was insistent on the pediatrician's providing the proof. Jacqueline herself was sullen and uncommunicative with her father. She revealed to the pediatrician that she did have a boyfriend whom she saw secretly, but Dr. McHale's impression was that either Jacqueline was withholding the full story—she denied having intercourse—or she was truly not understanding the pediatrician's vocabulary.

Dr. McHale was surprised and uncomfortable about the degree of involvement of this father in his daughter's intimate development, and confused about how to relate either to his position of total control or to Jacqueline's reticence and distrust. She explained to Jacqueline and Mr. Bernard that an examination would not provide the proof that he sought. She suggested that the family needed to find a way to manage the parents' concern for and surveillance of their daughter's social and physical maturation. In addition, she pointed out that they needed to find a way to support Jacqueline's inevitable independence and social development in this very different culture from what the parents had experienced in their own youth.

Mr. Bernard only reluctantly accepted this idea, and subsequent attempts by Dr. McHale and the child mental health consultants to work on a plan with the family failed. Several times over the next 2 years Mr. Bernard returned with Jacqueline to request pregnancy testing or culture for sexually transmitted disease. Communication between father and daughter had not improved and Mr.

Bernard remained angry. Jacqueline was still sullen but obviously was making her own way in the local adolescent culture. Shortly before graduating from high school, Jacqueline became pregnant and soon after married her second cousin, the father of the baby.

This case illustrates, first, cultural differences in the management of adolescent sexual behavior and, second, the clash of cultures not only between the Haitian parental generation and the American peer culture of their children but also between the parents' expectations of the pediatrician and what the pediatrician saw as her proper role. Strict control of adolescent sexual behavior, especially in girls, is normative in many cultures including Hispanic, Italian, and Asian Indian. In these cultures, it is often the father rather than the mother who has the most difficulty in adjusting to less restrictive American norms and who makes strenuous but unsuccessful attempts to control the daughter's behavior. The conflict over control of sexual behavior also reflects more general differences in authority relations within the family in patriarchal societies, in which men maintain a higher degree of control over both their wives and daughters. When such families move to a different societal environment such as in the United States, there can be significant disruption of family life.

The most striking aspect of this case, however, is the way it illustrates the dilemma faced by the pediatrician when asked to apply her expertise in a way that she finds personally and socially unacceptable. In this case, the pediatrician suggested an alternative strategy involving a change in power relationships among family members. The father, however, was apparently equally uncomfortable with this solution: he wanted help, but on his own terms. The failure in communication between the pediatrician and the father was mirrored in the failure of both the parents and the pediatrician to prevent the occurrence of pregnancy in the unwed adolescent daughter.

In retrospect, Dr. McHale thought that she might have done more to reach Jacqueline herself and learn her perspective on the situation; alternatively, perhaps Dr. McHale could have worked through Haitian community institutions such as the church. Perhaps, however, the outcome was not entirely inappropriate: Jacqueline had finished her education, had married within the community, and could begin a new, more independent stage of her life as a young married woman.

DIMENSIONS OF CROSS-CULTURAL VARIABILITY IN THE CLINICAL CONTEXT

A summary overview of the three cases described herein reveals how each of them relates to some of the dimensions of cross-cultural variability in environments and development set forth in the preceding section. The dimension of *social density*, first, is illustrated in the Portuguese case, in which the extended family lived in close proximity and the grandmother was intimately involved in care of the child. In the Haitian case, likewise, the family's social networks were organized by kinship ties, and the teenaged daughter married a relative. In the Anglo-American case, in contrast, the family lived more on their own and the loss of the mother's mother and foster mother accentuated this relative isolation. All three cases illustrate that both high and low social density can be sources of either support or stress. In relation to *privacy versus sharing*, the Haitian case is particularly striking in the way the father's stance regarding his adolescent daughter's sexual behavior contrasted to American norms of privacy. The dimension of *individual achievement versus group responsibility* is implicit in the Anglo-American case, in which the parents found that they had erred in the direction of providing too much individual stimulation to their baby. The issue of *independence versus interdependence* comes to the fore in both the Portuguese and Haitian cases as a topic that needed to be addressed in the clinical setting. For the Portuguese parents, the idea of independence as a desirable developmental goal was liberating, whereas for the Haitian father, independence in the domain of adolescent female sexuality was unacceptable. In addition, the Haitian case also clearly illustrates the dimension of *hierarchy versus equality* in family relations, including both marital and father-daughter relations. As this summary indicates, both the Portuguese and Haitian families would be categorized as *collectivistic* in their orientation, in contrast to the *individualistic* orientation of the Anglo-American family.

CULTURAL THEMES IN THE CLINICAL CONTEXT: SYMPTOM PRODUCTION AND REPORTING BY PARENTS

The three cases presented herein also illustrate three ways that cultural themes can be manifested in the clinical context of pediatric care. First, behavior problems often reflect cultural themes. Parents are likely to present specific developmental-behavioral problems that are manifestations of larger cultural themes, but usually without conscious awareness of this. In the Anglo-American case, for example, sleep problems are often construed as conflicts having to do with the child's (or the parent's) issues around separation from the other at night, relating to the larger theme of independence. Furthermore, the American cultural model of providing stimulation and attention to the child can create a conflict with the parents' need for the child to learn how to go to sleep and stay asleep without excessive parental intervention, as in the case of David and his parents. Unless the pediatrician understands the symbolic aspects of the situation, even advice based on solid developmental or temperamental information is likely to fail.

Second, problem domains vary cross-culturally. Particular behavioral domains—for example, sleeping, eating, and language or motor development—are especially resonant with the dominant cultural themes of different societies, and this variation is reflected in the kinds of "problems" that parents report to pediatricians. In the Anglo-American case, sleep seems to capture several important themes—independence, privacy (for parents), and regularity of scheduling. In the two first cases presented, it is notable that the Anglo-American and Portuguese parents labeled their problems rather differently, even though similar behavioral issues were involved in both.

Third, cultural themes relate differentially to developmental transitions. These may be particularly important points for the pediatrician to learn about cultural themes and to intervene, because they have different meanings in different cultural contexts. In Africa, for example, the culturally defined transition from infancy to early childhood (which generally happens at around age 2 years, when the next baby is born) signals an end to the baby's favored position as focal point of the family's nurturance and playfulness. In such societies characterized by differential authority relationships within the household, children must learn to take their place at the bottom of the hierarchy once they pass successfully beyond infancy. In American middle class culture, on the other hand, the same developmental transition, coinciding with the onset of rapid language development, relates to the cultural theme of individual achievement, providing parents with opportunities to help their child feel "special" through verbally mediated interactions. In the Haitian case described herein, the developmental transition to adolescence was evidently problematic for the father in the new cultural environment of the United States, although it may have been less so in the home culture.

A Culturally Sensitive Practice of Pediatrics

Bringing cultural sensitivity, in the sense of a nonprejudiced attitude toward unfamiliar practices, to a clinical assessment of behavior and development is not sufficient. In a culturally sensitive practice, the pediatrician approaches the family and the presenting problem with general knowledge of how cultures normally organize beliefs, values, and practices into a consonant whole, with specific knowledge of both the foreign culture and his or her own, and with flexibility in the manner of negotiating information and authority during the clinical communications. Examples of culturally relevant questions that the clinician must consider in the pediatric setting are listed in Table 10–1. This section describes the more profound changes in attitude, assessment, and intervention that, in combination with cultural knowledge, form the basis of a culturally sensitive practice. Table 10–2 summarizes important steps in this process.

A CULTURALLY SENSITIVE ATTITUDE

A culturally sensitive attitude in general and in developmental-behavioral pediatrics is both neutral and alert. Neutrality requires awareness of and perspective on one's own cultural beliefs and biases; alertness requires awareness of the possibility that any practice, problem, or response to pediatric assessment and management may have a cultural basis. This basis may be found at the level of family culture, ethnic community, or the dominant culture. Achieving and practicing with such a culturally neutral and alert eye requires knowledge of various cultures and ethnic groups. It can be attained through continued dialogue with patients themselves, interviews with community or religious leaders, searching the medical and social science literature on relevant ethnic groups, and even reading novels and biographical accounts by cultural insiders. A knowledgeable perspective on one's own ethnic beliefs and biases, those of the dominant, contemporary American

Table 10–1 • Aspects of Culture and Ethnicity in the Pediatric Setting

Principles	Questions
There is wide cultural variability in sleep practices.	Is the baby expected to fall asleep independently and sleep alone at night or do the parents feel the baby should have a caretaker nearby throughout the night?
There is a range of cultural beliefs and practices regarding infant/child feeding.	At what age is the child expected to have control over its own feeding?
Cultures vary in the extent to which independent and dependent behavior are considered normal and desirable.	Are the child's bids for a hug or a snuggle considered "clingy" behavior or the expression of a normal need?
There is cultural variability in ideas about children's needs for parental attention.	Do the parents feel that they should provide "stimulation" for the child's cognitive development or do they believe that children's cognitive competence develops naturally on its own?
Definitions of a "good mother" vary cross-culturally.	How does the developmental-behavioral issue at hand relate to the mother's sense of her own competence?
Fathers' roles relative to authority over childrearing vary across cultures.	Which of the parents is considered more "expert" about children? How is authority for decision making about the child shared?
Cultures vary in terms of how "child-centered" versus "family-centered" they are.	Do parents alter their own schedule to fit the child's perceived individual needs or is the child expected to adapt to the schedule of the family?
Families in different cultures vary greatly in their use of informal or family-based sources of information and support versus formal or "expert" sources.	Who beyond the parents is considered an appropriate child care provider? Whom do the parents call upon first for advice on a behavioral issue?
Parents' presentation of children's problems are often built around culturally salient themes and behavioral domains.	What culturally symbolic themes does the presenting problem relate to? How does this domain of behavior (e.g., feeding, sibling relations) or developmental transition (e.g., self-dressing, starting school) figure in the larger traditional culture?

culture, and the medical system as a culture must also be attained. The sources are similar to those for knowledge of others' cultures. Many medical education centers and private and professional societies offer postgraduate courses for enhancing one's cultural learning, not only for knowledge but also for skill and attitude.

A culturally sensitive attitude is adaptable and clarifying, and its goal is to support parents in making effective choices in harmony with their cultural goals and beliefs. In some ways it is antithetical to the usual medical approach,

Table 10–2 • Seven Steps to the Development of Culturally Sensitive Attitudes, Assessment, and Intervention

1. Acquaint yourself with the child's developmental niche, including daily routines, caretaking practices, and the cultural beliefs that give these meaning for the parents.
2. Use the six dimensions of cross-cultural variability (social density, privacy-sharing, achievement-responsibility, independence-interdependence, hierarchy-equality, and individualism-collectivism) to "place" the child and family in cultural perspective.
3. Explore with the parents how particular developmental-behavioral issues relate to their own cultural and personal backgrounds.
4. Use standard assessments (e.g., motor, language, cognitive, social, temperament, and attachment measures) to better understand the parents' presentation of "problems" regarding the child's behavior and development.
5. Be aware that standard developmental assessment tools reflect the cultural biases of the population for which they were developed.
6. Use your knowledge of the parents' practices, beliefs, and goals in formulating advice for handling developmental-behavioral issues.
7. Use the six dimensions of cross-cultural variability to place your own personal and cultural beliefs and values in perspective, and apply this knowledge to increase your cultural sensitivity with all patients, including those from similar backgrounds to yours.

because the pediatrician in this situation must listen attentively and must work to elicit the patient's own meaning, rather than impose a ready-made structure on the communication. People of differing cultures vary in intimate ways of being and thinking. Language shortcuts, slang, and even medical jargon can carry shared meanings efficiently between doctor and patient of the same culture, but they cannot be used with patients of different cultures without risking the flow of mutually meaningful information (Pedersen, 1985). To avoid this, the pediatrician must often be in a receptive rather than an active mode when assessing behavioral and developmental problems; certainty must be put aside for searching. Ballotting the abdomen and waiting for the informative return of the spleen is a close medical analogy to this sort of work. When resuming an action mode after such an attentive pause, the pediatrician should use other interactive skills such as problem solving, rather than answer-giving, in the traditional diagnostic phase, and negotiation, rather than prescription-giving or unilateral decision making, in the treatment or management phase. Both of these skills require holding open several options while exploring the benefits, limitations, and possible consequences of each one. In addition, pediatric adaptability must relate not only to choices of childrearing patterns and developmental outcomes but also to differences in utilization of medical services and definitions of problems. Patients must play an active role in shaping appropriate care.

Because culture is an organized and meaningful system, as indicated by the niche framework, a culturally sensitive approach in pediatric practice can be systematized along the same lines. Of particular significance to the practitioner is an understanding of how cultural beliefs and goals held by parents are used to organize children's daily environments and in customary childrearing practices. In general, as previously discussed, the beliefs of a culture support customary practices, which, if successfully carried out, lead to actualization of the shared values.

For example, the customs for infant sleep in Japan are different from those of the Euro-American middle class families in the United States. Japanese newborn infants sleep with their parents and continue to do so well into the school years. In the United States, on the other hand, newborns are customarily placed in a cradle near their parents' bed and are soon moved into their own bedroom. Parents in these two cultural settings can usually talk about the theory that supports their use of the local pattern for infant sleeping arrangements. Japanese mothers typically believe that the newborn is quite separate as an individual, even unconnected to others, so caregiving behaviors are chosen that lead to close physical contact between parent and infant. Euro-American parents often state the belief that the newborn infant is totally dependent on the mother, so caregiving behaviors that progressively leave the infant on his or her own are more often chosen.

These theories lead parents to choose (consciously or unconsciously) patterns of caregiving with their infants that are more likely to lead to the ideal adult in their own culture. The custom of sleeping with the newborn is an early actualization of the Japanese ideal of interdependence, just as it is an expression of a cultural model for what children need for proper development. Similarly, the Euro-American practice of putting down newborns in their own beds, and even in their own rooms, is a realization of the US ideals of independence and self-actualization.

Many individual customs or parental practices of childrearing are based on beliefs and values that are often not made explicit by the parent. When parents have a problem with their child's behavior, discovery of their underlying beliefs is important; those beliefs often support a continued practice that may not fit that particular child's temperament or that may not be suitable to the child's developmental stage. Reassuring or advising parents will probably fail unless their own beliefs and values are uncovered and tested. Once these are made explicit, other means of actualizing them can be sought. Taking a cultural perspective at the family level can alert one to a path of inquiry that opens up new possibilities

CULTURALLY SENSITIVE ASSESSMENT

Standardized tests normally offer the pediatrician a powerful and efficient method of assessing the nature and degree of developmental disturbance. However, variation in the cultural environments of children and their corresponding developmental differences point to the importance of considering culture and ethnicity when the pediatrician assesses behavioral development.

The application of standard tests of assessment to populations beyond the one for which norms were developed is problematic (American Psychological Association, 1992), and cross-cultural psychologists have been especially concerned with the possibilities for misuse and misunderstanding (Irvine and Carroll, 1980). The most obvious problem, that differences in experience will produce differences in norms, is not the greatest one. More serious is the fact that items in the test are usually chosen in light of cultural values and frequency of behaviors in Euro-American children. There is little conceptual (as opposed to empiric) basis for the most popular tests, including the Bayley Scales and the Denver Developmental Screening Test (Super, 1981). What children are seen to do and the age that they are seen to do it are captured in these tests, but when the tests are used on a new population, the developmental skill underlying the specific behavioral items may not be captured; in short, the construct validity may be threatened. Thus when children of a different culture do not perform a test item, it is not known whether they have merely failed in a specific act or whether they lack the social, representational, or motor skills that the item was designed to tap.

For example, 9-month-old Gusii infants in rural Kenya, when presented with a doll in the context of the Bayley examination, characteristically exhibit negative responses rather than the social responses (e.g., cuddling) that this part of the test was designed to elicit; to the Gusii mothers, the inert doll looked strange, too much like a dead baby (Keefer et al, 1990). It would be difficult to assess the social development of Gusii infants based on their response to this item of the Bayley scale. Moreover, other potential items in the Bayley examination that would reflect culturally significant aspects of development in other ethnic groups (e.g., sharing in the African context) do not appear on these American tests at all—the test as a collection of items is biased. Thus, until the behavioral scope of such tests is widened or culture-specific adaptations are made, the pediatrician should be cautious about their application and interpretation with children of other ethnic groups (Miller, Onotera, and Deinard, 1984).

CULTURALLY SENSITIVE INTERVENTION

The pediatrician can use cultural knowledge and sensitivity, together with thoughtful use of developmental assessments, to establish a strategy of intervention relevant to the needs of both the child and the parents. In this context, understanding the issues that parents face in their own cultural environments can help the pediatrician to intervene most effectively on behalf of the child's developmental needs. A recent immigrant family, for example, may have trouble adjusting to a change from a large extended family household living around a courtyard to a small nuclear household living in an apartment among strangers. In this situation, the mother may be feeling depressed and the young child may not be receiving adequate attention and care. Understanding the nature of this problem is central in helping the parents to reorganize their new environment and their own behavior constructively.

The pediatrician must also be alert to issues of "fit" between the child's culturally structured home environment and the wider environments of school, peer groups, and ultimately work settings. Anthropologists have noted that parental goals are oriented to the needs of adult life as parents have experienced them in the past or imagine them to be in the future (LeVine, 1973). For different cultural or ethnic groups, this orientation may not be compatible with success in middle class American society, and this presents particular problems to the pediatrician. For example, as discussed previously, the Puerto Rican children in Thomas and Chess' New York Longitudinal Study who had irregular sleep patterns presented no behavioral difficulties during the preschool years, but they did encounter problems with the structure of public school schedules when they started kindergarten. In such situations, pure cultural relativism—accepting all cultural systems as equally valid—is an inadequate response. Instead, the pediatrician faces a double challenge: (1) to understand the child's home environment and development as culturally structured phenomena and (2) to help the parents and child negotiate a successful relationship with the wider world.

Cultural Advocacy Issues: The Right to Be Different

A culturally sensitive attitude in diagnosis and intervention is an essential tool in clinical pediatrics. Children's development is shaped, in part, by the settings of their daily lives, the customs of care used at home, and the psychology of the caretakers. These three aspects of the developmental niche are, in turn, regulated by larger aspects of the culture in which the children and parents live. The broadly middle class, Euro-American environment, which forms the basis for the culture of medicine, differs in important ways from the environment of many modern pediatric patients. To hear the meaning of behaviors behind parents' depiction, to see the development underlying possibly biased standardized assessments, and to intervene in ways that are accepted and effective: these are the challenges in creating a culturally appropriate developmental-behavioral pediatrics. To meet this challenge, the pediatrician must turn an ethnographer's eye not only toward the patient but also toward his or her own personal beliefs and to those of the medical system itself. Just as the pediatrician must be an advocate for the right of the individual child to be different, he or she must also be an advocate for the right of particular cultures or subcultures to be different, even in the face of pressures from the dominant culture. Clarity and certainty, when an action is based on solid scientific data, are most useful when combined with cultural knowledge and a culturally sensitive perspective that allow for the rich varieties of normal human behavior and development.

REFERENCES

American Psychological Association: Ethical principles for psychologists and code of conduct. Washington, DC, American Psychological Association, 1992.

Chess S, Thomas A: Origins and Evolution of Behavior Disorders. New York, Brunner/Mazel, 1984.

DeGenova MK: Families in Cultural Context: Strengths and Challenges in Diversity. Mountain View, CA, Mayfield, 1997.

Giordano J: Ethnicity and Mental Health: Research and Recommendations. New York: National Project on Ethnic America of the American Jewish Committee, 1973.

Greenfield PM, Cocking RR (eds): Cross-Cultural Roots of Minority Child Development. Hillsdale, NJ, Lawrence Erlbaum, 1994.

Harkness S, Super CM (eds): Parents' Cultural Belief Systems: Their Origins, Expressions, and Consequences. New York, Guilford, 1996.

Harkness S, Super CM: Culture and parenting. In Bornstein MH (ed): Handbook of Parenting: Biology and Ecology of Parenting, Vol 2. Hillsdale, NJ, Lawrence Erlbaum, 1995.

Harkness S, Super CM: The developmental niche: a theoretical framework for analyzing the household production of health. Soc Sci Med 38:217, 1994.

Holland D, Quinn N (eds): Cultural Models in Language and Thought. New York, Cambridge University Press, 1987.

Irvine SH, Carroll WK: Testing and assessment across cultures: issues in methodology and theory. In Triandis HC, Berry JW (eds): Handbook of Cross-Cultural Psychology: Methodology, Vol 2. Boston, Allyn & Bacon, 1980.

Kagan J: Canalization of early psychosocial development. Pediatrics 70:474, 1982.

Kagitçibasi C: Individualism and collectivism. In Berry JW, Poortinga Y, Pandey J (eds): Handbook of Cross-Cultural Psychology: Social Behavior and Applications, 2nd ed, Vol 3. Boston, Allyn & Bacon, 1997.

Keefer CH, Dixon S, Tronick E, Brazelton TB: Cultural mediation between newborn behavior and later development: implications for methodology in cross-cultural research. In Nugent JK, Lester BM, Brazelton TB (eds): The Cultural Context of Infancy: Multi-Cultural and Interdisciplinary Approaches to Parent-Infant Relations, Vol 2. Norwood, NJ, Ablex, 1991.

Kermoian R, Leiderman PH: Infant attachment to mother and child caretaker in an East African community. Int J Behav Dev 9:455, 1986.

Killen M, Wainryb C: Independence and interdependence in diverse cultural contexts. In Harkness S, Raeff C, Super CM (eds): Variability in the social construction of the child. New Dir Child Dev, in press.

LeVine RA: Culture, Behavior, and Personality. Chicago, Aldine, 1973.

McGoldrick M, Pearce JK, Giordano J (eds): Ethnicity and Family Therapy. New York, Guilford Press, 1982.

Miller V, Onotera RT, Deinard AS: Denver Developmental Screening Test: Cultural variations in Southeast Asian children. J Pediatr 104:481, 1984.

Pedersen P (ed): Handbook of Cross-Cultural Counseling and Therapy. Westport, CT, Greenwood Press, 1985.

Schwartz T, White GM, Lutz CA (eds): New Directions in Psychological Anthropology. New York, Cambridge University Press, 1992.

Super CM: Behavioral development in infancy. In Munroe RH, Munroe RL, Whiting BB (eds): Handbook of Cross-Cultural Human Development. New York, Garland Press, 1981.

Super CM, Harkness S: The cultural structuring of child development. In Berry JW, Poortinga Y, Pandey J (eds): Handbook of Cross-Cultural Psychology: Basic Processes and Human Development, 2nd ed, Vol 2. Boston, Allyn & Bacon, 1997.

Super CM, Harkness S, van Tijen N, van der Vlugt E, Fintelman M, Dijkstra J: The three R's of Dutch child rearing and the socialization of infant arousal. In Harkness S, Super CM (eds): Parents' Cultural Belief Systems: Their Origins, Expressions, and Consequences. New York, Guilford, 1996.

Whiting BB, Edwards CP: Children of Different Worlds: The Formation of Social Behavior. Cambridge, MA, Harvard University Press, 1988.

11 Variations in Family Composition

John Sargent

 In recent decades family structures have changed somewhat toward fewer "traditional" families and more dual-career, unmarried, or single-parent families and living with nonparental relatives, as well as situations with two gay parents. Children today are being raised in more varied settings. This chapter wisely advises pediatricians to evaluate parenting quality in terms of commitment and appropriateness rather than with regard to preconceived criteria as to what structure is right. See Chapter 16 for discussion of the content of healthy and dysfunctional parenting.

The pediatrician sees children from families of varying composition and varying cultural backgrounds on a daily basis. Over the past 40 years, the typical family environment within which children grow up in the United States has changed dramatically. No longer are most children raised in two-parent families in which the father works outside the home and the mother is the homemaker with primary responsibility for the children. There are now all varieties of family composition. Children may live with two working parents, both of whom pursue careers; with unmarried parents; with single parents of either gender; with grandparents; with gay parents; or in state-supported living situations (Table 11–1).

The central requirement of parenting, regardless of who is carrying out the parenting role, remains the conscious commitment of these individuals to be responsible for the child's physical and emotional well-being and successful development (Goldstein, Freud, and Solnit, 1973, 1979). This chapter reviews the strengths, weaknesses, and risks for effective child development that are inherent in varying family structures and also presents a model for pediatric family assessment in relationship to childrearing that can be used for different family situations. In conclusion, I also propose specific concerns for pediatric advocacy to further prevent problems for children living in nontraditional families. (Adoptive and foster families are discussed in Chapter 13 and stepfamilies are discussed in Chapter 15. Specific family dysfunctions are presented in Chapter 16.)

The Traditional Family

The traditional family of 40 years ago was one in which two adults entered into a marriage that lasted throughout their lifetimes and from which children were born. The father worked outside the home and the mother worked primarily as a homemaker who took care of the children and ensured their health and daily safety. The mother also provided nurturing and encouraged socialization, school attendance, and academic involvement. Two myths remain prevalent concerning this form of traditional family: (1)

that this traditional father-breadwinner, mother-homemaker family is rare and is found in fewer than 10% of American households; and (2) that this form of family structure is idyllically happy and satisfying for all participants—father, mother, and children. In fact, recent data indicate that at least 35% of American preschoolers currently live in two-parent households in which the father works and the mother is not employed outside the home, works as a homemaker, and cares for the children (Popenoe, 1989). This percentage decreases as the children begin full-time attendance at school and get older, but at present fully one third of American children are raised in this form of family.

Although this traditional nuclear family had many strengths, it was never as satisfying for all the participants as myth would have it. In a successful traditional family, the availability of the mother provided consistency for the children and concern for their development, their happiness, and their achievement. If childrearing was satisfying for a woman, the children enjoyed her presence and thrived from her attention. Problems might be noticed earlier, roles and responsibilities were clear, and insofar as there was adequate recognition within the family of the contributions of both the father and the mother, this traditional family structure was successful. Several problems were present in many traditional families, however. As work became more complicated and more demanding, the father became less and less available to the family. He was involved outside the family in an activity that was respected, brought in external rewards, and was potentially stimulating and interesting. In this form of American family, the father had more economic power than the mother, whereas he had little direct input with the children (Leupnitz, 1988). They missed his attention, support, encouragement, and role modeling. Meanwhile, the mother worked daily at physical tasks that were often repetitive, not stimulating, and not rewarded through external remuneration. She was often isolated, especially as the American family grew more mobile and nuclear families grew more geographically and emotionally distant from the extended family. In these situations, the mother frequently came to rely on her children for praise, involvement, friendship, and support. In the more problematic situations, the children frequently

Table 11-1 • Changes in Family Composition, Roles, and Structures

Frequent changes in family membership and family structure
Increase in single-parent families
Enhanced role of grandparents and extended family
Increased use of day care
Rise in female-headed households with woman working
More two-career families
Nontraditional families:
    Unmarried parents
    Community-raised children (e.g., kibbutz, commune)
    Gay parents
Children living with other relatives

had difficulties separating from their mother and had little direct involvement with their father. As the children grew older and needed less of the mother's nurturing and direct involvement, it was often difficult for her to decide on a career or to re-enter the work force. In these situations, the woman often overtly taught her daughters to be like her while implying covertly that her life was dissatisfying and unrewarding. Sons learned from their fathers that excitement existed outside the family and that women were to be relied on as caretakers rather than as collaborators and equals.

With increasing awareness of these difficulties, many two-parent families have attempted to develop greater flexibility. They have increased involvement of the father in childrearing and made possible more options for the mother even if she chooses to stay home with the children and take care of the home. If problems develop with the children or with other areas of the family's life, a rigid role structure can inhibit the flexibility needed to respond to these problems and develop creative solutions. If roles are more flexible and both parents are actively involved in childrearing, the choice of one parent to remain home with the children to enjoy time with them and to be available for them can be a positive, rewarding, and exciting choice and one that is made with the knowledge that the choice can be changed at any time it seems necessary or appropriate. This flexibility can provide significant self-esteem for the children as they experience their importance in their parents' eyes and the ways in which family members can be in charge of themselves and make choices concerning their time and the direction of their lives. Respect for the choice of the parent who stays at home, appreciation of the value of childrearing, and the flexibility to change are necessary components of successful traditional families. If these things exist, the degree of attention, affiliation, and support that the children receive from both parents can be truly nurturing and can create strong bonds of affection, connection, and commitment. When parents feel locked into exclusive, separate, and constricted roles—father-breadwinner and career person, mother-homemaker and primary child care provider—the members of these families can become overwhelmed, unhappy, and unrewarded.

Dual-Career Families

The variety of childrearing situations in modern America now includes increasing numbers of dual-career families (approximately 10% of couples with children; Holder and Anderson, 1989). In these families, childrearing is often stressful for both parents and child. The need for effective child care and flexibility on the part of the parents to attend to the requirements of their careers and those of their children, as well as their activities and academic pursuits, can lead the family to be perpetually in motion and always busy. Children can feel pressure to contain themselves and manage their own lives independently, especially "latch-key" children who are alone after school until their parents come home from work (Elkind, 1983). There may be ambivalence in both parents concerning the balance among work activities, career advancement, and childrearing. Parents who divide their time between a career or profession and childrearing also have to deal with the pressures associated with work and the demands inherent in career advancement. Travel away from the home on business is commonly a problem in these families, requiring tight scheduling, close communication, and mutual support.

The husband and wife in dual-career families require a strong commitment to their marriage and marked flexibility in planning and being with their children. These families are most successful when there is significant mutual support between the parents, joy in being with the children, and a healthy sense of competence and effectiveness on each parent's part (Holder and Anderson, 1989). Parents can be unprepared for problems with discipline and can be unaware of difficulties that children may have in overestimating their capacity to manage themselves. Intercurrent illnesses and major life transitions, such as chronic illness or development of the children, often pose serious difficulties for these families, requiring flexibility and the capacity to re-evaluate and modulate career activity based on family needs (Libow, 1989; Rosman, 1988). Parents in dual-career families will often feel pressure from their jobs to demonstrate commitment, loyalty, and availability, which pulls them away from the children and increases any lingering ambivalence they may have about their choice of career and the balance of their activities between job and childrearing. This is often particularly difficult for the woman of the family who may feel that she is missing time with her children or that if she chooses a part-time position, she is endangering her opportunities for career advancement and exciting and fulfilling work. Effective role modeling for the woman is often lacking. Her mother may have been home with her when she was growing up and may not support the woman's choice to both pursue a career and have children. Special problems for children in dual-career families are summarized in Table 11-2.

Unmarried Parents

Households in which the child lives with two parental figures who are not married make up 28% of all households. This form of family composition can include partners who have never married and are living together, have made a commitment to stay with each other, and choose to have children as part of their lives together. Unmarried parental figures also frequently live with children who are the product of one or the other parent's previous marriages

Table 11–2 • Special Problems for
Children in Dual-Career Families

Need for effective child care
Need to support child's academic and social achievement and
    participation in activities and peer relationships
Stress associated with career concerns, tight scheduling, and
    travel
Possible lack of opportunities for recreation and child-focused
    family activities
Parents' possible lack of energy for the rigors, tensions, and
    uncertainties associated with childrearing
Difficulty with illness management and for children with special
    needs and handicapping conditions

or previous relationships. These families can work well for children if there is a strong bond between the parental figures, and their commitment to the children is warm, caring, and strong. In some situations these families are transitional families in which the parental figures plan to marry at some point in the future. The strength of the parental relationship in these situations often grows, and the family situations becomes increasingly permanent for the children. Issues inherent in raising children in stepfamilies are discussed further in Chapter 15.

The major developmental risk in families with unmarried parents or parental figures is the lack of permanence and the sense of stress engendered by conflicts concerning the relationship between the parental figures. Children easily experience the tenuousness and uncertainty inherent in some unmarried parents' relationships and can find this anxiety-provoking and uncomfortable. The stress associated with plans that are made and not followed through, ruptures in the parental figures' relationship, whether temporary or permanent, or conflicts between parental figures about what direction their relationship is going can be quite difficult for the children. These problems also are consuming for the parents, withdrawing their attention from the children and requiring that the children be more responsible for themselves than they are able to be. Children also react strongly to signs of distress in their parents if there are problems in the parental relationship. The relationship between unmarried parental figures can be difficult for grandparents and other involved relatives, including the noncustodial parent from a previous marriage, creating further stress and conflict within the family and for the children. If the parents are committed to one another and if changes in their relationship—whether they remain together, marry, or terminate the relationship—are planned and carried out in a compassionate and nonexplosive manner, children can find living in these families comfortable and quite successful. When family life is disrupted by conflict, inconsistency in who lives in the home, and painful ruptures of adult relationships, things become much more problematic. These difficulties can also involve the children's experiencing economic changes, moving frequently, and being uprooted from community, friends, and school. The children may also recognize that their parents' relationship is different, leading to further confusion and causing insecurity as well as taunts and teasing from peers.

Single-Parent Families

It was correctly projected that 70% of children born in 1980 would live for a time with a single parent by the time they reached 17 years of age. The divorce rate has increased to 21 divorces per 1000 marriages/year, leading to a projection that as many as 45% of marriages formed today will end in divorce. Births to unmarried women in 1985 totaled 22% of all children born (Popenoe, 1989). Other factors significantly influence the impact of these figures; children living with single mothers have lower incomes and a lower standard of living. Divorced or unmarried fathers are increasingly uninvolved in their children's lives—emotionally, physically, or financially. Eighty percent of divorced women work outside the home (Holder and Anderson, 1989). African American families demonstrate higher rates of unmarried births (now 60%), with some period of single parenthood for children (now 94%) in greater rates of poverty and homelessness (Popenoe, 1989).

Single parenting is a difficult process. The parent frequently works, often faces economic hardships, readily becomes tired, and often has difficulty establishing effective and rewarding social contacts. Numerous writers have highlighted the risks inherent in single parenting and have outlined features of successful single-parent families (Boyd-Franklin, 1989; Brown, 1988; Fulmer, 1988; Hines, 1988; Lindblad-Goldberg, 1987, 1989). Of major importance are the emotional and physical well-being of the parent and the parent's ability to develop and maintain a level of energy, optimism, and commitment to the children. Discipline is often difficult to maintain with consistency, and unexpected stresses such as illness in the children can be particularly problematic. Single parents who work must rely on alternative sources of child care, including day care when the children are young (Bradt, 1988). Older siblings often have significant responsibilities within the family that may interfere with peer relationships and their attention to academic and nonacademic interests. The single parent shares the child with many other adults who may be verbally praised by the child, whereas the parent who lives with the child receives the child's anger, frustration, and criticism. Single parents must be sensitive and self-confident enough to realize that this anger and criticism may reflect the fact that the child feels safe enough to voice these feelings only with the single parent. The single parent should also find methods of supporting the child's relationship with the other parent (Brown, 1988). This can be particularly difficult when it is emotionally painful for the parent living with the child, as in the case of divorce, abandonment, criminal behavior, abuse, or parental death. The child's statements can never be the sole indication of the parent's adequacy. If this occurs, the child becomes excessively responsible for the parent's self-esteem, limiting the parent's flexibility and options by his or her opinion, which may represent developmentally immature judgment. The child also cannot consistently be the parent's primary source of social contact or emotional support. If this occurs, separations, changes in the child's activities, or interests or difficulties of concern to the child become threats to the parent's emotional well-being. The parent may then respond to his or her distress by attempting to control rather than guide or support the child. Major concerns in single-parent families are listed in Table 11–3.

Single-parent families more often are headed by women. Economic difficulties in female-headed households are greater (Holder and Anderson, 1989). The mother may feel more conscious ambivalence about working and the amount of time she spends with her children. If the father or male figures have abandoned the family, acted abusively, or proved not to be trustworthy, it may be difficult for the children (male or female) to learn to appreciate, trust, and act assertively with men. Extended family, especially grandmothers, may find it difficult to be supportively involved, and their criticism of the single mother can lead to her worsening isolation, stress, and a sense of being overwhelmed. Lack of time for a social life and personal enjoyment can further burden the single mother. In these situations, the mother can become depressed, exhausted, and "burned out," leading to further self-recrimination, isolation, and frequently mistrust of helping figures.

The primary risks to the development of children living in single-parent homes generally arise from this cycle of burden, exhaustion, depression, and isolation experienced by the family. Young children are at risk for social withdrawal and depression if their primary caretaker is frequently unavailable because he or she is exhausted and depressed. Socialization can suffer if discipline is erratic and rules are inconsistently enforced. Often minor misbehaviors go unnoticed for a time until a threshold is reached and then an excessive (pent-up) response is delivered. The parent later recognizes that this response was excessive, feels guilty, and the discipline is undone, rendering the child confused and without effective limits. Single-parent families are more likely to have difficulties at points of change in child development without the supportive assistance of other adults. Chronic illness, physical disability, and intellectual academic or emotional difficulties caused by a need for special attention and treatment place increased demands on single-parent families (Libow, 1989; Rosman, 1988). Single mothers may have more problems disciplining adolescent sons, whereas single fathers may have more difficulties with adolescent daughters, especially in situations in which the parent has had seriously troubled and painful relationships with members of the opposite sex. Significant emotional difficulty or physical illness in the custodial single parent always requires the involvement of alternative adults in childrearing.

Frequently middle class families do not live near extended family and are self-reliant and somewhat isolated. Divorce or death of a parent requires that these single-parent families develop effective social support networks (Barth, 1989; Walsh and McGoldrick, 1988). Alternatively, as often occurs, the family moves closer to extended family, or a new spouse enters the household, requiring further adjustments from the child and creating further stresses.

In the face of these difficulties, it is important to remember that single-parent families can raise children successfully. The central features that lead to effective childrearing in these families include (1) most importantly, the willingness of the parent to organize and direct sources of support and the ability of these support persons to collaborate effectively with the parent; (2) the parent's capacity to be open, direct, and understanding with his or her children, recognizing their contributions to family life and supporting their need for enjoyment and accomplishment outside the family; (3) one or more strong personal friendships for the parent and available and supportive adults concerned about the child's life (teacher, coach, day care teacher, extended family member); (4) a level of economic well-being that is *perceived* as adequate by the family; (5) trusted resources (pediatrician, school personnel, and mental health professionals) who assist the parent and children in identifying problems rapidly and implementing effective solutions while supporting the single parent (Lindblad-Goldberg, 1989).

Children Living With Grandparents or Extended Family

Whether because of parental incapacity, parental wish, or the absence of parents resulting from abandonment or death, many children grow up, for a time or throughout childhood, in families headed by grandparents or other members of the extended family. Children usually come to these living situations after a period with one or both biological parents and after experiencing significant stress, hardship, or emotional turmoil. At times, a child's move to extended family occurs because of legal intervention and the efforts of social service agencies; at times, it occurs because of the wishes of the biological parents. Sometimes there may have been family conflict or legal conflicts over where a child should live, and often the parents, grandparents, or extended family may be disappointed when the child lives with a particular relative. The child may have had to move, leaving friends, neighborhood, and school behind, and he or she may be moving into a home with other children whom the child may not know well. Both the child and the caretaking relatives may be ambivalent or directly antagonistic toward the child's biological parents, and there may be emotional turmoil within the family because of the biological parents' difficulties. If this change in living situation has occurred because of the death of one or both parents, the children and relatives will be grieving in addition to experiencing the stress caused by the child's move (Barth, 1989). The pediatrician may learn of this change in living situation only when a child is brought for evaluation of an acute illness or for a physical examination mandated by school. Many of these children may have had developmental delay or emotional or behav-

---

Table 11–3 • Key Issues in Single-Parent Families

Emotional support from social network
Quality of alternative sources of child care
Financial status
Capacity to maintain appropriate discipline
Interest and enjoyment of child's strengths and accomplishments
Ability to develop own rewarding social life and relationships
Capacity to parent when exhausted or overwhelmed
Capacity to support child's relationship with noncustodial parent
Capacity to collaborate effectively in childrearing with other
    involved adults (noncustodial parent, grandparents, and so on)

ioral problems prior to moving in with the relative, and these pre-existing difficulties can make adjustment to a new living situation even more difficult.

It can be an extraordinarily taxing experience for grandparents to again parent children (Boyd-Franklin, 1989). New children require attention, nurturing, and discipline. They require patience as they deal with the stress of moving and adjusting to a new living situation, and they require support as they deal with their emotional reactions and feelings about their parents. These difficulties can vary as the children develop, with older children requiring more energy and flexibility, especially in managing discipline and socialization. Grandparents may not know other families in their community with children the age of their grandchildren. They may also be physically ill or have less energy than their grandchildren require, and they may have very different ideas about childrearing and discipline than the parents or previous caretakers. Grandparents also may experience marital stress and diminished social ties when raising grandchildren (Minkler and Roe, 1993; Minkler, Roe, and Robertson-Beckley, 1994). In situations in which the parents have emotional problems of their own, especially substance abuse or a major psychopathologic condition, grandparents may be concerned about their ability to parent their grandchildren more effectively and they may also wonder about the genetic influence of the emotional difficulties of the parents. Often the grandparents can become alarmed by mild behavioral difficulties in these children and may react critically, inhibiting emotional connections between them and the children. As this emotional connection is weakened, the authority of the grandparents to effectively discipline the children can be further diminished. The children may also withdraw, sensing further rejection and family problems. Children who have experienced multiple living situations or who have been in and out their parents' homes over many years will be more wary and less trusting, expecting further rejection and making the adjustment to a new living situation more difficult (Schwartz, 1994).

These families require significant support from social service agencies, day care, and the educational system and may require additional financial support if their earning power is diminished or if they are living on fixed income (Burton, 1992). These children, like all children, require attachment, a sense of consistency, and encouragement to develop self-esteem and confidence (Table 11–4).

In many situations, however, children do adapt well to living with grandparents or other extended family members for either limited periods or throughout their childhood. Good adjustment on the part of the children and the family often depends on (1) good pre-existing relationships between the child and the new caretakers, (2) legal sanctions that support the role of the parental figures, that ensure adequate financial support, and that maintain consistent involvement of the biological parents in the children's lives, and (3) professionals who recognize the courage and strength of extended family members who choose to raise children who cannot live with their parents. It is also essential that the choice to raise children who are not one's own be made in a direct and unambivalent fashion and communicated clearly with the children.

Table 11–4 • Special Challenges When Children Do Not Live With Their Parents

Emotional reaction to separation from parents, including sense of failure and shame
Repeated moves and multiple living situations
Capacity of caretakers to maintain discipline, concern, and commitment to the child
Need for support from social service agencies, day care teachers, educational system, and other professionals
Legal confusion about when biological parents can resume parenting
Need to support child's requirement for attachment, consistency, and competence
Need to support children's affection for and interest in their parents

Children Living With Gay Parents

Some parents find that they are homosexual after participating in a heterosexual relationship or marriage. As these parents identify and live according to their sexual identity, the children may then live with or visit a homosexual parent and a gay or lesbian step-parent. These children may have good relationships with both parents and may have been effectively nurtured prior to the change in living situation. The separation and divorce of their biological parents, if they had been married, may have been emotionally stressful for them, and they also need to adjust to the presence of a new adult in their household. Also, increasing numbers of gay and lesbian adults are choosing to have and raise children within their homosexual lifestyle. These adults may pursue adoption or lesbian women may have children through sperm donor insemination. Increasingly over the past 20 years, research reports are being published reviewing the development of children being raised by gay or lesbian parents (Flaks et al, 1995; Gottman, 1989; O'Donnell, 1993; Patterson, 1992; Ross, 1988; Tasker and Golombok, 1995; Victor and Fish, 1995).

These studies have identified similar psychosocial adjustment between children and adolescents raised by lesbian mothers and those raised by heterosexual mothers. There is no increased incidence of offsprings' becoming homosexual or having same-sex preferences than in the general population. Gender identity and gender role behavior have been normal for age and gender among children raised in homes with a lesbian mother and lesbian step-parent. These results appear similar for children born prior to their mothers' assuming a lesbian lifestyle and those born through donor insemination.

General mental health, development, and peer social relationships among these children and adolescents also have been noted to be satisfactory. In some studies, self-esteem in adolescence was higher among adolescents living with lesbian mothers than those living with divorced single heterosexual mothers (Tasker and Golombok, 1995). Overall adaptation of the children of gay and lesbian parents seems to depend on the homosexual parent's psychological adaptation, degree of participation, and support from the nonhomosexual parent (in divorced families) and the degree of community support (Patterson, 1992).

Parental divorce appears to generate more emotional difficulties for these children than the parent's homosexuality. Based on these studies, there appears to be no reason to deny visitation or custody to a parent or to refuse adoption purely on the basis of a parent's homosexual lifestyle. Further research is necessary in understanding the diversity of homosexual families with children, especially among homosexual parents of different ethnic and socioeconomic groups.

As children grow older, they are generally able to understand their parents' relationship and learn through their attachment with the biological homosexual parent to respect this parent's courage in living according to his or her sexual identity. However, problems can arise because of teasing by peers, a negative reaction within the community, secrecy of parents, or a negative reaction of the noncustodial biological parent. Raising children in this type of living situation often requires great sensitivity, compassion, and patience on the part of both the homosexual parent and the homosexual step-parent. With this commitment to the child, the direct support of the other parent, sensitivity to the child's feelings, and comfort with their living situation, gay parents can quite successfully raise children and help them to develop their own independent sexual preference as they grow into adolescence (Ross, 1988; Patterson, 1992; Tasker and Golombok, 1995).

Parental Commitment to Childrearing—The Essential Feature

In all family variations, common difficulties in childrearing emerge. The commitment to the child throughout the course of development is the central core of parenting. This commitment is challenged in all the forms of varied family composition discussed in this chapter. It can be challenged by career, by the death of a parent, by divorce or separation, by economic hardship, by a change in parental health or family strife, or by ambivalence or lack of support from a parent's social network. This commitment is the foundation of a parent's capacity to maintain the consistency and flexibility necessary for parenting. Family variations also challenge the parent's ability to help a child master painful feelings (Joselevich, 1988; Montalvo, 1982). The absence of a father, the distinct difference in a child's living situation from that of many of his or her peers, and the inability of the child to live with his or her own parents all create emotional reactions on the part of the child. These reactions change and are reworked as the child grows older. Openness of communication among all involved adults assists the child in adjusting to his or her different living situation. Resolution of conflict among these important adults also maximizes the adults' ability to attend to the child's needs. The child needs help in responding to peer concerns and questions as well as those raised by school personnel. Children who have been damaged or are untrusting will gradually respond to the affection of adults, but they require patience and a consistent feeling of belonging. The capacity of parental figures in varied family situations is stressed, particularly at times of transition across developmental stages and when the child has chronic illness, physical disability, intellectual inadequacy, learning disability, or emotional or behavioral problems. These special difficulties will create a further need for these families to create and maintain consistency in their lives and establish effective relationships with professionals treating their children.

Pediatric Evaluation and Interventions

The pediatrician has a special role with children who live in different family situations. He or she is capable of supporting the family's functioning, ensuring adequate attention to the child's needs, and promoting and encouraging the family's involvement with the community, social agencies, other professionals, and school professionals. Pediatricians can support the capacity of families to raise children effectively, appreciate and encourage the commitment of parental figures to childrearing, identify difficulties the family is experiencing at an early stage, and recommend appropriate and effective interventions. The pediatrician always needs to identify accurately who lives in the home, who is involved in child care, who provides emotional support for parental figures, where the biological parents are and how involved they are in the childrearing, how adequate the economic resources of the family are, and how rewarding childrearing is for this family. These questions need to be asked in a direct fashion. The pediatrician should also ascertain how the child came to be in the current living situation. This may include exploration of the role of the father, the circumstances of the child's being placed out of the biological parents' home, or the circumstances of a dual-career family. The pediatrician should pay attention to any hesitancy in the answers, signs of evasiveness, distrust, or emotional upset on the part of the parental figures, and any reluctance to divulge important information. Legal guardianship should always be clarified. The role of a noncustodial parent in the child's life should be ascertained. Legal difficulties and involvement with social services agencies should also be identified clearly.

In a primary care visit, the pediatrician can review the child's development, the aspects of his or her daily life and peer activities, the relationship of the child with parental figures, and any pre-existing problems the child may have. The effectiveness of pediatric support depends on the formation of an effective collaborative relationship between the pediatrician and the primary caretakers. He or she will also want to identify the nature of emotional support, setting of limits, and discipline for the child. The pediatrician can also gain important information about how the family functions by identifying how decisions are made in the family, who is involved, and who supports the parental figures, as well as who might disagree when these decisions are made (Sargent, 1990). The pediatrician can evaluate the emotional status of the child and determine the degree of his or her openness, self-confidence, and willingness to engage in the relationship with the caretakers. He or she should also talk with the child in a developmentally appropriate fashion about the living situation. The family re-

Table 11–5 • Pediatric Evaluation of Family Adequacy

Formation of collaborative relationship with primary caretaker or
    caretakers
Inquire about
    Living situation
    Who is involved in child care
    Adequacy of economic support
    Sources of emotional support for parental figures
    Location and involvement of biological parent or parents
Review development, daily life, and peer activities of child
Review family response to stressful situations or problems
Identify quality and appropriateness of emotional support and
    discipline for child
Review how important decisions are made in the family and how
    differences of opinion are resolved
Inquire about particular needs family has and how family is
    addressing them

sponse to stressful situations and the family's ability to attend to economic and emotional concerns further provide the pediatrician with information about the family's effectiveness and the degree of competence of the parental figures (Table 11–5).

It is especially important that the pediatrician begin contact with a family with an expectation that the members of the family can effectively raise their children and recognize that it is the pediatrician's responsibility to support that commitment. If the pediatrician approaches these families in a positive fashion, this respect and support for the family will foster a sense of trust in him or her so that they can discuss difficulties as soon as they arise. Families that are more guarded and disconnected have more difficulty maintaining consistent pediatric care and may be less open about their living situation or their lives. The pediatrician's openness, respect, and patience often help the parental figures discuss conflictive situations and reveal when they feel overwhelmed by the responsibilities of childrearing. The relationship with the pediatrician will enable the family to obtain social support and mental health treatment.

Children with limited curiosity and enjoyment; children who appear withdrawn, isolated, or depressed; and those with poor responses to stress manifested by increased temper tantrums, behavioral disturbances, or emotional withdrawal should receive further intervention. Poor adaptation to or management of chronic illness, disability, or learning difficulties also requires further investigation and a plan for remediation. If parental figures appear exhausted, angry, or disconnected and remote from the child, they may need assistance in gaining further support, especially within their social network. As the pediatrician pays attention to the parental figures' lives as adults, he or she also helps them appreciate the importance of attending to their own needs while they care for their children. The pediatrician can also identify areas of conflict between parental figures and other important adults in the child's life. Often a grandparent may disagree with how a single parent is parenting or may disagree with how a parent is pursuing his or her own life. Frequently the noncustodial biological parent may disagree so much that it interferes with both parents' commitment to childrearing and the consistency

the child experiences. The pediatrician might ask to meet with the parent and grandparent or a noncustodial parent. He or she should also discuss concerns with social service or mental health professionals or school personnel who are involved with the family. In these situations as well, mental health counseling for the entire family may be particularly effective. The pediatrician should inform parental figures that the difficulties they are having may worsen the developmental, emotional, or behavioral problems of the child and that changes in their lives may be stressful. Anticipatory guidance to assist parental figures with questions the children might ask about their living situation and to aid them with effective discipline is often helpful for these families as the children grow older.

Advocacy Issues for Pediatricians Concerning Alternative Families

There is a prominent role for pediatricians in assisting nontraditional families. Many families need adequate child care. They require babysitting networks and assistance when the children are sick so that the parents can get to work and not lose necessary economic support. They require afterschool activities that are both affordable and emotionally and physically adequate for the children. These parental figures require encouragement to enlist support and diminish their sense of isolation in their communities and with extended families. The adults may need encouragement to develop a sense of cohesion, a sense of the joy and enhanced confidence that comes from effectively raising children, and encouragement in achieving satisfaction in their lives and dealing with the ever-present threat of feeling overwhelmed, overburdened, or "burned out." The pediatrician can enlist school and social resources in their community to provide this assistance consistently. This can be done through clinical contacts, community network organizations, lectures, and other professional and personal contacts.

Pediatricians can communicate respect, support, and encouragement for these families in their roles with other professionals in the community and work to ensure that parental figures care adequately for the children. In particular, the pediatrician should support and promote the role of the father with his children, especially if the father does not live with the children, as well as support the personal success and satisfaction of mothers. The support of the

Table 11–6 • Advocacy Issues for Pediatricians Concerning Alternative Families

To promote the view that children can be raised successfully by
    nontraditional families if adequate support is provided
To enlist community groups, social agencies, and schools in
    supporting these families
To identify and support adequate child care resources
To help children, families, and communities maintain a balanced,
    tolerant, and forgiving view of parents who cannot live with
    their children
To remember that family life always involves balancing the
    child's needs with those of important adults

pediatrician and other community professionals can help children tolerate the stresses they have experienced and grow with greater optimism, openness, and possibilities (Table 11–6).

REFERENCES

Barth JC: Families cope with the death of a parent. *In* Combrinck-Graham L (ed): Children in Family Contexts. New York, Guilford Press, 1989.

Boyd-Franklin N: Black Families in Therapy. New York, Guilford Press, 1989.

Bradt JO: Becoming parents: Families with young children. *In* Carter B, McGoldrick M (eds): The Changing Family Life Cycle. New York, Gardner Press, 1988.

Brown FH: The postdivorce family. *In* Carter B, McGoldrick M (eds): The Changing Family Life Cycle. New York, Gardner Press, 1988.

Burton, L: Black grandmothers rearing children of drug-addicted parents: Stressors, outcomes and social service needs. Genotologist 32:744, 1992.

Elkind D: The Hurried Child. Reading, MA, Addison-Wesley, Publishing, 1983.

Flaks DK, Fisher I, Masterpasqua F, Joseph G: Lesbians choosing motherhood: A comparative study of lesbian and heterosexual parents and their children. Dev Psych 31:105, 1995.

Fulmer R: Lower-income and professional families: A comparison of structure and life cycle process. *In* Carter B, McGoldrick M (eds): The Changing Family Life Cycle. New York, Gardner Press, 1988.

Goldstein J, Freud A, Solnit AJ: Before the Best Interests of the Child. New York, Free Press, 1979.

Goldstein J, Freud A, Solnit AJ: Beyond the Best Interests of the Child. New York, Free Press, 1973.

Gottman JS: Children of gay and lesbian parents. Marriage Family Rev 14:177, 1989.

Hines PM: The family life cycle of poor black families. *In* Carter B, McGoldrick M (eds): The Changing Family Life Cycle. New York, Gardner Press, 1988.

Holder DP, Anderson CM: Women, work and the family. *In* McGoldrick M, Anderson CM, Walsh F (eds): Women in Families: A Framework for Family Therapy. New York, Norton, 1989.

Joselevich E: Family transitions, cumulative stress and crises. *In* Falicov CJ (ed): Family Transitions. New York, Guilford Press, 1988.

Leupnitz DA: The Family Interpreted. New York, Basic Books, 1988.

Libow J: Chronic illness and family coping. *In* Combrinck-Graham L (ed): Children in Family Contexts. New York, Guilford Press, 1989.

Lindblad-Goldberg M: Successful minority single-parent families. *In* Combrinck-Graham L (ed): Children in Family Contexts. New York, Guilford Press, 1989.

Lindblad-Goldberg M (ed): Single Parent Families. Vol 23. *In* Hansen JC (ed): The Family Therapy Collections. Rockville, MD, Aspen Publishers, 1987.

Minkler M, Roe KM: Grandmothers as Caregivers: Raising Children of the Crack Cocaine Epidemic. Newbury Park, CA, Sage Publications, 1993.

Minkler M, Roe KM, Robertson-Beckley RJ: Raising grandchildren from crack-cocaine households: Effects on family and friendship ties of African-American women. Am J Orthopsychiatry 64:20, 1994.

Montalvo B: Interpersonal arrangements in disrupted families. *In* Walsh F (ed): Normal Family Processes. New York, Guilford Press, 1982.

O'Donnell A: Voices from the heart: The developmental impact of a mother's lesbianism on her adolescent children. Smith College Studies in Social Work 63:281, 1993.

Patterson CJ: Children of lesbian and gay parents. Child Dev 63:1025, 1992.

Popenoe D: The family transformed. Family Affairs 2:1, 1989.

Rosman BL: Family development and the impact of a child's chronic illness. *In* Falicov CJ (ed): Family Transitions. New York, Guilford Press, 1988.

Ross J: Challenging boundaries: An adolescent in a homosexual family. J Fam Psychol 2:227, 1988.

Sargent J: Child and family psychosocial assessment. *In* Schwartz MW, Charney EB, Curry TA, et al (eds): Pediatric Primary Care: A Problem-Oriented Approach, 2nd ed. Chicago, Year Book Medical Publishers, 1990.

Schwartz LL: The challenge of raising one's non-biological children. Am J Family Ther 22:195, 1994.

Tasker F, Golombok S: Adults raised as children in lesbian families. Am J Orthopsychiatry 65:203, 1995.

Victor S, Fish MC: Lesbian mothers and their children. School Psych Rev 24:456, 1995.

Walsh F, McGoldrick M: Loss and the family life cycle. *In* Falicov CJ (ed): Family Transitions. New York, Guilford Press, 1988.

12 *Brothers and Sisters*

David J. Schonfeld • Elin R. Cohen

 Siblings have a unique and unparalleled lifelong relationship that helps to shape their development and behavior. A variety of factors in the family and in the children themselves determine the character of the interaction. There is much more to consider clinically than just sibling rivalry, which is usually the most common concern of parents. This chapter reviews the multitude of benefits as well as risks experienced by children in their sibling relationships, especially effects on language and social development.

"He (she) is like a brother (sister) to me" is a common means of expressing an extremely close relationship—one that exceeds even that of friendship. Yet the most common subject for discussion of sibling relationships within pediatric practice is sibling rivalry, in which antagonistic behaviors are the focus. The sibling relationship is a unique and unparalleled interpersonal relationship that is characterized by both intimacy and rivalry; a sibling provides strong social support but is, at times, also antagonistic. It is a lifelong relationship that begins at the moment of birth of the younger sibling and helps to shape the cognitive, language, and social development of both siblings. The sibling relationship is also a social context that is uniquely suited as an opportunity to practice and learn interpersonal and social skills, both positive and negative. The importance and intensity of the sibling relationship may not be readily apparent, because the social behaviors and strong feelings they engender often occur within the privacy of the family setting and may not be readily known to health care providers unless there is direct inquiry of families about peer relationships and the overall impact on the family.

Effects of Birth Order on Development and Behavior

LANGUAGE AND COGNITIVE DEVELOPMENT

The process of language development is qualitatively different for first and only children than for later siblings because of the impact of older children on the language environment of later-born siblings. The parent-child speech dyad is characteristically responsive, nondirective, and questioning. This type of language environment promotes the acquisition of vocabulary. Because parents generally spend more time directly speaking to first-born and only children than they spend speaking to later-born siblings, the rate of acquisition of vocabulary is enhanced for first-born and only children. To the extent that many traditional measures of speech that are used to assess young children's language skills are heavily influenced by measures of vocabulary size, first-born and only children may appear to be in an advantaged position for language development.

Although it is true that later-born siblings spend less time in dyadic conversation with the parent and therefore benefit less from responsive, nondirective conversation, they do have more opportunity to speak to other children within the family and engage instead in more directive, less responsive conversational patterns. The more complex conversational patterns that typify parent-child-sibling conversations foster distinct and more sophisticated conversational skills. Barton and Tomasello (1991) studied triadic conversation involving mothers, preschool-aged siblings, and 19- to 24-month-old children. The triadic conversations involving the mother and both children were longer in length and involved more turn-taking in the conversational course than were the dyadic conversations involving the mother and either sibling. Participation in the triadic conversation also fostered the skill of joining an ongoing discussion. To be successful in joining a discussion, the child must understand the nature of the ongoing conversation and be willing to participate in discussing a topic that is not necessarily of the child's own choosing.

In assessing the language skills of second or later-born siblings, it is important to appreciate the qualitative differences in the pattern of language development. First-born children may be relatively more proficient in learning what to say, whereas later-born siblings may be more skilled in how to conduct a more complex conversation. Language development may therefore take a qualitatively different, although not necessarily inferior, course for later-born siblings who are raised in a multichild language (and social) environment. These qualitative differences in the rate of acquisition of language skills between first-born or only children and later-born children are small in absolute magnitude, especially when compared to the variability found within the two groups. Parents and health care providers should therefore be cautious in dismissing true delays in language acquisition, such as expressive vocabulary, by attributing it to the myth that later-born children are characteristically delayed in achieving language milestones.

Many researchers have also reported on the relationship between intelligence quotient (IQ) and ordinal position of siblings. The results are highly variable, with advantages being attributed to the elder or younger sibling related to age, gender, and spacing intervals between the siblings. IQ differences may partly reflect a nonshared environment within the family, which may differentially encourage intellectual development among children within the family (McCall, 1983; Rowe and Plomin, 1981).

SOCIAL DEVELOPMENT

Piaget and Sullivan described two general characteristics of interpersonal relationships: reciprocity and complementarity (Dunn, 1983). Reciprocity highlights the similarities and shared experiences between like children, such as between friends. Complementarity, in contrast, involves a child's response when interacting with an individual with differing perspectives and experiences, such as between parent and child. The sibling experience is unique among most social relationships in the extent to which aspects of both complementarity and reciprocity simultaneously characterize the relationship. Siblings raised within the same home still experience a nonshared environment. The children's differing perspectives and experiences are, in part, a result of their different ages and ordinal positions within the family, as well as the influences of the genetics of each child and each parent (Plomin, 1995). Despite these differences, siblings still maintain an intense and intimate relationship such as is seen among peers. This unique combination of reciprocity and complementarity contributes to the richness of the sibling relationship and its impact on social development (Dunn, 1983).

Within American culture, the only child is often stereotyped as a socially maladjusted, self-centered, unhappy child. In contrast, a more positive impression of being an only child is endorsed by children without siblings, as well as by their parents. While siblings have a significant impact on the social development of other children within the family, it is necessary to look more broadly at the family constellation and other factors that may contribute to social development. For example, to the extent that parents can choose to have only one child, there may be characteristics of these parents that have an independent influence on the social development of their offspring (Falbo, 1982). Several recent studies regarding only children have found no overall significant differences in achievement or on measures of various behavior and psychological traits between only children and children with siblings. The increasing use of out-of-home group child care arrangements, such as day care and preschool, may mediate the impact on social development of being an only child.

Other Sibling Factors Affecting Development, Behavior, and Relationships

SPACING

How much time is optimal to space between children is a question that is often asked of pediatric health care providers as parents plan their families. The answer most likely depends on the unique characteristics of the individual parents and family.

On a short-term basis, the nature of children's re-

sponse to the birth of a sibling is to a large extent based on the age and developmental level of the older child. If the first-born child is 12 to 15 months of age, he or she may exhibit more clinging behaviors with the introduction of the new sibling. Toileting and feeding problems may characterize the behavioral response of a 2-year-old child, whereas a 3- to 4-year-old child may exhibit demanding behavior and temper tantrums. Therefore, the behavioral response is likely more an indication of the age and developmental level of the older child than it is the actual spacing between the two children, an unavoidable confounder (Dunn, 1985).

The gap in age between siblings does not affect positive interest during the newborn period in the new sibling. Whether the gap is less than a year or is greater than 4 years does not, in isolation, affect the amount of play, affection, hostility, or aggression between young children. As children grow older, though, the age gap between siblings may have a greater impact on their relationship, in that the *relative* gap in ages between the two children narrows and more opportunities for shared activities occur, bringing a greater potential for conflict and rivalry. Several studies have found that an age gap of 4 years or greater may diminish the degree of rivalry and conflict manifested between siblings as they grow older.

After a comprehensive review of studies examining the effect of siblings on cognitive development, Wagner, Schubert, and Schubert (1985) concluded that, after controlling for many potential confounders (including age, gender, ordinal position, parents' age at time of marriage, and socioeconomic status), research suggests that spacing siblings more widely than 24 months may confer an advantage for the IQ of both the younger and older sibling. The impact is greater in verbal than in math skills, and the patterns shown in different studies are somewhat inconsistent, most likely because of the impact of confounding variables, such as the varieties of spacing intervals among the studies. In addition, most studies focused on sibling relationships of two children in middle class suburban settings, suggesting caution should be used when attempting to generalize these findings to other groups.

FAMILY SIZE

The average number of children within an American family in 1865 was more than 7. In 1950 this number had decreased to 3.4, and in 1994 the average number of children had decreased to less than 2. Even though family size has decreased on average within the United States, a couple's decision of how many children to raise varies greatly and may depend on factors such as personal experience within the parents' extended families of origin, cultural or religious beliefs, or economic circumstances.

Within larger families, particularly those with more than three children, there is often less dyadic interaction between adult and child. Among the siblings, group processes of alliances and exclusions may form. Parents should be advised to be attentive to group dynamics that may place one child in a disadvantaged role as the "underdog" and to give careful consideration to the timing and appropriateness of interventions on behalf of this child. Fostering friendships for children outside of the family, especially for a child who is somewhat marginalized within the sibling group, may help ameliorate the impact of exclusions by siblings. The large family size often results in large age gaps, at least between the youngest and oldest siblings. Siblings may therefore take on various roles and responsibilities for care of siblings, including disciplining, teaching, or caregiving. Pediatric health care providers should assist parents in exploring the extent to which the children should be expected or allowed to assume these roles.

MULTIPLE BIRTHS

With increasing maternal age and medical interventions for infertility, there has been an increase in the incidence of multiple births. Multiple births are associated with an increased risk of complications, especially prematurity (54% of twins are born prematurely versus 9.6% of singletons) and the need for cesarean delivery. Even when twins and other multiples are born at term and healthy, parents face greater stress in caring for multiple infants. The babies' sleeping and feeding schedules are more challenging to coordinate than those of a single infant, and the parents may have more difficulty finding and paying for child care. In general, mothers of infant twins are less responsive to their infants and talk less and use less verbal reasoning than do mothers of singleton infants (Vandell et al, 1988).

Siblings from twin and other multiple gestations, even when they are not monozygotic, have a unique relationship wherein they are both siblings and same-age peers. This increases the tendency for others (and the children themselves) to make comparisons between the siblings and may, therefore, accentuate the risk of rivalry. However, it also affords a greater opportunity for shared experiences and the possibility of an especially close relationship between the siblings. Clinicians can help families identify relevant issues to consider in parenting twin and other multiple births (Table 12–1), and they can provide advice and support.

STEP-, ADOPTIVE, AND FOSTER SIBLINGS

Nearly half of all children born in the United States in the 1980s are expected to experience parental divorce, and one third are expected to live with a step-parent before they are 18 years of age. The stepfamily may become the most common family structure in the United States. Parental divorce, remarriage, and the creation of a blended family result in many potential stressors for the family (see Chapter 15), which can directly impact on the sibling relationships. Children within recently formed blended families often have to adjust to a different parent, home, neighborhood, school, and friends, while simultaneously being faced with new siblings, a change in the number or ratio of children of various genders in the family, and a change in their ordinal position within the family. They must adjust to the intimacy of living with these stepsiblings without the benefit of a shared experience of having grown up together. New alliances and exclusions may develop within the enlarged group of siblings. This generally occurs in a context of recently remarried parents who may need to withdraw some attention from their biological children in

Table 12–1 • Issues to Consider in Parenting of Twin and Other Multiple-Birth Children

To minimize stress on parents
  Identify means to organize and structure day-to-day care of children.
  Develop plans for help and support from extended family, friends, and alternative caregivers.
  Offer referral to parent support groups for parents of twin and other multiple births.
To help foster development of individual identity
  Avoid naming children with similar sounding names.
  Minimize dressing the children in matching outfits.
  Encourage and help each child to pursue individual interests.
  Do not discipline both for transgressions of one child; direct praise for individual achievements.
  Provide opportunities for separation from siblings, such as encouraging unique friendships, to minimize separation problems at time of enrollment within day care or school.
  Enroll children in separate classrooms.
To assist other (nonmultiple-birth) siblings within the family
  Recognize that multiple-birth children may receive a disproportionate share of attention from family members, friends, and strangers, and encourage these individuals not to exclude or ignore the other siblings.
  Be sure to spend quality time with other siblings individually.
  Minimize the assignment of child care responsibilities to other siblings.

order to attend to their new spouse and their spouse's children. An added tension may develop with visiting stepsiblings who may not have to abide by the same family rules or may be treated more leniently during their stay, potentially causing resentment between stepsiblings. The birth of a biological sibling in a blended family may foster resentment toward the new baby within the new marriage. On the other hand, the birth of the sibling, who is related to all family members, may help to unify the entire family.

Foster and adoptive children may experience similar changes in sibling relationships as those described for stepsiblings, but these children often come into a family with the added disadvantage of having no prior relationship or alliance with any member of the family. In the situation of foster care, there is also the added uncertainty in the length of placement. Pediatric health care providers can assist families considering and entering into foster or adoptive arrangements. Parents should be advised to discuss the planned arrival of new children with all children currently within the home and ask for their input regarding the sharing of toys, belongings, bedrooms, and so on, with their new siblings. The meaning of adoption or foster care should be discussed with all children in the family starting at a young age. In foster care situations, parents should give as much information as possible about planned departures of children to assist children with the transition (see Chapter 13).

TEMPERAMENT

The quality of a child's relationship with his or her siblings and parents is strongly influenced by the nature and compatibility of the temperamental traits of all members of the family. As seen in studies of friendship relationships, it is the "goodness of fit" or "match" of temperament between siblings, more than the individual temperamental traits in isolation, that affects the quality of the sibling relationship. Variations in level of conflict and aggression within sibling pairs have been related to the degree of mismatch in temperament. This is especially true of conflicts seen within older sibling pairs, which are more likely manifested in verbal, rather than physical, aggression (Munn and Dunn, 1989).

Health care providers who work with families should help them understand that even though people can choose their friends and spouses, siblings are placed within a lifelong and intense interpersonal relationship without their choice or input, simply by virtue of birth or family restructuring. The greater likelihood of incompatibilities poses a challenge for families. Parents should recognize the inherent conflict this can create and learn to frame their children's temperamental differences as acceptable variations without yielding to the temptation to judge individual children as "good" or "bad." Instead, helping children learn to interact with people of different temperamental profiles (whether they are siblings or parents) can be seen as a positive learning experience for social growth and development. Parents may also benefit from advice from health care providers regarding the limited capacity to modify children's temperamental qualities, which may be the basis of ongoing conflicts among siblings (see Chapter 8).

CHRONIC ILLNESS

The impact of having a child with a chronic illness or other special needs (such as developmental delay or mental illness) is multifactorial (see Chapter 34) and may affect the sibling relationships. Parents have limited reserves of energy, time, and money, and a child's chronic illness or other special needs may further strain the emotional and psychological resources of all family members, contributing to marital discord or impairments in sibling relationships. The well child may be expected to be more self-sufficient or independent than same-aged peers. Parents should be advised that even though it is important to keep all family members informed and involved in the ongoing care of the child with the chronic illness or other special needs, they should not overburden the well siblings with excessive responsibilities for the care of the affected sibling or younger siblings, or with responsibilities for maintenance of the home. To the extent possible, siblings should be encouraged to maintain their peer groups and continue involvement in activities outside of the family. Whereas the extra demands of caring for a child with a chronic illness or other special needs are potential stressors for families, including siblings, some studies have shown that children who grow up with a sibling with special health care needs may develop a greater capacity for empathy.

DEATH OF A SIBLING

Terminal illness and death of a child are major stressors for parents and siblings (see Chapter 14). After the death of a child, surviving siblings may be angry at the child who has died or experience guilt over having survived. Families may need help as they reorganize after the death of a child, so that siblings do not become the focus of projected defenses, often a result of unresolved guilt, that may impair further the surviving children's ultimate personality development. For example, guilt over the death of a child may cause parents to protect excessively the surviving children, which may interfere with their normative attempts to achieve independence (Krell and Rabkin, 1979).

IMPACT OF PARENTAL BEHAVIORS

How parents interact with their children affects the development of the relationship between siblings. Dunn and Kendrick (1982) found that how a mother talks to a first child about a new sibling has a major impact on how the relationship between siblings is formed. Mothers who talk about the baby as a person with feelings and needs for whom they both could take responsibility are able to more effectively draw the older child into the discussion about the baby. Within weeks of the baby's birth, older siblings in these families comment on the baby as a person with wants and desires. In follow-up 14 months later, these siblings demonstrate more friendly interactions.

Sibling Interactions

PROSOCIAL INTERACTIONS

The sibling relationship is an enduring peer relationship, generally lasting longer than any other relationship in life including spousal, parental, or friendship. The potential bond created by sharing experiences from childhood through adulthood is thus deep and unique.

The common perception often holds "sibling rivalry" as the pivotal element of the relationship between siblings. However, siblings also demonstrate emotionally charged positive interactions that are distinctive to the sibling relationship (Fig. 12–1). More than with friends who are peers, siblings during early childhood demonstrate imitation in their play and show an increased ability to comfort each other (Dunn, 1983). Particularly in societies in which girls

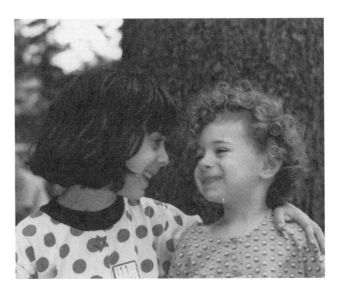

Figure 12–1. Prosocial interactions.

Table 12–2 • Minimizing Sibling Rivalry

Discuss with the child the anticipated birth of a sibling by the second trimester of the pregnancy.

Present the new baby as a person with feelings and needs.

Plan how an older sibling can take a role in helping to care for the new baby.

Recognize temperamental differences between children without labeling a "good" or "bad" sibling.

Intervene in conflict to protect a less dominant child without scapegoating one of the siblings.

Recognize and encourage positive interactions between siblings.

continue to be socialized as caretakers, younger male and female siblings show a tendency to seek out older sisters more often than older brothers for comfort and aid.

In early childhood, siblings are the most consistent and reliable playmates for one another. In later childhood and adolescence, the sibling may take on the role of confidant and socializing agent—setting standards, imitating, and giving advice. Furthermore, among brother/sister relationships, the sibling relationship may be the only nonsexualized context in which adolescents and adults can express closeness and affection with a member of the opposite gender (Lamb and Sutton-Smith, 1982).

ANTAGONISTIC INTERACTIONS

The sibling relationship has potential for deep or frequent conflict as well. The psychoanalytic view focuses particularly on the intense rivalry for parental attention, love, and approval. However, the origins and impact of other sibling conflicts should not be minimized. That "similarity of worlds," which allows for the unique empathy and closeness between siblings, can also form the basis for effective and hurtful teasing, competing, and insulting behaviors. Although conflict among siblings is in many ways normative, there is a potential for physical or emotional injury to a child in the course of sibling fighting. The challenge for parents is to protect a younger or less dominant sibling while being wary of constantly scapegoating or blaming one of the siblings.

Parents' responses to sibling altercations are varied and may reflect cultural and socioeconomic differences, as well as the parents' own personal experiences with their siblings. While some parents actively intervene and "referee" fights between siblings, other parents expect the children to resolve conflicts on their own. For some parents, the choice of response varies based on whether the conflict results in physical fighting or verbal insulting. Parents may be reluctant to seek advice on how to handle sibling fighting because of prevailing social pressures to keep conflict among family members private, thus creating the misconception that other families experience less conflict (Dunn, 1985). Direct inquiry about fighting among siblings can help the family to address this common source of family conflict.

Parents may be inclined to focus on the sibling rivalry and conflict that may be more readily apparent among young children, without appreciating the enduring and rich qualities of a sibling relationship that may develop over years and with maturity. Even though much has been written about the short-term "costs" of sibling rivalry and conflict, there is less attention given to the long-term benefits of the sibling relationship. In addition to offering anticipatory guidance on how to minimize sibling rivalry (Table 12–2), pediatric health care providers can help families maintain an appropriate perspective and realize that, with time, brothers and sisters may develop one of the most enduring and profound relationships that can be achieved between two individuals.

REFERENCES

Barton M, Tomasello M: Joint attention and conversation in mother-infant-sibling triads. Child Dev 62:517–529, 1991.

Dunn J: Sisters and Brothers. Cambridge, MA, Harvard University Press, 1985.

Dunn J: Sibling relationships in early childhood. Child Dev 54:787–811, 1983.

Dunn J, Kendrick C: Siblings and their mothers: developing relationships within the family. *In* Lamb M, Sutton-Smith B (eds): Sibling Relationships: Their Nature and Significance Across the Lifespan. Hillsdale, NJ, Lawrence Erlbaum, 1982, pp 39–60.

Falbo T: Only children in America. *In* Lamb M, Sutton-Smith B (eds): Sibling Relationships: Their Nature and Significance Across the Lifespan. Hillsdale, NJ, Lawrence Erlbaum, 1982, pp 285–304.

Krell R, Rabkin L: The effects of sibling death on the surviving child: a family perspective. Fam Process 18:471–477, 1979.

Lamb M, Sutton-Smith B (eds): Sibling Relationships: Their Nature and Significance Across the Lifespan. Hillsdale, NJ, Lawrence Erlbaum, 1982.

McCall R: Environmental effects on intelligence: the forgotten realm of discontinuous nonshared within-family factors. Child Dev 54:408–415, 1983.

Munn P, Dunn J: Temperament and the developing relationship between siblings. Int J Behav Dev 12:433–451, 1989.

Plomin R: Genetics and children's experiences in the family. J Child Psychol Psychiatry 36:33–68, 1995.

Rowe D, Plomin R: The importance of nonshared (E1) environmental influences in behavioral development. Dev Psych 17:517–531, 1981.

Vandell D, Owen M, Wilson K, Henderson V: Social development in infant twins: peer and mother-child relationships. Child Dev 59:168–177, 1988.

Wagner M, Schubert H, Schubert D: Effects of sibling spacing on intelligence, interfamilial relations, psychosocial characteristics, and mental and physical health. *In* Reese H (ed): Advances in Child Development and Behavior. Orlando, FL, Academic Press, 19:149–206, 1985.

BOOKS FOR PARENTS

American Academy of Pediatrics: Sibling Relationships: Guidelines for Parents [brochure]. Elk Grove Village, IL, American Academy of Pediatrics, 1996.

Faber A, Mazlish E: Siblings Without Rivalry: How to Help Your Children Live Together So You Can Live Too. New York, Avon Books, 1988.

Reit S: Sibling Rivalry. New York, Ballantine Books, 1985.

13 Adoption and Foster Family Care

S. Norman Sherry • Steven L. Nickman

 The adoption of an unrelated child by parents usually results in the raising of a person with normal development and behavior, but there are some special considerations to which pediatricians should be sensitive—issues such as obtaining adequate medical records, when to tell the child about the adoption, and the possible search for the biological parents. In the past 25 years or so, the situation has become more complex with more independent placements of children, more adoption of children with special needs, more subsidized care, more single-parent families, more intercountry adoptions, and more open adoptions. This chapter gives guidance on these matters and on the even more complex practices of surrogacy and artificial insemination. The special needs of the half million children in foster care in the United States are also discussed.

The family structure of adopted children and children in foster care is significantly varied from the usual biological family structure and can affect the child's development and behavior. The primary care physician who is aware of the social, emotional, legal, and medical implications of these variations is in a unique position to help families of these children.

Adoption

Approximately 2% of the child population in the United States is adopted. Adoption is a lifelong process; it is an important issue to children, parents, and physicians throughout childhood and adult life. Although adoption presents children with challenges that may lead to a life trajectory that differs slightly from that of their nonadopted peers, research has shown that most adoptions work out well and that most adoptees have a satisfactory life adjustment as adults.

Adoption is a legal and social process that gives full family membership to children not born to the adoptive parents. It has not always been so. Moses was adopted by Pharaoh's daughter without such privileges. In Caesar's day, adoption was a reward for great public service. Despite the long history of adoption, only recently have adopted persons become "complete and equal members of a family constellation, with all the privileges and responsibilities accrued to children born to their parents" (American Academy of Pediatrics, 1973).

A working knowledge of the terms used in adoption is necessary. Birth parents, adoptive parents, and the adopted child constitute the *adoption triad*. The *adoption agency* offers professional services, including counseling, to each member of the triad.

Many changes have occurred in adoption practices in the last 30 years. Many of these changes have their roots in a single social phenomenon—the shortage of healthy newborn babies available for placement. These changes include the increasing number of independent adoptions,

the adoption of children with special needs (once thought to be unadoptable), subsidized adoptions, and intercountry adoptions. Other changes are the result of shifting cultural trends—openness in adoption, single-parent adoption, and the use of surrogate parents.

The total number of adoptions in the United States in 1992 was 127,441. Of these, 42% (53,525) were by step-parents or relatives. Of the remaining 58% (73,916), other types of adoption were represented as follows (expressed as percent of the total adoptions):

- A total of 15.5% (19,753) were conducted by public agencies, that is, they were adoptions of children from the foster care system.
- A total of 5% (6536) were from other countries. The largest numbers were from Korea (1787), Colombia (403), and Chile (403).
- A total of 37.5% (47,627) were arranged either by a private agency or as independent adoptions, in approximately equal numbers.

The number of international adoptions varies with world events; for example, in 1995, there were 9384 such adoptions, the increase being brought about by political changes in Russia, Romania, and other former communist areas of Europe and by the Chinese government's new policy of allowing infants to be adopted in North America and Europe.

The number of completed adoptions from the US foster care system does not give a full picture of the numbers of children waiting to be adopted. For example, in 1993, approximately 18,000 adoptions from foster care were finalized. However, in the same year, an additional 86,000 children had a permanency plan of adoption, as follows:

- A total of 17,000 children were legally free for adoption and waiting in nonfinalized adoptive homes.
- A total of 21,000 children were legally free but still waiting to be placed in adoptive families.
- A total of 48,000 children were not yet legally free

for adoption; some of these children were living in preadoptive foster placements, but most were not.

AGENCY ADOPTION AND INDEPENDENT ADOPTION

In a traditional agency placement, a licensed voluntary agency or an authorized public agency places a child who is legally free for adoption. The child is placed with a family that has undergone careful social casework study. The licensed agencies, both public and private, continue services throughout the adjustment period and beyond, and all agency resources are made available to the adoption triad (American Academy of Pediatrics, 1973). Agencies share medical and social data with the adoptive parents.

An increasing number of parents find children through other avenues—physicians, attorneys, or clergy. Without the expertise of a licensed agency, privately arranged adoptions can have serious drawbacks. The birth mother rarely receives professional counseling. There may be no careful evaluation of the adoptive parents' physical and mental health. Both parties run the risk of legal complications arising from shortcuts often taken by independent facilitators of adoption. Most important, ongoing support services and crisis management for the adoptive family are not readily available. Ideally, the agency acts as a home base for the adoption triad. New information about problems, such as an inherited disease in the birth parents, can be reported to the agency.

Agencies often have a consulting physician whose expertise is available to families if children manifest physical, emotional, or developmental problems that require expert advice. An adopted adolescent or young adult desirous of further nonidentifying information about the circumstances of his or her placement can go to the agency. A young adult who decides to search for his or her biological parents can seek guidance from this source. The thrust toward "openness in adoption" may alter the circuit described; however, it does not alter the objective of serving the best interest of all in the adoption triad.

CHILDREN WITH SPECIAL NEEDS

The term "children with special needs" refers to those children needing adoption who are of school age, who are part of a sibling group, who are of color, or who have special physical, emotional, or developmental needs.

With careful social casework planning, adoption social supports after placement, and subsidies when appropriate, many more children with special needs are being successfully adopted. These children and their families may need more time with the physicians for support, guidance, and intervention.

SUBSIDIZED ADOPTION

Federal and state financial support—in the form of monthly cash payments and Medicaid coverage—has helped to encourage the adoption of children with special needs. These children, whose medical and special educational expenses can be burdensome, may more easily acquire a family of their own if subsidies are available to them after adoption.

Armed with this knowledge, physicians may be more effective advocates for their adoptable patients with special needs.

CHILDREN OF ETHNIC MINORITY DESCENT

Ethnic minorities are overrepresented among the children who need adoption placement. Many professionals believe that children who need adoption do best in a family that reflects their own racial heritage. However, adoption should not be denied or significantly delayed when adoptive parents of other races or cultures are available (National Adoption Task Force, 1987). Ultimately, the most important fact is that all children need permanent, nurturing families. Pediatricians should be alert to any special concerns that minority children adopted by white families may express, especially during adolescence.

SINGLE-PARENT ADOPTION

In the 1960s, only healthy newborns were considered candidates for adoption and only married couples were considered acceptable as adoptive parents. Currently, infants and older children are increasingly adopted by single men or women. The child and his or her needs are paramount and at the center of the adoption process. These needs can be successfully met in a single-parent family (Sherry, 1986).

OTHER ALTERNATIVES

There are other variables to the traditional adoptive process. An *identified adoption* is one in which birth parents have agreed to place their baby with specified adoptive parents and an agency provides full preparation, evaluation, and counseling to members of the triad before placement and provides supervision to the adoptive family after placement. A *legal risk adoption* is one in which a child is placed in foster care with parents interested in adopting the child if reunification does not prove feasible. There is an understanding that the child's legal adoption cannot be guaranteed to the prospective adoptive family because of continuing rights of birth parents or other legal action (National Adoption Task Force, 1987). Legal risk adoption can avert a change in parenting and environment in the early months of life and is of benefit to the infant and adoptive parents if the placement becomes permanent.

INTERCOUNTRY ADOPTION

Preliminary estimates indicate that 11,340 foreign-born children were adopted by Americans in 1996, with the largest numbers of children coming from the following countries: China (3388), Taiwan (3333), and regions of the former Soviet Union (2797) (CRS Report for Congress, 1997).

A preadoption visit between the prospective parents and the pediatrician is an important event for all adoptive parents. In intercountry adoptions, it is essential. The parents need professional guidance in obtaining and evaluating medical and developmental data. Accumulating accurate information is often difficult. The physician can offer to speak with or write to the local medical doctor with the aid of an interpreter, if necessary, to gather up-to-date reports of the health status of the infant to be adopted. Problems such as chronic otitis media or minor orthopedic problems can be discussed, and plans to set up a treatment program can be initiated before the child leaves his or her native country. Agencies working in the international field should gather as much medical and social data as possible to pass on to adoptive parents. Parents and pediatricians need to be aware that medical information about adopted children is often lacking or inaccurate. A newly adopted child from another country needs a comprehensive medical examination as soon as possible after arrival in the United States.

Contact with parent support groups can be useful for children and parents. Planned counseling visits with the physician can be of value, especially during these critical early years. Questions of personal identity can be especially sensitive during adolescence, and referral to an adoption-sensitive child psychiatrist or other therapist can be helpful.

SURROGACY

Surrogacy refers to an arrangement in which a woman agrees to be artificially inseminated with the spermatozoa of a man who is not her husband and then delivers the infant to him at birth to raise as his own child. If he is married, his wife usually adopts the infant. Contractual arrangements may vary. Payment to the woman is customarily part of the process.

There are many problems associated with surrogacy. Most social welfare groups oppose any form of baby selling. Often counseling is not available to the woman who is to bear the infant or to the couple that plans to raise the baby. Most social welfare groups think that surrogacy does not serve the best interest of the child; rather, it is designed to be self-serving for the adults involved in the plan (Child Welfare League of America, 1988).

Although some physicians may be opposed to surrogacy, they may care for children who were born from this practice. All of the pediatrician's behavioral skills may be needed to provide care for and to support the best interests of the child.

At each developmental stage, the pediatrician should consider the impact of surrogacy on each family member and be prepared to make a therapeutic intervention when necessary.

When other nontraditional reproductive techniques, such as artificial insemination by donor and in vitro fertilization, are used, the skills of the pediatrician are further challenged. Disclosure to the child or adolescent may be important to consider.

OPENNESS IN ADOPTION

An open adoption is one in which the biological and the adoptive parents agree in advance to interact. The degree of openness ideally is set by the birth parents, the prospective adoptive parents, the agency acting as the agent of society, and the person being adopted, if of appropriate age. To clarify the changing views on openness and confidentiality in the field, the Child Welfare League of America, the standard-setting organization for major child welfare ser-

vices, convened a National Adoption Task Force in 1987. They established the principle that, starting with children adopted in 1986, confidentiality shall no longer be in effect once the adopted child reaches 18 years or the age of majority and that agencies shall assist such adopted persons in establishing contact with the birth parents, siblings, and other members of their birth family, as long as these persons are willing to have an involvement with the adopted person. According to the National Adoption Task Force, members of the adoption triad shall be encouraged to exchange updated medical and social information through the agency for potential mutual benefit (National Adoption Task Force, 1987). When older children are adopted, "open" arrangements make possible a new permanent family while respecting ongoing birth family relationships. However, state legislatures are slow to enact the laws that would permit such free exchange of information; only two states permit such an exchange, and others are considering the matter. In closed-record states, individuals must either rely on informal searches or ask a judge to open birth records.

TELLING

Adoption revelation is a process involving the gradual disclosure of adoption information over time (Brodzinsky, 1984; Dewoody, 1993). All children should be told that they were adopted. Information should be imparted in an open, matter-of-fact way, with feelings of love and respect. "Telling" is a process that can span a considerable period. The information often must be repeated and modified, depending on the child's emotional reaction (Schechter and Holter, 1975). Discovering what the child wants to know and what the child can understand affects what and when the child is told.

Some adoption authorities recommend that this process begin between the ages of 2 and 4 years. Others encourage parents to use the term freely with family and friends right from the start. Parents are encouraged to begin with the simplest facts and add information appropriate to the child's growing understanding. At the same time, it is important that parents know that most preschool children "do not understand the adoption information presented to them. It is not that parents are doing a poor job at explaining the relevant information to children. On the contrary, it is a cognitive limitation of the child that precludes a realistic understanding during these early years" (Brodzinsky, 1984). For these reasons, it is important that the pediatrician help the parents understand how the child's thought processes change with age and how to adapt to the child's changing cognitive and emotional development.

Many of these tenets are applicable to children born of a surrogacy pregnancy or conceived by artificial insemination using donor spermatozoa. In these cases, the pediatrician should work with the parents early on to arrive at a specific plan for each family and its unique situation.

IMPACT OF ADOPTION ON PARENTS AND CHILD

A successful adoption experience should follow a natural sequence: separation from birth parents, union with adoptive parents, and finally independence and autonomy for the young adult adopted person (Dukette, 1984).

Yet the adoption experience has an impact on all members of the adoption triad throughout the child's life. Birth mothers describe myriad "sensitive areas" that trigger memories. Three such events are the child's birthday, the birth mother's meeting a child of the same age as hers, and attending a baby shower (Roles, 1989). Adoptive parents struggle with their own feelings and with those of their child when, for example, the child announces that tomorrow's assignment at school is to present a genealogical chart.

Many adopted children think about their roots infrequently. Some children, however, have difficulty coming to terms with the fact that they are adopted. These children may have learning problems, difficulties with peer and sibling relationships, and problems accepting limits and discipline, especially in adolescence. Many of these problems may be directly related to their preoccupation with thoughts about their birth parents and the reasons for their adoption.

EXAMPLE

Sarah A., age 6 years, was adopted soon after birth. She had recently begun first grade with a competent, business-like teacher. She complained to her parents that she did not like her new teacher and wished she were still in kindergarten with the warm young teacher she had had last year. She resisted going to school, then one day asked whether her new teacher could take her away from her parents the way she had been taken from her birth parents.

Her parents consulted a therapist with whom Sarah played out her feelings and ideas about adoption. She said, "I'm going to do Adoption if I can." Using puppets, she had a dog steal a baby rabbit from the mother rabbit. This was repeated until she reached a new insight: "You're going to laugh, but last year I thought my kindergarten teacher might be my real mother." The therapist assured her that such thoughts are natural and that it is hard knowing that there is a birth mother but not know who she is. She demonstrated the puppet play to her parents and seemed proud of her achievement in understanding what lay behind her reluctance to leave the kindergarten teacher behind. School attendance proceeded with no further problem.

Adoptive parents experience the same pleasures and tribulations of childrearing as do parents who raise their own biological children. Adoptive parents' openness and acceptance of the child as truly theirs, although not biologically so, is of significant importance to the child's adaptation.

Various studies of children referred for psychiatric intervention have revealed that about twice as many adopted children are seen as would be expected from their numbers in the general population (Kostopoulous et al, 1988). Part of this psychiatric liability may harken back to biological or social influences that existed before the adoption rather than the adoption process itself. Many children with special needs suffer emotional and physical deprivation before their adoption. Even so, a number of studies of these children with special needs show success rates (parents felt rewarded and children benefited) of 73% or better (Kadushin, 1967; Nelson, 1986). In a recent study of 927 older child adoptions in which the average age at the time of adoption was 7 years and the children had been in foster care nearly 3 years before being adopted, the success rate was 90% (Rosenberg, 1989).

It is convenient to use the word "losses" as a way to refer to the particular experiences of adopted persons that are not shared by their nonadopted peers. These losses fall into three general categories: overt losses, covert losses, and status losses.

Overt losses such as changes of caretaker, loss of a familiar home and surroundings, loss of possessions or pets, and loss of emotional and bodily integrity from neglect or abuse are often the predominant form of loss in children who are adopted from the foster care system.

Covert losses are those inner experiences that an adopted person undergoes as a result of learning about adoptive status and subsequently undergoing an emotional process akin to grieving. Typical concerns giving rise to sadness and preoccupation include "Why did she give me up?" "Was there something wrong with me?" "How can I learn more about my birth parents?" "Will I ever see them?" Covert losses are usually the most important type of loss in children adopted in infancy by parents of the same ethnic group. Children and adolescents deal best with these feelings of sadness and confusion when these feelings are accepted and tolerated within the family.

Status losses are occasions of discomfort in social situations when attention is drawn to the adopted person's "different" status. Children on the playground—perhaps themselves threatened in some way by the idea of adoption—may tease an adopted child, saying, "Your mother didn't love you or she would have kept you." International families are often singled out for comment in public places. Adopted children often need special understanding from the teacher when given school assignments to prepare a family tree. Status losses are experienced by most adopted persons at times, but they are perhaps most acutely felt by children placed transracially or placed from abroad when there is an obvious difference between the child's appearance and that of the parents.

Adopted children, especially those with special needs, and their parents benefit greatly from the skills that physicians and social agencies can bring them. Anticipatory guidance is especially helpful to inexperienced parents.

Adolescent adopted persons and their families often are seen when they are in crisis. Professionals may be strongly impressed by the negative emotions shown, but they may fail to recognize the long-term commitment of the parents and the adolescent's attachment to them. Parents and adolescents are helped most by sympathetic listening and by recommendations for services that can help stabilize the family (Nickman and Lewis, 1994).

EXAMPLE

Kevin B. was adopted from foster care at age 4 years after being neglected and abused. He showed serious behavior problems for the first 2 years after adoption, including negativism, food hoarding, aggression, and self-in-

jurious behavior. Mr. and Mrs. B. expended much effort to make him a part of their family emotionally, and by second grade he was settling down and beginning to make friends and take responsibility in the home. Psychotherapy was a regular part of the family's life for several years. At age 12 years, Kevin began stealing and saying he hated the family.

The situation got worse and Kevin's behavior began to affect his younger siblings. They complained that if Kevin got away with his behavior, then they should not have to follow family rules either. The parents considered terminating the adoption and consulted their pediatrician. After listening carefully to the parents and Kevin, together and separately, she advised that they not act on any wishes to terminate the family arrangement, but instead return to the therapist they had used in the past so that he could help them understand how the current crisis had arisen. In so doing, the family successfully weathered the storm. Current information about the birth family was obtained, which was helpful to Kevin, who confessed that he had been worried about them but was also angry at them and confused by his conflicting feelings. By age 15 years, Kevin had become a competent student and athlete with some social success, and was behaving responsibly within his family.

ROLE OF PHYSICIAN (Table 13–1)

A permanent family that intends to provide a lifetime relationship is the primary need for all children. Adoption is a positive process that provides such permanency for children whose biological parents cannot do so. It also gives adoptive parents a personal fulfillment probably not available otherwise.

Adoption is a lifelong process for children and parents. The problems that arise are sometimes confusing, and parents need objective, intelligent, and sensitive help in negotiating it. Some adoptive parents of infants want to

Table 13–1 • Guidelines for Working With
Adoptive Parents

To work effectively with adoptive families, physicians can
Learn about the adoption process and the changes taking place in the adoption field.
Set up a preadoption visit to get to know the parents and to be able to anticipate problem areas.
Offer to review and interpret information concerning pregnancy, labor, delivery, and family medical history.
Identify adoptees' charts and listen for specific adoption-related problems.
Consider adding time to each adoptee's yearly visit to deal with special concerns.
Advise parents to disclose the fact of adoption gradually with love and respect.
Help adolescents deal with identity problems, which can be especially acute in the adopted teenager.
Encourage teenaged patients to wait until they are older to search for birth parents.
Reassure adoptive parents that the search for biological identity is not a rejection of them.
Refer promptly for psychiatric consultation if necessary.
Seek out and work reciprocally with community social service agencies. Most public and private agencies welcome a physician's opinion.

---

forget, avoid, or erase memories of the adoption, wishing the child had been born to them. Early in the physician's relationship with the adoptive parents, it may be wise to introduce the concept of *difference* in rearing adopted children. For example, an adoptive mother may express a desire to attempt to breast-feed her adoptive infant, with the wish to form a close early relationship. Some devices can help produce small quantities of thin milk, but rarely in significant quantities to fully breast-feed an infant.

As with the biological mother who decides not to breast-feed, reassurance by the physician that the adoptive mother can form just as close a union with her infant with a bottle can be very meaningful. Also, the time and energy required for attempts at breast-feeding may be better spent on other vital areas of adjustment (Carey, 1981). The physician's recognition that the adoptive state is different from the biological state and that the differences are permanent is essential. The pediatrician can then make use of his or her knowledge of growth, development, temperament, and understanding of family dynamics and introduce the added variable of the adoptive state in assessing the child at each well-child visit. Neither an exaggeration nor a denial of adoption is a healthy sign in parent or child (Kirk, 1964). Wegar (1995) speaks to the importance of recognizing the stigmatization of adopted children and their parents by society.

To work effectively with adoptive families, pediatricians should become familiar with the adoption process, the adoptive triad, and innovations in the adoption field. A preadoption visit with the parents enhances the physician-parent relationship and allows parents to ask questions. The pediatrician should offer to review and interpret information relevant to the pregnancy, labor, and delivery. If the child to be adopted is in another state or country, an offer should be made to contact the child's physician.

In preadoption counseling, major medical problems need careful exploration. Hostetter and Johnson (1989) suggest the following:

> In counseling individuals or couples who are anguishing over the decision of whether to accept a child with significant medical problems, it is helpful to frame the discussion in the context of what is best for the child rather than what, one might paternalistically believe, is best for the parents. If, after examining their capabilities, the parents feel incapable of caring for the child, the physician can gently suggest that the child might be better off with another family who may have the needed resources. Adoptive parents must be made to feel that they are protecting rather than abandoning their child.

In domestic adoptions, a careful review of the prenatal information and labor and delivery record should be carried out. It is important to review with the adoptive parents all medical and social data. A careful examination of the infant should be performed in the presence of the adoptive parents. An appropriate developmental examination to measure social, cognitive, and motor skills should be carried out for older infants and children.

Soon after arrival in the United States, all intercountry adopted children must have a careful, comprehensive physical examination, including hearing and vision screening if possible. Other screening tests should include testing for human immunodeficiency virus, a hepatitis B profile, tuberculin testing, and fecal examination for ova and parasites. Testing for syphilis, complete blood counts with indices, and urinalysis and urine culture for cytomegalovirus are also necessary (Hostetter et al, 1989).

In brief, all adoptive parents should be urged to insist on all medical and nonidentifying social information at the time of placement. Uncertainties cannot be eliminated, but they can be minimized. Parents should write down the medical and social information as it is presented unless it is provided fully in a written form. The pediatrician should consider adding time to the adopted child's yearly visit to explore any special concerns. Adolescents may need help dealing with identity problems, and teenagers' wishes to explore their biological roots should be supported, but they should be encouraged to wait until they are older to search for their birth parents. Adoptive parents should be reassured that the child's wish to search is not denial of their adoptive ties; rather, it is a desire to understand more about the adopted child's early life. Pediatricians should work reciprocally with adoptive agencies and consider being active advocates for these children.

Foster Care

In the past 5 decades, agencies that offer child welfare services have sought to protect children from any harm, including that of inadequate parenting. The services most commonly used have been "child protective," that is, investigating cases of neglect and abuse and removing children from such an environment to a protective one, as in substitute care in a family foster home. Traditionally, agencies have attempted to support children and families in their own homes if that is a viable alternative (Child Welfare League of America, 1988). When services are offered in response to a crisis, there is rarely cohesion, and services are often fragmented. Prevention and early case finding to allow early intervention are ideal.

Foster care, also known as out-of-home care, is a child welfare service in which children must be placed away from their families to ensure their physical and emotional well-being. An estimated 90% of these children are reunited with their rehabilitated families. If reunification cannot occur and it is otherwise indicated, most children can be placed in adoptive homes. Most children needing out-of-home care are placed in family foster care. Group and residential care are used primarily for children with special emotional and behavioral needs that cannot be addressed in a family setting. Therapeutic family foster care provided by specially trained foster parents is often used as an alternative.

The need for foster placement and the placement experience itself have lifelong implications for children. When managed appropriately, foster care is a healing and helpful service to children and their families. Conversely, understaffed and underfunded programs may allow a child to live in an environment similar to that from which he or she was removed (McDonald et al, 1996).

Children enter foster care for a variety of reasons. In a longitudinal study of 624 foster children, Fanshel (1976) found that children who enter foster care because of their behavioral difficulties return home far more frequently than do children who are abandoned or deserted. Children who

entered out-of-home care when they were younger than 2 years of age stayed in care longer than did older children. Ethnicity and race were powerful predictors: African American and Hispanic children remained in care longer.

FOSTER CARE STATISTICS

In 1993, there were more than 448,000 children in foster care, many of whom would not return to their families. The corresponding figure for 1990 was approximately 400,000, and the following figures for that year indicate demographic characteristics and placement status:

Age
  5% younger than 1 year
  31% between 1 and 5 years
  32% between 6 and 12 years
  32% age 13 years or older
Ethnicity
  39% Caucasian
  40% African American
  12% Hispanic
Placement status
  75% in foster family homes
  16% in group homes and facilities or emergency shelters
  3% in adoptive settings that were not yet finalized
Status of parental rights
  88% had not had a relinquishment or termination of parental rights
  12% had had parental rights relinquished or terminated
Agency's placement goals
  Family reunification, 60%
  Adoption, 15%
  Independent living, 5%
  Guardianship, 2%

In 1980, a series of reforms were introduced through federal legislation (Public Law 96-272). Home-based and family preservation services were developed for foster care prevention and family reunification. Adoption subsidies increased the number of adoptions of children with special needs by their foster parents or other families. Preservice and in-service training for foster parents and casework staff was initiated. Programs began to consider the ethnic, racial, and cultural identities of children. Independent living programs were established for older children who could not return home and for whom adoption was not an option.

Kinship care is the full-time care, nurturing, and protection of children by relatives, members of their tribes or clans, or other adults who have a family relationship to a child (Child Welfare League of America, 1995). Thirty percent of all children in out-of-home care are living with relatives. Kinship care does the following:

- Enables children to live with persons whom they know and trust
- Reduces the trauma children may experience when they are placed with persons who are initially unknown to them
- Reinforces children's sense of identity and self-esteem, which flows from knowing their family history and culture

- Facilitates children's connections to their siblings
- Strengthens the ability of families to give children the support they need (Child Welfare League of America, 1995)

The dramatic increase in homelessness, drug addiction, acquired immunodeficiency syndrome (AIDS) cases, and deinstitutionalization of persons with mental illness has led to an increase in the number of children in foster care (Paztor, 1988). Many of the children in out-of-home care have been sexually abused, are more violent at a younger age, and have difficulties in school. One major goal of this child welfare service is to ensure permanency for children through "the systematic process of taking prompt, decisive, goal-directed action to maintain children in their own homes or place them permanently with other families" (Maluccio et al, 1986).

ROLE OF THE PHYSICIAN

The special training of the pediatrician may be called for to enhance prevention and for early case finding and appropriate intervention. Early recognition of parental depression, addiction, or excessive loss of control could enable early intervention. Understanding the value of specialized homemakers and parent aide programs, or referring parents for parenting education classes or other family support services, may well avert abusive behavior. The physician who is skilled in diagnosing behavioral disturbances in parents and in children and who is skilled in making successful referrals for treatment of such problems plays a crucial role in the child welfare continuum.

Foster children often receive erratic health care both before and after placement (American Academy of Pediatrics, 1993, 1994). Medical records are often unavailable. The incidence of chronic physical and mental health problems is high in this group of children (Schor, 1982). Certain innovative approaches to the care of these children may ease their passage.

1. When infants or toddlers go to family foster care, every effort should be made to send with the child those personal possessions that may ease the change. We recommend that the infant's own mattresses, diapers, washcloths, and schedule of daily activities be sent with the child.
2. When treating school-aged children, the physician can carefully explain what illness is being treated or what immunization is being administered. Children may well understand allergy, especially foods and medications that they should avoid.
3. The use of a medical "passport" containing all significant medical information is invaluable in tracking growth, health, and physical and emotional development. The agency responsible for the child's care should initiate this file, which accompanies a child to every placement and includes all data concerning immunizations as well as medical, surgical, and psychiatric problems and procedures.
4. Children who have experienced disruptions are at risk for depression and identity confusion in adolescence. One valuable protective step is the preparation of a "life book," containing snapshots and narrative material about the child and all caretakers, beginning with the birth family. Pediatricians can suggest that agency workers prepare such a scrapbook if they have not already done so.
5. Children in long-term family care, including those in kinship care, may best be served by the physician who cares for their foster family. The relationship with the parents has already been established. Some foster children prefer to be seen for yearly visits with their foster siblings. Others may wish to see the physician privately. Both options should be offered, allowing adequate time for a full discussion of medical and psychosocial problems.
6. Lines of communication with foster care service providers, such as agency supervisors, individual caseworkers, and foster parents, should be established. Physicians should consult with and advise agencies and legislative bodies regarding medical and psychosocial issues surrounding family foster care.
7. Because children cannot be their own advocates, physicians caring for children with special needs may wish to assume this role.

Advocacy can be offered in a number of ways. One method is by tithe—by contributing funds to a child welfare group of one's choice. Another method is by time—by contributing services to an agency or group of one's choice. Some persons prefer to work as political activists and encourage the passage of laws that are beneficial to children. This requires an understanding of the interrelationships of poverty and the lack of education, housing, family life, and health care, among others, and how these factors can influence the healthy growth and development of children.

Managed care is becoming a dominant factor in the organization of health care services. It is important to be sure that health care delivery and financing for this group of youngsters is addressed in light of the realities of managed care and that managed care must be examined in light of how it can be made to work effectively for children in foster care (Battistelli, 1996). The principles enumerated above are important regardless of the medical delivery system in place.

REFERENCES

American Academy of Pediatrics: Health care of children in foster care: Committee on Early Childhood, Adoption and Dependent Care. Pediatrics 93(2):335, 1994.

American Academy of Pediatrics: Developmental issues in foster care for children. Pediatrics 91(5):1007, 1993.

American Academy of Pediatrics: Adoption of Children, 3rd ed. Elk Grove Village, IL, 1973.

Battistelli ES: Making managed health care work for kids in foster care: a guide to purchasing services. Washington, DC, Child Welfare League of America, 1996.

Brodzinsky DM: New perspectives on adoption revelation. Early Child Dev Care 18:105–118, 1984.

Carey WB: Induced lactation. Am J Dis Child 135:973, 1981.

Child Welfare League of America: A View of Child Welfare in 1988 and Beyond. Policy Statement. Washington, DC, Child Welfare League of America, 1988.

Child Welfare League of America: Standards of Excellence for Family Foster Care. Washington, DC, Child Welfare League of America, 1995.

Congressional Research Service: CRS Report for Congress, The Library of Congress, Jan. 15, 1997.

Dewoody M: Adoption and Disclosure, a Review of the Law. Washington, DC, Child Welfare League of America, 1993.

Dewoody M, Ceta K, Sylvester M: Independent Living Services for Youths in Out-of-Home Care. Washington, DC, Child Welfare League of America, 1993.

Dukette R: Value issues in present day adoption. Child Welfare 63(3):233, 1984.

Fanshel D: Status changes of children in foster care: final results of the Columbia University Longitudinal Study. Child Welfare Vol. LV, No. 3, March, 1976.

Hostetter M, Johnson D: International Adoption. Am J Dis Child 143:325, 1989.

Hostetter M, Iverson S, Dole K, et al: Unsuspected infectious diseases and other medical diagnoses in the evaluation of internationally adopted children. Pediatrics 83(4):559, 1989.

Kadushin A: Reversibility of trauma: follow up of study of children when older. Soc Work 12(4):22, 1967.

Kirk HD: Shared Fate: A Theory of Adoption and Mental Health. New York, Free Press of Glencoe, 1964.

Kostopoulous S, Cote A, Joseph L, et al: Psychiatric disorders in adopted children. J Am Orthopsychiatry 58:608, 1988.

Maluccio AN, Fein E, Olmstead K: Permanency Planning for Children (Concepts and Methods). New York, Tavistock Publications, 1986, p IX.

McDonald TP, Allen RI, Westerfeld A, et al: Assessing the long term effects of foster care. Washington, DC, Child Welfare League of America, 1996.

National Adoption Task Force: Report of the Child Welfare League of America. Washington, DC, Child Welfare League of America, 1987.

Nelson K: On the Frontiers of Adoption. Washington, DC, Child Welfare League of America, 1986.

Nickman SL, Lewis BG: Adoptive families and professionals: when the experts make things worse. J Am Acad Child Adolesc Psychiatry 33:5, 1994.

Paztor EM: Foster Parent Ownership of Permanency Planning Tasks and Its Effect on Placement Outcomes and Role Retention. Doctoral Dissertation, National Catholic University School of Social Services, The Catholic University of America, Washington, DC, 1988.

Roles P: Saying Goodbye to a Baby. Washington, DC, Child Welfare League of America, 1989.

Rosenberg J: Ensuring the Survival of Families Who Adopt Special Needs Children–A Report. Washington, DC, National Committee for Adoption, 1989, p 38.

Schechter M, Holter RR: Adopted children in their adopted families. Pediatr Clin North Am 22(3):653, 1975.

Schor EL: The foster care system and health status of foster children. Pediatrics 69:521, 1982.

Sherry SN: Helping families adapt to adoption. Contemp Pediatr 3:96, 1986.

Wegar K: Adoption and mental health: a theoretical critique of the psychopathological model. Am J Orthopsychiatry 65(4):540–548, 1995.

BOOKS TO RECOMMEND TO ADULTS ABOUT ADOPTION

Brodzinsky D, Schechter MD, Henig RM: Being Adopted. The Lifelong Search for Self. New York Anchor Press, 1993.

Lindsay C: Nothing Good Ever Happens to Me: An Adoption Love Story. Washington, DC, Child Welfare League of America, 1996.

Melina LR: Raising Adopted Children: A Manual for Adoptive Parents. New York, Harper, 1986.

Watkins M, Fisher S. Talking With Young Children About Adoption. New Haven, CT, Yale Press, 1993.

BOOKS TO RECOMMEND TO CHILDREN ABOUT ADOPTION

Blomquist GM, Blomquist PB. Zachary's New Home. New York, Magination Press, 1990. (For young foster children entering adoptive families).

Nerlove E: Who Is David? New York: Child Welfare League of America, 1985. (The story of an adopted adolescent and his friends.)

Powledge F: So You're Adopted. New York, Scribner's, 1982. (Children who are in their middle years can benefit from this book.)

BOOK TO RECOMMEND TO BIRTH PARENTS

Roles P: Saying Goodbye to a Baby, Vols 1, 2. Washington, DC, Child Welfare League of America, 1989–1990.

BOOK ABOUT BIOLOGICAL PARENTS FOR FOSTER PARENTS

Lee J, Nisivoccia D: Walk a Mile in My Shoes. Washington, DC, Child Welfare League of America, 1989.

14 Critical Life Events: Sibling Births, Separations, and Deaths in the Family

W. Thomas Boyce • Lauren Heim Goldstein

 In all kinds of cultural and family settings, children experience critical life events such as births and deaths of family members and separations from their primary caregivers. Their responses to these stressful events can vary widely and may have considerable impact on their development and behavior. Because pediatricians are often involved directly as physicians or as family medical advisors, opportunities are extensive for monitoring the success of children's reactions and offering anticipatory guidance or counseling.

Children encounter many critical events, transitions, and crises that challenge their coping skills and resources. These events may become turning points in a child's life and can provide new opportunities for growth and development. The developmental, family, and community contexts in which children experience these events largely shape a child's psychological experiences and understanding of the events. Physicians serve as a principal source of assistance for a family and child during periods of challenging transition. In helping families and children adjust to critical life events, health care professionals should have a broad understanding of the child, family, and environmental factors that may contribute to a child's ability to cope with challenges and adversities (Table 14–1).

Critical life events such as the birth of a sibling, separation from a primary caregiver, and death of a parent or grandparent can require a qualitative reorganization of key relationships and behaviors in a child's life and may alter a child's perceptions of self and the surrounding world. Such events expose the child to novelty and challenge. For example, when a boy with a secure sense of self and a basic trust in his parents loses a parent, he must re-evaluate existing relationships and his view of the world as a safe place. For a child without a secure sense of self or basic trust, the loss of a parent may confirm the view of the world as a dangerous and untrustworthy place. Parents and health care professionals can help children understand and cope with life transitions and challenges by providing empathic care, developmentally appropriate explanations, and sensitive encouragement.

Whether a life event is normative or nonnormative, expected or unexpected, has an important impact on how a child experiences the event. Normative events are those that are experienced by most children, at the same age, under ordinary childhood conditions, and within a specific cultural context, such as entering kindergarten. Nonnormative events are those that represent threatening, unexpected, and often dramatic changes in life circumstances, such as the death of a parent. Nonnormative events are more difficult to explain to children and are more difficult challenges to coping for adults and children alike. Critical life events can be planned, such as separations during vacations or

scheduled medical procedures, or unplanned, as in the case of a parent's sudden death. Adults can exert some degree of control over certain family transitions, such as the birth of a sibling, but from a child's perspective, there is little control over the occurrence or timing of many such events.

How children respond to critical life events varies widely. Some children who experience stressors in their lives exhibit few negative responses and remain in generally good health, whereas other children experiencing similar levels of stress become frequently ill and show more negative behavioral and emotional responses. The consequences of stressful events in the lives of individual children are thus quite variable. Laboratory-based work on children's psychobiological reactivity to challenging or mildly stressful tasks has shown a wide range of responses, with a subgroup of children demonstrating significantly larger changes in measurable physiologic parameters, such as blood pressure or heart rate (Boyce et al, 1995). Children who exhibit this exaggerated "reactivity" to stress may be at higher risk for health problems during periods of stressful or unsettling change. Physicians and other care providers working with children should be aware that there is extensive and clinically important variability in children's psychological, biological, and behavioral responses to stressful life events. When working with families undergoing major transitions, it is important to assess the individual child's responses, as well as the personal meaning of the transition for the child and family. (See Chapter 8 regarding individual differences in temperament.)

Children experiencing critical life events may exhibit one or several nonspecific behavioral signs of stress (Table 14–2). Parents should be aware of the characteristic signs of distress for children within a given age range. Whereas some children may exhibit developmental regression such as a return to thumb-sucking or loss of toilet training, others may show sadness or withdrawal, and some children may exhibit more aggressive behavior.

This chapter discusses the impact of three types of critical events in the lives and development of children: the birth of a sibling, separation from a primary caregiver, and the death of a parent. The role of the physician is discussed and guidelines are suggested for helping families

Table 14–1 • Child, Family, and Environmental Factors to Assess in Reacting to Critical Life Events

Child factors
    Age, developmental level, temperament
Family factors
    Level of stress and conflict in the family
    Stability
    Family routines
    Security of parent-child relationships
Environmental factors
    Resources from friends, family, community
    Level of stability and stress in the neighborhood and
        larger community

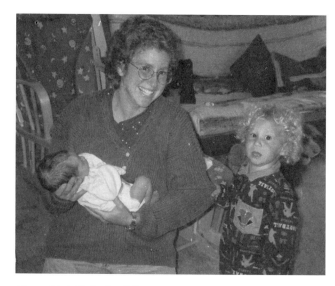

Figure 14–1. Birth of a sibling.

to cope with stressful events and transitions. The physician's ability to assist children and families through such events requires knowledge of the developmental context for major transitions, a capacity for eliciting and responding to children's emotional concerns, and an understanding of which coping strategies may be helpful to children during periods of stress and adversity. In the midst of such periods, it is crucial to assess the resources available to the child, the developmental skills required to master the transition, and the family's appraisals of the event or transition.

Birth of a Sibling

Although the birth of a sibling is generally viewed as an exciting and positive event in the life of a family, it also brings important losses in an older child's experience of his or her parents and position in the family. Family processes and the parent-child relationships are fundamentally changed by the addition of a new sibling. Parents must work to establish new relationships and to integrate the new sibling into an existing set of relationships (Fig. 14–1) (Kreppner, 1988). Especially for first children, but even for second, third, or fourth children in a large family, a newborn sibling brings an end to life as they have known it and the beginning of new relationships, expectations, and constraints. Parents' attention and reassurance become less accessible to the older child, as time and personal concern are increasingly focused on the new, more dependent infant. Before the new baby is born, it is common for the older child to be ambivalent about the pregnancy; after the baby arrives, feelings of jealousy and anxiety are normal

reactions. The older child may feel displaced, unsettled, or abandoned because of changes in the family and the reconfiguration of roles and expectations (see Chapter 12).

In helping a family prepare for the arrival of a new sibling, the developmental and social context into which the infant will be born should be carefully considered. For example, an older child's age, temperament, and developmental competencies should be assessed, as well as the home environment. A 5-year-old child who is adaptable to novel situations and people and who lives in a relatively stable home environment responds differently to the birth of a sibling than does a 2-year-old child who is inhibited and has a low tolerance for change. A 4-year-old child experiencing difficulty self-regulating aggressive impulses in preschool may feel anxiously out of control following the birth of a sibling. Parents should be told that the older sibling's emotional and behavioral responses to a birth depend crucially on aspects of both temperament and development.

Whether a child is capable of perspective-taking also influences how he or she reacts to the addition of a new sibling. Preschool children display egocentric patterns of thought and do not recognize that other people have different intentions and motivations; children who are cognitively egocentric have difficulty understanding the needs of a new sibling. When focus on self becomes less pronounced, children begin to appreciate that other people have perspectives that differ from their own. Children able to understand the thoughts and feelings of others may have an easier time adjusting to the birth of a sibling (Dunn and Kendrick, 1982).

The first 8 to 9 months after the arrival of a new sibling is a time for nearly continuous readjustment in family relationships. Changes in the mother-child and father-child relationship are likely to occur while new demands are placed on the parents and older sibling. During this transition, an older child may have difficulties adapting to new interactions and relationships, and to the changes in maternal attention and behavior. There is evidence that during this time period, fathers can usefully provide the

Table 14–2 • Behavioral Signs of Stress in Children

Externalizing behaviors
    Aggression, hostility, increased irritability
Internalizing behaviors
    Sadness, social withdrawal, inhibition, altered eating patterns
Sleep problems
Regressive behaviors
    Returns to bedwetting or thumb-sucking, difficulty with routine
        separations, speech disturbances, bowel problems
Increased neediness for comforting and reassurance
School/academic difficulties
    Problems with school behavior, decreased academic performance

older sibling with more attention, thereby compensating for the mother's preoccupation with the new infant (Kreppner, 1988). There is typically a marked dimunition in maternal attention to the older sibling, as well as an increase in punitive and restrictive maternal behavior.

Parents must also adjust to a new set of responsibilities and expectations following the birth of another child. In addition to caring for a newborn and an older child (or two, three, or more older children), parents can expect changes in sleep patterns, new financial obligations, and disruptions in family routines and patterns. Parents need to facilitate the new relationships between siblings and help teach the older siblings how to behave around the newborn. Because this is a stressful time for parents, eliciting help from friends and family with everyday tasks such as cooking, cleaning, and child care may ease the transition. (See Chapter 15 regarding addition of stepsiblings; see Chapter 13 regarding adoption and foster child placement.)

ROLE OF PHYSICIAN

Some recommendations for clinicians working with families during the transition include the following:

- Parents should be encouraged to be open with older children about the pregnancy and expected birth. Allowing children to share in the anticipation of a new birth helps them find ways to understand the upcoming event.
- The older child should be allowed to participate in the care of the baby. During pregnancy, the older child should be invited to come to obstetric appointments, listen to the fetus' heartbeat or watch it on an ultrasound image, and feel the baby move. After delivery, the older child can be involved by holding, feeding, and comforting the newborn under parental supervision.
- To foster a positive relationship between the older sibling and the new infant, parents should talk to the older child about the infant's wants, needs, and feelings. It is helpful to reinforce the older child's sensitivity and empathic feelings toward the newborn. Parents can be encouraged to avoid demanding too much of the older child in anticipation of the new sibling.
- Parents can help the older child prepare for the arrival of the baby by reading the child appropriate books on the birth of a younger sibling. This may offer an opportunity to begin thinking and talking about what the transition will mean.
- After the baby arrives, parents can encourage the older child to express emotions and reactions to the birth of the baby. Older siblings' feelings should be acknowledged and respected. Role play, fantasy play, and drawing may help children cope with their new emotions during this time. Parents can help the older child to understand the advantages and benefits of becoming a big sister or brother by emphasizing the behaviors and privileges of which the newborn is incapable.
- Whether the older child attends the birth of the new sibling is a decision for parents and the child. Pedia-

tricians can help parents weigh the advantages and disadvantages of having an older child at the delivery. Parents should consider the age and interest level of the child and discuss in detail with the child the events that will occur. If the child expresses any revulsion, fearfulness, or lack of interest, parents should respect this as an indication against attendance. If the child expresses interest, a videotape or photographic book on labor and delivery could be reviewed with the child, and any questions or fears discussed in detail. An older child's attendance at the birth should be cleared with the obstetrician or midwife and with the hospital or birthing center staff. In case the child changes his or her mind before or during the delivery, contingency plans should be made.

- Pediatricians should encourage fathers to use the postnatal period as an opportunity to spend more intensive time with the older child and attend to that child's individual needs during this sensitive period. The older sibling often needs more comforting and reassurance than usual in coping with the new addition to the family.
- Changes in the configuration of the older child's bed or bedroom should be carried out well in advance of the newborn's arrival (Boyce, 1996). Parents should emphasize positive aspects of this change. Switching the older child to a regular bed, for example, should be accompanied by statements of pride in the child's growth.
- It may be helpful for parents to minimize as much as possible other changes in the daily or weekly routine, and to defer other events such as residential moves or changes in preschool or child care arrangements until at least 4 to 6 months after the birth.

Separation From a Primary Caregiver

Young children may experience a variety of separations from their primary caregivers, ranging from daily separations to attend day care or preschool, to planned separations for a parent's business trip or military service, to unplanned separations resulting from parental hospitalization. The social context of the separation, the age and developmental level of the child, and the individual and interpersonal resources available to the child are all factors that help determine the impact of a separation on the child's development. Separation affects different children in different ways, and these individual differences may reflect variations in temperament as well as attachment security. Even though separations are often emotionally difficult for both parents and children, some separations can facilitate developmental growth by providing opportunities for learning and adaptation that would not otherwise occur.

In helping parents manage separation experiences and minimize children's distress responses, physicians should evaluate the following issues related to the context of the separation: (1) Will the separation be of short or long term? (2) Is the separation planned or unplanned? (3) Will the child be left in a familiar environment, with familiar caregivers, or in unfamiliar surroundings? (4) What is the quality of the child care arrangements? Will there be consistent care by primarily one person? (5) Is the separation occurring within a cohesive or a chaotic family environment? (6) What is the child's age and developmental status? (7) How has the child been prepared for the separation?

Certain cognitive and emotional skills that are gained with development enable older children to cope with short-term, planned separations better than younger children. For example, a 5-year-old girl who is separated from her parents for a few days has available to her a wide array of coping strategies (e.g., looking at a picture of her parents each day, counting the days until her parents return, talking about her feelings to other close adults, drawing pictures to express herself, and using a transitional object for comfort), as well as the ability to understand her parents' explanations upon separation and anticipate their return. A 10-month-old infant experiencing a similar separation has a more challenging adaptation to the separation because of a lack of coping strategies and other skills.

Brief separations from primary caregivers are not necessarily stressful for infants, especially if the quality of substitute care provided is high (Gunnar et al, 1992). Research has shown that 9-month-old infants experiencing a 30-minute separation from their primary caregivers in a new environment with an unfamiliar caregiver do not exhibit heightened physiologic stress responses if the caregiver is sensitive, warm, and attentive. The quality of the environment and the substitute care is of great importance in moderating the effect of the separation on the infant.

Longer separations (at least a few days) in the 1st year of life are generally disorienting for infants, especially after 6 months of age, because separation anxiety intensifies. Common responses to separation are protest, feelings of abandonment and despair, searching for the parent, and withdrawal. Bowlby (1973) describes the sequence of behaviors exhibited by a child separated unwillingly from his mother:

> At first he protests vigorously and tries by all the means available to him to recover his mother. Later he seems to despair of recovering her but nonetheless remains preoccupied with her and vigilant for her return. Later still he seems to lose interest in his mother and to become emotionally detached from her.

Upon reunion with the primary caregiver, the child may be sullen and angry and may turn away from the parent rather than seek contact. For a few days to weeks after the separation, the child may appear excessively clingy and in need of more comfort and reassurance than usual. The longer the separation between the child and the primary caregiver, the longer the time it takes for the dyad to resume normal interactions. Two conditions that have been found to alleviate the distress responses of young children are (1) receiving care from a familiar "substitute mother" (e.g., a well-known grandmother or aunt) and (2) having familiar possessions (e.g., a favorite blanket, toy, or pictures of parents) or a familiar companion (e.g., a sibling) (Bowlby, 1973).

Although older children may be more cognitively equipped to cope with separations from primary caregivers,

they may also be more aware of the anticipation and tension in the family environment before a separation. It is helpful to recognize and discuss this anticipatory tension with children before the separation, if possible. Research on military duty–induced separations in families has shown that the period directly preceding the separation is the most difficult time for children (Kelley, 1994). Mothers who maintain warm, supportive relationships with their children and create a cohesive family environment before the separation have children who cope better with separation (e.g., have fewer behavior problems).

Separation anxiety (i.e., apprehension and distress regarding separation from primary caregivers and resistance to separation) is a normal developmental phenomenon from approximately 7 months of age to the early preschool years (Bernstein and Borchardt, 1991). Some degree of separation anxiety during this time period may be regarded as a sign of healthy parent-child attachments, because it is in the best interest of the child to be in proximity to his or her primary caregivers. Developmentally inappropriate and excessive anxiety about separation from attachment figures, however, can become separation anxiety *disorder* if symptoms exist for at least 4 weeks based on criteria in the *Diagnostic and Statistical Manual of Mental Disorders IV (DSM-IV)* (American Psychiatric Association, 1994). Separation anxiety disorder is the most common of the childhood anxiety disorders. The frequency of various symptoms changes with development (Francis, Last, and Strauss, 1987). Children aged 5 to 8 years with separation anxiety disorder often report persistent worries about harm to primary caregivers, and they may refuse to attend school. Children aged 9 to 12 years more frequently report excessive distress at times of separation, and adolescents exhibiting separation anxiety disorder frequently display school refusal and report physical complaints. Physicians working with families on separation issues should be aware of the symptoms commonly exhibited by children diagnosed with separation anxiety disorder.

ROLE OF PHYSICIAN

The following recommendations may help parents and children effectively manage separation experiences:

- Parents should be encouraged to prepare the child for separation. Parents can explain why they are leaving and when they will be back to assure the child that his or her behavior did not cause them to leave. Parents can also give the child a concrete and comforting task to do in their absence (e.g., crossing off each day in the calendar).
- The use of a transitional object may help ease separation anxiety. Leaving a special toy or blanket with the child may comfort the child during the separation.
- If possible, the child should be left in a familiar environment with a warm, responsive caregiver. If the child must be left in a novel environment, it is important to leave familiar toys and other objects from home with the child.
- Parents should be encouraged to communicate openly with the child before, during, and after the separation via visits, telephone calls, and letters.

- Consistency of care should be maintained as much as possible. If possible, one substitute caregiver should consistently care for the child, rather than having a number of alternating caregivers. Having the child spend time with this substitute caregiver before separation may also help the child cope with the separation.
- Daily routines and rituals should be followed, if possible, during the separation to give the child a sense of continuity and sameness. Parents should leave instructions with the caregiver about routines surrounding bedtime, because this may be an especially difficult time for children.
- Parents can be prepared for the child's possible reactions of anger and avoidance upon reunion and be ready to accept the child's emotions and increased needs for comfort and reassurance.
- The birth of a sibling commonly involves separation when the mother goes into labor and leaves for the hospital. Plans for the care of the older child should be arranged well in advance of the delivery, and the child should be told about the arrangements, for example, who will care for him, where he will stay, and how long the parents will be away.
- Camp experiences and overnight stays at friends' houses are another form of parent-child separation that begins usually in the middle childhood years. The appropriate age at which overnights away from home should be allowed varies from child to child, and physicians may be asked to assist parents in deciding when to consent, when to defer, and when to encourage a reticent child. Homesickness is an emotionally painful experience that can occur during periods away from home and family at any age. Another important physician role is thus weighing the severity of homesickness and helping families to formulate developmentally appropriate responses. Homesickness may particularly trouble a child during a difficult developmental transition, such as school entry or early puberty.

Death of a Parent

The death of a parent is nearly always a profoundly sad and wrenching life event for people of all ages, especially children. For a child, a parental death is experienced as an unparalleled catastrophe: the dissolution and falling away of the world and its goodness. How a child reacts to and copes with this enormous loss varies widely and depends in part on the child's age, developmental competency, and temperament, and on the family and broader social context. After losing a parent, a child's daily life and routines, attachments, and emotional and instrumental support may be irreversibly changed. A child's ability to overcome bereavement and move on to a healthy developmental track depends on a number of interacting factors, including the security of the child's relationships with both parents before the loss, availability of prompt and accurate information about what has happened, opportunity for open grieving, and the continuing presence of nurturing, supportive adults in the child's environment (Bowlby, 1980). Specific needs

vary from child to child and with age and developmental status.

Although many school-aged children think about death, adults are often hesitant to talk about death with children (Lazar and Torney-Purta, 1991). Children younger than age 5 years generally have only a rudimentary and cognitively incomplete interpretation of death. Because of their egocentric views of the world, children of this age may feel that they did something to cause their parent's death, and feelings of guilt are common. Preschool children may also believe that death is reversible; if a parent dies during this developmental period, children may focus their concerns on imagined physical and concrete needs of the deceased person. Between 5 and 10 years of age, children gradually begin to understand, cognitively and emotionally, four central subconcepts about death: (1) death is permanent and irreversible, (2) all biological, emotional, and cognitive functions cease when a person dies, (3) death is inevitable, and (4) there are certain objective causes of death. There is evidence that children understand the subconcepts of irreversibility and inevitability earlier than they do the subconcepts of cessation and causality (Lazar and Torney-Purta, 1991).

In middle childhood, there is a gradual abandonment of egocentric thought and an increased ability to take the perspective of others; these developmental changes allow children to comprehend death more clearly. Children of this age may be increasingly fearful of death. If a child loses a parent, involvement in mourning activities may be particularly important to provide concrete information about the process of death and bereavement. The conditions or events occurring immediately before and after the death should be explained in clear and simple terms to help reduce fears. One of the main tasks of middle childhood is to develop peer relationships; development is facilitated by having a secure base at home on which to rely while developing competencies and friendships outside the family. If the secure base is disrupted by the death of a parent, children may have difficulties achieving a sense of autonomy and competence in the world outside the family.

During adolescence, a fully mature cognitive understanding of death is usually completed. Adolescents may often exhibit anxiety and denial about death as a result of their understanding of death's universality. As part of their normal developmental process, adolescents often fluctuate between independence and dependence. Losing a parent at this time may be particularly difficult, emotionally and cognitively, because of the child's developmental struggle over independence.

Research has shown that when young children (ages 4 to 8 years) are taught about the concept of death in school settings, their cognitive understanding is greatly increased over a short time span (Schonfeld and Kappelman, 1990). Children who have a better conceptual grasp of death may have increased coping abilities in response to the death of a parent. Parents, educators, and health professionals should use naturally occurring events such as the death of a pet or the death of a well-known actor or public figure to teach children about death.

Children's external responses to the death of a parent vary widely. Children grieve differently from adults (Osterweis, Solomon, and Green, 1984), and children's external behaviors may not reveal the intensity of their internal sadness. Some children show minimal symptoms and few behavioral changes, whereas others have difficulty functioning in school and at home. Many preschool children at first may exhibit little visible reaction to the loss and may return readily to normal activities of daily life. Some children may appear externally happy or undisturbed but be internally grieving in their own way. Other children may show regressive behaviors, expressions of inconsolable sadness or despair, or increased behavioral problems. Parents and other adults in the child's life should be encouraged to help the child express his or her emotions either indirectly through symbolic play and drawings, or directly through verbal expressions. Children should be encouraged to ask questions and to talk about the parent's death. As children develop new cognitive and emotional skills, they may repeatedly review and work through their reactions to the loss.

The means and effectiveness with which a child copes with the death of a parent depend on many factors, including the child's age and temperament, prior stress in the family, the surviving parent's mourning responses, and support from other family members and friends. The bereavement process is more difficult for children who have experienced long-term separations from the deceased parent before the death, who have witnessed high levels of family conflict before the death, and who do not have adequate support to help them through the difficult transition. Children living in unstable family environments before the death of a parent have a more difficult time adjusting than do children living in stable family homes (Elizur and Kaffman, 1983).

A child's temperament partially determines his or her style of coping with the death of a parent. Children who do not adapt well to change and who have poor impulse control may have more emotional and behavioral problems following the death of a parent than children with more positive temperamental characteristics. Children who have difficulty coping with frustration may have more difficulty accepting the reality of a parent's death. The surviving parent and other supportive friends and relatives should be made aware of temperamental characteristics that may hinder the child from grieving.

A child's reaction and adjustment to the loss of a parent is closely associated with how the surviving parent copes with the loss (Weller and Weller, 1991). If the surviving parent does not have adequate social support or does not allow himself or herself to express grief in front of the child, then the child may also hide emotions. Emotional restraint on the part of the surviving parent makes it more difficult for the child to express feelings and may increase the child's anxiety. The surviving parent must have the time and space to grieve so that the child may be included in the mourning process. A parent may believe that by hiding emotions, the child is being protected, but the child also needs to express emotions in order to cope with the loss. If the parent is able to share his or her reactions to the loss, then the child feels less alone in grieving.

HOW TO EXPLAIN DEATH TO THE CHILD

Adults are often unsure of how to tell children about the death of a parent or other close relative. Depending on the age of the child, a simple, concrete, and honest explanation should be given in a fairly calm manner; death should not be hidden (Crenshaw, 1990). When explaining death to children, especially to young children, parents should avoid giving false or misleading information such as "Daddy has gone to sleep." A comparison of death to sleep, for example, may increase a child's anxiety about sleep. Discussing death as the cessation of bodily functions is often useful (e.g., "Mommy's body has stopped working"). Children need to be told two important truths: (1) that the dead parent will not return and (2) where the body is and what has been done with it. To reduce feelings of guilt, children should be reminded that their behavior did not cause the parent to die; this is especially important for toddlers because their thoughts and actions are egocentric in character. It is also important for the surviving parent to provide children with explanations that they can believe. A child is likely to sense the parent's doubt in an explanation that does not coincide with parental beliefs, and the child may, in turn, feel greater anxiety and confusion.

DECIDING WHETHER CHILDREN SHOULD ATTEND THE FUNERAL

Many children find it helpful to attend the funeral, because this experience may make the death become more real. The decision of whether a child should attend the funeral should be left to the family and the child. Many children younger than age 4 years have trouble sitting through a funeral service. A child who is entirely unwilling and uninterested in attending or is frightened should not be forced to attend. It is likely, however, that the experience of attending the funeral will assist the child in understanding more about how people cope with death, providing the child with an opportunity to witness other people's grief and perhaps to share grief with others. Attending the funeral may provide the child with a way of formally saying good-bye to the deceased parent. Relatives should tell the child the reason for the funeral, what will occur, how long it will take, and who will be there. It may also be important for the family to develop other rituals after the death or on the anniversary of the death to provide opportunities for discussing feelings and memories about the loved one who was lost.

CHANGES THAT OCCUR WITH LOSS OF A PARENT

Many other changes and stressors may occur at the same time or within several months of the loss of a parent. If the deceased parent was working outside of the home, there will likely be changes in socioeconomic status. The surviving parent may have to change his or her employment situation to support the family, possibly by working outside of the home for the first time or taking on an additional job. Because of changes in financial status, the family may have to relocate to a new home or new community. A residential move often requires children to adapt to a new neighborhood, new friends, and a new school. There will most likely be a change in the emotional availability of the surviving parent, as that parent learns to cope with the loss. Children often rely on continuity and familiarity, especially during times of stress. Other changes to which a child must adapt following the loss of a parent may be especially difficult. As much as possible, the surviving parent should therefore try to limit the number of other changes occurring in the family for at least 6 months after the death.

LOSS AND PSYCHOPATHOLOGY

Losing a parent in childhood has been considered a risk factor for adult psychopathology, especially under the following circumstances: (1) the loss occurs when the child is younger than 5 years or during early adolescence, (2) for girls younger than 11 years, the parent who dies is the mother or, for boys in adolescence, the deceased parent is the father, (3) a child has prior psychological problems, (4) there is a conflictive prior relationship with the deceased parent, (5) an unstable family or community context is characterized by lack of support, (6) an inconsistent environment is characterized by multiple shifts in caregivers, and (7) the death is sudden as in suicide or homicide. Individuals who lose a parent in childhood are considered to be most at risk for development of subsequent depressive disorders.

ROLE OF PHYSICIAN

Some recommendations for physicians helping families cope with parental loss include the following:

* The surviving parent and other relatives should be told that efforts to "protect" children from the emotional pain of a family's grieving most often are ineffective. Children need to be able to observe other family members expressing their emotions. Children should be encouraged to express their feelings verbally or through play and drawing.
* Children need to feel safe and secure during a time of intense loss. Adults should assure the child that he or she will be taken care of and loved. Support, reassurance, and affection should be continuously available.
* Bereavement support groups for children may serve an important function. Children are given the opportunity to meet others their age who have experienced similar losses. Bereavement support groups provide children with a safe place where feelings can be shared.
* Children experiencing the loss of a parent need a stable, predictable environment. It is important to maintain family routines and structure as much as possible, because the familiarity of routines may be comforting to children during times of severe stress. As soon as the child is ready, resuming regular activities, such as sports, should be recommended to provide structure and familiarity to the child's daily life.
* Adults who have developed a long-standing basis of mutual trust and love are most able to help a child cope with the loss of a parent. It is important to have a substitute father or mother figure to whom the child can turn.
* Children who have lost a parent are likely to be more

sensitive in subsequent years to various kinds of natural disasters and sad events that occur in their community or in the world. Because one terrible, unexpected event happened in their lives, they may fear that a tragedy may be more likely for the surviving parent or for other loved ones. The surviving parent and other close relatives should be aware of this possible response and be sensitive to the child's perspective.

Death of Other Family Members

Many of the concerns and issues surrounding the death of a parent are also relevant to the death of other close family members, such as grandparents and siblings. How a child responds to these losses varies greatly depending in part on the child's age, developmental competency, and temperament, and on the family and broader social context. Although the death of a grandparent or sibling can have an enormous impact, these losses do not threaten the continuity of care for the child as does the death of a parent. How parents cope with these deaths greatly influences how children respond to the loss. Parents have the double burden of coping with the loss of either their own parent or child and of helping their surviving children. Because parents may be emotionally and physically unavailable to help their children cope, it may be important to have other adults available for support.

Grandparents can play important, nurturing roles in the lives of young children. The degree of emotional closeness between the child and the grandparent naturally affects the child's bereavement. The loss of a grandparent may be especially difficult if the grandparent lived with the family or was a primary caretaker. If the grandparent was ill for a prolonged period of time, parents may have had more time to prepare their children for the impending death. On the other hand, if the death was unexpected, children may have more difficulty coming to terms with the loss.

When a child's sibling dies, generally more attention is paid to the parents' loss of a child than to the sibling's loss. It is important for the family to recognize the feelings of the surviving child and to allow the child to mourn in his or her own way. If the sibling was ill for a prolonged period, the surviving child may feel neglected by the family and need extra attention and support after the death of the sibling. The surviving child may also have fears of experiencing similar illnesses or accidents that the deceased sibling encountered; these fears should be discussed. A decrease in physical health and feelings of anger, guilt, and depression are also common in children after losing a sibling. Family communication and emotional closeness may help ease children's bereavement process. (See Chapter 12 regarding death of siblings).

Conclusion

Although these three critical events in the lives of children—sibling birth, separation from primary caregivers, and death of a parent—differ greatly from one another, many commonalities exist in children's behavioral responses, in how families cope with the changes, and in how physicians can assist families and children. Similar behavioral signs of stress may be exhibited by children experiencing any one of these three critical life events. Physicians helping families during periods of stressful change need to assess the child, family, and environmental factors that may contribute to children's adaptations to challenges and adversities. How children respond to major transitions and stressors varies widely, and physicians must be sensitive to this variability and to the characteristic responses of an individual child.

REFERENCES

American Psychiatric Association: Diagnostic and Statistical Manual of Mental Disorders: DSM-IV. Washington, DC, American Psychiatric Association, 1994.

Bernstein GA, Borchardt CM: Anxiety disorders of childhood and adolescence: a critical review. J Am Acad Child Adolesc Psychiatry 30:518, 1991.

Bowlby J: Attachment and Loss. Loss, Vol 3. New York, Basic Books, 1980.

Bowlby J: Attachment and Loss. Separation, Vol 2. New York, Basic Books, 1973.

Boyce WT: Major family transitions: birth of a sibling and bereavement. *In* Rudolph AM, Hoffman JIE, Rudolph CD (eds): Rudolph's Pediatrics, 20th ed. Stamford, CT, Appleton & Lange, 1996, p 185.

Boyce WT, Chesney M, Alkon A, et al: Psychobiologic reactivity to stress and childhood respiratory illnesses: results from two prospective studies. Psych Med 57:411, 1995.

Crenshaw DA: Bereavement: Counseling the Grieving Throughout the Life Cycle. New York, Continuum Publishing, 1990.

Dunn J, Kendrick C: Siblings: Love, Envy, and Understanding. Cambridge, MA, Harvard University Press, 1982.

Elizur E, Kaffman M: Factors influencing the severity of childhood bereavement reactions. Am J Orthopsychiatry 53:668, 1983.

Francis G, Last CG, Strauss CC: Expression of separation anxiety disorder: the roles of age and gender. Child Psychiatry Hum Dev 18:82, 1987.

Gunnar MR, Larson MC, Hertsgaard L, et al: The stressfulness of separation among 9-month old infants: effects of social context variables and temperament. Child Dev 63:290, 1992.

Kelley ML: The effects of military-induced separation on family factors and child behavior. Am J Orthopsychiatry 64:103, 1994.

Kreppner K: Changes in dyadic relationships within a family after the arrival of a second child. *In* Hinde RA, Hinde JS (eds): Relationships Within Families: Mutual Influences. New York, Oxford University Press, 1988.

Lazar A, Torney-Purta J: The development of the subconcepts of death in young children: a short-term longitudinal study. Child Dev 62:1321, 1991.

Osterweis M, Solomon F, Green M (eds): Bereavement: Reactions, Consequences, and Care. Washington, DC, National Academy Press, 1984.

Schonfeld DJ, Kappelman M: The impact of school-based education on the young child's understanding of death. J Dev Behav Pediatr 11:247, 1990.

Weller EB, Weller RA: Grief. *In* Lewis M (ed): Childhood and Adolescent Psychiatry: A Comprehensive Textbook. Baltimore, Williams & Wilkins, 1991, p 389.

15 Separation, Divorce, and Remarriage

Judith S. Wallerstein

 With divorce the outcome of about half of the marriages in the United States, a large proportion of children experience this major disruption of family life, sometimes more than once. Although pediatricians do not become involved in the divorce negotiations themselves, they are expected to help parents deal with the inevitable effects on the children. This chapter provides helpful descriptions of and advice about the effects on the parents, the varying impact on children of different ages, the interferences with medical care, and assorted other pertinent issues including the challenges of remarriage.

Changes in family relationships wrought by divorce and remarriage have significantly altered the typical experience of growing up.

Certain consequences of these changes are relevant to the physician's task and role. Divorce-engendered stress and changes in parent–child interactions bear directly on the psychological health and development of the child at the time of the marital rupture and during the years that follow, extending well into adolescence and adulthood.

Demographics of Divorce

Since the mid-1970s, more than 1 million children each year have experienced the divorce of their parents. One researcher concluded in 1992 that at least 40% of young adult women were likely to divorce, 30% to remarry, and 16% to divorce twice if current divorce rates continued. Formal divorce statistics underreport the number of children who have separated parents, both because many couples separate without officially divorcing and because many couples who are not married break up their relationship after they have had a child. In 1988, 15% (9.7 million) of all children younger than age 18 years lived with a divorced or separated parent. An additional 7.3 million (11%) lived with a step-parent. Overall, 26% of children in the United States have already experienced their parents' separation or divorce (Furstenberg and Cherlin, 1991).

Most children live with their mothers after divorce. Approximately 13% of children live with their fathers. Although joint custody is a legal option in 40 states, the number of children in joint physical custody varies widely from a high of 19% reported in a recent study of two California counties to an estimated low of 5% in Massachusetts (Shiono and Quinn, 1994). The single mother or the remarried mother-stepfather family unit provides the dominant family structure for the child after the marital break-up. Because half of first divorces occur by the 7th year of the marriage, there is a preponderance of young children in the divorce population. Given the high incidence of remarried and redivorced families as well as the numerous brief and long-term informal liaisons that occur, many youngsters grow up in several different households with a changing cast of parents, step-parents, and live-in lovers for their parents.

Research Findings About Outcomes

Although many children weather the stress of marital discord and family rupture without psychopathologic sequelae, a considerable number falter along the way. As a result, the high divorce rate has also had a notable effect on the makeup of clinical populations. Children of divorce are greatly overrepresented in outpatient psychiatric, family agency, and private psychiatric practice populations relative to their presence within the general population. Parental divorce and parental loss are significantly linked to mental health referrals for school-aged children. A national survey of adolescents whose parents had separated and divorced by the time the children were 7 years old found that 30% of these children had received psychotherapy by the time they reached adolescence, compared with 10% of adolescents in intact families. By young adulthood, 40% had received psychological help. The representation of children from divorced families is even higher among inpatient populations. Although national figures are unavailable, many inpatient psychiatric facilities for adolescents report informally that 75% to 100% of their parents are from nonintact families. Overall, recent national data have shown that young people from single-parent homes or stepfamilies have a two to three times greater likelihood of experiencing emotional or behavioral problems as well as a higher incidence of learning problems than those living with both biological parents (Zill and Schoenborn, 1990).

The divorce literature, which scarcely existed before the 1970s, has proliferated as a growing number of investigators in psychiatry, psychology, and sociology have examined the processes involved in family separation and marital dissolution. As a result, knowledge is being accrued in many critical areas: the nature of the divorce process, the responses of children and adolescents by age and gender, the impact of divorce and parental conflict on parent–child relationships, factors in good and poor outcome in the short- and long-term perspectives, patterns of custody and visitation, the role of the father, the roots and dimensions of interparental conflict, and some of the issues that children and adults confront in remarriage. As findings from longitudinal studies have become available, light has been shed on divorce-specific anxieties that emerge belatedly in the lives of children of divorce when they enter young adulthood (Wallerstein and Blakeslee, 1989).

By and large, professional interest has not been directed toward issues of treatment. Except for mediation programs and school-based groups that have been developed in scattered areas of the country as well as a few pilot and demonstration projects (some clinical, others primarily educational), there has been a paucity of preventive or clinical services specifically designed to respond to the new stress points of change in divorcing families or to the special needs of children and adolescents whose family structure has been temporarily or more lastingly weakened by marital distress and breakdown. Most families struggling with divorce have relied perforce on the traditional medical and mental health services available in the community. As a consequence, the role of the pediatrician in helping parents make appropriate plans has become more salient.

Custodial Arrangements

The changing roles of men and women are mirrored in the courts and in legislation regarding custody and visitation. Early in the 1980s, the courts relied extensively on the concept of "the psychological parent," assuming that except in unusual circumstances or for older children, the mother would fulfill this role. Society has moved away from the expectation that single-parent custody, combined with reasonable visitation with the noncustodial parents, is the legacy of divorce. Attention has increasingly focused on the contribution of the father as parent and as potential primary parent. Custodial arrangements have changed over the past 15 years (Maccoby and Mnookin, 1992), although sufficient information is still lacking regarding the extent of this change in the direction of joint custody. During the 1980s, however, more than one half of the states enacted legislation that permits joint custody. In several instances, the public policy has leaned toward a presumptive preference for joint custody. In California, recent legislation, while acknowledging the importance of both parents for the child, emphasized the necessity of matching the custody arrangement to the needs of the individual family. Clearly, community attitudes and social policy are in flux.

Joint custody remains a variously defined arrangement, differing not only between states but also between local jurisdictions. Joint *legal* custody typically refers to an equally shared responsibility between parents for major decisions regarding their children's lives and well-being. Joint *physical* custody indicates that the child actually resides for substantial periods of time in each parent's home, although the proportion of time spent and the schedule of transitions between households varies widely. Joint physical custody can be properly regarded as a new family form. The motivation for its choice varies widely. Some parents select joint custody out of commitment to the child's continuing relationship with both parents; others, however, select this custody form out of the demands of the workplace; still others select joint custody because neither parent truly wishes to take responsibility for the child. The experience of the child varies with the parents' motivations and emotional investment in parenting.

Researchers have raised the question as to how important the custody arrangement by itself is to the psychological adjustment of the child. Kline, in a sample of 93 white middle and upper class divorcing families, compared the psychological adjustment of those 38% of the children who were living in joint custody with that of the remaining group who were in sole custody (Kline et al, 1989). She and her colleagues found that neither the custody arrangement itself nor the frequency of access and visitation with the father influenced the child's psychological and social adjustment. The factors affecting the child's psychological and social adjustment, regardless of custody arrangement, were the prior psychological functioning of the parents and the degree of postdivorce hostility and conflict between the parents.

One well-controlled longitudinal study of intensely conflicted families, for whom the court had ordered joint custody over the opposition of one or even both parents, showed that children in involuntary joint custody seriously deteriorated in their psychological and social adjustment, their school performance, and peer relationships. Both boys and girls seemed to suffer when frequent access to both parents was imposed on families locked in ongoing disputes (Johnston, Kline, and Tschann, 1989). This work addressed the serious issue that has been raised in many jurisdictions as to whether the courts should award joint custody in the event of one parent's strong opposition. Findings from this study are in accord with the clinical opinions that mental health practitioners have held over many years.

There is also evidence from a number of studies that some children prefer joint custody to sole custody and that they may benefit from this arrangement (McKinnon and Wallerstein, 1986). It seems that when it is entered into voluntarily by both parents with dedication and conviction, joint physical custody can be regarded as a viable family form. Under appropriate circumstances, it serves well, especially in the transition from divorce to remarriage. Joint custody does demand special effort and commitment from the parents, the ability of the formerly married partners to remain in close touch with each other without suffering undue distress, and considerable flexibility from both child and parents. There is an insufficiency of research on the long-term effects of joint physical custody. Findings from study of infants and young children are expected to shed light on how the frequency of going back and forth from one home to another affects bonding and development.

Under the following conditions joint custody appears to be a helpful arrangement for children:

- When both parents assign high priority to their parenting roles and are willing to make important life decisions in accord with this commitment
- When both parents are sensitive observers and respectful of the child's wishes, and are willing to accommodate living arrangements in response to the

child's changing needs and priorities as he or she matures

- When both parents respect each other as parents and are able to communicate effectively with each other about the child
- When both parents can live with the ambiguities and differences that inevitably arise and can work together cooperatively, especially around such day-to-day issues as bedtime, toilet training, and television watching
- When both parents can really help the child in making the transitions between households
- When the child can go back and forth between the two homes without disruption of his or her own psychological adjustment or social and educational activities

Elementary school children seem better able to tolerate these changes. Preschool children and adolescents are more likely to find the arrangement disruptive to their development (Table 15–1). Individual differences among children are salient in the success or failure of joint custody.

Economic Consequences of Divorce

After a divorce, many families face problems that involve diminished financial resources, unemployment, child care arrangements, and social isolation—difficulties similar to those encountered by single-parent families. One major problem related to divorce that has been approached uneasily and with mixed success in different legal jurisdictions is how to enforce the collection of child-support payments from resistant, unreliable, or absent parents. Despite new legislation and improved collection methods, delinquency in the regular payment of child support is widespread. The lives of a significant proportion of the current generation of American children are being deprived by financial impoverishment directly attributable to divorce.

Levels of income and education are generally much higher among parents in two-parent intact or remarried families than among parents in families with only one parent present. In middle class families as well, the decline in the standard of living for divorced mothers and their children is striking. Also, because in most states, child support stops when the child reaches 18 years of age, the child of divorce is disadvantaged. We found that in a middle class and affluent population, only 10% of the

Table 15–1 • Issues Affecting Children of Divorcing Parents

Continued fighting between parents
Abandonment by one parent
Continued litigation over custody and visitation
Emotional/mental disturbances in parents
Diminished parenting
Poor relationships with step-parents
Little support from outside nuclear family
Economic hardships

---

young people were helped financially by their fathers to attend college (Wallerstein and Corbin, 1986).

Dynamics of Divorce

DECISIVE SEPARATION

The central event of the divorce from the standpoint of the child is the decisive separation of the parents and the departure of one parent from the home. The legal divorce is of little moment either to children or to most adolescents. The child's acute response to the family rupture, as well as early efforts to cope, commences with the parents' announcement of the impending divorce and one parent's departure. Thus, parents who announce their decision to separate but continue to reside together are apt to confuse their children needlessly, burdening them with an ambiguous situation that they have great difficulty comprehending. Such parents should be advised to separate if indeed divorce is their intention.

IMPACT OF DIVORCE ON PARENTS

There has been insufficient recognition of the disabling impact of divorce itself on the psychological functioning of the adult and particularly on the adult's capacity to carry on with his or her expected roles or responsibilities during the months immediately preceding the marital rupture, the height of the divorce crisis, and the year or more that follows the separation. Many adults who can live alongside each other for years without open anger become openly hostile as the marriage ends. Others who suffer from chronic or moderate depression may become severely depressed or agitated. In most households, feelings of bitterness and scenes of conflict increase. Much of the anger and depression reflects the fact that in a family with children, the decision to divorce is rarely mutual. Most often the divorce is sought by one member of the couple and is opposed or is reluctantly accepted by the other. This difference between the adults and the humiliation engendered by the one-sided decision set the stage for the interaction at the time of the divorce and during the years that follow.

Perhaps centrally important from the child's perspective is the bizarre, although short-lived, behavior frequently exhibited by the parents, such as verbal accusations and threats as well as rage accompanied by violence and depression, and possibly suicidal ideation. A marriage that has been humdrum for years is likely to spring to life with the decision to divorce, and the unrestrained expression of aggressive sexual impulses and intense feelings tends to dominate households that were accustomed to a more circumspect way of life before the divorce decision. Children are at high risk for witnessing violence and spousal abuse at this time. Also, young children are more likely to be left alone without adult supervision.

DIMINISHED CAPACITY TO PARENT

The acute phase of the divorce is characterized by diminished physical and psychological availability of the parents. Newly employed parents are likely to leave children alone after school or for long periods with new baby-sitters in a strange setting. Sometimes the burden of work for the parent is such that very young children prepare their own lunches, get themselves to school, and put themselves to bed. The practical changes of life take an immense toll in reducing the time and attention available for children and so increase a child's anxiety and anger.

In addition, new relationships become important and demand considerable time. The flurry of social or sexual activity that often immediately follows the marital rupture is likely to absorb weekend time and evenings and to take custodial and noncustodial parents out of the home or to bring new sexual partners into the home.

At the outset, the noncustodial parent's house is often poorly equipped for the child's visits, and early visits tend to be uneasy, tense, or on the run. Also, new partners, some of whom have children, are likely to be present during these early visits, and children may feel aggrieved because their access to the parent has been blocked.

The household disorder that prevails in the aftermath of divorce, the rising tempers in both mother and child—especially between mothers and small sons—seem to eventuate in a sense of reduced competence and a greater sense of helplessness in the mother, provoking a continuing cycle of mutually interactive destructive behaviors (Hetherington, Cox, and Cox, 1979). Further cause for household deterioration can be found in the parents' fear of reproach by their children. Fearful of invoking the children's anger, a parent may retreat from requiring certain standards of behavior or meeting ordinary household standards.

These problems, added to the preoccupation with his or her own decisions and concerns, cause the custodial parent to be less competent as a parent and less able to maintain the structure of the household. As a result, there is mounting disorder, less discipline, less caregiving, more time spent by the parent away from home, at work or school or in resuming dating, and a sense among the children that the divorce has led to the loss of not one but both parents.

ABSENCE OF SUPPORT AT THE SEPARATION

One of the more striking findings of the California study was the loneliness of the child in the divorcing family. More than half the children studied felt that their father was entirely insensitive to their distress at this critical time, and one third of the children felt that their mother was entirely unaware of their distress. Children age 9 and older were acutely aware of the lapses in parenting and felt neglected and aggrieved, whereas the younger children felt in danger of imminent abandonment (Wallerstein and Kelly, 1980).

The children experienced an extraordinary lack of support outside the family. Only 25% were helped by grandparents or other members of the extended family. Those children who did have the support of grandparents appeared to benefit considerably from special concern and attention. Outside of the school, few institutions touched these children's lives, according to the California findings. Fewer than 5% were approached by a member of a church or synagogue, although half the families in the study were

active members of religious establishments. All in all, less than 10% of the children received any help or support from adults outside the family. It is particularly relevant that although most of the children were regularly under the care of pediatricians, none of these physicians was contacted at the time of the crisis and none talked to the children.

It is often useful to encourage parents to seek help from members of the extended family, including grandparents. Although grandparents often are unavailable, there is evidence that a significant number of grandparents are hesitant about intruding at the time of crisis but, if called upon, would happily make themselves available as a resource for their grandchildren. Grandparents and members of the extended family can be especially helpful in visiting regularly, providing a special treat, baby-sitting, and giving other forms of support. In addition, parents should be encouraged to take their concerns about the children directly to the school and to enlist the teacher's help during the crisis, requesting perhaps some special attention for the child or some special words of encouragement, or suggesting an assignment related to the child's interest that might provide both pleasure and recognition at this difficult time.

The physician who knows the child can directly convey a compassionate recognition of many feelings, fears, and concerns. Such acknowledgment of the stress resulting from family rupture can be beneficial in allaying the child's sense of loneliness and of diminished adult support and availability, and may allay the child's fears of being lost or overlooked in the welter of sudden family changes.

Telling the Child About the Divorce

Children who are told of the divorce before the parent's departure from the household and who are also assured that they will continue to see the departing parent are significantly calmer than those who must confront the divorce without any preparation. It is essential that parents inform the child and allow time for several discussions so that the child may come to both believe and understand the impending break-up of the family.

Parents often experience difficulty in telling their children about the decision to divorce, not knowing how much to reveal about their marital intimacy. They are confused about when or where to tell their children, how soon to tell their children before one parent's departure from the household, or whether they should tell the children together or separately. Moreover, parents are apprehensive that their children may be unhappy, frightened, or angered by their decision and, feeling themselves somewhat battered and depleted by their own ordeal, are often reluctant to take on this issue. As a result, children—especially young children—are often not made aware of the final rupture and many wake up one morning to find that one parent has left. They remember this day for many years as a devastating time in their young lives. Sometimes it is hard for them to regain any trust in their parents.

Ideally, informing the child about the divorce is not a single, separate announcement but part of a supportive process over time, which the parents provide for the child and which enables the child to understand the divorce and thus begin to cope with the family changes. The purpose of the initial discussion is to begin to explain the divorce so that it appears as a rational step to the child and at the same time to prepare the child for the changes to come. Because this is only the first step in the process of overall support for the child, communication about the divorce should be kept open, and the parents should expect and encourage continued questions and repetitions in the normal course of the household routines and especially during times of particular intimacy between parent and child. The pediatrician can be helpful in explaining this process to parents.

WHAT SHOULD CHILDREN KNOW?

Children should understand what divorce means, what the family structure will be like in the immediate future, and what immediate changes they can expect in their living arrangements and daily routines. They need to be told emphatically that they will continue to be cared for in the present and into the future and that their needs will be considered and their wishes given some priority in the new postdivorce family. They need the explicit assurance that they will not be "lost in the shuffle."

Moreover, children need to believe that their relationship with each parent will endure and that they will not be abandoned by either parent. The pattern of visiting that will be established with the noncustodial parent should be explained to them. If the father is to leave the home, they need to feel confident that he has not disappeared, and they need to be protected from their worry that he has no place to sleep and no one to care for him. (It is helpful for children to see as soon as possible where the father is residing in order to help allay specific worries about him.) The frequency of the visiting should be based on the child's needs and the quality of the father-child relationship and should not be determined by the degree of conflict between mother and father, nor should it be governed by the father's "right to access."

Children should be apprised of the reasons for the divorce and assured that their parents are rational people who thought carefully before making such a weighty decision that would so powerfully affect all their lives. Children need to know that their parents have tried and exhausted every resource before coming to the divorce. They should be offered an explanation appropriate to their age and level of understanding. Young children can be told that the parents are unhappy and fighting, and that the purpose of the divorce is to bring an end to both the fighting and the unhappiness. Older children should be informed of the various attempts the parents made to resolve their conflicts and the parents' disappointment and sorrow with the marital failure. Details of sexual infidelity are not helpful to children. On the other hand, if the child is aware of an extramarital relationship, it should not be misrepresented but should be presented as symptomatic of the unhappiness within the marriage.

Finally, children need to understand clearly that they did not cause the divorce, even when there has been open parental discord over the management of the child, that their efforts cannot mend the broken marriage, and that the divorce represents the parents' decision and is entirely

separate from the children's involvement. They need to be assured that neither parent expects them to take sides against the other. They need permission to love both parents and to experience fully their feelings of sadness, anger, and disappointment. They need to understand that their family structure has not been destroyed and that they can expect a return to order and familiar routine in their lives following the transitional instability and difficulty of the immediate future. As they grow older, the children will need to understand that the parental failure in marriage does not presage failure in their own future intimate relationships. This is a long-lasting fear that causes children of divorce great suffering; it becomes central in their lives when they enter young adulthood (Wallerstein and Blakeslee, 1989).

Impact of Separation and Divorce on Children and Adolescents

It is important to distinguish the initial responses to and the impact of divorce from its long-lasting effects. Initial responses are more observable, whereas the long-lasting impact on development is complex and impossible to predict. Developmental factors are critical in the response of children and adolescents at the time of the marital rupture. Even though there may be significant differences among individuals, the child's age and developmental stage appear to be the most important factors governing the initial response. The child's stage of development profoundly influences his or her need for and expectation of the parents, the perception and understanding of the divorce, and the child's available armamentarium of defensive and coping strategies.

One of the major findings of research on divorce has been the recognition of patterns of response within different age groups. The age groups identified were preschool (2½ to 5 years of age), early school-age (6 to 8 years), later school-age (9 to 12 years), and adolescents. Rather than a priori categories, these groupings reflect the unexpected commonalities that were discovered in the children's responses.

ROLE OF THE PEDIATRICIAN

In general, (1) a child's illnesses can put an unexpected strain on a marriage, (2) the stress of marital conflict may increase the demand for medical service because of more concern, greater amount of illness, or both, (3) healthier divorce proceedings are better for the child, (4) a pediatrician can help coordinate child's health care after separation, (5) referral to a mental health professional is indicated when a child's suffering and symptoms continue over several months, and (6) stress of marital conflict may also decrease parental attention to a child's physical health and psychological condition. Table 15–2 lists some specific ways a pediatrician can be helpful.

PRESCHOOL CHILDREN

Preschool children are most likely to show regression following the decisive separation. This regression usually

Table 15–2 • Assistance Related to the Age of the Child

Age	Common Reactions of Child	Role of Physician
2 to 5 years	Regression, irritability, sleep disturbance	Encourage restabilization of household and bedtime routines. Reassure child. Urge restoration of contact with departed parent.
6 to 8 years	Open grieving, feelings of rejection	Support maintenance of child's relationship to both parents. Reassure child.
9 to 12 years	Fear, anger at one or both parents	Express interest and availability to child.
Adolescence	Worried about own future, depressed and/or acting-out behavior	Offer opportunity for private discussion.

affects the most recent developmental achievement of the child, for example, in toilet training, going to nursery school, venturing into car pools unattended by the parent, playing with peers, or remaining at nursery school unattended by the mother. Youngsters may return to thumb-sucking, to security blankets, and to increased masturbatory activity. Intensified fears are evoked by routine separations from the custodial parent during the day and at bedtime. Sleep disturbances are particularly frequent and appear to be linked to the young child's terrifying preoccupation with the thought of awakening to an empty household and to fear of abandonment by both parents. Indeed, the central concerns of many young children are abandonment and starvation. Many play out elaborate scenes that portray adults caring for children and children caring for children. These children are also likely to become irritable and demanding with parents and to behave aggressively with younger siblings and with their peers (Wallerstein and Blakeslee, 1989).

The physician can help by providing the parent with direct guidance. Whenever possible, household routines should be maintained and the child's life should be stabilized to the extent that the parent is able to do so. In addition, the young child should be assured repeatedly that the parent loves the child and will continue to care for him or her. At each separation, the child should be told when the parent will return. At bedtime, the parent is well advised to spend additional time with bath rituals and bedtime stories. The child should be told where the parent will be when the child goes to sleep and awakens. It is helpful for the parent to arrange to be present throughout the evening hours during the first few weeks after the separation.

It is of utmost importance that the child visit with the departed parent whenever possible. Very young children fear that disasters have overtaken the parent whom they do not see daily. Children at a very young age are more likely to feel that they have caused the divorce. The child should be told explicitly that this is not so and that the parents decided to divorce to improve the quality of life for the entire family.

The young child is easier to reassure and to comfort directly than are older siblings. Often the new symptoms disappear in a few weeks with direct assurance by the parent and the reinstating of stable routines that enhance the child's sense of predictability and order in the household. If the child is fearful about leaving the home or going to nursery school, the parent may either go with the child for a few days and then gradually leave or permit the child to remain at home temporarily in recognition of the child's fear of abandonment. All such parental behavior should be accompanied by verbal assurance and an explanation that the child's fear is unfounded.

CHILDREN AGED 6 TO 8 YEARS

Children in the 6- to 8-year-old group are likely to show open grieving, including sighing and sobbing. They are preoccupied with feelings of rejection, with longing for the departed parent, and with the fear that they will never see him or her again. They share the terrifying and humiliating fantasy of being replaced: "Will my Daddy get a new dog? a new Mommy? a new little boy?" Children are likely to weave "Madame Butterfly" fantasies, asserting that the departed father will some day return—"he loved me the best"—and are unable to believe that the divorce will endure. Children in this group feel torn by conflicting loyalties and by guilt if they turn toward one parent. In the California Children of Divorce study, half the children in this age group suffered a precipitous decline in their level of schoolwork and reported difficulty in concentrating and worry about their parents. A few children at this age, however, appeared untroubled and were able to maintain their usual composure and their full range of activities.

During the visit with the noncustodial parent, the children are likely to be well behaved out of fear that the visiting parent may not reappear if they are naughty; upon their return home, they may be irritable with the custodial parent as a reaction to having been on such strained good behavior during the visit. On the other hand, they may become fearful of expressing anger with either parent. Boys are likely to feel especially vulnerable to the mother's anger and may be fearful of being "thrown out." They are likely to assume that the divorce occurred because of a fight in which the father was ejected from the household, and they fear that the same fate will befall them if they disobey their mother.

The physician can be helpful to parents of children in this age group by requesting to see both parents in order to explain the importance of allowing the child to love both parents without feeling that he or she is called upon to make choices in the marital conflict. Parents should be urged to make it easy for the child to cross back and forth between the parents and, in fact, should try to help the child with these different transitions. In addition, each parent should make an effort to reduce the child's worry about herself or himself and about the parents. The child should be repeatedly and simply reassured by each parent that the conditions of life will improve and that the child should not worry about either of them but should try to concentrate on customary activities and on school.

The physician can also meet the child to hear his or her concerns directly and to help diminish worry about the present and the future. The physician can directly address the child's loyalty conflict and assure the child that love for *both* parents continues after divorce.

CHILDREN AGED 9 TO 12 YEARS

Children in the 9- to 12-year-old group are frightened by the divorce and often worried about entering puberty and adolescence without the supportive structure of the intact family. They may feign nonchalance or disinterest in the family events. School performance and peer relationships are likely to deteriorate during the year following the separation.

More characteristic of this age, however, is intense anger at one or both parents for the divorce decision. As these children mourn the loss of the intact family and struggle with anxiety, loneliness, and a sense of their own powerlessness, they often cast one parent in the role of the "good" parent and the other as "bad." They are vulnerable to the blandishments of one or another of the parents who are actively engaged in fighting with the other and are easily co-opted as allies in strategies designed to harass and humiliate the other parent. Children in this group are also often helpful to a troubled parent and can show enhanced maturity and greater compassion as a response to the divorce.

It may be difficult to speak directly with children in this age group, because they are likely to deny discomfort or to remain silent. Nevertheless, it is helpful for the physician to express a continuing interest in and specific concern for the child who may feel lonely and beleaguered; this also indicates to the child that the door is open for future conversation, which the child can initiate as needed.

Parents should be advised not to involve children in their disputes and to realize that children probably do not understand the issues, despite their pseudosophisticated remarks. They should also be helped to perceive the unhappiness that underlies the child's surface bravado, anger, or false disinterest. Children at this age are vulnerable to sexual overstimulation and should not be given the role of confidant regarding parental love affairs.

Children should be assured that the parents are working hard to stabilize the family, and they should be directed to the importance of continuing with their schoolwork and other customary activities.

ADOLESCENTS

The incidence of disturbance among adolescents faced with their parents' divorce is higher than has been generally expected. A large number of adolescents become worried about their own future entry into young adulthood and are concerned about the fate of their own marriages and the possibility that they, too, may experience sexual and marital failure. They also become concerned with issues of morality and respond in a global way to what they experience as a need to reorganize their opinions about the world around them and to rethink values.

Of particular interest for the physician is the high potential for acute depression with accompanying suicidal preoccupation in adolescents who seemed in good psychological health before the family rupture. Such a response should be taken very seriously, especially if the depression is acute or lasts more than a few weeks. There is a high potential in this age group for acting-out behaviors such as truancy, new sexual activity, alcohol or drug abuse, or even a suicide attempt.

The physician can be helpful in initiating contact directly with the adolescent when a prior relationship has existed. These children are likely to welcome the opportunity for a serious, wide-ranging discussion of the impact of the divorce on their future expectations and plans. At that time the physician can ascertain whether the young person is depressed and whether he or she is taking appropriate or too much responsibility in the home, and can respond accordingly.

The parents should be advised that although the adolescent can be helpful to them at this critical time, the young person also needs some protection and encouragement to pursue his or her age-appropriate interests. Parents should be urged not to depend heavily on their adolescent son or daughter but to seek support for their own needs from their family therapist or friends.

GENDER DIFFERENCES

Although it had been widely accepted by researchers that boys are more vulnerable than girls in both initial and long-term responses to divorce, this finding has been called into question by a critical analysis of the methods used in a range of studies (Zaslow, 1988, 1989). The picture is confusing, in part because the comparative developmental course of boys and girls in intact families, from infancy to young adulthood, is far from being clearly understood. The current state of knowledge of divorce populations links gender differences to the different developmental stages. Thus major differences between preschool boys and girls at approximately 4 years after separation have been observed on a wide range of cognitive, social, and developmental measures (Hetherington, Cox, and Cox, 1982). Although traditional sex-role typing in girls did not appear to be disrupted by divorce, boys scored lower on male preference and higher on female preference on the sex-role preference tests at this same time. The boys were also spending more time playing with girls and with younger children. They showed affective narrowness and a constriction in fantasy and play and were more socially isolated than their female peers.

Gender differences were observed as well in the California Children of Divorce study. Although boys and girls did not differ in their overall psychological adjustment at the time of the marital break-up, 18 months later the boys' psychological adjustment had deteriorated, whereas that of the girls had improved, making for a significant gap between the two groups. Guidubaldi and Perry (1985), in a national survey of elementary school-aged children 6 years after divorce, found that boys, but not girls, tested significantly below a matched control group from intact families in academic achievement and social relationships. Other evidence suggests that in general, marital turmoil has a greater impact on boys than on girls, both in divorced families and in intact, discordant families. One report from a national longitudinal study of divorce effects on children suggests that, at least for boys, negative symptoms that are usually considered divorce sequelae are actually apparent before the marital break-up (Cherlin et al, 1991).

A critical question is how much of the reported differential response between the sexes, if it does exist, is mediated by mother custody. One small study from the late 1970s found that school-aged children in the custody of the same-sex parent showed greater sociability and independence than did those boys and girls in the custody of the opposite-sex parent (Santrock and Warshak, 1979).

Finally, there is increasing evidence that adolescent girls in divorced and remarried families confront particular difficulties. Kalter has described special problems that girls from divorced families face in their relationships with their mothers, especially the difficulties of separating at adolescence (Kalter et al, 1985). Wallerstein's California Children of Divorce study, at the 10-year mark, also reported that young women from divorced families often have a turbulent adolescence and a conflict-ridden entry into young adulthood. A significant number of young women at the 10-year mark were caught up in a web of short-lived sexual relationships, some with much older men. They described themselves as fearful of commitment, anticipating infidelity and betrayal. Many of the young women who encountered difficulties in late adolescence had done well during the early years after the divorce, when they were preschool and elementary school–aged children. It may be that boys, especially preschool and school-aged boys in mother-custody homes, have a more difficult time during the years immediately following the divorce, whereas girls in mother custody find adolescence and entry into young adulthood particularly difficult. Clearly, gender differences need to be explored further for the various age groups and within different family structures.

FACTORS IN OUTCOME

The initial responses of children do not predict long-term consequences for psychosocial adjustment, either for those who did well at the time of the divorce or for those who fared poorly. Nor do preliminary findings at the 15-year mark of the California Children of Divorce study indicate that even 10-year outcomes have remained stable. There appears to be considerable shifting in individual adjustment as the young people, in their 3rd decade of life, either seek psychotherapy for themselves after several relationship failures or succeed in building gratifying heterosexual relationships and marriages. No single theme appeared among the children in this study who were functioning well immediately following the separation and divorce or over the years that followed, nor was there a single thread associated with poor outcome. Many of the children who were doing well at the 10-year mark were well-parented or had had considerable help along the way from at least one parent or grandparent. Very few were well-parented by both parents. Visiting frequency or patterns of visiting were unrelated to outcome, but whether the child felt rejected by the father remained a critical factor. Some had found adult mentors, and those who did showed particular promise in scholarship or athletics. Many had taken a great deal of responsibility for bringing themselves up. Those who did assume this responsibility felt aggrieved at their parents but proud of their own achievement.

Although in remarried families the step-parent can on occasion play a critical role in the child's development, the extent to which this occurs is unclear. In the cited 10-year study, few step-parents took on a central role in the child's life. Also, in a significant number of remarried families, the children felt excluded from the orbit of the remarriage. The latest national figures provide no clear support for the protective or mitigating influence of remarriage for children of divorce, although when divorce had occurred early in the child's life, parental remarriage seemed to offer benefit to the child (Zill, Morrison, and Coiro, 1993).

In Wallerstein's California Children of Divorce study, the amount of stress observed in the postdivorce family was considerable. One of two children experienced a second parental divorce. One of two children continued to live with intense anger between their parents that did not subside over the years. Three of five felt rejected by one or both parents. There were additional economic stresses, and one fourth of the children experienced a significant decrease in their standard of living, which they did not recoup during the postdivorce decade.

In effect, in investigating the long-term adjustment of the child of divorce, there is a rich mix of individual issues in the resiliency and vulnerability of child and parent, the individual talents and staying power of the child, the nature of the relationship between the child and each parent (especially the custodial parent), the extent to which the postdivorce coparenting relationship is relatively free from continued conflict that involves the child, and the encouragement and support available to the child from whatever other sources are available within or outside the family.

Briefly stated, components that seem central to the course and outcome in varying combinations of importance include the following:

- The extent to which the parents have been able to resolve and put aside their conflicts and angers and to make use of the relief from conflict provided by the divorce
- The psychological intactness of the custodial parent and his or her emotional and physical availability to the child
- The quality of the custodial parent's handling of the child and the resumption or improvement of parenting within the home
- The extent to which the child does not feel rejected in the relationship with the noncustodial or visiting parent and the extent to which this relationship has continued on a regular basis and has kept pace with the child's growth
- The individual assets, capacities, and deficits that the child brings to the divorce

- The availability to the child of a supportive human network, including siblings and extended family members, and the child's ability to make good use of it
- The absence of continuing anger and depression in the child
- The developmental needs of the child relative to sex and age

Although the initial break-up of the family is profoundly stressful, the eventual outcome depends in large measure not only on what has been lost but also on what has been constructed to replace the failed marriage. The effect of the divorce ultimately reflects the success or failure of the parents and children to master the immediate disruption, to negotiate the transition successfully, and to create a more gratifying family to replace the family that failed.

Parents and Children After Divorce

The relationship between parents and children following the divorce undergoes many significant changes. The visiting parent's relationship with the children is especially likely to change. Poor—even impoverished—relationships may improve, whereas others that have been close and affectionate during the marriage may dwindle unexpectedly. Young children are more likely to be visited over the years than are older ones. On the other hand, some adolescent boys and girls develop and maintain a close friendship with the visiting father—especially when the mother is depressed or unavailable.

Similarly, the custodial parent and children move into new roles. Many children, some very young, become closer to their mothers as proud helpers and confidants. Others move precipitously away from a closer involvement out of fear of engulfment. Altogether the divorce emerges as a nodal point of change in parent–child relationships in many of the families.

There is considerable evidence that the relationship between children and both divorced parents does not lessen in emotional importance over the years. Although the mother's caregiving and psychological role becomes increasingly central in families in which the mother has custody, there is no evidence that the father's psychological significance declines correspondingly. Even in remarriage, the biological father's emotional significance does not disappear or diminish markedly, and the children appear to face little conflict in creating a special slot for the stepfather in addition to their relationship with the biological father. It is strikingly apparent that whether the children maintain frequent or infrequent contact with a noncustodial parent, they would consider the term "one-parent family" a misnomer. The self-image of children who have been reared in a two-parent family appears to be firmly tied to the continuing relationship with both parents, regardless of a parent's physical presence within the family.

INTERVENTIONS BY PHYSICIANS

Many families need professional advice and guidance in negotiating their way through the complex and tangled pathway of divorce and the postdivorce years. Moreover, it is important not only to provide the services that they need but also to find ways to reach both adults and children at the appropriate times, namely, at the marital rupture and at critical turning points along the arduous road that lies ahead. Essentially, divorcing families confront two sets of divorce-related issues that fall within the domain of the physician: those associated with the acute crisis engendered by the marital break-up and those associated with rebuilding the family, and subsequent families, that will provide a "holding environment" for children and adults during the postdivorce years. These two sets of issues translate into two separate preventive and clinical agendas: one addressed primarily to the amelioration of the psychological disequilibrium of the separation crisis and its immediate aftermath and a second addressed to building or restoring family structure and parent–child relationships within the postdivorce or remarried family (Wallerstein, 1990).

Finally, there is considerable likelihood that children in these families have witnessed severe verbal abuse or physical violence between the parents. Often the effects of such experiences do not show up initially in the symptoms of the child; however, they may be associated with serious conscience deficits and skewed expectations regarding relationships between men and women, which, although they may not become manifest during childhood, may, if left untreated, come to the fore at subsequent developmental stages, especially at adolescence. The physician is well advised to make appropriate inquiries about parental conflict in the child's history that may not be readily forthcoming and to attempt to engage the child in an exploration of his or her reactions to what may have been searing incidents.

Duration of the Divorce Process

The timetable of the divorcing process is considerably longer than most people realize. The decision to divorce leads to many changes—both intended and unintended—that affect the adults, the children, and their relationships with each other. The drama, complexity, and scope of these changes exceed the expectations of many of the participants. Often the period of disequilibrium in the lives of the family members lasts several years, and even 5 years after the marital separation, divorce-related issues continue to evoke strong feelings in children and adults. In the California Children of Divorce study, the average time needed by the newly divorced woman to reestablish a sense of continuity and stability in her life was 3 to 3½ years. The men required 2 to 2½ years to establish or reestablish a sense of order in their lives. The divorce remained a live issue for half the adults at the 10-year mark. Only rarely did both parties achieve the same degree of psychological closure, and for at least one partner, the divorce was often still a painful issue 10 years later.

Similarly, as a group, the children remained strikingly aware of their family and its vicissitudes over the decade. One consequence of divorce appears to be that the family becomes a focus of the conscious—even hyper-alert—attention and consideration of the children. As the youngster matures, she or he reassesses the divorce and makes an effort to explain and master the march of family events in ways consonant with an enhanced maturity. In this way, the intellectual and emotional efforts of the youngster to cope with the family rupture appear to be reorganized at each developmental stage and extend throughout the growing-up years, including young adulthood.

Many families need professional advice and guidance in negotiating this complex and tangled pathway through the divorce and the years that follow. It is equally evident that many parents do not know where to turn for help with their children.

Remarriage

Most remarriage involves children from the former marriage of one or both partners. If both adults have been divorced, it is likely that their former marital partners maintain a presence in their lives as they continue to share parenting, to visit the children, and to provide economic support for the children. In addition, the former marital partners may have remarried, and their partners' children or children from the new marriage may further extend the already complex kinship system. The network of relationships created by the remarried family, referred to variously as blended, reconstituted, or binuclear, has been poorly defined and insufficiently studied. As Furstenberg (1980) observed, "We have no set of beliefs, no language, and no rules for a family form that has 'more than two parents,' yet a substantial minority of the population of the United States will participate or already is participating in such a family system."

The remarried family begins with a past history that is often overlooked both by the adults within the family and by those who counsel remarried families. The period of single parenthood, which for women averages 2½ to 3½ years following the divorce, is a major part of the remarried family's history. During the period of single parenthood, specific patterns of parent–child interaction are likely to arise. It is not uncommon, for example, for the single parent to relate to one or more children with a special closeness and mutual dependency. These patterns are likely to change suddenly with the entry of a new parent into the family system, leaving the children with strong feelings of having been rejected by the biological parent and with intense anger at the step-parent as intruder.

There is encouraging evidence from social agencies, parent self-help groups, life education courses, adult education classes, and some preliminary research that adults enter the second marriage more realistically. They bring an eagerness to work at the marital relationship and a greater willingness for compromise. It has been shown that remarried couples practice greater flexibility in the division of household tasks, more shared decision making, and a greater degree of emotional exchange between husband and wife than occurred in their first marriages. In general, there is less adherence to a marital bond built along strictly defined sex roles. In the California Children of Divorce study, most of the men, and even more of the women, expressed approval and a sense of increased contentment with the second marriage.

The changes required by remarriage are nevertheless formidable and extend well beyond creation of the family structure and relationships. As expected, remarriage sometimes leads to geographic relocation. Such a move introduces disruption and discontinuity, including greater physical distance between the noncustodial parent and the child. As family units combine, different lifestyles need to be integrated. Perhaps the greatest changes occur in the new family unit with the parent–child and step-parent–stepchild relationships. Several myths associated with remarriage identify the step-parent–stepchild relationship as hampering the formation of the new family unit. Three conflicting myths are (1) that stepfamilies are essentially the same as nuclear families, (2) that stepmothers are wicked and cruel to the children, and (3) that step-parents and children will love each other instantaneously (Visher and Visher, 1979).

STEP-PARENTS AND CHILDREN

Special attributes attach to parent–child relationships in the remarried family. Prior histories of both step-parent and stepchild represent ever-present "ghosts." Children deal with a range of conflicting feelings concerning their relationship with the step-parents as well as with a new and sometimes overwhelming network of new relationships with half siblings and stepsiblings of various ages.

In the California Children of Divorce study, the stepfathers were older than their wives and had been married before. Having traveled a lonely road, they were eager for a home and a gratifying marriage. They were a sober and committed group who were supportive of their wives. With few exceptions, they expected to assume the role of parent to the wives' children. Encouraged by the women, most men took this responsibility seriously and moved quickly into the role of the man of the household with the purposes, prerogatives, and authority accorded this position in traditional homes.

The precipitous entry of the stepfather into the role of husband and father generated anxiety in the children. Several of the new husbands had lived in the household previously as lover and companion. During that time, their relationship with the children was different and more inclined to be friendly, casual, or uninvolved. Occasionally, the men were especially pleasant or generous with the children while they were courting the mother. Perhaps in reaction to their own insecurity in the new role, a substantial number of stepfathers assumed a fairly rigid, disciplinary stance with the children, especially with the older ones. Stepfathers were variously described by complaining children as "stern," "cold," or "too strict." Other comments reflected the child's attitude of submission: "When he says something he never changes his mind," "He has a temper," or "He only likes things his way."

Fewer children live with their stepmothers because fewer fathers have obtained custody. Nonetheless, this relationship can be as complex as that with a stepfather. One major difference is that the stepmother is likely to be younger—sometimes too young to maintain appropriate distance and discipline with an adolescent child of a prior marriage. The tugs and tensions between adolescent and stepmother are formidable. Sometimes these conflicts are exacerbated by the youth's perception of the stepmother as the person who is responsible for the marital break-up. In a significant number of homes in which the adolescent lives with the father, the young person has been ejected by the mother for misbehavior and banished to the father's household for the control that the mother feels the father is better able to provide. All these circumstances burden the new and growing relationship between stepmother and stepson or stepdaughter. Nevertheless, there is also the potential for a close and sisterly relationship, especially between stepmother and stepdaughter, for whom the relationship may remain very important over many years.

UNREALISTIC EXPECTATIONS

Not surprisingly, many of the problems in the remarried family that center on the children derive from the adults' failure to recognize that relationships are created over time with children as well as with adults. Thus adults who fully anticipated the gradual development of the marital relationship may, in contrast, expect instant love, respect, and obedience from the children. Few adults appear sensitive to the need to cultivate a relationship with the child gradually and to allow for the child's suspiciousness and resistance in the initial phase. Such expectations of instant response are especially disturbing for children, who feel they are being called upon to betray their love for their parent and to substitute the step-parent in his or her place. Even young children need to be reassured that the new adult is not being presented as a substitute for the departed parent. Generally, it is better and easier for all concerned if the step-parent is given a special name—*not* "mother" or "father."

CRITICAL VARIABLES IN ADJUSTMENT

Age of the child is a significant factor in the interaction between stepchild and step-parent. The relationship with the younger children, mostly those younger than 8 years old, takes root fairly quickly and is likely to become happy and gratifying to both child and adult. Young girls and boys alike are responsive to the affection and interest of the new step-parent.

The relationship between the step-parent and an older child tends to follow a more conflicted course and is also much influenced by the gender of the child. There is mounting evidence that girls feel much more threatened by the entry of a stepfather into the family than boys do. This is in part because girls in divorced families often form very close relationships with their mothers and this closeness is clearly changed by the mother's remarriage (Hetherington, 1987). Older children and adolescents may continue to resent the step-parent's presence and may ultimately fail to develop a positive attachment. Youths in remarried families are likely to leave home earlier. Others gradually change their minds. In the California Children of Divorce study, some youngsters eventually sought to emulate the step-parent and placed him or her as the central figure with whom they could identify. Often the troubled relationship takes an important turn at a particular moment in time, following an incident or even a confrontation, when the child suddenly changes her or his attitude and decides to accept the step-parent as an authority figure and a parent.

At the outset of the remarriage, children may be both eager and anxious. They welcome the arrival of the step-parent because of the greater security that the presence provides, and they are relieved to be part of a two-parent household again. At the same time, children may resent the new adult's special place in their parent's affection and the instant authority conferred on this person. They are concerned that they might be replaced by or excluded from the new relationship. As they worry, they watch tensely for evidence of acceptance or exclusion.

Even when children feel reassured by the remarriage, they may continue to worry whenever friction develops between the new parents. The new marriage evokes the memories of the early experience, and children report retiring in anxiety in their rooms or crying at night when the newly married couple quarrels. Their view of the seriousness of family friction is sometimes at odds with the adult perspective and is often surprising to the adults.

The child's relationship with the step-parent and the parent and the various ways in which this issue is resolved by the child and the adults, or continues as a source of open conflict, are of central importance in the psychological development and adjustment of the child within the remarried family. Many children are able to maintain and enjoy both relationships. Father and stepfather, mother and stepmother do not occupy the same slot in the child's feelings, and the child does not confuse the relationships. These children are well able to enlarge their view of the family and to make room for all the major parental figures. All the adult relatives may be considered by the child to be of importance in providing figures for imitation and identification. Thus, the general expectation that children necessarily experience conflict as they turn from parent to step-parent as they are growing up is not borne out by observation, nor is the expectation that in the happily remarried family, the biological father is likely to fade out of the children's lives. Children with step-parents whom they love and admire do not turn away from parents whom they continue to visit.

Many adults, however, are less successful than the children in defining the different roles. Rivalries between father and stepfather and between mother and stepmother in the remarried families are often bitter and long-lasting. When the child experiences painful psychological conflict and feels torn between the love for the father and the love and loyalty to the stepfather or between mother and stepmother, the adults are likely to be pulling in opposite directions or failing to help the child.

The relationships between the step-parent and parent can easily become charged with the unresolved anger regarding the divorce and the aggravated jealousies of the remarriage. Such problems of competing parents and step-parents are especially difficult to resolve because communication is limited and there is no proper forum for discussion. Feelings may then be exacerbated as both find new grounds for accusations and counteraccusations. Often the child becomes the hapless scapegoat of adult anger and is placed in grave psychological danger by the unremitting conflict of the major adults in his or her life.

REMARRIAGE—SUMMARY

Overall, remarriage appears to enhance the lives of many children, particularly those who have not yet reached adolescence. These children are better parented by happier parents and by step-parents who take their responsibility seriously and try hard to fulfill a parental role. Such children are also content with their relationship with their visiting parent when the adults are not in conflict over the child's loyalty and affection.

The needs of older youth often diverge from those of the remarried parents, and the remarriage that brings contentment and greater maturity to the adults may not enhance the lives of the children. In some families, the relationship is not satisfactorily resolved, and the conflicts generated between step-parent and stepchildren can lead to rupture of the remarriage. Nevertheless, many adolescents and preadolescents, after an initial resistance and with the passage of time, are able to develop strong, close, and meaningful attachments to their step-parents, who then greatly influence their consolidation of values and choice of lifestyle and career (Table 15–3) (Wallerstein and Blakeslee, 1995).

ROLE OF THE PHYSICIAN

The physician can be helpful to adults on the threshold of remarriage. Most families welcome both encouragement and competent guidance. Moreover, there is considerable evidence that adults benefit from anticipatory guidance, which enables them to discuss the impact of major events before their occurrence and to look ahead constructively to the tasks that need to be mastered. The concerns of children and adolescents that can be expected can be explained by the physician to the new parent. The physician can call special attention to the differences in age and temperament among the children and to the children's hopes and fears regarding the anticipated changes within their lives.

Furthermore, the physician can help family members distinguish the remarried family from the earlier family, which can never be recovered or reconstituted. Fortunately, there is clear evidence from guidance of remarried families that many adults and children alike can benefit significantly from even brief advice emphasizing that the relationships in the remarried family are likely to be different, less intense, and perhaps, therefore, longer lasting than those of the initial family.

Perhaps the central issue is the honest recognition that the needs of the children and the needs of parents do not necessarily converge at all times. Different needs and wishes require careful balancing and sensitive consideration. The family may need help in learning how to provide adequate time, place, and opportunity for the continuing communication of feelings, concerns, and conflicts that inevitably arise in the course of daily living and especially during periods of great change or crisis.

Thus the couple should be encouraged to find time to be together without the children and, at the same time, to provide for activities for the family as a whole. The couple needs to be mindful that the children have already sustained the trauma of their parents' divorce and understandably need to be reassured, in words and behavior, that they will not be excluded from the new relationship. With all of these issues, the pediatrician can provide sympathetic listening and guidance, especially in counseling the parents that building a new family unit takes patience and time.

Table 15–3 • Issues for Children in Stepfamilies*

Complex relationships with new family members
Altered relationships with own family, especially change in mother-daughter closeness
Geographic relocation and separation
Unrealistic expectations for new harmony
Harder for older children and adolescents
New family tensions raise fears of further destabilization
Rivalries between parents and step-parents
Establishing new family ceremonies and shared values while continuing to respect earlier family history and loyalties

Role of physician: When asked for guidance, consider these issues and support the needs of the child.

REFERENCES

Cherlin AJ, Furstenberg FF, Chase-Lansdale PL, et al: Longitudinal studies of effects of divorce on children in Great Britain and the United States. Science 252:1386–1389, 1991.

Furstenberg FF Jr: Reflections on remarriage. J Family Issues 1:443, 1980.

Furstenberg FF Jr, Cherlin A: Divided Families: What Happens to Children When Parents Part. Cambridge, MA: Harvard University Press, 1991.

Guidubaldi J, Perry JD: Divorce and mental health sequelae for children: a two-year follow-up of a nationwide sample. J Am Acad Child Psychiatry 24:531–537, 1985.

Hetherington EM: Family relations in six years after divorce. In Pasley K, Ihinger-Tollmant M (eds): Remarriage and Stepparenting Today: Current Research and Theory. New York, Guilford Press, 1987, pp. 185–205.

Hetherington EM, Cox M, Cox R: Effects of divorce on parents and children. In Lamb ME (ed): Nontraditional Families: Parenting and Child Development. Hillsdale, NJ: Lawrence Erlbaum, 1982.

Hetherington EM, Cox M, Cox R: Family interaction and the social, emotional and cognitive development of children following divorce. In Vaughan VC III, Brazelton TB (eds): The Family: Setting Priorities. New York, Science and Medicine, 1979.

Johnston JR, Kline M, Tschann JM: Ongoing postdivorce conflict: effects on children of joint custody and frequent access. Am J Orthopsychiatry 59:1–17, 1989.

Kalter N, Reimer B, Brickman A, et al: Implications of divorce for female development. J Am Acad Child Psychiatry 24:538–544, 1985.

Kline M, Tschann, JM, Johnston JR, et al: Children's adjustment in joint and sole physical custody families. Dev Psychol 25:430–438, 1989.

Maccoby E, Mnookin R: Dividing the Child: Social and Legal Dilemmas of Custody. Cambridge, MA: Harvard University Press, 1992.

McKinnon R, Wallerstein JS: Joint custody and the preschool child. Behav Sci Law 4:169–183, 1986.

Santrock JW, Warshak RA: Father custody and social development in boys and girls. J Soc Issues 35:112, 1979.

Shiono P, Quinn L: Epidemiology of divorce. The Future of Children 4:15–28, 1994.

Visher JS, Visher EB: Stepfamilies and stepchildren. In Berlin IN, Stone LA (eds): Basic Handbook of Child Psychiatry, Vol 4. New York, Basic Books, 1979.

Wallerstein JS: Preventive interventions with divorcing families: a reconceptualization. In Goldston SE, Heinicke CM, Pynoos RS, et al (eds): Preventing Mental Health Disturbances in Childhood. Washington, DC: American Psychiatric Press, 1990, pp 167–185.

Wallerstein JS, Blakeslee S: The Good Marriage: How and Why Love Lasts. New York, Houghton Mifflin, 1995.

Wallerstein JS, Blakeslee S: Second Chances: Men, Women and Children a Decade After Divorce. New York, Ticknor & Fields, 1989.

Wallerstein JS, Corbin SB: Father-child relationships after divorce: child support and educational opportunities. Fam Law Q 20:109–128, 1986.

Wallerstein J, Kelly J: Surviving the Breakup: How Children and Parents Cope With Divorce. New York, Basic Books, 1980.

Zaslow MJ: Sex differences in children's response to parental divorce. II:

Samples, variables, ages, and sources. Am J Orthopsychiatry 59:118–141, 1989.

Zaslow MJ: Sex differences in children's response to parental divorce. I: Research methodology and postdivorce family forms. Am J Orthopsychiatry 58:355–378, 1988.

Zill N, Morrison DR, Coiro MJ: Long-term effects of parental divorce on parent-child relationships, adjustment and achievement in young adulthood. J Fam Psychology 7:91–103, 1993.

Zill N, Schoenborn CA: Developmental, learning and emotional problems: Health of our nation's children, United States, 1988. Advance Data, Vital and Health Statistics of the National Center for Health Statistics. Washington, DC: National Center for Health Statistics 190, November 16, 1990.

BOOKS FOR PARENTS

Kalter N: Growing Up with Divorce. New York, The Free Press, 1990.

Wallerstein JS, Blakeslee S: Second Chances: Men, Women and Children a Decade After Divorce. New York, Ticknor & Fields, 1989.

16 *Family Function and Dysfunction*

Stephen Ludwig • Anthony Rostain

 The child's family is obviously the primary influence of the psychosocial environment on her or his development and behavior. This chapter encourages the reader to think of the family's effects in terms of the specific tasks of supplying physical requirements; providing developmental, behavioral, and emotional needs; and socializing the child by furnishing and teaching about normal social relationships. Also described here are the consequences when there is a dysfunctional inadequacy or excess in the fulfillment of these roles, and their clinical management. The results of variations in family structure, rather than function, are discussed in Chapter 11.

The family's influence on a child is perhaps the single most significant determinant of a child's development. Clearly, there are important genetic and constitutional factors that are present at birth and that continue to influence the child through life. Yet in the process of helping children grow and develop, the family and its functioning stand out as the single strongest environmental factor. Although family structures, styles, and behavior patterns are varied in our culture (Bronfenbrenner, 1986) and around the world, the family is still the central social institution in all human societies.

A precise definition of family is difficult to construct, because our concepts are in a state of change. In 1965, a standard definition of *family* was "a social group characterized by common residence, economic cooperation, and reproduction" (Murdoch, 1965). The family includes adults of both sexes, at least two of whom maintain a socially accepted sexual relationship, and there are one or more children born to or adopted by the sexually cohabitant adults. However, this definition would not include many of the families rearing children today. This chapter does not explore the anatomy or structure of the family but rather its physiology, or function. (For a description of variations in family structure, see Chapter 11). We explore the specific tasks of a family and then review the nature and impact of various family dysfunctions on the child.

Family Functioning

It is important to remember that there are many variations not only in family form but also in family functioning. All families have strengths and weaknesses. All families place different emphasis on different tasks at different points in the family's life cycle (Walsh, 1982).

Although there are many specific and specialized family functions, we can condense those pertaining to childrearing into three general categories: (1) to supply physical needs; (2) to provide developmental, behavioral, and emotional needs; and (3) to socialize or teach about relationships. In the realm of supplying physical needs, the family must provide protection, food, shelter, health care, and other material goods. In the second area, the family should stimulate development and intellectual growth, provide guidance through approval and discipline, and meet needs for affection. The third category of function is socialization or teaching. This involves helping the child relate initially with family members and later with external social networks (extended family, peers, school, and neighborhood) and with society in general. This last function may be termed the promotion of citizenship. These family functions are listed in Table 16–1. There are also some families that suffer from pervasive parental dysfunction. The nature of this kind of dysfunction threatens all areas of family function and the integrity of the family unit.

Given the multitude of complex tasks that families strive to accomplish, it is reasonable to ask what constitutes normal family functioning. The answer depends on one's definition of the term *normal*. From the child's point of view, normal means that a family is meeting the child's needs.

Family Dysfunction: Specific Forms

The concept of dysfunction usually suggests lack of something important. For example, with regard to the family function of providing food, inadequate function is considered to be lack of food, malnutrition, or failure to thrive. It is equally injurious to the child when there is excess—for example, oversupplying food. Table 16–2 lists various forms of dysfunctional inadequacy and excess, such as too little or too much health care. There can also be a qualitative dimension; lack of protection may range from placing the child at risk for injury to active physical abuse by the parent. Although these forms are listed as distinct entities, they often overlap. Thus the child who is physically abused is also likely to be psychologically abused. With each blow there is an unspoken (and at times spoken) message to the child: You are bad, worthless, and unloved.

The factors responsible for and related to dysfunctional parenting are numerous, including personal problems

Table 16–1 • Family Tasks in the Care of Children

Supply physical needs
    Protection
    Food
    Housing
    Health care
Provide developmental, behavioral, and emotional needs
    Stimulation—developmental and cognitive
    Guidance—approval and discipline
    Affection
Socialize: provide and teach social relationships
    Training for family life
    Training for citizenship

of the parents, a variety of acute and chronic social stresses, and challenges presented by the child. Rather than present a list of these factors at once, we introduce them in the following sections, where they are most pertinent.

PHYSICAL NEEDS

Protection

Perhaps the most easily recognized and best documented form of family dysfunction is lack of protection. Lack of

Table 16–2 • Family Dysfunction

Task	Dysfunctional Inadequacy	Dysfunctional Excess
Supplying Physical Needs		
Protection	Failure to protect Child abuse	Overprotection and overanxiety
Food	Underfeeding Failure to thrive	Overfeeding, obesity
Housing	Homelessness	Multiple residences "Yo-yo"/vagabond children
Health care	Medical neglect	Excessive medical care Munchausen syndrome by proxy
Providing Developmental Behavioral, Emotional Needs		
Stimulation: developmental and cognitive	Understimulation Neglect	Overstimulation "Hothousing" Parental perfectionism
Guidance: approval and discipline	Inadequate approval Overcriticism Psychologic abuse	Overindulgence, "spoiled child"
Affection: acceptance intimacy	Inadequate affection Emotional neglect Rejection Hostility	Sexual abuse Incest
Socialization		
Intrafamilial relationships	Attenuated family relationships Distanced parents	Parenting enmeshment Overinvolved relationships
Extrafamilial, community relationships	Boundary-less families Deficiency in training in extrafamilial relationships	Insular families Excessive restriction from extrafamilial relationships

protection may range from parents who simply do not think of or provide a safe environment for their children (e.g., free of toxins, pests) to those who are actively abusive. In this type of dysfunction, parents, rather than being protective, become destructive of their children.

Physical Abuse

Because there are state laws and sophisticated reporting systems for protecting children from this kind of injury, we now have some idea of its incidence. The term *Child Abuse* is used as if it were a diagnosis when it really describes a category or class of disorders that represent many different forms of family dysfunction. The 1995 report of the National Center on Child Abuse and Neglect Data System (NCCANDS) indicates that there were over 3 million reports of abuse and over 1 million substantiated reports. The rate of reports was 43 per 1000 population. Physical abuse was documented in 24.5% of the cases. However, it is believed that there is gross underreporting of physical abuse and that official reports may represent only one half of the actual number of cases. The breakdown of the forms of abuse is shown in Figure 16–1.

Definition. Part of the problem of accurate reporting is the difficulty of uniformly defining physical abuse. Each state designates physical abuse in its own child protective laws. Each person may interpret abuse in his or her own way, based on a number of individual factors such as age, sex, religion, cultural group, experiences as a child, experiences as an adult, professional training, and the like. Giovannoni and Becerra (1979) showed that physicians and attorneys differ in their perceptions of abuse. Furthermore, notions that child abuse exists and that each child has a right to societal protection from injury are evolving concepts. One must recall that the first child abuse laws did not appear until as recently as the late 1960s. With all the nuances involved, clearly and precisely defining abuse as a risk factor is difficult. We know that child abuse is injury

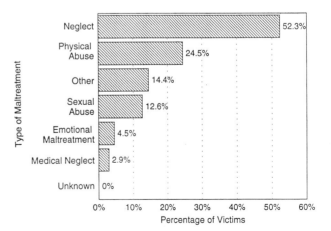

Figure 16–1. Types of maltreatment. N = 1,000,502 victims in 49 states. Note: Percentages total more than 100 percent because some states report more than one type of maltreatment per victim. (From United States Department Health & Human Services, National Center on Child Abuse & Neglect. Child Maltreatment 1995: Report from the States to the National Child Abuse & Neglect Data System. Washington, DC, US Government Printing Office, 1997.)

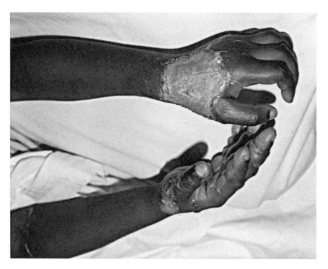

Figure 16–2. Six-year-old boy with history of firesetting who was overdisciplined by his mother's touching his hands to fire, producing second degree burns of both hands.

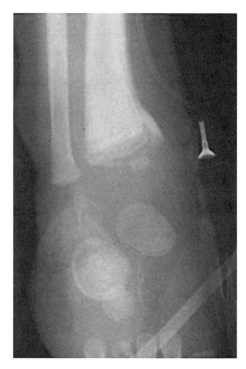

Figure 16–3. Bucket-handle fracture of distal tibia consistent with child abuse.

of a child by a parent or other caregiver either deliberately or by omission. Within a group of children captured by such a broad definition are those who have been murdered or repeatedly tortured by a deviant criminal parent and those who have on a single occasion been overzealously punished for a misbehavior (Fig. 16–2). Thus at our current level of sophistication, it is difficult to meaningfully define the risk in terms of developmental or behavioral effects. We use the term *child abuse* as if it were a solitary diagnosis when in reality it reflects a spectrum of disorders.

Contributing Factors. Just as definitions and forms of abuse vary, so do reasons for child-harming behavior (Ludwig, 1993). Many factors are relevant. Why would a parent hurt a child? Table 16–3 lists these and divides them into personal, familial, community-, and society-based fac-

tors. Overall, parental stress stands out as the single most important factor. The factors shown in Table 16–3 mediate through increasing parental stress levels. When stress becomes too great, the abuse-prone parent loses control. Children are always provocative and ready victims for parental explosive behavior. Physical injury results. The influence of societal violence is also an important contributing factor to the dynamics of violence against children.

Effects on the Child. The impact of physical abuse is both physical and psychological. Each time a parent physically abuses the child, the potential exists for physical injury (e.g., broken bones, blindness, brain injury; Fig. 16–3) and for psychological injury (e.g., "You are worthless; I can destroy you") that may seriously impede normal development and behavior (Table 16–4).

Table 16–3 • Factors Contributing to Physical Abuse

Parental factors
  Lack of knowledge about child development
  Lack of preparation for parenting
  Unrealistic expectations of child
  Proclivity to violence in other forms—poor impulse control
  Stress: marital/housing/economic
  Use of drugs or alcohol
  Emotional disorders—depression
Child factors
  Temperamental difficulty in the child
  Child fails to meet parental expectations
  Child is symbolic of something negative
Family factors
  Family pattern of physical violence
  Isolation: absent or unhelpful extended family
Community factors
  Lack of support and community resources for parents
  Factors that contribute to social isolation
Societal factors
  High rate of family mobility
  Tolerance of corporal punishment
  High level of violence in society
  Devaluation of children

Table 16–4 • Behavioral, Developmental, and Emotional Consequences of Physical Abuse

Situational, short-term consequences
  Depression, anxiety
  Avoidance behavior
  Aggressive behavior
  Scapegoating and self-pity behavior
  Developmental delay
  Academic difficulty
  Social maladaptation
Profound, long-term consequences
  Borderline personality
  Distorted self-concept and self-esteem
  Antisocial, delinquent behavior
  Self-destructive behavior
  Mental retardation

In its worst form, physical abuse results in homicide. Indeed, studies by the Centers for Disease Control (1982) show that the child homicide rate has increased sixfold since the 1930s. The 1995 NCCANDS report indicates that 45 states reported 996 child fatalities caused by abuse. The report estimates the rate of 110 per 100,000 population. Seventy-seven percent of the homicides involved children less than 3 years old. The consequences are experienced not only by the victim but by siblings and other family members. Studies of families that have lost a child show the profound effect of this type of loss even when the manner of death was other than homicide. Fortunately, most abuse victims do not die.

The number of physical manifestations that result from abuse are many and need not be detailed, as they are in references that focus on the diagnosis and physical management of abuse (Figs. 16–4 and 16–5) (Ludwig, 1993; Ludwig and Kornberg, 1992; Reece, 1994; Wissow, 1990; Giardino, Christian, and Giardino, 1997). Although any organ system or body part may be affected, a large number of head and sensory organ injuries are reported. Some authors have suggested that the head is a prime target for abuse since it is the body part that cries, that talks back, and that holds the personality the parent wishes to injure. Head trauma unfortunately carries with it the greatest potential for neurodevelopmental impairment. Martin's (1976) 5-year follow-up study of abused children found 53% of the 58 children studied to have some type of neurologic abnormality. Of those followed, 31% had moderate to severe injury that handicapped the everyday functioning of the child. Buchanan and Oliver (1979) estimated that 3% to 11% of children residing in hospitals for the retarded and handicapped were there as the result of violent abuse. Other studies (Sandgrund, Gaines, and

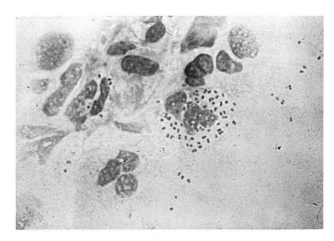

Figure 16–5. Gram stain of vaginal secretions showing gram-negative intracellular diplococci suggestive of sexual abuse.

Green, 1975; Frank, Zimmerman, and Leeds, 1985; Appelbaum, 1977) have documented similar findings. In addition to brain injury, there are many instances of damage inflicted upon sensory organs, particularly the eyes (Fig. 16–6). The resulting sensory deficits have the potential for chronic, severe physical disability.

The developmental and behavioral consequences are extensive (Egeland, Stroufe, and Erikson, 1983). A long-standing belief in the concept of the "cycle of abuse" is well articulated by Helfer (1974) in his notion of "the abnormal rearing cycle." Widom (1989) demonstrated that a cohort of abused children manifested more antisocial behaviors in adolescence and young adulthood than did a control group. Anecdotal studies have shown a high rate of histories of child abuse among the prison population and among those seeking psychiatric care in adulthood. It also appears that today's abused children have a greater chance of becoming tomorrow's abusing parents, although this is certainly not an inevitable consequence. Children who are chronically abused appear to either accept the role of the victim or become the aggressor themselves.

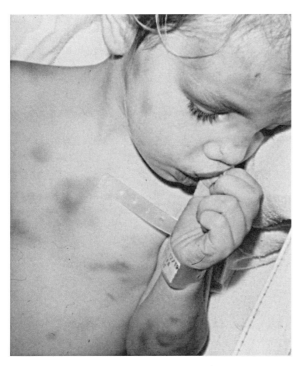

Figure 16–4. Child with multiple bruises secondary to inflicted trauma.

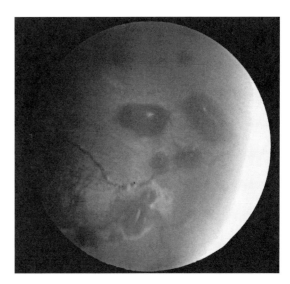

Figure 16–6. Retinal hemorrhages secondary to shaking.

The more immediate developmental and behavioral effects of physical abuse are probably dependent on several factors, among them (1) the age of the child, (2) the severity and duration of abuse, (3) the extent of positive parenting behaviors that are present in nonabusive periods, and (4) individual strengths or vulnerabilities in the child. It is apparent that some children tolerate extreme amounts of abuse yet seem intact. Other children may find one assault at the hands of a temporary family member quite devastating. The specific developmental and behavioral manifestations of physical abuse (Martin, 1976) are shown in Table 16–4. Some can be classified as specific psychiatric diagnoses, others are effects on speech and language development and intelligence, and still others represent abnormal or undesirable patterns of child behavior that may be attempts at adaptation (Kline, 1977).

Management. The first step in any management scheme is the identification of abuse. Health care providers need to be alert to the high incidence of abuse and to the fact that any traumatic injury must be suspected to be abuse if only for a moment's consideration (Ludwig, 1993). Some pediatricians may have difficulty in drawing the line between discipline and abuse. Most traumatic injury will be found to be nonintentional, but some injuries are more indicative of abuse. Evaluating a suspected injury comes from seeing it, trying to match the injury to a plausible history, using diagnostic tests and radiographs to under-

stand it further, and observing the interactions and interrelationships of family members. By using all four of these categories of information, the physician may arrive at a level of suspicion requiring a report of abuse. Wissow (1995) has published a compact list of the common signs and symptoms that should alert one to consider the diagnosis of abuse (Table 16–5). Indeed, each state has a reporting law mandating physicians to report suspected abuse and legally protecting them for doing so. The steps in case management are shown in Fig. 16–7. What should follow the report of suspected abuse is an investigation by the local Child Protective Services (CPS) agency. It is the responsibility of such agencies to evaluate the strengths and weaknesses of the family and to determine a plan for remediation. When the extent and nature of abuse has reached a criminal level, the physician needs to report this directly to the police to obtain immediate attention and protection for the child.

In addition to the identification and reporting of abuse, the physician must make an assessment of the child's safety. If the home is not safe, hospitalization is indicated, even without serious physical injury. Whether or not hospitalization is needed, the fact that the case is being reported to the CPS should be explained directly to the parents. This step would be easy for the physician to omit, but such an omission sets up a difficult and nontherapeutic situation for the workers who must follow up. Police,

Table 16–5 • Signs and Symptoms That Should Arouse Concern About Child Abuse or Neglect

Subnormal growth
   Weight, height, or both less than the 5th percentile for age
   Weight less than the 5th percentile for height
   Decreased velocity of growth
Head injuries
   Torn frenulum of upper or lower lip
   Unexplained dental injury
   Bilateral black eyes with history of single blow or fall
   Traumatic hair loss
   Retinal hemorrhage
   Diffuse or severe central nervous system injury with history of minor-to-moderate fall (<3 m)
Skin injuries
   Bruise or burn in shape of an object
   Bite marks
   Burn resembling a glove or stocking or with some other distribution suggestive of an immersion injury
   Bruises of various colors (in various stages of healing)
   Injury to soft-tissue areas that are normally protected (thighs, stomach, or upper arms)
Injuries of the gastrointestinal or genitourinary tract
   Bilious vomiting
   Recurrent vomiting or diarrhea witnessed only by parent
   Chronic abdominal or perineal pain with no identifiable cause
   History of genital or rectal pain
   Injury to genitals or rectum
   Sexually transmitted disease
Bone injuries
   Rib fracture in the absence of major trauma such as a motor vehicle accident
   Complex skull fracture after a short fall (<1.2 m)
   Metaphyseal long-bone fracture in an infant
   Femur fracture (any configuration) in a child <1 year old
   Multiple fractures in various stages of healing
Laboratory studies
   Implausible or physiologically inconsistent laboratory results (polymicrobial contamination of body fluids, sepsis with unusual organisms,
     electrolyte disturbances inconsistent with the child's clinical state or underlying illness, wide and erratic variations in test results)
   Positive toxicologic tests in the absence of a known ingestion or medication
   Bloody cerebrospinal fluid (with xanthochromic supernatant) in an infant with alerted mental status and no history of trauma

From Wissow LS: Child abuse and neglect. N Engl J Med 332(21):1423–1431, 1995.

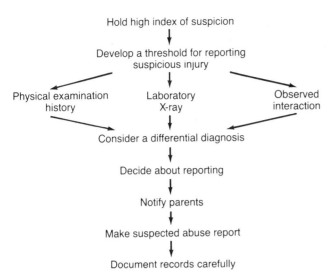

Hold high index of suspicion

Develop a threshold for reporting
suspicious injury

Physical examination
history

Laboratory
X-ray

Observed
interaction

Consider a differential diagnosis

Decide about reporting

Notify parents

Make suspected abuse report

Document records carefully

Figure 16–7. Steps in the management of child abuse.

courts, and even some CPS workers judge the severity of the child's abuse by the severity of the physical injury sustained. Unfortunately, such a relationship between extent of physical abuse and seriousness of family dysfunction does not exist. Thus the physician should also assess the assets and deficits in other areas of family functioning. An assessment of the child's mental health and developmental level is also important. Obviously, a child who has regressed, is developmentally delayed, and is bruised may be more at risk than the child with intact functioning who has sustained multiple fractures. Unfortunately, the court may make the opposite determination, as the number of broken bones is easy to count and constitutes concrete evidence.

The physician seeing a child for the developmental or behavioral manifestations of abuse may not know of the preexistent abuse. Thus in the evaluation of any child with a developmental or behavioral problem, the physician should inquire about abuse. Abuse is so common a phenomenon that it deserves constant consideration in these settings, just as it does in situations in which acute trauma is the presenting sign.

Parental Overprotection and Overanxiety

Overprotective parents are pervasively afraid that some terrible disaster will befall their child. They call the physician for even the most minor complaints, conveying tremendous anxiety about every physical symptom or ailment. They express a great deal of concern about normal developmental transitions and behavioral variations in the child. There is often a history of an adverse event (or series of events) having affected the child (or another family member). Unresolved feelings about these stressful events leads to a general pattern of behavior first described by Green and Solnit (1964) as *the vulnerable child syndrome* (see Chapter 33). Perhaps a better term for this pattern of parental behavior would be *the overprotective parent syndrome*. Overprotective parents often display an excessive preoccupation with bodily functioning and with potential

threats to health, occasionally to the point of being hypochondriacal. Minor illness episodes become family crises, with the parents becoming incapable of carrying out their usual daily activities. Avoidance of all possible risks (and by extension, avoidance of conflict) is the general rule guiding family life. Such parents are themselves likely to be overanxious individuals who are insecure about their own parenting skills, who consult many experts for advice about parenting, and who are likely to have grown up in overprotective families with overanxious parents. Occasionally, these parents are overwhelmed, depressed, lonely, or unfulfilled. Their overprotectiveness brings them into close proximity with their children, who function as emotional supports. When there is marital distress, focusing on the child's vulnerability serves to defuse tensions between the spouses. Finally, in extreme cases, overprotective parents fail to formulate rules, set limits, or discipline their children for fear of hurting or upsetting them.

The primary care physician can play an important role in helping overprotective families become less fearful. Once the overprotective pattern is recognized, the physician should invite the parents to discuss their concerns about their child and their own previous experiences with illness and other adverse events. The next step is gently but firmly to challenge the parents' perceptions that their child is sickly or at increased risk of harm. Such parents will need a great deal of reassurance that they are doing a good job of caring for their child but that their anxiety is both unwarranted and potentially harmful. They will also need a fair amount of education regarding the appropriate use of health care resources. This may require repeated conversations over the course of several months, since certain parents may have trouble believing medical opinion and need time to develop a trusting relationship with the physician. The goal of these discussions is to get the parents to realize they are excessively fearful and to help them take steps to reduce their anxiety level. If they persist in their overprotectiveness, it may be necessary to confront them directly and to insist they change their inappropriate behaviors. Enlisting the help of another family member who views the behavior as overprotective and dysfunctional may stimulate the parents to reconsider their attitudes. In cases in which the parents are intransigent, referral for mental health intervention is indicated. If the parents resist this recommendation, it may be necessary for the physician to make this a major condition for continuing his or her relationship with the child and family.

Food

Underfeeding: Failure to Thrive and Starvation

Failure to thrive is a term that is used to describe children who are not growing according to normal standards. This problem, which is described in detail in Chapter 41, is often an outcome of family dysfunction.

Parents may also underfeed children for a variety of other reasons ranging from poverty to inappropriate selection, as in food fads (see Chapter 40). Some parents may succumb to media stereotypes of beauty and strive to keep their child fashion-model thin. When underfeeding to the point of death occurs, it is termed *starvation*. There are many unfortunate clinical examples of this degree of family dysfunction.

Parental Overfeeding: Obesity

An undersupply of food is not the only form of family feeding dysfunction. The opposite is overprovision of food, leading to obesity in the child. As a society, we tend not to consider obesity in the same way we view failure to thrive or starvation, yet to the child the consequences may be just as debilitating (see Chapter 38 for further discussion).

Housing

Homelessness

In the past few years, the number of children being raised in families without housing has risen dramatically. It is estimated that single mothers and young children constitute over one third of the 2.5 million homeless persons in the United States (Bassuk and Rosenberg, 1990). The plight of these families has only recently begun to be documented. Although the root causes of homelessness lie in society's failure to provide adequate economic assistance to families living in poverty, its dire effects on psychological well-being and social relationships are many. Family integrity is undermined, family life is disrupted, and family relations are strained and torn apart. Life in homeless shelters is chaotic and stressful. Families are often crowded into a single room and are obliged to share toilet and eating facilities with dozens of other families in similar circumstances. Parents often feel inadequate, ineffective, and overwhelmed by a sense of powerlessness. Hopelessness, helplessness, apathy, confusion, and uncertainty are also common. (See Chapter 17 for further description of the consequences of homelessness for children.)

Multiple Homes

Children with an oversupply of homes have been described by the terms *yo-yo* and *vagabond* children. These are children who have too many homes, as may occur in privileged wealthy families who may not appreciate the adverse effects of not having a single home. It also occurs while the parents fight over who has custody and authority. Moore (1975) has described a series of 23 such cases, but the number of families experiencing this type of dysfunction is growing ever larger as divorce rates increase.

The effects of such custody relationships are many. Children are unsettled, knowing neither where they live nor who is making the rules. Sometimes, a child is abducted from one parent by the other. Children feel themselves to be pawns in a parental chess game. The result is anxiety, frustration, and depression. There have been no large or long-term studies of this phenomenon.

The physician must be aware of marital status and custody arrangements and must serve as an active child advocate. Sometimes parental rights are placed at a higher level than what is good for the child. This is when the pediatrician must step forward to speak for the needs of the child. Parents who continue to be destructive to their child in the process of being destructive to one another may need to be reported to the child protective services or referred for counseling.

Health Care

Medical Neglect

The distinction between medical neglect and nonadherence is a fine one. Nonadherence is the act of not following medical advice. There may be a good reason (e.g., the wisdom of the patient) or it may simply be a lack of motivation, resources, or understanding. Studies of rates of compliance for simple antibiotic regimens show them to be quite low even for intelligent and educated parents consulting pediatricians in private practice. When lack of compliance results in actual injury to the child, it falls into the category of medical neglect. Since providing for a child's health is an important family function, failing to do so represents a form of dysfunction.

There are no official reports on the incidence of medical neglect. Increasing numbers of children do not receive regular well-child care. Immunizations have also been documented as being inadequate in substantial segments of the population. Some children die because their parents have not sought appropriate care for them. This pattern may begin in the prenatal period. Investigators have shown that women who do not get adequate prenatal care are also less likely to obtain care for their newborns postnatally.

In managing medical neglect, physicians need to explain carefully their recommendations to parents. Where nonadherence is occurring, the physician should document the treatment recommendation and clarify again the rationale for the therapy. Some physicians may even wish to develop a formal contract with the parents. When a child is injured by medical neglect, the issue needs to be brought to the child protective service agency. In this circumstance, outside intervention is required to remediate the family dysfunction.

Parental Overuse of Medical Care: Munchausen Syndrome by Proxy

Munchausen syndrome by proxy (Rosenberg, 1987) refers to a parental fabrication or induction of illness in young children so that the parent gains recognition and support from a medical institution and its health care providers. The term is an outgrowth of a psychiatric disorder described in adults who subject themselves to multiple diagnostic evaluations and surgical treatments to derive the care and comfort extended to a patient. Thus the Munchausen syndrome by proxy may be seen as opposite of medical neglect. Instead of the family's underproviding medical services, it overprovides them, sometimes by exaggerating symptoms or sometimes by falsifying symptoms and laboratory findings. It is questionable whether Munchausen syndrome by proxy represents a distinct psychiatric problem or whether it is the extreme end of a spectrum that begins with parents' prolonging an acute minor illness (Libow and Schreier, 1986), doctor shopping, making an excess number of doctor visits, or using a child's illness to postpone their own return to work. Many forms of Munchausen syndrome by proxy have been reported, including administration of insulin, false hematuria, false fevers, suffocation, and intravenous administration of feces, causing polymicrobial infections, to name a few (Levin and Sheridan, 1995). Meadow (1977) has named the syndrome the "hinterland of child abuse."

In its full-blown form, Munchausen syndrome by proxy is an extremely serious disorder that produces significant morbidity and mortality. Rosenberg (1987) reported two deaths in a series of 10 reported cases, along with 10 unexplained sibling deaths. Other authors described a 5% to 15% mortality. In less serious cases, morbidity takes the form of children learning the benefits of the "sick child role." This may lead to future Munchausen behaviors or simply to hypochondriacal and dependent behaviors exhibited by many adults. The children may undergo unnecessary procedures, laboratory tests, and operations. They may also become involved in the falsification of signs, symptoms, and laboratory data. There have been scant long-term studies of these children to document either the long-term manifestations or the possible cyclic nature of the problem.

As with the management of frankly abusive behavior, the clinician's first step is to suspect a medical problem that stumps all the experts. The parents involved are usually described as cooperative to excess. Usually there is a family pattern in which only one parent is an active caretaker while the other is often absent, either physically or emotionally. Another clue may be that the parent may have a complex medical history or may have a professional background in nursing or in allied medical professions. If Munchausen syndrome by proxy is suspected, hospitalization may be required to finalize the diagnosis. It will not be difficult to convince the parent of the need for the hospitalization, because this ties in with his or her existing needs. Once the child is in the hospital, either through close monitoring of the parent, through covert videotaping, or through restricting the parents' visiting pattern, a diagnosis can be confirmed. Once the diagnosis is established, it must be presented to the parents and to the local child protective service for the creation of a management plan. In some cases, separation of the child from the family may be necessary. The long-term outcome with therapy is not known.

DEVELOPMENTAL, BEHAVIORAL, AND EMOTIONAL NEEDS

Stimulation: Developmental and Cognitive

Understimulation; Neglect

On occasion, pediatricians encounter parents who do not exhibit sufficient developmental or intellectual stimulation for their children. Such parents are likely to have been raised in families with similar difficulties. They may strike the physician as uncaring, uninvolved, indifferent, or intellectually impaired. They may appear to be unresponsive to their child's social cues, unaware of their emotional needs, or lacking in skills to play with or talk to their babies in ways that might promote their intellectual development. They may seem preoccupied, apathetic, self-absorbed, depressed, or uninterested in caring for their children. At one

extreme, such parents may be completely neglectful of their children's need for protection, nurturance, and guidance. This situation is generally easy to detect and requires the immediate attention of child protective services. In less severe cases, understimulating or neglectful parents may provide adequately for the child's physical needs but are unable to engage in intellectually stimulating forms of interaction with their children. Hugging, kissing, holding, rocking, cuddling, and other forms of affectional exchange may also be rare or absent. Playing with age-appropriate toys and games, conversing about why and how things work, engaging in creative activities such as art and music, reading stories aloud, taking trips to explore the outdoor environment, and discussing issues that are interesting to the child may be missing from the parents' repertoire of behaviors. Strong dependence on television or radio is also typical of these families.

Children raised in understimulating or neglectful families may suffer a host of adverse consequences, both immediate and long-term. Intellectually, such children are prone to become functionally mentally retarded or to exhibit learning difficulties. Emotionally, they may be prone to depression, anxiety, behavior disturbances, and personality disorders. Socially, these children may develop peer interaction difficulties, poor impulse control, or frank conduct disorders.

Children in understimulating or neglectful families may present to the pediatrician as dull, apathetic, emotionally bland, or indifferent. In severe cases, they can present with failure to thrive or developmental delay (see Chapter 41). In the office, the physician may observe limited or stilted parent-child interactions. There may be very little eye contact, spontaneous conversation, or signs of mutual emotional connection. The parents may perform their caretaking functions in a mechanical fashion or may interact with their children primarily around control of behavior and discipline. Indicators of this kind should prompt the physician to open a line of discussion with the parents regarding the child's needs for developmental and intellectual stimulation. If the parents demonstrate an interest in discussing these issues, it can be helpful to describe a few simple activities to promote parent-child interaction, to recommend a practical parenting guide, and to schedule a revisit in the near future to focus on the child's developmental and intellectual needs. If the situation is more severe, or if the parents are unwilling to discuss the concerns the physician is raising, referring the family to early intervention, child care and parenting programs, and reporting the case to child protective services may be indicated.

Parental Overstimulation or Perfectionism

In recent years, there have been a number of social factors contributing to "hothousing" (Katz and Becher, 1987), or overstructuring of the lives of children. Elkind (1981) has written *The Hurried Child: Growing Up Too Fast Too Soon*. A suggested definition of this problem is inducing knowledge that is usually acquired at a later developmental level. In terms of family function, overstimulation of this kind may be just as deleterious as the understimulation discussed in the previous section. Several societal factors may play a part in the growth of this phenomenon, including the increase of parental age, number of two-career families, maternal career development, divorce rates, and competition in the educational system and society in general.

There have been no thorough studies of the effects of hothousing. Some authors (Katz and Becher, 1987) have pointed to the possible consequences. They suggest that overstructuring may be done by parents who feel inadequate and guilty about the amount of time they can spend with their children. Unfortunately, hothousing may result in even less time being spent together. A second consequence may be that the child gets the subtle message that achievement is important to receiving parental love. Hills (1987) has stated, "In affluent, upwardly striving, middle-class families, children may be alternatively indulged and pressured for early, high, and sustained levels of achievement. Such children may come to believe that parental love and social acceptance are invariably conditional upon their achievement." (See Chapter 17.) Structured learning also takes away from unstructured play, an activity that is vital for normal development.

It is important for the physician to assess how much of the child's life is being structured for him or her. When reviewing the child's growth and development, it is essential for the pediatrician to inquire about activities. Children should be asked about their own desires and inclinations and about nonschool undertakings. Parents who discuss their children in terms of their accomplishments rather than their qualities indicate possible overstructuring. School-aged children who present with vague complaints such as fatigue or prolonged sleeping or toddlers with temper tantrums may also be the victims of hothousing. If such symptoms are related to excessive parental pressure to achieve, the physician can help the family to attain a healthier equilibrium.

Guidance: Approval and Discipline

Inadequate Approval; Overcriticism; Psychological Abuse

Psychological or emotional abuse involves a repeated pattern of disapproval, excessive discipline, hostility, criticism, scorn, and ridicule in the interactions among family members. In emotionally abusive families, relationships are charged with negative emotions, which are readily expressed or acted out in ways that undermine the trust, self-esteem, and a sense of security. Psychological abuse can occur among spouses, siblings, parents, and children, or other family members. Relationships become marred by frequent and constant conflicts, arguments, "put-downs," scapegoating, blaming, and derision. There is often a history of substance abuse, inadequate parenting in the parents' families of origin, and physical abuse, abandonment, or both during periods of stress or emotional crisis. It is not uncommon for individuals to state openly their hatred of and their wish to be rid of the individual with whom they have the greatest amount of conflict. Spouses may remark they wish they had never married, and parents may disclose to their children the wish that they had never been born. Emotional abuse may also take place in school (Krugman and Krugman, 1984).

Children in psychologically abusive families may react in any number of ways. Those prone to internalize their feelings may present with generalized anxiety, clinginess, inhibitions, phobias, perfectionism, depression, and profound feelings of shame. They may be overly compliant and excessively self-controlled for fear of rejection or scorn. Those with a tendency to externalize may demonstrate aggressiveness, hyperactivity, defiance of rules and authority, irresponsibility, provocative behavior, and oversensitivity to criticism. This group may present as undersocialized, uncontrollable, and rebellious in social situations. Children from abusive families may appear "starved for affection," may display an inappropriate need for acceptance and reassurance, and may be excessively eager to please adults, often going to great lengths to receive any positive attention they can solicit from others. If they can verbalize their emotions, these children may reveal deep-seated anger and resentment toward the emotionally abusive family members, along with profound feelings of shame, rejection, inadequacy, and self-doubt. Many express a sense of being unloved and unwanted. Some feel guilty for burdening their families with having to care for them. Children who are raised in emotionally abusive families tend to have chronic feelings of diminished self-worth and persistent problems with intimate personal relationships. They are at increased risk for developing marital and occupational difficulties, parenting problems, and psychiatric disorders.

When faced with evidence of emotional abuse within the family, the physician needs to respond in a straightforward and honest fashion. After expressing a deep concern for the emotional well-being of the child, the physician should emphasize that emotional abuse harms everyone in the family and that it needs to be brought under control as quickly as possible. Parents may not be aware they are being critical of the child to a point that is harmful. Or they may acknowledge the presence of tensions in the family that are causing them to be unsupportive. The prognosis for change is always better when there is eventual recognition of the problem. A referral for family therapy is strongly indicated in more serious cases. If there is evidence of moderate to severe psychological distress in the child and if the physician's attempts to be helpful are met with strong resistance by the parents, consideration should be given to contacting child protective services to pressure the family to seek help.

Parental Overindulgence

Parents in overindulgent families smother their children with an overabundance of love and nurturance but are unable to set suitable limits or enforce restrictions. There is excessive approval and insufficient discipline. Whether out of fear of harming the child, anxiety about being disliked or rejected by the child, discomfort with being in authority, or discomfort with feelings of anger and aggression, or in reaction to a sense of being insufficiently loved by their own parents, overindulgent parents avoid conflicts with their children at all costs. They constantly give in to their children's demands and seem incapable of effectively setting limits on their behavior. This pattern is often seen in families in which parents are older, are working, are divorced or unmarried, or are not functioning effectively as a team. In families with marital distress, overindulgence of the children may function either to divert attention away from or to intensify the spousal conflict.

Commonly viewed as "spoiled" (McIntosh, 1989), overindulged children are able to exert tremendous control over their parents by whining, complaining, demanding, threatening, screaming, and throwing temper tantrums. They may not exhibit these behaviors with adults who can set limits effectively (e.g., grandparents or teachers), but they can and will embarrass their parents in a variety of social settings (e.g., restaurants, stores, friends' homes) whenever their wishes or desires are not met instantly. When others express criticism of these manipulative behaviors, parents either agree with them (and feel terribly guilty and ineffective) or they defend their children and yield to their demands. Overindulged children tend to be immature, selfish, insecure, and easily bored and frustrated. They have trouble delaying gratification and give up easily when faced with difficult tasks. They may have grandiose opinions or unrealistic expectations of themselves and often become extremely disappointed when they fail to achieve their own goals. They have difficulty with self-control and are prone to misbehavior, particularly when conformity requires them to subordinate their wishes to those of others. They have problems with peers who may view them as "stuck-up," snobbish, and vain.

Physicians can be helpful to overindulgent parents by teaching them to become more assertive with their children. Techniques such as Parent Effectiveness Training have been successful in helping parents to feel less guilty, to overcome their sense of powerlessness, and to effectively set limits and enforce discipline with their children. After validating the parents' right to say "no" to their children's demands, and after emphasizing how important it is for children to learn to respect their parents' rules, the skillful physician can help overindulgent parents develop specific household rules with clear rewards and consequences. By starting with something relatively simple and straightforward (e.g., picking up toys after playing with them), parents can be instructed to monitor the behavior they are trying to modify and to practice giving rewards and enforcing consequences around one particular rule before moving on to developing other ones. If the parents appear particularly ineffective or are unwilling to stick to their decisions in the face of their children's opposition, then a referral for more intensive counseling is indicated.

Affection, Acceptance, Intimacy

Emotional Neglect or Rejection

Emotional neglect can be defined as a relationship pattern in which an individual's affectional needs are consistently disregarded, ignored, invalidated, or unappreciated by a significant other. People in neglectful families are emotionally disconnected from one another, behaving as if they were living on different planets. Parents may have trouble understanding their children's needs for love, affection, closeness, and support, or they may simply feel too overwhelmed or powerless to meet these needs on a consistent basis. Neglectful parents usually come from families in

which, as children, they were ignored or neglected by their parents. They also may suffer from a lack of emotionally satisfying adult relationships. Forced to rely on themselves for support, afraid of their own dependency needs, and reluctant to admit their pain, these parents are highly ambivalent about their children's needs, particularly when their children are hurting, crying, or looking for emotional support. They may feel jealous or resentful of their children and may perceive them as excessively demanding and impossible to satisfy. They may be so preoccupied with their own needs that they never consider the children's point of view. Or they may feel so angry and resentful about having children that they simply ignore them.

For children, affectional neglect may have devastating consequences: failure to thrive, developmental delay, hyperactivity, aggression, depression, low self-esteem, running away from home, substance abuse, and a host of other emotional disorders are associated with parental neglect. These children feel unloved and unwanted. They may strive to please others, or they may misbehave to receive the attention they crave. They may withdraw from people and appear uncaring and indifferent. They may be afraid of emotional closeness and may shun intimacy in relationships. In short, they are at risk for emotional problems throughout the rest of their lives. The degree of neglect and the individual vulnerability apparently affect the magnitude of the consequences.

Severe cases of neglect are generally easy to spot (e.g., when the child's development is grossly delayed or shows evidence of failure to thrive), but more subtle examples are harder to detect. If the primary care practitioner observes a relative lack of spontaneous, positive, parent-child interactions in her or his office, if the parent seems uninformed and apathetic about the child's development and behavior, or if the child is exhibiting signs of emotional distress without an obvious cause, emotional neglect should be suspected. Questions about daily routines and sources of support to the parent should precede any direct queries into the parent-child relationship. Encouraging the parent to describe the child's positive attributes, and focusing the discussion on these strengths can serve as an opening to raising matters of concern. It is important for the parent to hear these concerns directly from the practitioner. Vague, general, or indirect comments should be avoided, and specific recommendations should be made regarding the child's need for more sustained and positive interactions with the parent. How important the parent is to the child and how vital it is for the parent to receive more support from his or her social network so as to be more emotionally available to the child are also important issues to emphasize. Most neglectful parents feel isolated and unsupported in their own families and feel that their own emotional needs are not being met. Encouraging the parent to talk directly with the physician about her or his view of parenting is another way of opening up the discussion.

Often it is helpful to obtain additional information from other family members, particularly other caregivers. This will enable the practitioner to assess the availability of emotional support to the parent and child from within the family system. Finally, whenever possible, a home visit and a family interview should be conducted. This may require the services of an experienced clinical social worker, who can help make the decision to contact Children and Youth Services should emotional neglect be substantiated.

Sexual Abuse and Incest

The dysfunctional opposite of inadequate affection is what occurs when the family fails to maintain sexual boundaries between the generations. When this happens, there is an inappropriate excess, and sexual abuse or incest results. Sgroi (1984) has suggested that the term *sexual misuse* replace sexual abuse. This term more accurately reflects the misuse of the power of the perpetrator. The perpetrator is usually known to the child and has legitimate access to him or her. The child is coerced by positive rewards, destructive threats, or blackmail. The abuser begins by using casual touching, caressing, or kissing. This steadily increases to more advanced and overt sexual activities, often to the point of sexual intercourse. The type of sexual contact has been correlated with the age of the child victim. The victim may have a positive relationship with the abuser in many nonsexual realms of interaction. The victim may be told to "listen to your elders" and may repeatedly be placed in contact with the perpetrator. Until recently, many children have tried to tell adults about their sexual contacts only to be unheard or ignored. Since the early 1980s, professionals have urged parents to listen to their children, and reports of child sexual abuse have increased strikingly. Several prevalence studies (Finkelhor, 1979; Russell, 1983) indicate that this form of family dysfunction is extremely common, involving up to one in five girls and one in ten boys.

All states have laws that define incest as well as other forms of sexual abuse. It is noteworthy that this form of family dysfunction is so societally unacceptable that its definition is established by the tenets of criminal law.

The impact of child sexual abuse has never been fully or carefully documented. Paradise (1984) reviewed many of the existing studies and found that those that have been published often lack the necessary scientific rigor. We know that in the short term, sexual abuse causes many and varied physical and behavioral symptoms. Some of these are alleviated when the children disclose their histories of abuse. In addition, some studies document the long-term effects of this type of abuse through work with adult patients seeking psychiatric care. We know also that the effects of sexual abuse may depend on several cofactors, such as the age of the child victim, the duration of the abuse, the disturbance of existing family life resulting from disclosure, the vulnerability of the child, and heterosexual versus homosexual abuse. Whether or not sexual abuse leaves a distinctive set of behavioral or developmental problems has yet to be proved. The consequences of sexual abuse may be confounded by other factors–for example, parental divorce. When sexual abuse is intrafamilial, its disclosure may lead to parental divorce. Faller (1991) reported several distinct interaction patterns of these variables.

Finkelhor and Browne (1985) have characterized the aftermath of sexual abuse into four possible *traumagenic dynamics*. The first is *traumatic sexualization*, in which the child's introduction to sexuality becomes distorted, leaving the child with excessive fears or feelings about sexuality and sexual behavior. Second, the child may feel powerless. Third, some children indicate that they feel different from other children (stigmatization). They may even feel that they can be picked out of a group of other children because of their experience. Fourth is a sense of betrayal and the feeling that adults cannot be trusted. These dynamics are clearly present in many victims of sexual abuse with whom we have worked. However, they are certainly not constants. Issues of sexuality, power, stigmatization, and trust are all a part of the normal developmental process. One can easily imagine the tremendous impact an abusive experience might have on a child who is already struggling.

Some authors have suggested that there may be a sex difference in the way the risk factors affect boys compared with girls (Farber, Showers, and Johnson, 1984). For example, the Minnesota longitudinal study (Erikson and Egeland, 1987) indicates that girls may react by becoming more quiet and dependent. Male victims on the other hand may tend to act out their abuse on younger children and thus identify with the aggressor. We have been impressed by the number of young adolescent males who have been perpetrators of sexual abuse involving young girls. We hypothesize that this may result from the adolescents' being stimulated and "instructed" by readily available pornographic magazines, books, and films as well as by having been themselves victims of abuse.

Beyond the developmental and behavioral effects of child sexual abuse, there are serious physical consequences. About 5% to 10% of child sexual abuse cases are diagnosed by the documentation of a sexually transmitted disease. Pregnancy may also be the result of sexual abuse. There are documented cases of HIV infection as a consequence of sexual abuse.

In managing sexual abuse, the physician must open his or her mind to the possibility that the sexual abuse exists and that it appears to be a common phenomenon in our society. When one is willing to believe that sexual abuse of children occurs, the recognition of cases will be easier. Children may draw attention to their diagnosis by telling about their abuse or more likely by showing their distress in trying to keep it secret. The signs and symptoms may be specific or may be nonspecific and vague. Many of the behavioral problems presented throughout this volume may be manifestations of abuse. The list of nonspecific symptoms (Ludwig, 1993) includes enuresis, encopresis, school avoidance, runaway behavior, development of phobias, and others. When children manifest any change in behavior or personality, child sexual abuse should be considered.

Once the suspicion of sexual abuse has been raised, the next step in management is its reporting. The reporting criteria for each state are determined by law. Reports may need to be made to the police, the child protective service agency, or both.

The child should undergo a complete physical examination, and cultures for sexually transmitted diseases should be obtained. Other aspects of evidence collection have been reviewed elsewhere. Usually, once the child reveals the "secret" of abuse there may be a temporary relief of symptoms. Once parents learn of the abuse, they are burdened with the terrible weight of the problem. The physician has a role in working with both parents and child to monitor their respective adjustments to the problem. In many cases, referral to mental health workers will be necessary. The need for such services may be based on the continuation of existing symptoms or the development of new problems.

SOCIALIZATION

Intrafamilial Socialization

Dysfunctional Inadequacy in Socialization Within the Family: Distant, Disengaged, or Absent Parents

Functional families provide and teach about family social relationships. Parental distancing or attenuated family relationships result from a variety of conditions. Parents may suffer from psychiatric disorders such as schizophrenia, manic depressive illness, recurrent depressions, alcoholism, substance abuse, and a host of personality disorders. They may be emotionally unavailable to their children as a result of separation, divorce, abandonment, military service, incarceration, or physical illness. They may lack the ability to empathize with their children or to understand and respond to their basic emotional needs. They may be so consumed by excessively demanding jobs, by their own emotional difficulties, or by conflicts with their partners that they cannot provide their children with love and a sense of safety and security. Leaving aside situations of frank abuse or neglect (discussed in earlier sections), disengaged parents are frequently inconsistent, erratic, and ineffective in their approaches to childrearing. It is likely that this inconsistency itself is most detrimental to the child's development.

Children in families with distant or disengaged parents do not learn by experience about normal family social roles and are at heightened risk of developing emotional and behavioral problems. This risk is further increased if the child possesses a particularly difficult temperament, is physically disabled or intellectually limited, or has limited coping skills. Children may exhibit signs of depression, anxiety, somatization, hyperactivity, conduct problems, or emotional maladjustment in response to parental dysfunction. These tend to ameliorate when parental functioning improves and to worsen when parental dysfunction increases. For example, when parents with psychiatric disorders experience an exacerbation of their symptoms, it is not unusual for their children to become more anxious or depressed. When children experience repeated separation from or abandonment by a particular parent, they usually exhibit signs of intense distress during the transition period immediately following the separation. Repeated loss of contact with a parent is generally extremely traumatic.

Physicians who encounter families with distanced or disengaged parents have three tasks: (1) to develop a helping relationship with the parents on behalf of providing care to the children, (2) to gain the trust of parents and learn about their difficulties, and (3) to support parents in their efforts to obtain treatment or help for their problems. Without gaining familiarity with the parents' issues, it is difficult to avoid becoming judgmental and critical of them. Parents who are dysfunctional usually appreciate the physician's efforts to help them become more effective in their

parental roles. In situations when there is a serious split between the parents (e.g., where one parent is reporting on the dysfunctional behavior of the other), it is imperative that the clinician meet both parents and get to know their strengths and weaknesses. If their trust can be gained, it will be easier to win their cooperation in efforts to improve their parenting. Obviously, it is also important for the physician to have access to mental health and social service resources to refer dysfunctional parents for treatment. When making such referrals, it is important that the physician maintain an ongoing relationship with the family and continue to support them in their attempts to cope with the dysfunctional aspects of their lives.

Dysfunctional Excess of Relationships Within the Family: Overinvolved or Enmeshed Families

Overinvolvement of parents with their children can create serious difficulties for all family members. The most extreme example of such overinvolvement is termed *enmeshment*, a situation in which the ego boundaries among individuals are so poorly defined that they cannot separate or individuate from one another without experiencing tremendous anxiety, anger, or other forms of emotional distress. The preconditions for overinvolvement include intergenerational patterns of overinvolvement, insufficient separation and individuation of parents from their own parents, parental disharmony, situational or developmental crises, perhaps temperamental predisposition, and other related factors. The primary characteristic of these families is the extreme emotional closeness that exists between parents and children. Although this may be a normative aspect of parenting during infancy, as the child begins to separate from her or his parents, they usually respond by "pulling back" emotionally and allowing the child to become a separate individual. If parents feel threatened by the child's move toward autonomy, they may undermine this process by focusing all their attention on the child, conveying to him or her the message that it is not all right to be a separate individual. In some cases, the parents may continue to perform functions long past the age when the child is capable of self-care, such as feeding or dressing. In other situations, the child may withdraw from facing normal developmental tasks (e.g., going to school, sleeping over at friends' homes) and may exhibit overt signs of separation anxiety. As with other forms of dysfunction, this ranges from minimal to severe.

Children whose parents are overinvolved also do not experience and learn normal family roles. Anxiety about normal developmental tasks and preoccupation with their parents' emotional well-being leads some children to avoid developing friendships or to resist going to school. In the most severe cases, children can present with anxiety disorders, depression, and somatization disorders.

The physician's approach to overinvolved or enmeshed families is outlined in the section on overprotective families. The most important function the physician can play is to firmly challenge the parents to invest their emotional energy in areas other than their children. Emphasizing that the children need to separate from them to become healthy, independent, and self-reliant adults can help parents to relax their grip and to allow their children some emotional freedom. If discussion of these issues fails to result in change, the family should be referred for psychotherapy.

Extrafamilial Socialization

Deficient Training in Extrafamilial Relationships: Undercontrolling, Boundary-less Families

Functional families provide experience and instruction in extrafamilial relationships: what they are and how they differ from intrafamilial ones. Undercontrolling families appear to have no boundaries with the outside world. There is a tendency for family members to be overly sociable, friendly, and emotionally accessible to nonfamily members. At times, relationships outside the family take precedence over those within the family. Romantic involvements, intense friendships, business relationships, neighbors, and acquaintances seem to occupy the bulk of family members' time. Parental roles and executive functions are de-emphasized, and children are given unusual freedom and latitude to come and go and do as they please. The term *hurried children* has been used to describe those with excessive freedom and insufficient supervision who become responsible for themselves before they are emotionally prepared.

Children in undercontrolling families do not experience and learn appropriate extrafamilial relationships. They are extremely conscious of their social standing and are constantly in search of social acceptance. At the same time, these relationships may be so numerous that they fail to form any deep attachments and ultimately end up without a foundation for true citizenship or friendship. Such children often experiment with sex, drugs, and alcohol at a young age and may first be exposed to these activities by observing their parents. Beneath their pseudomature appearance, children from unrestricted families are likely to be anxious, insecure, and unhappy. In severe cases, these children may become depressed, withdrawn, or apathetic about life. Family conflicts, school failure, indiscriminate sexual relations, and other forms of acting-out behavior may also be seen.

Excessive Restriction From Development of Extrafamilial Relationships: Isolated or Insular Families

Insular families have few external social supports and a very limited social network. Adults in these families have few friends and spend little time with nonfamily members. There is a tendency to see the outside world as unfriendly or threatening and to view outsiders in a way best described as "us against them." It is often difficult to learn what happens in these families since access to them is limited. Where there are excessively strong bonds of family loyalty, it is expected that children will stay in the household (or in the nearby vicinity) even as adults. At times, dysfunctional relationships and behavior patterns (e.g., incest or alcoholism) as well as health and psychosocial problems in these families are hidden and maintained through secrecy and denial. Although it would be incorrect to conclude that insular families have a higher incidence of disturbance than noninsular families, it is clear that when dysfunctional relationships or psychosocial problems are present, these families are more difficult to treat.

Children in insular families do not learn appropriate extrafamilial relationships. They are usually discouraged from having friendships or from engaging in activities that take them out of the home. They may be shy or socially immature and may appear to others to be loners or marginal individuals. Problems may surface when the child attempts to separate from the family and starts to form friendships outside the home. If the family attempts to stifle these relationships, the child may begin to defy parental authority by going out without parental permission or even by running away from home.

Physicians who encounter insular families need to be aware of the difficulty involved in forming trusting relationships with them. If the child appears to be developing normally, is reasonably well adjusted, and is not exhibiting emotional or behavior problems, then consistent encouragement of the child's developing peer relationships and outside activities is indicated. If there is evidence of family dysfunction or of a disturbance in the child, it is most helpful to begin by understanding the parents' views and concerns before offering any advice. If it appears that the parents are resisting the physician's recommendations, it is best to enlist help from other family members and to gain insight into the family's perceptions of the problem before proceeding to involve mental health professionals. By spending extra time winning the trust of key family members, the physician is more likely to succeed in getting the family to accept a recommendation for counseling or family therapy.

Pervasive Parental Dysfunction: Threats to Family Integrity

All too commonly, clinicians will be faced with situations in which there is evidence of severe and pervasive parental dysfunction, often to the point where the integrity of the family is threatened. These include families in which parents suffer from severe psychiatric disturbances, personality disorders, mental deficiency, or alcohol or substance abuse, and those in which there is evidence of chronic and severe family discord leading to domestic violence. Although the incidence of serious psychopathology in parents is difficult to measure, epidemiologic studies report that 20% of the general population suffers from alcoholism, 5% from other substance-related disorders, 6% from depression, 1% from bipolar affective disorder, 1% from schizophrenia, and 5% from mental deficiency. Given these statistics, it is reasonable to conclude that a substantial number of children are being raised by parents who are mentally ill or mentally impaired.

There is considerable evidence from research and clinical literature that mental disorders in parents have deleterious effects on child development. For example, in an early study from the 1920s, children of parents with affective disorders or psychosis had a 21% incidence of behavior disorders, and those whose parents had antisocial personality disorders had a 45% incidence of problems (Minde, 1991). A more recent study of children of schizophrenics found the incidence of conduct disorder to be 9.5%, as compared with 1.6% of control subjects (Rutter and Quinton, 1984). Among children with parents suffering from affective disorders, the rate of behavior problems when there was one affected parent was 24%; with two affected parents, the rate jumped to 74% (Beardslee et al., 1983; Weissman et al, 1987). It appears that the combined effects of genetic loading, disordered parenting, and family discord account for these childhood disturbances.

The precise mechanisms by which children in families with severe dysfunction become themselves afflicted with mental disorders is still the subject of intense research. Current theories emphasize several important aspects: decreased parental responsiveness to the child's needs (due to excessive preoccupation with themselves), inadequate protection of the child from extremes of affect (e.g., excitement, anger, distress), inconsistent supervision, ineffective disciplinary practices, excessive conflict and hostility in the family (much of which may be directed at the child), frequent separations and disruptions to family life (e.g., hospitalizations, departures from the family, migration), and unpredictable or erratic behavior. Regardless of the nature of the psychiatric disturbance itself, parenting is an extremely difficult responsibility for individuals who are mentally ill. The effects on the child are mediated by factors such as the duration and intensity of the parent's mental disorder, comorbid conditions (such as depression and alcoholism), the effectiveness of treatment, parent adherence to treatment, and the availability of social support. If the child does not have other parenting resources readily available, the negative is greater. It also appears that younger children and boys are at greater risk of developing psychiatric disorders.

Two patterns of parenting are particularly deleterious to child development: the detached and unresponsive pattern, and the hostile and overcontrolling pattern. In the former case, children are left neglected for long periods of time, often leading to an insecure pattern of attachment to the parent and to understimulation of cognitive functioning. In the latter case, children are frequently subjected to intense parental anger and to coercive forms of discipline, often leading to aggressive, defiant, and antisocial behavior. A third important pattern of pervasive parental dysfunction is the violence-prone family. Domestic violent behavior between parents has been shown to have a pervasive deleterious effect on all the family members (Straus and Gelles, 1990; Fantuzzo et al, 1991). Even when not directly engaged in the physical conflict, children raised in a violent family suffer severe long-term consequences.

It is important that clinicians recognize the signs of severe parental dysfunction as early as possible, both to assist the parents in getting treatment for themselves and to closely monitor the child for signs of developmental, emotional and/or behavioral disturbances. If the pediatrician approaches these situations with a nonjudgmental but direct approach, there is a greater likelihood that positive steps will be taken by the family to ensure that the child's safety and well-being are not being compromised. In the most severe cases, collaboration with mental health and social service providers will be required, especially when the family's survival is threatened.

Conclusion

Physicians tend to speak in terms of "good families" and "bad families." In doing so, they are really applying a broad qualitative judgement about family function. In working with families, a more helpful approach is to look more precisely at family structure (anatomy) and function (physiology) and to evaluate for areas of strengths and areas of weakness. In doing so, we can build on the functional parts, that is, the strengths, and aid in the correction of dysfunction.

REFERENCES

Appelbaum AS: Developmental retardation in infants as a concomitant of physical child abuse. J Abnorm Child Psychol 5:417–422, 1977.

Bassuk EL, Rosenberg L: Psychosocial characteristics of homeless children and children with homes. Pediatrics 85:257–261, 1990.

Beardslee WR, Bemporad J, Keller MB, et al: Children of parents with major affective disorder: A review. Am J Psychiatry 140:825–832, 1983.

Bronfenbrenner U: Ecology of the family as a context for human development. Research perspectives. Dev Psychol 12:723–742, 1986.

Buchanan A, Oliver JE: Abuse and neglect as a cause of mental retardation. Child Abuse Negl 3:467, 1979.

Centers for Disease Control: Child homicide in US. MMWR 31:292–293, 1982.

Cicchetti D, Carlson V: Child Maltreatment: Theory and Research on the Causes and Consequences of Child Abuse and Neglect. Cambridge University Press, New York, 1989.

Egeland B, Stroufe A, Erikson M: The developmental consequences of different patterns of maltreatment. Child Abuse Negl 7:459–469, 1983.

Elkind D: The Hurried Child: Growing Up Too Fast Too Soon. Reading, MA, Addison-Wesley, 1981.

Erickson MR, Egeland B: A developmental view of the psychological consequences of maltreatment. School Psychol Rev 16:156–168, 1987.

Faller KC: Possible explanations for child sexual abuse: Allegations in divorce. Am J Orthopsychiatry 6(1):86–91, 1991.

Fantuzzo JW, DePaola LM, Lambert L, Martino T, et al: Effects of interpersonal violence on the psychological adjustment and competencies of young children. J Consult Clin Psych 59(1):1–8, 1991.

Farber ED, Showers J, Johnson CF: The sexual abuse of children: A comparison of male and female victims. J Clin Child Psych 13:294–297, 1984.

Finkelhor D: Sexually Victimized Children. New York, Free Press, 1979.

Finkelhor D, Browne A: The traumatic impact of child sexual abuse. Am J Orthopsychiatry 55:530–541, 1985.

Frank Y, Zimmerman R, Leeds N: Neurologic manifestations in abused children who have been shaken. Dev Med Child Neurol 27:312–316, 1985.

Giardino AP, Christian C, Giardino ER: A Practical Guide to the Evaluation of Child Abuse and Neglect. Thousand Oaks, Sage Publications, 1997.

Giovannoni JM, Becerra RM: Defining Child Abuse. New York, Free Press, 1979.

Green M, Solnit AJ: Reactions to the threatened loss of a child: A vulnerable child syndrome. Pediatrics 34:58–64, 1964.

Helfer RE: World of Abnormal Rearing. Unit 1. In Self-Instructional Program on Child Abuse. Elk Grove Village, IL, American Academy of Pediatrics, 1974.

Hills TW: Children in the fast lane. Early Child Res Q 2:265–273, 1987.

Katz LG, Becher RM: Hothousing of young children. Early Child Res Q 2:1–299, 1987.

Kline DF: Educational and psychological problems of abused children. Child Abuse Negl 1:301–308, 1977.

Krugman RD, Krugman MK: Emotional abuse in the classroom. Amer J Dis Child 138:284–286, 1984.

Levin AV, Sheridan M: Munchausen Syndrome by Proxy. New York, Lexington, 1995.

Libow JA, Schreier HA: Three forms of factitious illness in children: When is it Munchausen syndrome by proxy? Am J Orthopsychiatry 56:602–611, 1986.

Ludwig S: Child abuse. In Fleisher G, Ludwig S (eds). Textbook of Pediatric Emergency Medicine, 3rd ed. Baltimore, Williams & Wilkins, 1993.

Ludwig S: Child abuse: Its causes and solutions. In Luten R (ed). Problems in Pediatric Emergency Medicine. New York, Churchill Livingstone, 1988.

Ludwig S, Kornberg AE (eds). Child Abuse: A Medical Reference, 2nd ed. New York, Churchill Livingstone, 1992.

Martin HP: The abused: A multidisciplinary approach to developmental issues and treatment. Cambridge, Ballinger Publishers, 1976.

McIntosh BJ: Spoiled child syndrome. Pediatrics 83:1;108–115, 1989.

Meadow R: Munchausen syndrome by proxy: The hinterland of child abuse. Lancet 2:343–345, 1977.

Minde K: The effect of disordered parenting on the development of children. *In* Lewis M (ed): Child and Adolescent Psychiatry: A Comprehensive Textbook. Baltimore, Williams & Wilkins, 1991, pp. 394–407.

Moore JG: "Yo Yo children," victims of matrimonial violence. Child Welfare 54:557–566, 1975.

Murdoch G: Social Structure. New York, Free Press, 1965.

Paradise J: Personal Communication, 1984.

Reece RM (ed). Child Abuse: Medical Diagnosis and Management. Philadelphia, Lea & Febiger, 1994.

Rosenberg DA: Web of deceit: A literature review of Munchausen syndrome by proxy. Child Abuse Negl 11:547–563, 1987.

Russell D: The incidence and prevalence of intrafamiliar and extrafamiliar sexual abuse of female children. Child Abuse Negl 7:133–146, 1983.

Rutter M, Quinton D: Parental psychiatric disorder: Effects on children. Psychol Med 14:853–880, 1984.

Sandgrund A, Gaines RW, Green AH: Child abuse and mental retardation: A problem of cause and effect. J Ment Defic Res 19:327–336, 1975.

Sgroi S (ed): Handbook of Clinical Intervention in Child Sexual Abuse. Lexington, KY, Lexington Books, 1984.

Straus MA, Gelles RJ: Physical Violence in American Families: Risk Factors and Adaptations to Violence in 8,145 Families. New Brunswick, NJ, Transaction Publications, 1990.

United States Department Health & Human Services, National Center on Child Abuse & Neglect: Child Maltreatment 1995: Report from the States to the National Child Abuse & Neglect Data System. Washington, DC, United States Government Printing Office, 1997.

Walsh F: Conceptualizations of normal family functioning. *In* Walsh (ed). Normal Family Processes. New York, Guilford Press, 1982.

Weissman MM, Gammon D, John K, et al: Children of depressed parents: Increased pathology and early onset of major depression. Arch Gen Psychiatry 44:847, 1987.

Widom LS: The cycle of violence. Science 244:160–166, 1989.

Wissow LS: Child abuse and neglect. N Engl J Med, 332(21):1423–1431, 1995.

Wissow LS: Child Advocacy for the Clinician: An Approach to Child Abuse and Neglect. Baltimore, Williams & Wilkins, 1990, pp 1–242.

17 The Neighborhood: Poverty, Affluence, Geographic Mobility, and Violence

George L. Askew • Paul H. Wise

 In addition to the family, schools, and general culture, the characteristics of the child's dwelling and neighborhood are potent biopsychosocial influences affecting development and behavior. This chapter discusses several of the principal components: economic circumstances that vary from poverty to affluence, housing accommodations ranging from frequent moves to homelessness, and diverse amounts and types of violence and danger in the immediate environs. Discussion focuses on the ways clinicians can help children and their families manage the stresses of these situations. Other elements of the home and neighborhood (e.g., toxins and electronic media) are discussed in other chapters.

Defining the Neighborhood

The neighborhood for children is the relatively small environmental range and inherent relationships of home, school, and community that, together, determine the fabric of a child's daily life. Although this sphere often widens as children grow older and become more independent, this definition is intended to recognize the central importance of a child's functional environment in determining the material resources and human interaction so necessary to child health and social well-being. Family relations are discussed primarily in Chapters 11 and 16. (For the larger cultural setting, see Chapter 10.)

Poverty

Despite being a common focus of discussion and research, poverty has defied a single definition. In large measure, this lack of agreement reflects variation in the perceived origins of poverty and the intended use of the definition. Most often, for purposes of policy formulation and research, poverty is defined as a measure of subsistence: that level of resources that permits the maintenance of physical efficiency. Here, the measure of poverty takes on an absolute quality, concerned with the basics of food and shelter, and it changes only in response to changes in prices. An example of this absolute definition of poverty is the official "poverty line" for the United States, which is derived from the US Department of Agriculture's estimate of food costs for a basic, but nutritionally adequate, diet. This figure is then multiplied by three, because studies indicated that, at the time of the inception of the index several decades ago, a typical family spent approximately one third of its income on food. In 1995, the official poverty level for a family of four was $15,569. Calls for a more refined official measure of poverty continue to be advanced. In 1995, a special panel commissioned by the National Academy of Sciences recommended a new method for defining poverty (Citro and Michael, 1995). This new poverty measure would consist of a budget for the three basic categories of food, clothing, shelter (including utilities), and a small additional amount to allow for other needs (e.g., household supplies, personal care, non–work-related transportation). Although a more refined method of determining poverty, this approach remains based on the determination of some absolute figure with little reference to how it would relate to the general distribution of income and wealth in the rest of society. In this manner, such absolutist definitions do not respond to human needs beyond subsistence nor to concerns of equity in the distribution of income. Alternatively, some authors have proposed definitions of poverty that are based on the concept of relative deprivation (Townsend, 1979). Here, poverty implies a level of resources so inadequate that participation in expected, customary, community, or societal activities is prohibited. Although somewhat more difficult to use in a standard manner, this relativist concept recognizes the important difference between economic hardship and poverty as well as the fundamental power of poverty to threaten health, distort human interaction, and preclude participation in even the most fundamental of societal activities (Huston, McLoyd, and Coll, 1994).

RECENT TRENDS IN CHILDHOOD POVERTY

Despite the common belief that childhood poverty has been a relatively stable phenomenon in American history, rates of childhood poverty are sensitive to economic and social trends. After 2 decades of falling poverty rates, there was a disturbing increase in the percentage of children living in poverty in the early 1980s, the rate climbing to more than 22% in 1983, based on the official poverty index. In 1995, the portion of American children living below the poverty line remained more than one in five for children younger than 18 years of age and nearly one in four for children younger than age 6 years. This is the highest poverty rate among any age group in American society.

The primary reasons for increases in childhood poverty are the demographic changes and decline in the earning power of the young American family. Children are more likely to be raised in single-parent, female-headed households, which have a greater likelihood of being poor. In addition, real wages for young adults, particularly those with limited education, have decreased dramatically over the past 2 decades. For children, the alternative to the family for income distribution is the state. Here, too, support for children in families with insufficient earnings has deteriorated significantly. Between the mid-1970s and early 1990s, family benefits for the Aid to Families with Dependent Children (AFDC) program, the primary public mechanism dedicated to this purpose, when adjusted for inflation, declined by 40% (Brown, 1995). In 1996, however, the AFDC program was replaced by the Transitional Assistance for Needy Families legislation. This new program ended a poor child's entitlement to income support, embraced time limits for enrollment, and granted far more control over eligibility criteria, benefit levels, and oversight to the individual states. Although the impact of this legislation remains unclear, it is likely that the emphasis on greater state control will lead to greater heterogeneity in the nature and adequacy of welfare programs in the years to come.

CLINICAL EXPRESSION OF POVERTY

The clinical impact of poverty lies as much in its pervasiveness as it does in its deadening persistence. Children living in poverty experience elevated rates of developmental and medical problems and a greater likelihood that these problems will produce deleterious outcomes. This "double jeopardy" (Parker, Greer, and Zuckerman, 1988) characterizes a number of disorders and represents a dual injustice; poverty distorts the promise of life by erecting biological obstacles to health, while at the same time sapping the social capacity to respond. The elements of this interaction are complex and remain poorly defined. However, there are several considerations that are fundamental. Severe material deprivation lies at the heart of poverty's effects on child health. Even when material resources may be sufficient under normal circumstances, material reserves may not exist, making financial emergencies both more frequent and more threatening when they do occur. Maternal stress factors are both more frequent and more severe among poor women, and emotional supports may be inadequate for families isolated by their poverty and social alienation (Roghmann, Hecht, and Haggerty, 1975). Informational supports in the form of frequent access to community resources and referrals may be lacking in poor families. In addition, social support systems—a critical component of resilience—are commonly far weaker and more constrained for poor children and their families. Structural aspects of the neighborhood and the quality and breadth of school-based educational programs can also help determine the dimensions of the impact of poverty (Rutter, 1981). Together, material deprivation, heightened stress, reduced social supports, and debilitating neighborhood and school conditions can affect the full spectrum of essential developmental needs of children, including stability, security, and the maintenance of a nurturing, stimulating home environment.

Childhood poverty has been linked to a variety of specific emotional, developmental, and health problems with both direct and indirect implications for child development and behavior. As discussed, its mechanisms of action are multiple and complex. Nevertheless, to respond clinically to this diverse presentation, the influences of poverty can be viewed as elevating the likelihood of poor health by two broadly defined mechanisms: the enhancement of risk for poor health and the reduction of access to those interventions effective at minimizing the impact of elevated risk.

Enhancement of Risk

Elevated risk can affect health by increasing the probability that an illness or traumatic event will occur and by increasing the severity with which the illness or injury affects the child. This can take the form of increased exposure or the suppression of protective mechanisms.

Reduction of Access

Risk can be modulated by intervention. When a capacity to alter the impact of risk exists, then disparities in access to this capacity can create inequities in outcomes. The essential element in this relationship is efficacy, because interventions without efficacy are not likely to cause differences in outcome regardless of differences in access. The interaction of elevated risk and reduced access is manifest in a variety of health conditions and defines, in tragic terms, the clinical expression of poverty.

DISPARITIES IN MORTALITY

The starkest manifestation of the impact of poverty on child health lies in its capacity to shape disparities in survival. From birth, poor children are at higher risk of death than nonpoor children, although the dimensions of this disparity and the implications for clinical intervention vary considerably by age and cause of death.

Neonatal and Infant Mortality

Neonatal and infant mortality rates have long been recognized as sensitive indicators of social conditions. The influence of poverty on mortality during the neonatal period (<28 days) can take the form of elevated rates of low birth weight (<2500 g) or elevated rates of mortality among newborns of comparable birth weight groups (Starfield et al, 1991; Wise et al, 1985). The influence of poverty on birth weight distribution is mediated primarily by the health of the mother both before and during pregnancy, which may reflect the adequacy of nutrition; maternal age; parity; maternal behaviors, including smoking, alcohol use, and illicit drug use; and a range of social stresses. In addition to elevating the chance that an infant will be born at low birth weight, poverty can also increase the risk that an infant will die, even among neonates of comparable birth weights. This occurs primarily when poverty, often accompanied by inadequate health insurance coverage, affects access to tertiary care facilities, including neonatal intensive care, and access to new techniques. Recent studies show that death in the 1st year of life is greater than 1.6 times more likely for infants of women living below the poverty level. For infants between the ages of 28 days and 1 year, the death rate doubles for infants of women living in poverty (Centers for Disease Control, 1995). The effects of poverty in the postneonatal period (28 through 365 days of age) are mediated by increased deaths from infectious diseases, sudden infant death syndrome (SIDS), injuries, and the serious sequelae of high-risk neonatal conditions. Although recent efforts to educate parents regarding infants' sleep position have been associated with major reductions in SIDS mortality rate, it remains unclear whether these improvements have occurred equally in all social groups.

Mortality From Trauma

Trauma claims the life of more children than any other cause. Because the occurrence of life-threatening injury is so closely tied to the activities of daily life, the adequacy of social conditions plays an important role in shaping childhood patterns of trauma and resultant mortality.

Fire

There are few causes of death more closely related to the adequacy of daily living conditions than is fire. House fires are the source of the overwhelming portion of childhood fire deaths. The leading cause of fatal house fires is the adult use of cigarettes, accounting for approximately 30% of all such fires. However, the second and third leading causes are directly related to the adequacy of housing, that is, fires caused by heating and electrical equipment.

Motor Vehicle

Injury associated with the use of motor vehicles represents the largest contributor to traumatic mortality in childhood, affecting occupants of motor vehicles as well as pedestrians struck by motor vehicles. With some variation, particularly in some urban areas, motor vehicle occupant mortality rate is higher for children living in poverty. The reasons for this association have not been well defined. However, there appear to be significant social influences on the development of relevant health and risk-taking behaviors, including alcohol use. Pedestrian mortality is heavily influenced by social status. Because poor neighborhoods are often located in seriously congested inner city areas, the risk of pedestrian injury to children in this setting is likely to be elevated substantially. The importance of the street as a play area and the lack of engineered barriers that separate children from motor vehicle thoroughfares contribute to the functional proximity of young children and moving vehicles, an association that guarantees high rates of pedestrian injury and death.

Homicide

Homicide is among the most important causes of death among American children. In some urban communities, homicide is the leading cause of injury-related mortality in children from birth through adolescence. The tragedy of homicide in children has defied clear understanding. However, its concentration in poor communities has been documented repeatedly. Child homicide can be grouped into three general categories, all of which reveal sharp social gradients: (1) infanticide related to violent anger directed at the child by a caretaker in response to persistent crying or other anxiety-producing behavior; (2) in toddlers and preschool-aged children, fatal child abuse and neglect as a result of harsh punishment for the child's failure to meet unrealistic demands; and (3) among older children, community-based homicide, in which the dangers of the adult world confront the increasing independence of the preadolescent and adolescent. In a clinical setting, family-based approaches to reducing the risk of violence against children are often useful (Dubowitz and King, 1995).

DISPARITIES IN MORBIDITY

Preventable death may be the ultimate expression of poverty, but a variety of less severe emotional, developmental, and health problems may also affect poor children. In broad terms, children of poor families experience more days of restricted activity owing to health problems and more days absent from school than do their wealthier counterparts.

Intellectual Development and Socioemotional Functioning

Poor children are at increased risk for problems of cognitive and behavioral development. Reports from the long-term follow-up studies of children in Kauai, HI, revealed profound socioeconomic effects on intelligence quotient (IQ) (Werner and Smith, 1977). In a recent examination of economic deprivation and early childhood development, family income and poverty status were powerful correlates of cognitive development and behavior in children. The greatest effect was found for duration rather than timing of poverty. IQs at age 5 years were found to be higher in neighborhoods with greater concentrations of affluent neighbors, whereas increased prevalence of low-income neighbors was related to increases in externalizing behaviors (Duncan, Brooks-Gunn, and Klebanov, 1994). Empiric insights have also underscored the interactive quality of social status and biological impairments in shaping developmental outcome. In general, children of affluent families with biological disabilities are far more likely to overcome the developmental implications of their conditions than are poor children. The Kauai studies revealed that poor children with no apparent perinatal sequelae had IQ scores similar to those of more affluent children with significant perinatal complications. The worst developmental risks are generally seen in children with perinatal insults who are also poor (Escalona, 1982).

Chronic Medical Conditions

Poor children experience disproportionately high rates of serious chronic conditions. Hearing loss is more prevalent among poor children, at least in part a reflection of elevated rates of chronic otitis media and an increased likelihood that it will lead to subsequent hearing impairment and associated developmental and behavioral problems. Visual acuity is similar for poor and nonpoor children. However, nonpoor children are considerably more likely to have any visual deficit diagnosed and corrected early, resulting in an increased rate of functional visual impairment among poor children. Reports on the prevalence of asthma among poor children are variable. However, there is evidence that the impact of asthma on poor children is greater, with a higher frequency of attack, a greater limitation of activity, and an increased requirement for hospitalization.

Nutrition and Growth

Growth retardation, generally associated with chronic undernutrition, is more prevalent among poor children and is independently associated with poorer cognitive function (Miller and Korenman, 1994). Iron deficiency anemia, which is associated with low development scores in infancy and, later, decreased attentiveness and a higher incidence of behavioral disorders, is three times as prevalent among the poor as among the nonpoor in age groups 1 to 5 years and 12 to 17 years. Intake of vitamins and other essential nutrients is also far more likely to be inadequate (Cook and Marti, 1995). Although the causes are complex, poverty can exert its influence on nutrition through the maldistribution of otherwise adequate resources in the family or by the absolute inadequacy of family resources. Poverty can also create profound social stress and can interrupt the provision of adequate nutrition to young children through the distortion of healthy family relationships. It can also force children into marginal care-taking situations that can complicate adequate nutrition. Yet, the most direct impact of poverty on child nutrition is the primary lack of resources to acquire adequate food. For many poor families, income available for food may represent merely the remaining portion of income once the less flexible costs of housing, utilities, and transportation are met. The absolute inadequacy of resources that leads to poor child nutrition, indeed child hunger, remains an alarming phenomenon in the United States and is one that may remain hidden from the clinician until frank clinical signs emerge (Brown and Pizer, 1987).

Lead Poisoning

Lead poisoning causes a variety of significant health, developmental, and educational problems and is highly associated with poverty. Data from the early 1990s suggested that the prevalence of elevated lead levels among children aged 1 to 5 years from low-income families (16.3%) is approximately four times higher than the prevalence for children from high-income families (4.0%). African American children from low-income families had the highest proportion of elevated lead levels (28.4%) (Brody et al, 1994). There is also evidence that rates of elevated lead levels during pregnancy are higher in poor women. Heightened exposure in old, deteriorating housing, surrounding soils, and contaminated air is closely associated with poverty. Beyond broad measures, such as the elimination of lead from gasoline, the principal approach to combating lead poisoning is screening children for elevated lead lev-

els. Although it is effective in identifying children with high lead burdens, screening represents a deformed public policy whereby children are used to identify lead-containing homes, rather than identifying such homes directly and eradicating lead before poisoning can occur. Furthermore, lead screening is a mandatory component of the Early and Periodic Screening, Diagnosis, and Treatment component of Medicaid, but less than half of all children covered by Medicaid receive such screening and less than half of all poor and near-poor children are currently enrolled in Medicaid (see Chapter 30).

Sequelae of Low Birth Weight

The dramatic improvement in the survival of low–birth weight newborns has been accompanied by a growing population of survivors at high risk for serious neurodevelopmental and medical problems. However, for poor children, the sequelae of low birth weight can be particularly severe. The most common medical conditions found in low–birth weight children are asthma, upper and lower respiratory infections, and ear infections. In an examination of the long-term developmental outcome of low–birth weight infants, those from disadvantaged backgrounds were found to fare worse than socially advantaged children (Hack, Klein, and Taylor, 1995). In addition, when compared with more affluent newborns of similar birth weight, poor infants have greater postneonatal mortality rates, lower IQ scores, and a higher prevalence of educational difficulties. This reflects the pervasive character of poverty and confronts the clinician with the too common quandary of sending a clearly high-risk child into an obviously suboptimal environment.

Acquired Immunodeficiency Syndrome

Acquired immunodeficiency syndrome in children is another problem that is intimately linked with poverty. Primarily the result of maternal transmission, infection with human immunodeficiency virus (HIV) generally implies significant morbidity and mortality risks in early childhood. Similar to high-risk neonatal survivors, children with HIV infection require a level of comprehensive and multidisciplinary services that can easily overwhelm the already inadequate local health service capacity in areas of concentrated poverty. Unlike low birth weight, however, HIV infection in a child implies the coexistence of a chronic, life-threatening illness in at least one parent. This affects profoundly the interaction between clinicians, child welfare agencies, and foster caretakers. Recent advances in interrupting maternal transmission and in treating infection in children have the potential to alter the risk and impact of infection. The burden remains, however, to ensure that these and all future therapeutic strides are provided equitably to all those in need.

HOMELESSNESS

An extreme manifestation of poverty and failed societal provision is homelessness. Although precise numbers of homeless children have been difficult to establish, estimates have ranged from 200,000 to 3 million nationally. Beyond the problems inherent in measuring a population defined by a lack of residence, these estimates tend to vary owing to differences in definition, in particular the length of time a child must be without formal shelter before being considered homeless, and the political and social agenda of the group performing the count. Nevertheless, there is substantial evidence that the population of homeless children in the United States has grown since the mid-1980s. Indeed, the fastest growing component of the homeless population has been families with children; it is estimated that between 25% and 40% of the nation's homeless are families, most often headed by single women with two to three young children. Another population of homeless children is older children and adolescents often labeled "runaways" or "throwaways," estimated to number almost 500,000 nationwide. Generally the product of troubled families with high rates of physical and sexual abuse, these children are concentrated in major urban centers and often are compelled to rely on illegal and self-destructive means of subsistence including petty crime, drug trade, and prostitution.

Compared with the general population of children, homeless children have twice as many health problems, are more likely to go hungry, have higher rates of developmental delay, and possibly have higher rates of depression, anxiety, and behavior problems. School performance among homeless children is affected drastically, with seriously elevated rates of school failure and requirements for special education. While overall cognitive functioning of homeless children is comparable to that of housed children, academic achievement in the areas of reading, spelling, and arithmetic are dramatically lower for homeless children (Rubin et al, 1996). In addition to elevated risk, homeless children have drastically reduced access to comprehensive services. Immunization rates, vision and hearing assessment, and lead screening among homeless children have been shown to be seriously inadequate. Confronting the psychosocial toll of homelessness requires coordinated social service, psychological, and educational intervention, although these services are rarely available in the scope and intensity that are needed. As for all poor children, the primary task for the clinician caring for homeless children is the provision of appropriate clinical services. However, to an extent greater than for virtually all other children, the manifold risks associated with being homeless are likely to overwhelm the capacity of clinical intervention to assure optimal outcomes. The fundamental imperative remains the establishment of decent shelter—a task that clinicians can pursue by assisting individual families with their care, by linking them to other sources of support, and by participating in the development of effective long-term solutions.

CONFRONTING THE IMPACT OF POVERTY ON CHILD HEALTH: ROLE OF THE CLINICIAN

Ultimately, those who provide care to children must confront the clinical expression of poverty. Even though clinicians who care for poor children can make significant contributions through the direct provision of clinical services, the needs of poor children can never be fully met by clinical intervention alone. Rather, the role of the clinician is defined by dual recognition of the considerable efficacy of medicine and its inherent limitations. A complete reliance on clinical services does not address the larger social forces that determine the dimensions and character of clinical need. But the importance and relevance of clinical care should not be discounted. Alternatively, clinicians can address the needs of their patients through the linkage of clinical intervention to a spectrum of community-based services and an informed involvement in the formulation of public policies that promote the well-being of children (Table 17–1).

Provision of Health Services

In a setting of poverty, the purpose of health care is to uncouple poverty from its implications for health. Although far from complete, the capacity of medical care to meet this objective is considerable. Accordingly, the primary responsibility of the clinician is the provision of high-quality health services to all children in need. This often requires the refinement of clinical practices to meet the specific needs of poor children in local communities. This in turn may require knowledge gained from community-based epidemiology and needs assessment activities. Nevertheless, there exists a series of specific services that hold particular promise for ameliorating the detrimental effects of poverty on optimal health and development.

Lack of Health Insurance and Decreased Access to Care

Lack of health insurance is a well-documented obstacle to the receipt of adequate health care. In 1992, 21% of children living in families with incomes less than 200% of the federal poverty level had no health insurance (Newacheck, Hughes, and Cisternas, 1995). Fewer poor children (85.3%) have a reported usual source of care when compared with

Table 17–1 • Interventions of Special Importance in Caring for Poor Children and Their Families

Provision of health services
  Family planning and health services for women
  Prenatal care
  Nutrition supplementation
  Prevention of nonintentional and intentional injuries
  Comprehensive care for infants, children, and adolescents
Community-based services
  Outreach
  Home visiting
  Developmental and behavioral services
  Community advocacy
Formulation of public policy
  General
  Economic and employment
  Minimum wage
  Education and job training
  Special programs
  Aid to Families with Dependent Children (AFDC)
  Medicaid
  Supplemental Food Program for Women, Infants, and Children (WIC)
  Food stamps
  Title V (Maternal and Child Health)
  Linkage with nonhealth services

nonpoor children (92.1%). In addition, children without Medicaid coverage are less likely than those with Medicaid coverage to have a usual source of care (78.2% versus 90.9%) (St. Peter, Newacheck, and Halfon, 1994). In 1987, 37.8% of poor whites, 29.9% of poor blacks, and 49.2% of poor Hispanics were uninsured (Cornelius, 1993).

Social disparities in patterns of immunization in the United States illustrate how differences in access can influence the provision of highly effective services. Children living below the poverty level are less well vaccinated than those living at or above the poverty level. In 1992, 80.2% of children below poverty level and 84.3% at or above poverty level received measles vaccine, 66% of children below poverty level and 74.7% of children at or above poverty level received polio vaccines, and 79.7% of children below poverty level and 84.6% of children at or above poverty level received diphtheria-pertussis-tetanus vaccines (Centers for Disease Control, 1994). Several factors may account for this phenomenon, including decreased access to primary care services, missed opportunities to vaccinate, and vaccination beliefs and practices among pediatric providers in poor communities that run counter to standard vaccination recommendations (Askew et al, 1995).

Maternal Health and the Health of Women

To an important extent, inequities in the rate of poor birth outcomes are a legacy of inequities in women's health status before conception. Poor women suffer from elevated rates of a number of chronic and acute conditions, many of which affect maternal and fetal health during gestation, as well as child health in subsequent years. High-quality general health care for women is essential, and clinicians who care for children should do all they can to ensure that women bringing their children for services also have health care. Gynecologic and obstetric conditions noted during previous pregnancies may require significant medical management before conception. Timely access to high-quality family planning services, including counseling and reproductive health screening, helps ensure that a child is wanted and will enter a home environment that is nurturing and supportive of normal growth and development. Family planning services provide women with control over their reproductive lives and a capacity to plan for their economic responsibilities. Family planning services can reduce infant mortality rate, incidence of low birth weight, and number of stillbirths and can increase the probability that timing of birth, interval between births, and family size will serve to enhance the infant's healthy development (Institute of Medicine, 1996). Despite the importance of family planning, approximately 30 million women in the United States who are at risk for unwanted pregnancy do not receive adequate health and family planning services. Almost 3 million unplanned pregnancies occur each year, with half of them being terminated by abortion. Contact with the medical system during the birth experience provides a special opportunity for clinicians to link women with appropriate reproductive and family planning services. Primary care for young children also affords ongoing contact with young mothers and a continuing clinical capacity to ensure adequate reproductive care.

Prenatal Care

Prenatal care represents a critical component of comprehensive health services for women of childbearing age. A range of services for women during the prenatal period have been shown to enhance maternal health before, during, and after delivery and represents a critical mechanism to optimize the health of the newborn and its early development. Although the precise mechanisms of effect remain poorly understood, late or no prenatal care is associated with an increased incidence of low birth weight, prematurity, and death of normal–birth weight infants (Institute of Medicine, 1988). Despite this demonstrable efficacy, there remain substantial disparities between poor and nonpoor women in the use of prenatal care services. National data reveal that approximately one in five women giving birth in the United States begins prenatal care later than the first trimester and that late initiation is heavily concentrated among poor and young women. Barriers to appropriate use are multiple: high out-of-pocket costs for uninsured women, too-narrow eligibility criteria for publicly funded programs such as Medicaid, failure of some local practitioners to accept patients covered by Medicaid, cultural and language barriers, inadequate transportation to clinical facilities, long waits for care, and lack of awareness of early pregnancy. In addition, the content of prenatal care services should be refined to address directly the true needs of women living in poverty. Nutritional supplementation, social service support, counseling, and referral with follow-up for appropriate and accessible interventions to reduce smoking and use of illicit drugs and alcohol may prove to be major contributors to effectiveness of prenatal care in a setting of poverty.

Nutrition

Throughout the course of life, but particularly in pregnancy and childhood, growth and healthy development depend on adequate and balanced nutrition. For families living in poverty, limited resources can constrain both the variety and amount of necessary foods. In response, clinicians can assist such families by referrals to publicly supported nutrition programs. A primary resource is Supplemental Food Program for Women, Infants, and Children (WIC), which provides food supplements to low-income pregnant lactating women, to infants, and to children younger than age 5 years. In addition, the food stamp, school lunch, and breakfast programs and a variety of Title V (Maternal and Child Health)–supported projects have proved beneficial to enrolled families. However, serious underfunding of these programs has meant that they can provide services to only a small fraction of all families in need. Despite repeated evaluations that show the efficacy of the WIC program, only about half of all children that meet eligibility criteria nationwide actually receive WIC services. Another important element of the effort to improve child nutrition is support for breast-feeding. Culturally sensitive, hospital-based programs that encourage breast-feeding, particularly when linked with supportive primary care involvement during the first few months after delivery, can significantly increase breast-feeding by women who are poor and possess little formal education.

Injury Prevention

The occurrence of serious injury is directly tied to the social conditions of everyday life. However, there is a growing capacity to alter the probabilities of traumatic injury through clinical intervention. Because injuries are the most important contributors to social disparities in childhood mortality beyond infancy, injury prevention represents a critical element of clinical practice in poor communities.

In many urban areas, falls from open windows represent an important danger to young children. The use of window gratings or reinforced screens is an important preventive intervention. There is good evidence that the presence of a working smoke detector can reduce the likelihood of mortality once a fire has begun. In many communities, education and legislation have increased the number of homes in which smoke detectors have been installed. However, access to working smoke detectors may be hindered by several factors common to poor families. The cost of the units may be prohibitive; legislation mandating the installation of detection equipment by landlords tends to focus on new construction and tends to ignore the need in older housing; and, particularly when housing is scarce, the fear of eviction tends to overpower incentives to report violations of detector ordinances. Also, detectors require the periodic replacement of batteries, a task that may be less commonly performed in poor neighborhoods. Over the past decade, the importance of restraint systems in reducing injury and death from motor vehicle collisions has become widely appreciated. The provision of appropriate car seats at low cost is designed to overcome the financial barrier to car seat usage. However, ongoing discussion and education efforts are often required to ensure that available child restraint systems will actually be used on a consistent basis.

Comprehensive Care

Despite the efficacy of a number of specific interventions, nothing can substitute for high-quality comprehensive care in assuring optimal child health, especially for poor children who are at elevated risk for a multitude of often interrelated health problems. Comprehensive care strategies include the following:

1. Primary preventive services that attempt to eliminate causative factors before the occurrence of illness or injury. These services include immunization, window bars to prevent falls, and provision of contraceptives to sexually active teens.
2. Secondary prevention that addresses pathologic conditions that are present but not yet clearly expressed as recognized symptoms is particularly important in reducing the functional impact of medical problems in poor children. Such prevention often involves screening procedures, including those implemented at birth and the early detection of vision and hearing deficits.
3. Tertiary prevention that is implemented after failure of primary and secondary prevention, which, for poor children, is common. This aspect of care involves limiting the suffering and disability associated with chronic illness and requires a strong and continuous coordination of a range of clinical services.

Comprehensive care must also include a strong commitment to anticipatory guidance, school performance monitoring, and counseling. The process of providing and exchanging information regarding the development and social functioning of the child can lead to enhanced understanding, competence, and confidence in their own perceptions and concerns on the part of parents. Poverty breeds isolation, but clinical guidance can play an important role in supporting parental efforts to address temperamental differences in their children, unrealistic expectations, unfounded anxieties, and the debilitating stresses of low income, crowded housing, poor education, and a climate of crime, violence, and scant hope for the future.

It is the nature of poverty to reduce access to services as much as it is to increase need. Therefore, in poor communities, clinicians must play an enhanced role in ensuring that families receive needed care. Follow-up care takes on new significance in that clinical deterioration is far more likely in poor children as a product of both elevated risk of severe illness and the layers of practical problems that undermine poor families' ability to comply precisely with medical advice; that is, financial costs for specialty consultation or medications may be prohibitive, access to medical advice by telephone may be limited, parents may be hesitant to seek care owing to dehumanizing interactions with the medical system in the past, and the child's clinical status may not be known owing to multiple caretakers or a chaotic social situation.

Community-Based Services

Community-based programs provide a crucial range of services and represent an important resource for clinicians caring for poor children. Such services often take the form of programs designed to serve children who have specific conditions or children with special requirements for a broad range of coherent community-based services. Others attempt to enhance access to medical and social services through intensive home visiting, follow-up care, and social supports.

Outreach

Outreach bridges the gap between the apparent availability of a service and actual use by a family in need. Parents may have a poor understanding of some of the health benefits and services available to their children. Furthermore, even if they understand the benefits of services available, they may not be aware of the nature or severity of their child's problem or may have a poor understanding of the processes by which the service can be received. However, at least as common are the problems families may encounter when dealing with a medical and human service system that is often poorly coordinated, inconsistent in both eligibility and benefit criteria, and characterized by layers of complex bureaucracy. Outreach services can enhance clinical practice because outreach personnel can provide focused expertise in overcoming these barriers and free physicians, nurses, dentists, and other health professionals to focus on providing clinical care. Perhaps most important, however, is the role of outreach workers in ensuring that cultural, language, and other social barriers to care are diminished and that professional staff are responsive and accountable to the community they serve. Despite the utility of outreach efforts, even massive outreach cannot make up for the absence of high-quality, accessible, and appropriate services.

Home Visiting

Home visiting services may be an effective means of delivering and linking families to needed services in poor communities. Although programs vary considerably, most provide a broad range of responses to family needs. They provide information and assistance in making the home a safe and nurturing environment, they address nutritional concerns and ensure that families are linked with clinical and other relevant human service programs, and they offer social support for families isolated from relatives or community activities. Many home visiting programs focus on children with specific conditions or health care needs, providing physical therapy, home intravenous therapy, or respiratory support. Regardless of the specific need, home visiting services are most effective when they are coordinated with local clinicians and agencies and are closely integrated into a comprehensive system of care.

Developmental and Behavioral Services Beyond the Health Care System

The distinctive needs of poor children can best be met by coordinated efforts that tie clinical expertise to the skills and commitment of professionals whose work extends beyond the health system to other settings where children live, work, play, and study. Teachers, day care workers, juvenile correctional officers, foster parents, social workers, guidance counselors, and others working with disturbed and distressed young people represent important resources for children, their families, and clinicians who care for children. Their insights and informed energy should be integrated into individual care plans and communitywide efforts to improve the developmental outcomes of poor children. Schools offer a particularly important arena for coordinating services, because school personnel are often the first to identify children in need of help and may represent a critical component of any therapeutic response. In addition, the effort to engage children with significant chronic illness in regular school settings requires a close relationship between educational and clinical personnel.

Clinician as Community Advocate

Clinicians can act as powerful advocates for the development of needed community-based programs and the expanded support for those already in place. Clinicians may possess a special capacity to speak to the need and nature of services such community-based programs could provide. Politically, local health professionals can provide significant legitimacy and strength to advocacy calls for improved local services. Social networks, both formal and informal, can be important sources of support to poor families in need and can be strengthened by local professionals. This might include the collaboration of local neighborhood groups, business organizations, labor unions, religious assemblies, and a variety of other community-based institutions in addressing a specific set of local health problems. In this role, clinicians must reach out and lend their expertise and commitment to the larger arena of service development and community empowerment.

Clinician and Formulation of Public Policy

Beyond clinical care and community-based services, the promise that all children will be afforded an environment to grow and develop depends on development and implementation of effective public policies. Most fundamental are those that shape the nature and dimensions of elevated risk for poor outcomes. This relates directly to primary determinants of child poverty, which, in turn, relate to policies that affect the economic well-being of young families and the adequacy of ameliorative public programs. The determination of economic policies, including the minimum wage, earned income tax credits, income support, employment and job training programs, and community development strategies, relates directly to the scope of child poverty.

State and federal policies that address child poverty through specialized services and resource transfers, such as welfare programs, Medicaid, Supplemental Security Income (SSI), supplemental nutrition programs (WIC and food stamps), and Title V (Maternal and Child Health) programs, are of major importance to clinical practice in poor areas, particularly during a period of enormous programmatic revision. Rapidly changing eligibility criteria, benefit levels, and administrative practices increasingly become more heterogeneous and may exclude previously covered groups, particularly foreign citizens residing in the United States. Policies that forge new linkages between local education, social service, and health care agencies always benefit from a significant involvement of the clinical community, particularly in areas of concentrated poverty and social dislocation.

Responsibility for advocacy for improved public policy does not fall directly within the clinical domain, yet its impact has fundamental clinical implications. Clinical intervention remains of critical importance to children living in poverty. However, the complex spectrum of risk associated with poverty will never be addressed entirely by clinical practice. At some level, people who care for children must respect the dual currency of activity that ties the search for expanded clinical efficacy to the struggle for equity in social well-being. This linkage of purpose and energy will best assure that the clinical and public commitment to optimal child development will prove both effective and just.

Affluence

The inclusion of affluence as a potential deterrent to healthy development is not to imply that the role of affluence might be analogous to that of poverty. It is not. Poverty implies hardship and barriers to healthy development that are difficult to overcome without some combination of individual, familial, or community strengths and appropriate, accessible services. Affluence, on the other hand, implies access to full societal participation that is not constrained by basic material concerns. Affluence is discussed in this chapter in consideration of environmental influences on normal development to call attention to aspects of the affluent environment that may prove deleterious despite their occurrence in a framework generally thought to provide the most promising environment for healthy development.

Affluence, like poverty, can be defined in a number of ways. Because the influence of family resources on child well-being can take different forms in different settings, herein affluence is understood simply as an abundance of available material resources.

Relationship Between Affluence and Development

Among the negative outcomes in which growing up in affluence may be implicated are alcohol and drug abuse, juvenile delinquency, motor vehicle occupant injuries, suicide, cult membership, severe narcissism, profound alienation, and eating disorders. Yet it remains unclear whether the primary risk is great wealth, a rapid ascendancy into wealth, or an exclusivity of social relations that precludes peer contact with the nonwealthy. Wealth may serve as only a proxy for risk in that it may be associated with more potent influences, such as the fame, power, lack of traditional family interactions, and intense emphasis on extraordinary achievement, which may characterize a significant proportion of wealthy families.

Aspects of Affluence With Possible Negative Effects

Aspects of the environment that may be present in a significant number of affluent families and that may be deterrents to healthy development are listed in Table 17–2. However, the suggested associations have not been subjected to repeated systematic investigation, and empiric insight into significant causal relationships remains almost entirely lacking.

Parental Absence or Neglect and Weakened Family Ties

A significant portion of affluent parents live in a style that may demand, and certainly permits, long absences from

Table 17–2 • Aspects of Affluence With Possible Negative Effects

---

Circumstances may lead to absence of strong, consistent parental presence and weakening of family ties
Role of substitute caretakers may be variable and transient
Unrealistic or destructive parental expectations
An overabundance of possessions with diminished need for choice and effort
Relatively easy access to cars, drugs, and alcohol

---

home and children. Parents who find parenthood burdensome have the means to circumvent childrearing tasks in a socially sanctioned manner. Preoccupations with professional or recreational interests may eliminate protected time for parent-child involvement, nurturance, and communication. Constant professional and social demands may undermine a daily structure for family interaction and create a marked failure in the systematic transmission of family concerns, traditions, values, role expectations, and expressions of love based on everyday events.

A constellation of psychosocial problems, rooted in a profound and harmful narcissism, has been noted in the youth of affluent families. Described as the "silver spoon syndrome," it is characterized by narcissistic tendencies associated with a poor sense of nurturance, depression, a compelling sense of public self, but a low regard for private self (LeBeau, 1988). Poor parent-child interaction has been suggested as the primary etiology of this complex of problems, and its resolution is best approached through family-based therapeutic strategies.

Role of Substitute Caretakers

The decline of the extended family and the rapid increase of women in the work force have made child care by adults other than the parents a common component of current day childrearing. However, among some affluent families, childrearing can be left primarily to others and particularly to in-home servants. In such situations, the opportunity for the creation of a strong bond between parents and children may be considerably diminished. Although there are governesses, nannies, housekeepers, and other servants who provide extraordinarily consistent and profound caring and nurturance, the potential lack of close parental supervision may allow inappropriately harsh forms of punishment or extreme permissiveness. There may be repeated turnover of employed caretakers, and when such caretakers have been the principal loving adults in the child's life, such departures can be painful and debilitating. The potential for conflict and even jealousy to emerge between parent and caretaker can also lead to destructive inconsistencies and tension in disciplinary practices and daily routines. A primary reliance on employed caretakers requires a close and independent relationship between the parents and child and an informed alliance between the parents and caretaker.

Unrealistic or Destructive Parental Expectations

Goals and standards set by affluent parents for their children may include extraordinary pressures to measure up to the success of the parents and a narrow definition of what is acceptable. Scholastics, sports, and social achievements that are good may not be good enough; they may have to be "best." The message that love and acceptance are contingent on high achievement can be particularly harmful to children with average abilities. In addition, the child's perception of parental standards may be far more stringent than the true feelings of the parents—a situation that can lead to unnecessary, but real, pressure on the child.

Overabundance of Possessions

Most children in wealthy families are surrounded by a wealth of possessions. This may be part of a general expression of wealth in a consumer-based society, or parents may buy expensive gifts to assuage a sense of guilt for not spending enough time with their children. Regardless, these children may have little experience with having to delay gratification or with the frustration that comes from having to do without a coveted object. This may compound the harmful effects of growing up with little contact with children from a diversity of backgrounds and social class. Furthermore, such children may develop unrealistic expectations of the extent to which one need not adapt to life but can make the world adapt to one's whims. The expectation that familial resources will pave the way for them in life and eliminate the need for personal accomplishment may so characterize children of certain affluent families. Easy access to automobiles, drugs, and alcohol may so be implicated in high rates of automobile-related injuries and substance abuse among some wealthy adolescents.

Preventing Detrimental Effects of Affluence

Health professionals can be especially alert to the specific signals that may characterize abnormal development in affluent families. A frank discussion of these issues can be integrated into the anticipatory guidance component of primary care, and when concerns do arise, appropriate advice or referrals can be provided. Because family interactions tend to play the primary role in shaping developmental problems in affluent children, family-centered therapy is often most helpful. Clinicians can also support school and community efforts to provide organized service projects and other substitutes for the challenges of fighting for economic survival, including demanding outdoor activities in which children encounter the impartial realities of nature.

Most important perhaps is the role health professionals can play in emphasizing the critical and unique function of parenthood to those parents with the resources to leave childrearing to others. The clinician can serve as an advocate for the child, stressing the role that parents have in providing nurturance, love, and support; in setting firm and realistic limits to behavior; and in conveying to their children a clear set of traditions, values, and moral precepts.

Geographic Moves

A child's ability to thrive can be greatly enhanced by stable and familiar surroundings. Stability and familiarity breed opportunities to master developmental tasks and to develop secure relationships. Changing neighborhoods, especially frequent changes, places the child at risk for academic, behavioral, emotional, and potentially health problems. For example, a recent analysis of data from the 1988 National Health Interview Survey of Child Health revealed that school-aged children who moved three or more times were at increased risk for emotional/behavioral and school problems (Simpson and Fowler, 1994). The magnitude of concern increases when considering that nearly 40% of all school-aged children have moved three or more times and that poor children are more likely to move frequently.

Geographic moves also increase the likelihood that a child does not have a specific site for health care (Fowler, Simpson, and Schoendorf, 1993). This, in turn, may place the child at risk for poor physical health and reduced receipt of health care services. In addition, delayed receipt of prior medical records often makes it difficult for new health care providers to know exactly what services, such as age-appropriate vaccinations, are needed and what physical and mental health problems deserve attention. Parents may not be familiar with the details of the physical and emotional ailments of their children, including current therapies and past evaluations. It is therefore necessary for child health care providers to create effective systems to gather prior medical record data and to be vigilant in obtaining information regarding children and families who have moved and are seen for the first time.

Neighborhood Violence and Danger

Violence in the lives of American children, as victims, perpetrators, and witnesses to violence, has grown to epidemic proportions (Prothrow-Stith, 1995) (see Chapter 51). Neighborhoods, which should provide a sense of familiarity and protection to children, often do the opposite. Nationwide surveys have shown widespread fear among children of the potential for physical harm in their neighborhoods. The seductive lure of the drug trade and the widespread availability of guns have exposed children of the inner cities to assaults that may be unprecedented in their degree of physical and psychological violence. Children in suburban areas may also harbor significant fears of violence in their schools and on neighborhood streets.

The research literature focusing on the prevalence and impact of children's exposure to violence has grown substantially in the past few years. A large percentage of children are exposed to violence as witnesses or victims within their home in the forms of domestic abuse and television violence, and on the streets and in schools in the form of assaults, attempted assaults, and physical threats (Schooler and Flora, 1996). Victimization from some form of direct violence for children between the ages of 6 and 17 years has recently been reported in the range of nearly 20% to more than 50%, and witness to violence rates, including muggings, rapes, shootings, and stabbings, have ranged from 10% to 90%, depending largely on the intensity of neighborhood poverty and drug use. Violence exposure crosses socioeconomic strata yet is more prevalent among low-income children. The prevalence of violence exposure is extraordinary, and most reported figures are likely to be underestimates. Exposure to violence has important physical, developmental, and emotional sequelae; that is, children become perpetrators of violence or have poor school functioning, emotional instability, symptoms of posttraumatic stress disorder or depression, and altered world view. When children come to view the world as a dangerous and unpredictable place, their exploration of the world around them may be restricted dramatically (Augustyn et al, 1995). This, in turn, can further compromise a child's ability to address and conquer the physical, developmental, and emotional challenges necessary for normal progression to adulthood.

ROLE OF PUBLIC HEALTH CLINICAL SERVICES

For all people who provide care for poor children, the menace of violence and intentional injury remains a source of enormous frustration. Clearly, fundamental solutions lie outside the health care system, but health professionals can play a constructive role as influential advocates for larger ameliorative public policies (Sege and Dietz, 1994). Because many of these exposures to violence go unreported by children and their parents, it is incumbent upon those who work and care for children to be cognizant of potential at-risk situations and to explore this profound threat to the health and well-being of children in the context of providing comprehensive care. This forum allows an opportunity for discussions regarding discipline practices, the use of verbal means of expressing anger, and strategies to address inappropriate television viewing; these discussions can also help frame a home environment that supports nonviolent resolution of conflict. The removal or absolute separation of children from household guns is essential. Clinicians can also help to identify young children whose environment puts them at high risk for violent behavior or victimization, including those with a family or peer history of violence, school failure, substance abuse, or gang membership (Graham, 1996). New efforts to use the clinical pediatric encounter to address the risk of violence have been promising. The expressed inclusion of violence prevention discussions and education within routine clinical practice may prove useful. Tightly coordinated, early referral to counseling or other supportive services may strengthen family and community-based efforts to reduce the risk of exposure to violence.

REFERENCES

Askew GL, Finelli L, Lutz J, et al: Beliefs and practices regarding childhood vaccination among urban pediatric providers in New Jersey. Pediatrics 96(5):889–892, 1995.

Augustyn M, Parker S, Groves BM, Zuckerman B: Silent victims: children who witness violence. Contemp Pediatr 12(8):35–57, 1995.

Brody DJ, Pirkle JL, Kramer RA, et al: Blood lead levels in the U.S. population, Phase 1 of the Third National Health and Nutrition Examination Survey (NHANES III, 1988–1991). JAMA 272(4):277–283, 1994.

Brown JL: Statement on Key Welfare Reform Issues: The Empirical Evidence. Medford, MA, Tufts University Center on Hunger, Poverty and Nutrition Policy, 1995.

Brown JL, Pizer HF: Living Hungry in America. New York, Macmillan, 1987.

Centers for Disease Control and Prevention: Poverty and infant mortality—United States, 1988. MMWR 44(49):922–927, 1995.

Centers for Disease Control and Prevention: Vaccination coverage of 2-year-old children—United States, 1991–1992. Morb Mortal Wkly Rep 42:985–998, 1994.

Citro CR, Michael RT: Measuring Poverty: A New Approach. Washington, DC, National Academy of Science Press, 1995.

Cook JT, Marti KS: Differences in Nutrient Adequacy Among Poor and Non-poor Children. Medford, MA, Tufts University Center on Hunger, Poverty, and Nutrition Policy, 1995.

Cornelius LJ: Barriers to medical care for white, black, and Hispanic American children. J Natl Med Assoc 85(4):281–288, 1993.

Dubowitz H, King H: Family violence. A child-centered family-focussed approach. Pediatr Clin North Am 42:153–166, 1995.

Duncan GJ, Brooks-Gunn J, Klebanov PK: Economic deprivation and early child development. Child Dev 65;296–318, 1994.

Escalona S: Babies of double hazard: early development of infants at biologic and social risk. Pediatrics 70:343–350, 1982.

Fowler MG, Simpson GA, Schoendorf KC: Families on the move and children's health care. Pediatrics 91(5):934–940, 1993.

Graham P: Violence in children: the scope for prevention. Arch Dis Child 74(3):185–187, 1996.

Hack M, Klein NK, Taylor HG: Long-term developmental outcomes of low birthweight infants. The Future of Children 5(1), 1995.

Huston AC, McLoyd VC, Coll CG: Children and poverty: issues in contemporary research. Child Dev 65, 275–282, 1994.

Institute of Medicine: Best Intentions. Washington, DC, National Academy of Science Press, 1996.

Institute of Medicine: Prenatal Care. Washington, DC, National Academy of Science Press, 1988.

LeBeau J: The "silver-spoon" syndrome in the super rich: the pathologic linkage of affluence and narcissism in family systems. Am J Psychother 42(3):425–436, 1988.

Miller J, Korenman S. Poverty and children's nutritional status in the United States. Am J Epidemiol 140:233–243, 1994.

Newacheck PW, Hughes DC, Cisternas M: Children and health insurance: an overview of recent trends. Health Affairs (Millwood) 14:244–254, 1995.

Parker S, Greet S, Zuckerman B: Double jeopardy: the impact of poverty on early child development. Pediatr Clin North Am 35:1227–1240, 1988.

Prothrow-Stith DB: The epidemic of youth violence in America: using public health prevention strategies to prevent violence. J Health Care Poor Underserved 6(2):95–101, 1995.

Roghmann K, Hecht P, Haggerty R: Coping with stress. In Haggerty R, Roghmann K, Pless I (eds): Child Health and the Community. New York, John Wiley & Sons, 1975.

Rubin DH, Erickson CJ, San Augustin M, et al: Cognitive and academic functioning of homeless children compared with housed children. Pediatrics 97(3):289–294, 1996.

Rutter M. The city and the child. Am J Orthopsychiatry 51(4):610–625, 1981.

Schooler C, Flora JA: Pervasive media violence. Ann Rev Public Health 17:275–298, 1996.

Sege R, Dietz W: Television viewing and violence in children: the pediatrician as agent for change. Pediatrics 94(4 pt 2):600–607, 1994.

Simpson GA, Fowler MG: Geographic mobility and children's emotional/behavioral adjustment and school functioning. Pediatrics 93(2):303–309, 1994.

Starfield B, Shapiro S, Weiss J, et al: Race, family, income, and low birth weight. Am J Epidemiol 134:1167–1174, 1991.

St. Peter RF, Newacheck PW, Halfon N: Access to care for poor children, separate and unequal? JAMA 267(20):2760–2764, 1992.

Townsend P: Poverty in the United Kingdom. Berkeley, CA, University of California Press, 1979, p 31.

Werner E, Smith R: Kauai's Children Come of Age. Honolulu, HI, University of Hawaii Press, 1977.

Wise PH, Kotelchuck M, Wilson ML, et al: Racial and socioeconomic disparities in childhood mortality in Boston. N Engl J Med 313:360–366, 1985.

18 *Electronic Media*

Henry L. Shapiro

 We are all likely to be baffled by the virtual tidal wave of advances in the electronic media. Electronic games, interactive CD-ROM, and innovations in television are among the many advances that may represent a rather mixed blessing for developing children and their parents. This chapter offers a systematic review of what we know about the promises as well as the threats inherent in these innovative modes of communication and stimulation. It is likely that in the future, primary care physicians will be asked increasingly about the effects of the media on children. This chapter provides valuable background information to help clinicians become more responsive to these critical contemporary issues.

When television is good, nothing—not the theatre, not the magazines or newspapers—nothing is better. But when television is bad, nothing is worse. I invite you to sit down in front of your television set. . . . I can assure you that you will observe a vast wasteland.
—FEDERAL COMMUNICATIONS COMMISSIONER NEWTON MINNOW, 1961. (MINNOW AND LAMAY, 1995)

We are all the product of mass media culture—Gutenberg, Morse, Marconi, Edison, Zworykin, and Gates—we live in a sea of mediated communications. Less in a global village than a vast bazaar of messages, we are more in contact with the thoughts and intentions of others than at any other time in history. Electronic media can positively influence social behavior, knowledge, and understanding. Exposure to programming showing prosocial and empathetic themes can increase these behaviors in viewers. On the other hand, electronic media have been accused of increasing aggression and having negative effects on learning. This chapter explores electronic media, particularly television, and the newest media of electronic games and computers and their impact on the development and behavior of children.

Background

Children (and adults) watch a great deal of television. Viewing peaks between the ages of 2 and 5 years and declines briefly on school entry, before increasing until adolescence, when viewing is at a minimum, displaced by listening to music and other peer activities (Bryant and Rockwell, 1994). Children watch much of their television alone, and 80% of their viewing is developmentally inappropriate adult fare (Huston et al, 1992). Family television viewing peaked at over 7 hours a day in 1985–1986 and has declined to about 4 hours (Andreasen, 1994).

Adult programming contains about five violent acts per hour. Children's Saturday morning programming con- tains 20 to 25 depictions of violence per hour. A typical child watches 15,000 to 18,000 hours of television by age 18 years (compared with attending 12,000 hours of school) and witnesses 200,000 acts of television violence, including 18,000 murders. Other media children are exposed to include newspapers, magazines, music recordings, film, and videotape (Huston et al, 1992), constituting massive media exposure for the average child.

Neurodevelopment and Learning

There is a growing literature about the impact of electronic media exposure on attention, memory, executive functions, language and communication, visual-spatial processing, reasoning, and social and emotional functioning. This literature focuses on television more than on other media. Huston and colleagues (1992) report on the attentional and cognitive aspects of children's television viewing. The evidence does not support the assertion that television has a negative effect on attention. Children's ability to attend to television increases until about age 9 years, when it reaches about 70% of viewing time. Attention to television appears to be closely related to the child's understanding of the content. Humor, character movement, sound effects and auditory changes, children's and women's voices, and animation are most effective at getting and maintaining children's attention. Violent content per se does not seem to differentially improve children's attention when other interesting content is present.

Children watch television strategically, focusing on salient content just like good readers. Pacing of a show has less of an effect on subsequent behavior than program content. Neuman (1991) reviews the possible effects of television on different constructs of attention and motivation. One concern about television is that the amount of invested mental effort may be less than reading or other activities, resulting in less depth of processing. However, this viewpoint does not have much support. Neuman points out that television, "like text, offers a panoply of social actions, events and situations. Viewers must select and transform these experiences into synthesis or interpretation, which is integrative and satisfying" and therefore does require active mental effort. The impact of television on visual processing and language appears to be neutral. Families often watch television together, and video games provide social opportunities.

Print literacy is hard-won. Building on everyday language, it draws on metalinguistic and metacognitive skills that come directly out of the education experience. Is visual literacy analogous to print literacy? Studies of individuals with little or no exposure to modern pictorial and cinematic material do not show major gaps in their ability to "read" the explicit content of film or video. Comprehension differences seem to be related to cultural differences and prior knowledge. Unlike the phonologic code of written language, visual mass media do not require training in a formal notational system. Formal conventions such as camera angles and flashbacks, spatial and distance cues (such as perspective and movement parallax) apparently require only minimal exposure in terms of perception (Messaris, 1994).

Other research (Sprafkin, Gadow, and Abelman, 1992) shows a developmental trajectory in children's understanding of more complex story elements such as deception, characterization, narrative, and cultural references; children with learning differences often have difficulty in these areas, but this is not limited to television. Children with learning disabilities watch more television than their peers, have more difficulty distinguishing fiction from reality, and have difficulty with drawing inferences and narrative continuity.

Sprafkin, Gadow, and Abelman (1992) reported on attempts to teach media literacy to regular and exceptional students and showed positive results, but they cautioned that these skills may not generalize to other environments where other social factors are probably more important. Children with mental disabilities may benefit from educational television, but they appear to have difficulty following stories and need repetition to learn effectively.

There is a strong negative correlation between amount of television viewing and school achievement (Huston et al, 1992). Television displaces other entertainment media (e.g., film, comic books) but it does not necessarily decrease reading time. For example, in the average range of viewing (less than 4 hours a day), reading achievement appears unaffected (Neuman, 1991). Parental expectations and the child's reading confidence are much better predictors of academic success than total viewing time. Neuman quotes a 1986 Swedish study that indicated that higher school achievement was associated with the use of television as a complement to learning when children were encouraged by parents to ask appropriate questions about content.

Negative Media Influences

Research on aggression in children related to electronic media has taken several forms (Singer and Singer, 1981; Strasburger, 1995). Early studies focused on aggressive behavior after exposure to television violence in the laboratory. These studies have been criticized because they did not occur in natural settings. Another line of research looked at the introduction of television into formerly isolated communities. Finally, there are a variety of naturalistic studies. Even though they are difficult to compare because of their various designs and different cultural environments, these studies have documented an increase in aggression immediately following exposure to violence, as well as an apparent increase in aggression in children following communitywide introduction of television (Huston et al, 1992). These effects are seen most in children with higher baseline levels of aggression and appear to be short-lived. There is some "modeling" effect, such as repetition of violent acts. There also seems to be a general "arousal" effect, leading to a greater tendency to act aggressively when provoked or predisposed to aggression.

The notion of general arousal leading to aggression is supported by observations that highly arousing but nonviolent shows also increase aggression. Other research findings include evidence of desensitization to violence after viewing violent television. Research into pornography yields similar findings, particularly in regard to desensitization to violence against women and the relationship of general arousal to aggression (Weaver, 1994). There are contrasting studies showing an increase in prosocial behavior after viewing prosocial content.

In summary, numerous studies have shown that there is an increase in aggression in children immediately after viewing violent content. Research on attention, cognition, and learning does not support the hypothesis of a strong television effect. Television displaces other leisure activities but may have less impact on other constructive activities such as hobbies, sports, family activities, and reading.

Educational Potential of New Media

The "new media" include computer games and the Internet. Their defining characteristics are interaction and multimedia potential. Instructional technology and connectivity within schools has been fairly well funded recently. Starr (1996) recently noted that "past efforts to improve education with better technology have not lived up to their promise," but new technologies may offer a level of richness of content and interactivity not seen in previous technologies. Starr reviews the history of computer-assisted instruction, which experienced only mixed success, but notes the potential advantages of distance learning. The demise of schools resulting from introduction of new technologies has been falsely predicted many times. Access to the new media remains a major problem.

Computer software intended to develop specific processing skills shows great promise. Software of this kind often features either simulations involving problem-solving situations, or drill and practice with periodic entertaining "rewards" (Torgeson and Barker, 1995). Newer programs can track and adapt to individual performance and offer reporting capability. Children seem to enjoy both simulations and drill and practice approaches as long as they are sufficiently interesting.

Violence on the Internet has been less of a concern than sexually explicit material and exposure to predatory

Table 18–1 • Taking a Television History

1. How do you decide what shows to watch? Movies?
2. What are the rules about watching shows or movies?
3. How many hours a day do you watch television?
4. Is there a limit to how many hours are allowed per day?
5. Must any activities be done before television is allowed?
6. Who watches the television?
7. Where is (are) the television(s)?
8. Do you eat meals in front of the television?
9. Do you snack while watching? What do you eat?
10. How late do you watch television?
11. What are the most-watched shows in the house?
12. What did you watch yesterday? The day before?
13. Are there rules regarding music videos? Video games?
14. Do you use Internet-blocking software?

From Walsh D, Goldman LS, and Brown R: Physician Guide to Media Violence. Chicago, American Medical Association, copyright 1996.

adults. Violence might become more of a problem when Internet connection speed increases. It is possible for a parent to monitor a child's Internet usage and to limit access to undesirable content using password protection for access and software that blocks connection to sites containing sexually explicit material. A new threat comes in the form of commercial interests, in which deceptive methods are used to get personal information from children in order to target them for marketing. Current technology allows commercial World Wide Web sites to create a profile of child users, observing every action they take on the site (Furger, 1997). There is no substitute for parental supervision and monitoring.

Video Games

Video games have rapidly penetrated all socioeconomic groups. Technology is advancing. Games have evolved from relatively simple eye-hand coordination exercises to immersive worlds, frequently with violent content. Funk (1993) surveyed 357 middle class seventh- and eighth-graders and found that 66% of the girls played video games at least 1 to 2 hours a week at home, compared with 90% of boys. Boys played in arcades more often than girls did. Girls were estimated to play for an average of 2 hours a week compared with 4.2 hours a week for boys, although 15 children reported playing games for 15 or more hours a week. Of five categories, the two violent categories accounted for half of the preferred games; only 2% of children in the sample preferred educational games. There are no conclusive studies linking video game playing to problems with behavior or learning.

Seizures associated with video games are rare. Ferrie and colleagues (1994) report 15 such cases and comment on 20 other cases in the world literature. Photic stimulation was thought to contribute to many of the seizures, but excitement, fatigue, sleep deprivation, cognitive processing, and diurnal variation in seizure susceptibility were thought to be contributing factors. The main diagnoses were idiopathic generalized epilepsy, with or without photosensitivity, and partial (occipital) seizures. Television-associated seizures share similar characteristics.

Clinical Issues and Advocacy

Electronic media have been heavily politicized since their invention. Despite the federal mandate to serve the public interest, electronic media have been minimally regulated in the past and are currently effectively deregulated. With deregulation, there was a significant decrease in children's television programming and a return to so-called program-length commercials with deceptive practices aimed at children (Minnow and Lamay, 1995). This was partially reversed by the Children's Television Act of 1990.

Table 18–2 • American Medical Association Recommendations for Parents

1. Be alert to the shows your children see. These suggestions are important for all children, and most important for young children: the younger the child, the more impressionable he or she is.
2. Avoid using television, videos, or video games as a baby-sitter. It might be convenient for busy parents, but it can begin a pattern of always turning to media for entertainment or diversion. Simply turning the sets off is not nearly as effective as planning some other fun activity with the family.
3. Limit the use of media. Television use must be limited to no more than 1 or 2 quality hours per day. Set situation limits, too: no television or video games before school, during daytime hours, during meals, or before homework is done.
4. Keep television and video player machines out of your children's bedrooms. Putting them there encourages more viewing and diminishes your ability to monitor their use.
5. Turn the television off during mealtimes. Use this time to catch up and connect with one another.
6. Turn television on only when there is something specific you have decided is worth watching. Don't turn the TV on "to see if there's something on." Decide in advance if a program is worth viewing. Identify high-quality programs, using evaluations of programs in your selection process.
7. Don't make the TV the focal point of the house. Avoid placing the television in the most prominent location in your home. Families watch less television or play fewer videos if the sets are not literally at the center of their lives.
8. Watch what your children are watching. This will allow you to know what they're viewing and will give you an opportunity to discuss it with them. Be active: talk and make connections with your children while the program is on.
9. Be especially careful of viewing just before bedtime. Emotion-invoking images may linger and intrude into sleep.
10. Learn about movies that are playing and the videos available for rental or purchase. Be explicit with children about your guidelines for appropriate movie viewing and review proposed movie choices in advance.
11. Become "media literate." This means learning how to evaluate media offerings critically. First learn yourself and then teach your children. Learn about advertising and teach your children about its influences on the media they use.
12. Limit your own television viewing. Set a good example by your moderation and discrimination in viewing. Be careful when children are around and may observe material from "your" program.
13. Let your voice be heard. We all need to raise our voices so that they are heard by program decision makers and sponsors. We need to insist on better programming for our children.

From Walsh D, Goldman LS, and Brown R: Physician Guide to Media Violence. Chicago, American Medical Association, copyright 1996.

Questions about electronic media exposure should be part of a complete developmental and behavioral history (Table 18–1). Prosocial aspects of television viewing, particularly the family context in which shows are viewed and discussed, are as important as quantity. The American Medical Association has taken a leadership role in helping physicians counsel parents about television (Table 18–2).

Recent public debate has focused on using technology to censor television with much less emphasis on funding excellent content development for children. Pediatricians need to support better choices for children as well as educate parents about potential harmful effects of media. Several authors have suggested ways of advocating for children (Charren, Gelber, and Arnold, 1994; Shelov et al, 1995). These include direct contact with industry, local stations, and music producers; communication with government; advocacy for media literacy curricula within schools; promoting organizations that develop quality children's programming; and working through existing professional groups to lobby industry and Congress.

Conclusion

Electronic media are unavoidable artifacts of modern life. An epiphenomenology about pervasively harmful effects on children needs to be replaced with an accurate understanding of mediated communication and its messages as well as its formal properties. It is crucial for clinicians to use judgment about problems associated with electronic media and their effects on children so they can focus their energies appropriately. New media not only provide new opportunities but also present a new predicament for children affected by developmental differences, problems with self-regulation, and negative environmental influences including abuse, neglect, and poverty. Pediatricians also need to understand the emergence of new media and the promise it offers for revolutionizing education, provided that there is adequate access to this expensive technology.

Pediatricians can promote positive change by informing the public about quality programming, ways of using media effectively, and advocating for access to quality media. Previous successes have included eliminating misleading vitamin advertisements and passage of the Children's Television Act of 1990. With successful campaigns in the past to promote bicycle helmet safety, prevention of poisoning and drowning, and motor vehicle safety, pediatricians now need to address the pervasive effects of media violence on children and youth.

REFERENCES

Andreasen MS: Patterns of family life and television consumption from 1945 to the 1990s. *In* Zillman D, Bryant J, Huston AC (eds): Media, Children, and the Family: Social Scientific, Psychodynamic, and Clinical Perspectives. Hillsdale, NJ, Lawrence Erlbaum, 1994, pp 19–36.

Bryant J, Rockwell SC: Effects of massive exposure to sexually oriented prime-time television programming on adolescents' moral judgment. *In* Zillman D, Bryant J, Huston AC (eds): Media, Children, and the Family: Social Scientific, Psychodynamic, and Clinical Perspectives. Hillsdale, NJ, Lawrence Erlbaum, 1994, pp 183–195.

Charren P, Gelber A, Arnold M: Media, children, and violence: a public policy perspective. Pediatrics 94:631–637, 1994.

Ferrie CD, DeMarco P, Grünewald RA, et al: Video game induced seizures. J Neurol Neurosurg Psychiatry 57:925–931, 1994.

Funk JB: Reevaluating the impact of video games. Clin Pediatr 32:86–90, 1993.

Furger R: Your children are talking to strangers. PC World 15(6):35–39, 1997.

Huston AC, Donnerstein E, Fairchild H, et al: Big World, Small Screen: The Role of Television in American Society. Lincoln, NE, University of Nebraska Press, 1992.

Messaris P: Visual Literacy: Image, Mind, & Reality. Boulder, CO, Westview Press, 1994.

Minnow NM, Lamay CL: Abandoned in the Wasteland: Children, Television, and the First Amendment. New York, Hill and Wang, 1995.

Neuman SB: Literacy in the Television Age: The Myth of the TV Effect. Norwood, NJ, Ablex, 1991.

Shelov S, Bar-on M, Beard L, et al: Media violence (statement of the American Academy of Pediatrics Committee on Communications). Pediatrics 95:949–950, 1995.

Singer JL, Singer DG: Television, Imagination, and Aggression: A Study of Preschoolers. Hillsdale, NJ, Lawrence Erlbaum, 1981.

Sprafkin J, Gadow KD, Abelman R: Television and the Exceptional Child: A Forgotten Audience. Hillsdale, NJ, Lawrence Erlbaum, 1992.

Starr P: Computing Our Way to Educational Reform. The American Prospect 27:50–60, 1996 (http://epn.org/prospect/27/27star.html).

Strasburger VC: Adolescents and the Media: Medical and Psychological Impact. Thousand Oaks, CA, Sage Publications, 1995.

Torgeson JK, Barker TA: Computers as aids in the prevention and remediation of reading disabilities. Learning Disability Q 18:76–87, 1995.

Weaver JB: Pornography and sexual callousness: the perceptual and behavioral consequences of exposure to pornography. *In* Zillman D, Bryant J, Huston AC (eds): Media, Children, and the Family: Social Scientific, Psychodynamic, and Clinical Perspectives. Hillsdale, NJ, Lawrence Erlbaum, 1994, pp 215–228.

19 Disasters

Max Sugar

The impact of disasters on children can be great and lasting, whether they are natural like hurricanes or floods, industrial like airplane crashes or toxic spills, or societal like neighborhood shootings or warfare. This chapter describes the range of disasters, the factors affecting their impact on children's development and behavior, and the resulting reactions. Because pediatric training and textbooks have little instruction on these matters, this chapter is particularly valuable, especially on matters of diagnosis and management.

Despite the ubiquity of disasters, they are painful to consider and people quickly relegate them to the recesses of their minds unless they are personally involved. This must be viewed as avoidance and denial, which is a major recognition problem for the family and possibly for the physician. This chapter provides data and assistance for pediatricians in preparing for, assessing the effects of, and responding to the emotional needs of children and adolescents in disasters.

Prevalence and Variety of Disasters

In 1996, there were 23 wars around the world. Between 1971 and 1980, there were 326 major natural disasters (e.g., floods, and hurricanes) in the United States (Gordon, 1982), not including industrial and societal disasters such as toxic fumes, airplane crashes, train wrecks, and nuclear disasters.

Beginning with the Spanish Civil War in the 1930s, detailed studies have shown that children under fire have increased disturbances, along with acute and chronic posttraumatic stress disorder (PTSD), whether from terrorist attacks, war, civil disruption, or witnessing of violence between parents (Arroya and Eth, 1985).

Meijer (1985) found that boys who were born within 6 months after the end of a war had developmental delays that affected their speech, walking, and sphincter control, and they had "regressive nonaffiliative dissocial behavior" at 7 years of age. He thought that this was related to their deviant attachment resulting from a disturbed mother-child relationship based on the mother's war trauma. In their review of the literature on war and children, Jensen and Shaw (1993) concluded that children may be overwhelmed by massive wartime trauma but that, in low to moderately intense situations of military activity, the child's innate adaptive capacities, cognitive immaturity, and plasticity may reduce the effects of war on their effective functioning.

McCloskey and Southwick (1996) focused on the problem of war refugee children and especially on the risk factors of (1) their ethnic background being in cultural conflict with their hosts', (2) perception of illness, (3) death

of a parent, and (4) mother diagnosed with depression or PTSD.

Among 25 "normal" children and adolescents (those not in disasters) aged 9 to 17 years, Terr (1983) found 10 who exhibited aftereffects of some severe fright, and five of these children had been psychically traumatized years before. She concluded that in many children, the emotional effects of trauma are not observed and are much more common than had previously been assumed. Sugar (1992) observed accurate memories of disaster events in toddlers diagnosed with PTSD. These findings indicate that trauma from disasters can affect children emotionally, beginning prenatally as a result of parental reactions, and even when parents are unaware that the child was exposed to such reactions.

Nuclear disasters present a potent global annihilating risk (e.g., Hiroshima, Nagasaki, and Chernobyl). Even when there is no dangerous level of radiation, the threat of such radiation along with evacuation caused PTSD in children, adolescents, and adults at Three Mile Island in Middletown, PA (Handford et al, 1986).

Although fires often make local headlines, they are soon forgotten despite being the fifth leading cause of death in persons younger than age 19 years. Furthermore, they cause injuries, death to all ages, family disruption, and property loss (Centers for Disease Control, 1990).

Children's Reactions to Disaster

Children have a specific postdisaster clinical presentation, along with some varying symptoms. Among immediate nonspecific effects are marked anxiety, confusion with a shocklike state, disorganization, frozen or inhibited movement, apathy or crying and screaming, a sense of hopelessness, and withdrawal with disturbed sleeping and eating (Table 19–1).

In a few days or weeks after the disaster, nonspecific reactions may include sleep difficulty (insomnia, nightmares, somnambulism), clinging to parents, a lack of personal responsibility, poor school performance, withdrawal, loss of usual interests, concentration and attention problems, nausea, vomiting, loss of appetite and weight, hostility, irritability, anxiety, encopresis, enuresis, violent behav-

Table 19–1 • Children's Reactions to Disasters

Causes of Varying Symptoms	General Nonspecific Reactions			Disaster-Specific Reactions
	Immediate	*Later (Days or Weeks)*	*Month(s) Later*	
Type of disaster, age and sex of victim	Shock	Loss of recent development	Posttraumatic stress disorder (PTSD)	Recall and re-experiencing disaster
Physical trauma	Fear	Eating disturbance	Delayed PTSD	Phobias
Psychic trauma or threat, helplessness, family disruption, breakdown of community organization	Acute anxiety	Sleep disturbance	Anxiety disorder	Reenactment
	Acute distress disorder	Clinging to parents	Depressive disorder	Disaster play
		Lack of personal responsibility	Multiple personality disorder	Repetitive talk of the disaster
		Withdrawal		
		Irritability		
		Time distortion		
		Guilt about survival		
		Dissociative reactions		
		Hostility and violent behavior		
		Encopresis		
		Enuresis		
		Brooding		
		Foreshortening of future		
		Pessimism		
		Posttraumatic play		
		Development of omens		

ior, setting of fires, brooding, development of omens with negative predictions, lesser goals and shorter life expectancy (i.e., foreshortening of their future), pessimism, and guilt about survival (Sugar, 1989).

Grade school children and younger children may have regressive symptoms, such as losing recently acquired developments in speech, behavior patterns, and sphincter control. Dissociative reactions (sudden temporary altered states of consciousness, identity, or motor behavior) can develop early, and multiple personality can develop later.

Among specific reactions to a disaster may be (1) recall and re-experiencing of the disaster in response to various stimuli, (2) phobias about these experiences with startle (diffuse motor) responses, (3) reenactments resembling some aspect of the disaster, (4) risky, bizarre features in their play, called disaster play (e.g., "burying in the sand play" or "tornado play"), (5) repetitive talk, and (6) posttraumatic play. The latter consists of play about the disaster that has excitement without pleasure and does not relieve the child's anxiety (Terr, 1981). There are also distortions and misperceptions in time, with sequencing, duration, and time skew, but not amnesia.

Adolescents exhibit the same symptoms but usually do not engage in posttraumatic play. In the United States, adolescents manifest higher rates of unwed pregnancy, vandalism, belligerence, substance abuse (Adams and Adams, 1984; Erikson, 1976), delinquency, guilt about survival, and hypertension (Gleser, Green, and Winget, 1981). There are significant cultural differences among whites, African Americans, Hispanics, immigrants, and native Americans in the expression of their emotions and in diagnosing and treating problems associated with reaction to disaster. For example, southeast Asian youngsters were more often seen with symptoms of PTSD and depression years after the Cambodian genocide. In contrast, adolescents in the United States more often manifest postdisaster symptoms as behavior or conduct disorder (Sack et al, 1986).

Children's responses result from their own percep-

tions of the disaster, based on their cognitive, psychosexual, and physical developmental level. If the children are separated from their parents or if their parents are unable to cope, this complicates and augments, but does not initiate, the child's symptoms. When a child must deal with a disaster in the parents' absence, it does not mean that separation anxiety is the source of the reaction to the disaster.

There are conflicting reports (Sugar, 1989) about whether sex differences affect reactions, but boys seem to be more affected than girls. In my experience, after a disaster adolescent boys tend to discharge angry and anxious feelings in a hostile and antisocial fashion, even if this was not the boy's previous pattern. Compared with girls, boys use significant denial and experience more difficulty in engaging in and remaining in therapy.

There is a more extreme or severe reaction in older than in younger children, in those who are closer to the disaster, in those who are injured, in those whose parents are injured, dead, or missing, in those with poor and disorganized living conditions, and in those whose response is to intrusions by strangers.

Frequency and Duration of Reactions

If a child remains with the family during and after the disaster, there is no separation effect and there may be decreased confusion and disruption, with the opportunity to reintegrate the child sooner, with the guidance and support of the parents, into a more "normative" routine. However, this depends on the parents' ability to be clear, supportive, and not confused or disorganized in the midst of a disaster. This means not that the children's reactions to the disaster depend on the parents, but that the presence of parents provides a more supportive environment and decreases anxiety. Children have their own reaction to disaster, which may be augmented or moderated by their parents' reactions.

Frederick (1985) noted that 40% to 68% of children had long-term effects several years after various disasters. In my experience with disasters (including hurricanes, a plane crash, a refinery explosion, and a sunken ship) as well as that of others, it appears that when an individual psychiatric evaluation is made following the disaster, almost all children show an immediate disturbed reaction (e.g., acute stress disorder or anxiety reaction). When the assessment of the disaster reaction is based on a questionnaire done months or years later, the percentage of such reactions found decreases considerably.

Factors Affecting the Impact on the Child

The impact of a disaster on the child is due to multiple factors. Disasters can cause death, leading to bereavement or grief reactions in the survivors; injuries, physical pain, and disability; and emotional disturbance.

Children's dependency on parents or others makes them vulnerable to further trauma following the disaster. After a disaster, adults experience a confused state, with shock, disruption of their daily lives, and threats to their integrity (physically, socially, and emotionally), which affects their handling of the children. When there is a breakdown of community organization, parents are further disturbed, and their functioning is disrupted even more. A disaster is accompanied by multiple traumatic events during and afterward, with a consequent upheaval of family life that causes disruption in the children's development.

An acute distress disorder is evident immediately in some children. Various reactions and disorders may continue for months or years afterward. Their symptoms may not be obviously connected with the disaster and can go unnoticed for many years. This leaves the child to suffer on his or her own, which is more likely if the parents do not deal suitably with their own posttraumatic difficulties. Prior individual or family psychopathologic conditions compound the clinical picture.

Diagnostic Considerations

Children in a disaster may have an acute distress disorder, a generalized anxiety reaction, a depressive reaction, an adjustment reaction, PTSD, or another psychiatric condition. Each child does not necessarily show disaster play or reenactment, but most of these children have some disaster reactions. The diagnosis of PTSD is a frequent accompaniment of disasters and refers to the "development of characteristic symptoms following exposure to an extreme traumatic stressor" (*Diagnostic and Statistical Manual of Mental Disorders IV,* 1994). If these symptoms last for a month, the diagnosis of PTSD may be made. (See Chapter 64 for further description of PTSD.)

Children have variable abilities to cope, and some children with better defenses (resilient ones) may have no evidence of the emotional residua of a disaster. However,

among these children are some with unobserved reenactment behavior and delayed effects, such as continued and repeated nightmares of the trauma, repetitious posttraumatic play, dissociated episodes, fugues, or multiple personality.

Management Considerations

A major difficulty in assessing children who have experienced disaster is that the parents may be so confused and disturbed or have such perceptual distortions immediately after the disaster that they are not aware of their child's troubles. This may result from their shock reaction in the initial postdisaster stage. However, many adults (e.g., parents and school principals) (Blom, 1986; Handford et al, 1986) tend to minimize the effect on children because of their own denial. Adult disaster victims (more men than women) tend to minimize or deny the need for psychiatric help for themselves, their spouses, and their children. When the significant and responsible adults do not bring matters to the attention of the pediatrician, the problem may be unattended.

The pediatrician may be part of the team that is involved immediately in assessing the victims of the disaster. Assessment includes doing triage and deciding who needs immediate care or referral for physical injuries or emotional disturbances. The pediatrician could assist with arrangements in matters of public health (hygiene and prevention), such as providing shelter, food, and potable water, along with attention to general medical needs. In addition, the media presence should be kept to a minimum because it intrudes on public health.

The pediatrician should try to help the family avoid making any permanent major decisions immediately after the disaster until the confusion and anxiety have decreased and an increase in stabilization of routine daily life takes place. An immediate component of this strategy is to keep lawyers and insurance adjusters away until the family has stabilized.

Attention should be paid to the basic needs of the disaster victims, with care being given to their physical state using medical intervention and by keeping the family together, if possible, after the emergency. The family needs to be given support, reassurance, and guidance, especially because they may be in denial.

When the pediatrician is alert to adult denial (which is a major hindrance to psychiatric case finding) and the effects of disasters on children and adults, the child's needs can be more readily detected. The pediatrician can provide the emotionally symptomatic child with reassurance and, if needed, a sedative or anxiolytic, along with guidance for the parents or immediate psychiatric referral. At a minimum, every child and family should be able to avail themselves of the local state or community group support services for ventilation of concerns and support to help with the immediate general reactions, as provided by the 1974 Disaster Relief Act—PL 93-288 (US Government, 1976).

Psychiatric consultation is indicated if the child's symptoms continue unabated for several weeks after the family has stabilized despite reassurance, support, and medication. Immediate psychiatric attention is in order

Table 19–2 • Management of Disasters by Pediatricians

Predisaster
Prevention of disasters
Training rescue workers for disaster
Emergency response and care
Physical
Emotional
Triage
Support, sedation
Referral
Community care
Attention to safety, hygiene, water, food, shelter, sleep
Aftercare
Provide support groups
Minimize intrusions
Expect emotional reactions
Expect denial by parents
Provide psychiatric referral

when there is risky or dangerous reenactment or posttrauma play (Table 19–2).

In a substantial number of children, the effects of a disaster are likely to be an acute and chronic disturbance with extensive impairment of long duration that is highly resistant to change. For those requiring treatment, time and effort are needed.

Reactions of the Disaster Relief Workers, Including Medical Professionals

Troubled feelings often arise in disaster relief workers who are exposed to the suffering and bizarre, frightening scenes of destruction and death. They often experience "burnout" and various disturbed behaviors after a disaster.

Wraith (1988) noted that children of relief workers in a disaster may respond to the professional experience of their parents and suffer PTSD because of their marked anxiety about the parents' at-risk activities.

Denial occurs in the adults who are involved as victims, observers, or helpers, including parents, teachers, relief workers, and physicians. There is often a feeling of helplessness in the helpers as they witness the child's struggle to deal with the effects of the disaster. These feelings can intrude on the pediatrician's ability to assess the child's or parents' need for psychiatric help. This is a major issue to be considered by anyone dealing with children in a disaster. When an adult relief worker is feeling overburdened or is given indications that this is occurring by colleagues, staff, or family, then professional support should be sought.

Advocacy and the Pediatrician

The pediatrician is in a prime and prominent position to help in disasters by arranging for and promoting a crisis plan before disaster occurs in any municipality. This should include regular training programs for the significant people in the community who work with disaster victims (Frederick, 1985). This makes the pediatrician an advocate of preparedness. In his or her position in the community, the pediatrician has a major contribution to make in helping to plan and arrange for predisaster training and care, as well as in giving care during and after the disaster.

A general guideline for disasters that might be helpful for pediatricians and all physicians is *Psychosocial Issues for Children and Families in Disasters* (US Department of Public Health and Human Services, 1995). It is available gratis from National Mental Health Services Knowledge Exchange, P. O. Box 42490, Washington, DC, 20015, or by telephone (800) 789-2647.

Some pediatricians may be more inclined to publicly express their concerns about environmental hazards, and speak out about them both as physicians and as private citizens. Too often risks are not voiced publicly. The pediatrician can voice hopefulness to patients and the community about controlling risks.

REFERENCES

Adams PR, Adams GR: Mount Saint Helens's ashfall: evidence for a disaster stress reaction. Am Psychol 39:252, 1984.
Arroya W, Eth S: Children traumatized by Central American warfare. *In* Eth S, Pynoos RS (eds): Post-traumatic Stress Disorder in Children. Washington, DC, American Psychiatric Press, 1985.
Blom GE: A school disaster—intervention and research aspects. J Am Acad Child Psychiatry 25:336, 1986.
Centers for Disease Control. Childhood injuries in the United States. Am J Dis Child 144:627, 1990.
Diagnostic and Statistical Manual of Mental Disorders, 4th ed. Washington, DC, American Psychiatric Press, 1994.
Erikson K: Everything in Its Path. New York, Simon and Schuster, 1976.
Frederick CJ: Children traumatized by catastrophic situations. *In* Eth S, Pynoos RS (eds): Post-traumatic Stress Disorder in Children. Washington, DC, American Psychiatric Press, 1985.
Gleser GC, Green BL, Winget TC: Prolonged Psychosocial Effects of Disaster: A Study of Buffalo Creek. New York: Academic Press, 1981.
Gordon P: Special Statistical Summary—Deaths, Injuries and Property Loss by Type of Disaster, 1970–1980 (A127645). Washington, DC, Federal Emergency Management Agency, 1982.
Handford HA, Mayes SD, Mattison RE, et al: Child and parent reaction to the Three Mile Island nuclear accident. J Am Acad Child Psychiatry 25:346, 1986.
Jensen PS, Shaw J: Children as victims of war: current knowledge and future research needs. J Am Acad Child Adolesc Psychiatry 32:697, 1993.
McCloskey LA, Southwick K: Psychosocial problems in refugee children exposed to war. Pediatrics 97:394, 1996.
Meijer A: Child psychiatric sequelae of maternal war stress. Acta Psychiatr Scand 72:505, 1985.
Sack WH, Angell RH, Kinzie JB, Rath B: The psychiatric effects of massive trauma on Cambodian children. II. The family, home and school. J Am Acad Child Psychiatry 25:377, 1986.
Sugar M: Toddlers' traumatic memories. J Infant Ment Health 13:245, 1992.
Sugar M: Children in a disaster—an overview. Child Psychiatry Hum Dev 19:163, 1989.
Terr LC: Life attitudes, dreams, and psychic trauma in a group of 'normal' children. J Am Acad Child Psychiatry 22:221, 1983.
Terr LC: "Forbidden games" post-traumatic child's play. J Am Acad Child Psychiatry 20:741, 1981.
US Department of Health and Human Services: Psychosocial Issues for Children and Families in Disasters. Washington, DC, US Government Printing Office, 1995.
US Government, Federal Register: Washington, DC, Office of Federal National Archives and Record Service, November 6, 1976.
Wraith R: Experiences in children of workers in emergency services and disaster situations. Presented at the International Conference on Dealing with Stress and Trauma in Emergency Services, Melbourne, Australia, 1988.

20 Schools as Milieux

Carl W. Swartz

 School-aged children may be thought of as school-*caged* children. Throughout their years of academic education, boys and girls are perpetually under the influence of the school environment. Its structure, its governance, its politics, its culture, and its social dynamics together constitute potent forces that significantly influence a child's pattern of development and learning. This chapter reviews some of the critical contemporary issues regarding the school as a backdrop for the scenarios of school-age progression. Much of the material contained herein is not included in traditional medical literature, yet it certainly has a significant bearing on a clinician's ability to understand the daily life of a school-aged child under her or his care.

Jeremy

"No! Already? I can't believe that it's time to get up for school. I'm tired . . . I feel like I just went to sleep." Jeremy did finally fall asleep after an hour of lying in bed wondering if he would ever fall asleep. Each night is the same for Jeremy; incomplete homework sitting on his desk, his class study guides still sitting in his backpack when he goes to bed sometime between 9:00 and 10:00 PM, asleep 60 to 90 minutes later, a restless sleep (as evidenced by his pillow and blankets starting off on his bed and ending up on the floor), and finally being awakened between 5:45 and 6:00 AM. As Jeremy struggles out of bed he sighs, "I hope Mom did the laundry last night."

Jeremy's second challenge of the day is quite possibly his most important, at least to him: creating his armor for the day. ". . . for sure not that shirt . . . Oh man, I CANNOT believe Mom DID NOT do the laundry . . . I guess this one will have to do . . . the pants I need are dirty . . . I'll wear 'em anyway . . . where are my new shoes? I can't wear those raggedy old shoes I had on yesterday . . . Mom!" Jeremy's ensemble of clothes is selected not so much to gain favor from his peers as to deflect any of their unwanted looks and unneeded negative comments. Unfortunately, his clothes will not protect him from his teachers, who will at some point expose him to his peers for his obvious menu of shortcomings—lack of social skills, poor academic performance, attention deficits, and inappropriate behavior—which Jeremy knowingly uses to cover up his other difficulties. Jeremy possesses a great many strengths: he is a computer aficionado, having already authored some creative software programs, and he is an excellent athlete. Jeremy's problem is that computer time, physical education, and recess are taken from him when his academic work is not completed, when he does poorly on a test, or when he behaves inappropriately. Jeremy does not know when his day will be ruined, or even why; he just knows the day will end up like the others, and he wonders why he can't find some success. Jeremy

longs to be like the other kids who arrive at school with everything they need—completed homework, pencils, pens, paper, clothes and hair just right, friends, and no problems. On the bus Jeremy anxiously hopes, "My study guide and homework better be in my backpack . . . I can't go to summer school . . . Oh man . . . no lunch, no money, and Jones said she won't lend me anymore lunch money!"

Jeremy's Parents

"Is Jeremy up?" Mr. Lee mutters to his wife.

"Yeah, for now. You'll have to go in and check on him in a few minutes to make sure he is moving around."

"I can hear him. Do you think he finished his homework and studied for his science test?"

Ms. Lee sighs, "I hope so. I hope the letter from his teachers saying he will have to go to summer school if he does not improve his performance during the next grading period put some fear into him, especially because he'll be retained if he doesn't pass summer school."

"I don't know if all of that will get him going. It seems to me that the school threatens him but does not give him the help he needs to do well. Look at all of the meetings we have been to about one thing or another. Besides, I was just like him when I was his age."

Ms. Jones

On her drive into school, Ms. Jones ponders her dilemma: "I have too much content to cover during the next few weeks and I still need to get my classes ready for those "all-too-important" end-of-course exams and minimum competency tests! I could teach if I did not have to deal with so many problem students who don't want to be in school: the ADD kid, the LD kid, LD/GT students, the BED kid. How can I teach to so many different types of students when many of them can't read and write . . . I have a master's degree in biology . . . I'm the science teacher."

Dr. Walters

At a breakfast meeting of community business leaders and legislators, the superintendent of schools confidently speaks: "We will have world-class schools where every student is literate, not only in reading and writing, but in the sciences, mathematics, and technology as well. Our students will meet the responsibilities of the next century as informed citizens, able to consume and use information for the betterment of their community. Our teachers will be as well educated in their disciplines as any in the state, if not the country. But we need your help."

As Dr. Walters speaks, buses are running and the schools are already filled with teachers and administrators and are filling with children and adolescents. Dr. Walters' administrative assistant is taking a message from the president of the local Learning Disabilities Association regarding the district's noncompliance in the delivery of services for students with learning disabilities. The message will be placed on top of the one from a community activist wanting an appointment to discuss curriculum issues, and messages from two different principals who are warning him that their middle schools will not be able to physically accommodate the eighth grade students who are at risk of being retained if they do not pass the minimum competency test after attending summer school, given the number of rising seventh graders.

These vignettes depicting the early morning lives of the key players who create, maintain, and can modify the milieux of schools are not atypical, although it should be acknowledged that the viewpoints about school and schooling, even within the same school, range from the extremely positive to even more pessimistic than these vignettes. These vignettes merely provide a window into the inherent complexity of schools.

The purpose of this chapter is to build on pediatricians' unique knowledge about child and adolescent development by providing an overview of the influences and context in which children and adolescents spend significant portions of their lives. The goal is for pediatricians to use this information to (1) frame questions and issues to discuss with parents and children about the context in which they may find themselves experiencing varying degrees of success, failure, and anxiety; and (2) become key members of collaborative efforts to shape schools as a milieu that is positive for child growth. The content of this chapter is not so much a summary of empiric research that has established relationships about school-related factors and classroom performance (e.g., class size and achievement) as it is an overview of the external and internal influences that currently shape and will influence the context of education into the next century. The information may be common knowledge to those within education, but the information may not be as well known to persons who have not historically been directly involved in shaping the educational milieu. The current needs of teachers, parents, and children require that those disciplines become key members of collaborative efforts to improve schools for individual students, and if possible, other students as well.

Overview of Schools as Milieux

Mission Statement:
College Park Middle School
Hickory, North Carolina

The mission at College Park Middle School is to unite the educational community in a common quest for excellence in: curriculum, academics, character, and citizenship.

WE BELIEVE:
- All members of the school community are continuous learners.
- Through the efforts of school, home, and community, a safe and inviting school can address the diverse needs of students and encourage success and self-worth.
- The continuing development and enhancement of the curriculum is necessary to meet the needs of society.
- Educators must model the learning process.

Reprinted with permission from Ms. Martha Hill, Principal of College Park Middle School, Hickory, NC.

The mission statement from College Park Middle School, although easy to comprehend, in practice reflects the increasingly complex nature of formal education. No longer is it only the role of the schools to assume the responsibility for educating our youth in the three R's. Today, it is the school's role to "unite the educational community" in the search for attaining standards of excellence in "curriculum, character, academics, and citizenship." Members of the educational community with their disparate backgrounds, needs, and expectations work in concert from a foundation of a common set of beliefs to meet the diverse needs of students, and ultimately for the betterment of society. But, is there a role for physicians and other health care providers? If so, what is their niche?

The complexities of schools and schooling is attributable to the interaction between external sources and internal sources of influence that operate to create a tension that supports or stresses the educational system, even though these sources should be united in a common quest. External sources of influences on the educational system include familial, cultural, economic, political, and religious. Each source may possess hidden agendas that manifest themselves in attempts to exert some pressure on the nature of the educational setting, such as accountability and services, control of curriculum, and level and funding of educational programs. Internal sources of influence on education include school boards and administrators who develop school-district policy and procedures, and administrators and teachers who organize schools, classrooms, and curricula based on these policies and procedures, and then teach based on their expectations and their differential beliefs about their students' ability to meet these expectations.

Each day, children and adolescents themselves contribute a significant stress to the system. Students bring to classrooms a plethora of positive and negative experiences from home and school, unique profiles of neurodevelopmental functions and dysfunctions (e.g., attention, memory, language), varying levels of academic skills and motivation for learning, and their personal belief about the value of education for enhancing their present and future well-being.

Often the student's belief about the value of an education is not one shared with the adults in his or her life because an individual student's belief can be shaped by a more powerful influence, the peer group. The dynamic interplay and interdependency between the general public outside of education, school personnel, parents or caregivers, and students that make up an "educational community" together affect an individual's current classroom performance, immediate and future development, and personal and professional trajectories.

Influences on the Milieux of Schools

EDUCATION REFORM EFFORTS

> *[T]he educational foundations of our society are presently being eroded by a rising tide of mediocrity that threatens our very future as a Nation and a people.*
> —NATIONAL COMMISSION ON EXCELLENCE IN EDUCATION, 1983; p. 5.

With that statement, significant and sweeping reforms were initiated to reinvent schools in some systematic manner. The Goals 2000: Educate America Act of 1994 represents the foundation from which local school reform efforts spring and the standards to which these efforts aspire. Goals 2000 includes the following goals:

By the year 2000
1. All children in America will start school ready to learn.
2. The high school graduation rate will increase to at least 90%.
3. All students will leave grades 4, 8, and 12 having demonstrated minimum competency in challenging subject matter in the core academic subjects, including English, mathematics, science, foreign languages, civics, government, economics, arts, history, and geography; every school will ensure that all students learn to use their knowledge and skills so they will be prepared for responsible citizenship, further learning, and productive employment.
4. Teachers will have access to programs for their ongoing professional development in order to better prepare students.
5. American students will be first in the world in science and mathematics achievement.
6. All adults will be literate, be able to compete in the economy, and exercise their rights and responsibilities of citizenship.
7. Every school will be free of alcohol, drugs, violence, and firearms, and teaching and learning will occur in a disciplined environment favorable to learning.
8. All schools will promote partnerships that will increase parental involvement and active participation in enhancing the intellectual, academic, and affective growth of students.

Goals 2000 is important not only because the legislation sets an agenda for education but also because the language presents an implicit summary of the current milieu. The most recent National Education Goals Report (1995) provides a sober summary of each state's progress, and therefore our national performance in terms of attaining goals based on legislation such as Goals 2000. The report stated that as a nation, performance has been improved in the following areas:

1. General health status of infants has improved.
2. Ratio of preschoolers regularly read to and told stories has increased.
3. Mathematics achievement in Grades 4 and 8 has increased.
4. Reported episodes of threats and injuries to *students* has declined.
5. The number of females receiving degrees in mathematics and science has increased.

The report also stated that as a nation, performance has declined in the following areas:

1. Reading achievement at Grade 12 has decreased.
2. Student drug use has increased.
3. Sale of drugs at school has increased.
4. The gap between those adults who have a high school degree or less and those who have furthered their education in postsecondary schools has increased.
5. The percentage of high school teachers who hold a degree in their content area teaching assignment has declined.
6. More teachers are reporting incidents in their classrooms that disrupt teaching and learning.
7. Threats and injuries to *teachers* have increased.

Furthermore, as a nation, no discernible progress has been made in the following areas:

1. Reducing the gap between rich and poor who have access to quality day care
2. Improving the high school graduation rate
3. Increasing reading achievement in Grades 4 and 8
4. Increasing mathematics achievement in Grade 12
5. Reducing the number of students who reported using alcohol
6. Reducing student reports of classroom disruptions that interfere with their learning
7. Increasing the number of mathematics and science degrees awarded to minority students
8. Reducing the gap in college enrollment and completion between minority students and white students

These findings were based on aggregated data from every state. Many states are making progress in selected areas that are creating more positive instructional milieux, whereas other states are not making the same degree of progress or are actually doing worse in the same areas. Federal reports such as the one cited provide annual updates describing national and state progress toward attaining federally mandated goals. Each state's Department of Public Instruction provides annual reports that describe an overall picture of that state's and local education agency's or individual city or county schools' progress toward meeting educational goals mandated by state legislation.

In summary, federal and state governments have legislated educational goals and standards with the purpose of creating schools in which students and teachers are safe and high expectations for performance are maintained at the same time that the academic, social, and affective needs of students are met. It is important to note that for many students, legislators did not account for "law of unintended consequences" in their educational mandates. For example, classroom teachers and parents may not have the knowledge base about child and adolescent development to entertain the many reasons why a student is not doing well. Regardless, the student may have to attend summer school or be retained because he or she is not meeting the standards of his or her present grade level. Should this occur, possible unintended effects on the student might include (1) an increased passivity towards school until the time he or she can legally drop out, (2) the development of work patterns that lead to lifelong underachievement, and (3) the development of behavior problems as a cover for academic deficiencies. In short, there is no evidence to support the myths surrounding the benefits of retention, and a plethora of evidence supporting the negative impact that retention has on students. For schools, the retention of these students at grade levels in which minimum competency examinations are given will create bottlenecks in which schools will have too many failing students and too few professionals who can effectively manage their education.

Importantly, legislators realize that schools as milieux cannot be transformed to meet these goals unless individuals with their unique knowledge and skills work in concert. In this era of standards and testing, developmental-behavioral pediatricians can use their understanding of child and adolescent development and behavior, patterns of normal variation, and dysfunctions to collaborate with content-area specialists to shape more positive instructional milieux for individual students or the student body as a whole. For example, given patterns of academic achievement and behavior provided by teachers and parents, a pediatrician can begin a process of trying to uncover the neurodevelopmental functions that underlly such patterns. Teachers, pediatricians, parents, and the student can develop a menu of accommodations and interventions at the breakdown points after a thorough description of a child's profile of strengths and dysfunctions is developed.

SCHOOL ORGANIZATION AND MANAGEMENT

In an attempt to create instructional milieux that better meet the needs of teachers, students, and parents and caregivers, many schools have modified their organization and management procedures, including the following:

1. *Site-based management*, which allows individual schools to develop policy and procedures for school governance and selection of professional development programs with teachers having significant control in making school-based decisions, as opposed to decisions being made in a central office at the school district level.

2. *Middle schools*, such that traditional junior high schools, which were focused on the delivery of content, are transformed into middle schools that are focused on the unique developmental needs of early adolescents.

3. *Inclusion*, or the integration of students with handicapping conditions into general education classrooms with special education providing support to students in need.

4. *Charter schools*, which are schools developed by members of the community, open to all students, that receive public tax dollars based on per pupil enrollment and can receive waivers from many legislated mandates.

Because each of these modifications in school organization and management is relatively new, there is little empiric evidence to support their effectiveness in meeting mandated educational standards. The research that does exist is equivocal as to the benefit of these different models of school organization and management. Clearly, developmental-behavioral pediatricians can have a better impact on the milieu of schools when school-level organization and management reflect a philosophy of student needs first, standards and testing second, and a respect and tolerance for differences.

CLASSROOM ORGANIZATION AND MANAGEMENT

Optimally, classroom organization and management should reflect the developmental and behavioral needs unique to each age-band and individual students who may not fit those developmental trajectories. Unfortunately, the results of recent survey research suggest that classroom teachers do not receive the necessary instruction at the university level to manage the developmental, individual, and cultural differences that students present to them each day in the classroom (Berninger, 1996). Furthermore, future classroom teachers are not well trained in the processes and skills underlying their students' acquisition and sophisticated use of reading and writing strategies and mathematic computation and problem solving. In general, preservice classroom teachers are taught to deliver content, although this statement is probably more true for teachers in the middle and secondary schools than for elementary school teachers. Given this context, classroom teachers and students may become adversarial in their relationships because teachers will attribute student failure to the student's not exerting enough effort or to his or her not being intellectually able to perform, whereas students will attribute their failure to their "being dumb" or to teachers' not being willing to help them.

Pediatricians may have the greatest impact on the milieu of education at the classroom level by alleviating these misconceptions. Pediatricians who possess an awareness of the context of schools (which can be different for each school) and who are also well-versed in neurodevelopment and patterns of neurodevelopmental variation and dysfunction can collaborate with teachers to develop effective management plans based on an individual student's profile of neurodevelopmental strengths and dysfunctions and level of academic skill development given the milieu of that school and classroom. Importantly, individuals with the expertise can work to shape a school district's or school's selection of in-service professional development programs that enhance teachers' knowledge about the developmental and individual differences related to classroom performance, to balance most teachers' content expertise. Individual pediatricians with both the time and expertise can provide a useful service to schools by providing classroom teachers with topical workshops.

PEER GROUP MEMBERSHIP

The description of schools as milieux has thus far focused on the external and internal influences on schools as a milieu beyond the level of student. Other chapters in this book provide thoughtful descriptions characterizing the familial, cultural, developmental, and behavioral impacts on school-related outcomes. As important as each of these factors is on educational outcomes, a final factor plays a unique role in shaping the current milieux of individual students and can also mediate developmental trajectories and adult-related outcomes: the peer group to which one is affiliated. Peer group affiliation seems to exert significant influence during the ages of 11 to 18 years (Lee, Bryk, and Smith, 1993):

1. Peer interactions, both inside and outside of schools, foster a climate characterized as nonacademic or antiacademic.
2. The amount of time spent with peers has a significant negative impact on achievement.
3. African American adolescents avoid "acting white," which means working hard and doing well in school.
4. Students, regardless of their own ability level, who affiliate with low-achieving peers have significantly lower achievement scores than students who affiliate with high-achieving peers.
5. Peer influence on misconduct seems to increase with age; the degree of perceived pressure on misconduct varies as a function of peer group membership (e.g., tough kids vs. athletes vs. popular students).

These results indicate that peer group membership can have a significant effect on educational outcomes yet is often overlooked during the assessment process. In many cases, the implementation of a management plan designed to help a student may be facilitated if the student is a member of a group that values success in school or inhibited if the student is affiliated with a group of peers that does not value success in or out of school. Therefore, peer group membership should be accounted for during the assessment process with ongoing support and counseling during the process of monitoring student academic and behavioral progress.

Conclusion

Physicians and other health care providers have at the current time their greatest opportunity to work with others to directly influence the present and future context of education. Physician involvement in the educational community is critical because schools are the common setting shared by every child and family, with all of the many risk factors students bring to school that affect their health as well as their learning and development. Developmental-behavioral pediatricians possess a unique understanding of child and adolescent development that they can use to both inform and shape educational policy and help children and their families understand and manage the educational setting.

REFERENCES

Berninger VW: Reading and Writing Acquisition: A Developmental Neuropsychological Perspective. Boulder, CO, Westview Press, 1996.

Goals 2000: Educate America Act of 1994, Pub. L. No. 103–382, Title III, 361, 384(a), 394(f), 108 Stat. 3974, 4018, 4027, 1994.

Lee VE, Bryk AS, Smith JB: The organization of effective secondary schools. Rev Res Educ 19:171–267, 1993.

National Commission on Excellence in Education: A Nation At Risk: The Imperative for Education Reform. Washington, DC, US Department of Education, 1983.

National Education Goals Panel: The National Education Goals Report: Building a Nation of Learners. Washington, DC, US Government Printing Office, 1995.

SUGGESTED READINGS

Levine MD: Developmental Variations and Learning Disorders, 2nd ed. Cambridge, MA, Educators Publishing Service, 1998.

Levine MD: Educational Care. Cambridge, MA, Educators Publishing Service, 1994.

21 Child Care

Bettye M. Caldwell

 People who were unaware of the need for child care 2 decades ago, and people who denounced it as a family-weakening influence 1 decade ago, now advocate it—and use it.

As of the autumn of 1993, there were approximately 10 million children in the United States under the age of 5 who required child care while their mothers worked.

Results of the studies lend no credibility to the charge of a reduced likelihood of secure attachment associated with the use of infant child care.

Probably no milieu for the development of children has so captured the public's consciousness within the past decade as has the field of day care, or *child care*, as it is now more commonly labeled. This service has been used ever since there have been children to rear; it has taken the form of extended family members, wet nurses and nannies, baby-sitters, and sibling care. It has taken the form of a formal public service for more than a century. For some reason, however, perhaps because people did not want to accept the existence of child care, few seemed aware of it until recently.

Today, however, day care has been very much discovered and for the most part accepted—at least on the surface. People who were relatively unaware of the need for it 2 decades ago, and people who denounced it as a family-weakening influence 1 decade ago, now advocate it—and use it. Media coverage is extensive and is no longer limited to horror stories and sensationalism. Female protagonists in film and television dramas are not infrequently depicted as working in child care—an unofficial but significant indicator of public acceptance. The provision of more care of a higher quality is an item on the agenda of all state legislatures and the US Congress. Major corporations often include child care as part of their benefits package and either provide on-site care for employees' children or offer subsidies for the purchase of care elsewhere. Most importantly, however, many young parents simply do not think of rearing their children without it. It has become an experience almost as universal as primary and secondary education.

How would one describe child care in America today? Is it a comprehensive, integrated, growth-fostering, well-financed, and clearly conceptualized service system? Hardly. Rather it is a patchwork of services offered in multiple settings by persons with differing levels of training and experience and with different motives for working in the field. Although it is now regulated in all states, and one hopes does not fall to less than a minimal level of quality necessary to support the development of children, the field as a whole cannot claim collectively to provide the kind of environment young children need and parents expect. Much of it takes place in informal settings that are poorly monitored, if they are monitored at all. It still has a long way to go.

Brief History of Child Care

Child care, as an alternative to maternal care, began the first time a relative (perhaps not a grandmother, for they did not live long enough) helped care for a young child while the mother participated in some other task assigned to women in that culture. But as a formal service, it is probably accurate to state that it began in 1816 with the efforts of a wealthy industrialist, Robert Owen, to provide a service for the children whose parents worked in his textile mills. The ideas reached America shortly thereafter, finding proponents in people who held one or both of two convictions: (1) that low-income parents could not adequately train and socialize their children and (2) that experiences in settings attuned to the developmental needs of young children would result in educational benefits to the children and the gradual improvement of society, a very modern-sounding concept.

As is generally the case, a few daring mothers among the affluent challenged the appropriateness of having such programs only for the poor (Cahill, 1989) and, as early as 1825, encouraged the establishment of "infant schools." This movement did not last long, however. It succumbed to the pressures against any externalization of primary socialization for young children, with warnings that such programs might cause physical illness or even insanity (Tank, 1980). Thus began a refrain that has echoed for at least the past 150 years and which led to the development of a dual set of programs—early childhood education and day care—which, though separate, were never equal. From the time of the American Civil War until approximately 1970, day care in America, later redesignated as child care, was a service for the poor and for dysfunctional families, was underfunded, was researched not at all, and was largely ignored by the professions generally concerned with the development of children.

The Phenomenal Growth of Child Care

The exponential growth over the past 2 decades in the acceptance of child care as a developmental environment can be attributed primarily to two factors. The first is derived from *child developmental theory*, which for 3 decades has stressed the importance of the early years of life for the fulfillment of a child's genetic potential. The second is purely pragmatic—the dramatic *demographic changes* in entry into the work force by mothers of very young children.

INFLUENCE OF DEVELOPMENTAL THEORY

In the early 1950s, powerful clinical and experimental data forced developmental theorists to pay attention to the early years of life. Beginning perhaps with the clinical studies of Spitz (1945, 1946) of infants separated from their mothers, and buttressed by the scientific investigative reporting of Bowlby (1952) of the subsequent life histories of individuals who spent the early years of their lives in orphanages, data indicative of the critical importance of the first months and years of life began to accumulate. During the same era, experimental animal studies of either severe deprivation (such as chimpanzees being reared in total darkness) or enrichment (such as rats being kept in cages containing a rich variety of objects for both stimulation and response) forced consideration of the role of experience during early life on brain development. Brilliant summaries of such work (Hunt, 1961; Bloom, 1964), and the increasing acceptance of the work of Piaget (1952), stressing the importance of sensory-motor experiences for the development of intelligence, had profound influence on American scientists of the period. However, in spite of its persuasiveness, such work might not have given as clear direction to research of the era had it not been for the timely political attention suddenly given to the needs of children growing up in poverty. With the declaration of the War on Poverty in 1965 and the launching of Head Start as its primary weapon, the field of early childhood came into its own—but not day care. That still needed another catalyst. And that catalyst was found in demographic changes occurring in American families.

DEMOGRAPHIC CHANGES

Evidence of these changes can be found in census and survey data obtained by the Bureau of the Census and other groups concerned with population statistics. Such statistics tend to become obsolete almost by the time they are published, so rapid have been changes in maternal employment over the past several decades.

As of the autumn of 1993, there were approximately 10 million children in the United States under the age of 5 who needed care while their mothers worked (US Bureau of the Census, 1996). Thus, when we talk about child care, we are not talking about small numbers.

The greatest concern about possibly deleterious effects of child care is directed toward care for infants and toddlers. And this is precisely the age group in which the increase has been most dramatic in recent years. Figure 21–1 describes changes from 1980 to 1990 in the percentage of working mothers with children younger than 1 year. The overall increase is from 38% to 53%; however, the most dramatic changes occurred in women with higher education, from 44% to 68%. In that decade, mothers with less than a high school education showed almost no increase at all. The better-educated women represent the trend-setters for our culture, and this dramatic rise indicates a paradigm shift in the way young parents now think about employment while their children are still infants. And it mandates ever greater professional and public concern about making quality child care available on a larger scale.

Early Transition to Respectability

The earliest American programs that attempted to help give child care more respectability as a legitimate and badly needed service to children and families were clearly influenced by both of these trends. The Syracuse Project (Caldwell and Richmond, 1964), generally cited as the first infant day care center in America, is a clear example of

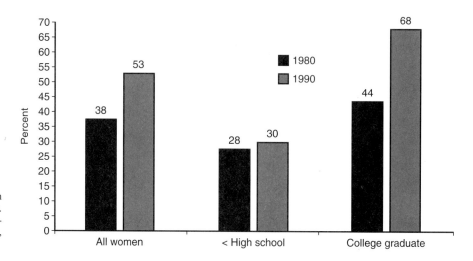

Figure 21–1. Percent of working mothers with infants younger than 1 year in 1980 and 1990. (Data from Current Population Reports, Special Studies Series P-23. Washington, DC, 1992.)

this. It was planned as a means both of optimizing the development of poor children, as prevailing theory suggested was possible, and of addressing the needs of working mothers, as contemporary demographics said was necessary, by creating a high-quality alternative environment for infants and young children. Although this project originated after Salk and Sabin vaccines were available and epidemics of measles and other major childhood diseases were no longer major threats, possible health risks associated with bringing very young children together in groups could still be identified. Thus it was no accident that this first "officially sanctioned" infant child care program was located in a Department of Pediatrics. The same was true for a similar program in Chapel Hill, NC, which began shortly thereafter (Robinson and Robinson, 1971).

Although both of these programs hypothesized gains for participating children associated with the day care experience, the climate of public and professional opinion at that time was such that the research burden laid on the program developers was to prove that they did not harm the participating children. Such evidence quickly began to appear. From the Syracuse project came evidence of cognitive gains associated with attendance at the center, with the more deprived children showing the greatest gains (Caldwell and Richmond, 1968); evidence that attachment to the mother need not be impaired (Caldwell et al, 1970); and proof that children whose early years had included experience in the day care environment showed no more signs of emotional maladjustment than did children without this experience (Braun and Caldwell, 1972). From the Chapel Hill project came similar evidence about cognitive gains (Robinson and Robinson, 1971) and reassurance that infants in the group did not have significantly more respiratory illnesses than did comparable control subjects (Loda et al, 1972).

In retrospect, one can see that it took a lot of courage to design those early programs. (Fortunately at the time we did not realize that.) No one had the expertise or knew what kind and amount of training should be required; most decisions were simply "best guesses." The research was of shaky quality, as the indentification of appropriate control groups was difficult, if not impossible. The very fact that some parents were willing (and sometimes eager) to enroll their children in the programs identified those families as "different" from the remainder of the population in ways likely to influence the development of their children as much as or more than participation in day care. Random assignment, and all the design elegance that goes with it, was out of the question. Even so, what these and other early projects accomplished was to offer reassurance to professionals and parents and to help identify parameters of risk and benefit that have guided subsequent programs and research in the field.

Improved Methodology and Strengthened Knowledge Base

Since roughly the beginning of the 1970s, child care has been brought into the domain of behavioral science research in a big way. After the early wave of research demonstrated that risks associated with early day care could

be minimized and that there could possibly be associated benefits, program expansion and professional, if not public, acceptance increased markedly. Research on outcomes began to be conducted by individuals who were not associated with program operation, and more exemplary procedures were devised. Since this chapter is not intended as an exhaustive review of the literature on the subject, only studies that illustrate major findings and key issues are cited. The three major areas in which effects have been sought are (1) cognitive functioning, (2) socioemotional behavior, and (3) health. The more exemplary projects have been concerned with more than one area, often all three.

COGNITIVE FUNCTIONING

The effects of early child care on cognitive and intellectual development appear to be a function of the type of sample studied and perhaps of the extent to which a given program emphasizes this area of development. As already indicated, cognitive enhancement for socially disadvantaged children was a major objective of some of the early centers; this has not been a major objective of much of the more recent child care research. Furthermore, in much of the literature that is cited in support of lasting cognitive gains for children who have participated in high-quality early childhood programs, it is not clear whether the intervention involved only half-day or full-day programs. It is the long day, day after day, that has been worrisome to most people. Perhaps the most objective summary that can be offered is that, *if quality is at all reasonable, no published study has given support to the fear that young children in day care are at risk for intellectual decline.* Furthermore, at least two major studies have demonstrated that substantial intellectual gains are possible in high-quality child care settings. These two studies are the Abecedarian Study (Ramey, Bryant, and Suarez, 1985; Campbell and Ramey, 1994), which was targeted at *socially* high-risk children, and the Infant Health and Development Program (1990), which was concerned with *biologically* high-risk infants.

In the Abecedarian study, which began in 1972 and has probably not officially ended even now, the children were recruited shortly after birth. The last major published assessment was when the subjects were 15 years old. After parental permission was obtained, the infants were randomly assigned either to an intensive intervention program (57 children) or to a control group (54 children). Beginning at 6 weeks, the intervention children participated in a full-day program that focused on language development, general cognitive enrichment, and adaptive social behavior. In addition, social services for the parents were provided. Controls had the social work services but not the day care. All subjects were from low-income African American, mainly one-parent families. Results of carefully controlled assessments of the children in the two groups revealed consistent intelligence quotient (IQ) difference in favor of the enriched children from 18 months onward. Originally about 19 points, by 5 years the difference was about 14 points. The discrepancy continued to attenuate, although it was still statistically significant at age 12 (6 IQ points). At age 15 there was still a 5-point difference, but it was not statistically significant. However, differences in favor of the experimental children remained in achievement test scores, in grade retention, and in numbers referred for special education. Clearly the high-quality early day care had a positive effect.

The Infant Health and Development Program (1990), surely one of the most carefully conducted studies in the entire domain of the behavioral and health sciences, dealt with the question of whether the behavioral deficits often reported in low–birth weight children could be avoided and ameliorated by high-quality infant intervention that included health surveillance, parent education, and day care. The subjects included 985 low–birth weight infants from eight research sites; 377 of these infants participated in the intervention and 608 infants served as control subjects. From birth to 1 year of age, a home visitor went weekly into the homes of the intervention infants, demonstrating simple teaching activities to be carried out with the children and helping the mothers deal with the problems the families might be having. When the infants were 1 year old, they entered a day care program with very favorable adult to child ratios (1:3), highly trained staff, careful curriculum supervision, health monitoring, and exemplary sanitation and nutrition practices. Biweekly home visits continued during this period.

Measures of intellectual development made when the children were 3 years of age showed significant advantages for the intervention group, with the difference being greater for the heavier (>2000 g) than for the lighter (<2000 g) low–birth weight babies. The heavier intervention children scored on the average 13.2 IQ points higher than did the control subjects, and the lighter intervention babies scored 6.6 points higher. Both differences were statistically significant. One cannot separate the effects of the day care from the parent contacts in this study, as both were part of the intervention package. However, this study adds support to the reassurance provided by the earlier wave of infant day care research: Infant day care is not the same as the dreaded institutional care of previous eras, and critics should not continue to imply that it is.

SOCIOEMOTIONAL DEVELOPMENT

Along with worries that early day care would stunt intellectual development were concerns that it would adversely affect socioemotional development, especially the security of children's attachment to their own mothers. Attachment theory has been a major influence on child development research for some 30 years. Following an early publication (Blehar, 1974) suggesting that children who had been in day care as infants were less likely to be securely attached to their mothers, a flurry of studies attempting either to substantiate or to refute those findings appeared in the literature. The Blehar study used the Ainsworth and Wittig (1969) Strange Situation Test, a laboratory procedure in which infants and toddlers are observed with their mothers and then separated from them, with ratings made of the disturbance during separation and reunion behavior. Although there were methodologic flaws in the Blehar study, including the use of 3- and 4-year-old children in a procedure standardized on infants, and although most of the replication attempts failed to substantiate these early findings, questions have persisted about whether there was an association between the use of early and extensive day care

and attachment security. The debate centering on this issue was refueled with the publication of a very provocative article by Belsky (1986), suggesting that unpublished studies and findings of close-to-significant differences suggested that there was indeed a risk of insecure attachment behavior and also a likelihood of more aggression with peers and less compliance to adults.

The Belsky article has been debated in the popular press, in the media, and in professional publications (Phillips et al, 1987). The debate has been beneficial in that it has highlighted the importance of the issue. If cognitive gains should occur at the expense of socioemotional functioning, there would be no real developmental advantage. This debate has also caused researchers to consider the wisdom of exclusive reliance on a procedure that may be inappropriate for children in the age range in which it has often been used and that might have an entirely different impact on a child accustomed to daily separations and reunions (as is true of children in child care) than it does on one for whom this is a rare experience. On the basis of the research that was available to fuel the debate at the time it raged, no definitive statement could be made. Contemporary data, however, (to be presented in a later section), offer highly relevant information and reassurance on this issue.

HEALTH

In the more than 3 decades of child care primarily dealt with in this chapter, there have been several cycles of reassurance and alarmism in regard to health maintenance in group programs. The ground-breaking work done in the early North Carolina project (Loda, Glezen, and Clyde, 1972) tended to be reassuring, showing that children under 5 years of age in group care had no more upper respiratory infections than a comparable group of control subjects (about 8 1/2 per year). For infants younger than 1 year, the incidence was slightly but not significantly higher in the day care children. Following this early work came analyses alerting caregivers and parents to the increased possibility of hemophilus-B influenza, hepatitis A, diarrhea associated with a variety of pathogens, and cytomegalovirus infection affecting both infants and caregivers (Osterholm, 1994). Several pediatricians, perhaps most notably Aronson and her colleagues (Aronson, 1994), have made special efforts to translate complex information about health maintenance into language that can be easily understood by caregivers in both group- and family-based programs (Aronson and Aiken, 1980). Such materials have had profound effects on preventive practices in licensed and monitored group programs. Whether they have reached and influenced family day care providers and others whose alternative care is unmonitored remains unknown.

The Infant Health and Development study cited previously (1990) offers the most impressive contemporary data on health maintenance in child care. The low–birth weight subjects in this study would have to be considered at high risk for morbidity, thus suggesting caution about bringing them together in groups. Findings from the study showed no major differences in health status between the day care and the control groups. The only measure on which health differences were found was a morbidity index based on maternal reports. On this instrument, the lighter (<2000 g) day care babies were reported to have had significantly more minor illnesses, although the numeric difference was very small and not really meaningful (7.9 compared with 7.0 in controls). There were no differences in minor health problems for the heavier (>2000 g) babies nor in serious health problems in either subgroup.

It should be noted here that results from this study should not be thought of as typical of what might be found in most alternative care settings, as the eight centers maintained exemplary sanitary procedures, and the health of the children was monitored constantly. Rather, these results should serve as a model of what is possible—even with a high-risk sample—when the care offered is of high quality and when maintaining health of the children is a major program objective.

Contemporary Research

It is difficult to appreciate the role of child care in pediatrics without understanding the modern history of the field. Similarly, it is important to realize that the research history, skimpy though it might have been until recently, has made its own contribution to the confusion existing in the public consciousness about child care effects.* Analyses and syntheses of research data have been characterized more by polemics and partisanship than by reason and objectivity. Nobody, including the researchers themselves, appears to be neutral on the subject. As a consequence, findings are sometimes discussed out of context; titles alarm more than inform; and potential consumers of the service remain confused and anxious. Furthermore, samples are generally small and sometimes haphazardly assembled, and evaluation methods are less than definitive. For example, the Strange Situation Test, on which most of the studies on day care and attachment depend, is probably not an appropriate measure for children older than 18 months of age, and yet it has often been used well beyond this point in day care research.

Most importantly, however, even the best of the more modern studies have looked at day care as though it were an isolated experience in the young child's life, not one that interacts with other simultaneous influences in the total developmental milieu. For example, children go into day care from "good families," from "mediocre families," and from "disastrous families" who are barely able to keep a child alive, much less facilitate development. Likewise, children go into day care that may be high quality, mediocre, or a totally unfit environment for children. Furthermore, the matching up of these environments to the children is probably not random—that is, the "good families" are more likely to obtain high-quality care for their children. Finally, children of different degrees of robustness and vulnerability spend time in these various environments. What is needed in child care research is an ecologic model that considers at least these three variables simultaneously:

the family environment, the day care environment, and the personal characteristics that the child brings to the situation.

THE NICHD STUDY OF EARLY
CHILD CARE

A large-scale research project funded by the National Institute of Child Health and Human Development (NICHD), based on this kind of ecologic model, is currently underway in 10 American cities (NICHD Early Child Care Research Network, 1994). Beginning in 1991, each site recruited 120 newborns and measured family, child, and child care variables when the children were 1, 6, 15, 24, 36, and 54 months of age, using a wide variety of tests and observations. Parental attitudes and feelings about their own lives and about potential value or detriment associated with maternal employment, and indications of depression or other emotional problems are assessed in the mothers; in addition, observations are made of their interactions with their children under both controlled and naturalistic conditions. Various temperament indicators, as well as performance on outcome measures (looking at both products and processes), are obtained on the children. Live observations are made in the child care settings regarding the nature of input the children receive from their caregivers, along with structural indicators of quality such as training of caregivers and adult-to-child ratios. Data collection will continue at least until the children reach first grade. Major objectives of the study include determining the relationship between infants' child care experiences (quantity and quality) and concurrent and long-term development; determining how the social ecology of the home and individual differences among children moderate the effects of child care; evaluating the consequences of maternal employment and child care choices on family relationships, parental mental health, and family stress; and examining demographic characteristics and parental characteristics associated with families' child care decisions.

In such a large-scale study, with its massive burdens of selecting and developing procedures, training data collectors, demonstrating cross-site comparability, and preventing lapses in reliability, data collection has to be given priority over data analysis. Accordingly, at this point in time, the project is far from having achieved all these objectives. However, within the past year, several major reports have emerged. An early report (NICHD-ECCRN, 1997a) indicated that by the time the infants were 6 months old, 38% of the mothers worked full-time and 25% worked part-time, thus mandating access to some type of nonmaternal care. During the first year of life, 80% of the children received some regular child care, with 3 months being the average age of entry. By 1 year, 58% of the infants were receiving more than 30 hours of care per week. Figure 21–2 shows the care arrangements of the 831 children in care at 1 year. Care by the fathers and in child care homes (what is usually called *family day care*) accounted for almost half of the placements. Use of child care centers was quite limited (about 14%). Less than 20% of the total sample spent the entire first year with only the mother as primary caregiver.

This description of characteristics of the child care

---

*Readers needing a more comprehensive review of the research literature dealing with one or another aspect of child care might wish to check the special supplement to the January, 1993 (Vol. 91, #1) issue of *Pediatrics,* entitled *Pediatrics and Child Care.*

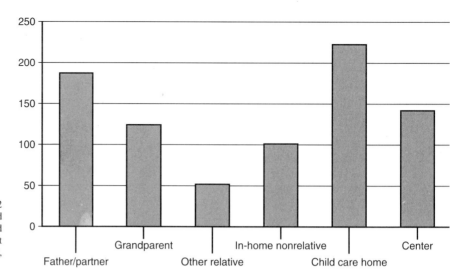

Figure 21–2. Primary type of care at 12 months. (Data from National Institute of Child Health and Human Development Early Child Care Research Network: Child care in the first year of life. Merrill Palmer Q 43:340–360, 1997a.)

patterns found during the first year of life in the NICHD study was amplified by an examination of structural characteristics associated with observed caregiver behavior. For this purpose, an observational procedure—the Observational Record of the Caregiving Environment (ORCE)—was developed and used in two 44-minute observation cycles in the care setting of each child. During the observations, specific behaviors designated as quality (e.g., talking, smiling, teaching, responding) were noted in 30-second intervals, and ratings of overall quality were made at the end of the sessions. At the 6-month assessment, 576 infants and their caregivers were observed in this meticulous way (representing close to 1000 hours, without considering travel and set-up time). Results revealed that caregivers were rated as providing more positive caregiving when group sizes and child-to-adult ratios were smaller and when caregivers held less authoritarian beliefs about childrearing. In general, these findings held in all types of care (fathers, grandparents, in-home sitters, child care homes, and centers).

In keeping with the ecologic model of the study, the investigators examined family characteristics associated with type and timing of child care (NICHD-ECCRN, 1997b). Family income is obviously a critical selection factor. Children placed in care between 3 and 5 months of age were likely to have highly educated and better-salaried mothers; nonmaternal family income also tended to be higher. In addition, children of mothers who were more extroverted and outgoing and who believed that maternal employment had benefits for children tended to be placed in care earlier. When in-home care (family home or family day care) was used, quality tended to be higher in the settings used by higher-income families. For center care, a curvilinear relationship was observed, with highest-quality care found in settings used by high- and low-income families and lower quality care found in those used by moderate-income families. These findings strengthen the realization that parental factors likely to influence child development will also influence child care choice patterns. Thus it is naive to ignore such variables when attempting to assess the effects of child care. Choices of age of enrollment, hours used per week, and type—variables gen-

erally considered as inputs or causative forces in child care research—are themselves outcomes associated with family variables.

The most recent publication from the NICHD study (NICHD-ECCRN, 1997c) deals with one of the most theoretically relevant outcomes and one which is of great practical concern: attachment security. As indicated earlier, the issue of whether early and extensive child care participation increased the likelihood that children would be less securely attached to their mothers has been heatedly debated for more than a decade. In the NICHD study, this was examined with 1153 mother-child pairs when the infants were 15 months old, using the Strange Situation procedure. All sessions were videotaped at the site and then coded from the tapes at one site by highly trained coders uninformed about child care histories, with repeated reliability checks. The generally accepted classification of Secure (B), Insecure/avoidant (A), Insecure/anxious (C), Disorganized/disoriented (D), or Unclassifiable (U) was used. Results lent no credibility to the charge of reduced likelihood of secure attachment associated with use of infant child care. There were no significant effects of child care experience (amount, age of entry, stability, type, or quality) on attachment security classification. However, when attachment classification was examined in relation to certain family variables (maternal sensitivity and responsiveness as observed in a play setting and on the HOME [Home Observation for Measurement of the Environment] Inventory), there were significant effects. Infants of mothers who were more sensitive and responsive were more likely to be classified as securely attached. In addition there was an interaction between insecure attachment and low maternal sensitivity combined with poor-quality child care, larger amounts of care, and unstable care. The overarching conclusion from the attachment analysis is that the nature of the interaction between the mother and the child is a far more powerful influence on attachment security than is child care.

Several other child outcomes are currently being examined in the NICHD study. A recent one of great interest to pediatricians deals with cognitive and language functioning (NICHD-ECCRN, 1997d). Many parents feel secure in their emotional relationships with their children and thus experience little anxiety about attachment. However, they may well seek reassurance from their pediatricians that their children will either benefit or not suffer intellectually as a result of their child care experience. Again, the NICHD study offers such reassurance. At 24 months the Bayley Scales of Infant Development and the MacArthur Communicative Development Inventory were administered, and at 36 months the measures were the Bracken Scale of Basic Concepts and the Reynell Developmental Language Scale. The analysis revealed no relation between number of hours in care and any of the cognitive or language measures; thus child care, per se, was not a significant influence. However, when quality was added, clear and meaningful associations appeared. Child care of higher quality was consistently associated with better cognitive and language outcomes. This finding was primarily accounted for by the frequency of language stimulation (as measured in the ORCE). The relationship held for children in different types of care, from families of different income and stimulation levels, from different ethnic groups, and of both genders.

As so much space has been devoted to the NICHD study (and as I am one of the participating investigators), perhaps a brief comment on the advantages and disadvantages of this type of mega-research—undoubtedly the wave of the future in many disciplines and topical areas—would be in order. Clearly the ecologic design is needed to help unravel some of the simultaneously operating influences on the development of children that come from parental and nonparental sources. The NICHD study is able to handle that. On the other hand, ecologic models yield associations and relationships, not the clear cause-effect channels delineated by experimental models with random assignment (as the Infant Health and Development Program had). Furthermore, although such a gloriously large sample size increases confidence in results, it also leads to statistically significant differences and correlations that, in terms of the range and robustness of the measures, may be of only trivial magnitude. Even so, such studies offer the best hope of arriving at reasonably definitive answers to the legitimate questions that linger in the minds of parents and professionals about the effects of child care on our children.

Policy Issues

Although day care has come a long way in terms of professional and public acceptance, it still has a long way to go. At least three key policy issues for the immediate future can be identified: the economic base, the conceptual base, and the question of quality.

THE ECONOMIC BASE

Day care of high quality is expensive. It is people-intensive, and people who are trained enough to know what they are doing do not and should not come cheaply. In 1993, the average weekly cost was $74 per week, with care for infants being about $10 higher (US Census Bureau, 1996). Some of the more prestigious programs charge about $200 per week. And, of course, in families that hire resident nannies, the cost is about twice that amount. Poor families spend about 18% of their income on care, whereas nonpoor families spend only about 7%. As is often the case, financial problems associated with purchasing day care are greater for low- and middle-income families; the poor and the wealthy have less of a problem.

The passage in late 1990 of the Child Care and Development Block Grant bill has helped low-income families somewhat. This bill provides tax credits for low-income working families and directs block grant money to the states on a population and income status basis that can be used both to increase availability and to improve quality. Although the final version of this bill did not contain everything its advocates had worked for, its passage represents significant progress.

In recent years, corporations have come to recognize the importance of quality day care as a service to employees and have begun to offer financial support through activities such as information and referral services, the provision of on-site care, or voucher payments for care selected by the workers. To have child care come to be considered an economic issue and be recognized as part of the infrastructure necessary for business and commerce represents a major step forward.

THE CONCEPTUAL BASE

I have been stressing for 2 decades the need to reconceptualize day care and, in the process, to rename it with a more appropriate label: *educare*. Both the terms *day care* and *child care* communicate nothing about what the service provides and are only one step up from the even more pejorative term *baby-sitting*. Some professionals have struggled to make a distinction between *early childhood education* and *day care* or *child care,* stressing that they are two different services with different goals and procedures. Such an assertion implies a false dichotomy, however, when in reality these terms merely represent endpoints of a single continuum. One cannot educate young children without also caring for them, and one cannot provide appropriate care and protection without including education in the process.

Regardless of whether the field is given or accepts the neologism *educare* as its label, it needs to endorse the concept of a comprehensive, integrated service offered in an environment that supplements, but does not substitute for, the family environment. Anything less is neither accurate nor honest.

THE ISSUE OF QUALITY

Day care varies in quality, just as health services, social services, legal services, and family life vary in quality. It is no more homogeneous than the children and families it serves. Yet the quality of the environments investigated in most child care research has rarely been examined or reported. State licensing standards vary widely, and resistance to any sort of national or federal standards has been impassioned and unwavering. The development of better ways to assess and then to ensure quality remains a major issue.

Two important developments in this area have occurred in recent years. One is the establishment of an accreditation system by the National Association for the Education of Young Children (NAEYC), which follows procedures not unlike those that hospitals wishing to be accredited must go through. This procedure has been in place since 1985, and more than 5000 centers have now been accredited. Once this procedure is more widely accepted, it will become an assurance indicator that parents can look for before enrolling their children. Instead of beginning their search for educare by asking whether a facility is licensed by the state—which ensures that a basement of quality will be present—they will begin to inquire about whether it is accredited. When a certain critical mass of accredited centers is present in every community, those that do not meet accreditation criteria will have to upgrade quality in order to survive.

The other new development that will improve quality is the preparation of a new set of standards by the American Public Health Association and the American Academy of Pediatrics (APHA-AAP, 1992). These standards were given to the licensing agencies throughout the country in 1991, and most states have made genuine efforts since that time to improve caregiver training to the point that they will follow the guidelines. Offering a strong emphasis on health and illness-prevention, they have become benchmarks against which all states can now examine their own programs as a means of upgrading quality in the area of health maintenance. Wide-scale adoption of these APHA-AAP standards for health and the NAEYC standards for programs will help usher in a new era for child care in which no one should have to apologize for poor quality.

Conclusion

Within the past decade, child care has come into its own as one of the major environmental influences on the lives of young children. Every practicing pediatrician needs to be familiar with some of the basic research on the effects of child care, as parents will ask, early and often, "When is it safe to enroll my baby?" "Will she get sick more often?" "Will he still love me?" Within the past decade, appropriately designed research has appeared that provides up-to-date answers to these questions. As current knowledge is always at best penultimate, waiting to be amended by new knowledge acquired via better methods, the practicing pediatrician must always stay tuned to ever more current findings pertaining to this extremely important developmental milieu.

REFERENCES

Ainsworth MDS, Wittig BA: Attachment and exploratory behavior of one-year-olds in a strange situation. *In* Foss BM (ed): Determinants of Infant Behavior, Vol 4. London, Methuen, 1969.

American Public Health Association and the American Academy of Pediatrics: Caring for our children: national health and safety performance standards: guidelines for out-of-home child care programs. Washington, DC, American Public Health Association, 1992.

Aronson SS: The science behind the American Public Health Association/ American Academy of Pediatrics National Health and Safety Guidelines for child-care programs. Pediatrics 94(6):1101–1104, 1994.

Aronson SS, Aiken L: Compliance of child care programs with health and safety standards: impact of program evaluation and advocate training. Pediatrics 65:318–325, 1980.

Belsky J: Infant day care: a cause for concern? Zero to Three 6:1–6, 1986.

Blehar MC: Anxious attachment and defensive reactions associated with day care. Child Dev 45:683–692, 1974.

Bloom BS: Stability and Change in Human Characteristics. New York, John Wiley, 1964.

Bowlby J: Maternal Care and Mental Health. Geneva, Switzerland, World Health Organization, 1952.

Braun SJ, Caldwell BM: Emotional adjustment of children in day care who enrolled prior to or after the age of three. Early Child Dev Care 2:13–21, 1972.

Cahill ED: Past Caring. New York, Columbia University, National Center for Children in Poverty, 1989.

Caldwell BM, Richmond JB: The Children's Center in Syracuse, New York. *In* Dittman L (ed): Early Child Care: The New Perspectives. New York, Atherton Press, 1968, pp 326–358.

Caldwell BM, Richmond JB: Programmed day care for the very young child: a preliminary report. J Marriage Family 26:481–488, 1964.

Caldwell BM, Wright CM, Honig AS, Tannenbaum J: Infant day care and attachment. Am J Orthopsychiatry 60:690–697, 1970.

Campbell FA, Ramey CT: Effects of early intervention on intellectual and academic achievement: a follow-up study of children from low-income families. Child Dev 65:684–698, 1994.

Hunt J McV: Intelligence and Experience. New York, Ronald Press, 1961.

Infant Health and Development Program: enhancing the outcomes of low-birth-weight premature infants. JAMA 263:3035–3042, 1990.

Loda FA, Glezen WP, Clyde WA Jr: Respiratory disease in group day care. Pediatrics 49:428–437, 1972.

National Institute of Child Health and Human Development Early Child Care Research Network: Child care in the first year of life. Merrill Palmer Q 43:340–360, 1997a.

National Institute of Child Health and Human Development Early Child Care Research Network: Factors affecting parental selection of infant child care. J Marriage Family 59:389–409, 1997b.

National Institute of Child Health and Human Development Early Child Care Research Network: The effects of infant child care on infant-mother attachment security: results of the NICHD Study of Early Child Care. Child Dev 68:860–879, 1997c.

National Institute of Child Health and Human Development Early Child Care Research Network: Mother-child interaction and cognitive outcomes associated with early child care. Poster symposium presented at the Biennial Meeting of the Society for Research in Child Development, April, 1997d.

National Institute of Child Health and Human Development Early Child Care Research Network: Child care and child development: the NICHD Study of Early Child Care. *In* Friedman SL, Haywood HC (eds): Developmental Follow-Up. New York, Academic Press, 1994.

Osterholm MT: Infectious disease in child day care: an overview. Pediatrics 84(6):987–990, 1994.

Phillips D, McCartney K, Scarr S, et al: Selective review of infant day care research: a cause for concern! Zero to Three 7:18, 1997.

Piaget J: The Origins of Intelligence in Children. New York, International Universities Press, 1952.

Ramey CT, Bryant DM, Suarez TM: Preschool compensatory education and the modifiability of intelligence: a critical review. *In* Detterman EK (ed): Current Topics in Human Intelligence, Vol 1, Research Methodology. Norwood, NJ, Ablex, 1985.

Robinson HB, Robinson NM: Longitudinal development of very young children in a comprehensive day care program: the first two years. Child Dev 42:1673–1683, 1971.

Spitz R: Hospitalism: an inquiry into the genesis of psychiatric conditions in early childhood. Psychoanalytic Studies of the Child 1:53–74, 1945.

Spitz R: Hospitalism: a follow-up report. Psychoanalytic Studies of the Child 2:113–117, 1946.

Tank RM: Young children, families, and society in America since the 1820s: the evolution of health, education, and child care programs for preschool children. Unpublished doctoral dissertation, University of Michigan, Ann Arbor, 1980.

US Bureau of the Census: How we're changing: demographic state of the nation, 1996.

PART III
Biological Influences

22 Genes, Behavior, and Development

Robert M. Greenstein • Elisabeth M. Dykens

Although individual genetic maladies are relatively infrequent, collectively they constitute over 15,500 recognized disorders and affect 13 million Americans.

If the pedigree analysis is not compatible with a single gene pattern, yet it still reveals familial transmission, then multifactorial inheritance is strongly suggested.

Indeed, over 750 known genetic causes of mental retardation have now been identified. A number of these syndromes have characteristic cognitive or behavioral profiles and trajectories, often referred to as *behavioral phenotypes*.

Within-syndrome variability refers to the fact that not all people with a given syndrome show that syndrome's characteristic behavior to the same degree, or at the same point in development.

Webster's New Collegiate Dictionary defines *behavior* as "anything that an organism does involving action and response to stimulation." The definition implies that human behaviors are the result of interactive processes between the individual and the environment. In this chapter we are interested in the biology of the individual, specifically the manner by which genes contribute to normal and abnormal behavior. We also cannot ignore the fact that a person's behavior, especially abnormal behavior, will affect the behaviors of those around him or her, making it difficult at times to separate genetic or biological factors from environmental influences. And these environmental factors will in turn modify or shape the behavior of the affected person, perhaps to an even greater extent than his or her own genetic factors. This interaction asks the age-old question of nature versus nurture. Our purpose in this chapter is to remain more focused on the *nature*, or biological issues.

Behavior and the Development of Modern Genetics

In the past 30 years, there has been a virtual explosion of new knowledge about molecular structure, the function of genes and their location on specific chromosomes, and the impact of heredity on the incidence and prevalence of human disease. Although individual genetic maladies are relatively infrequent, collectively they consitute over 15,500 recognized disorders and affect 13 million Americans (McKusick, 1994; Borgaonkar, 1994). The Human Genome Project is well on its way to identifying the chromosomal location of all of the 50,000 or more human genes, and this effort acts as a wellspring for identifying

the role and function of both normal and mutated genes. The influence of molecular biology and molecular genetics on development and behavior now permits us to link patterns of heredity within families and populations with specific alterations in gene function. Genetic linkage studies on mental health disorders, such as schizophrenia and manic-depressive disorder (Hall, 1996), or the identification of probable syndrome-specific behaviors in Prader-Willi, Williams, and Smith-Magenis microdeletion syndromes (Dykens and Kasari, 1997; Pober and Dykens, 1996), suggest that genetic mechanisms contribute significantly to the etiology of behavior. Thus the biological explanation of certain behaviors becomes more understandable when the genetic and metabolic contributions affecting them are more precisely illustrated and illuminated.

In an effort to link genes, behavior, and heredity in this chapter, we first present a classification of biological factors and a series of model systems that enable us to further analyze the effect of disturbances of these factors on behavior. We then review the principles of genetic inheritance and the associated risks for transmission of mutant genes in parents to offspring. The reader is encouraged to seek more detailed information from standard medical genetics texts. The second section of this chapter deals briefly with the interaction of these biological and genetic factors with environmental influences that subsequently lead to the development of distinct patterns of behavior in children. This section addresses the question posed by Plomin (Plomin and Daniels, 1987): "Why are children in the same family so different from one another?" The emerging discipline of behavioral genetics is beginning to offer answers to this question. The third section of this chapter deals with the contribution of genetics and heredity to abnormal behaviors, including "syndrome-specific behaviors" and unusual behavioral phenotypes related to specific genetic or molecular abnormalities. This information implies that there are discrete genetic mechanisms that may explain unique or abnormal behaviors, such as mental retardation syndromes, psychopathology, or even dyslexia. This information has important implications for recurrence risk counseling and reproductive planning for families. The third section of the chapter also deals briefly with issues of treatment and interventions, including genetic counseling and emotional support for parents whose children are found to have disabilities related to genetic disorders.

Classification of Biological Factors

Multiple factors must be considered in the biological causation of, or contribution to, behavioral disorders. These are divided into genetic and nongenetic categories (Table 22–1). There is considerable overlap among the categories, as well as between categories of biological and environmental factors. For the most part, the essential target for the impact of these biological factors is the central nervous system and its development, organization, integrity, and function (Volpe, 1995). Although it is true that many of these factors affect the individual systemically, it is the effect on the brain that focuses our attention on the resultant behaviors of the individual. The genetic factors are discussed subsequently. They reflect the manner in which genetic and molecular processes contribute to both normal and abnormal development. The nongenetic factors are divided into prenatal and postnatal time frames and reflect to a greater extent the various causes of central nervous system abnormality or dysfunction. Subsequent chapters in this volume explore their individual effects in greater detail.

MODEL SYSTEMS TO EXAMINE BIOLOGICAL EFFECTS

In an effort to further explore the effects of biological factors on behavior, it is useful to examine models developed for the purpose of evaluating the dynamics of multiple, interrelated biological effects. No one model explains all the variation of abnormal behaviors seen in clinical settings, but each one helps us to better understand the complex nature of the interaction between genetic and nongenetic factors.

Critical Periods of Embryologic Development Model

The convergence of developmental biology, molecular genetics, and anatomic pathology helps us understand the complex and rapidly changing phases of embryologic development. These are timed, serial processes that are intimately integrated and usually successfully accomplished. The organ systems develop at different critical time periods. When these processes are disrupted, the result will be different patterns of physical features and clinical phenotypes, depending on the timing and duration of their disturbance during embryologic development (Fig. 22–1).

In maternal insulin-dependent diabetes mellitus, for example, if the control of the disorder is poor at conception and during the first trimester, with elevated fasting morning glucose levels over 120 mg/dL and HgbA1C levels greater than 10, then the risk for birth defects will be high (Reece and Hobbins, 1986). This condition is referred to as the *diabetic embryopathy* syndrome and presents with a recognizable pattern of malformations and an increased risk of mental disability. On the other hand, a discrete exposure to thalidomide at days 37 to 39 will produce a highly characteristic pattern of limb reduction malformations, but sparing of the central nervous system (McBride, 1961). These clinical patterns suggest when disturbances may have occurred during critical periods of embryologic development. Identifying the timing of these malformations may also identify their specific cause.

Fetal-Maternal-Placental Model

In studying the multiple factors that contribute to the cause of small for dates infants, Andrews and coauthors (1970) developed a fetal-maternal-placental model to address the contributions of each of these components individually as well as interactively (Fig. 22–2).

The Andrews model examines the contributions that each domain makes to the etiology of intrauterine growth disturbance and serves as a dynamic model for their possible interaction. It addresses primary growth delay in Down syndrome as a fetal abnormality, maternal infection with rubella as a secondary cause of fetal growth delay and malformation, and placental insufficiency as a cause of third trimester intrauterine growth retardation. All of these conditions may result in cognitive disturbance of prenatal origin and subsequent behavioral abnormality.

Cellular Growth and Nutrition Model

Growth of any organ may be caused by an increase in the number of cells (hyperplasia), by an increase in the size of the existing cells (hypertrophy), or by both processes occurring simultaneously. Winick, Brasel, and Rosso (1972) developed a useful construct that reflects the critical

Table 22–1 • Biological Factors in Behavior

Genetic factors
    Single gene (mendelian)
    Polygenic/multifactorial
    Chromosomal
    Mitochondrial
    Nontraditional
Nongenetic factors
    Prenatal
        Anatomic/deformations
        Nutritional
        Maternal disorders
        Infection
        Hypoxic/vascular
        Toxins/teratogens
    Postnatal
        Accidents/trauma
        Vascular
        Infection
        Toxins
        Nutrition

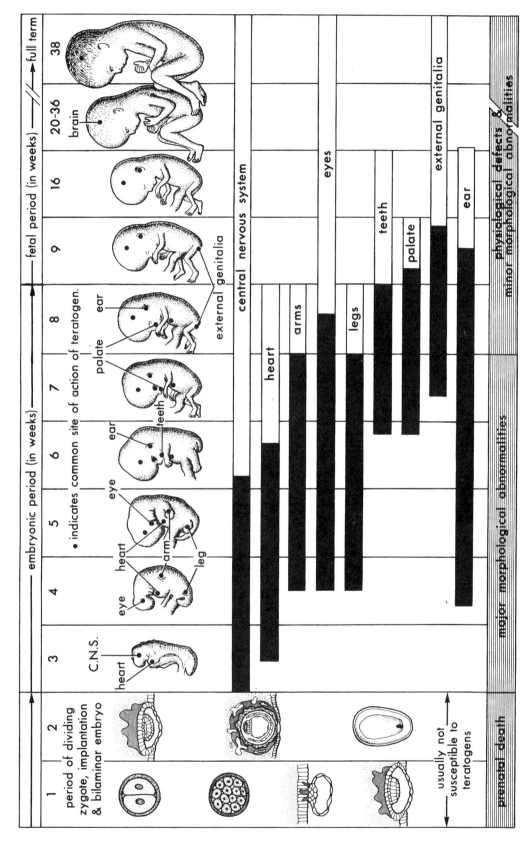

Figure 22–1. Model for critical periods of embryologic development. (From Moore KL: Causes of congenital malformations. *In* The Developing Human, 6th ed. Philadelphia, WB Saunders, 1998.)

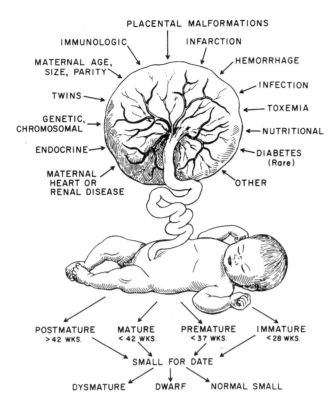

Figure 22–2. The "small for dates" baby. (From Andrews BF: Pediatr Clin North Am 17:185–198, 1970.)

stages of growth of the fetus and neonate in relation to abnormalities in nutrition. Early growth of the embryo and fetus occurs mainly by rapid mitotic increase in cell number. By mid-trimester, growth proceeds by increases both in cell size and in cell number at the tissue and organ levels, and continues on thereafter into postnatal life (Fig. 22–3).

Disruptions that interfere with the hyperplastic or cell number phase of growth may result in irreversible effects. For example, primary microcephaly may be of genetic or environmental (vascular, nutrition, viral) etiology and consequently may reflect an irreversible reduction in the number of neuroblasts produced during their critical period of fetal growth, at approximately 8 to 20 weeks of gestation. On the other hand, disturbances in nutrition via placental dysfunction or by postnatal malnutrition may result in the reduction in cell size (hypertrophy). Under these circumstances, the problem may be reversible if nutrition is re-established in a timely fashion. An example of this process is intrauterine growth retardation in the third trimester following normal growth in the first two trimesters. The resulting small for dates infant will resume normal growth when provided adequate nutrition, but should the child continue to experience postnatal malnutrition, the prenatal effects will be intensified, particularly affecting brain growth and cognitive development.

Development of the Central Nervous System

Volpe (1995) comprehensively described the intricate details and interrelated organization of the developing central nervous system. These phases include neuronal proliferation, migration, organization, and myelination. These events span a time frame beginning at about 2 months of gestation and continuing into adult life. Abnormalities in the various steps and processes that would otherwise lead to a fully integrated and normally functioning central nervous system are reviewed in Table 22–2. For example, *microcephaly*, defined as a head circumference measurement more than 2 standard deviations below the mean for postnatal age, may be viewed as a disorder with multiple etiologies, depending on the timing of the insult and whether it is acquired or genetic. The specific neuropathology of microcephaly will reflect disturbances during a particular phase or phases of central nervous system development. Autosomal recessive microcephaly *(microcephaly vera)* reveals a marked decrease in the number of neurons in cortical neuronal layers II and III without evidence for a destructive process or migrational defect. On the other hand, in type I lissencephaly, as seen in Miller-Dieker syndrome, there is a "smooth brain" with very few or no gyri that resulted from a defect in neuronal migration. This finding is associated with a submicroscopic deletion at

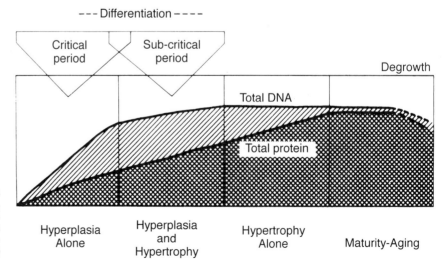

Figure 22–3. Cellular growth and nutrition model. (Adapted from Winick M, Brasel JA, Rosso P: Nutrition and cell growth. *In* Winick M [ed]: Nutrition and Development. New York, John Wiley & Sons, 1972. Copyright © 1972. Reprinted by permission of John Wiley & Sons, Inc.)

Table 22–2 • Developmental Disorders of the Central Nervous System

Normal Processes	Developmental Disorders
Neuronal proliferation, peak 3–4 months; ventricular zone proliferation from stem cells symmetrically, then asymmetrically	Neuronal proliferation 1. Microcephaly (familial, teratogenic) 2. Macrocephaly (neurocutaneous syndromes, chromosomal disorders, familial)
Neuronal migration, peak 3–5 months; radial migration of cerebral and cerebellar cells; neurons migrate along radial guides	Neuronal migration 1. Schizencephaly 2. Lissencephaly 3. Agenesis of the corpus callosum 4. Polymicrogyria 5. Heterotopias
Organization, peak 5 months to postnatal; differentiation of neurons, lamination, neurite outgrowth, glial proliferation	Organization 1. Primary disturbance (mental retardation, Down syndrome) 2. Associated disturbance (rubella, phenylketonuria) 3. Potential disturbance (ventilator-dependent premature infant)
Myelination, peak birth to postnatal; oligodendroglial proliferation, differentiation, alignment to myelin sheath	Myelination 1. Primary disturbance (cerebral hypoplasia, aminoacidopathies, postnatal malnutrition) 2. Associated disturbance (rubella, Down syndrome) 3. Potential disturbance (perinatal insult)

Data from Volpe JJ: Neuronal proliferation, migration, organization, and myelination. *In* Neurology of the Newborn, 3rd ed. Philadelphia, WB Saunders, 1995.

17p13.3 in about 90% of affected infants. Thus, two infants with the same microcephalic head measurement postnatally may have completely different etiologies. Understanding neuropathologic features therefore assists in relating behavioral phenotypes to disturbances in developmental differentiation of anatomic regions.

Classification of Genetic Disorders

In the discipline of medical genetics, categories of heritable traits are generally classified as diseases, inborn errors of metabolism, or congenital abnormalities, usually on the basis of a mutation or chromosome abnormality (Table 22–3). This classification system is functionally useful because it is inclusive of most conditions and also reflects clinical applications. The single gene disorders are usually mutations inherited in autosomal dominant or recessive patterns or sex-linked dominant or recessive patterns, the recurrence of which reflects specific statistical probabilities. *Polygenic*, or multifactorial, inheritance includes additive or quantitative traits, such as behavior, cognition, and intelligence, and represents complex characteristics along a measurable continuum that does not conform to mendelian probabilities. *Dysmorphic* syndromes are included because there are a number of well-recognized syndromes—some with submicroscopic deletions but others without as yet a specific genetic mechanism—that also exhibit possible syndrome-specific behaviors. The *nontraditional* category is included because of the increasing identification of these mechanisms in the cause of birth defects and associated behavioral disorders. Finally, the *teratogens and toxins* category is included because a number of disorders, such as fetal alcohol syndrome, fetal dilantin syndrome, and other exposures, must be distinguished from genetic causes when evaluating a patient's clinical presentation for a medical genetic disorder.

PRINCIPLES OF GENETIC INHERITANCE

Family History and Pedigree

To begin an analysis for possible genetic, familial, or hereditary factors in the cause of a particular disorder or disease, it is first necessary to collect the relevant information in the graphic format of a genetic or family pedigree. This involves at least a three-generation history of all living and deceased individuals from both the maternal and paternal sides, including miscarriages, stillbirths, causes of death, birth and death dates, and notation of possible consanguinity (inbreeding, cousin mating). Figure 22–4 shows the common symbols used in pedigree drawing. Figure 22–5 demonstrates a model three-generation pedigree for Marfan syndrome, an autosomal dominant disorder of connective tissue with full penetrance and variable expressivity. Marfan syndrome demonstrates multiple organ

Table 22–3 • Classification of Genetic Disorders

Category	Description
Single gene	Follow mendelian inheritance patterns, 1 in 2000 to 1 in 200,000 incidence
Polygenic	Multifactorial, quantitative traits, complex inheritance, 1–5 in 1000 incidence
Chromosomal	Abnormalities of number or structure; 1 in 200 live births
Dysmorphic syndromes	Recognizable phenotypic patterns but genetic cause not always certain
Mitochondrial	Maternally transmitted, usually energy metabolism (oxidative phosphorylation) disorders
Nontraditional	Includes triplet repeat expansions, imprinting, and uniparental disomy
Teratogens/toxins	Included because these effects must be distinguished from genetic causes

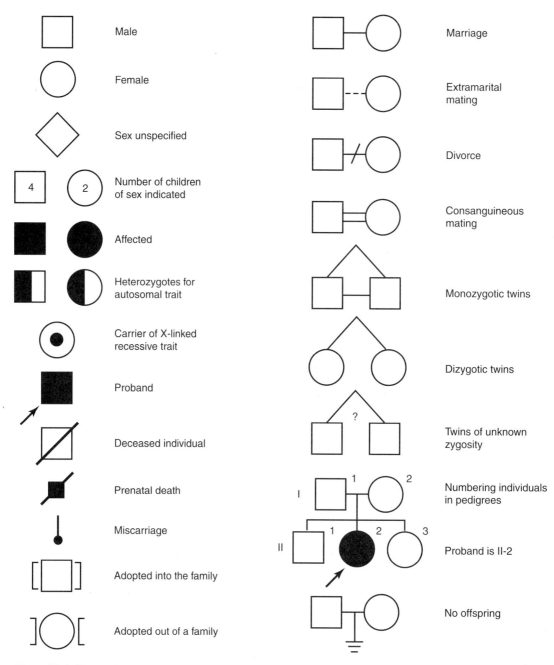

Figure 22–4. Commonly used pedigree symbols.

effects, principally the skeletal, visual, and cardiovascular systems.

Obtaining the family history by a graphic pedigree provides the opportunity to get to know the family and help reduce the natural tension and anxiety involved in attempting to diagnose a child with a disability or addressing the issue of reproductive risk. Analysis of the pedigree also reveals what additional information may be needed from other family members, such as medical records, autopsy reports, laboratory results, and family photographs. Finally, the graphic pedigree provides the opportunity to identify a possible pattern of inheritance for a particular disorder, as shown in Figure 22–5.

Patterns of Inheritance

There are 46 chromosomes in the nucleus, or 23 pairs, 22 of which are homologous or identical plus one pair of sex chromosomes, either XX female or XY male. Each parent contributes a *haploid* set of 23 chromosomes. At conception, there are 23 pairs, or 46 chromosomes, established, which is the *diploid* number. A gene located on one chromosome of a pair will have an identical location, or *locus*, on its homologous pair. Therefore genes for any product, such as a protein or clinical trait, are paired; pairs of genes at the same locus are referred to as *alleles*. The distribution of alleles into gametes (sperm and eggs) is the basis for single gene inheritance, and mutations of these alleles is

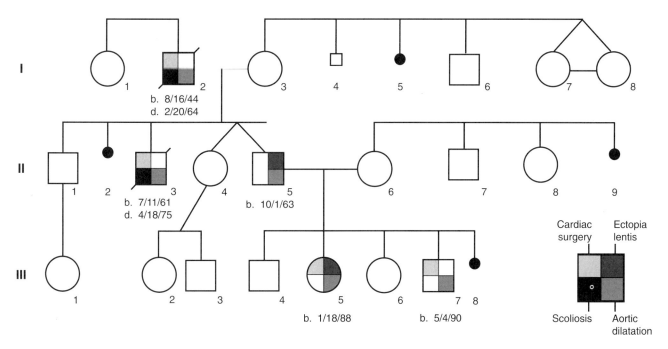

Figure 22–5. Family pedigree: Marfan syndrome.

the basis for the expression of disease in individuals or populations. The two alleles at each locus separate during gametogenesis and segregate into different gametes (Mendel's first law). Alleles along a single chromosome assort independently of each other during meiosis unless they are tightly linked to each other (Mendel's second law).

When a mutation occurs in one allele of a pair and is responsible for the appearance of a clinical disorder in that individual, the effect is termed *dominant*. When a disorder occurs on the basis of a deleterious or disease mutation of both alleles of the pair, essentially resulting in the absence of the normal gene, the effect is termed *recessive*. The clinician needs to understand these patterns of the distribution of single genes from parent to offspring, especially when mutations that result in a disease or clinical disorder have occurred. Understanding the *genotype* (allele or gene function) will help to elucidate the *phenotype* (clinical appearance).

Autosomal Dominant Inheritance

An *autosomal* (non-sex chromosome) dominant disorder occurs when only one allele of the pair is mutated and the mutation is expressed as a disorder. This may occur as a new mutation for that conception when neither parent carries the mutant gene. More commonly, the mutation is inherited from an affected parent, who has one chance in two, or 50%, of passing the mutation on for each conception. It may affect males or females equally, and in pedigree analysis it usually occurs in each generation without skipping a generation. Figure 22–6 depicts the recurrence risks for offspring when a parent expresses an autosomal dominant mutation. Whether an individual at risk for inheriting the mutation exhibits it depends on the *penetrance* of the gene, that is, the expression of the disorder when the mutation is present. Some disorders, such as neurofibro-

matosis and Marfan syndrome, are usually fully penetrant, but other disorders may exhibit *incomplete penetrance*, that is, when a person carries the gene but does not phenotypically express the disorder. These individuals may then pass this "silent" mutation on to their offspring, who may then express it as the disorder; the pattern essentially skips a generation. The reasons for this are not well understood but may involve genetic loci from other chromosomes, so-called *epigenetic factors*, gonadal mosaicism, or perhaps prenatal and postnatal environmental effects. Figure 22–7 demonstrates a model pedigree for autosomal dominant inheritance.

Dominant inheritance may also demonstrate *variable expressivity* among affected family members, usually more evident within the same generation. Thus, each of three siblings in the same family, all of whom inherit the same mutation, may exhibit the disorder but to varying and even subtle degrees. All the same, a subtly affected person could pass the mutation on to an offspring who will be severely affected. Other reasons for variable expression are early versus later age of onset and *imprinting effects*; that is, specific maternal versus paternal DNA methylation patterns of the mutation-bearing chromosome influence the expression of the disorder in a differential manner.

Autosomal Recessive Inheritance

When both alleles (genes) at the same locus of a pair of homologous autosomal chromosomes are mutated, the resulting disorder is considered recessive, that is, occurring in the absence of the modifying effect of the normal gene at that locus. A mutant gene at that locus was inherited from both parents, who are referred to as *obligate heterozygotes* or unaffected carriers for the disorder. Examples of autosomal recessive inheritance include many metabolic and biochemical disorders, such as cystic fibrosis, Tay-

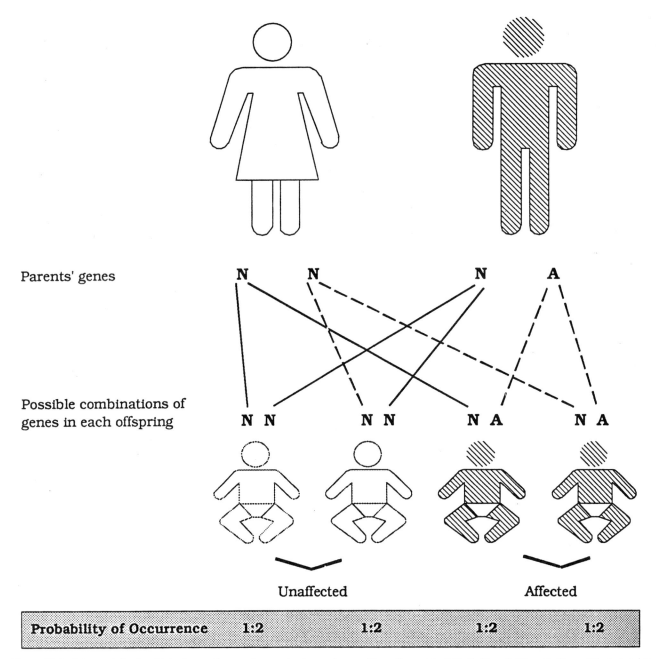

Parents' genes

Possible combinations of
genes in each offspring

Unaffected   Affected

Probability of Occurrence   1:2   1:2   1:2   1:2

Figure 22–6. Autosomal dominant inheritance. N, normal gene; A, abnormal gene. (From Greenstein RM, Haddow P, Kloza E, Young DL: Improving Access to Medical Genetics Services: An Education Manual on the Reimbursement Process. Monograph published by Department of Pediatrics, University of Connecticut Health Center, MCH #MCJ-009107010, June 1989.)

Sachs disease, sickle cell anemia, and thalassemia. It is possible that a number of mutations with a wide range of differential effects may exist at a single locus and result in variable phenotypic effects. This is referred to as *allelic heterogeneity* and explains why it is possible to have variable expressivity for the same autosomal recessive disorder among many families. These autosomal recessive mutations are distributed among individuals in the general population with different frequencies, depending on geography, mating patterns, and the effect of the mutation on fertility. Deleterious recessive genes may be carried in families for generations without detection because of the low back-

ground frequency of the heterozygote and the cultural pattern of discouraging cousin marriages (consanguinity). It is estimated that all individuals carry approximately five to eight deleterious recessive genes. Cousin marriages, however, increase the likelihood that rare recessive mutations may appear as a disease *(homozygous for the mutation)* for the first time in unsuspecting families.

The pattern for autosomal recessive inheritance is illustrated in Figure 22–8. Males and females may be carriers, noncarriers, or affected. Obligate heterozygote parents, frequently identified only after the birth of an affected child, have a one in two, or 50%, chance of having

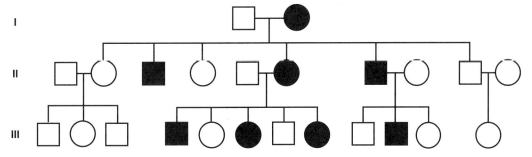

Figure 22–7. Model pedigree for an autosomal dominant disorder. The dark circles and squares represent affected individuals. The pattern depicts both affected males and females, does not skip a generation, and exhibits male-to-male transmission.

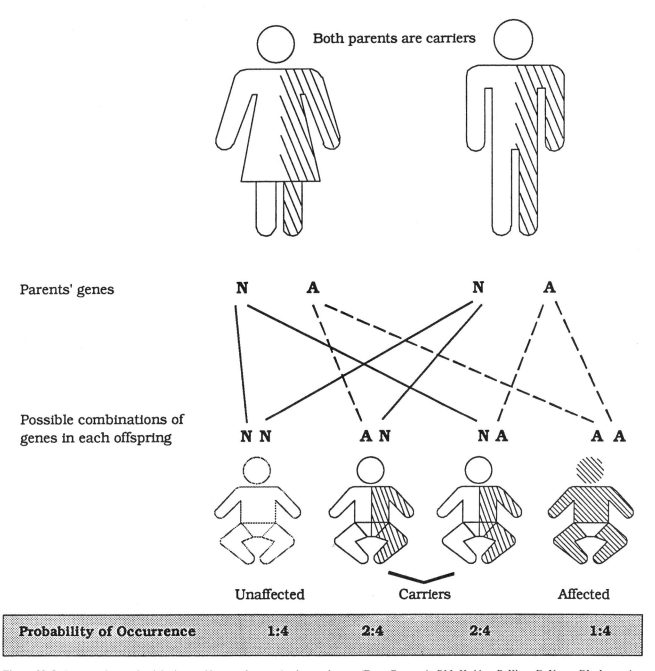

Figure 22–8. Autosomal recessive inheritance. N, normal gene; A, abnormal gene. (From Greenstein RM, Haddow P, Kloza E, Young DL: Improving Access to Medical Genetics Services: An Education Manual on the Reimbursement Process. Monograph published by Department of Pediatrics, University of Connecticut Health Center, MCH #MCJ-009107010, June 1989.)

a heterozygote offspring with each conception, a one in four, or 25%, chance of having a homozygote normal offspring, and a one in four, or 25%, chance of having an affected offspring. It is possible to screen for the presence of some recessive mutations, especially if they are found in the general population with a carrier frequency of 1 in 20 to 1 in 40, such as cystic fibrosis, Tay-Sachs disease, and sickle cell trait. The purpose of such population or community screening programs is to alert couples to their potential risk for having a child affected with a recessive disorder and to initiate treatment early enough to prevent a permanent disability. Figure 22–9 depicts a typical model pedigree for an autosomal recessive disorder. Note that the affected child appears only after several generations of carrier "out-marriages" have occurred; that is, the disorder is unknown to the family.

When trying to identify whether a particular pattern of congenital malformation, mental retardation, or an abnormal behavioral complex is caused by a single gene mutation, such as an autosomal recessive mutation, however, the uncertainty of the counseling becomes all the more challenging if we are dealing with rare occurrences or small families who cannot "demonstrate" the typical pattern. Under these circumstances, the risk of recurrence may be as high as 25%, but could also be much lower.

Sex-Linked Recessive Inheritance

An X-linked disorder occurs when the mutant gene is located on the X chromosome. Females have two X chromosomes; males have one and are therefore referred to as *hemizygous*. X-linked disorders are usually recessive because the disorder is generally expressed in the *absence* of the normal gene. Males will be affected but females will be heterozygotes, or carriers. It is possible, however, that carrier females may also express an X-linked disorder, perhaps to a lesser degree. This is because of the *X-inactivation* phenomenon. In each cell, one of the two X chromosomes is randomly inactivated, leaving only one active, or expressing, X chromosome. Thus, females are naturally occurring *mosaics* or mixtures of their maternal and paternal originated X chromosomes. If, however, one

of the X chromosomes carries a mutant gene, such as Duchenne muscular dystrophy or hemophilia A, then the risk for an affected offspring will depend on which one of the female's X chromosomes is passed to the egg and whether it is fertilized by an X- versus Y-bearing sperm. Because of X inactivation, it is statistically possible that a larger proportion of mutant-bearing X chromosomes will be active and express the mutation, thus establishing a mildly affected female phenotype.

Figure 22–10 illustrates the risk for recurrence of affected males, as well as the occurrence of carrier females. The pattern indicates that there is no male-to-male transmission and that 50% of sons born to a carrier mother will be affected and 50% of the daughters will be carriers. If the father is affected, then 100% of his daughters will be carriers. It is important to look for normal females with affected brothers or maternal uncles in pedigrees suspected of transmitting an X-linked recessive disorder.

Figure 22–11 depicts a typical pedigree for the transmission of a sex-linked recessive disorder. The presence of an X-linked recessive disorder may have resulted from either transmission of the X-linked mutation from the mother or a new X-linked mutation for that conception only. There are notable exceptions to this pattern, such as *germ line* or *gonadal mosaicism*; that is, the mutation is found only in a proportion of germ cells in the ovary but not in other somatic cells of the mother. Another exception occurs when the gene mutation mechanism is itself unusual, such as for the fragile X syndrome, in which interference with gene expression depends on the expansion of the number of CGG triplet repeat sequences on the X chromosome in either males or females. Therefore, females with greater than 200 repeats and with loss of expression of the normal gene on the active X chromosome will be affected and likely exhibit cognitive impairment.

Sex-Linked Dominant Inheritance

X-linked dominant disorders are rare and resemble autosomal dominant inheritance, except there is no male-to-male transmission (Fig. 22–12). One hundred percent of the daughters of an affected male will also be affected, but

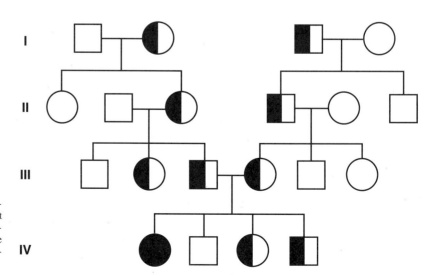

Figure 22–9. Model pedigree for an autosomal recessive disorder. Half-shaded squares and circles reflect carrier or heterozygous individuals. Fully shaded circle is an affected person, or homozygous for the mutation or mutations. Carriers are usually phenotypically normal.

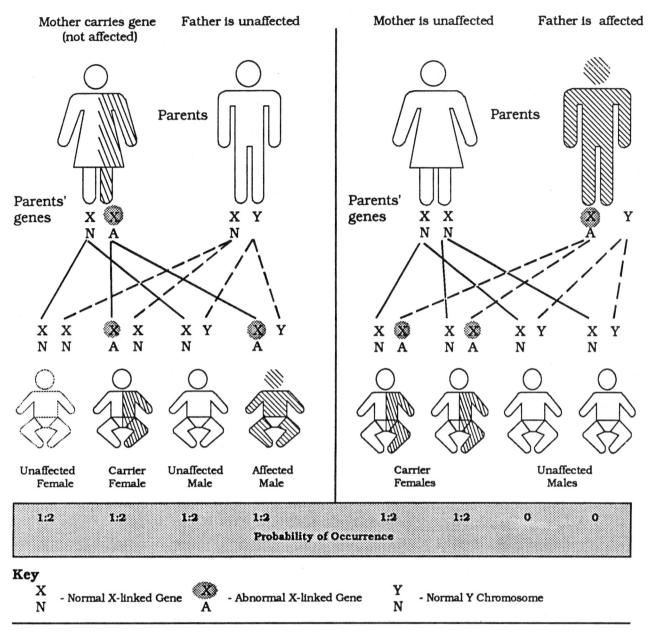

Figure 22–10. X-linked recessive inheritance. (From Greenstein RM, Haddow P, Kloza E, Young DL: Improving Access to Medical Genetics Services: An Education Manual on the Reimbursement Process. Monograph published by Department of Pediatrics, University of Connecticut Health Center, MCH #MCJ-009107010, June 1989.)

with an affected female, there is a 50% risk to male and female offspring, similar to that described for autosomal dominant inheritance. Families with small numbers or incomplete ascertainment of family members make identification of this pattern difficult.

Mitochondrial Inheritance

Most genes are nuclear in location, distributed over the 46 chromosomes. Mitochondria are cytoplasmic structures that contain their own DNA, called mtDNA. The mtDNA has been completely sequenced and it codes for two types of ribosomal RNA, 22 transfer RNAs and 13 polypeptides, that are important for oxidative phosphorylation, whereas

other subunits of the same enzymes are coded from nuclear DNA. Mitochondrial inheritance is exclusively maternal because the sperm neither carries nor transmits mitochondria. There are multiple mitochondria in each cell and there may be thousands of mitochondria per cell. Therefore, when mutations in mtDNA occur, the expression of a disorder of energy metabolism (oxidative phosphorylation) will depend not only on the frequency of the mutation within each cell's mitochondria but also on the total number of cells or tissues, or both, involved. Disorders of lactic acid metabolism, such as MELAS (myoclonic epilepsy, lactic acidosis, and stroke) or Leber hereditary optic neuropathy, may present with variable expression associated with mental retardation or episodic abnormal behaviors.

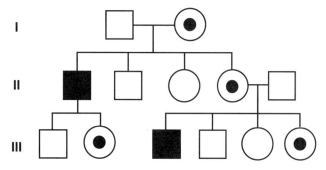

Figure 22–11. Model pedigree for a sex-linked recessive disorder. The circles with a shaded dot depict a carrier female, or heterozygote for the mutation. The shaded squares reflect affected males. There is no male-to-male transmission, but carrier females may have affected brothers.

This expression depends on the *heteroplasmic* versus *homoplasmic* distribution of the mtDNA mutations.

Nontraditional Inheritance

In the past 10 years, enhanced understanding of previously unusual or misunderstood patterns of inheritance has emerged from the new technologic developments in molecular biology and genetics. Three of these mechanisms are briefly reviewed because they will likely become more important to the understanding of behavioral syndromes in the future.

Imprinting is the differential expression of genomic information, either chromosomal or allelic, that depends on whether it is inherited from the maternal or paternal parent (Barlow, 1995). A number of human chromosome regions have been identified that require genetic material from both parents to be represented for normal development to occur. For example, Prader-Willi syndrome occurs when there is selective loss of the paternal 15q11–13 chromosomal region, leaving the maternal region intact but "unbalanced." The reverse of this situation, loss of the maternal 15q11–13 chromosomal region, results in a completely different disorder, Angelman syndrome. For selected regions, a balance of both maternal and paternal contributions is necessary for normal development.

Uniparental disomy occurs when both chromosomes of a pair originate from a *single parent,* such as two maternal chromosomes but no paternal chromosome (Ledbetter and Engel, 1995). This occurrence is determined by using molecular mapping and tracking technologies to determine the parental origin of the chromosomes. The loss of an entire parental chromosome is somewhat similar to loss through imprinting of the balance between maternal-paternal genes and may lead to loss of appropriate genetic expression with subsequent disruption of developmental processes. This problem may occur prenatally during *confined placental mosaicism,* for example, leading to intrauterine growth retardation. In Prader-Willi syndrome, about 3% of occurrences are a meiotic result of the presence of two maternal chromosomes 15 but no paternal chromosome 15 (Dykens and Cassidy, 1996).

Expansion of trinucleotide repeated sequences, such as CGG or CAG repeats, occurs normally throughout the human genome, and these sequences are located within or near active genes. Their length is usually between 22 and 37 repeats in the normal individual; however, when these sequences are expanded to lengths that interfere with the normal expression of the gene, a clinical disorder ensues. This is seen in the fragile X syndrome (>200 repeats) (McKusick, 1994: MIM 309550), Huntington disease (>42 repeats) (McKusick, 1994: MIM 14310), and myotonic dystrophy (>100 repeats) (McKusick, 1994: MIM 160090). These syndromes exhibit unusual phenomena in addition to their single gene inheritance: "anticipation" in myotonic dystrophy with increasing severity in younger individuals in subsequent generations, or an increased risk of affected fragile X offspring from women who carry an intermediate number (premutation, 50–200) of repeats.

Toxin or Teratogen Effects

Prenatal exposure of the fetus to certain chemicals (alcohol), drugs (phenytoin), infectious agents (rubella), or maternal disorders (maternal phenylketonuria) may be responsible for causing either isolated or multiple malformations, depending on the timing of the embryonic phase, the duration of the exposure, and the dose of the teratogen. Agents such as these, as well as others, may cause patterns of malformations associated with cognitive disability and behavioral abnormalities that must be distinguished from genetic or hereditary causes. These agents are essentially environmental influences that interact with genetic mechanisms at critical periods of fetal development.

Polygenic or Multifactorial Inheritance

A number of disorders appear to be inherited or familial but do not follow established patterns of single-gene (mendelian) or chromosomal inheritance. These disorders, such as the common congenital malformations of infancy (cleft lip and palate, pyloric stenosis, spina bifida) or common adult diseases (diabetes mellitus, rheumatoid arthritis, arteriosclerotic heart disease), are felt to be caused by multiple factors. This *multifactorial* or *polygenic* inheritance suggests that there are both genetic and environmental elements in the causation or recurrence of disorders in families or the population at large. In particular, when we consider the cause of behavioral syndromes or the many complex causes of mental retardation, understanding the analysis for multifactorial inheritance becomes essential.

Many normal characteristics, such as height, blood pressure, and intelligence, demonstrate multifactorial inheritance because their measurement exhibits continuous variation throughout the population. The trait is affected by both heritable and environmentally modifying elements and exhibits a measurable set of variations into a normal range. Measurements that fall outside of these normal ranges are considered "abnormal." Because these values are measurable, they are considered to be *quantitative* in their distribution in the population, frequently described as a Gaussian or normal distribution, which exhibits 2 standard deviations around the mean for a particular measurement. Because we are dealing with multiple genes that contribute to a single trait in heritable fashion from parent to offspring, the contributions by individual genes or alleles are considered to

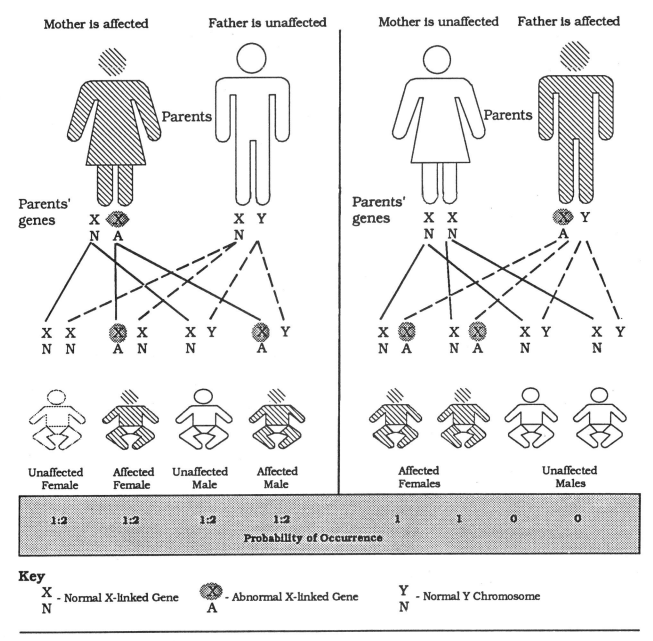

Figure 22–12. X-linked dominant inheritance. (From Greenstein RM, Haddow P, Kloza E, Young DL: Improving Access to Medical Genetics Services: An Education Manual on the Reimbursement Process. Monograph published by Department of Pediatrics, University of Connecticut Health Center, MCH #MCJ-009107010, June 1989.)

be *additive* (Fig. 22–13). The more genes that are separately recruited to contribute to the expression of a particular trait, the greater will be the continuum of variation experienced by the population.

There are some traits or phenotypes that will exceed the range of normal variation for that trait and appear as a disease or disorder. The continuous variation of the trait and the quantitative factors that contribute to its appearance have been described as displaying a *variation of liability* that exceeds a given threshold dividing the population into unaffected and affected individuals (Fig. 22–14).

The characteristics of multifactorial inheritance include (1) a familial pattern of recurrence that does not

follow single gene probabilities; (2) the recurrence risk to offspring of an affected parent, or for recurrence to parents already with an affected offspring, significantly greater than the background incidence for the disorder in the general population; (3) a greater recurrence risk when other first-, second-, or third-degree family members are affected; and (4) the more severe the expression of the disorder, such as unilateral versus bilateral cleft lip and palate, the greater the risk of recurrence, suggesting that there is more genetic or additive loading from both parents. When considering environmental factors, however, such as in the situation of neural tube defects, its recurrence in affected families is significantly reduced when 4.0 mg of folic acid is taken daily by the mother preconceptionally and throughout pregnancy. This intervention is successful for the general population and suggests that in spite of well-demonstrated heritable factors, alterations in the environment also play an important role.

The analysis for the existence of a multifactorial trait is aided by using several data-based instruments. Studying the rate of concordance (both twins affected with the same disorder) of a particular trait, such as congenital heart disease or schizophrenia among monozygotic and dizygotic twins, is useful in identifying genetic versus nongenetic factors in the etiology of these traits. A higher rate of

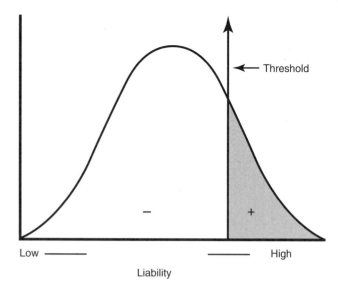

Figure 22–14. Multifactorial threshold liability model. Individuals at the low end of the distribution have a reduced risk of developing the condition, while those at the high end have more disease-producing genes. When combined with other factors, these individuals have now exceeded the threshold and will express the condition.

concordance may identify a greater genetic contribution for monozygotic twins; that is, monozygotic twins should share an identical contribution of their parental DNA, whereas dizygotic twins should share, on average, only 50% of the parental contribution. The theoretical rate of concordance for monozygotic twins is 1.0, and for dizygotic twins it is 0.5. For example, the concordance rate for schizophrenia in monozygotic twins is 0.46 and in dizygotic twins is 0.14 (Table 22–4). The lower-than-expected rate of concordance for monozygotic twins would suggest that nongenetic as well as genetic factors are important in the cause of schizophrenia.

In addition, studying multiple families with the same disorder through pedigree analysis serves as a form of proof to include or exclude the presence of an autosomal dominant or recessive pattern of inheritance. For a possible

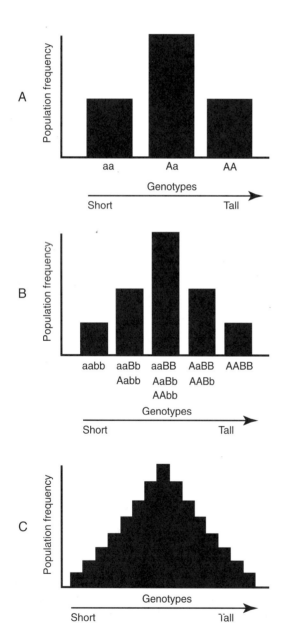

Figure 22–13. Additive genes contribute to a continuum of variation. *A*, Distribution of height in a population assuming that height is controlled by a single gene locus, resulting in genotypes AA, Aa, and aa. *B*, Distribution of height assuming that height is controlled by two gene loci, A and B, resulting in nine genotypes and five phenotypes. *C*, Distribution of height assuming that each of multiple factors is contributing a small effect to the trait.

Table 22–4 • Proband-wise Concordance Rates for Schizophrenia in Recent Identical and Fraternal Twin Studies

Study	Concordance Rate/ No. of Pairs	
	Identical Twins	*Fraternal Twins*
Finland 1963, 1971	.35/ 17	.13/ 20
Norway 1967	.45/ 55	.15/ 90
Denmark 1973	.56/ 21	.27/ 41
United Kingdom 1968, 1987	.58/ 22	.15/ 33
Norway 1991	.48/ 31	.04/ 28
United States 1969, 1983	.31/164	.06/268
Overall	.46/310	.14/480

Data from Gottesman II: Schizophrenia Genesis: The Origins of Madness. San Francisco, Freeman, 1991.

autosomal dominant disorder, the proportion of affected to nonaffected siblings should approximate 50%. For an autosomal recessive disorder, the proportion of affected to nonaffected siblings should approximate 25%. If the pedigree analysis is not compatible with a single gene pattern, yet it still reveals familial transmission, then multifactorial inheritance is more strongly suggested.

Empiric Risk Assessment for Multifactorial Traits. The assignment of a recurrence risk to a complex trait, behavior, or birth defect may sometimes be based on observed population data rather than theoretical predictions. This type of *empiric risk assessment* requires careful population data collection on that specific disorder, and being sure that all affected individuals in fact have the same disorder. Empiric risk assessment also requires that geographic distribution and ethnic or racial elements are considered, and that the family data analysis includes all affected and unaffected members. This is a very labor-intensive process and involves providing families with probabilities and odds ratios as an expression of their at-risk and recurrence risk status (Table 22–5).

Molecular Genetics and Linkage Studies

Brock (1993) notes that "all genetic variation depends ultimately on mutation: physical and chemical alterations in the hereditary material." A full explanation of the technology of molecular genetics is beyond the scope of this chapter, but the reader is referred to Thompson, McInnes, and Willard (1991), Gelehrter, Collins, and Ginsburg (1997), or Brock (1993) for more in-depth information. An increased understanding of the structure and function of human genes has been generated by the new technology developments from the Human Genome Project. Figure 22–15 depicts a typical gene structure and its function. DNA is transcribed to RNA, then the introns are spliced out to produce mature RNA, which is then translated into the protein product, which may then be further modified by posttranslational processes at specific tissue or organ locations. As more human genes are mapped, cloned, and sequenced, particularly those related to complex traits and behavioral disorders, the relationship between genotype and phenotype should become clearer, as will, ultimately, our understanding of the contribution of heredity to behavioral syndromes. Some of the laboratory tools that have been developed for the purposes of performing direct and indirect (linkage) mutation analysis include southern and northern blotting, polymerase chain reaction, allele-specific oligonucleotide analysis, and DNA sequencing. These technologies permit evaluation of molecular pathology, the creation of linkage maps for the association of complex traits to DNA markers, the identification of candidate genes to explain patterns of inheritance in families with disability conditions, and the potential for applications of more specific pharmacomolecular therapy to address the result of DNA and RNA abnormalities (Kidd, 1993; Crowe, 1993).

Modern molecular genetics has developed the laboratory and statistical tools to evaluate genetic risks that previously depended on the tedious collection of family pedigree data and biological observations. The use of linkage markers for family studies has permitted the mapping of genes to chromosomes and subsequently clinical behaviors to these genes. The DNA linkage map identifies when two traits or genes may be observed together more often than would occur by chance alone. This approach uses the fact that linkage maps have been developed with normally occurring DNA markers no more than 5 to 10 centimorgans apart along the length of all 46 chromosomes. Thus the occurrence of a disease or disorder within families may be linked to known DNA markers and thereby permit localization of the gene on the chromosome and subsequent cloning and sequencing of that "candidate" gene. Cytogenetic maps have permitted the association of syndrome-specific features with critical regions of the chromosome, such as for Down syndrome (21q22) or DiGeorge syndrome (22q11). This has accelerated the understanding of how contiguous genes in these regions may modify the clinical presentation. These technologies have reduced the need for acquiring large numbers of similarly affected families, since a single, large, extended family will now permit a similar degree of pertinent analysis.

RISK COUNSELING

The genetic counseling process must take into account the ability of the counselee to understand these complex ge-

Table 22–5 • Empiric Recurrence Risks for Common Multifactorial Disorders

Disorder	Incidence (per 1000)	Unaffected Parents With a Second Affected Child (%)	Affected Parents With an Affected Child (%)
Cleft lip with or without palate	1–2	4	4
Club foot (talipes)	1–2	3	3
Congenital heart defects	8	1–4	2 (affected father)
			6 (affected mother)
Congenital hip dislocation	1	6	12
Manic-depressive psychosis	4	10–15	10–15
Neural tube defect			
Anencephaly	1.5	4–5	—
Spina bifida	2.5	4–5	4
Mental retardation (idiopathic)	3	3–5	10
Schizophrenia	10	14	16

Adapted from Mueller RF, Young ID: Emery's Elements of Medical Genetics, 9th ed. New York, Churchill Livingstone, 1995.

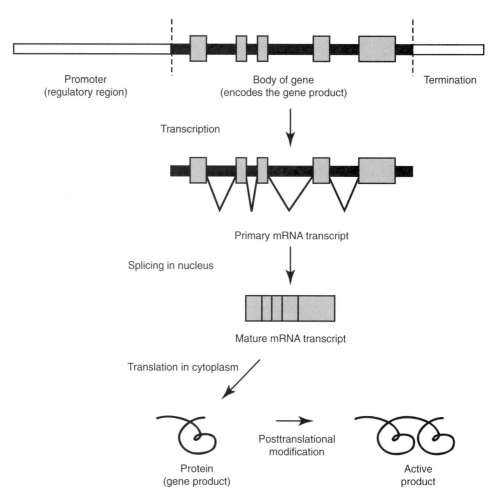

Figure 22–15. Model for gene structure and function. Exons in the open reading frame are transcribed, the introns are spliced out, and the mature mRNA transcript is translated to the protein gene product.

netic concepts, as well as the ability of the counselor to present quantitative and empiric information in as many different modalities as necessary to ensure understanding.

Genetic counseling is a communication process that deals with the human problems associated with occurrence, or the risk of occurrence, of a genetic disorder in a family. The process involves an attempt by one or more appropriately trained persons to help the individual or family to (1) comprehend the medical facts, including the diagnosis, probable course of the disorder, and available management; (2) appreciate the way heredity contributes to the disorder, and the risk of recurrence in specified relatives; (3) understand the alternatives for dealing with the risk of recurrence; (4) choose the course of action that seems to them appropriate in view of their risk, their family goals, and their ethical and religious standards, and to act in accordance with that decision; and (5) make the best possible adjustment to the disorder in an affected family member or to the risk of recurrence of that disorder ("Genetic Counseling," 1975).

Of equal importance is the manner in which this information is transmitted. It is often associated with giving bad news and should be carried out with sensitivity and compassion. Parents often are in awe of how health care professionals are able to "know" what is going to happen to their child or that we are able to predict the future so accurately with our tests and examinations. Explaining

patterns of inheritance to families is an essential skill for the pediatrician, especially if the pediatrician deals with the occurrence and interpretation of complex behavioral traits and disorders.

Behavioral Genetics: Nature and/or Nurture

Differences among individual members within populations and families, particularly behavioral differences, are of great scientific and social interest. These differences include variations in body characteristics, physical skills, intellectual and artistic abilities, personality, attitudes, and motivation. Social scientists and psychologists believed at one time that most of the fabric of human behavior was woven under the influence of environmental experience. Recent behavioral-genetic research indicates that for many traits, genetic effects *increase* throughout early childhood and adolescence (McCartney, Harris, and Bernieri, 1990), but environmental influences are subsequently shared by all family members. In contrast, Plomin and Daniels (1987) believe that environmental influences are more responsible for making family members different from one another than genetic influences are. Their research on personality, psychopathology, and cognition indicates that environment, more so than heredity, makes two children in the same family as different from one another as are pairs of children selected randomly from the population. Although this chapter is devoted to the consideration of biological factors in shaping behavior, it is nevertheless essential to understand the role of environment in the etiology of normal and abnormal behaviors.

The techniques and methodologies used to arrive at these conclusions are built on the theories of quantitative genetics (multifactorial inheritance) as applied to populations, already discussed in this chapter. The quantitative approach examines the fact that some genes distributed over population groups may be independent of the effects of other genes and may have *additive* effects. The effects of other genes may also be *nonadditive* and represent epigenetic influences at other gene loci. These statistical techniques are useful to analyze the causes of individual differences within the normal range of population variation, as well as the identification of contributing causes to abnormal behaviors.

Family studies use the resemblance among family members as a function of shared or additive genes interacting with common environments.

Twin studies permit us to examine the extent to which family resemblance is caused by shared genes (heredity) and the extent to which it is caused by shared environments. Twin studies contrast monozygotic pairs in similar or separate environments, as well as contrasting monozygotic and dizygotic twin pairs.

Adoption studies are used in several ways to illustrate differences between heredity and environment. Genetic factors are studied by comparing monozygotic twins adopted separately and reared apart. It is also possible to study environmental effects by examining the behaviors of nonrelated children adopted into the same family over time.

There are other newly developed statistical methods to study genetic and environmental effects on behavioral phenotypes. These include *quantitative-trait loci analysis* and *biometric model fitting*. Quantitative-trait loci analysis addresses the identification of susceptibility genes for common, complex disorders such as mental retardation or schizophrenia. This approach uses molecular linkage technology to assign behavioral phenotypes to specific chromosomal regions. These methods use exclusion mapping of qualitative traits, maximum-likelihood mapping of qualitative traits, and quantitative trait mapping, all of which are well suited to computer software applications (Kruglyak and Lander, 1995; Sherman et al, 1997).

In *biometric model fitting*, statistical methods of path analysis and structural equation modeling are used to study genetic-environmental effects. These quantitative techniques have evolved to include analysis of consistency over populations (Loehlin, 1992), analysis of traits over time (McArdle, 1986), and analysis of multiple phenotypes whereby two or more disorders are influenced by the same candidate gene (Reus and Freimer, 1997).

These techniques measure differences in phenotypic expression attributable to both genetic and nongenetic factors. When the contribution of heredity is controlled for, adoption and twin studies attempt to separate the environmental effects on behavior into two components: shared and nonshared environment (Plomin and Daniels, 1987). Shared environment (common environmental variance or

between-family differences) include those factors that make children in a family similar to one another beyond recognized genetic endowment. Nonshared environment tends to make family members different from one another based on within-family, individual, unique, or specific factors. Because both adoption and twin studies estimate variance related to heritability and shared environment, nonshared environment may be estimated as variance not experienced by heritability or shared environment.

Plomin and Daniels conclude dramatically that "children in the same family experience practically no shared environmental influence that makes them similar for behavioral traits." In addition, they contend that most of the variability in personality arises from environmental differences among siblings, *not* from the differences among families. This concept is also applicable to the genesis of abnormal behaviors among siblings. Research on nonshared environment has begun to identify those environmental influences that are specific to each child in a family and not shared by other siblings (Table 22–6).

The results from applied interventions suggest that the importance of the nonshared environment on children works through a mechanism or mechanisms within the family that permit individual differentiation even when the same environmental influences are presented "equally" to all siblings. From an interactive point of view, the differences experienced by children in the same family create the environmental factors that drive their behavioral development. One advantage of the concept of nonshared environment is that it prompts us to develop individual child-specific interventions. Genetic factors may indeed play an important role in shaping behavioral phenotypes, and they may even be responsible for the underlying psychopathology or mental retardation that results from single gene or multiple gene mutations. In fact, metabolic or dietary treatment may modify the genetic defect, but it is ultimately the interactive family environment that shapes the evolving personality and behavior of the child, as well as influencing the behaviors of the adults differentially to their children (Plomin, 1996). This idea is explored further below, where we examine the concept of syndrome-specific behaviors in selected disorders of known genetic etiology.

Syndrome-Specific Behaviors

Thus far, we have identified that important contributions are made by biological and genetic factors to the develop-

Table 22–6 • Categories of Environmental Influences That Cause Children in the Same Family to Differ

Categories	Examples
Error of measurement	Test-retest unreliability
Nonshared environment	
Nonsystematic	Accidents, illnesses, trauma
Systematic	
Family composition	Birth-order, gender differences
Sibling interaction	Differential treatment
Parental treatment	Differential treatment
Extrafamilial networks	Peer groups, teachers, television

Adapted from Plomin R, Daniels D: Why are children in the same family so different from one another? Behav Brain Sci 10:1–16, 1987.

ment of normal and abnormal behavior, such as mental retardation and psychopathology. The modifying role of environment in the nature/nurture behavioral paradigm has also been described, particularly through the use of quantitative and statistical methodologies. The genetic-environment correlation is therefore viewed as dynamic and interactive and has been described as passive, reactive, and active (Plomin, DeFries, and Loehlin, 1977). The *passive correlation* occurs when parents and offspring continuously share both genes and environment. The *reactive correlation* refers to experiences that result from reactions of other people to an individual's genetic phenotype or syndrome. The *active correlation* occurs when individuals themselves modify or select experiences that are related to their own genetic phenotype or syndrome. Research on the active correlation group as it relates to syndrome-specific behavior provides us the opportunity to develop more effective and specific interventions for children with behavioral disorders.

THE BEHAVIORAL PHENOTYPE

Over the past 30 years, chromosomal and molecular technologies have permitted the identification and etiology of a growing number of clinically recognizable syndromes. Indeed, over 750 known genetic causes of mental retardation have now been identified (Opitz, 1996). A number of these syndromes have characteristic cognitive or behavioral profiles and trajectories, often referred to as *behavioral phenotypes*. Salient behavioral features in some of these syndromes are presented in Table 22–7.

In studying these characteristic profiles and trajectories, Dykens (1995) defined a behavioral phenotype as the "heightened probability of likelihood that people with a given syndrome will exhibit certain behavioral or developmental sequelae relative to those without the syndrome." Viewing phenotypes as a probability has implications for variability within and between syndromes, as well as for total versus partial specificity.

Within-syndrome variability suggests that not all people with a given syndrome show that syndrome's characteristic behavior to the same degree, or at the same point in development. For example, although hyperphagia is invariably seen in people with Prader-Willi syndrome, the strength of the drive for food varies considerably across individuals, as well as within the same person over time. Environmental factors such as dietary management or increased stress are likely to be associated with this variability, and preliminary findings suggest genetic contributions as well. In particular, less overeating and lower values for body mass index are found in children with Prader-Willi syndrome associated with maternal uniparental disomy as opposed to paternal deletion (Dykens and Cassidy, 1996). Both genetic and environmental factors are thus implicated, and Prader-Willi syndrome and other mental retardation syndromes are emerging as a particularly promising avenue for sorting out complex gene-environment interactions.

Total and partial specificity refers to how mental retardation syndromes are both the same and different across various behavioral domains. Total specificity involves a unique behavioral outcome, such as hyperphagia in Prader-Willi syndrome (Holm et al, 1993), hand wringing in Rett syndrome (Van Acker, 1991), self-mutilation in Lesch-Nyhan syndrome (Ernst, 1996), and self-hugging in Smith-Magenis syndrome (Finucane et al, 1994). Yet it is more often the case that syndromic behaviors are not unique, and that two or more different genetic syndromes share similar types of cognitive profiles or maladaptive behaviors; this is referred to as *partial specificity* (Hodapp, 1997). For example, stubbornness is routinely noted in people with Prader-Willi and Down syndromes; temper tantrums and impulsivity are seen in fragile X and Prader-Willi syndromes; and difficulties with sequential-based, short-term memory tasks are relative weaknesses in people with Smith-Magenis, fragile X, and Prader-Willi syndromes. Studies of between-syndrome similarities and differences are needed to clarify the issue of specificity.

In addition to the *direct effects* related to genetic

Table 22–7 • Syndromes With Specific Behavioral Phenotypes

Syndrome	Chromosome Location	Behaviors	References
Smith-Magenis	17p11.2	Hyperactivity, inattention, sleep disturbance, self-stimulation (hugging), self-injury: pulling out fingernails, object insertion, head banging	Juyal, 1996
Prader-Willi	15p11.2	Hypotonia, hyperphagia, food seeking, stealing, hoarding, skin picking, obsessive-compulsiveness, stubbornness	Dykens & Cassidy, 1996
Williams	7q11.23	Hyperacusis, poor balance, social disinhibition, heightened social ability, anxiety, compulsiveness	Greer, 1997
Rett	X-linked	Dementia, loss of language, sleep disturbance, hyperventilation, lip smacking, hand wringing	Braddock, 1993
Neurofibromatosis	17q11.2	Verbal and motor disinhibition, inattention, social awkwardness	Chapman, 1996
Turner	45,XO	Sensory-motor disintegration, visual-motor problems, low performance IQ, spatial and math deficits	El Abd, 1995
Klinefelter	47,XXY	Impaired verbal memory, low self-esteem, dependency, social reticence, depression	Bender, 1995
Lesch-Nyhan	X-linked	Intense self-mutilation, socially outgoing, fearfulness, panic reactions	Ernst, 1996

abnormalities, there are also *indirect effects* that relate to environment: parents, siblings, families, peers, and communities. These indirect effects are reminiscent of the concept of nonshared environment described by Plomin (1996) and discussed earlier. Scarr and McCartney (1983) refer to these issues as *evocative genotype-phenotype interactions*, which implies that a person's genotype may evoke unique environmental responses or that a person may seek environments that reinforce his or her unique genotypes.

The idea of indirect effects is seen in a relatively new line of research on stress levels in the families of offspring with different types of mental retardation syndromes. For example, relative to Prader-Willi or cri du chat syndrome, consistently lower rates of stress are found among families with a member with Down syndrome (Hodapp, Dykens, and Masino, 1997; Hodapp, Wijma, and Masino, 1997). This is attributed, in part, to the easy-going and charming personalities and lower rates of behavioral problems in many younger children with Down syndrome. These syndromic predispositions, in turn, likely facilitate more positive interactions with others in their environment.

In an effort to consolidate these concepts, we offer a model system to account for syndrome-specific behaviors that also permits within-syndrome variability and partial specificity as it is related to genetic-environment modifications (Fig. 22–16). Genetically driven abnormalities impart early and significant specificity in the development of the syndrome's clinical phenotype. The most important "behavioral target" is the central nervous system, which controls and directs unique responses from genetic and environmental insults to the structure and organization of the brain and spinal cord. These alterations thereafter result in both specific and nonspecific syndrome behaviors that are further modified by the nature of the interactive interven-

tions and other environmental factors. Future research will need to examine correlations between syndrome-related behaviors and specific anatomic-neuropathologic regions of the central nervous system.

The evolution of syndrome-specific behaviors over the lifetime of the affected person is subject to ongoing biological and health-related complications, as well as to changing social environments, including the specificity and continuity of treatments and interventions. Because the behaviors are specific to the syndrome, it is essential that we identify more effective, specific, and unique interventions to improve developmental outcomes.

INTERVENTIONS

Similar to people with mental retardation in general, those with specific disability syndromes are more likely to experience psychiatric disorders or behavioral or emotional dysfunction, relative to the population at large (Borthwick-Duffy, 1994; Dykens, 1998). Most studies on psychopathology in people with mental retardation use a mixed-group approach, lumping together subjects with known and with nonspecific etiologies (Dykens, 1996; Hodapp and Dykens, 1994). As a result, we know more about psychopathology in the heterogeneous population of people with mental retardation than we do in people with specific mental retardation syndromes. Even so, psychiatric studies in specific mental retardation syndromes have already shed new light on gene-brain-behavior relationships (Dykens, Leckman, and Cassidy, 1996; Reiss et al, 1995), as well as generating guidelines for intervention and treatment (Dykens and Hodapp, 1997). Because syndrome-specific interventions will be increasingly identified and applied, we offer two examples that exhibit different behavioral pheno-

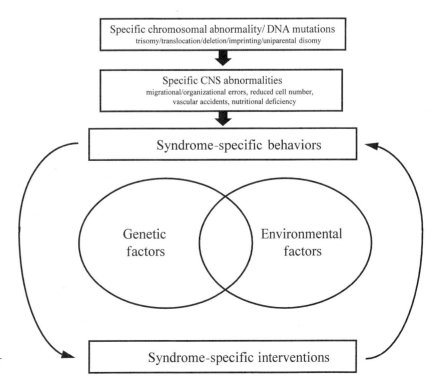

Figure 22–16. Model for the development of syndrome-specific behaviors.

types and predispositions to psychopathology and therefore lead to different treatment implications.

Williams Syndrome

The incidence of Williams syndrome is approximately 1 in 20,000, caused by a deletion at 7q11.23, the region that includes the elastin gene. The phenotype includes increased sensitivity to noise, infundibular aortic stenosis, neonatal hypercalcemia, hypertension in adults, and characteristic facial features (Pober and Dykens, 1996). The cognitive profile includes mild to moderate mental retardation; relative weaknesses in visual-spatial skills, especially integrating parts into a whole; and unusual linguistic functioning (Dilts, Morris, and Leonard, 1990). Many persons with Williams syndrome show remarkable linguistic strengths, especially in expressive language, and these skills often exceed overall mental age. The representativeness of this linguistic profile, however, is open to debate. Behaviorally, people with Williams syndrome are often keenly interested in others, excel at facial recognition, and show an engaging, overly friendly personality. High rates of inattention, over-activity, and anxiety are also common. Anxiety is also manifest in specific fears, somatic complaints, or excessive worry about uncertainty (Pober and Dykens, 1996).

The treatment implications include the following syndrome-specific recommendations:

- Ensure that charming style does not mask sadness or anxiety
- Assess increased risk of exploitation
- Teach more effective social skills, e.g., making friends
- Emphasize people-oriented jobs
- Evaluate linguistic strengths for verbal therapies
- Be aware of increased sensitivity to loss
- De-emphasize written tasks
- Emphasize computers, calculators, verbal ability

Prader-Willi Syndrome

Prader-Willi syndrome affects about 1 in 15,000 people and is associated with mild mental retardation (Dykens and Cassidy, 1996). The syndrome is caused by either a deletion of the paternal 15q11.2 region or maternal uniparental disomy (exclusion of the paternal chromosome 15). The clinical phenotype includes central hypotonia, feeding problems, and developmental delays during infancy. This is followed by hyperphagia after the age of 2 years and leads to truncal obesity and food-related maladaption. There are characteristic facial features, small hands and feet, hypopigmentation of the skin, and short stature. Males have hypogonadism and require replacement therapy to augment behavioral strategies.

In addition to the problem of hyperphagia, there is food seeking, food stealing, and hoarding that may result in severe obesity and carbohydrate intolerance. Other salient maladaptive features include many nonfood, compulsive-like behaviors such as skin picking, inflexibility in routines, and concerns with symmetry and exactness. Indeed, increased risks of obsessive-compulsive disorder are seen in people with this syndrome (Dykens, Lechman, and Cassidy,

1996). Temper tantrums, emotional lability, and stubbornness are also highly prevalent, and depression and low self-esteem tend to increase with advancing age (Dykens and Kasari, 1997; Dykens and Cassidy, 1996).

The treatment implications include the following syndrome-specific recommendations:

- Ongoing role of nutritionist is critical
- Encourage regular exercise
- Restrict access to food, supervise school cafeteria
- Appreciate impact of nonfood behaviors on family
- Provide consistent behavioral limits at home
- Assess for obsessive-compulsive, impulse control, and depressive disorders
- Provide extra support with transitions
- Treat hypogonadism with replacement medication

These examples reveal how different genetic syndromes and their characteristic psychopathologies lead to very different treatment recommendations. Each syndrome has a behavioral phenotype that plays an important role in shaping the key elements of the intervention. However, there are several caveats to consider about the uniqueness of the interventions.

1. Not all of the interventions are explicitly unique to the syndrome, but certain treatment approaches are more relevant than others.
2. Syndrome-specific treatment approaches have not yet been systematically evaluated, in part because many advocates and practitioners in the mental retardation field prefer generic, noncategorical interventions that de-emphasize genetic labeling of their patients.
3. There may be significant within-syndrome behavioral variability, and therefore responses to syndrome-specific therapies may show wide variation.
4. Not every mental retardation syndrome necessarily shows distinctive behavioral phenotypes. Yet even when little is known about the genetic etiology of a particular disorder, if it is usually a recognizable clinical phenotype, then a behavioral phenotype can be sought.
5. The success of therapeutic interventions may also depend on the impact of the syndrome on family systems, that is nonshared or indirect effects.

Conclusion

The purpose of this chapter was to illustrate how behavior is shaped by both biological and environmental forces. In particular, biology is dominated by its basic genetic or hereditary contributions. There is an essential "genetic blueprint" that serves as the basis for subsequent environmental experiences. The quality and quantity of these experiences further shape the day-to-day behaviors of the individual and thus interactively shapes the behaviors of others around him or her. Children with developmental disabilities may have altered genetic or biological blueprints that are then expressed in the form of syndromes, birth defects, or disorganized neuroanatomy. These disorders are associated with maladaptive or impaired behaviors, the genesis of which may arise from altered neuroanatomic structures and result in syndrome-specific psychopathology.

It is essential that professionals who diagnose, treat, and manage patients with these disorders become familiar with the basic principles of single and polygenic inheritance, chromosomal disorders, and especially molecular biology and molecular genetics. But it is abundantly clear that environmental factors also play essential and significant roles in modifying, shaping, and redirecting these biological mechanisms. The inferences we have gained from studying syndrome-specific behaviors lead us to the conclusion that more research is needed to clarify the linkage between abnormal molecular function, disorganization of the development of the central nervous system, and specific behaviors that are generated when these events ensue.

REFERENCES

Andrews BF et al: Small for dates babies. Ped Clin North Am 17:185–198, 1970.

Barlow DP: Gametic imprinting in mammals. Science 270:1610–1613, 1995.

Bender BG: Psychological adaptation of 39 adolescents with sex chromosome abnormalities. Pediatrics 96:302–308, 1995.

Borgaonkar DS: Chromosomal Variation in Man, 7th ed. New York, Wiley-Liss, 1994.

Borthwick-Duffy SA: Epidemiology and prevalence of psychopathology in people with mental retardation. J Consult Clin Psychol 62:17–27, 1994.

Braddock SR: Rett syndrome: an update and review for the primary pediatrician. Clin Pediat 32:613–626, 1993.

Brock DJH: Molecular Genetics for the Clinician. Cambridge, UK: Cambridge University Press, 1993.

Chapman CA et al: Neurobehavioral profiles of children with neurofibromatosis 1 referred for learning disabilities are sex specific. Am J Med Genet 67:127–132, 1996.

Crowe RC: Candidate genes in psychiatry: an epidemiological perspective. Am J Med Genet 48:74–77, 1993.

Dilts CV, Morris C, Leonard CO: Hypothesis for development of a behavioral phenotype in Williams syndrome. Am J Med Genet 6:126–131, 1990.

Dykens EM: Maladaptive behavior and dual diagnosis in people with genetic syndromes. In Burack J, Hodapp RM, Zigler E (eds): Handbook of Mental Retardation and Development. New York, Cambridge University Press, 1998.

Dykens EM: DNA meets DSM: the growing importance of genetic syndromes in dual diagnosis. Ment Retard 34:125–127, 1996.

Dykens EM: Measuring behavioral phenotypes: provocations from the "new genetics." Am J Ment Retard 99:522–532, 1995.

Dykens EM, Cassidy SB: Prader-Willi syndrome: genetic, behavioral and treatment issues. Child Adolesc Psychiatr Clin North Am 5:913–927, 1996.

Dykens EM, Hodapp RM: Treatment issues in genetic mental retardation syndromes. Professional Psych Res Pract 28:263–270, 1997.

Dykens EM, Kasari C: Maladaptive behavior children with Prader-Willi syndrome, Down syndrome, and nonspecific mental retardation. Am J Ment Retard 102:228–237, 1997.

Dykens EM, Leckman JF, Cassidy SB: Phenomenology of obsessive-compulsive disorder in Prader-Willi syndrome. J Clin Psychol Psychiatr 37:995–1002, 1996.

El Abd S: Psychological characteristics of Turner syndrome. J Child Psychol Psychiatr 36:1109–1125, 1995.

Ernst M et al: Presynaptic dopaminergic deficits in Lesch-Nyhan disease. N Engl J Med 334:1569–1572, 1996.

Finucane BM et al: The spasmodic upper-body squeeze: a characteristic behavior in Smith-Magenis syndrome. Dev Med Child Neurol 36:70–83, 1994.

Gelehrter TD, Collins FS, Ginsburg D: Principles of Medical Genetics, 3rd ed. Baltimore, Williams & Wilkins, 1997.

Genetic Counseling. Am J Hum Genet 27:240–242, 1975.

Gottesman II: Schizophrenia Genesis: The Origins of Madness. San Francisco, Freeman, 1991.

Greer MK et al: Cognitive, adaptive and behavioral characteristics of Williams syndrome. Am J Med Genet 74:521–525, 1997.

Hall LL: The human implications of psychiatric genetics. In Hall LL (ed): Genetics and Mental Illness. New York, Plenum Press, 1996.

Hodapp RM: Direct and indirect behavioral effects of different genetic disorders of mental retardation. Am J Ment Retard 102:67–79, 1997.

Hodapp RM, Dykens EM: Mental retardation's two cultures of behavioral research. Am J Ment Retard 98:675–687, 1994.

Hodapp RM, Dykens EM, Masino LL: Families of children with Prader-Willi syndrome: stress-support and relations to child characteristics. J Autism Develop Disorders 27:11–24, 1997.

Hodapp RM, Wijma C, Masino L: Families of children with 5p- (Cri Du Chat) syndrome: familial stress and sibling reactions. Dev Med Child Neurol 39:757–761, 1998.

Holm VA et al: Prader-Willi syndrome: consensus diagnostic criteria. Pediatrics 91:398–402, 1993.

Juyal RC: Molecular analysis of 17p11.2 deletions in 62 Smith-Magenis syndrome patients. Am J Hum Genet 58:998–1007, 1996.

Kidd KK: Associations of disease with genetic markers: déjà vu all over again. Am J Med Genet 48:71–73, 1993.

Kruglyak L, Lander ES: Complete multipoint sib-pair analysis of qualitative and quantitative traits. Am J Hum Genet 57:439–454, 1995.

Ledbetter DH, Engel E: Uniparental disomy in humans: development of an imprinting map and its implications for prenatal diagnosis. Hum Mol Genet 4:1757–1764, 1995.

Loehlin JC: Genes and Environment in Personality Development. Newbury Park, CA, Sage Publishing, 1992.

McArdle JJ: Latent variable growth within behavior genetic models. Behav Genet 16:163–200, 1986.

McBride WG: Thalidomide and congenital abnormalities. Lancet ii:1358–1360, 1961.

McCartney K, Harris MJ, Bernieri F: Growing up and growing apart: a developmental meta-analysis of twin studies. Psychol Bull 107:226–237, 1990.

McKusick VA: Mendelian Inheritance in Man: A Catalog of Human Genetics and Genetics Disorders, 11th ed. Baltimore, MD, Johns Hopkins University Press, 1994.

Mueller RF, Young ID: Emery's Elements of Medical Genetics, 9th ed. New York, Churchill Livingstone, 1995.

Opitz JR: Historiography of the causal analysis of mental retardation. Presented to 29th Annual Gatlinburg Conference on Research and Theory in Mental Retardation, Gatlinburg, TN, 1996.

Plomin R: Beyond nature versus nurture. In Hall LL (ed): Genetics and Mental Illness. New York, Plenum Press, 1996.

Plomin R, Daniels D: Why are children in the same family so different from one another? Behav Brain Sci 10:1–16, 1987.

Plomin R, DeFries JC, Loehlin JC: Genotype-environment interaction and correlation in the analysis of human behavior. Psych Bull 84:309–322, 1977.

Pober BR, Dykens EM: Williams syndrome: an overview of medical, cognitive and behavioral features. Child Adolesc Psych Clin North Am 5:929–944, 1996.

Reece EA, Hobbins JC: Diabetic embryopathy: pathogenesis, prenatal diagnosis and prevention. Ob Gyn Survey 41:325–335, 1986.

Reiss AL et al: Contributions of the FMR1 gene mutation to human intellectual dysfunction. Nat Genet 11:331–334, 1995.

Reus VI, Freimer NB: Understanding the genetic basis of mood disorders: where do we stand? Am J Hum Genet 60:1283–1288, 1997.

Scarr S, McCartney K: How people make their own environments: a theory of genotype-environment effects. Child Dev 54:424–435, 1983.

Sherman SL et al: Behavioral genetics 1997: ASHG statement. Am J Hum Genet 60:1265–1275, 1997.

Thompson MW, McInnes RR, Willard HF: Genetics in Medicine, 5th ed. Philadelphia, WB Saunders, 1991.

Van Acker R: Rett syndrome: a review of current knowledge. J Autism Dev Dis 21:381–406, 1991.

Volpe JJ: Neuronal proliferation, migration, organization and myelination. In Neurology of the Newborn, 3rd ed. Philadelphia, WB Saunders, 1995.

Winick M, Brasel JA, Rosso P: Nutrition and cell growth. In Winick M (ed): Nutrition and Development. New York, John Wiley & Sons, 1972.

23 Chromosomal Disorders

Randi Jenssen Hagerman

 Over the course of the last 2 decades, we have gained an appreciation for chromosomal disorders that may cause only minor physical variations coupled with mild developmental problems, such as learning disabilities or behavioral difficulties.

The behavioral features are usually more helpful in making the diagnosis than are the physical features in the prepubertal child with fragile X syndrome. A short attention span is always present, and hyperactivity complicates the picture in more than 70% of such boys.

The usual patient with an XXY karyotype has an intelligence quotient score (IQ) in the normal range, but the verbal IQ is often lower than the performance IQ.

Longitudinal follow-up studies of unselected patients with an XYY karyotype are limited in number, although the prevalence of this disorder is approximately 1 in 1000 individuals.

Persons with Prader-Willi syndrome usually present in early infancy with severe hypotonia, a poor suck reflex, and failure to thrive. As the hypotonia improves at approximately 2 years of age, problems with overeating begin to develop and the appetite can become insatiable.

Disorders of chromosome number and structure can cause a range of developmental disabilities and structural defects. Patients can present with profound retardation and severe malformations or with minor learning disabilities and subtle physical features. The common trisomies, including trisomy 21 (Down syndrome), trisomy 18 (Edward syndrome), and trisomy 13 (Patau syndrome), were identified in 1959 and 1960. Down syndrome is reviewed in Chapter 24. Trisomy 13 and trisomy 18 are associated with multiple congenital malformations that are usually incompatible with life beyond the first 6 months to 1 year of age. Perhaps because of these severe disorders, chromosomal testing was not typically done in the 1960s and 1970s unless significant dysmorphic features or severe mental retardation, or both, were present. Over the course of the last 2 decades, we have gained an appreciation for chromosomal disorders that may cause only minor physical variations coupled with mild developmental problems, such as learning disabilities or behavioral difficulties. Advances in cytogenetic technology have made it possible to identify subtle chromosomal structural defects, such as small interstitial or microdeletions, duplications, or the fragile site at Xq27.3, which could not be consistently identified before the 1980s. Advances in molecular biology have led to the identification of numerous genes that are associated with developmental disorders, including the fragile X mental retardation 1 gene *(FMR1)*, the FRAXE gene *(FMR2)*, the myotonic dystrophy gene *(DM)*, the elastin gene *(ELN)*, which when deleted is associated with Williams syndrome, the gene associated with Angelman syndrome *(UBE3A)*, and numerous others. Direct DNA testing can now be carried out for many disorders, and molecular testing has been incorporated into cytogenetic testing with fluorescent in situ hybridization (FISH) techniques, such that a fluo-

rescent DNA probe can detect deletions that are too small for visualization even with high-resolution studies. The clinician must therefore become familiar with syndromes associated with chromosomal or specific gene defects so that the appropriate studies can be requested to confirm specific diagnoses.

This chapter reviews disorders of chromosome structure that are often identified in the clinical evaluation of a child with developmental or behavioral problems. Of all the studies that are performed on peripheral blood, a cytogenetic study that includes high resolution for subtle structural defects in addition to *FMR1* DNA testing will give the best yield for positive findings in the work-up for any child with mental retardation or autism of unknown cause. Cytogenetic studies or *FMR1* DNA testing, or both, are also indicated for individuals with borderline intellectual functioning or significant hyperactivity when they also have dysmorphic features, particularly if these features are suggestive of a specific syndrome, such as fragile X syndrome. The clinician's index of suspicion must be high, particularly for sex chromosomal disorders and the fragile X syndrome, so that chromosomal and DNA studies are readily ordered. It is important to confirm the diagnosis by these studies because genetic counseling issues can be important for the patient and extended family members. Identifying the syndrome can also clarify the prognosis and treatment issues, which is discussed later in the chapter.

Chromosomal abnormalities are not uncommon, and approximately one third to one half of all fertilized ova have such an abnormality (Gilbert and Opitz, 1982). The vast majority are incompatible with life and lead to spontaneous abortion within the first few weeks of pregnancy.

The most common chromosomal abnormality is Down syndrome, with an incidence of 1 in 700, although prenatal diagnosis for advanced maternal age has lowered the prevalence at birth to approximately 1 in 1000. The fragile X syndrome is the next most frequent, with a prevalence of approximately 1 in 4000 to 1 in 2000 in the general population, although the carrier rate may be as high as 1 in 259 in women and approximately 1 in 700 in men. This disorder is, however, the most common *inherited* cause of mental retardation, and it usually affects several individuals in a pedigree.

Fragile X Syndrome

The fragile X syndrome is associated with an inducible cytogenetic fragile site. A fragile site consists of a constriction of the chromatin, which occurs at specific locations in the genome. The fragile site at Xq27.3 (Fig. 23–1) was first reported in 1969, but it was not consistently identified by cytogenetic laboratories until the 1980s because of the need for folate- or thymidylate-deficient tissue culture media.

In 1991, through an international collaborative effort the gene for fragile X syndrome was identified and sequenced and named the *fragile X mental retardation 1 gene (FMR1)* (Verkerk et al, 1991). A remarkable trinucleotide repeat expansion was discovered, specifically a CGG repetitive sequence at the 5' end of the gene. Normal individuals have approximately 5 to 50 CGG repeats, with a mean of 30. Individuals who are carriers but unaffected intellectually have a small expansion, specifically 54 to 200 repeats, which is termed the *premutation*. Individuals who are clinically affected by fragile X syndrome have a full mutation, which consists of a much larger CGG expansion ranging from approximately 230 repeats to over 2000 repeats. The full mutation is usually associated with methylation of the *FMR1* gene that blocks the transcription of this gene and therefore the *FMR1* protein (FMRP) is not produced. It is the lack, or a deficiency, of FMRP that causes the clinical and intellectual features that are associated with fragile X syndrome. FMRP is normally found in most tissues, but it is present in high levels in all neurons. This protein is thought to be important for neuronal development and

maturation and its absence is thought to be associated with a lack of the normal pruning process in development. Therefore, individuals with fragile X syndrome usually have a large brain, and specific areas in the brain including the hippocampus, caudate, and thalamus are associated with a significantly increased size compared with control subjects (Abrams and Reiss 1995). The neurobehavioral phenotype of fragile X syndrome described further is associated with the neuroanatomic changes in the brain related to the lack of normal FMRP levels.

There is a broad clinical spectrum of involvement in fragile X syndrome ranging from severe mental retardation to a state in which individuals have normal cognitive abilities but experience behavioral problems and learning difficulties. The molecular findings are associated with the variability of clinical involvement. For instance, males who have fragile X syndrome but who are not retarded usually have a variant DNA pattern, such as a full mutation, that lacks complete methylation; therefore, a limited level of FMRP is produced. Higher functioning males may also be found to have a mosaic pattern on DNA testing of blood, which means some cells with the premutation that are producing FMRP and other cells with the full mutation that are not producing FMRP. Males with a mosaic pattern or with a lack of full methylation in a full mutation usually have a higher IQ than typical fragile X males who have a full mutation that is completely methylated (Merenstein et al, 1996).

Females are less affected by fragile X syndrome because they have two X chromosomes and only one carries the *FMR1* full mutation. The degree of involvement in females is related to the percentage of cells that have the normal X chromosome as the active X chromosome (activation ratio). DeVries and coworkers (1996) found that the activation ratio in females with the full mutation correlates with the performance IQ and the full scale IQ but not with the verbal IQ. Approximately 50% to 70% of girls with the full mutation have cognitive deficits in the borderline or mentally retarded range. Those females with the full mutation who have a normal IQ often have executive function deficits caused by a mild deficiency of FMRP. Individuals with executive function deficits can present with attentional problems, disorganized behavior, tangential speech, and often denial of more significant emotional or learning problems (Sobesky et al, 1996).

The degree of executive function deficits also correlates with the activation ratio in females with the full mutation. It is important to realize that other background genes can also influence the IQ in females with fragile X syndrome. Reiss and coworkers (1995a) found that the mean parental IQ predicted 26% of the variance in the IQ of girls with fragile X syndrome, whereas the activation ratio predicted 33% of the IQ variance. In addition, environmental factors can be important for ultimate IQ. Clearly, IQ is influenced by both genetic and environmental factors.

A typical boy with the fragile X syndrome is born full-term but demonstrates hypotonia and language delays within the first 2 years of life. A short attention span is always present, and hyperactivity complicates the picture in more than 70% of such boys. Hyperactivity is often the presenting complaint. In more than 80% of affected boys, other features typical of children with pervasive develop-

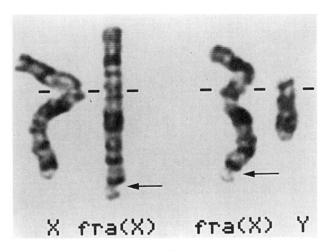

Figure 23–1. The fragile sites at Xq27.3 are marked by arrows.

mental disorders are also present, including hand flapping when excited or anxious, hand biting when upset, poor eye contact with friends and acquaintances, and tactile defensiveness or an aversion to touch. A delay in onset of language is usually seen, with subsequent development of perseverative speech. The speech can also be cluttered and tangential with poor topic maintenance related to the attentional problems and significant impulsivity.

The behavioral features have been termed *autistic-like* because they are typical of children with a pervasive developmental disorder or autism. Although the majority of boys with fragile X syndrome have difficulties with interpersonal interactions in the sense of anxiety, odd mannerisms, shyness, and poor eye contact, they usually want to relate and are friendly without a pervasive lack of relatedness. Therefore most children with fragile X syndrome are not autistic, although some autistic-like behaviors are common. Conversely, fragile X syndrome is frequently diagnosed in children with autism. The screening of small numbers of autistic boys has yielded a low percentage or none with the fragile X chromosome, whereas larger screening endeavors have yielded 13% to 16% with the fragile X syndrome. Averaging these results shows that approximately 7% of boys with autism have the fragile X syndrome (Brown et al, 1986; Hagerman 1996). Preliminary studies in autistic females suggest that 5% have the fragile X syndrome. Therefore cytogenetic studies should be performed in children with autism for which there is no known cause, to identify fragile X syndrome or other cytogenetic abnormalities.

Although autism has occasionally been described in females with fragile X syndrome, affected girls with the full mutation more typically present with learning disabilities or borderline to mild mental retardation. Shyness and social anxiety are common and attentional problems, usually without hyperactivity, are seen in 30% of those girls. Deficits in mathematic ability are the most common academic problem, and special education help is usually required. Language delays often require individual or group therapy and include difficulties with auditory processing, comprehension, abstract reasoning, memory, and topic maintenance. They are usually milder versions of the deficits found in boys. Motor incoordination and sensory-motor integration deficits require occupational therapy in approximately one third of affected girls. Sisters of boys with fragile X syndrome require *FMR1* DNA studies and detailed developmental testing if the *FMR1* mutation is found. Appropriate treatment, including special education, therapy, and medication when indicated, can lead to significant improvements in development with an overall better prognosis than that of their brothers.

The behavioral features are usually more helpful in making the diagnosis than are the physical features in the prepubertal child with fragile X syndrome. The most common physical features seen in young boys are wide and prominent ears sometimes with no antihelical folds so that the ears cup forward (Fig. 23–2). A long, narrow facial structure is more common after puberty in affected boys and girls. Hyperextensible finger joints (metacarpophalangeal joint extension to greater than or equal to 90 degrees), double-jointed thumbs, flat feet, a high arched palate, and soft velvet-like skin, especially on the hands

(on which the palms are often wrinkled), are common findings and appear to be secondary to a connective tissue dysplasia. Macroorchidism, or large testicles, is present in 80% of postpubertal boys with fragile X syndrome but is seen in only approximately 20% of prepubertal boys. Macroorchidism is more difficult to identify in young boys, and an orchidometer is helpful for comparing the testicular size to the normal volumes. Figure 23–3 demonstrates mild macroorchidism in a 10-year-old boy whose testicular volume is 12 mL. Other features that should be observed during the physical examination include a single palmar crease (seen in 30% of patients), hand calluses secondary to repetitive hand biting, and hand mannerisms, or stereotypies.

Seizures occur in 20% of affected children. They can be partial complex seizures with staring spells, arm or face jerking, unusual sensory experiences, falling episodes, or grand mal seizures. The seizures are usually infrequent, are well controlled with anticonvulsants such as carbamazepine, and often disappear after puberty. In approximately 50% of boys with the fragile X syndrome, the electroencephalogram demonstrates spike wave discharges in the central or temporal regions, or in both regions.

Recurrent otitis media is common in these boys, perhaps because of the facial structure or floppy eustachian tubes related to loose connective tissue. Nevertheless, recurrent infection and the chronic presence of fluid in the middle ear can further exacerbate the language problems because of a fluctuating conductive hearing loss. Therefore aggressive treatment is warranted to normalize hearing, often with placement of pressure-equalizing tubes.

Strabismus is also seen in approximately 30% of these boys, and therefore ophthalmologic evaluation is mandatory in early childhood to avoid amblyopia. Mitral valve prolapse is also seen in approximately 50% of affected adult males. When it is detected, subacute bacterial endocarditis prophylaxis is recommended for dental or surgical procedures that involve bacterial contamination of the blood. An occasional patient will demonstrate significant mitral insufficiency that requires careful follow-up. Patients with a click, murmur, or arrhythmias should be referred for cardiologic follow-up.

The treatment for behavioral problems in this syndrome is mainly focused on attentional deficits and hyperactivity. Stimulant medication, particularly methylphenidate, is usually helpful for children 4 years of age or older. It must be used cautiously because higher doses (greater than 0.6 mg/kg) are often associated with an increase in irritability or temper outbursts. The use of folic acid is controversial, although some reports suggest that it can be helpful for a limited number of prepubertal children, with an effect similar to that of stimulant medication. Other medications, including clonidine, tricyclic antidepressants, selective serotonin-reuptake inhibitors, valproic acid, risperidone, lithium, and thioridazine, may also be helpful in improving hyperactivity, mood lability, aggressive behavior, and violent outbursts, although controlled studies of their efficacy are not yet available. Medication should always be considered only one aspect of an integrated treatment program. The boys always require speech and language therapy, occupational therapy, and special education to maximize their development. Whenever possible,

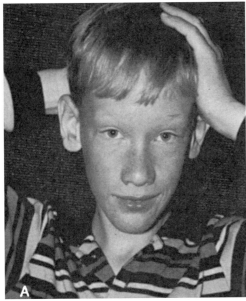
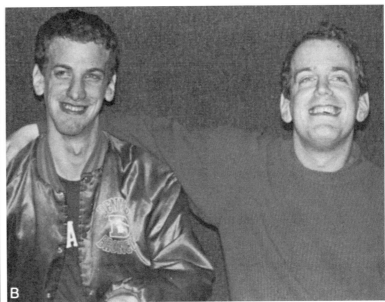
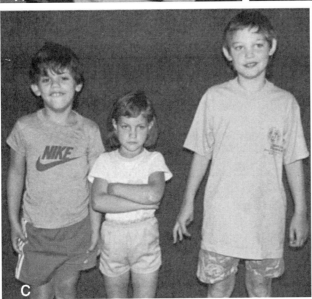

Figure 23–2. *A*, Prepubertal boy with fragile X syndrome. *B*, Two affected adult brothers. Note the long, narrow faces and prominent ears. *C*, A learning disabled girl with fragile X syndrome who has mildly prominent ears, standing between her two brothers who also have fragile X syndrome. (Reprinted with permission from Hagerman RJ: Physical and behavioral features. *In* Hagerman RJ, Silverman AC [eds]: Fragile X Syndrome: Diagnosis, Treatment, and Research, 2nd ed. Baltimore, Johns Hopkins University Press, 1996.)

mainstreaming or integration into the regular classroom is warranted; the boys tend to imitate the behaviors to which they are exposed, and appropriate modeling is helpful.

Longitudinal studies have shown a decrease in IQ over time in affected boys and in some girls with the full mutation. In the preschool years, developmental testing often demonstrates low-normal or borderline intellectual functioning. This is because the tasks that are emphasized in testing at this age, such as single-word vocabulary skills and visual matching, are generally strengths for children with fragile X syndrome. In middle childhood and adolescence, however, reasoning and problem-solving skills are emphasized in testing, and these areas are significant weaknesses in these boys. Children with fragile X syndrome do not lose skills, nor do their cognitive abilities degenerate. They continue to gain abilities over time but not at the same pace that their early childhood IQ would predict.

The diagnosis of fragile X syndrome is important to make not only for organizing appropriate treatment but also to provide genetic counseling to immediate and extended family members. A high risk (approximately 50%) of passing on the *FMR1* full mutation is present in premutation female carriers, and prenatal diagnosis and new reproductive technologies can prevent the recurrence of fragile X syndrome (Cronister, 1996). In addition, new families can receive educational information and link up with a local parent support group by contacting the National Fragile X Foundation at (800) 688–8765.

Other Trinucleotide Repeat Disorders

Fragile X syndrome is only one of many disorders that have been discovered since 1991 and are associated with a

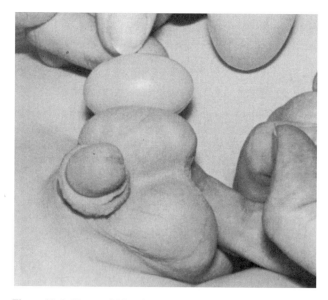

Figure 23–3. Macroorchidism in a prepubertal male. Testicle is compared to a 12-mL orchidometer volume.

trinucleotide repeat. Two other genes have been identified just distal to the *FMR1* gene on the bottom end of the X chromosome. One is the FRAXE gene, which has been named the *fragile X mental retardation 2 gene (FMR2)* (Gecz et al, 1996). Mutation at the FRAXE location is consistently associated with mental retardation and it is also associated with a cytogenetic fragile site that is hard to distinguish from the *FMR1* fragile site. The *FMR2* gene also has a CGG repetitive sequence that expands into a full mutation that is associated with clinical disease. The phenotype of FRAXE mutation appears to be quite variable, but only a handful of cases have been reported and the prevalence is estimated to be at 1 per 50,000 males in the general population (Brown, 1996). Patients with FRAXE mutation usually have only mild mental retardation and less prominent ears than those with fragile X syndrome but there has not been consistent documentation of the phenotype. FRAXF is an additional fragile site distal to *FMR1* and the FRAXF gene also has a CGG repetitive sequence, but the FRAXF mutation is not consistently associated with mental retardation.

Other trinucleotide repeats that have been associated with recently discovered genes include Huntington disease at 4p16.3 associated with CAG repeat; cerebellar ataxia types I, II, and III, all with CAG repeats; spinobulbar muscular atrophy, or Kennedy disease, at Xq11 associated with a CAG repeat; dentatorubral pallidolusyian atrophy (DRPLA) associated with a CAG repeat; Machado-Joseph disease associated with a CAG repeat, myotonic dystrophy at 19q13 associated with a CTG repeat; and the most recent finding of a GAA repeat in the gene for Friedreich ataxia on chromosome 9.

Most of these disorders with trinucleotide repeats, including fragile X syndrome, are associated with anticipation, which means greater involvement or earlier involvement in subsequent generations. Other disorders that feature anticipation, including some psychiatric disorders such

as bipolar disease or other forms of depression, may also turn out to have a trinucleotide repeat mutation.

Sex Chromosome Abnormalities

Abnormalities in the number of sex chromosomes are the only numeric chromosomal problems that are consistently associated with learning disabilities rather than with significant mental retardation. The prevalence of these disorders is high (Table 23–1) in the general population, and yet they are not usually identified in childhood. Although early reports documented severe behavioral problems in selected groups, particularly in individuals with the XYY karyotype, our understanding of their prognosis has improved in the last decade with well-designed follow-up studies of unselected infants with sex chromosome abnormalities. Each of these disorders is considered in detail.

MALES WITH 47,XXY, INCLUDING KLINEFELTER SYNDROME

Klinefelter and colleagues described Klinefelter syndrome in 1942 in nine men with small testes, aspermia, gynecomastia, and elevated gonadotropin levels. Most patients are diagnosed in adulthood because of infertility, or in late adolescence because of small testicles secondary to hyalinization of the seminiferous tubules or gynecomastia. The prevalence of Klinefelter syndrome is approximately 1 in 1000 individuals, and the phenotypic appearance occurs with one or more extra X chromosomes in addition to a Y. Mosaicism is common, and the presence of cell lines with XX or XY in addition to XXY is associated with less severe physical features. However, individuals with a larger number of X chromosomes, such as XXXY, have more significant cognitive and social deficits.

The usual patient with an XXY karyotype has an IQ in the normal range, but the verbal IQ is often lower than the performance IQ. Moderate problems exist in language skills, including auditory processing abilities, auditory memory, and expressive language, that often require speech and language therapy. Reading problems occur in approximately 50% of these patients and require special education help. Mild to moderate problems are frequently seen in motor coordination, and these individuals are often de-

Table 23–1 • Incidence of Sex Chromosome Abnormalities in Newborn Surveys

Chromosomal Abnormality	Incidence
XYY	1/1000
XXY	1/1000
XXX	1/1000
Turner phenotype	1/2000
Trisomy 13	1/20,000
Trisomy 18	1/8000
Trisomy 21	1/700
Other trisomies	1/50,000
Balanced rearrangement	1/500
Unbalanced rearrangement	1/2000

scribed as awkward in their early motor development. Psychosocial development is often hampered by a poor self-image, and more significant emotional problems can occur, particularly if the family environment is dysfunctional. Hyperactivity is uncommon, but impulsive behavior has been reported. Treatment with testosterone at puberty can be helpful in improving behavioral difficulties, self-image, and physical appearance in more than 70% of these boys (Winter, 1991).

MALES WITH XYY

Early studies in Scotland identified persons with an XYY karyotype who had antisocial behavior. Other studies of selected populations have found hyperactivity, impulsiveness, aggression, and difficulties with relatedness and interpersonal interactions. Longitudinal follow-up studies of unselected patients are limited in number, although the prevalence of this disorder is approximately 1 in 1000 individuals. Language deficits are usually mild when compared with males who have an XXY karyotype, but hypotonia and sensory-motor integration deficits are common (Berch and Bender, 1990). Males with XYY are usually tall with long fingers, and there is a high incidence of behavioral and psychiatric problems although hypogonadism is not present. Facial acne is also a frequent problem and is perhaps related to the elevated testosterone levels. Treatment is usually focused on the aggressive, impulsive, and inattentive behavior, and stimulants are usually helpful, although additional medications such as clonidine or risperidone are sometimes necessary in complex cases.

POLYSOMY OF X: 47,XXX, 48,XXXX

Females with additional X chromosomes have more serious cognitive deficits than do persons with other sex chromosome abnormalities, though the IQ can be in the low-normal to borderline range. The IQ is inversely related to the number of X chromosomes. Receptive and expressive language problems occur, and auditory comprehension and articulation deficits are severe. In a prospective study of 11 unselected girls with an XXX karyotype, all had speech problems by the first grade and four girls were nonverbal. Shyness and immaturity were frequent problems, and the girls tended to be tall and poorly coordinated compared with control subjects (Linden et al, 1988). Typical physical features are not usually seen, though problems with menses and ovarian failure are not uncommon. The prevalence is again 1 in 1000 individuals. Problems with balance, diadochokinesia, motor planning, hypotonia, visual perception, and sensory integration are typical (Linden, Bender, and Robinson, 1995).

TURNER SYNDROME: 45,X GONADAL DYSGENESIS

In 1938 Turner described a phenotype that included short stature, broad neck, widespaced nipples, and gonadal dysgenesis or streaked gonads. Cardiovascular malformations occur in one fourth of these individuals, and shortening of a metacarpal is common. Approximately 1% of all fertil-ized ova are XO, and less than 5% survive to birth. Mosaicism is common in those that survive, and this leads to significant variability in the phenotype. Those girls with a significant normal cell line are taller and may menstruate normally.

Girls with Turner syndrome usually have a lower performance IQ, compared with a relatively preserved verbal IQ. A visual-spatial deficit is present and involves difficulties with drawing, design copying, handwriting, and spatial orientation such as map reading or finding one's way through a building (Reiss et al, 1995b). Attentional problems associated with hyperactivity are seen in 30% of the girls, and stimulant therapy may be required (Rosenfeld and Grumbach, 1990). Motor deficits are present in 80% of girls with Turner syndrome and include hypotonia, retention of some primitive reflexes, and dysfunctional sensory-motor integration, which may improve with occupational therapy.

Autosomal Abnormalities

TRISOMIES

The most common chromosomal disorder, trisomy 21, is discussed in Chapter 24. Trisomies 13 and 18 are associated with multiple congenital malformations, severe mental retardation, and usually early death (Table 23–2). The other trisomies cause death before birth unless mosaicism exists with a normal cell line, as seen in trisomy 22 and trisomy 8. Trisomy 8 causes a range of abnormalities because of mosaicism. The IQ is usually between 50 and 80, although a normal female with mosaic trisomy 8 has been reported (Kurtyka et al, 1988). Dysmorphic facial features, osteoarticular anomalies, and typical dermatoglyphic findings were also present.

Partial trisomies are more common than are full trisomies, and they can arise by the segregation process in a translocation carrier, from crossing over in a pericentric inversion carrier, or de novo. It is important to obtain parental chromosomes to clarify the origin and the risks for recurrence in subsequent children. Consistent clinical features are seen in many of the partial trisomies, and a limited list of the more common ones is given in Table 23–2.

A duplication of genetic material can also occur as a repeat or tandem duplication on a single chromosome. These tandem duplications arise from unequal crossing over and may not be deleterious.

DELETIONS

Advances in high-resolution technology for cytogenetic assessments have enhanced our appreciation of chromosomal deletions as a cause of developmental disabilities. Although many of the large deletions listed in Table 23–3 have been identified for years and are associated with dysmorphic features, significant retardation, and organ malformations, more subtle deletions have been appreciated recently and are associated with less severe developmental disabilities. A few of the microdeletion syndromes are described.

Table 23–2 • Trisomies

Cytogenetic Features	Clinical Features	Cognitive or Behavioral Features
Trisomy 13	Multiple congenital malformations, polydactyly, microcephaly, microophthalmia, cleft lip and palate, death usually in first 3 months of life, incidence 1 in 20,000	Severe mental retardation
Trisomy 18	Multiple congenital malformations, hypoplastic nails, overlapping fingers, death usually in first 6 months of life, incidence 1 in 8000	Severe mental retardation
Mosaic trisomy 8	Prominent forehead, hypertelorism, low-set prominent ears, camptodactyly	IQ 50–80, more severe mental retardation with less mosaicism
Partial trisomies		
4p	Microcephaly, synophrys, flat nasal bridge, camptodactyly, hypoplastic nails, micropenis	Severe mental retardation with language affected more severely than motor skills
6p	Microcephaly, small mouth, hypotelorism, failure to thrive	Mental retardation, autism
9p	Macrocephaly, hypertelorism, short fingers and toes, skeletal anomalies, cupped ears	Moderate to severe mental retardation
20p	Hypotonia, tremor brachycephaly, hypotelorism, large ears, cryptorchidism	Mild to severe mental retardation

Smith-Magenis Syndrome: Deletion at 17p11.2

More than 100 patients with Smith-Magenis syndrome (SMS) have been described since the initial report in 1982 describing two patients with mental retardation, cleft palate, and cardiac malformations. SMS is considered to be a contiguous gene deletion syndrome with 10 genes identified in the region 17p11.2 so far (Chen, Potocki, and Lupski, 1996). Hyperactivity with aggression and developmental delays are usually the presenting problems, but the craniofacial features, including midface hypoplasia, brachycephaly, frontal bossing, prognathia, and abnormal ears, in addition to short broad hands and short stature, characterize the syndrome. There is a typical behavioral phenotype that includes unusual self-injurious behavior such as onchotillomania (pulling out of fingernails and toenails), polyembolokoilamania (insertion of foreign bodies into body orifices), head banging, and wrist biting, all of which may be related to features of peripheral neuropathy seen in 75% of SMS patients. Sleep disturbances, including difficulty falling asleep and frequent night wakenings, in addition to tan-

trums and mood lability, add to a high level of parent distress associated with this disorder.

The frequency of SMS is 1 per 25,000 in the general population, and the diagnosis can be confirmed by high-resolution cytogenetic studies that identify the deletion at 17p11.2. Smaller submicroscopic deletions can be identified by FISH studies using molecular probes for the SMS critical region. The medical work-up includes echocardiogram and cardiac consultation to assess possible heart disease; ophthalmologic assessment because structural anomalies of the eye such as microcornia, iris anomalies, strabismus, and myopia are common; ear, nose, and throat evaluation for velopharyngeal incompetence, submucous cleft, and sensorineural or conductive hearing loss; and a renal ultrasonogram to rule out structural anomalies of the urinary tract that can be seen in approximately 35% of patients with SMS (Greenberg et al, 1996). Most children with SMS have mental retardation, although some may have severe learning disabilities with receptive and expressive language deficits. Both motor and language therapy are essential in SMS, and behavioral therapy or counseling,

Table 23–3 • Selected Autosomal Deletions

Cytogenetic Features	Physical Features	Cognitive or Behavioral Features
4p − Wolf-Hirschhorn syndrome	Defect of midline fusion involving mouth, nose, lips, palate, penis, growth deficiency	Profound mental retardation, seizures
5p − Cri du chat syndrome	High-pitched cry, growth retardation, hypertelorism, epicanthal folds, down-slanting palpebral fissures	Severe speech and language delays, moderate mental retardation
11p − Wilms tumor–aniridia	Aniridia, ambiguous genitals, deletion of 11p13 segment involves Wilms tumor	Mental retardation
15q11-q13 deletion Prader-Willi syndrome or Angelman syndrome ("happy puppet syndrome")	Hypotonia, FTT, short stature, cryptorchidism, insatiable appetite or wide mouth, ataxia, and puppet-like arm movements	Low-normal IQ to severe retardation
Interstitial deletion of p11.2 band of 17 Smith-Magenis syndrome	Brachycephaly, broad nasal bridge, short broad hands	Severe hyperactivity, mental retardation, self-abuse, autism, hearing loss
17p − Terminal deletion Miller-Dieker syndrome	Microcephaly, lissencephaly, growth deficiency	Severe mental retardation, seizures

FTT = failure to thrive.

or both, is usually helpful for the patient and the family. Medication interventions include stimulants for hyperactivity, clonidine for aggression and sleep disturbances, and mood stabilizers such as lithium, valproic acid, or carbamazepine for severe aggression and mood lability. Interested families and professionals can contact PRISMS (Parents and Researchers Interested in Smith-Magenis Syndrome) at (703) 709–0568 for further educational information.

Velocardiofacial Syndrome and 22q11 Deletion

In recent years, the detection of microscopic or submicroscopic deletions at 22q11 has helped to lump several previously described disorders into this deletion syndrome. DiGeorge syndrome (DGS), originally described in 1965, includes conotruncal cardiac defects and aplasia or hypoplasia of the thymus and parathyroid glands leading to immune deficiency and hypocalcemia. In addition, DGS is also associated with hypertelorism, low-set and prominent ears, micrognathia, and learning problems. The majority of patients with DGS have a deletion at 22q11. Patients with conotruncal anomaly face syndrome have been shown to have the 22q11 deletion, and 20% to 30% of newborns with truncus arteriosus, tetralogy of Fallot, or interrupted aortic arch also have the 22q11 deletion. Several patients with Opitz syndrome involving hypertelorism, hypospadias, cardiac defects, and cryptorchidism have also been found to have the 22q11 deletion (Driscoll and Emanuel, 1996). Lastly, velocardiofacial syndrome (VCFS), also called Shprintzen syndrome after the man who reported it in 1981, is associated with the 22q11 deletion. VCFS includes palatal abnormalities leading to hypernasal voice and early feeding difficulties, and characteristic facial features including a long face, prominent nose with a bulbous tip and narrow alae, almond-shaped eyes, large or malformed ears, and long fingers (Jones, 1996). The verbal IQ in people with VCFS ranges from normal to borderline, but the performance IQ is often lower, reflective of significant visual-spatial perceptual deficits. Attention-deficit hyperactivity disorder (ADHD) is seen in 50% and bipolar disorder in 70% of children and adolescents with VCFS (Morrow et al, 1996). Individuals with VCFS are also at higher risk to develop schizophrenia in late adolescence or adulthood. Several genes are present in the 22q11 deletion region, including the gene for catechol-O-methyl-transferase (COMT), which is important for the metabolism of norepinephrine and dopamine and may play a role in the development of psychiatric illness, including psychosis, in VCFS.

The phenotype can be quite variable in the 22q11 deletion syndrome, depending on the size of the deletion. Patients with findings including the cardiac and facial features described earlier should be tested with high-resolution studies with the addition of the FISH probe for this region to detect the deletion. Subsequent cognitive, learning, and language studies are indicated to organize an appropriate educational and therapy intervention program.

Williams Syndrome: Deletion at 7q11.23

Williams syndrome (WS), first described in 1961, includes elfin-like facies, gregarious personality, congenital heart disease, and infantile hypercalcemia. Recently a submicroscopic deletion that is detectable by FISH studies has been observed in 96% of patients with the classic WS phenotype (Lowery et al, 1995). The elastin gene *(ELN)* is within the deletion, and absence of one allele causes the cardiac defects, including supraventricular aortic stenosis, peripheral pulmonic stenosis, or mitral valve prolapse, and the connective tissue problems, including joint hyperelasticity, lordosis, hypertension, inguinal hernias, and diverticula of bladder and intestines, that are associated with WS. Some of the craniofacial features may also be secondary to *ELN* hemizygosity, such as periorbital fullness, epicanthal folds, short upturned nose, long smooth philtrum, and full lips. Pérez-Juardo and colleagues (1996) reported that more severe growth retardation occurs when the deletion is of maternal origin, suggesting an imprint effect on a gene that influences growth in this region.

The cognitive profile in WS ranges from low-normal to moderate mental retardation with relative preservation of expressive language skills, short-term auditory memory, and facial discrimination skills (Wang et al, 1995). However, visual-spatial perceptual deficits and visual-motor incoordination are severe problems for patients with WS. ADHD is seen in 80% of children, and anxiety or depression, or both, is common in adults. Hypersensitivity to sound or hyperacusis is also a unique feature of the behavioral phenotype in WS (Udwin and Dennis, 1995). Two other genes involved with the deletion, *LIMK1* and replication factor C subunit 2 *(RFC2)*, are possible candidates for causing the cognitive and behavioral problems associated with WS. The incidence is estimated at 1 per 20,000 live births, and the diagnosis is made by assessing the clinical phenotype with confirmation by FISH studies to document the submicroscopic deletion. Treatment includes stimulants and special education help for the ADHD and learning deficits, and counseling and selective serotonin-reuptake inhibitors for the anxiety and depression.

Prader-Willi Syndrome and Angelman Syndrome: 15q11-q13 Deletion

Angelman syndrome (AS) and Prader-Willi syndrome (PWS) are caused by deficient gene expression in the 15q11 to q13 region, which is maternally derived in AS and paternally derived in PWS. In AS, approximately 70% of patients have a de novo maternal deletion at 15q11-q13, 2% have paternal uniparental disomy, and 2% to 3% have imprinting mutations, that is, a paternal pattern of methylation on both chromosomes even though there is biparental inheritance. These three patterns lead to an absence of gene expression from maternally inherited genes in this region. The clinical appearance of severe mental retardation, nonexistent speech, a large mouth, widely spaced teeth, prognathism, abrupt inappropriate laughter, ataxia, and jerky arm movements led to the term *happy puppet syndrome*. In the remaining 25% of AS cases, there is no deletion, abnormal methylation, or uniparental disomy. Matsuura and colleagues (1997) and Kishino, Lalande, and Wagtstaff (1997) recently detected several different mutations in the *UBE3A* gene that is in the AS critical region within the 15q11 to q13 deletions. This is strong evidence that the absence of the *UBE3A* gene product, which is predicted to be expressed exclusively from the maternal allele because of imprinting, is the cause of AS. This gene product has a role in ubiquitin-mediated proteolysis, which appears to be important in central nervous system development through alteration of synaptic connectivity in animal studies (Kishino, Lalande, and Wagtstaff, 1997).

In an adjacent area to the AS region within 15q11-q13 there are five genes that are thought to be critical for the PWS phenotype, including the small nuclear ribonucleoprotein-associated polypeptide N, which is involved with alternative splicing of DNA. In approximately 60% to 70% of patients with PWS, a paternally derived de novo deletion is detected by FISH studies. In most of the remaining patients, maternal uniparental disomy is present.

Prader-Willi syndrome was first reported in 1956, and individuals usually present in early infancy with severe hypotonia, a poor suck reflex, and failure to thrive. As the hypotonia improves at approximately 2 years of age, problems with overeating begin to develop and the appetite can become insatiable. Obesity develops in addition to other dysmorphic features, including small hands and feet, short stature, small penis and cryptoorchidism. Mild mental retardation is typical, although cognitive abilities can range from normal to severe mental retardation. Recent behavioral studies have demonstrated that obsessive-compulsive behavior involving a variety of areas in addition to food foraging is common in patients with PWS (Dykens and Cassidy, 1996).

The overall prevalence of PWS is approximately 1 in 10,000, and treatment involves an intensive behavior modification program to control the eating behaviors in addition to medications such as serotonin-reuptake inhibitors to help with the obsessive-compulsive behavior. In addition, children with Prader-Willi and Angelman syndromes require special education services for their unique cognitive and behavioral needs (Dykens and Cassidy, 1996).

OTHER SYNDROMES

Recombinant 8 Syndrome

An interesting combination of both deleted and duplicated material is found in the recombinant 8 syndrome. Sujansky and colleagues reported this problem in families of Hispanic background in Colorado in 1981. Affected children have mental retardation and growth deficiency with characteristic facial features, including a wide face, hypertelorism, slanted palpebral fissures, a long philtrum, and congenital heart disease. On cytogenetic testing, the parents were found to carry a pericentric inversion of chromosome 8 without clinical problems. In the pairing for replication of this inverted segment, however, there is a crossover that creates a recombinant chromosome with duplication of the distal segment of the long arm and deficiency of a small portion of the distal end of the short arm [rec(8),dup q,inv(8)(p23q22)], which gives rise to the affected children. Families that are involved in this syndrome have been identified throughout the western United States, but their ancestors have come from the San Luis Valley region in southern Colorado and northern New Mexico. It appears that there was a common single origin for this inversion.

Conclusion

The variations of chromosomal structural abnormalities are limitless. With newer technology, including FISH studies, we can recognize even single-gene deletions that are associated with central nervous system dysfunction. These discoveries are furthering our understanding of brain development and expanding our diagnostic abilities. The families benefit from improvements in genetic counseling and treatment. The next century will reap the benefits of the Human Genome Project, including the use of gene therapy; however, patients will not benefit from these advances unless they are diagnosed. Therefore, clinicians must be sensitized to pursue chromosomal and DNA studies when clinically indicated, which is more frequently than they are performed at present.

REFERENCES

Abrams MT, Reiss AL: The neurobiology of fragile X syndrome. Ment Retard Dev Disabil Res Rev 1:269, 1995.

Bender BG, Linden M, Robinson A: Cognitive and academic skills in children with sex chromosome abnormalities. Read Writ Interdis J 3:315, 1992.

Berch D, Bender B (eds): Sex Chromosome Abnormalities and Behavior. Psychological Studies. Westview Press for AAAS. Washington, DC, 1990.

Brown WT: The FRAXE syndrome: is it time for routine screening? Am J Hum Genet 58:903, 1996.

Brown WT, Jenkins EC, Cohen IL, et al: Fragile X and autism: a multicenter survey. Am J Med Genet 23:341, 1986.

Chen K-S, Potocki L, Lupski JR: The Smith-Magenis syndrome [del (17) p11.2]: clinical review and molecular advances. Ment Retard Dev Disabil Res Rev 2:122, 1996.

Cronister A: Genetic Counseling. In Hagerman RJ, Cronister AC (eds): Fragile X Syndrome: Diagnosis, Treatment and Research, 2nd ed. Baltimore, MD, Johns Hopkins University Press, 1996, pp 251–282.

deVries BBA, Wiegers AM, Smits APT, et al: Mental status of females with an FMR1 gene full mutation. Am J Hum Genet 58:1025, 1996.

Driscoll DA, Emanuel BS: DiGeorge and velocardiofacial syndromes: the 22q11 deletion syndrome. Ment Retard Dev Disabil Res Rev 2:130, 1996.

Dykens EM, Cassidy SB: Prader-Willi syndrome: genetic behavioral and treatment issues. Child Adoles Psychiat Clin North Am 5:913, 1996.

Gecz J, Gedeon AK, Sutherland GR, Mulley JC: Identification of the gene FMR2, associated with FRAXE mental retardation. Nat Genet 13:105, 1996.

Gilbert EF, Opitz JM: Developmental and other pathologic changes in syndromes caused by chromosome abnormalities. In Rosenberg HS, Bernstein J (eds): Perspectives in Pediatric Pathology, Vol 7. New York, Masson, 1982.

Greenberg F, Lewis RA, Polocki L, et al: A multi-disciplinary clinical study of Smith-Magenis syndrome (deletion 17p11.2). Am J Med Genet 62:247, 1996.

Hagerman RJ (eds): Fragile X Syndrome: Diagnosis, Treatment and Research, 2nd ed. Baltimore, Johns Hopkins University Press, 1996.

Jones KL: Smith's Recognizable Patterns of Human Malformation, 5th ed. Philadelphia, WB Saunders, 1996.

Kishino T, Lalande M, Wagtstaff J: UBE3A/E6-AP mutations cause Angelman syndrome. Nat Genet 15:70, 1997.

Kurtyka ZE, Krzykwa B, Piatkowska E, et al: Trisomy 8 mosaicism syndrome. Clin Pediatr 27:557, 1988.

Linden MG, Bender BG, Harmon RJ, et al: 47,XXX: what is the prognosis? Pediatrics 82:619, 1988.

Linden MG, Bender BG, Robinson A: Sex chromosome tetrasomy and pentasomy. Pediatrics 96:672, 1995.

Lowery MC, Morris CA, Ewart A, et al: Strong correlation of elastin deletions, detected by FISH, with Williams syndrome: evaluation of 235 patients. Am J Hum Genet 57:49, 1995.

Matsuura T, Sutcliffe JS, Fang P, et al: De novo truncating mutations in E6-AP ubiquitin-protein ligase gene (UBE3A) in Angelman syndrome. Nat Genet 15:74, 1997.

Merenstein SA, Sobesky WE, Taylor AK, et al: Molecular-clinical correlations in males with an expanded FMR1 mutation. Am J Med Genet 64:389, 1996.

Morrow B, Carlson CG, Goldberg R, et al: Psychiatric illness in children with velo-cardio-facial syndrome with/without 22q11 deletions. Am J Hum Genet 59(suppl):A89, 1996.

Pérez-Juardo LA, Peoples R, Kaplan P, Hamel BCJ: Molecular definition of chromosome 7 deletion in Williams syndrome and parent-of-origin effects on growth. Am J Hum Genet 59:781, 1996.

Reiss AL, Freund LS, Baumgardner TL, et al: Contribution of the FMR1 gene mutation to human intellectual dysfunction. Nat Genet 11:331, 1995a.

Reiss AL, Mazzocco MMM, Greenlaw R, et al: Neurodevelopmental effects of X monosomy: a volumetric imaging study. Ann Neurol 38:731, 1995b.

Rosenfeld RG, Grumbach MM (eds): Turner Syndrome. New York, Marcel Dekker, 1990.

Sobesky WE, Taylor AK, Pennington BF, et al: Molecular/clinical correlations in females with fragile X syndrome. Am J Med Genet 64:340, 1996.

Sujansky E, Smith ACM, Peakman DC, et al: Familial pericentric inversion of chromosome 8. Am J Med Genet 10:229, 1981.

Udwin O, Dennis J: Psychological and behavioral phenotypes in genetically determined syndromes: a review of research findings. *In* Obrien G, Yule W (eds): Behavioural Phenotypes. London, MacKeith Press, 1995, pp 90–208.

Verkerk AJ, Pieretti M, Sutcliffe JS, et al: Identification of a gene (FMR-1) containing a CGG repeat coincident with a breakpoint cluster region exhibiting length variation in fragile X syndrome. Cell 65:905, 1991.

Wang PP, Doherty S, Rourke SB, Bellugi U: Unique profile of visuoperceptual skills in a genetic syndrome. Brain Cognition 29:54, 1995.

Winter SD: Androgen therapy in Klinefelter syndrome during adolescence. Birth Defects 26:235, 1991.

24 Down Syndrome: Care of the Child and Family

William I. Cohen

Health care for the child with Down syndrome combines standard well-child care protocols, awareness and detection of specific medical situations that occur with greater frequency, and screening protocols to prevent secondary conditions.

In one recent study, more than 64% of children between the ages of 2 months and 3 1/2 years had evidence of hearing loss—conductive, sensorineural, or mixed.

There is significant risk to children for cord compression at the time of surgery (especially for ear, nose, and throat procedures) and with anesthesia in general (related to neck manipulation).

In the current decade, individuals with special needs are being educated in inclusive settings, that is, in regular education classes alongside their age-mates.

Down syndrome (DS) is the most common genetic disorder causing mental retardation. This discussion of its diagnosis and management serves the dual purpose of reminding the clinician of the important features of this condition and providing a model for the management of other developmental disabilities, combining a comprehensive understanding of the biological disorder and an appreciation of how the parents, extended family, and community respond to the child and his or her unique needs (Fig. 24–1).

The first clinical identification of the disorder was given by John Langdon Down in 1865. In 1959 Jerome LeJeune discovered the presence of an extra chromosome 21 (trisomy 21) in individuals who fit Down's description. DS occurs in 1 of 800 live births, or 1 of 1000 conceptions. The higher rate for conceptions reflects the fact that one of four spontaneous abortions are of fetuses with trisomies of various kinds.

Genetics

Three different chromosomal abnormalities are associated with individuals who have the phenotypic appearance of DS: translocations, mosaicism, and trisomy 21.

Ninety-five percent of individuals with the physical appearance of DS have *trisomy 21*, which is the presence of an extra chromosome 21 produced by nondisjunction. In this situation, the chromosomes fail to pair or fail to exchange genetic material, or both. These events usually occur at the first meiotic division, although they can occur at the second meiotic division. Most often the extra chromosome is of maternal origin, but paternal origin occurs as well. In one study of infants with trisomy 21, 7% received the extra chromosomal material from their fathers. Nondisjunction occurs sporadically in individuals of all ages, but the association of increasing maternal age with

trisomy reflects a well-known age-related increase in meiosis I nondisjunction. At maternal age of 35 years, the risk is approximately 1 in 250. By the age of 48 years, the risk of trisomy 21 is 1 in 11. The recurrence rate for trisomy 21 is reported to be 1%.

This association, however, has been the cause of some confusion. Most babies with DS are born to mothers younger than 35 years. Women 35 years and older account for only about 7% of births overall each year and approximately 20% to 25% of babies with DS. Consequently, the other 75% to 80% are born to younger women.

Of individuals with DS, 3% to 4% have a *translocation*, with the extra chromosomal material "stuck" to another chromosome. The extra chromosome 21 is commonly attached to chromosome 14 or 21. Half of the translocations occur de novo and have a low risk of recurrence in subsequent pregnancies. The other half, however, are inherited from a normal parent with a balanced translocation. In the families of children with DS of the latter pattern, there is a high risk of recurrence in subsequent pregnancies. Therefore, parents of children with translocations should be offered a karyotype if they wish to be able to predict the risk of recurrence in subsequent pregnancies.

Mosaicism, in which only some of cells in the body have the extra chromosome, occurs in 1% to 2% of children. This usually represents nondisjunction in an early postzygotic mitosis, and the effect of having some tissues in the body with an extra chromosome 21 varies with the time of the event. The greater the proportion of tissues with an extra chromosome 21, the greater likelihood that the individual will have the characteristic DS phenotype. On the other hand, individuals with only a small proportion of tissues affected may never be detected, since they would be unlikely to be karyotyped.

Mosaic forms of DS appear to cause much confusion to both the families and physicians, who often assume that children with mosaicism have a milder form of DS. This

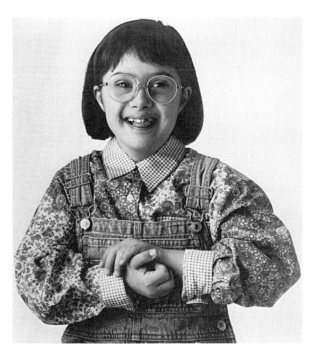

Figure 24–1. Katie, then 10 years old and a third-grade student in a regular class. At that time she wanted to become a doctor, but now, at 14 years, she wishes to be a singer. Katie studies ballet and has won a gold medal in Special Olympics for figure skating.

statement is partially correct: depending on the tissues involved, an individual who has some cell lines with an extra chromosome 21 may be indistinguishable from the typical child. However, most children with mosaicism and the full phenotypic expression of DS will show the typical characteristics of this disorder. On the other hand, children with subtle physical features of DS or with minimal developmental delay are sometimes thought by their physicians to have mosaic DS, even when their karyotype is consistent with trisomy 21. This reflects the fundamental nature of any syndrome: a varying collection of findings that together lead to a common diagnosis. The confusion seems to stem from a failure to realize the enormous biological variability (the full spectrum) of trisomy 21: from significant hypotonia requiring assistance in feeding at birth to normal muscle tone; from significant development delay to mild variations in learning styles.

In current practice, definitive prenatal testing for DS (via amniocentesis or chorionic villus sampling) is recommended for women 35 years of age and older. Screening tests, such as maternal serum alpha-fetoprotein, widely used to detect neural tube defects, may under certain specific circumstances suggest the likelihood of DS in a fetus. Unfortunately, many parents and not a few obstetricians have mistaken this as a definitive test for DS. It has been demonstrated that measurement of maternal serum alpha-fetoprotein, unconjugated estriol, and human chorionic gonadotropin, correlated with gestational age, will provide suggestive risk information about 60% of fetuses with DS with a 6.7% false positive rate. Unfortunately, in the absence of specific counseling, the 30% of women carrying a fetus with DS may interpret the statement that "the test was negative for DS" to mean that definitive testing had

been done. Medical geneticists and genetic counselors can provide a wealth of information on age-adjusted risk, screening, and prenatal testing methods. In addition to amniocentesis, which is usually performed at 16 weeks' gestation and has a 0.5% risk of spontaneous abortion, chorionic villus sampling is now available. This test can be done at 9 to 12 weeks' gestation and has a risk of spontaneous abortion that, though somewhat higher, is close to that of amniocentesis. Genetic counselors are trained to provide information that allows parents to make the best decision possible. Other sources of information include local DS clinics and parent groups. These should be kept in mind as options for the pediatrician who finds himself or herself counseling parents (Stein, 1997).

Making the Diagnosis in the Newborn Period

The diagnosis of DS is first suggested by a variety of physical characteristics that together indicate the probability of this diagnosis. The facial appearance of the child is often the first clue: flat profile, upslanted palpebral fissures, epicanthal folds, flat nasal bridge, small auricles (external ears), nuchal fat pad, short head (brachycephaly). In reality, babies born vaginally often have edema of the face and eyelids, making it more difficult to notice the eye findings. On the other hand, central hypotonia, manifested as poor muscle tone, may make the diagnosis easier, whereas relatively normal tone will confound the picture. Many clinicians have learned one or two findings that they invariably associate with DS. A single palmar crease seems to be one of the most commonly considered, and the absence of this finding may cause doubt about the clinical diagnosis. Interestingly, this finding, which also occurs in the general population, occurs in only 50% of individuals with DS. On the other hand, a wide gap between the first and second toes occurs in approximately 95%.

The only way to make the diagnosis definitively is to carry out a chromosomal karyotype. In some hospital laboratories, the preliminary results may be ready within 48 hours. Ordinarily, the results take up to 2 weeks, even longer if they are sent out to a commercial laboratory. A physician or nurse in the delivery room who suspects that an infant has DS can do a great service to the family by obtaining a heparinized sample of cord blood that can subsequently be sent to the cytogenetics laboratory if the clinical suspicion is strong enough.

Informing the Family

The challenge that next arises is how and when to communicate the physician's concerns to the family. We are fortunate that much investigation has been accomplished on this subject, for disabilities and congenital malformations in general and for DS in particular (Cooley and Graham, 1991; Cunningham, Morgan, and McGucken, 1984; Holan and Cohen, 1992). Most of the published studies report parents' perceptions of the informing interview. The interaction between the physician and the family can be complex and subtle.

Parents want to be told by someone who is positive and knowledgeable. However, despite the incidence of DS, most practitioners are likely to have had limited experience with children with developmental disabilities, including DS. This may lead the physician to speak more out of personal experience than from current information. Most of our opinions and beliefs reflect what we have learned in training or in the course of our years in practice. It is both unfortunate and true that physicians trained some time ago may advise families to place the child for adoption or even to seek residential programs for the baby. On the other hand, physicians trained more recently often have had exposure to families of individuals with DS and other developmental disabilities and have been able to appreciate the societal changes that have occurred over the last 20 years leading to the appreciation of the value of all individuals.

If DS is suspected in the newborn period, the practitioner should explain his or her concerns to the parents as soon as possible. A karyotype (chromosomal analysis) will confirm or deny the suspicions. Parents sense when doctors and nurses have a secret. The diagnosis need *not* be certain. In fact, this lack of certainty often gives families an opportunity to consider the possibility while maintaining hope. The unexpected birth of a baby with DS deprives the family of the normal child they had hoped for and imagined. The time it takes to get the karyotype results from the laboratory is often helpful to ease the shock.

DILEMMAS FOR PHYSICIAN IN INFORMING

None of us wish to cause distress to the families of our patients, and yet there is little doubt that breaking this news can cause significant emotional distress—feelings that are experienced by both the parents and the physician. As the parents react to the discovery that their child is not the one that they expected, the physician is responding to the fact that he or she directly caused the parents' upset. Our intellectual certainty of the diagnosis may waver in view of our desire to avoid facing the grief of a new family. Some clinicians try to avoid discussing the issue and seek a genetic consultation. Others rely heavily on positive forecasts for the future of this child: "Things have never been better for children with DS." Others who suspect the diagnosis and are not certain may choose to wait for a few weeks. As we find a way to tolerate our own sense of bewilderment, we are challenged to acknowledge the emotions of the parents: "I can understand why you're feeling this way."

Medical Conditions in Down Syndrome and Health Care Guidelines

Health care for the child with DS combines (1) standard well-child care protocols, as described by the American Academy of Pediatrics; (2) awareness and detection of specific medical situations that occur in greater frequency; and (3) specific screening protocols to prevent secondary conditions. This is particularly true of those occurrences that can exacerbate a developmental problem attributable to the underlying disorder itself. For example, children with DS generally have delays in acquiring verbal language. They also are at greater risk for hearing loss. The clinician who attributes the delay in spoken language to the general developmental disabilities of DS and fails to detect and treat or habilitate this hearing loss will further compromise the achievement of language function. What follows is a systematic review of health concerns in individuals with DS.

Cardiovascular Disorders. The incidence of congenital heart disease has been estimated at 46% to 62% in individuals with DS. The most commonly occurring conditions are atrioventricular septal defect (previously called endocardial cushion defect), ventricular septal defect, atrial septal defect, and tetralogy of Fallot. The only reliable way of detecting the presence of structural abnormalities is echocardiography. A serious cardiac defect may be present in the absence of a murmur. Children with DS are likely to develop early increased pulmonary vascular resistance that reduces the left to right intracardiac shunt, minimizes the heart murmur, and prevents symptoms of heart failure and respiratory problems. Children with DS who have a significant cardiac defect, and who in the first 6 months of life seem to be doing clinically well or getting better, may actually be developing serious pulmonary vascular changes. Timely surgery, frequently during the first 8 months of life, may be necessary. Infants should have an evaluation before 3 months of age by a pediatric cardiologist and this should include an echocardiogram.

Gastrointestinal Disorders. Congenital gastrointestinal malformations such as duodenal atresia and imperforate anus occur in approximately 5% of children with DS. Vomiting and the inability to pass stool in the first 12 hours of life warrant immediate investigation. (Interestingly, the diagnosis of intestinal obstruction may be the first clue to the diagnosis of DS. Likewise, the prenatal ultrasonographic findings of a "double bubble" may suggest the diagnosis in utero.) These conditions are rarely occult, and the obvious need for intervention makes it impossible to overlook. Hirschsprung disease is 25 times more likely to occur in individuals with DS than in the typical child. Failure to pass meconium in the first 24 hours of life may be the initial sign of this condition. Severe constipation in infancy is an indication for evaluation for Hirschsprung disease because of the high mortality associated with enterocolitis. Chronic constipation is reported in 30% of individuals with DS. It is often successfully treated with stool softeners, such as Karo syrup or Maltsupex. Failure to respond should suggest further evaluation for Hirschsprung disease or hypothyroidism. Celiac disease (gluten enteropathy) has been estimated to occur in 7% of children with DS, most likely on an autoimmune basis. Failure to thrive and symptoms of vomiting and diarrhea should lead to an evaluation by a pediatric gastroenterologist.

Ophthalmologic Difficulties. It is important to check for optimal visual function in children with DS. Cataracts are estimated to occur in 11% to 46% of individuals with

DS. There are a variety of types, which range from minor and visually insignificant to those that seriously impair vision. Dense congenital cataracts occur more frequently in individuals with DS than in the general population. The absence of a red reflex on fundoscopic examination is an indication for emergent ophthalmologic referral. Cataract extraction is critical because amblyopia (loss of vision) can occur rapidly, within 7 days in children less than 1 year of age. Children with DS have an increased incidence of strabismus, nasolacrimal duct stenosis, and nystagmus. The detection of these conditions warrants timely referral. Because refractive errors occur in 50% of children with DS, they should regularly be referred for pediatric ophthalmologic evaluation by 6 to 12 months of age, even in the absence of obvious ocular pathology.

Audiologic and Ear, Nose, and Throat Abnormalities. DS is considered a condition with high risk for hearing loss, and according to the Joint Committee on Infant Hearing, children with DS should be screened between 3 and 6 months of age. In one recent study, over 64% of children from the ages of 2 months to 3 1/2 years had evidence of hearing loss—conductive, sensorineural, or mixed (Roizen et al, 1992). The developmental disabilities of children with DS make it particularly difficult to use subjective measures in children under 12 months of age. Therefore, an objective measure, such as auditory brainstem response testing or evoked otoacoustic emission testing, is necessary.

DS is characterized by midfacial hypoplasia. Most of the airways and passages are narrower than in typical children. This predisposes children with DS to a variety of infections, such as otitis media and recurrent croup. Eustachian tube dysfunction is common. Furthermore, stenotic external auditory canals make visualization of the tympanic membranes difficult, if not impossible, and consultation with an otolaryngologist may be necessary. Serous otitis media occurs frequently and often requires vigorous treatment (antibiotics or tympanostomy tube placement or both) to address associated conductive hearing loss. Purulent nasopharyngitis or sinusitis is common and usually requires antibiotic treatment. Prophylactic use of antibiotics may be considered for the child who has recurrent infections throughout the winter months.

The narrow nasopharyngeal and oropharyngeal airways can be obstructed with adenoidal and tonsillar tissue. Furthermore, hypotonia and collapse of the airway can lead to obstructive upper airway problems. When a story consistent with sleep apnea is described, intervention is clearly indicated. However, some children do not snore, but rather are particularly restless sleepers. They may wake themselves up many times during the night when they experience obstruction or hypoxemia. These children may present with irritability and hyperactivity because of sleep deprivation. Careful questioning will indicate the need for further evaluation by otolaryngology or pulmonology services.

Infectious Disease. In addition to ear, nose, and throat infections, some individuals with DS have been shown to have deficiencies of cellular and humoral immunity. The most clinically relevant condition is a deficiency of immunoglobulin G subclasses 2 and 4 in the presence of normal total immunoglobulin G. Children with repeated serious pyogenic infections, such as pneumonia, should have quantitative immunoglobulins measured and be considered for intravenous immunoglobulin treatment (Ferrante et al, 1991; Loh et al, 1990). In addition to the usual complement of immunizations, the physician should consider adding influenza and pneumococcal vaccinations.

Hematologic Disorders. Children with DS account for 2% of all instances of acute childhood leukemia. There is a 10- to 30-fold increased incidence of leukemia in DS over typical children. Most of the children under 3 years of age get nonlymphocytic leukemia, which is most often megakaryocytic. In children older than 3 years of age, only 20% of leukemias are nonlymphocytic; the rest are lymphocytic. An unusual, severe, transient myelodysplastic syndrome is seen in some newborn children with DS. This disorder, also called transient leukemia or leukemoid reaction, is characterized by elevated peripheral leukocyte count and predominance of megakaryoblasts. In the majority of these children, the condition resolves by 2 to 3 months without treatment; however, 20% of these children develop nonlymphocytic leukemia several years later.

Endocrine Disorders. Congenital hypothyroidism has been reported to occur 27 times more frequently than in the typical population, so that diligent attention to the results of newborn screening is mandatory. Any concerns, such as an equivocal test or a lost screening, should prompt a repeat laboratory evaluation with a measurement of serum thyroid-stimulating hormone. In addition, acquired hypothyroidism occurs with increased frequency in children and adults with DS, finally reaching between 14% and 20%, depending on the series. The diagnosis is frequently autoimmune thyroiditis; investigation of elevated thyroid-stimulating hormone levels should therefore include thyroid antibodies. Early diagnosis and treatment are indicated to promote optimal physical growth and learning. Other autoimmune endocrinopathies, such as juvenile diabetes mellitus, occur with greater frequency.

Musculoskeletal Conditions. The central hypotonia of DS that is often noted at birth can interfere with the establishment of successful feeding. This can be particularly difficult for those mothers who wish to nurse their babies. Fortunately lactation specialists can provide specific techniques to overcome these difficulties.

Poor muscle tone and ligamentous laxity is a common feature of DS. Children often show remarkable flexibility of the hips. This ligamentous difference has been of significant interest regarding the craniocerebral junction, where it causes atlantoaxial instability (i.e., at the first and second cervical vertebrae). Fifteen percent of the population of individuals with DS have greater than 5.0 mm of space between the posterior arch of the atlas and the odontoid process. This condition has been called *asymptomatic atlantoaxial instability* (AAI). Approximately 2% of individuals with DS have neurologic signs consistent with spinal cord compression. Most of these individuals have greater than 7.5 mm of space.

Concern that asymptomatic AAI may predispose individuals with DS to develop symptomatic AAI led to the recommendation by Special Olympics to require those participants with DS to have lateral cervical spine radiographs (in flexion, neutral, and extension positions). Individuals found to have asymptomatic AAI are forbidden to participate in activities that put them at theoretical risk of injury (e.g., contact sports, diving, tumbling). This recommendation has been generalized to all children with DS aged 3 years and older. Current practice recommends re-examining the child at 12 years and 18 years.

In July 1995, a subject review by the Committee on Sports Medicine and Fitness of the American Academy of Pediatrics once again raised concerns about this issue. The committee concluded that the current screening is a poor method and that the frequency of the disorder is low. More importantly, most individuals are symptomatic before cord catastrophes occur. However, since the Special Olympics has no plans to remove the requirement that all athletes with DS receive radiographs of the cervical spine, the committee closed its review with the call for a multicenter study to document the true incidence of AAI, and the development of a more appropriate screening mechanism to prevent sports injury.

Pediatric anesthesiologists are aware that neck manipulation during induction of anesthesia and especially during otolaryngologic procedures puts children at risk for cord compression, and they usually take appropriate precautions (Litman, Zerngast, and Perkins, 1995; Mitchell, Howard, and Facer, 1995).

Growth and Development. Children with DS grow at a slower rate than typical children. The mechanism is multifactorial, including metabolic and endocrine abnormalities related to the presence of extra genetic material, and the growth retardation begins prenatally. The growth of children with DS should be plotted on DS-specific growth charts, which exist for both boys and girls from birth to 18 years of age. Growth charts for head circumference are available up to age 36 months. Most children with DS produce sufficient growth hormone. DS children with growth hormone deficiency cross percentile lines on the DS growth charts.

Most children with DS have mild to moderate mental retardation. They have delays in all areas of development: gross and fine motor, cognitive, language, and personal-social. There is one important distinction: in general, expressive (verbal) language abilities are more delayed than cognitive and receptive language.

Children with DS from birth to 3 years of age are eligible for Early Intervention services. This partially federally funded program provides a range of developmental services, carried out by child development specialists, occupational therapists, physical therapists, and speech-language pathologists. We encourage teaching children some elements of sign language to overcome problems in verbal expression and to improve communication in general. Learning sign language does not interfere with the subsequent development of spoken language. Interestingly, adolescents with DS show continued verbal language development. Nevertheless, a few children do not develop appreciable verbal expressive language, and they should be considered as candidates for augmentive communication devices.

Most new parents have no frame of reference to understand what mental retardation or developmental delay means. They may believe that the child may never walk or talk or be toilet trained. The use of information such as that given in Tables 24–1 and 24–2 can be very comforting to parents.

Table 24–1 • Developmental Milestones

	Children With Down Syndrome		"Normal" Children	
Milestone	Average (months)	Range (months)	Average (months)	Range (months)
Smiling	2	1½–4	1	½–3
Rolling over	8	4–22	5	2–10
Sitting alone	10	6–28	7	5–9
Crawling	12	7–21	8	6–11
Creeping	15	9–27	10	7–13
Talking, words	16	9–31	10	6–14
Standing	20	11–42	11	8–16
Walking	24	12–65	13	8–18
Talking, phrases	28	18–96	21	14–32

From Pueschel SM (ed): Down Syndrome: Growing and Learning. Kansas City, Andrews, McMeel & Parker, 1978.

After the child has reached 3 years of age, services are provided by local school districts. Individuals with disabilities are eligible for educational programming at least through the age of 21 (see Educational Issues).

The Health Care Guidelines for Individuals With Down Syndrome

In 1981, Mary Coleman published the first compilation of recommendations designed to ensure optimal health and well-being for individuals with DS. Originally named the "Preventive Medical Checklist," these recommendations have evolved over the last 15 years. The most recent version, published in the journal *Down Syndrome Quarterly* in June 1996, was renamed "Health Care Guidelines for Individuals with Down Syndrome," reflecting its expanded content, as it addresses developmental, adaptational, and social aspects of caring for individuals of all ages with DS (Cohen, 1996). The Guidelines are revised by members of the Down Syndrome Medical Interest Group (DSMIG), an ad hoc organization of medical professionals and other interested parties who provide clinical services to individuals with DS. The Guidelines are designed to be distributed

Table 24–2 • Self-help Skills

	Children With Down Syndrome		"Normal" Children	
Skill	Average (months)	Range (months)	Average (months)	Range (months)
Eating				
Finger-feeding	12	8–28	8	6–16
Using spoon/fork	20	12–40	13	8–20
Toilet training				
Bowel	42	28–90	29	16–48
Bladder	48	20–95	32	18–60
Dressing				
Undressing	40	29–72	32	22–42
Putting clothes on	58	38–98	47	34–58

Table 24–3 • Health Care in the Newborn
Period for Children With Down Syndrome

Establish the diagnosis: karyotype
    Offer genetic counseling to parents
Examine for serious medical problems
    Gastrointestinal malformations
        Intestinal obstruction
    Congenital cataracts
        Look for red reflex
    Cardiac disease
        Echocardiography
Be alert to feeding problems
    Involve feeding or lactation specialists, if needed
Check results of thyroid screen to detect congenital hypothyroidism
Use specific growth charts for children with Down syndrome
Refer for early intervention services
Discuss family support
    Individual parent-to-parent contact, support groups, community and family support

Table 24–5 • Health Care for Children 1 to 12
Years Old With Down Syndrome

Thyroid function testing (thyroid-stimulating hormone and thyroxine)
    annually
Periodic vision evaluations: every 2 years, or as recommended by vision
    professional
Periodic hearing evaluations: yearly until age 3; then every 2 years
Regular dental evaluations, starting at age 2 years
Radiologic screening for atlantoaxial instability at ages 3 to 4 years and
    12 years
Assess for obstructive sleep apnea and other disorders

widely to parents and professionals, to be used in a partnership to provide care to individuals of all ages. DSMIG believes that these preventive services can be offered by the primary care physician. Other resources include developmental-behavioral pediatricians, medical geneticists, and specialized Down syndrome centers or clinics. A current list of these centers is available on the World Wide Web (see Internet References). Tables 24–3 through 24–6 summarize the recommendations for children from birth to age 18 years.

Educational Issues

Most children with DS are eligible for special education services, under federal Public Laws 94–142 (passed in 1975) and 99–457 (1986), renewed in 1997 as PL 105–17. In the not-too-distant past, most children with special needs were educated in special classes, sometimes, but not always, located in neighborhood schools. In the current decade, individuals with special needs have been educated in inclusive settings, that is, in regular education classes, alongside their age-mates. This has been accomplished by providing supportive services within the regular education

setting, through a combination of assistive personnel to the pupil and support for the instructional staff from an inclusion specialist. The spread of this form of educational programming reflects the efforts of the parents of these children who realized that their children participated in the community alongside typical children in all activities except schooling. In addition to providing role models for the children with special needs, this method of education has an enormous benefit in leveling differences between the typical children and those with special needs. If we believe that the goal of education is to prepare all individuals to function in our communities, it makes sense that we begin the process of integration earlier rather than later in the life of the individual.

Alternative Therapies

Over the years, a large number of controversial treatments have been proposed for individuals with DS. Often the claims made in support of such regimens are similar: that it will result in improved intellectual function, alter physical or facial appearance, decrease infections, and generally improve the well-being of the child. Analogous claims are

Table 24–4 • Health Care for Infants 2 to
12 Months Old With Down Syndrome

Perform established well-child care protocols
Use specific growth charts for children with Down syndrome
Refer for objective hearing evaluation by 6 months of age (auditory
    brainstem response test or evoked otoacoustic emissions test)
Refer for ophthalmologic evaluation by 6 months of age
Monitor for history of otitis media and upper respiratory infections
    Refer to otolaryngologist as needed
Inquire about constipation
    Consider the diagnosis of Hirschsprung disease in severe situations
        that do not respond to dietary interventions
Discuss developmental progress
    Refer for early intervention if child is not receiving services
Discuss family support

Table 24–6 • Health Care for Adolescents
With Down Syndrome

Thyroid function testing (thyroid-stimulating hormone and thyroxine)
    annually
Periodic vision and hearing evaluations
Regular dental evaluations
Radiologic screening for atlantoaxial instability at 18 years
Assess for obstructive sleep apnea and other disorders
Provide educational information about sexuality, especially abuse
    prevention
Sexually active teenage girls should have a pelvic examination by an
    experienced practitioner (adolescent medicine physician or
    gynecologist with experience dealing with individuals with
    developmental disabilities)*

*Sexually active women should have a cytologic screening (Pap smear) every 1 to 3 years, starting at the age of first intercourse. Those women who are not sexually active should have a single-finger "bimanual" examination with a finger-directed cytologic screening every 1 to 3 years. Transabdominal pelvic ultrasonographic screening should be performed every 2 to 3 years for women who have a baseline bimanual examination but refuse to have or have inadequate follow-up bimanual examinations of adnexa and uterus.
From Cohen WI (ed): Health care guidelines for individuals with Down syndrome. Down Synd Q 1:1, 1996.

currently being made for other untested therapies purported to cure autism and other developmental disorders (see Chapters 60 and 84).

Interventions such as patterning and chiropractic manipulation have had varying popularity. Sicca cell treatment (also called fetal cell therapy) consists of injections of freeze-dried fetal animal cells and has not been shown to be of any benefit. It also has potential side effects of allergic reactions and the risk of the transmission of slow virus infections.

Nutritional supplements, including vitamins, minerals, amino acids, enzymes, and hormones in various combinations, represent one form of intervention, and these treatments have had a long history. A number of earlier well-controlled scientific studies failed to show any benefit from megadoses of vitamins. Neverthelsss, there has been a recent resurgence of interest in nutritional mixtures, featuring especially the provision of antioxidant materials.

There is also interest in piracetam, a drug that is classified as a cerebral stimulant or noötropic. It has been tried in adults with Alzheimer disease without any benefit and has been shown to improve the reading abilities of typical boys with dyslexia. However, piracetam is not approved by the Federal Drug Administration for use in the United States, and there have been no published scientific studies reporting its use in children with Down syndrome. The recommendation to use piracetam in newborns has been a source of concern to clinicians, although to date there have been no substantial reports of adverse effects, either of the nutritional regimen or of this noötropic drug.

Some parents decide that they wish to proceed with newer treatments and merely inform the physician of their decision. They do not look to the primary care provider for approval. Other parents are skeptical but ask the physician because they do not wish to miss something that could be helpful. These parents seem to understand that in the absence of controlled studies, it is not possible to give approval for or recommend these treatments. A third group presses for the physician's approval. When these parents sense a lack of enthusiastic support they are disappointed and question why the necessary studies have not been organized to demonstrate what has been reported anecdotally. The striving of these families to better their child's future is a challenge to conventional care providers. Maintaining a trusting, collaborative relationship with the family allows respect for the family's intent and simultaneously honors the status of scientific knowledge.

Issues for Adolescents

Parents and health care providers are often startled by the discovery that the adorable little children who needed love and protection have now grown into adolescents and young adults with mature bodies and with interests in members of the opposite sex. Unfortunately, failing to anticipate this inevitable progression can invite disaster. Therefore, early and frequent discussion about social-sexual training will help families recognize and advocate for appropriate educational programming within their schools. We must be mindful that the training provided for children should focus on

the kind of life we would like them to have as adults: independent, safe from sexual exploitation and maltreatment, with companionship needs met, and aware of the rules of society (Edwards and Elkins, 1988).

Caring for Families of Children With Down Syndrome

The tremendous societal change in attitudes toward individuals with disabilities has created a sense of positive expectation that continues to challenge what used to be minimal expectations. The celebrity of Chris Burke, who played the role of Corky on the television program *Life Goes On,* is but one example of the way in which thinking about DS has changed. Inclusive educational programs and participation in community activities such as scouting and camping have likewise helped develop a positive sense of expectancy.

Ironically, the positive imagery from media and local and national organizations that may buoy one family's flagging spirits may inadvertently cause anxiety in another. Children with DS, like those with every other biological disorder, have a spectrum of abilities and behavioral characteristics. There are indeed those who function in the severe to profound range of mental retardation. There are children with significant neurobehavioral disorders such as attention-deficit hyperactivity disorder and autism, which make them difficult to manage, despite expert pediatric and subspecialty care. There can be great emotional stress in having a child with a chronic condition, for which the family must anticipate future living arrangements, protection from maltreatment, and financial security. The extraordinary sense of optimism expressed by the aforementioned sources may leave little room for parents to be able to openly complain about how trying it is to raise a child with special needs. Our enthusiasm can blind us to specific experiences of individual families. Parents may even experience notable competitive feelings. One couple reported: "We heard about another little girl with Down syndrome who was potty trained at 4 years of age. We were devastated. Our son is 4 and is barely interested. Then we found out that it took 6 months to train her, and we were relieved. It was amazing, we were competing against this child, and, what's more, we hadn't been given the whole story."

These parents had sought help in dealing with issues that were very distressing to them. Sam was a charming 4-year-old who was showing behaviors appropriate for a 2 1/2-year-old. However, on occasion, he would stare at his parents and not respond. Further questioning revealed that in the community and in his educational program, Sam was experiencing no difficulty whatsoever. The parents expressed great concern: "We know Sam will not be smart. It's clear that he is going to have to make his way in the world on the basis of his personality. And that's what really scares us. We're afraid that these misbehaviors he is having are going to really keep him from being successful." This fueled their fears for his future and resulted in their overly stern discipline. Obviously it is necessary to carefully look and listen for indicators that a family is experiencing distress. One must be mindful of the effect of the birth of a child with a developmental disorder on the marital equilibrium and on sisters and brothers. Doherty (personal communication, 1994) describes the dual process of "making a place for the disorder and putting the disorder in its place." An overly roseate approach may make it difficult for families to put the disorder in its place.

Down Syndrome as a Model for Developmental Disorder

The presence of persons with DS in our world has had multiple ramifications. The last 25 years has seen a proliferation of information about DS that appears to be directly related to societal changes, such as access to free and public education, the closing of public institutions for the care of persons with disabilities, and the advocacy of parents and organizations such as the Arc (formerly the Association for Retarded Citizens). These individuals refused to believe the dire predictions made for their babies: they dreamed of a future of broad possibilities. The initiative for the emergence of individuals with DS from the recesses of their family's homes sprang from the passionate commitment of those parents who never doubted that their children had a future in society, their physical, developmental, and behavioral features notwithstanding. Trusting their own intuition, parents such as Frank and Marian Burke, Emily and Charles Kingsley, and Barbara and Jack Levitz, among hosts of others, challenged the conventional wisdom of the day and devised programs of supportive services that were then enhanced and replaced by a variety of educational opportunities. And their children, Chris Burke, Jason Kingsley, and Mitchell Levitz, have now embarked on the next phase of this remarkable journey from despair to confidence. They serve as role models for youngsters with DS and provide visible proof that the possibilities open to our children may not be a fantasy if we choose to maintain hope, love, and support.

Indeed, these families, with the instrumental support of local and national parent organizations, including the two main organizations in the United States (the National Down Syndrome Congress and the National Down Syndrome Society), have helped spearhead the growth of a powerful partnership between consumers, on one hand, and the professional community of health care professionals, basic scientists, educators, therapists, and public policy advocates on the other. The advances in inclusive education, the founding of regional Down Syndrome Clinics and Centers, and the regional and national meetings for parents and professionals alike have given great impetus to both basic and applied research.

Conclusion

Children with DS provide a multifaceted opportunity to integrate our expertise about the medical, developmental, and emotional issues surrounding the diagnosis and management of a common condition. Our ability to minimize the impact of the medical aspects in the service of promoting maximal functional adaptation of the individual and optimal rewards for the family makes this endeavor both challenging and satisfying.

REFERENCES

Cohen WI (ed): Health care guidelines for individuals with Down syndrome. Down Synd Q 1:1, 1996.
Committee on Sports Medicine and Fitness (American Academy of Pediatrics): Atlantoaxial instability in Down syndrome: subject review. Pediatrics 96:151, 1995.
Cooley WC, Graham JM: Down syndrome: an update and review for the primary care physician. Clin Pediatr 30:233, 1991.
Cunningham CC, Morgan PA, McGucken RB: Down's syndrome: is dissatisfaction with disclosure of diagnosis inevitable? Dev Med Child Neurol, 26:33, 1984.
Edwards JP, Elkins TE: Just Between Us. Austin TX, Pro-Ed, 1988.
Ferrante A, Beard LJ, Thong Y, Vuddhakul V, Rowan-Kelly B, Goh D, Mai GT, Loh RKS, Harth SC, Pearson C, Roberton D: Immunodeficiency in Down's syndrome. In Imbach P (ed): Immunotherapy With Intravenous Immunoglobulins. London, Academic Press, 1991.
Holan JE, Cohen WI: Reflections on the informing process: "Why are these people angry with me?" Down Synd Papers Abstr Prof 15:4, 1992.
Litman RS, Zerngast B, Perkins FM: Preoperative evaluation of the cervical spine in children with trisomy-21: results of a questionnaire study. Paediatr Anaesth 5:355, 1995.
Loh RKS, Harth SC, Thong YH, Ferrante A: Immunoglobulin G subclass deficiency and predisposition to infection in Down's syndrome. Pediatr Infect Dis J 9:547, 1990.
Mitchell V, Howard R, Facer E: Down's syndrome and anaesthesia. Paediatr Anaesth 5:379, 1995.
Roizen NJ, Wolters C, Nicol T, Blondis T: Hearing loss in children with Down syndrome. Pediatr 123:S9, 1992.
Stein M (ed): Challenging case: responding to parental concerns after a prenatal diagnosis of trisomy 21. J Dev Behav Pediatr 18:42, 1997.

RESOURCES FOR PARENTS AND FAMILIES

Kingsley J, Levitz M: Count Us In: Growing Up With Down Syndrome. New York, Harvest Books, 1994.
McDaniel JB: A Special Kind of Hero: Chris Burke's Own Story. New York, Doubleday, 1991.
Stray-Gundersen K: Babies with Down Syndrome, 2nd ed. Bethesda, MD, Woodbine House, 1995.
Van Dyke DC, Mattheis P, Eberly SS, Williams J (eds): Medical and Surgical Care for Children with Down Syndrome: a Guide for Parents. Bethesda, MD, Woodbine House, 1995.

RESOURCES FOR PROFESSIONALS

Down Syndrome Quarterly is a multidisciplinary journal that began publication in 1996. For information about subscriptions, contact Samuel Thios, PhD, Editor-in-Chief, *Down Syndrome Quarterly*, Denison University, Granville, OH 43023.
Pueschel SM, Pueschel JK (eds): Biomedical Concerns in Persons with Down Syndrome. Baltimore, Paul Brookes, 1992.
The Down Syndrome Medical Interest Group (DSMIG) addresses aspects of the medical care of persons with Down syndrome. DSMIG wishes to promote the highest quality care for children and adults with DS by (1) fostering and providing professional and community education; (2) disseminating tools for clinical care and professional support, such as the Health Care Guidelines; and (3) engaging in collaborative clinical research of issues related to the care of individuals with Down syndrome. DSMIG schedules its meetings in conjunction with a variety of national organizations, such as the National Down Syndrome Congress (NDSC), the National Down Syndrome Society (NDSS), the American Association on Mental Retardation. For more information on DSMIG, contact William I. Cohen, MD, at Children's Hospital of Pittsburgh, 3705 Fifth Avenue, Pittsburgh, PA 15213, (412) 692-7963, email: cohenb@chplink.chp.edu.

INTERNET REFERENCES

Canadian Down Syndrome Society home page: http://home.ican.net/~cdss/index.html

Down Syndrome Clinics in the US home page: http://www.davlin.net/users/lleshin/clinics.htm

"Health Care Guidelines for Individuals with Down Syndrome" on the Down Syndrome Quarterly home page: http://webby.cc.denison.edu/dsq/

National Down Syndrome Congress home page: http://members.carol.net/ndsc/ Telephone: 1–800–232-NDSC

National Down Syndrome Society home page: http://www.ndss.org/ Telephone: 1–800–221–4602

25 Congenital Anomalies

Louanne Hudgins • Suzanne B. Cassidy

 Many congenital malformations can have more than one cause, often with different possible associated anomalies and different recurrence risks. Cleft lip and palate, for example, can be isolated or part of dozens of different syndromes and can be multifactorial, autosomal dominant, autosomal recessive, X-linked, chromosomal, or teratogenic in etiology.

Known teratogenic factors cause only 5% to 10% of congenital anomalies in spite of the ever-expanding list of potential teratogens in our increasingly chemical environment.

Routine chromosomal analysis is indicated in those individuals with ambiguous genitalia, two or more major anomalies, multiple minor anomalies, or growth or mental retardation in association with anomalies.

The Alliance of Genetic Support Groups, a national organization, serves as a resource to identify whether a designated consumer group exists for a specific condition and also lists more general associations.

Congenital anomalies, isolated or as part of syndromes, are a common cause of medical intervention, long-term illness, and death. They also have a major impact on families. Very frequently, congenital anomalies are accompanied by some degree of cognitive or behavioral dysfunction; therefore, the developmental pediatrician may be the first person to identify necessary evaluations and management and the first to have the opportunity to provide information for the parents about the cause and prognosis. Ideally the developmental pediatrician should be part of an interdisciplinary team that manages children with congenital anomalies to assess the whole child, not just the physical alteration and its consequences. It is thus important to recognize the etiology, associated problems, impact, and recurrence risks of these anomalies. This chapter reviews some of the significant etiologic and epidemiologic aspects of congenital anomalies and provides an approach to and framework for the evaluation of the child with congenital anomalies, with emphasis on those conditions that might be present in children evaluated by a developmental pediatrician.

Terminology

To ensure an understanding of the somewhat specialized terminology used in describing congenital anomalies, it is important to be familiar with terms in common use. Many people confuse the terms congenital and genetic. *Congenital* means present at birth and does not denote etiology. *Anomaly* is a structural defect that departs from the norm. A *major anomaly* is one that may require significant surgical or cosmetic intervention, or both, whereas a *minor anomaly* has no major surgical or cosmetic importance. Minor anomalies overlap with normal phenotypic variation

and are discussed later in this chapter. It is important to distinguish between a major and minor anomaly and a normal variant, because their implications are so different, both for the child and for the family.

One useful approach to identification of the etiology of a congenital anomaly is to consider whether it represents a *malformation, deformation*, or *disruption* (Spranger et al, 1982). A *malformation* is a primary structural defect in tissue formation, usually caused by abnormal development (morphogenesis) of the tissue for genetic or teratogenic reasons, such as a neural tube defect or congenital heart defect. *Deformations* result from abnormal mechanical forces, often related to intrauterine constraint, acting on normally developed tissues. Club feet or altered head shape is often due to deformation. Breech or other abnormal positioning in utero, oligohydramnios, and uterine anomalies are the most common causes of deformations. Observation of the position of comfort in early infancy, combined with a careful history of fetal movement, fetal position, and fluid volume, can be very helpful in identifying the anomaly as a deformation. *Disruptions* represent interruption of development of intrinsically normal tissue and often affect a body part rather than a specific organ. Vascular occlusion and amniotic bands are common causes of disruptions. Monozygotic twinning and prenatal cocaine exposure are common predisposing factors for disruptions on the basis of vascular interruption.

Disruptions and isolated deformations are most often sporadic, with negligible or low recurrence risks, and are unlikely to be associated with cognitive dysfunction. On the other hand, malformations may predispose to deformations, such as renal agenesis (a malformation) causing Potter sequence, in which facial and limb deformations and pulmonary hypoplasia result from oligohydramnios. A neural tube defect, also a malformation, predisposes to hip dislocation and club feet because of lack of movement below the level of the lesion.

Many congenital malformations can have more than one cause, often with different possible associated anomalies and different recurrence risks. Cleft lip and palate, for example, can be isolated or part of dozens of different syndromes and can be multifactorial, autosomal dominant, autosomal recessive, X-linked, chromosomal, or teratogenic in etiology (Gorlin, Cohen, and Levin, 1990).

If more than one anomaly is present in an individual, then one should consider whether it is part of a sequence, an association, or a syndrome, which have different implications for prognosis and recurrence risk. *Sequence* refers to a pattern of multiple anomalies arising from a single known or presumed cause. An example is the oligohydramnios sequence, often referred to as Potter syndrome, which consists of limb deformations; simple ears, a beaked nose, and infraorbital creases (Potter facies); and pulmonary hypoplasia. These features are seen when there is lack of amniotic fluid, be it secondary to chronic leakage of amniotic fluid or to lack of fetal urine (renal agenesis). The term *association* refers to a nonrandom occurrence of multiple malformations for which no specific or common etiology has been identified. An example is the VATER (or VACTERL) association, an acronym for a pattern of anomalies consisting of *v*ertebral abnormalities, *a*nal atresia, *c*ardiac anomalies, *t*racheo*e*sophageal fistula, and *r*adial (*l*imb) and renal dysplasia. Finally, the term *syndrome* refers to a recognized pattern of anomalies with a single specific etiology, such as Holt-Oram syndrome in which radial dysplasia and cardiac defects occur as a consequence of an autosomal dominant gene. For many syndromes, the etiology is unknown, although identification of the genetic basis of many syndromes has been rapidly occurring, in significant part as a result of the Human Genome Project.

Phenotype is the observable manifestation of *genotype*, that is, the genetic constitution of an individual. Therefore, when one speaks of the phenotypic features, reference is being made to the observable physical features present in that individual.

Epidemiology and Etiology

FREQUENCY AND ETIOLOGY OF MAJOR MALFORMATIONS

Approximately 2% of newborn infants have a serious anomaly that has surgical or cosmetic importance (Holmes, 1974; 1976). This figure is a minimum estimate, since it is based on examination of newborn infants only, and additional anomalies are detected with increasing age. The etiology of malformations can be divided into broad categories: genetic (multifactorial, single gene, chromosomal), teratogenic, and unknown. The terms *genetic* and *hereditary* are sometimes used interchangeably, but they are not truly identical. Genetic means determined by genes, whereas hereditary indicates transmission from parent to offspring. New gene mutations, for example, are genetic but not of hereditary origin.

Multifactorial

The largest number of congenital malformations (86%) are isolated (Holmes, 1974), and of this group the majority are believed to be the consequence of multifactorial inheritance involving the interaction of multiple genetic and environmental factors. The most common and familiar birth defects fall into this category, including congenital heart defects, neural tube defects, cleft lip and palate, club foot, and congenital hip dysplasia.

Single Gene (Mendelian)

Single major genes are responsible for causing 0.4% of newborns to have major malformations (Holmes, 1976). The most common mode of mendelian inheritance for major malformations is autosomal dominant, with a minority due to autosomal recessive or, more rarely, X-linked genes. Limb anomalies, including postaxial polydactyly, syndactyly, and brachydactyly, constitute the most prevalent major localized malformations and are frequently the result of a dominant gene. Any type of malformation, however, may be under the control of a single gene, including multiple anomalies arising in different structures or organ systems. Relatively little is understood about the biochemical defects underlying the production of malformations by mutant genes, although advances are being made. For example, Smith-Lemli-Opitz syndrome, characterized by mental retardation, genital abnormalities, syndactyly of the second and third toes, ptosis, and wide alveolar ridges, has been found to be associated with a defect in cholesterol biosynthesis. Although increasingly the biochemical or molecular basis is being recognized, specific diagnosis still relies heavily on the family history and clinical evaluation.

An excellent reference for all single gene conditions is *Mendelian Inheritance in Man* (McKusick, Francomano, and Antonarakis, 1994), which is also available online.

Chromosomal

About 0.2% of newborns have a major malformation as a result of a chromosomal disorder (see Chapters 23 and 24), and this amounts to 10% of all the major congenital malformations (Holmes, 1976). It is important to note, however, that approximately 0.6% of newborns have a noteworthy chromosomal anomaly, but 66% of these infants do not have any abnormalities detectable by physical examination at birth (Hook, 1982). Included among these early phenotypically undetectable chromosomal anomalies are common disorders of the sex chromosomes, such as 47,XXY, 47,XYY, and 47,XXX, conditions that might well be suspected first by the developmental pediatrician in the evaluation of cognitive or behavioral difficulties. The most prevalent malformation syndrome caused by an abnormal chromosomal constitution in newborns is Down syndrome, or trisomy 21, which occurs in about 1 in 800 births (see Chapter 24). The other relatively common trisomies are trisomy 18 and trisomy 13, occurring approximately once in 5000 to 10,000 and once in 10,000 to 20,000 births, respectively. All three trisomies are more frequent with increased maternal age. Other well-known chromosomal syndromes are Klinefelter syndrome, due to 47,XXY, occurring in 1 in 1000 male births, and Turner syndrome, due to 45,X or another X chromosome abnormality, present in 1 in 5000 female births. Many other types of chromosomal aberrations have been identified using chromosome banding techniques, including translocations, inversions, ring chromosomes, marker chromosomes, insertions, and deletions (Schinzel, 1983). Not all deletions are detectable by routine cytogenetic analysis, however. Fluorescence in situ hybridization (FISH) is a technique using fluorescently labeled DNA probes and chromosome metaphase spreads to identify microdeletions associated with such conditions as Prader-Willi syndrome (long arm of chromosome 15), Williams syndrome (long arm of chromosome 7), and velocardiofacial-DiGeorge syndrome (long arm of chromosome 22). This technique will undoubtedly continue to contribute to better definitive diagnosis for conditions involving multiple congenital anomalies caused by absence of a gene or genes.

EXAMPLE: VELOCARDIOFACIAL-DiGEORGE SYNDROME

Jane is a 4-year-old girl with mild developmental delay, particularly in speech, and her mother feels that she has a short attention span and is constantly in motion. She was noted to have a very nasal quality to her speech, which was diagnosed as being velopharyngeal incompetence due to a submucous cleft palate. Careful evaluation revealed that she had a long, straight nose with built-up sides and a bulbous tip, and horizontally small palpebral fissures (Fig. 25–1). A soft heart murmur was heard, and evaluation showed that she had a small ventricular septal defect. Jane's mother has similar facial features and also has a history of having had an interrupted aortic arch successfully repaired as an infant. Her mother has also had a diagnosis of schizoaffective disorder, which is well controlled with medication.

Jane underwent chromosome analysis, including evaluation with a FISH probe for deletion of chromosome 22q11. She was found to have this deletion, which con-

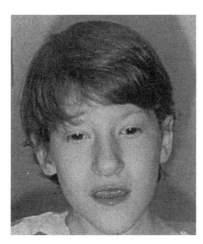

Figure 25–1. Velocardiofacial-DiGeorge syndrome. Characteristic facial features in velocardiofacial-DiGeorge syndrome include short, narrow palpebral fissures, long nose with prominent nasal bridge and/or nasal root, and bulbous nasal tip.

Table 25–1 • Causes of Human Malformations

Etiology	Frequency (%)
Genetic disorders	10–25
Teratogens	10
Maternal conditions	4
Infectious agents	3
Deformations and mechanical problems	1–2
Chemicals, drugs, radiation, hyperthermia	<1
Multifactorial and unknown	65–75

Data from Brent RL, Beckman DA: Prescribed drugs, therapeutic agents, and fetal teratogenesis. *In* Reece EA, Hobbins JC, Mahoney MJ, Petrie RH (eds): Medicine of the Fetus and Mother. Philadelphia, JB Lippincott, 1995.

firmed a diagnosis of velocardiofacial-DiGeorge syndrome. Evaluation of other family members revealed that her mother also had the deletion, as did Jane's now 3-month-old brother, in whom no abnormalities have yet been identified.

Because of this deletion, Jane, her mother, and her brother have a 50% risk with each child born to them that the child will have some abnormalities in the spectrum of velocardiofacial-DiGeorge syndrome, which can range from mild to severe and can include conotruncal cardiac defects, cleft palate and velopharyngeal incompetence, facial dysmorphism, immune deficiency, hypocalcemia, developmental disabilities, psychiatric problems, and a number of other less frequent abnormalities. Jane's siblings who do not have this deletion are at no increased risk for these anomalies. Prenatal detection is available.

Teratogenetic

A *teratogen* may be defined as anything external to the fetus that causes a structural or functional disability postnatally. Teratogens may be drugs and chemicals, altered metabolic states in the mother, infectious agents, or mechanical forces (Hoyme, 1990). Known teratogenic factors cause only 5% to 10% of congenital anomalies in spite of the ever-expanding list of potential teratogens in our increasingly chemical environment (Table 25–1). Before attributing malformations to a teratogenic agent, there must be one or only a few specific anomalies, or a recognizable pattern of anomalies, found to occur at increased incidence over the background risk in infants exposed at the appropriate developmental stage (usually 2 to 12 weeks' gestation). With only a few exceptions, teratogenic agents do not affect every exposed infant, which is probably related to genetic susceptibility factors. Dosage and timing of exposure also affect teratogenic potential.

Although many drugs may have teratogenic potential, some commonly used ones are worthy of some discussion. Alcohol is thought to be the most common teratogen to which a fetus may be exposed. Chronic maternal alcohol use during pregnancy is associated with increased perinatal mortality and intrauterine growth retardation, as well as congenital anomalies such as cardiac defects, microcephaly, short palpebral fissures, and other anomalies (Fig. 25–2). Long-term effects include mental retardation and behavioral problems. Alcohol carries serious risks when used at almost any time during pregnancy in sufficient quantities

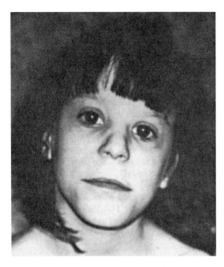

Figure 25–2. Fetal alcohol syndrome. This 8-year-old girl was born to a chronically alcoholic woman. She is mildly retarded and growth deficient with facial features typical of fetal alcohol syndrome (short palpebral fissures, flat nasal bridge with epicanthal folds, long smooth philtrum with thin upper lip). (From Graham JM, Jr: Manual for the Assessment of Fetal Alcohol Effects. Seattle, University of Washington Press, 1982.)

because the fetal central nervous system continues to develop throughout pregnancy. For this reason, it is recommended that women avoid alcohol, even in small amounts, throughout their pregnancy.

Anticonvulsants are a common category of teratogens to which a fetus is likely to be exposed. Fetal hydantoin syndrome is one well-recognized condition caused by an anticonvulsant drug (Fig. 25–3). Although the published medical evidence is somewhat controversial, clinical geneticists, dysmorphologists, and clinical teratologists generally identify a variable but recognizable pattern of anomalies and developmental defects that occur at significantly in-

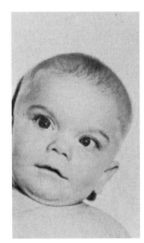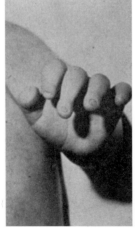

Figure 25–3. Fetal hydantoin syndrome. Facial features consistent with hydantoin exposure in utero include ocular hypertelorism, flat nasal bridge, and small upturned nose. The hands exhibit distal phalangeal hypoplasia with small nails. (From Jones KL: Smith's Recognizable Patterns of Human Malformation, 4th ed. Philadelphia, WB Saunders, 1988.)

creased frequency among fetuses exposed to all currently used anticonvulsants (Seaver and Hoyme, 1992).

Some altered metabolic states in the mother are also known to have teratogenic potential. One of the most common is maternal diabetes mellitus. Infants of diabetic mothers are at increased risk for congenital heart defects, sacral dysgenesis, and central nervous system abnormalities such as holoprosencephaly, as well as other anomalies. In this population, there is an approximately threefold increase in the risk for congenital anomalies over that of the general population. The risk for congenital anomalies seems to be lower in offspring of diabetic mothers who have better control of blood glucose, although this is not absolute and factors other than blood glucose levels are thought to play a role in teratogenesis.

Congenital anomalies may also be associated with certain infections during pregnancy. The most common and best understood infections are represented by the acronym TORCH, for *t*oxoplasmosis, *o*ther (including syphilis), *ru*bella, *c*ytomegalovirus, and *h*erpes. One should consider these congenital infections in individuals with intrauterine growth retardation, microcephaly, chorioretinitis, intracranial calcification, microphthalmia, cataracts, or any combination of these conditions. Confirmation of the specific diagnosis should be made by antibody studies and other evaluations such as ophthalmologic examination and imaging studies.

Mechanical forces may also be categorized as teratogens. Deformations, such as club feet, may develop because of intrauterine constraint secondary to mechanical forces such as uterine fibroids. Disruption of the amnion may also be associated with deformations as well as other limb anomalies.

Unknown

Approximately two of three major malformations have no recognized etiology, if one includes those of presumed polygenic and multifactorial etiology (see Table 25–1). It is likely that as our understanding of congenital anomalies increases, specific genetic and environmental causes will be identified. For example, in recent years, folic acid has been recognized to decrease the risk for neural tube defects, thus implicating folic acid deficiency in the etiology of the anomalies. Specific genes have been implicated in the multifactorial disorder Hirschsprung disease.

MINOR ANOMALIES AND PHENOTYPIC VARIANTS

Major malformations are often easy to identify. Minor anomalies, however, by their nature, are more subtle and may not be appreciated unless specifically sought. They are nevertheless significant for a number of reasons. First, they may be important as part of a characteristic pattern of malformations and thus may provide clues to a diagnosis. Second, their occurrence may be an indication of the presence of a more serious anomaly. In one large study of 4305 newborns, 19.6% of the 162 babies with major malformations had three or more minor anomalies. A single minor anomaly, on the other hand, is associated with a major malformation in only 3.7% of cases (Leppig et al, 1987).

Minor anomalies are most frequent in areas of complex and variable features, such as the face and distal extremities (Marden, Smith, and McDonald, 1964). Among the most common are lack of a helical fold of the pinna and complete or incomplete single transverse palmar crease patterns. Typical single transverse palmar crease (formerly called simian crease) occurs in almost 2% of normal newborns but appears in 45% of individuals with trisomy 21.

Among the most frequent phenotypic variants, defined as being present in 4% or more of the population, are an overfolded helix of the pinna and mongolian spots in African American and Asian children (Marden, Smith, and McDonald, 1964). Before attributing medical significance to an apparent minor anomaly or phenotypic variation, it is useful to determine whether it is present in other family members or whether it occurs frequently in that particular racial or ethnic group. It is common for isolated minor anomalies such as syndactyly of the second and third toes to be familial.

RACIAL DIFFERENCES

The prevalence of specific congenital malformations varies significantly between racial groups. This is most likely the consequence of differing genetic predispositions, as well as variable environmental factors operating in diverse areas. It is of interest that certain anomalies are especially common in a particular race, such as polydactyly in African American people and hypospadias and club foot in white people. Minor malformations may show an equally striking racial predisposition. Brushfield spots are common in white people but rare in African American people. Umbilical hernias, on the other hand, are common in African American infants but relatively infrequent in white infants. The widely varying frequencies of various traits in different races demonstrate that whether any given characteristic is considered a minor anomaly or a phenotypic variant may be strongly dependent on the race of the patient being studied. One of the best examples is mongolian spots, which occur in almost 50% of African American or Asian infants but in only 0.2% of white infants (Marden, Smith, and McDonald, 1964).

Evaluation of the Child With Congenital Anomalies

Every child with a congenital anomaly, as well as every child with a developmental abnormality, deserves a careful diagnostic evaluation. It is important to make an accurate diagnosis to identify the etiology of the anomaly so that the natural history of the condition as well as the recurrence risk for similarly affected future children can be determined.

When a child is identified as having one or more anomalies, a number of considerations should guide the physician in the evaluation. The most critical factors to be considered are the detailed *prenatal, medical, developmental*, and *family history*, the *dysmorphic physical examination* including careful observation and measurements of individual features, and the use of *appropriate diagnostic tests* and *evaluations*, particularly if there is more than one anomaly. It is essential to identify whether the malformation is *isolated* or part of a constellation of anomalies. This requires determination of whether there are other major or minor anomalies, including perhaps inapparent internal malformations, and the recognition of well-described *patterns of malformations*. Practice in such recognition, or consultation with others who have such expertise, may be required.

HISTORY

The evaluation of a child with congenital anomalies begins with a detailed history. The important goal is to attempt to identify a possible genetic predisposition, environmental factor, or other clue to the cause of the anomalies. It is useful to begin with the pregnancy and document fetal movement and vigor, complications, illnesses, maternal use of any medications, possible exposure to teratogens, and the timing of all complications and exposures. The extent of smoking and alcohol consumption should be determined, and every mother should be directly asked about illicit drug use.

Past medical history is also very important. The examiner should inquire about major medical problems requiring hospitalization, surgery, medication, or evaluation by a specialist. Medical records may be important in documenting the exact nature and extent of the problem.

A careful developmental history is always helpful and, whenever possible, formal evaluations should be used to document the degree and pattern of developmental delay or mental retardation. Atypical behavior should also be noted and may be helpful in the diagnosis. For instance, a child with Williams syndrome is likely to have relative sparing of expressive language skills, and an outgoing, friendly demeanor is common for this condition.

A careful three- to four-generation family history, charted in a concise manner in the form of a pedigree, should be constructed using squares for males and circles for females. Horizontal lines are used to indicate genetic union and vertical lines indicate genetic descent. All abortions and stillbirths should be noted. A question should always be specifically asked about possible consanguinity. A simple way to inquire is to ask if the affected child's parents are related in any way. If so, then the charting should indicate the exact relationship. The presence of other relatives with congenital anomalies of any type or with growth or developmental abnormalities should be recorded along with other pertinent information, such as the maternal and paternal ages. Family photographs are often very useful in clarifying questions of possible unusual facial features. The pedigree should, at a minimum, include all siblings and parents of the proband as well as aunts, uncles, cousins, and grandparents. In the case of possible dominant or X-linked disorders, a more extensive pedigree may be needed.

EXAMPLE: WILLIAMS SYNDROME

Jamie is a 4-year-old girl who was referred to the developmental clinic for evaluation of developmental delay and possible attention deficit disorder. The parents are also concerned about some of her unusual behaviors, such as being inappropriately friendly and talkative, even with total strangers, and expressing undue fearfulness and anxiety in new or stressful situations. Past history is significant for feeding difficulties in infancy that contributed to failure to thrive, surgical repair of bilateral inguinal hernias, and a ventricular septal defect that "closed on its own." On physical examination, the physician notes a small child with distinctive facial features, including periorbital fullness, bright blue irides with a stellate appearance to the iris, a small upturned nose with anteverted nares, a long philtrum, and a large mouth with full lips (Fig. 25–4).

Jamie's physical features and past medical history are compatible with a diagnosis of Williams syndrome. FISH using a probe for the elastin-Williams syndrome chromosome region showed hybridization of this probe to only one homologue of chromosome 7 in all cells examined, which confirmed this diagnosis.

This diagnosis is discussed with the family, and information from the Williams Syndrome Association is given to them, including material on the educational aspects. The parents state that this will be useful to the personnel at Jamie's preschool.

Williams syndrome is an autosomal dominant condition, but the majority of children represent de novo, or new, microdeletions. Because neither of the parents has findings suggestive of this condition, testing on them is not necessary and they are counseled that their recurrence risk is low. They are delighted, since they would like to have more children but feel that they could not handle another child with Jamie's behavioral and medical problems. Jamie, however, will have a 50% chance of passing on the microdeletion to each of her children, should she have any.

PHYSICAL EXAMINATION

The goal of the examination of a child with congenital anomalies is to determine whether the anomaly is isolated or to detect a recognizable pattern of malformations so that a specific etiologic diagnosis can be made. The usual physical examination forms the foundation for this assessment. In addition, careful attention must be directed not only to an exact description of the major anomalies but also to apparent minor anomalies or variations. Distinctive physical features may become clues in figuring out the puzzle of the child with multiple congenital anomalies. For the most part, this involves detailed inspection of various features of external anatomy and measurement, where appropriate. Objective description of anomalous features allows for accurate utilization of resources or consultants. In this section, an outline of the external examination is presented by region or structure and certain helpful points, as well as aspects of the differential diagnosis, are discussed. The reader is also referred to various resources in which the anomalies and syndromes mentioned in this section are discussed at length (Buyse, 1990; Gorlin, Cohen, and Levin, 1990; Jones, 1997; McKusick, Francomano, and Antonarakis, 1994; Stevenson, Hall, and Goodman, 1993).

Skin

A variety of lesions with altered pigmentation may provide useful clues to a diagnosis. Café au lait spots are characteristic of neurofibromatosis, which can be associated with learning difficulties. However, these hyperpigmented lesions can also occur in other conditions and may be isolated, especially in darkly pigmented individuals. Hypopigmented macules may be the earliest manifestation of tuberous sclerosis in the young child. Hypomelanosis of Ito, which can be associated with mosaicism for a chromosomal abnormality, is characterized by irregularly pigmented lesions.

Hair

The relative sparseness or prominence of body hair should be noted. Sparse hair is characteristic of an ectodermal dysplasia but occurs in other syndromes. "Kinky" hair is a characteristic finding in Menke syndrome. Generalized hirsutism is typical of Cornelia de Lange syndrome and the fetal hydantoin and alcohol syndromes but may also occur in trisomy 18. It also may be a racial (Hispanic, native American) or a familial characteristic.

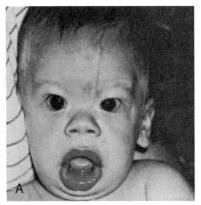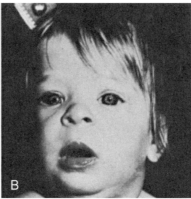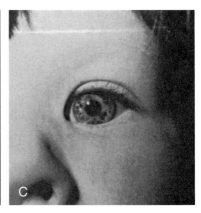

Figure 25–4. Williams syndrome. This condition is characterized by (*A* and *B*) periorbital fullness, flat nasal bridge, short upturned nose, long philtrum, macrostomia, full lips, and (*C*) a "stellate" pattern to the iris.

Abnormal scalp hair patterns may reflect underlying brain abnormalities. In microcephaly, there may be a lack of the normal parietal whorl, or it may be displaced more centrally or posteriorly. In addition, the frontal hair may show a prominent upsweep. A low posterior hairline occurs with a short or webbed neck, as in Turner syndrome and Noonan syndrome. Punched-out scalp lesions in the parietal occipital area (aplasia cutis congenita) are typical of trisomy 13, or may be seen in isolation and may be familial.

Head

The size of the head, measured by the maximum head circumference, and the sizes of the anterior and other fontanels, if still open, should be compared with appropriate standards. Head size varies with age, sex, and racial group and has a general correlation with body size. Macrocephaly as an isolated anomaly is often familial and inherited in an autosomal dominant fashion. Therefore, determining the head circumferences of the parents is helpful. On the other hand, macrocephaly may be a manifestation of a number of disorders, including hydrocephalus, storage disorders, neurofibromatosis, and various conditions affecting the skeletal system, such as achondroplasia. Microcephaly can also be familial, either autosomal dominant or recessive, but it is more commonly a manifestation of many syndromes and brain malformations that result in mental retardation. Large fontanels occur in hypothyroidism; trisomies 21, 18, and 13; and many bone disorders, such as hypophosphatasia and cleidocranial dysostosis. A small anterior fontanel may be a sign of failure of normal brain growth.

The normal shape of the head may vary from an increase in the anteroposterior diameter (dolichocephaly) to a decrease in this dimension (brachycephaly). Premature infants and those with trisomy 18 characteristically have dolichocephaly, but either type of head shape may be familial or racial. Many Asian and native American infants, for example, have relatively brachycephalic heads.

Premature fusion of cranial sutures (craniosynostosis) results in an abnormal configuration in head shape. Various types occur, depending on the sutures involved, and may be associated with abnormalities of the limbs. Torticollis or abnormal mechanical forces in utero can cause asymmetric head shape (plagiocephaly).

A common anomaly in head shape is frontal bossing, which is frequent in some skeletal dysplasias such as achondroplasia, in the mucopolysaccharidoses, and in some cases of hydrocephalus.

Face

The face is composed of a series of structures, each of which demonstrates considerable normal variation, providing a distinctive and particularly unique appearance to every human being. Since examination of the face is both complex and important, a systematic approach is necessary. It is never sufficient to merely describe the face as "funny looking" or unusual, although a gestalt diagnosis can sometimes be made at a single glance (Down syndrome, for example). Specific abnormalities must be analyzed and quantified, when appropriate, even though an overall gestalt impression may suggest a diagnosis in some instances.

Eyes

Hypotelorism occurs when the eyes are unusually close together; when they are too far apart there is hypertelorism. Clinically, hypotelorism and hypertelorism are defined by the interpupillary distance, which may be estimated in a relaxed patient by measuring between the midpoints of the pupils. This is often impossible in an infant or small child; therefore, two other relevant measurements that are useful and relatively easier to obtain are the inner canthal distance and the outer canthal distance. Telecanthus is manifested by an increase in the inner canthal distance and may occur in the absence of hypertelorism, such as in Waardenburg syndrome type I. Other factors may create an illusion of hypertelorism, such as epicanthal folds and a flat nasal bridge. For this reason, a subjective impression should always be confirmed by measurement of all three distances, if possible. From a prognostic and diagnostic point of view, it is important to identify hypotelorism, since it is often associated with holoprosencephaly. Holoprosencephaly is a major malformation of the central nervous system usually associated with severe disturbance of brain function and early death. It can be isolated or part of trisomy 13 and other chromosomal abnormalities. Hypertelorism, on the other hand, occurs in a number of syndromes, such as frontonasal dysplasia, and, even when severe, is less likely to be related to an underlying brain malformation.

Epicanthal folds are a feature of normal fetal development and may be present in normal infants. They are also characteristic of trisomy 21 (Fig. 25–5) but occur in many other malformation syndromes, especially those that include a flat nasal bridge.

Normally an imaginary line through the inner and outer canthi should be perpendicular to the sagittal plane of the face. An upward slant to the palpebral fissures is seen in trisomy 21 (see Fig. 25–5), and a downward slant is seen in conditions including Noonan syndrome. Either type of slant can be part of a number of other syndromes.

Palpebral fissure length is measured from the inner to the outer canthus. Short palpebral fissures may occur in association with other ocular anomalies, such as microphthalmia, and is characteristic of syndromes such as fetal alcohol syndrome and velocardiofacial-DiGeorge syndrome (see Fig. 25–1).

A coloboma is a developmental defect in the normal continuity of a structure and often is used in reference to the eye. Colobomas may involve the eyelid margin, as in Treacher Collins syndrome, or the iris and retina, as in CHARGE association (*c*oloboma, *h*eart disease, *a*tresia choanae, *r*etardation of growth and development, *g*enital hypoplasia, and *e*ar anomalies and/or deafness). Identification of a coloboma should lead to a formal eye evaluation. Other abnormalities of the irides should be noted, such as a stellate appearance, which is characteristic of Williams syndrome (see Fig. 25–4).

Synophrys, or fusion of the eyebrows in the midline, is common in hirsute infants and usually occurs in Cornelia de Lange syndrome (Fig. 25–6). It may also be familial.

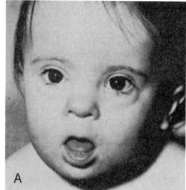
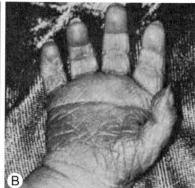

Figure 25–5. Down syndrome (trisomy 21). Typical features of Down syndrome include (*A*) upslanting palpebral fissures, broad flat nasal bridge with epicanthal folds, midface hypoplasia, prominent tongue, and (*B*) short fingers with fifth finger clinodactyly and a single transverse palmar crease. (*A* from Jones KL: Smith's Recognizable Patterns of Human Malformation, 4th ed. Philadelphia, WB Saunders, 1988.)

Ears

The external ear, or pinna, commonly shows great variation, but a number of anatomic landmarks can be identified and should be described when evaluating the anomalous ear. These include the helix, antihelix, tragus, crus, external meatus, and lobule (Fig. 25–7). If the ears appear to be large or small, they should be measured by obtaining the maximum length of the pinna from the lobule to the superior margin of the helix. Preauricular tags or pits may be isolated or associated with other abnormalities of the pinna.

Low-set ears are designated when the helix joins the head below a horizontal plane passing through the outer canthi perpendicular to the vertical axis of the head. It is critical that this condition be assessed with the head in vertical alignment with the body, since any posterior rotation of the head can easily create an illusion of low-set ears. The relative placement of the ears is more a function of head shape and jaw size than an intrinsic anomaly of the ear.

When the vertical axis of the ear deviates more than 10 degrees from the vertical axis of the head, the ears are posteriorly rotated. This anomaly is often associated with low-set ears and represents a lag in the normal ascent of the ear during development.

It is important to note that any significant abnormality of the external ear may be an indication of additional anomalies of the middle or inner ear and associated hearing loss. Therefore an early hearing assessment is indicated in such situations.

Nose

The nose, like the external ear, shows great individual variation, but certain alterations in shape are frequent in malformation syndromes involving the face. A depressed nasal bridge with an upturned nose occurs in many skeletal dysplasias, such as achondroplasia. When the depression is severe, the nostrils may appear anteverted and the nose shortened (see Fig. 25–3). A hypoplastic nose is often syndromic, and one with a single nostril is highly suggestive of holoprosencephaly. A prominent nasal root and bulbous nasal tip are characteristic of velocardiofacial-DiGeorge syndrome (see Fig. 25–1). Individuals with Rubinstein-Taybi syndrome have a characteristic beaked appearance to the nose (Fig. 25–8).

Mouth

The mouth is a complex structure with component parts, each requiring separate evaluation.

The size and shape of the mouth may be altered. A small mouth, or microstomia, occurs in trisomy 18.

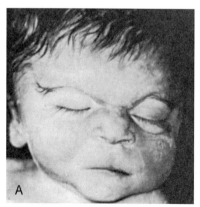
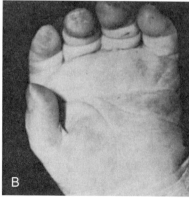
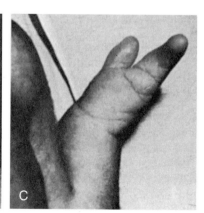

Figure 25–6. Cornelia de Lange syndrome. This syndrome can easily be recognized by the characteristic facial features (*A*), which are synophrys, prominent arched eyebrows, long eyelashes, small upturned nose, long philtrum, thin upper lip with cupid's bow appearance, and by characteristic limb anomalies (*B* and *C*) ranging from small hands to ulnar deficiency and oligodactyly.

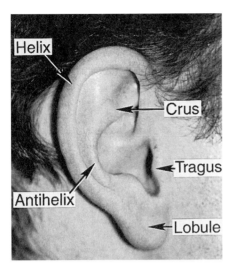

Figure 25–7. Normal pinna and its landmarks. It is helpful to describe which components of the pinna are unusual in the dysplastic ear.

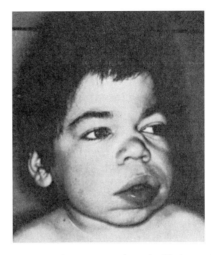

Figure 25–9. Hunter syndrome (mucopolysaccharidosis, type II). Characteristic facial features illustrated in this 14-year-old boy with Hunter syndrome include prominent eyebrows, fleshy nasal tip, and full prominent lips and cheeks.

Macrostomia, a large mouth, should be noted as well and may be present in such conditions as Williams syndrome (see Fig. 25–4) and Angelman syndrome. Severe macrostomia may result in association with a lateral facial cleft. The corners of the mouth may be downturned, as in Prader-Willi syndrome and other conditions with hypotonia. An asymmetric face during crying occurs with congenital deficiency in the depressor anguli oris muscle on one side, and this may be associated with other abnormalities, as in hemifacial microsomia.

Prominent full lips occur in various syndromes including Williams syndrome (see Fig. 25–4) and are part of what in the past have been referred to as "coarse" facial features, seen in many storage disorders such as Hunter syndrome (Fig. 25–9). A thin upper lip may be seen in Cornelia de Lange syndrome (see Fig. 25–6) and in fetal alcohol syndrome (see Fig. 25–2).

A cleft upper lip is usually lateral, as in the common multifactorial cleft lip/palate anomaly. The presence of pits in the lower lip associated with a cleft lip or palate, however, is suggestive of a different malformation syndrome

(Van der Woude syndrome), which is inherited in an autosomal dominant manner. A median cleft lip is very suggestive of holoprosencephaly. In fact, there are many diverse syndromes with cleft lip or palate that are important to identify, since they may have other associated malformations and relatively high genetic risks of recurrence. Therefore it is important to evaluate the infant with cleft lip or palate carefully for evidence of other malformations, to give accurate recurrence risk and prognostic information to the family.

Isolated cleft palate is different genetically from the cleft palate associated with cleft lip. Mild forms of cleft palate are represented by submucosal clefts, pharyngeal incompetence with nasal speech (velopharyngeal insufficiency), and bifid uvula. Velocardiofacial-DiGeorge syndrome (see Fig. 25–1) should be considered in individuals with cleft palate and velopharyngeal insufficiency. A high arched palate may occur normally but is also a feature of many syndromes, especially if hypotonia or another longstanding neurologic abnormality is present.

Macroglossia may be relative, as in Pierre Robin

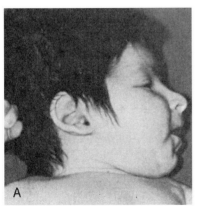
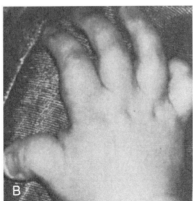
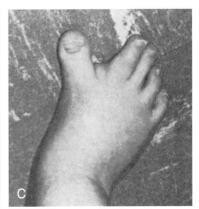

Figure 25–8. Rubinstein-Taybi syndrome. Findings in this condition include (A) beaked nose with the columella extending below the alae nasi and low anterior hairline, and (B) broad thumbs and (C) great toes that are often deviated.

syndrome, in which the primary abnormality is mandibular hypoplasia. In other instances, such as hypothyroidism, Beckwith-Wiedemann syndrome, and Down syndrome, the tongue appears protruding and enlarged. A cleft or irregular tongue or oral frenula occurs in various syndromes such as the orofaciodigital syndromes.

The lower portion of the mouth is formed by the mandible, which in young infants is relatively small. An excessively small mandible is termed *micrognathia,* which is a feature of many syndromes. In other syndromes, the maxilla likewise may be hypoplastic, decreasing the prominence of the upper cheeks (malar hypoplasia).

Neck

The neck may be short, and limitation of rotation should raise the suspicion of fusion of cervical vertebrae, as in a Klippel-Feil anomaly. Excessive skinfolds are characteristic of Turner syndrome, Noonan syndrome, and Down syndrome. In these conditions, the excess nuchal skin often represents resolution of a cystic hygroma that was present but resolved prenatally.

Chest

The thoracic cage may be unusually small as part of a skeletal dysplasia. The sternum itself may be unusually short, as is typical in trisomy 18, or it may be altered in shape, as in pectus excavatum or pectus carinatum. The latter anomalies are commonly seen in a variety of skeletal dysplasias and connective tissue disorders.

Abdomen

Hypoplasia of the abdominal musculature may occur in association with intrauterine bladder outlet obstruction and other anomalies of the urogenital system. It results in a characteristic "prune belly" appearance. An omphalocele, in which abdominal contents protrude through the umbilical opening, may be part of the Beckwith-Wiedemann syndrome or chromosome abnormalities such as trisomy 13. Gastroschisis, on the other hand, is usually an isolated disruption in which the abdominal contents protrude through the periumbilical abdominal wall. Anomalies of a more minor nature, such as inguinal or umbilical hernias, occur in normal infants but are more frequent in various syndromes, including Williams syndrome, velocardiofacial syndrome, and connective tissue disorders, in particular.

Anus

Imperforate anus may be isolated or may occur as the mildest expression of caudal regression sequence in which other anomalies such as sacral dysgenesis are seen. It is most commonly part of a constellation of anomalies, such as the VATER association. It can also be seen in a number of chromosomal abnormalities.

Genitalia

Hypogenitalism can be seen in association with hypotonia in Prader-Willi syndrome, or with low-set dysplastic ears,

syndactyly of the toes, and thickened alveolar ridges in Smith-Lemli-Opitz syndrome. Genital ambiguity is associated with renal anomalies and an increased risk for Wilms tumor in the Denys-Drash syndrome.

Spine

Among the most common congenital anomalies are the neural tube defects, which involve abnormalities of the central nervous system along with defects in the associated bony structures. Minor external anomalies, particularly of the lower spine, include unusual pigmentary lesions, hair tufts, dimples, and sinuses. Some of these changes, such as hair tufts and sinuses above the gluteal cleft, may be an indication of a more significant deeper anomaly and require further evaluation such as by magnetic resonance imaging.

Extremities

Extremities may be either relatively long, as occurs in Marfan syndrome or homocystinuria, or unusually short, as occurs in a diverse group of skeletal dysplasias, the most common being achondroplasia. A simple guide to evaluating relative extremity length is to determine where the fingertips are in relation to the thighs when the upper extremities are adducted alongside the body. In the normal child, the fingertips fall below the hip joint. A more precise and useful measurement is to determine the arm span, which should approximate the height within a few centimeters.

Paired extremities may be asymmetric either in length or in overall size, suggesting either atrophy of one or hypertrophy of the other. The distinction may be difficult to make at times, although it is often evident if an extremity is unusually large or excessively small. Hypertrophy of limbs may be a manifestation of Beckwith-Wiedemann syndrome or Klippel-Trenaunay-Weber syndrome. It is important to identify hemihypertrophy because individuals with this finding are at increased risk for intraabdominal tumors, such as Wilms tumor, and thus require close monitoring.

Foreshortening of long bones will lead to various limb abnormalities, depending on the segments involved. A number of terms have been used to describe such anomalies. *Rhizomelia* denotes proximal shortening of the limbs, such as in achondroplasia. *Mesomelia* refers to shortening of the middle segment, and *acromelia* to relative shortening of the hands or feet, or both.

The hands and feet have epidermal ridges and creases forming a variety of configurations. Normally there are two deep transverse palmar creases that do not completely cross the palm. In various conditions, such as trisomy 21, there may instead be a single transverse palmar crease, sometimes termed a four-finger line (see Fig. 25–5).

Dermatoglyphics, the study of configurations of the characteristic ridge patterns of the volar surfaces of the skin, can sometimes aid in the diagnosis of the child with congenital anomalies. This subject is beyond the scope of this chapter and therefore the reader is referred to other sources (Mulvihill and Smith, 1969).

The hands and feet may be enlarged as a result of lymphedema. This is characteristic of children with Turner or Noonan syndrome, in which the dorsum of the hands and feet may have a puffy appearance. Congenital lymphedema can also be an autosomal dominantly inherited condition with variable expressivity.

Rocker-bottom feet are manifested by a prominent heel and a loss of the normal concave longitudinal arch of the sole. They are common in trisomy 18 and other syndromes.

Significant anomalies of the underlying structure will produce alterations in the normal form of the hands and feet. Such abnormalities may be classified into the following categories: absence deformities, polydactyly, syndactyly, brachydactyly, arachnodactyly, and contracture deformities.

Absence anomalies are of various types, and the etiology and possible associated malformations vary with the type. Congenital absence of an entire hand is termed *acheiria,* whereas absence of both hands and feet is *acheiropodia. Ectrodactyly* refers to a partial or total absence of the distal segments of a hand or foot with the proximal segments of the limbs more or less normal. All such anomalies are examples of terminal transverse defects and may occur sporadically or as part of a syndrome. The term ectrodactyly is frequently misused for the lobster claw anomaly, which is best described as split hand/split foot. In this anomaly, the central rays are deficient and there is often fusion of the remaining digits. Split hand/split foot may be seen in isolation, when it is autosomal dominant, or may be seen with other anomalies.

It is useful to determine whether the defects involve primarily the radial, or preaxial, side of the limb, or the ulnar, or postaxial, side. For example, blood dyscrasias such as the Fanconi pancytopenia syndrome and the thrombocytopenia–absent radius syndrome commonly involve radial deficiency. Cornelia de Lange syndrome, on the other hand, is characterized by ulnar deficiency (see Fig. 25–6).

Polydactyly refers to partial or complete supernumerary digits and is one of the most common hand malformations. Postaxial polydactyly is more frequent than preaxial, particularly in black people. As an isolated anomaly, polydactyly may be inherited as an autosomal dominant trait. It also may be a manifestation of a multiple malformation syndrome. Postaxial polydactyly may occur in a variety of syndromes, including trisomy 13 and Bardet-Biedl syndrome.

Syndactyly refers to fusion of digits and is usually cutaneous but may involve bone as well. Minimal syndactyly of the second and third toes is common in normal newborns. More extensive syndactyly is seen in Smith-Lemli-Opitz syndrome and some of the craniosynostosis disorders such as Apert syndrome.

Brachydactyly refers to shortening of one or more digits owing to anomalous development of any of the phalanges, metacarpals, or metatarsals. Various clinical types may be distinguished, but most isolated forms of brachydactyly are inherited in an autosomal dominant fashion. Brachydactyly is also a component of numerous disorders, including skeletal dysplasias such as achondroplasia and syndromes such as Down syndrome (see Fig. 25–5).

Arachnodactyly refers to unusually long, spider-like digits and is characteristic of but not invariable in Marfan syndrome and homocystinuria. The appearance of brachy-

dactyly and arachnodactyly can be confirmed by measuring and determining a middle finger to total hand length ratio and comparing the ratio to normative date (Jones, 1997).

A variety of congenital joint deformities involving the limbs may occur. *Arthrogryposis,* that is, multiple congenital contractures, may be sporadic or genetic and may be associated with oligohydramnios or be the result of some underlying neuromuscular abnormality. Talipes equinovarus or calcaneovalgus deformities of the ankle are common isolated joint contractures. Contractures may also occur in numerous syndromes. Joint hypermobility is frequent in various connective tissue disorders, such as Marfan and Ehlers-Danlos syndromes.

Clinodactyly designates an incurving of a digit, most commonly the fifth finger. This is common in trisomy 21 (see Fig. 25–5) and some other syndromes.

Camptodactyly is irreducible flexion of the digits. In the hand, it usually involves the fifth finger but may affect other fingers as well. Isolated camptodactyly may be inherited as an autosomal dominant trait. Camptodactyly may also be part of a syndrome such as the mosaic trisomy 8, trisomy 10q, and Freeman-Sheldon syndromes.

More unique anomalies of the digits may prove to be diagnostic clues. For example, broad thumbs and great toes are characteristic of Rubinstein-Taybi syndrome (see Fig. 25–8).

Neurologic Exam

The fine points of a complete neurologic examination are not reviewed here, but one topic warrants discussion. Hypotonia is a common finding in many syndromes and is invariably found in Prader-Willi syndrome. In hypotonic infants without an identifiable cause, especially in males with undescended testes, Prader-Willi syndrome should be considered and the appropriate testing sought.

EXAMPLE: PRADER-WILLI SYNDROME

Bryan is a 16-year-old boy whose mother brought him to see the pediatrician because of failure to complete puberty despite having developed pubic and axillary hair at the age of 10 years. Although the family history is unrevealing, a past history of Bryan reveals that this is not his only problem. Prenatally, there was concern about the pregnancy because of poor fetal movement. In the perinatal period the baby had failure to progress and was in the breech position, and a cesarean section was required. At birth and for the next several months he was very hypotonic, with poor arousal, weak cry, and failure to awaken to feed. His testes had not descended. A routine chromosomal analysis and computed tomographic scan of the head at that time had normal results. The child had a very poor suck, not succeeding with breast-feeding and requiring gavage tube feeding for 3 weeks prior to slowly beginning to bottle-feed. He had a period of early failure to thrive but then seemed to do much better in terms of feeding and tone. By 9 months, he was eating well and beginning to put on weight. By 12 months, he sat unsupported, and he was walking by 24 months. Although he was also late in talking, he was very social and interactive from early in infancy, and by age 4 his parents felt

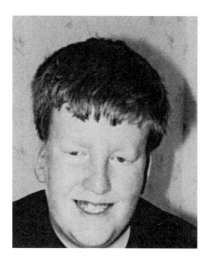

Figure 25–10. Prader-Willi syndrome. Bryan as a young man. The narrow bifrontal diameter, sharp nasal bridge, and thin upper lip with down-turned corners of the mouth are typical findings.

that he was talking a lot, although his articulation was poor.

At about that time, Bryan began to eat excessively. Although the parents were pleased that he no longer had poor gain, they were concerned that he became very plump. When they tried to restrict food he strenuously objected. By the age of 7, his demands for food and temper tantrums when it was denied had become a significant problem, and his food-seeking behavior at school was interfering with his schoolwork. He also had severe learning disabilities. He required extra help in several of his academic subjects, although he was mainstreamed for the remainder of his subjects. By high school, it was apparent that he had some intellectual limitations, and testing revealed an IQ of 79. He also had social difficulties because he was very controlling and stubborn.

At the age of 16 years, Bryan's height was at the 3rd percentile, weight well above the 95th percentile, and head circumference normal (Fig. 25–10). He had a narrow forehead, thick saliva with crusting on the lips, a thin and poorly rugated scrotum with testes in the upper scrotum, and scanty Tanner stage IV pubic hair. His hand and foot length were at less than the 3rd percentile, and his hands were slender and narrow, compared with his centrally obese body. Testosterone, luteinizing hormone, and follicle-stimulating hormone levels were low. The pattern was suggestive of Prader-Willi syndrome, and at the suggestion of the local cytogeneticist, the pediatrician obtained a methylation analysis, which indicated that Bryan has only maternal contribution to chromosome 15q11-13, consistent with that diagnosis. Additional testing revealed that he has maternal uniparental disomy, in which both chromosomes 15 are maternal in origin and there is no paternally contributed chromosome 15. Recurrence risk is negligible. Testosterone replacement therapy is effective in completing Bryan's pubertal development, and a low-calorie diet, a regular exercise regimen, strict enforcement of limits, and constant supervision to prevent his taking extra food help him in achieving a healthier weight and improved behavior.

DIAGNOSTIC TESTING AND INDICATIONS

Once the history and clinical findings are noted, various laboratory studies may be indicated to aid in making an accurate diagnosis.

In a child with one or more obvious major malformations or with multiple minor anomalies, imaging studies are often indicated to identify other anomalies. Ultrasonograms of the head and abdomen in infants are useful to screen for major structural anomalies of the brain and kidneys. Head ultrasonography is a very crude study for brain abnormalities, and if they are suspected, more definitive testing such as computed tomography or magnetic resonance imaging is indicated. Echocardiography is also helpful, as congenital heart defects are among the most common major malformations. Detection of major anomalies involving the brain, heart, and kidneys not only is useful for diagnostic purposes but also may allow for better management and more accurate prognostication.

Routine chromosomal analysis is indicated in those individuals with ambiguous genitalia, two or more major anomalies, multiple minor anomalies, or growth or mental retardation in association with anomalies. A routine karyotype from peripheral blood allows for better resolution than a karyotype from amniocentesis and will thus allow for detection of small deletions or duplications, so such a study should be performed even if the result of a prenatal chromosomal analysis was normal. In children who were found to have a normal karyotype more than 5 years previously, the study should be repeated, preferably at higher resolution, since technical advances may now allow a small chromosome anomaly to be identified. FISH will allow for identification of microdeletions that are not detectable by routine cytogenetic analysis in a number of disorders (Table 25–2).

Molecular genetic analysis is an increasingly useful tool in diagnosing the child with congenital anomalies. For example, in infants with unexplained hypotonia and contractures, DNA testing may identify an expansion in the myotonic dystrophy gene. As more disease-causing genes are identified, molecular analysis will undoubtedly become a cost-effective aid in diagnosis.

Table 25–2 • Common Microdeletion Syndromes Associated With Developmental Disability and Identifiable by Fluorescence in Situ Hybridization*

Syndrome	Clinical Features	Chromosomal Location
Williams	Supravalvular aortic stenosis, hypercalcemia, full lips, periorbital fullness	7q
Prader-Willi	Hypotonia, hypogenitalism, obesity	15q
Miller-Dicker	Lissencephaly (smooth brain), seizures	17q
Velocardiofacial-DiGeorge	Conotruncal heart defects, palatal abnormalities, ear anomalies, hypocalcemia	22q

*See also Chapter 23.

Another area of burgeoning research that is likely to result in useful diagnostic testing is that of metabolic disorders. These conditions were traditionally thought of as not being associated with congenital anomalies, but this concept is changing. A definitive diagnosis of Smith-Lemli-Opitz syndrome, which is associated with syndactyly of the second and third toes, ptosis, thick alveolar ridges, and other anomalies, can be made by obtaining a low serum cholesterol level and an elevated 7-dehydrocholesterol level. Presumably, many other conditions with congenital anomalies will be found to have a biochemical basis, allowing for more definitive diagnoses.

Ophthalmologic evaluation can also be useful in diagnosing the child with congenital anomalies, especially if brain malformations are present. This evaluation should also be performed if small genitalia are present in a male (septo-optic dysplasia) or if features of CHARGE association are present.

Once a thorough history and physical examination have been accomplished and appropriate testing is underway, the clinician should identify those features that are most unique. Sometimes a pattern is readily recognized, such as Down syndrome in a child with an atrioventricular canal, hypotonia, upslanting palpebral fissures, small squared ears, and fifth-finger clinodactyly. Often, however, a review of reference texts is required to determine whether the findings represent a previously described condition. A clinical geneticist or dysmorphologist may be especially helpful at this point as well. Other evaluations may be indicated, including those listed above.

Sometimes a diagnosis does not become apparent until later in the child's life, as the physical features change and other anomalies become apparent. Parents should be counseled about this possibility and told that even though a definite diagnosis may not be possible, the child's condition may very well have a genetic basis and recurrence in future pregnancies is possible. This is an important reason for ongoing, approximately annual re-evaluation of children in whom the cause of anomalies has not been identified.

Finally, if the child has a fatal disorder, the value of the postmortem examination cannot be overemphasized. A thorough evaluation by an experienced pathologist, particularly a pediatric pathologist, can yield findings that would not be identified otherwise and that may lead to a definitive diagnosis and thus information about recurrence risk and possible prenatal testing in future pregnancies. The role of the clinician is to educate the family in the importance of such an evaluation.

GENETIC COUNSELING

Genetic counseling is a communication process during which families are informed about the abnormalities present in the affected individual. During this process, medical and genetic knowledge is translated into practical information for individuals and families. A description of the anomaly, the natural history, associated abnormalities, and prognosis for the disorder are provided. The etiology of the abnormality (if known), whether genetic or nongenetic, is explained in such a manner that the family can understand it. The family is also given reassurance that the

condition in the affected individual is not the fault of any individual, and information about recurrence risk is provided. Those family members who are at increased risk of being affected or having affected offspring, as determined by pedigree analysis and etiology, are identified, and prenatal diagnostic testing, if possible, is described, including the complications and accuracy of the test. Assistance in reaching a decision about prenatal testing and in accessing it is offered. Genetic counselors provide supportive counseling to families, assist families in coping with a lifelong condition, and serve as patient advocates. Information about appropriate community services and family support organizations is also offered.

Genetic counseling can be done by anyone willing to take the time and make the effort. Genetic counselors, sometimes called Genetic Associates, are individuals with a masters degree who have been specifically trained to understand and be knowledgeable about genetic disorders and congenital anomalies, as well as in helping families with the psychological and emotional adaptation to having a child with a serious and chronic problem. Medical geneticists are physicians (or sometimes PhDs) who have received special training in the diagnosis and management of genetic disorders and birth defects and in genetic counseling.

SUPPORT ORGANIZATIONS AND EDUCATIONAL MATERIALS

Because most congenital anomalies and genetic disorders are relatively rare, usually occurring with a frequency of 1 in 1000 or less, family support organizations have been developed to help combat the isolation and grief felt by families who have an affected child. These groups usually offer support and empathy and serve as a clearing-house for information about the disorder and its management. Often, the group has a newsletter that is sent to members describing helpful coping mechanisms and keeping families updated on relevant resources and research.

Such organizations have often been started and are usually staffed by parents of affected individuals, or affected individuals themselves. As a result, they vary greatly in both the format and content of what they offer and in the accuracy of information they distribute. Organizations for more frequent disorders, such as Down syndrome and Prader-Willi syndrome, are generally large and professionally run; offer educational forums, such as an annual conference, Web sites, and lay literature; keep listings of resources locally and nationally; and may even offer grant funding for research on the disorder. Smaller organizations for less common conditions may serve primarily a social and support function. Because of this variability in the knowledge of support organizations and the resultant uncertainty concerning the accuracy of information provided, it is advisable for the physician to become familiar with a given support organization and its functions before referring a family to it.

A national organization called Alliance of Genetic Support Groups serves as a resource to identify whether a designated consumer group exists for a specific condition; it also lists more general associations. It will supply contact information and data about the organizations. The Alliance prints the *Directory of National Genetic Voluntary Organizations and Related Resources,* which it updates regularly. The Alliance can be reached by calling 1–800–336-GENE. Another group, the National Organization for Rare Disorders, or NORD, functions as a clearing-house for information on genetic disorders and for a small fee will send a summary of this information written for lay individuals, will match families, and will make medical referrals if appropriate. It can be reached at 1–800–999-NORD.

Conclusion

It is the role of the developmental pediatrician to evaluate the child with developmental delay or behavioral problems and to identify both major and minor congenital anomalies. Diagnostic testing and evaluations, along with consultation of references and specialists in the field, such as clinical geneticists and dysmorphologists, may be helpful. The goal is to identify the etiology of the condition so that accurate information on prognosis and recurrence risk can be shared with the family.

REFERENCES

Buyse ML (ed): Birth Defects Encyclopedia. Cambridge, MA, Blackwell Scientific Publications, 1990.

Gorlin RJ, Cohen MM Jr, Levin LS (eds): Syndromes of the Head and Neck. New York, Oxford University Press, 1990.

Holmes LB: Current concepts in genetics: congenital malformations. N Engl J Med 295:204, 1976.

Holmes LB: Inborn errors of morphogenesis: a review of localized hereditary malformations. N Engl J Med 291:763, 1974.

Hook EB: Contribution of chromosome abnormalities to human morbidity and mortality. Cytogenet Cell Genet 33:101, 1982.

Hoyme HE: Teratogenically induced fetal anomalies. Clin Perinatol 17:547, 1990.

Jones KL (ed): Smith's Recognizable Patterns of Human Malformation. Philadelphia, WB Saunders, 1997.

Leppig KA, Werler MM, Cann CI, et al: Predictive value of minor anomalies: I. Association with major malformations. J Pediatr 110:531, 1987.

Marden PM, Smith DW, McDonald MJ: Congenital anomalies in the newborn infant, including minor variations: a study of 4,142 babies by surface examination for anomalies and buccal smear for sex chromatin. J Pediatr 64:357, 1964.

McKusick VA, Francomano C, Antonarakis S: Mendelian Inheritance in Man: A Catalog of Human Genes and Genetic Disorders, 11th ed. Baltimore, Johns Hopkins University Press, 1994; and www.omim.org.

Mulvihill JJ, Smith DW: The genesis of dermatoglyphics. J Pediatr 75:579, 1969.

Schinzel A: Catalog of Unbalanced Chromosome Aberrations in Man. Berlin, Walter de Gruyter, 1983.

Seaver L, Hoyme HE: Teratology in pediatric practice. Pediatr Clin North Am 39(1):111, 1992.

Spranger J, Benirschke K, Hall JG, et al: Errors of morphogenesis: concepts and terms. J Pediatr 100:160, 1982.

Stevenson RE, Hall JG, Goodman RM (eds): Human malformations and related anomalies. New York, Oxford University Press, 1993.

26 Stresses and Interventions in the Neonatal Intensive Care Unit

Betty R. Vohr • William J. Cashore •
Rosemarie Bigsby

Survival rates for infants weighing less than 800 g at birth have improved from 0% in 1943 to 34% in 1987 to 70% in 1994.

Perhaps the greatest known risk for neurodevelopmental sequelae is the combination of intraventricular hemorrhage and periventricular leukomalacia.

Very low birth weight infants (<1500 g) have been shown to have adequate sucking ability and to tolerate breast-feeding at a mean age of 35 weeks.

Whatever is obviously painful at any other age is probably painful for the newborn (and possibly for the 2nd- and 3rd-trimester fetus) regardless of gestational age at birth.

Nesting has the added advantage of containing random movements, assisting the infant in returning to a calm state after startling or jerking.

Medical providers have for many years known of clear associations between specific maternal stresses (e.g., diabetes, epilepsy, syphilis, HIV infection) or fetal or neonatal factors (e.g., multiple pregnancy, severe acidosis, intraventricular hemorrhage) and nonoptimal infant outcome. The 1980s and 1990s, however, have brought an increasing awareness that infant outcome is the result of a complex intermingling of maternal and infant biological factors and environmental stresses and interventions. A number of well-designed clinical research studies have demonstrated the powerful interaction between biological and environmental risk and protective factors within the infant and the environment. In addition, many tertiary care centers that care for high-risk neonates currently maintain an in-house database of demographic variables, maternal and infant risk factors, and interventions. This collection facilitates maintenance of statistical data on multiple parameters that affect outcome and acts as a quality control for care provided in the nursery. In addition, neonatal follow-up programs provide a mechanism for monitoring growth, neurologic status, development, and behavior after discharge.

Although recent trends in vital statistics in the United States are consistent with a decrease in the number of births (estimated at 3,900,000 in 1995) and the infant mortality rate, the percent of low–birth weight infants weighing less than 2500 g continues to rise (7.3% in 1994). The multiple birth ratio of 25.7 per 1000 births in 1994 has increased 33% since 1980. As reported by Guyer and colleagues (1996), the estimated infant mortality rate in the United States in 1995 was 7.5 per 1000 births, the lowest ever recorded in the United States. Numerous advances over the past 10 years in perinatal and neonatal management have resulted in the increased survival of both full-term high-risk infants and premature infants. Among very

low birth weight (VLBW) infants (<1500 g and <30 weeks' gestation), the most significant increase in survival has occurred for the fragile extremely low birth weight (ELBW) infant (<1000 g). The use of prenatal steroids, surfactant for respiratory distress syndrome, prophylactic indomethacin for prevention of intraventricular hemorrhage, and improved nutritional management and ventilatory techniques has contributed to improved survival, especially for those infants with birth weights of 800 to 1200 g. Survival rates of infants weighing less than 800 g have improved from 0% (1943–1945 birth cohort) to 34% (1987–1988 birth cohort) to 70% in 1994 (Hack and Fanaroff, 1989; McCormick, 1993).

Maternal Biological Risk Factors

Hospitals have developed screening criteria for enrollment in high-risk prenatal clinics and criteria for categorizing the risk status of women admitted in labor. Hobel and colleagues (1973) developed a maternal prenatal and intrapartum scoring system used both as a clinical tool to modify patient management and in numerous research protocols to assess risks for neonatal mortality and neonatal and long-term morbidity. Specific tests commonly used for antepartum fetal surveillance include the nonstress test and the contraction stress test, both of which reflect heart rate changes. Use of the biophysical profile permits the clinician to score a combination of biophysical parameters, including acute markers of fetal distress (fetal breathing movements, fetal movements, fetal tone, and fetal reactivity) and a chronic marker (qualitative amniotic fluid volume), and has been determined to be efficacious in identifying the fetus experiencing stress. Nelson (1996) reported a weak association between abnormal fetal heart rate tracings and subsequent cerebral palsy.

MORBIDITY ASSOCIATED WITH IN VITRO FERTILIZATION

Couples with infertility problems in the 1990s have a wide array of reproductive techniques available to assist with conception. The recent increased incidence of multiple-gestation pregnancies is a direct result of these interventions. With in vitro fertilization, an egg is fertilized in vitro and transferred transcervically into the uterine cavity. Typically several embryos are transferred, and thus the multiple gestation rate is increased by as much as 20-fold. Pregnancies resulting from in vitro fertilization are associated with increased maternal complications, including pregnancy-induced hypertension, premature labor, and labor induction, and higher rates of fetal loss, low birth weight, premature delivery, multiple fetuses, neonatal morbidity, and duration of hospitalization (Tallo et al, 1995). Implantation of fewer embryos per cycle of in vitro fertilization to reduce the risk of high-order multiple gestation is currently recommended.

Maternal Environmental Risk Factors

A number of maternal social and environmental factors are known to affect not only the risk of prematurity and admission to the neonatal intensive care unit (NICU) but perhaps more importantly neurodevelopmental outcome. On the top of the list is poverty, followed closely by characteristics that may be highly correlated with one another, including African American or Hispanic ethnicity, teen pregnancy, single parenting, lack of prenatal care, and substance abuse.

Specific Neonatal Biological Factors

THE LOW–BIRTH WEIGHT INFANT

Whereas early studies in the literature described the outcome of low–birth weight infants of less than 2500 g, in the 1970s and 1980s, the interest was in VLBW infants of less than 1500 g, and in the 1990s, most studies report on ELBW infants of less than 1000 g. In fact, there is growing interest in so-called micropremies, those infants weighing less than 800 g. The timing of assessment of outcome of VLBW and ELBW infants is complicated by the fact that these infants often experience a turbulent and protracted neonatal hospitalization. During the first year of life, the VLBW infant experiences both maturational changes and recovery from neurologic insult. Findings vary significantly from infant to infant. Whereas an ELBW infant of 800 g may be ready for discharge at 35 weeks' corrected age, another infant of 1000 g may still be on multiple medications and oxygen when discharged at 45 weeks' corrected age. It is well known that abnormal neurologic findings present at term, including hypertonicity, tremors, and asymmetries, gradually resolve in the majority of infants in the

first year of life. This plasticity or ability to recover from insult is prevalent among infants.

INTRAUTERINE GROWTH RESTRICTION

Evaluation of the maturity and growth status of the infant at the time of delivery (Ballard Score; see Ballard et al, 1991) is a standard part of the newborn examination in the NICU. Growth impairment identified in utero with decreased fetal measurements is currently termed *intrauterine growth restriction.* When identified at birth by physical examination with resultant weight measurements plotted below the 10th percentile on standard intrauterine growth curves, it is referred to as *small for gestational age.* When weight, length, and head circumference measurements all plot below the 10th percentile, the findings are termed *symmetric growth restriction,* as compared with asymmetric growth restriction, in which growth of the head is spared. The findings in symmetric growth restriction are suggestive of more prolonged nutritional deprivation to the fetus and have been associated with less optimal neurodevelopmental and growth outcome.

RESPIRATORY DISTRESS

The initial problem leading to the admission of most newborns into special care or premature nurseries is respiratory distress or hypoxemia. Perinatal causes of neonatal respiratory distress include airway obstruction, fetal distress in utero, retention or aspiration of amniotic fluid, pulmonary immaturity, congenital heart disease, and pneumonia, whether caused by infection or meconium aspiration. In terms of outcome, neonatal respiratory disorders can be broadly classified in two groups: easily treatable, that is, mild and self-limited; or potentially life-threatening, that is, of longer duration and needing more intensive treatment. Retained lung fluid (transient tachypnea of the newborn), mild aspiration syndromes, and mild but treatable cases of tachypnea with pulmonary infiltrates generally classed as "pneumonia" are prominent in the first group of respiratory disorders. With respect to neonatal environmental stress, during a clinical course of 1 to 4 days, the newborn has tachypnea with minimal obvious distress and with minimal to no supplemental oxygen requirement and no need for mechanical assisted ventilation. By the second half of the first week, the tachypnea is resolving and care requirements are back to normal, or nearly so. The initiation of feeding may sometimes be delayed and the hospital stay prolonged 2 to 7 days. Many infants in this category receive several days of intravenous antibiotics but are usually fed normally and cared for by their parents after the first day or two of treatment.

RESPIRATORY DISTRESS SYNDROME, BRONCHOPULMONARY DYSPLASIA, AND SEVERE RESPIRATORY DISTRESS

A more serious group of disorders includes respiratory distress syndrome of prematurity, severe meconium aspiration syndrome, and severe perinatal pneumonia with sepsis. Also included in this second, more stressed group is the small number of infants with fixed anatomic upper airway obstructions or severe congenital heart disease presenting at birth. The biological stresses on these infants may include hypoxemia, acidosis, and circulatory derangements with periods of right to left shunting or hypoperfusion. Environmental stresses include more prolonged and invasive neonatal intensive care such as intubation with assisted ventilation, indwelling catheters, frequent blood sampling, and withholding of oral feedings until clinical conditions improve. Sicker infants with respiratory distress also have longer separation from parents and are often placed in noisy surroundings. Pulmonary treatments such as suctioning, chest physical therapy, steroids (Vaucher et al, 1988), and surfactant administration (Jones et al, 1995) are intended to improve pulmonary function but may be stressful when administered. These infants have a prolonged period of tachypnea with oxygen requirements and often need diuretics or respiratory stimulant medication to maintain adequate pulmonary function. Some have long periods of suboptimal feeding, and the worst cases require prolonged assisted ventilation.

Term infants with severe hypoxemia that persists despite conventional medical therapy may benefit from the use of extracorporeal membrane oxygenation. The first successful report of extracorporeal membrane oxygenation for term infants with severe respiratory failure was published in 1985. Primary diagnoses for which it is used include meconium aspiration syndrome, congenital diaphragmatic hernia, pneumonia, respiratory distress syndrome, and persistent pulmonary hypertension. Estimates are that approximately 1 in 3000 term infants will require this degree of therapy. Infants who receive extracorporeal membrane oxygenation are among the sickest in the NICU and are at increased risk of pulmonary, neurologic, and sensory sequelae. It is difficult, if not impossible, to determine whether sequelae are secondary to the preexisting disease process or to the intervention. It is important to note, however, that these infants would not survive with conventional management. A few infants with prolonged or chronic disorders of pulmonary function or control of respiration are sent home on cardiorespiratory monitors, oxygen, and medications including bronchodilators, respiratory stimulants, and diuretics. These infants and their families experience extended stress related not only to the underlying chronic illness but to the complex array of medical therapies and prolonged hospitalization. The overall survival and outcome of VLBW and ELBW infants with respiratory distress syndrome treated with surfactant, however, is improving (Vaucher et al, 1988).

HYPERBILIRUBINEMIA

The ordinary physiologic jaundice of infancy should not produce any particular stress on the newborn. Higher concentrations of bilirubin may create concern related to diagnosis and treatment or to the underlying cause of the jaundice itself. High uncontrolled levels of unconjugated bilirubin (generally >20 mg/dL indirect) may cause impairment of brainstem function or even produce permanent neurologic injury. However, a more common source of stress for newborn infants is the need to treat moderate levels of hyperbilirubinemia to keep them from becoming more severe. Treatments may include phototherapy to

lower serum bilirubin, intravenous hydration or formula changes to counteract the effects of underfeeding, and, occasionally, exchange transfusion if an infant has severe unconjugated hyperbilirubinemia or hemolysis as a source of the jaundice (Cashore, 1994). The last of these modalities, exchange transfusion, is a highly invasive procedure requiring catheterization of the umbilical vessels and multiple infusions and withdrawal of blood. During the procedure, many infants develop tachycardia and other signs of irritability. Posttransfusion recovery, however, is usually rapid. Phototherapy requires undressing the infant, often in a closed incubator, and patching the eyes during treatment. Typically, the infant will spend most of the phototherapy period undressed and under bright lights with the eyes patched. Occasional respites are given for feeding and care, but for each 24-hour period of phototherapy, usually 18 to 20 hours are consumed by the therapy, which tends to separate the infants from parents. Long-term recovery from hyperbilirubinemia is generally very good. A few infants show transient depression of auditory brainstem responses, but many make a prompt recovery during or after treatment, with no obvious long-term effects.

NECROTIZING ENTEROCOLITIS

Necrotizing enterocolitis is an inflammatory bowel condition characterized by ileus and pneumatosis, and occasionally by peritonitis and generalized sepsis. Its origin is probably multifactorial, although an infectious component is strongly suspected in many cases. A confirmed case of necrotizing enterocolitis requires bowel rest with intravenous feedings for 5 to 7 days, or sometimes longer. In most cases, the infant also shows evidence of abdominal distention, with pain and discomfort. Once again, an infant with this condition is separated from the parents for a time without being fed. Although the outcomes are generally favorable, a few infants require surgery and a few remain very difficult to feed after the resolution of necrotizing enterocolitis by physical and radiologic examination.

ASPHYXIA

Asphyxia is a term describing a complex condition of organ hypoxemia and hypoperfusion. Much of what is called "perinatal" asphyxia may derive from antenatal episodes of fetal circulatory insufficiency. It is often characterized by signs of fetal or neonatal distress, or both, and sometimes by neurologic abnormalities that may include sedation, coma, hyperirritability, and seizures. All four components may be present during the clinical evolution of hypoxic ischemic encephalopathy (Volpe, 1995). In addition, severe asphyxia may produce damage to other organs, such as liver, kidney, myocardium, and bowel. In milder cases, recovery is rapid. In more severe cases, recovery may be prolonged and only partial. The condition is highly stressful as a result of circulatory impairment, acidosis, and neurologic dysfunction.

Apgar scores are routinely obtained at deliveries in the United States. Persistently low Apgar scores are associated with a markedly increased risk of neonatal death. The largest outcome study to evaluate the relationship between Apgar scores and outcome was reported in 1981 (National

Collaborative Perinatal Project; see Nelson and Ellenberg, 1981). A group of 49,000 infants on whom standardized Apgar scoring had been completed underwent standardized neurologic evaluations at 1 and 7 years of age. Persistently low Apgar scores were, as expected, associated with cerebral palsy. One-minute Apgar scores alone, however, did not predict developmental outcome or risk of cerebral palsy. Only 12% of children with Apgar scores of 0 to 3 at 10, 15, and 20 minutes had later cerebral palsy, whereas 80% of the survivors were free of major handicap at school age. This finding probably reflects both the resistance of the immature central nervous system to asphyxial injury and its plasticity and ability to recover from insult.

INFECTION

Bacterial meningitis is an infection with inflammation of the meninges (the membranes that surround the brain and spinal fluid). Hristeva and colleagues (1993) reported that the rate of bacterial meningitis over a 7-year period was 2.5 per 10,000. Group B streptococcus was the most common cause of early-onset meningitis, and gram-negative organisms accounted for the majority of late-onset meningitis. Twenty-seven percent of the infants had neurologic sequelae. Bacterial meningitis in the neonatal period is currently stated to be the leading cause of acquired deafness in childhood. Infections that may develop prior to delivery (antepartum) or during labor and delivery (intrapartum) may have significant neurosensory and physical effects on the fetus and newborn. Screening for the TORCH (*t*oxoplasmosis, *o*ther infections, *r*ubella, *c*ytomegalovirus infection, and *h*erpes simplex) infections is done with appropriate blood and urine cultures and antibody titers. It is currently estimated that cytomegalovirus is the most prevalent viral infection causing hearing loss in the neonate. It is estimated to occur in 1% (30,000 to 40,000) infants born in the United States each year. About 90% of infants with cytomegalovirus infection are asymptomatic at birth. Hearing impairment is more common in infants with clinical signs, including petechiae, jaundice, hepatosplenomegaly, and central nervous system findings, including abnormal computed tomographic scans. Although hearing impairment occurs in 20% to 65% of symptomatic infants, it is also found in about 7% to 13% of the asymptomatic population.

Infants delivered vaginally to mothers with an active primary genital herpes simplex virus lesion have a 50% chance of getting the disease. Most infants with herpes simplex virus infection, however, are delivered from mothers without an active lesion and with a negative history. Infants suspected of the diagnosis are treated with varicella-zoster immune globulin and acyclovir. The incidence of syphilis in the United States since the 1980s has increased in at-risk populations. Identified mothers are aggressively treated with antibiotics to prevent transmission. In untreated mothers, congenital syphilis can occur through transplacental infection or direct contact with infectious lesions during delivery. Infants with congenital syphilis are treated with antibiotic therapy based on their serologic test results, cerebrospinal fluid status, and radiographic findings.

Toxoplasmosis is caused by exposure to the parasite *Toxoplasma gondii*. The infected neonate may manifest a rash, enlarged liver and spleen, enlarged lymph nodes, jaundice, and thrombocytopenia. Cerebral calcifications may be present on computed tomographic scan as a consequence of intrauterine meningoencephalitis. The sequelae may include mental retardation, vision impairment, learning problems, and hearing deficit.

Human immunodeficiency virus (HIV) infection in the neonate remains uncommon but varies depending on the geographic area. This population of infants is, however, increasing in number and is at high risk of multiple medical and neurosensory and developmental sequelae. All TORCH infections are more common in HIV-infected infants.

INTRAVENTRICULAR HEMORRHAGE

Hemorrhage into the germinal matrix tissues, with or without extension into the ventricular system and parenchyma of the developing brain, has been shown to be a serious neonatal morbidity of premature infants born at less than 32 weeks' gestation (Volpe, 1989). Papile and colleagues (1978) first reported a radiographic grading system for describing the severity of periventricular-intraventricular hemorrhage in 1978. This development permitted clinicians and researchers to place neonates into intraventricular hemorrhage (IVH) categories that reflected the severity of the insult, including grade I (subependymal hemorrhage), grade II (IVH without ventricular dilation), grade III (IVH with ventricular dilation), and grade IV (IVH with parenchymal hemorrhage).

Studies published prior to the 1980s reported incidence rates of IVH in neonatal intensive care units of 40% to 45%. Many centers have reported a decreasing incidence in the 1980s and 1990s, with rates between 12% and 30%. Treatment advances, including prenatal administration of steroids, surfactant, and prophylactic indomethacin, have contributed to the decline in the incidence of IVH, although it remains a significant risk factor for neurologic, neurosensory, developmental, behavioral, and educational sequelae (Ahmann et al, 1980; Ment et al, 1994; Papile et al, 1978). Dilated ventricles occur more frequently in association with moderate hemorrhage and may or may not be related to posthemorrhagic obstruction. Approximately 50% of infants with ventricular dilatation exhibit resolution of the condition in about 4 weeks. In contrast, an increasing fontanel size, increasing ventricular size, irritability, apnea, and poor feeding are signs suggestive of increased intracranial pressure. As soon as the medical team determines that the infant can tolerate a surgical procedure, a ventriculoperitoneal shunt should be placed. Placement of a coiled catheter into the peritoneal cavity is safe, accommodates the infant's growth, and decreases the frequency of shunt revision.

A number of studies suggest that ventriculomegaly at term is associated with an increased incidence of subsequent motor abnormalities (Allan et al, 1982; Hill and Volpe, 1981; Philip et al, 1989). It is important to note that although ventricular dilatation occurs most frequently with moderate to severe hemorrhage and posthemorrhagic obstruction, it may occur in association with small ependymal hemorrhage. Saliba and colleagues (1990) prospectively followed a cohort of low–birth weight infants born at less than 35 weeks' gestation with serial cranial ultrasonograms at weekly intervals during hospitalization and at 2, 4, 6, 9, and 19 months. Ventricular growth velocities were significantly higher in infants with a history of ventricular dilation or periventricular leukomalacia (PVL) and were associated with the poorest outcome at 18 to 24 months of age.

PERIVENTRICULAR LEUKOMALACIA

Periventricular leukomalacia is more often identified in premature infants with IVH than in those without IVH. It is believed to be secondary to the changes in cerebral blood flow that accompany IVH (Szymonowicz, Yu, and Bajuk, 1986). PVL is generally a symmetric injury of the periventricular white matter, which can be seen by cranial ultrasonography as cystic lesions located at the corners of the lateral ventricles in the frontal, parietal, and, less commonly, occipital regions. Risk factors for PVL include hypotensive, apneic, and ischemic events that are associated with decreased cerebral blood flow. Perhaps the greatest known risk for neurodevelopmental sequelae is the combination of IVH and PVL. This is compounded by the fact that PVL occurs most often in the sickest and smallest infants. Although all forms of spasticity, vision and hearing impairments, and developmental abnormalities may occur with PVL, the most frequent clinical correlate of PVL is spastic diplegia.

NEONATAL SEIZURES

The most common types of neonatal seizures seen in premature infants are subtle (oral-buccal or ocular-motor movements) or generalized tonic. The majority of premature infants with neonatal seizures do not develop epilepsy. Infants with neonatal seizures who have had grade III or IV IVH, moderately abnormal findings on an electroencephalogram, or neurologic findings, however, are at increased risk of this sequela and require follow-up with a neurologist. Infants discharged on an anticonvulsant medication (in most cases phenobarbital) should be re-evaluated by 3 months' corrected age to determine the need for continued medication. An acceptable approach in a stable infant with no abnormal neurologic findings is to allow the infant to "outgrow" the anticonvulsant dose. Those infants who continue to have seizure activity should be monitored by a pediatric neurologist.

METABOLIC DISORDERS

Although numerous rare metabolic disorders have been identified, there is wide variation among states regarding guidelines for screening. The American Academy of Pediatrics advocates universal screening for hypothyroidism and phenylketonuria. Diseases that are screened for in a limited number of states include galactosemia, homocystinuria, tyrosinemia, maple syrup urine disease, biotinidase deficiency, and congenital adrenal hyperplasia. It is recommended that the screening be done after the infant has begun feeding and after 24 hours of age.

GENETIC DISORDERS AND CONGENITAL DISORDERS

Infants with major chromosomal abnormalities, including trisomies 13, 18, and 21, and those with neural tube defects will be recognized in the delivery suite if the diagnosis has not already been made with cytogenetic or biochemical analyses using amniotic fluid samples. Other conditions that may rapidly manifest as a clinically distressed state include congenital cardiac or pulmonary anomalies, Pierre Robin anomaly, and osteogenesis imperfecta. Advances in mapping and sequencing of the human genome are gradually paving the way for the treatment of genetic conditions. Gene mapping technology can provide accurate diagnosis before symptoms become evident, sometimes permitting presymptom intervention and prevention.

APNEA

Apnea is usually defined as a cessation of breathing that may be short (6–10 seconds) and self-limited, or prolonged (>10 seconds) and associated with bradycardia. A variety of respiratory abnormalities associated with apnea can be found in premature infants. To fully understand their clinical significance, it is important to know their definitions. There are two primary types of apnea: central, which occurs when breathing effort is absent; and obstructive, which occurs secondary to a blockage, such as airway collapse or mucus. A combination of these two types of apnea is referred to as *mixed apnea*. Presence of pallor, cyanosis, limpness, stiffness, or unresponsiveness indicates a serious event. Any of these potentially life-threatening occurrences are called *pathologic apnea. Apnea of prematurity* is increased periodic breathing in association with pathologic apnea in a premature infant. It is a common finding and has been reported in 84% of infants with a birth weight of less than 1000 g. Apnea of prematurity is a problem when events are associated with bradycardia of less than 100 beats per minute, when oxygen desaturation is less than 90%, when the infant requires stimulation to recover, or a combination of these.

Since the control of respiration depends on maturity of both the central nervous system and the respiratory system, the premature infant is vulnerable to respiratory abnormalities. Before 28 weeks of gestation, 100% of premature infants have periodic breathing, and 50% of those infants have pathologic apnea. Although the majority of premature infants outgrow apnea of prematurity by 37 weeks of gestation, the presence of persistent clinically significant apnea in an infant who in other respects is ready for discharge from the NICU represents an important clinical management issue. This concern arises from the association between apnea of prematurity and sudden infant death syndrome (SIDS). Four percent of infants with a history of apnea of prematurity die of SIDS, and both prematurity and bronchopulmonary dysplasia have been associated with an increased incidence of SIDS.

GASTROESOPHAGEAL REFLUX

Reflux is another relatively common event often observed in association with central or obstructive apnea in small premature infants, particularly those with bronchopulmonary dysplasia, those with increased abdominal pressure, and those receiving steroids or theophylline. Gastroesophageal reflux normally occurs when infants burp or spit up. In a few cases, acid reflux produces lower esophageal irritation and pain and interferes with feeding and respiration. This condition is more common in preterm than in term infants but seems often to be overdiagnosed. It is difficult to obtain a clear idea of the incidence of serious gastroesophageal reflux that actually needs and responds to treatment. When gastroesophageal reflux is severe, it may impair feeding sufficiently to interfere with normal weight gain and growth. In a few situations, especially in children with neurologic disabilities who have an absent or impaired gag reflex, surgical treatment is required. Most patients can be treated conservatively by elevating the head of the bed, giving small feeds, and thickening the formula with rice cereal. Antacids and prokinetics may be beneficial when symptoms persist. Most reflux symptoms of premature infants resolve by 6 months of age. Infants with reflux may have apneic and bradycardiac events associated with feeds or following feeds, with or without spitting up, gagging, and choking. Severe reflux events can be life-threatening. Multichannel recordings of electrocardiogram, respiratory effort by impedance, nasal air flow, oxygen saturation, and esophageal pH can provide important information to the diagnostic process when uncertainties about the etiology of events exist. They are used as an adjunct to the clinical evaluation to assist in differentiating central apnea from obstructive problems and reflux.

NUTRITION AND GROWTH

Infants in the NICU have a variety of medical problems related to their underlying illness (e.g., asphyxia, infection, congenital abnormalities, cardiorespiratory illness, metabolic problems, prematurity) that have an impact on feeding ability, feeding tolerance, nutritional absorption, or nutritional intake. Infants with necrotizing enterocolitis or asphyxia or those requiring assisted ventilation may be unable to receive or tolerate feeds. In the premature infant or the neurologically impaired infant, gastrointestinal function may be impaired, and sucking and swallowing may be undeveloped or uncoordinated. All of these factors contribute to the risk of inadequate nutritional intake, weight loss, and secondary growth restriction. In addition, the intake in sick infants and premature infants is often administered primarily parenterally and does not meet the necessary requirements for growth. Premature infants lose 10% of body weight in the first days of life and do not achieve their birth weight until approximately 2 weeks of age. To achieve catch-up growth comparable to that of an infant born 2 weeks later of the same postconceptual age, the infant must have accelerated catch-up growth.

Good nutrition is an important biological component of normal neonatal development, and feeding is an important element of normal mother-infant interaction. The nutritional, psychological, and social benefits of normal feeding may be disturbed in high-risk infants. Many infants with respiratory distress or other signs of physiologic compromise receive nothing by mouth immediately after birth, and some are not fully or normally fed for several weeks. The most obvious stress related to lack of oral feeding is hunger. Short periods without oral nutrition seem to be tolerated without adverse long-term sequelae. Prolonged periods without adequate oral intake place the infant at risk of nutritional compromise and may also disturb the balance between nutritive and nonnutritive sucking and swallowing, as well as the normal cycles of hunger and satiety that well newborns experience. Conditions such as recurrent infections and bronchopulmonary dysplasia both compromise the infant's ability to eat and raise energy requirements. Energy requirements may also be high in the early stages of feeding VLBW infants, whose body configuration and lack of subcutaneous fat provide a high ratio of surface area to body mass, with high rates of insensible caloric and water loss. Prolonged periods without oral intake, especially if mechanical devices are placed in the oropharynx or upper airway for long periods, such as endotracheal tubes, tracheostomy tubes, or continuous positive airway pressure prongs, may render a few infants aversive to normal nipple-feeding and require subsequent retraining of the sucking and swallowing mechanism. A final question is the quality of growth in rapidly growing infants who cannot maintain normal oral nutrition. On some programs of technically assisted nutrition, such as prolonged parenteral nutrition, weight gain can be documented, but the distribution of calories and body composition of new growth may not be ideal. Breast-feeding of low–birth weight infants is usually initiated at the same time that the infant has developed the ability to nipple-feed. VLBW infants of less than 1500 g have been shown to have adequate sucking ability and to tolerate breast-feeding at a mean age of 35 weeks, although some may require supplemental feedings by bottle to obtain the necessary volume for weight gain.

PAIN-RELATED STRESS IN NEWBORNS

Pain is a potential source of pathophysiologic stress in the newborn infant. The newborn's inability to describe sensations or experiences of pain often causes the problem of pain in the newborn period to be misunderstood or overlooked. Skepticism or lack of information concerning the physiologic and developmental significance of neonatal pain, and concern about overtreatment or unintended consequences of pharmacologic pain relief, further combine to reinforce a common tendency to minimize the importance of pain as a separate medical problem in newborns. Sometimes, pain responses in sick newborns may even be relied on as informal guides to level of alertness, readiness for respirator weaning, and so on. This approach, formerly more common than now with all pediatric patients, may mean that commonly painful routines and procedures in newborns may be underestimated and not enough care taken to treat or avoid the associated pain.

Cutaneous receptors for tactile and painful stimuli are actively developing by the 17th to 18th weeks of gestation (Anand and Carr, 1989). Afferent fibers from the skin to synapses in the dorsal spinal nerve roots are linked to higher central nervous system (CNS) regions via the spinothalamic tracts and then to the sensory cortex. At 20 to 24 weeks, afferent connections from the skin to the sensory cortex are rapidly maturing, so that pathways for tactile and pain perception in the CNS are already developed at, or somewhat before, the gestational age of presumed fetal viability (Anand and Carr, 1989). The density of pain fiber endings per square centimeter of skin may be greatest at 20 to 22 weeks of gestation, although the level of conscious perception and memory for pain at this stage cannot be accurately estimated. In utero, fetuses of 20 to 24 weeks' gestation show reflexive responses to various stimuli during monitoring and diagnostic procedures, and ELBW infants of 23 to 24 weeks' gestation in the nursery regularly show aversive responses to diagnostic and therapeutic procedures (e.g., venipuncture) that are normally considered painful at any other age. It may be appropriate, then, to state as a first principle of understanding and managing pain in newborns that whatever is obviously painful at any other age is probably painful for the newborn (and possibly for the 2nd- or 3rd-trimester fetus), regardless of gestational age at birth.

Acutely painful procedures that adult caregivers can readily observe include injections, phlebotomy, closed thoracotomy, lumbar puncture, and circumcision (Anand and Hickey, 1987; Bell, 1994; Gottfried et al, 1981). Clinical signs of crying, withdrawal, or anticipation with these procedures (e.g., crying when the skin is prepared) correspond to signs of increased neurophysiologic instability, including tachycardia, O_2 desaturation, and increased catecholamine secretion (Bell, 1994).

Other procedures and clinical conditions may produce more chronic pain, sometimes with recurrent signs of physiologic disturbance or instability. These include prolonged invasive procedures and postoperative incisional pain, of which the most common form is pain after circumcision. Subtle behavioral changes, possibly pain-related, have been described within the first 12 to 24 hours after circumcision performed without analgesia.

Another likely source of pain in VLBW infants is cutaneous trauma. Examples include bruises acquired during phlebotomy or invasive procedures, abrasions and desquamation caused by tape or monitor electrodes, and heat injury from cutaneous oxygen and pulse oximeter probes. Superficial or deep injury to the skin is often painful in older patients and is probably painful to preterm infants, who have a higher density of pain fibers than older children and adults. Cutaneous trauma and desquamation are common in "borderline viable" 23- to 25-week preterm infants and may cause unrecognized chronic or recurrent pain. The effect of pain on postnatal adaptation or chances for survival in ELBW infants is not known.

Objective standards for interventions to prevent or treat pain in newborns are difficult to establish. Some procedures that cause momentary pain may not warrant administration of potent analgesics or slow-acting topical anesthetics, especially if delay of a procedure (e.g., a blood culture or lumbar puncture) while waiting for analgesia may further endanger the patient. Even if regional or local analgesics or anesthetics have only a small risk of adverse drug reactions, delay in the procedure or distortion of the sampling site (e.g., an artery or an intervertebral space) may be medically counterproductive. On the other hand, postoperative pain, or procedure-related pain that is more than transient and minor (as with, e.g., closed thoracotomy), may warrant consideration of local or systemic analgesia (Bell, 1994). Acetaminophen (Tylenol) appears useful for analgesia in many such situations, and pain relief with opiates is indicated after major surgery or for other persistently painful conditions.

Analgesia and sedation have been used more or less routinely for ventilatory management in some neonatal units, but seldom in others. There are no objective criteria to assess pain or to guide the practice of opiate administration or heavy sedation as routine adjuncts to ventilator care. In some respects, oversedation in ventilatory management may be counterproductive and perhaps even harmful, prolonging respirator dependence, increasing the risk of ventilator-related complications, obscuring the course of respirator weaning, and possibly risking a postventilator period of opiate tolerance and withdrawal.

In summary, pain is a potential cause of physiologic and psychological stress, which may often be underestimated and sometimes undertreated in the newborn. Practical problems include recognition of pain in nonverbal patients and balancing the risks and benefits of analgesia or sedation in particular clinical circumstances.

The Neonatal Environment: Developmental Intervention in the Neonatal Intensive Care Unit

Issues in developmental intervention in the NICU continue to emerge as the survival of infants of extremely low birth weight becomes more common. During the 1980s, the potentially adverse effects of environmental stimuli within the NICU on the physiologic stability of preterm infants were reported (Gottfried et al, 1981). Other studies reported favorable effects of specific types of sensory stimulation on the growth and development of preterm infants. The ELBW survivors of the 1990s, however, by virtue of their neurologic immaturity and medical fragility, possess behavioral and developmental needs that are likely to be different from those of preterm infants of the past. The current approach to developmental intervention in the NICU, in which individual needs of the infant and family dictate the plan of care, has evolved in response to the increasing diversity and vulnerability among preterm infants in neonatal intensive care (Gorski, 1991).

Just as medical status is continually reassessed throughout the infant's stay in the NICU, the need for and appropriateness of developmental intervention needs to be evaluated on an ongoing basis. Developmental care is initiated in response to the specific needs of the infant but quickly enlarges its focus to include caregivers and family members in as many aspects of assessment and planning as possible. Each plan for developmental care involves careful consideration of the infant's current medical and physiologic stability and assessment of the unique behavioral cues the infant provides. These behavioral cues, in combination with physiologic measures, can inform caregivers of the infant's tolerance for caregiving procedures and availability for social interaction. As one of the first avenues for communication between infant and caregiver, behavioral cues provide a vehicle for family participation in their infant's care (Fig. 26–1).

ACCOMMODATING THE NEEDS OF A DEVELOPING NERVOUS SYSTEM

By 17 weeks' gestation, the human fetus possesses all the neurons that will ever be produced within the CNS, and the process of establishing neural connections is occurring at a rapid rate. By 23 weeks, when some infants begin neonatal intensive care, the vestibular, tactile, auditory, and

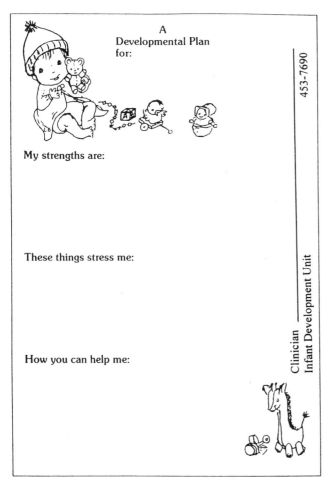

Figure 26–1. An individual developmental care plan developed by nursery staff and parents can be placed at the bedside to increase continuity of care. (From Cole JG, Grappier PA: Infant stimulation reassessed. A new approach to providing care for the preterm infant. J Obstet Gynecol Neonatal Nurs 14[6]:471–477, 1985.)

visual receptors are developed and capable of processing this sensory input. Although motor immaturity and the effects of neurologic compromise sometimes prevent the ELBW infant from responding to stimuli in an organized fashion, this does not negate the fact that sensory information is being received and processed. Through a mechanism that has been termed *neuronal sculpting,* processing of sensory experience forms the basis for development of neuronal pathways, solidifying some neuronal connections and allowing other unused or nonadaptive connections to degenerate (Als et al, 1994). Thus, caregiving experiences in the NICU have the potential to influence the formation of new neural pathways and can also be assumed to influence the process of CNS recovery after IVH. The challenge in providing appropriate interventions in the NICU is to optimize the potential for normal development in an environment that is, first and foremost, intended to provide intensive medical care.

REDUCING RISK OF PROGRESSION OF INTRAVENTRICULAR HEMORRHAGE: POSITIONING AND HANDLING

Birth position, mode of delivery, perinatal and neonatal medications, and mechanical ventilation have all been in-

vestigated for possible effects on the incidence and severity of IVH and developmental outcome. Potential effects of nursing care practices such as frequency of handling and positioning have also been explored. Although a direct relation between specific handling practices and progression of intracranial bleeding has not been shown, the effects of routine handling on stability in physiologic functioning, such as respiration, oxygenation, and blood pressure, are known. Therefore, minimal handling is generally considered to be prudent for preterm infants, especially those of extremely low birth weight, who may be at greater risk of intracranial hemorrhage. Avoidance of rapid changes in position to prevent undue fluctuation in intracranial pressure, and maintenance of unobstructed venous return from the head through elevation to approximately 30 degrees, may be beneficial to infants with posthemorrhagic hydrocephalus. Central apnea and bradycardia can sometimes be reduced through positioning in prone position. The prone position offers a mechanical advantage to immature musculature in the thoracoabdominal region that enhances respiration (Wolfson et al, 1992) and maximizes body contact with the supporting surface, reducing the tendency toward self-startles. However, prolonged positioning in prone presents some disadvantages, particularly while the infant is receiving respiratory support by ventilator or continuous positive airway pressure, as it necessitates asymmetric positioning of the head, with some associated flattening, and, occasionally, breakdown of skin around the ears. Commercially available gel pads that cushion the head uniformly can help maintain the contours of the skull and, when covered with soft flannel, prevent skin abrasion.

Positioning also results in soft-tissue changes that may influence postural development. Prolonged neck extension contributes to shortening of the neck extensors and prolonged overstretch of the flexors, inhibiting active neck flexion. While the infant is receiving ventilatory support, ventroflexion of the neck is not recommended, as this can interfere with the position of the endotracheal tube. However, once the infant is able to be treated with continuous positive airway pressure, there is greater opportunity to achieve alignment of the head with the body axis. This modification prepares the infant for breathing with the head partially flexed forward, a position that will be used for breast- or bottle-feeding, and, nearer to the date of discharge, when seated in an infant seat or car seat. Many infants continue to have poor neck and head control through the transition home; therefore, caregivers of preterm infants need to be informed prior to discharge of the possibility of airway obstruction secondary to excessive neck flexion, particularly when the infant is placed in a semiflexed, seated position. The American Academy of Pediatrics recommends a 90-minute trial in the infant's own car seat, with pulse oximetry, to assess the risk for obstructive apnea in this position (Committee on Injury and Poison Prevention and Committee on Fetus and Newborn, 1992). If the infant cannot be safely seated, an approved car-bed can be used as an alternative.

Postural alignment and active movement of the shoulder and pelvic girdles also may be affected by positioning in the NICU. Preterm infants are at increased risk for postural abnormalities, particularly related to midline control, some of which can be prevented through proper positioning. Preterm infants begin their stay in the NICU with very little body tone and little opportunity for active movement. Prolonged positioning in prone or supine position can result in shoulder girdle elevation and extension, along with excessive shoulder extension and external rotation. This position can lead to difficulty in horizontally adducting and flexing the arms toward midline. The typical lower extremity posture of the ELBW preterm infant is equally a problem, as a combination of gravity and diapering maintains the legs in a widely abducted, semiflexed, externally rotated position. One strategy for achieving shoulder and hip flexion and adduction in prone position is to place a thin layer of blanket supports beneath the infant in a T-shape, with the wide portion under the head and the vertical piece fully supporting the infant's chest and abdomen, leaving the pelvis free. The padding raises the infant just enough for gravity to assist the infant in bringing the arms more closely to the sides and permits hip flexion rather than abduction. Nesting, a curved roll of bedding surrounding the lower extremities and secured to the mattress for stability, can be used in prone or supine position to bring the legs into more flexion, adduction, and internal rotation. Or, a long, thin blanket roll may be tucked under the mattress of the Isolette and around the infant's buttocks in a ''sling,'' to maintain flexion in prone position. Nesting has the added advantage of containing random movements, assisting the infant in returning to a calm state after startling or jerking (Fig. 26–2). Side-lying is preferred over supine positioning, as gravity can be utilized in this position to bring the legs into more neutral alignment. A nest can be used in side-lying to keep the legs flexed, with an additional roll of padding placed under the top leg to maintain some abduction and for support. Waterbeds are used in some NICU settings to enhance flexion and reduce startles, thus increasing quiet rest and weight gain; however, results of studies demonstrating the effectiveness of these beds are inconclusive, as these studies lack controlled comparison groups.

Some preterm infants, especially those who have experienced oligohydramnios, have joint limitations at birth that require gentle passive range of motion exercises. These infants benefit most from a program that emphasizes hold-ing gently at the endpoint of the range for several seconds, rather than multiple repetitions. Infants with oligohydramnios may also show a clear persistence of lower extremity posturing in excessive leg and ankle flexion and abduction. A positioning aid that abducts the legs and provides a short horizontal bar on each side for positioning the feet can be used in prone or side-lying position with a soft, neoprene strap around the ankles to hold them in neutral alignment. Splints fabricated of thin (1/16 inch) thermoplastic material, lined with soft padding, have also been used successfully in positioning the ankle and foot in neutral position. These positioning aids are used in combination with passive range of motion exercises.

CONSIDERATIONS FOR ASSESSMENT OF NIPPLE-FEEDING

Nipple-feeding of infants with respiratory and neurologic involvement requires careful assessment to determine the optimal approach for each infant. State of arousal is an important consideration, as the infant must be sufficiently alert to participate in the process yet must not become overstimulated. Overstimulation may result in sucking disorganization, fatigue, or the need to actively avoid further interaction by falling asleep. Depending on the severity of involvement, infants with IVH may have greater difficulty than other preterm infants in learning to coordinate breathing with sucking and swallowing. Readiness for nipple-feeding is assessed through examination of infant state; postural tone; integrity of oral structures; presence of oral reflexes; size, shape, and firmness of the nipple; the position of the infant; and nonnutritive and nutritive sucking pattern and sucking rhythm, as all can contribute to bottle- or breast-feeding performance. The Neonatal Oral Motor Assessment Scale (Palmer, Crawley, and Blanco, 1993) and the Wolf and Glass protocol (1992) provide guidelines for assessment during the transition from gavage to nipple-feedings. The primary concern in a feeding assessment is the need to simultaneously monitor physiologic stability for signs of distress and to pace the flow of liquid and the duration of the feeding accordingly. Alternation of gavage and nipple- or breast-feeding is often used to allow for rest

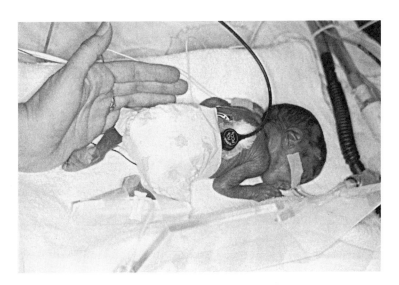

Figure 26–2. Soothing the premature infant by enhancing flexion and providing boundaries with bedding decreases extraneous movement and conserves energy.

and recovery between feedings and to conserve energy. Breast-feeding is well tolerated by some preterm infants with little effect on physiologic stability (Bier et al, 1996). Method of feeding should be selected only after careful evaluation, to obtain optimal nutrition and growth.

VISUAL AND AUDITORY PERFORMANCE

Preterm infants may exhibit delayed visual or auditory awareness or difficulties with focusing and conjugate eye movements. Although initial difficulties often subside, preterm infants with IVH have a higher incidence of hearing loss, functional visual deficits, and problems with ocular-motor control than preterm infants with no IVH. Thus, evaluating visual and auditory responsiveness in an environment with limited visual and sound contamination should be a routine part of the developmental assessment.

BEHAVIORAL ORGANIZATION

Although ultimately focused on function, appropriate developmental interventions for preterm infants in the NICU need to go beyond the medical and neurologic status of the infant to include social and behavioral factors. To facilitate behavioral organization, primary interventions should be directed toward maintenance or enhancement of physiologic stability. The infant's state of arousal and medical factors such as medications, the work of breathing, thermal regulation, noise, light, and postural support may all have an impact on sensory and motor responses and should be considered in interpreting the assessment. Close observations of infants prior to, during, and after caregiving procedures (Fig. 26–3) reveal vulnerabilities and strengths that

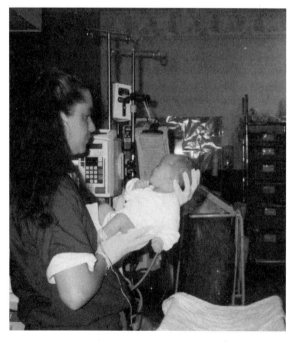

Figure 26–3. Attending to the infant's behavioral cues and pausing during care to accommodate physiologic recovery will enhance overall behavioral organization and energy conservation.

are unique to each infant and can be used as a basis for an individualized plan of developmentally supportive care.

Caring for the Caregivers: Supporting Parents and Siblings

As hospitals adopt the philosophy and goals of family-centered care (Harrison, 1993), parents can become more involved in providing care, and the potential for continuity during the transition from hospital to home is increased. Participation in behavioral observations and developmental interventions enables family members to join the multidisciplinary NICU team in formulating a care plan that meets the infant's needs while supporting their roles as parents. Such communication between family members and the medical team facilitates trust and prepares families for the transition from hospital to home.

Spending time with a preterm infant in the NICU necessitates some disruption to home routines. These disruptions can be especially difficult for young siblings, who find they must share their parents' time and attentions with an infant they may never have seen. In the past, sibling visitation was banned in most NICU settings because of concern for the spread of childhood illnesses. Recent studies have shown, however, that a simple health screening of sisters and brothers prior to each visit prevents the spread of infections. Moreover, having a program in which siblings are prepared for and supervised during their visits by hospital staff ameliorated most concerns on the part of NICU staff about sibling visits while enabling brothers and sisters to understand more about their preterm infant sibling and to participate in welcoming the infant into the family.

Concerns about developmental outcome are compounded among parents of ELBW preterm infants, as they include not only the effects of extreme prematurity but also the possibility of damage to neural structures that support future motor, sensory, and cognitive functions. Regardless of whether developmental interventions are facilitated by a therapist, nurse, or developmental pediatrician, it is important for this professional to have a total understanding of the process, beginning with NICU events, the transition home, follow-up needs, and early intervention and special education services. This perspective allows the professional to assist the family in preparing realistically and practically for the infant's future developmental needs.

Transition Home and Discharge Planning

For the family, the prospect of taking a premature infant home is often a combination of joy mixed with grief over the infant's prolonged illness and uncertainty about the infant's future health and development. After months of hospitalization, the future medical and neurodevelopmental status of the infant may be unclear. Therefore, families must assume greater responsibility for their fragile infant in the presence of continuing uncertainty. A discharge developmental assessment is helpful to identify, with the parents, ongoing vulnerabilities and considerations for preventive care, while also pointing out positive changes in the infant's sensory and motor performance. Daily routines are outlined, to discuss how the infant's care will be integrated into family life (see Chapter 33).

The period between 35 weeks' gestation and 1 month corrected age is a time of rapid change in postural tone for preterm infants, and thus it is important to involve an experienced neonatal occupational or physical therapist to monitor sensory and motor development and to discriminate atypical responses from those that are part of normal preterm development.

Neurosensory Screening

NEUROLOGIC STATUS

The neurologic assessment completed prior to discharge for all infants should include a standard evaluation of suck, swallow, vision responses, auditory responses, movement patterns, and deep tendon and primitive reflexes. If the infant has experienced a CNS insult, the evaluation may include the following: computed tomography scan, magnetic resonance imaging, electroencephalography, auditory brainstem response, and vision evoked response.

There are neonatal, neurologic, and neurobehavioral examinations, including the Brazelton (1984) and the Neonatal Network Neurobehavioral Scale (Lester and Tronick, 1994), which provide additional information about the infant's neurosensory and behavioral responses.

HEARING

It is currently recommended by the American Academy of Pediatrics and the Joint Committee on Hearing that all infants be evaluated for hearing impairment. All NICU infants should have a hearing screen prior to discharge. Screening may be done with transient evoked otoacoustic emissions, brainstem audiometric evoked response, or automated brainstem audiometric evoked response. Infants who do not have a clear pass in these tests are referred for diagnostic audiologic assessment. Middle ear disease and conductive hearing loss are also more common in premature infants. Management by an audiologist, assessment of speech and language, and intervention services are needed. All premature infants should have a hearing screen before being discharged from the NICU.

VISION

All infants with a birth weight of less than 1500 g who are cared for in an NICU should undergo a vision examination for retinopathy of prematurity (ROP) completed by an ophthalmologist skilled in examining neonates prior to hospital discharge. ROP is a disorder of developing retinal vessels in extremely premature infants. The abnormality may either heal completely or progress to sequelae. The examination should occur by at least 32 to 34 weeks postconception. The status of the infant's eyes is characterized with the criteria established by the International Committee for the Classification of Retinopathy of Prematurity (1997). Close monitoring of all infants with findings to

determine the need for ophthalmologic intervention (cryotherapy, laser therapy, buckle or vitrectomy procedures) is recommended. In addition, a follow-up visit by 3 to 6 months is recommended for infants with negative findings. Long-term ROP sequelae include retinal detachment, myopia, strabismus, and amblyopia and blindness. Infants with visual sequelae require ongoing monitoring by an ophthalmologist and early intervention services.

SOCIAL AND ENVIRONMENTAL RISK

Many states now screen families of infants for social and environmental risks such as teenaged parent, Medicaid dependence, no prenatal care, and parental substance abuse in an effort to identify candidates for early intervention programs or for developmental monitoring.

Neonatal Follow-up

An important component of postdischarge management of the high-risk patient is the long-term assessment provided by a neonatal follow-up program. The evolution of neonatal follow-up programs to monitor the growth and neurodevelopmental outcome of high-risk infants, as an adjunct to care provided by the primary physician, has provided a mechanism for maintaining quality control of the management and care techniques used in the NICU. To attain this objective, a follow-up program must have both service and research goals. The service goals include the following:

1. Follow the growth and development of at-risk infants.
2. Identify medical, neurologic, developmental, and behavioral abnormalities.
3. Make referrals to consultants, early intervention programs, and education programs where appropriate.
4. Provide prompt comprehensive reports of assessments to the primary physician.

Research goals include the following:

1. Maintain a structured database of high-risk populations as a quality control for nursery standards.
2. Develop research protocols to study the effects of medical morbidities, treatments, and interventions on outcome.

To accomplish these goals, it is necessary to develop a follow-up team composed of a director, a coordinator, physicians (neonatologists, developmental pediatricians, or neurologists), a nurse, a psychologist, and a data analyst. Other participants may include a pediatric occupational or physical therapist, a nutritionist, a respiratory therapist, a social worker, a secretary, and student volunteers.

Each hospital must establish risk criteria for which infants are eligible for the longitudinal assessments. This list should depend on the risk population served, the funding available, and the clinic staff and space available. It is important that the infants considered at greatest risk of sequelae (e.g., very low birth weight, asphyxia, neurologic problems) be followed.

IMMUNIZATIONS

Routine immunization with hepatitis B vaccine is recommended for all newborns. A preterm infant with a birth weight less than 2000 g whose mother is HbsAg-negative should receive hepatitis B vaccine by the age of 2 months. If the mother is HbsAg-positive, the preterm infant should receive the vaccine and hepatitis B immune globulin within 12 hours of birth. In addition, the American Academy of Pediatrics recommends that preterm infants receive full-dose diphtheria-tetanus-pertussis (DTP) vaccine and oral polio vaccine at routine intervals of chronologic ages 2, 4, and 6 months. Infants who remain hospitalized at an age appropriate for immunization may receive their first dose of either diphtheria-tetanus-acellular pertussis (DTaP) or DTP in the hospital. Morbidities such as bronchopulmonary dysplasia and IVH are not contraindications for immunization. Prevention of respiratory syncytial virus with intravenous respiratory syncytial virus immune globulin intravenous was licensed by the Food and Drug Administration in January 1996. It is currently recommended for infants less than 24 months of age with a history of premature birth (<35 weeks) or bronchopulmonary dysplasia. Because of short-term effects, monthly infusions are needed during the respiratory syncytial virus season (October to March) to prevent severe lower respiratory tract disease and rehospitalization. Parents who may be reluctant to expose their infant to the stress of repeated infusions need a full explanation of the risk of catching respiratory syncytial virus.

Follow-up Studies of Neurologic and Neurosensory Outcomes

Both neurologic maturation and neurologic recovery from insult are processes that occur in the first year of life in VLBW infants. It is well documented that neurologic findings such as hypertonicity, asymmetry, jerky movements, and tremors, which may be present at term, 3 months, or 6 months of age, may resolve by 12 months of age. In contrast, although a diagnosis of cerebral palsy may be impossible to make at 3 months of age, the characteristic findings become clear by 12 to 18 months of age. Allen and Alexander (1997) reported on the effective use of motor milestones (rolling, sitting, crawling, and cruising) in a multistep process to screen for cerebral palsy. Primary outcome measures for many studies continue to be cerebral palsy, blindness, deafness, and mental retardation. It remains important, however, to consider the family's socioeconomic profile when making predictions about outcome. Escalona (1982) was one of the first to clearly demonstrate less optimal social and economic factors that had negative effects on intelligence quotient scores by 3 years of age. Follow-up studies now all address the issue of study population characteristics.

EXTREMELY LOW BIRTH WEIGHT OUTCOME

Many recent follow-up studies have focused on ELBW infants, those at the limits of viability. Hack, Friedman, and Fanaroff (1996) compared two time periods (1982–1988 and 1990–1992) for cohorts of ELBW infants of less than 750 g, and, despite a significant increase in survival rates between the study periods, found no difference in neurodevelopmental outcomes. Casiro and colleagues (1995) evaluated the effects of surfactant on ELBW infants as part of the Canadian Exosurf Neonatal Follow-up Group and found comparable developmental outcomes with a significant decrease in the incidence of severe ROP in the surfactant group compared with the air placebo group. Zorn and colleagues (1996) examined 236 infants born at less than 29 weeks' gestation receiving prophylactic colfosceril palmitate (Exosurf) or calf lung surfactant extract (Infasurf). Severe cerebral palsy, defined as inability to sit at 2 years, was present in less than 5% of the infants. Severe mental retardation, defined as a Bayley Mental Developmental Index (MDI) less than 50, was present in 17.5% of Exosurf and 10.7% of Infasurf recipients. Blindness or deafness was present in less than 1% of either group.

Since the 1980s, there has been increased interest in evaluating and reporting the functional status of VLBW survivors. This change occurred after a proposal by the World Health Organization (WHO) (1980) of a model for classifying pathophysiology, impairment, disability, and handicap when assessing health status in adults. The National Center for Medical Rehabilitation Research (NCMRR) (National Advisory Board on Medical Rehabilitation Research, 1993) expanded the WHO model to include functional and social limitations. This type of assessment can easily be used for children and determines the child's ability to perform tasks of daily living and fulfill social roles of children of the same age and culture. Areas assessed include feeding, dressing, bathing, maintaining continency, mobility, communication, play, and social interaction. The Functional Independence Measure for Children (WeeFIM) Instrument was developed to assess and track neurodevelopmental disabilities and evaluate functional outcomes of children receiving developmental interventions. Studies using this instrument have shown that the overall functional status at 4 1/2 years of VLBW infants without major neurodevelopmental impairments was good. For instance, 100% were able to walk 150 feet, talk in sentences, maintain continency, and understand simple requests. Another important assessment time is kindergarten age to determine appropriate school placement for VLBW infants. Kindergarten readiness is dependent on the interaction of cognitive skills, language skills, perceptual skills, motor coordination, and attention. A single test should not be used and may result in misuse and misinterpretation. This necessitates the use of a multisource approach that incorporates parent reports, teacher reports, and independent psychoeducational assessments. VLBW survivors remain at increased risk of school achievement difficulties. Reports of school performance of VLBW infants indicate that they are more likely to need special education placement (23%–50%) and repeat a grade (37%). This is in contrast to national data in which 7.6% of children repeat kindergarten or first grade. As many as 30% to 50% of term infants from impoverished environments, however, are at risk of academic underachievement.

Conclusion

The outcome of VLBW infants is the result of contributions of numerous maternal, neonatal, and postneonatal factors affecting growth, neurologic status, developmental functioning, and behavior. The internal resiliency of the individual child, chronic illness, and the quality of the postneonatal environment are important factors that can modify early biological risks (Werner and Smith, 1992). Infants have been shown to have a certain internal plasticity or ability to recover from many biological perinatal and neonatal risk factors. Children residing within stressed environments, however, continue to be at increased risk of mental health problems and learning disorders. Comprehensive family case management and behavioral and developmental intervention provide an opportunity to identify and facilitate protective factors that will aid in the recovery of high-risk infants. It is reassuring that the majority of VLBW infants of less than 1500 g continue to survive free of major neurologic and sensory sequelae and mental retardation.

REFERENCES

Ahmann PA, Lazzara A, Dykes FD, et al: Intraventricular hemorrhage in the high risk preterm infant: incidence and outcome. Ann Neurol 7:118–124, 1980.

Allan WC, Holt PJ, Sawyer LR, et al: Ventricular dilatation after neonatal periventricular-intraventricular hemorrhage. Am J Dis Child 136:589–593, 1982.

Allen MC, Alexander GR: Using motor milestones as a multistep process to screen infants for cerebral palsy. Dev Med Child Neurol 39:12, 1997.

Als H, Lawhon G, Duffy FH, et al: Individualized developmental care for the very low birthweight preterm infant: medical and neurofunctional effects. JAMA 272:853, 1994.

Anand KJS, Carr DB: The neuroanatomy, neurophysiology, and neurochemistry of pain, stress, and analgesia in newborns and children. Pediatr Clin North Am 36:795, 1989.

Anand KJS, Hickey PR: Pain and its effects in the human neonate and fetus. N Engl J Med 317:1321, 1987.

Ballard JL, Khoury JC, Wedig K, et al: New Ballard Score, expanded to include extremely premature infants. J Pediatr 119:417–423, 1991.

Bell SG: The National Pain Management Guideline: implications for neonatal intensive care. Neonat Network 13:9, 1994.

Bier J, Ferguson A, Morales Y, et al: Comparison of skin-to-skin contact with standard contact in low-birth-weight infants who are breast-fed. Arch Pediatr Adolesc Med 150:1265, 1996.

Brazelton TB: Neonatal Behavioral Assessment Scale, 2nd ed. London, Spastics International Medical Publications, 1984.

Cashore WJ: Neonatal hyperbilirubinemia. *In* Oski FA, Deangelis CD, Feigin RD, et al (eds): Principles and Practice of Pediatrics, 2nd ed. Philadelphia, JB Lippincott, 1994, pp 446–455.

Casiro O, Bingham W, MacMurray B, et al: The Canadian Exosurf neonatal study group and the Canadian Exosurf neonatal follow-up group. One year follow-up of 89 infants with birth weights of 500–749 grams and respiratory distress syndrome randomized to 2 rescue doses of synthetic surfactant or air placebo. J Pediatr 126:553, 1995.

Committee on Injury and Poison Prevention and Committee on Fetus and Newborn: Safe transportation of premature infants. Pediatrics 87(1):120, 1992.

Escalona SK: Babies at double hazard: early development of infants at biologic and social risk. Pediatrics 70:670, 1982.

Gorski P: Developmental intervention during neonatal hospitalization: critiquing the state of the science. Pediatr Clin North Am 38(6):1469, 1991.

Gottfried AW, Wallace-Lande P, Brown SS, et al: Physical and social environment of newborn infants in special care units. Science 214(6):673, 1981.

Guyer B, Strobino DM, Ventura SJ, et al: Annual summary of vital statistics-1995. Pediatrics 88(6):1007–1019, 1996.

Hack M, Fanaroff AA: Outcomes of extremely low-birth weight infants between 1982 and 1988. N Engl J Med 321:1642–1647, 1989.

Hack M, Friedman H, Fanaroff AA: Outcomes of extremely low-birth weight infants. Pediatrics 98:931, 1996.

Harrison H: The principles for family-centered neonatal care. Pediatrics 92(5):643, 1993.

Hill A, Volpe J: Normal pressure hydrocephalus in the newborn. Pediatrics 68:623, 1981.

Hobel CJ, et al: Prenatal and intrapartum high-risk screening. Am J Obstet Gynecol 117:1, 1973.

Hristeva L, Booy R, Bowler I, et al: Prospective surveillance of neonatal meningitis. Arch Dis Child 69:14–18, 1993.

The International Committee for the Classification of the Late Stages of Retinopathy of Prematurity: An international classification of retinopathy of prematurity II. The classification of retinal detachment. Arch Ophthalmol 105:906, 1997.

Jones R, Wincott E, Elbourne D, et al: Controlled trial of dexamethasone in neonatal chronic lung disease: a 3-year follow-up. Pediatrics 96:897–906, 1995.

Lester BM, Tronick EZ: Neonatal Network Neurobehavioral Scale. Research Edition. *In* Zeskind S, Singer L (eds): Assessment of the Newborn and Young Infant. New York, Guilford Publications, 1994.

McCormick MD: Has the prevalence of handicapped infants increased with improved survival of the very-low-birth-weight infant? Clin Perinatol 20(1):263–276, 1993.

Ment LR, Oh W, Ehrenkranz RA, et al: Low dose indomethacin and prevention of intraventricular hemorrhage: a multicenter randomized trial. Pediatrics 93:543–550, 1994.

National Advisory Board on Medical Rehabilitation Research: Report and plan for medical rehabilitation research (NIH Publication No. 93-3509). Bethesda, MD, National Center for Medical Rehabilitation Research, 1993.

Nelson KB: Uncertain value of electronic fetal monitoring in predicting cerebral palsy. N Engl J Med 334(10):613–618, 1996.

Nelson KB, Ellenberg JH: Apgar scores as predictors of chronic neurologic disability. Pediatrics 68:36–44, 1981.

Palmer MM, Crawley K, Blanco I: The Neonatal Oral Motor Assessment Scale: a reliability study. J Perinatol 13:28, 1993.

Papile LA, Burstein L, Burstein R, et al: Incidence of evolution of subependymal and intraventricular hemorrhage. A study of infants with birth weight less than 1500 grams. J Pediatr 92:529–534, 1978.

Philip AGS, Allan WC, Tito AM, et al: Intraventricular hemorrhage in preterm infants: declining incidence in the 1980s. Pediatrics 84(5):797–801, 1989.

Saliba E, Bertrand P, Gold F, et al: Area of lateral ventricles measured on cranial ultrasonography in preterm infants: association with outcome. Arch Dis Child 65:1033–1037, 1990.

Szymonowicz W, Yu VYH, Bajuk B, et al: Neurodevelopmental outcome of periventricular hemorrhage and leukomalacia in infants 1250 g or less at birth. Early Human Dev 14:1, 1986.

Tallo CP, Vohr B, Oh W, et al: Maternal and neonatal morbidity associated with in vitro fertilization. J Pediatr 127:794–800, 1995.

Vaucher YE, Merritt AT, Hallman M, et al: Neurodevelopmental and respiratory outcome in early childhood after human surfactant treatment. Am J Dis Child L142:L927–930, 1988.

Volpe JJ: Hypoxic-ischemic encephalopathy: clinical aspects. *In* Volpe JJ (ed): Neurology of the Newborn, 3rd ed. Philadelphia, WB Saunders, 1995, pp 314–369.

Volpe JJ: Intraventricular hemorrhage in the premature infant: current concepts. Part 1. Ann Neurol 25(1):3–11, 1989.

Werner EE, Smith RS: Overcoming the Odds: High Risk Children From Birth to Adulthood. Ithaca, Cornell University Press, 1992.

Wolf LS, Glass RP: Feeding and Swallowing Disorders in Infancy: Assessment and Management. Tucson, AZ, Therapy Skill Builders, 1992.

Wolfson MR, Greenspan JS, Deoras KS, et al: Effect of position on the mechanical interaction between the rib cage and abdomen in preterm infants. J Appl Physiol 72(3):1032, 1992.

World Health Organization: International classification of impairments, disabilities and handicaps: a manual of classification relating to the consequences of disease. Geneva, Switzerland, WHO, 1980.

Zorn WA, Msall ME, Rogers BT, et al: Two year neurodevelopmental outcome of infants <29 weeks enrolled in a multicenter comparison trial of Exosurf (EXO) and Infasurf (INFA) prophylaxis for RDS [abstract 1696]. Pediatr Res 39(part 2):285A, 1996.

27 Central Nervous System Disorders

David L. Coulter

 When a patient presents with a history of episodes that may or may not represent seizures, the first step is to take a complete history. The past medical history and family history may suggest the etiology. A complete physical and neurologic examination is then performed, which may also suggest the etiology. If the history implies a reasonable possibility of seizures, then an electroencephalogram is indicated.

Head injury accounts for 6000 to 12,000 child deaths per year in the United States, most of which are entirely preventable.

The mortality rate for bacterial meningitis in children remains 1% to 5% despite modern antibiotics, and the rate of neurologic sequelae may be as high as 40%.

The most common sporadic viral encephalitis is caused by herpes simplex virus (HSV). Epidemic encephalitis is typically caused by enteroviruses or by arthropod-borne viruses.

The brain is the "organ of the mind" and so occupies a special place in our awareness of the body. Most parents believe that their child's brain mediates the child's sense of who she is, how she relates to others, and her aspirations for the future. The "black box" mysteries of how the brain does this adds to the sense of awe and fear with which parents consider real and potential threats to the child's brain. In some settings, a child with a brain disorder may be viewed as possessed by the devil (as when seizures occur), or defective (as when the child has mental retardation). Clinicians need to be sensitive to parents' perceptions of brain disorders, which may be quite different and dominated by personal and cultural beliefs. Clinicians also need to remember (and help the family remember) that the child with a brain disorder is a child first, a developing person who is a valued member of the family and the community.

The child's brain is growing and developing even as the effects of the brain disorder are manifesting themselves. This dynamic interplay involves both a vulnerability and a resiliency that is unique to childhood. The neurobiological processes involved include critical periods and plasticity, both of which are the subjects of intensive research. For example, a stroke in infancy may result in minimal residual hemiparesis, owing to the plasticity of the developing brain. On the other hand, aphasia acquired after middle childhood is less likely to resolve completely because the critical period for developing basic language skills has passed. The ongoing development of synaptic connectivity throughout childhood and adolescence underlies the resiliency of the child's brain, so that positive environmental, educational, and therapeutic efforts may permit substantial (and sometimes dramatic) recovery of function.

This chapter considers several common brain disorders of childhood and adolescence, including seizures, brain injury, and infections. Subsequent chapters consider other brain disorders, including cerebral palsy, mental retar-

dation, and congenital anomalies. Readers should not lose sight of the child and the family in attempting to make sense of all of this information, because the purpose of learning it is to help the child with a brain disorder to achieve the happiest, healthiest, and most productive life possible.

Seizures and Epilepsy

SEIZURES

A seizure is a distinct event during which an abrupt discharge of neurons in the brain is associated with a simultaneous alteration in motor or sensory function or consciousness, or any combination of these (Aicardi, 1994). The neuronal discharge can be detected by electroencephalographic recording (EEG) from the scalp in most seizures. In certain situations, the scalp EEG may fail to detect the discharge, however. In some partial seizures without altered consciousness (see later discussion), the discharge may be detectable only by electrodes inserted deep into the hippocampus or amygdala. This subcortical discharge may continue for some time before it spreads to the cortex and becomes detectable by scalp EEG. When consciousness becomes altered during a seizure (as in complex partial and generalized seizures), scalp EEG usually demonstrates the discharge. Scalp EEG may also fail to detect certain types of neonatal seizures, particularly subtle or fragmentary seizures occurring in premature infants (Mizrahi and Kellaway, 1987). The neuronal discharge in these infants may remain subcortical and never reach the cortex or scalp.

Partly for this reason, the diagnosis of seizures remains a clinical one and is not proved (or disproved) by scalp EEG. Seizures manifest themselves in a limited number of ways; not all abrupt behavioral alterations are necessarily seizures. An experienced clinician must elicit a thor-

Table 27–1 • Seizure Description

Precipitating events, if any (describe):
Usual time of day (if any):
Frequency:
Usual duration:

Behavioral observations (check all that apply):

1. General:	_____	Fall down
	_____	Go limp
	_____	Stiffen body/go rigid
	_____	Blue/gray color of lips or skin
	_____	Incontinent of urine
	_____	Incontinent of feces
2. Head:	_____	Arched back
	_____	Flexed forward
	_____	Turned to left
	_____	Turned to right
3. Eyes:	_____	Right eyelid twitch
	_____	Left eyelid twitch
	_____	Eyes deviated to right
	_____	Eyes deviated to left
	_____	Eyes deviated upward
	_____	Eyes staring straight ahead
4. Face:	_____	Left side jerking
	_____	Right side jerking
	_____	Eyes blinking
	_____	Lip smacking
	_____	Tongue movement
	_____	Sucking
	_____	Swallowing
5. Body:	_____	Right arm stiffened
	_____	Right arm jerking
	_____	Left arm stiffened
	_____	Left arm jerking
	_____	Right leg stiffened
	_____	Right leg jerking
	_____	Left leg stiffened
	_____	Left leg jerking
	_____	Body arched backward
	_____	Body flexed forward
	_____	No movement
6. After:	_____	Sleepy
	_____	Confused
	_____	Combative
	_____	Agitated
	_____	Headache
	_____	Vomiting
	_____	Usual self

Other features and comments:

ough description of the events and then decide whether the behavior resembles that known to occur during true seizures. In most cases, the diagnosis is as good (or as bad) as the history. Table 27–1 shows a checklist developed for use by the staff of a private residential school to facilitate a complete description of behavior during events that may or may not be seizures. Similar information can be elicited by careful history-taking from parents and patients. The clinician then evaluates this information and decides whether the behavior was likely to have been a seizure. If the description of the behavior is grossly inadequate and there is no other reason to suspect seizures, it is best to wait

until better information becomes available before making a diagnosis.

Seizures are classified according to the International Classification of Epileptic Seizures (ILAE, 1981) (Table 27–2). In this system, seizures are either partial or generalized. Partial seizures are divided into simple partial seizures, in which consciousness is not altered, and complex partial seizures, in which consciousness is altered. Since memory is preserved during simple partial seizures, patients may recall having an aura (visual, auditory, olfactory, or somatosensory hallucinations; epigastric sensations; feelings of fear or anxiety; or déjà vu) or experiencing twitching or jerking of an arm or leg. During complex partial seizures, patients may have a blank stare and do not recall what they do or what is said to them. They may have oral-motor automatisms (chewing, lips smacking, or swallowing) or engage in semipurposeful, automatic behavior. Because consciousness is impaired, a patient having a complex partial seizure is not able to initiate planned, goal-directed behavior.

A common problem in evaluating a behaviorally troubled youth is whether to attribute aggressive or disruptive behavior to complex partial seizure activity. The behavior is more likely to be a seizure if (1) it occurs

Table 27–2 • International Classification of Seizures

Partial seizures
  Simple partial seizures (consciousness not impaired)
    With motor signs
    With somatosensory or special sensory symptoms
      Somatosensory
      Visual
      Auditory
      Olfactory
      Gustatory
      Vertiginous
    With autonomic symptoms or signs
    With psychic symptoms
      Speech disturbance
      Memory disturbance (déjà vu)
      Cognitive disturbance (dreamy state)
      Affective disturbance (fear, anger)
      Illusions
      Structured hallucinations
  Complex partial seizures (with impairment of consciousness)
    Simple partial onset followed by impairment of
      consciousness
    With impairment of consciousness at onset
      With impairment of consciousness alone
      With automatisms
  Partial seizures evolving to secondarily generalized seizures
Generalized seizures
  Absence seizures
    With impairment of consciousness only
    With mild clonic components
    With atonic components
    With tonic components
    With automatisms
    With autonomic components
  Atypical absence seizures
  Myoclonic seizures
  Clonic seizures
  Tonic seizures
  Tonic-clonic seizures
  Atonic seizures
Unclassified seizures (inadequate or incomplete data)

randomly and not just when the child is frustrated or provoked; (2) there is a defined aura; (3) the motor activity consists of oral-motor automatisms, deviation of the eyes, face, or head to one side, or posturing or jerking of the limbs; (4) the pulse and blood pressure are increased; (5) the patient is unaware of and unresponsive to others during the episode; (6) the patient has no memory of what happened (except for the aura, if there was one); (7) the episode lasts for a few minutes (not for a half hour or more); and (8) the patient is tired or exhausted afterward. The presence of spike waves on the EEG between episodes (especially if located in temporal or frontal electrodes) supports a seizure diagnosis, but the EEG may be normal between episodes of true seizures. Other EEG findings (such as slow waves or sharp waves) are less specific and may occur in patients who do not have seizures.

Simple and complex partial seizures may spread and become secondarily generalized tonic-clonic seizures. More commonly, tonic-clonic seizures are primarily generalized (begin all over the body without a focal onset). Other types of generalized seizures include absence, tonic, clonic, atonic, and myoclonic seizures.

Episodes of blank starting with lack of awareness or responsiveness are more likely to be absence seizures if (1) they begin after the age of 2 to 3 years; (2) they occur several times a day; (3) they occur randomly at home as well as at school; (4) they occur during speech, play, or mealtime (not just when the child is bored or inactive); (5) there is no aura; and (6) the patient returns immediately to normal afterward (is not tired or lethargic). Episodes of blank staring may also be seen in children who have been abused (''dissociative'' episodes), in those who are anxious or confused, and, occasionally, in children with attention deficit. The EEG is helpful in evaluating the possibility of absence seizures, since generalized spike waves (typically during hyperventilation) are almost always present in children with absence seizure. These spike waves occur less frequently and may be missed in adolescents with absence seizure, however.

Tonic and atonic seizures are usually seen in patients with other disabilities such as mental retardation. Tonic seizures are often confused with tonic-clonic seizures, but they are much briefer (seconds rather than minutes), there is only tonic posturing of the limbs and no clonic jerking, and the patient is usually not cyanotic or incontinent. Atonic seizures are often associated with injury because the patient is unconscious during the fall and makes no effort at self-protection during the seizure. An atonic seizure may last for a minute or two, during which time the patient lies limply on the ground, or it may be very brief and the patient may get up right away. Myoclonic seizures may occur at any age and in patients with or without other disabilities. Patients with myoclonic seizures usually have other types of generalized seizures as well.

A number of conditions can cause behaviors that resemble seizures but that are not actually seizures as defined previously. Table 27–3 lists some of the more common nonepileptic paroxysmal disorders that may cause diagnostic confusion (Duchowny, 1996). When a child is thought to have seizures but the episodes do not respond to appropriate anticonvulsant treatment, the clinician should rethink the diagnosis and consider whether the behavior

Table 27–3 • Nonepileptic Behaviors

If the Behavior Resembles:	Also Consider:
Complex partial seizures	Confusional migraine
	Explosive disorder
	Hyperventilation
	Night terrors
	Paroxysmal vertigo
	Psychotic hallucinations
Tonic-clonic seizures	Conversion disorder
Absence seizures	Anxiety disorder
	Attention-deficit hyperactivity disorder
	Boredom/daydreaming
	Dissociative disorder
Tonic seizures	Paroxysmal dyskinesia
	Paroxysmal torticollis
	Sandifer syndrome
	Conversion disorder
	Breath-holding spells (cyanotic type)
Atonic seizures	Hypoglycemia
	Syncope
	Breath-holding spells (pallid type)
	Mitral valve prolapse
	Cataplexy
	Basilar migraine
Myoclonic seizures	Sleep myoclonus
	Tic disorder
	Shuddering attacks
	Essential myoclonus

may in fact be due to one of the disorders listed in Table 27–3. Electroencephalographic monitoring (see later) is often helpful in these situations.

EPILEPSY

It is undoubtedly true that anyone can have a seizure under certain conditions, such as electroconvulsive therapy. Not all seizures are caused by epilepsy, however. Seizures that are symptomatic of some acute process, such as a febrile illness or metabolic derangement (hyponatremia, hypoglycemia, or hypocalcemia), are true seizures as described previously but are not considered epileptic. *Epilepsy* is a relatively long-standing or chronic disorder of the brain that predisposes the patient to have seizures and has caused at least two or more seizures. A number of disorders fit this definition, so there are a number of different types of epilepsies. Some are sufficiently well-described to be considered syndromes, with each syndrome having a characteristic etiology, pathology, symptomatology, response to treatment, and prognosis. The International Classification of Epilepsies and Epileptic Syndromes is shown in Table 27–4 (ILAE, 1986). Detailed information about these syndromes is available (Aicardi, 1994; Roger et al, 1992).

One particularly common epileptic syndrome in childhood is benign childhood epilepsy, with centrotemporal spikes on EEG, also known as rolandic epilepsy. Onset of seizures is usually around 3 to 5 years of age, and remission (no seizures with no treatment) nearly always occurs by adolescence. Seizures typically occur at night and consist of unilateral jerking of the face and hands.

Table 27-4 • International Classification of Epilepsies and Epileptic Syndromes

Localization-related (partial) epilepsies and syndromes
  Idiopathic, with age-related onset
    Benign childhood epilepsy with centrotemporal spikes*
    Childhood epilepsy with occipital paroxysms*
  Symptomatic (frontal, temporal, parietal, occipital)
Generalized epilepsies and syndromes
  Idiopathic, with age-related onset
    Benign familial neonatal convulsions*
    Benign nonfamilial neonatal convulsions*
    Benign myoclonic epilepsy of infancy*
    Childhood absence epilepsy*
    Juvenile absence epilepsy*
    Juvenile myoclongic epilepsy*
    Epilepsy with tonic-clonic seizures on awakening*
  Idiopathic and/or symptomatic
    West syndrome (infantile spasms)*
    Lennox-Gastaut syndrome*
    Epilepsy with myoclonic-astatic seizures*
    Epilepsy with myoclonic absences*
  Symptomatic
    Nonspecific etiology
      Early myoclonic encephalopathy*
    Specific etiology (many identified causes)
Epilepsies and syndromes undetermined as to partial or generalized
  With both partial and generalized seizures
    Neonatal seizures*
    Severe myoclonic epilepsy of infancy*
    Epilepsy with continuous spike waves in sleep*
    Landau-Kleffner syndrome*
  Without clear-cut generalized or partial features
Special syndromes
  Situation-related seizures
    Febrile seizures*
    Seizures due to other identifiable causes
  Isolated, apparently unprovoked seizures
  Reflex epilepsies*
  Epilepsia partialis continua of childhood*

*Epileptic syndrome.

Generalized tonic-clonic seizures may also occur. Finding on neurologic examination and neuroimaging studies (computed tomography [CT], magnetic resonance imaging [MRI]) are normal, but a family history of childhood epilepsy is often present. The EEG is diagnostic and shows characteristic spike wave discharges in the centrotemporal area on one or both sides that dramatically increase in frequency during drowsiness and sleep. Many patients have only one or two seizures in their lifetime without treatment. Thus, treatment is often deferred until the patient has had three or more seizures. The prognosis is uniformly good.

In contrast, an especially severe epileptic syndrome in childhood is the Lennox-Gastaut syndrome. The onset may be as early as 1 to 2 years of age and may be preceded by infantile spasms in the first year of life. Virtually all patients have some form of static encephalopathy manifested as developmental delay, mental retardation, or cerebral palsy. Any type of seizure may occur, but tonic and atonic seizures are characteristic. Generalized myoclonic and tonic-clonic seizures are also common. The findings on neurologic examination are abnormal and reflect the static encephalopathy. The results of neuroimaging studies are often abnormal and may demonstrate a specific brain malformation, cerebral atrophy, or the results of previous brain injury. The EEG shows a typical pattern that includes slow and disorganized background activity, scattered multifocal spikes, and bursts of generalized 1- to 2 Hz high-voltage spike waves. The seizures are very frequent and may occur many times a day. Response to anticonvulsant treatment is often poor, although the ketogenic diet may be successful (Freeman, Kelly, and Freeman, 1996). The prognosis is poor for seizure control, and seizures typically continue into adulthood.

The advantage of making a diagnosis of an epileptic syndrome is that it predicts the response to treatment and indicates the prognosis. The same type of seizure may have a very different significance depending on the epileptic syndrome present. For example, a generalized tonic-clonic seizure may occur as part of rolandic epilepsy and may not require treatment, or it may occur as part of the Lennox-Gastaut syndrome and be refractory to treatment.

Two conditions included in Table 27-4 are not ordinarily considered forms of epilepsy. Neonatal seizures and febrile seizures are usually symptoms of an acute process rather than of a chronic disorder, and thus are not truly epileptic in nature. The acute events causing neonatal seizures (such as birth asphyxia) may of course result in chronic brain damage and predispose the child to later epilepsy. Further information about the etiology, symptoms, pathology, treatment, and prognosis of neonatal seizures is available (Volpe, 1995). Similarly, children with febrile seizures usually do not have a chronic neurologic disorder (by definition, febrile seizures exclude children with intracranial infections). The seizures are symptomatic of an acute febrile illness, and the risk of later epilepsy is usually quite low (Nelson and Ellenberg, 1978). Treatment is usually not indicated, although administration of diazepam at the first sign of a fever can prevent recurrences of febrile seizures in some children (Rosman et al, 1993).

EPIDEMIOLOGY

Approximately 1% of children will have at least one afebrile seizure by age 14. By age 11, 0.4% to 0.8% of children will have recurrent afebrile seizures (epilepsy), and 1% of the population can be expected to have developed epilepsy by 20 years of age. The prevalence of active epilepsy in preschool children is about 1.5 per 1000 and in school-aged children is about 5 per 1000. The etiology of childhood epilepsy is idiopathic in 40% of cases and symptomatic in 60% of cases. Eighteen percent to thirty-four percent of epilepsies are partial and 31% to 65% are generalized, the remainder being unclear. Mortality for children with epilepsy is slightly increased, particularly for those with symptomatic types of epilepsy. Death may be caused by the underlying condition, by prolonged tonic-clonic status epilepticus, by seizure-related accidents or injuries, or by the syndrome of sudden unexplained death in epilepsy (Hauser and Hesdorffer, 1990).

PATIENT EVALUATION

When a patient presents with a history of episodes that may or may not represent seizures, the first step is to take a complete history. This includes a detailed description of the events (see Table 27–1). The past medical history and family history may suggest the etiology. A complete physical and neurologic examination is then performed, which may also suggest the etiology. If the history suggests a reasonable possibility of seizures, then an EEG is indicated. For maximal diagnostic utility, the EEG should (1) be recorded following some degree of sleep deprivation; (2) begin with the patient awake and include recording during waking, drowsiness, and sleep; and (3) include recording during photic stimulation and hyperventilation (if the child will cooperate). Neuroimaging studies should be performed if (1) the history suggests that the patient is having partial seizures; (2) the neurologic examination results are abnormal; or (3) the EEG shows a focal abnormality. Neuroimaging studies may be unnecessary if the patient has had only generalized absence seizures, the neurologic examination results are normal, and the EEG shows only the typical generalized 3-Hz spike wave discharges characteristic of childhood absence epilepsy.

In cases of diagnostic uncertainty, the patient may have episodes that are not obviously true seizures and the EEG may show no or only nonspecific abnormalities. If the episodes are fairly frequent, prolonged electroencephalographic monitoring may be helpful. The purpose of this procedure is to record the electroencephalographic readings long enough to "capture" one of the episodes in question. If the behavioral episode occurs during prolonged electroencephalographic recording and the EEG shows an epileptic discharge during the behavior, then the behavior may be classified as a seizure. If no such behavior occurs during the procedure, then no conclusion can be made as to the nature of the behavior in question.

Several techniques for prolonged electroencephalographic recording are available. Ambulatory encephalographic monitoring (usually for 24 to 48 hours) involves continuous recording on a portable tape recorder while the patient is at home or at school. Simultaneous video-electroencephalographic recording involves recording of the patient's behavior with a closed-circuit television camera time-linked to continuous recording of the electroencephalographic reading. The patient is not as mobile (since he or she must remain visible to the camera) and the procedure is usually performed in the hospital or laboratory.

Prolonged EEG using one or the other of these techniques is especially helpful when the patient has static encephalopathy or mental retardation and is having unusual episodic behavior such as staring, jerking, or aggression. Studies using prolonged encephalographic monitoring in such patients have shown that these behaviors are usually not seizures (Donat and Wright, 1990; Holmes, McKeever and Russman, 1983; Neill and Alvarez; 1986).

Another technique that may be helpful in cases of diagnostic uncertainty is a therapeutic trial of anticonvulsant therapy. This may be considered if the behavioral episodes in question may well be seizures but are so infrequent (once a week or less) that prolonged monitoring is not likely to capture one of the episodes. The anticonvulsant drug should be selected based on the likely type of seizure present (Table 27–5). Careful documentation of the nature and frequency of the target behavior is essential,

Table 27–5 • Selection of Anticonvulsant Drugs

Seizure Type	First Choice	Alternatives

Partial
  Simple
  Complex
	Carbamazepine, phenytoin, phenobarbital (in infants)	Valproate, gabapentin, lamotrigine, topiramate, primidone, felbamate

Tonic-clonic	Phenytoin, carbamazepine, valproate	Phenobarbital, gabapentin, lamotrigine, topiramate, primidone, felbamate
Absence	Ethosuximide	Valproate, clonazepam
Atypical absence	Ethosuximide	Valproate, clonazepam

"Minor motor"
  Myoclonic
  Tonic
  Clonic
  Atonic
	Valproate	Lamotrigine, topiramate, felbamate, methsuximide, acetazolamide, ketogenic diet

first during a baseline period before starting treatment and then during the treatment once the drug selected has reached a therapeutic level in the patient. Anticonvulsant treatment should be continued only if there is a dramatic reduction in the frequency of the episodes (at least 50% or more). If the clinical response is uncertain or minimal, the drug should be discontinued and an alternative diagnosis pursued.

TREATMENT

If seizures are likely to recur, treatment to prevent recurrence is generally indicated. A number of anticonvulsant drugs are available for this purpose. The use of these drugs should follow the generally accepted guidelines (Aicardi, 1994; Coulter, 1997) shown in Table 27–6. Of particular importance is the need to individualize the assessment of risk and benefit (Guideline #1). One should treat the patient, not just the seizure. It may be better for some patients to have an occasional seizure than to experience significant adverse drug effects from the amount of drug therapy needed to prevent all seizures. On the other hand, parental anxiety about the possibility of seizure recurrence (and the attendant restriction on the child's activities) may warrant more drug treatment in some cases.

Selection of an anticonvulsant drug is based on the principle of using the drug that is likely to be the safest and most effective (Guidelines #2 and #3). The generally accepted first-choice drugs, as well as alternative drugs that may be considered, are shown in Table 27–5. Phenobarbital is a first-choice drug for newborns and young infants because of its safety and predictable pharmacology. It is not a first-choice drug in older children, however, because of

Table 27–6 • Guidelines for
Anticonvulsant Drug Therapy

1. On an individual basis, balance risks (seizures, adverse drug effects) and benefits (no seizures, no drug effects).
2. Select the preferred drug based on the type of seizure present, choosing the most effective and least toxic drug first.
3. Start with a single drug (monotherapy). Administer the drug at intervals equal to or less than one half-life.
4. If seizures persist after a fair trial at therapeutic levels of the chosen drug, add a second drug (follow principles 1–3).
5. Remove a drug if it did not help to control seizures.
6. Measure anticonvulsant drug levels*:
   A. After starting a new drug (wait for the drug to reach steady-state concentration, at least five times the half-life).
   B. Whenever toxicity is suspected clinically.
   C. If seizures are not yet controlled (level may be low).
   D. If seizures begin after having been controlled.
   E. If noncompliance is suspected.
   F. Routinely once or twice a year.
7. Watch for emerging adverse effects of drugs, which may be hard to recognize. All drugs have multiple effects (desired and undesired), and virtually any adverse effect is possible with any drug.

*Free (unbound) drug levels may be useful in certain situations and may be preferred when multiple drugs are prescribed.

the high rate of adverse effects and the availability of other equally effective drugs. Phenytoin and carbamazepine are equally effective for partial seizures, and either can be a first-choice drug for older children. Phenytoin, carbamazepine, and valproate are all effective for generalized tonic-clonic seizures, and the choice is based primarily on the risk of adverse effects. Either valproate or ethosuximide may be used as a first-choice drug for absence seizures, but valproate is generally preferred if the patient also has tonic-clonic seizures. Valproate is the most effective drug and is the first choice for patients with myoclonic, tonic, and atonic seizures. Anticonvulsant drug levels are often helpful in monitoring therapy (Guideline #6).

A number of new drugs have been released for use recently, including felbamate, gabapentin, lamotrigine, and topiramate. None of them is currently considered a first-choice drug. They can be used as alternatives if the first-choice drug is ineffective or causes unacceptable adverse effects (see Guidelines #4 and #5). Most are currently approved only as add-on therapy (in addition to another drug) but are likely to be effective as monotherapy in appropriate cases. Some are not yet approved for use in children. Experience with these drugs over time will likely result in some of the drugs' becoming approved and widely accepted as first-choice agents in children.

No anticonvulsant drug is perfect, and virtually any adverse effect is possible with any drug (Guideline #7). Clinicians should prescribe drugs with which they are familiar, since some of these adverse effects can be hard to detect, uncommon, or life-threatening. The pharmacology of commonly used drugs is shown in Table 27–7, and common or serious adverse effects of these drugs are shown in Table 27–8 (Levy, Mattson, and Meldrum, 1995; Wyllie, 1993).

Monitoring the response to anticonvulsant treatment over time is facilitated by the use of a flow sheet to track seizure frequency, anticonvulsant drug doses and levels,

other laboratory test results, clinical observations, and changes made in response to clinical events. An example of such a flow sheet is given in Table 27–9 (Coulter, 1997).

STOPPING TREATMENT

When a diagnosis of epilepsy is made and anticonvulsant treatment prescribed, the treatment is generally continued for at least 2 years. Once the patient has been seizure-free for 2 years, it is reasonable to consider whether continued treatment is necessary. Certain risk factors predict recurrence if treatment is withdrawn: (1) frequent seizures before achieving control; (2) multiple types of seizures before achieving control; (3) abnormal findings on neurologic examination; (4) the presence of a fixed, chronic brain abnormality causing the seizures; and (5) the continuing presence of spike waves in the EEG after seizure control has been achieved (Aicardi, 1994). If any of these risk factors are present, the risk of recurrence is approximately 50% and treatment is generally continued. If none of these factors are present, the risk of recurrence is approximately 20% and treatment may be withdrawn. The drug dosage is tapered over approximately 3 months to prevent withdrawal symptoms. Most recurrences occur during the first year after coming off medication, but recurrence may occur years later.

For patients who remain seizure-free on medication but who have at least one of the risk factors listed, treatment is usually continued until the patient has been seizure-free for at least 4 to 5 years. At that point, the patient and family may want to consider whether a trial off medication is worth undertaking. The risk of recurrence off medication remains approximately 50%, but the possibility of continuing to take medication unnecessarily is also approximately 50%. There is no right or wrong approach in this situation, so the clinician should discuss the available options with the patient and family and respect their decision.

Head Trauma

GENERAL CONSIDERATIONS

Head injury is an unfortunately common cause of death and disability in children. It accounts for 6000 to 12,000 deaths per year in the United States, most of which are entirely preventable (Kraus, Fife, and Conroy, 1987). One cannot emphasize enough the importance of such activities as identifying parents in need of support to prevent inflicted injury (abuse), education and training of parents and children to avoid household and pedestrian accidents, and requiring all children to wear adequate helmets while riding a bicycle, skateboarding, or in-line skating. The neurologist or trauma surgeon is glad when childhood head injury statistics decline, because this means that young lives have been saved and futures preserved through effective prevention.

Minor head injuries are generally reversible, and full recovery is the rule (Levin, Eisenberg, and Benton, 1989). When a severe head injury occurs, however, the functioning of the child and family is changed forever. It is useful to consider that rehabilitation following severe head injury

Table 27-7 • Pharmacokinetic Properties of Anticonvulsant Drugs

Parameter	Valproate	Carbamazepine	Phenytoin	Phenobarbital	Clonazepam	Ethosuximide	Felbamate	Gabapentin	Lamotrigine	Topiramate
Dose in mg/kg/day	15–30	10–20	5–10	2.5	0.1–0.15	10–40	15–45	15–30	4–7	30–60
Percent protein binding	70–93	75	90	45	85	10	25–35	0	55	13–17
Volume of distribution in L/kg	0.16	0.8–2.0	0.75	0.55	3.0	0.65	1.0	0.65–1.04	0.9–1.3	0.55–0.80
Time to maximal serum concentration in hours	1–2	4–12	4–12	0.5–4	1–4	1.4	6–20	2–3	1–3	1.8–3.5
Elimination half-life in hours	5–15	20–50	10–60	65–110	20–40	30–60	19	5–9	24*	23–29
Time to steady state in days	2	20–30	15–20	15–20	6	7–8	4–5	1–2	5–7	4–5

*Increases to 59 hours when given with Depakote (divalproex sodium).

Table 27–8 • Effects of Antiepileptic Drugs

Effects	Valproate	Carbamazepine	Phenytoin	Phenobarbital	Clonazepam	Ethosuximide	Felbamate	Gabapentin	Lamotrigine	Topiramate
Systemic/physical effects	Hepatitis Pancreatitis Low carnitine Low platelets Obesity Alopecia	Leukopenia Anemia Hepatitis SIADH Low vitamin D Rash	Hirsutism Gingival Hyperplasia Low folate Rash	NS	Drooling	Anemia Leukopenia Rash	Aplastic anemia Hepatitis Rash Body odor	Weight gain Leukopenia Rash Low platelets (rare) Electrocardiographic changes (rare)	Rash Hepatitis	Fatigue Anorexia Renal stones Weight loss
Central nervous system side effects (at usual levels)	Tremor Nausea	NS	NS	Sedation Depression Irritable Overactive	Sedation Disinhibition Hallucination Hypotonia Ataxia Nystagmus	Lethargy Nausea Dizziness	Anorexia Vomiting Insomnia Lethargy Headache	Lethargy Fatigue Dizziness Ataxia Headache Nausea Diplopia Tremor	Lethargy Blurred vision Dizziness Ataxia Headache Nausea Diplopia	Lethargy Dizziness Ataxia Nystagmus Tremor Anxiety Depression
Toxic effects	Sedation Vomiting Cerebral Edema	Diplopia Ataxia Nausea Sedation Dyskinesia Arrhythmia	Ataxia Nystagmus Vomiting Sedation Dyskinesia Arrhythmia Seizures	Sedation	Sedation Aspiration	Vomiting Lethargy Visual changes	Weight loss Insomnia Lethargy	Lethargy Ataxia Dizziness	Lethargy Dizziness Headache	Confusion Inattention Dysfluency

NS = None significant.

283

Table 27–9 • Anticonvulsant Medication Response Flow Sheet

Name: _____   Identification No: _____

Date of evaluation:			

SEIZURE FREQUENCY
Number of _____ type
seizures since last evaluation
Number of _____ type
seizures since last evaluation

ANTICONVULSANT DRUG TREATMENT
Drug name _____
   Dosage and serum level
Drug name _____
   Dosage and serum level

LABORATORY TEST RESULTS
Test name: _____
Test name: _____
Test name: _____
Test name: _____

CLINICAL OBSERVATIONS
Individual's weight
Describe individual's behavior since last evaluation (include observer's initials)

RESPONSE TO INTERVAL EVALUATIONS
Describe steps taken to respond to the findings of this interval evaluation (include respondent's initials)

should begin on the day of the injury and continues indefinitely. The pediatrician can help the family get through the acute phase and negotiate the long-term rearrangement of their lives. This includes timely referral for educational assistance, emotional support, and help with health care financing. Families can also be referred to the National Head Injury Foundation (1-800-444-NHIF) for more information and support.

CATEGORIES OF HEAD INJURY

- **Mild** head injury: initial and subsequent Glasgow Coma Scale (GCS) scores of 13 to 15, with no or brief (less than 30 minutes) loss of consciousness, no focal neurologic deficit, no intracranial hematoma, and no depressed skull fracture (linear skull fracture may be present).
- **Moderate** head injury: initial or subsequent GCS scores of 9 to 12, with variable loss of consciousness, focal neurologic deficit, intracranial hematoma, or depressed skull fracture.
- **Severe** head injury: initial or subsequent GCS scores of 8 or less with prolonged loss of consciousness, often with focal neurologic deficit, intracranial hematoma, or depressed skull fracture.

PATHOPHYSIOLOGY

The force of a blow to the head may be concentrated locally or spread diffusely. Both mechanisms are often present in severe head injuries. The consequences of localized trauma include skull fracture (which may be linear, comminuted, or depressed), hemorrhage at the site of the injury (which may be epidural, subdural, or intraparenchymal), and focal brain injury (which may consist of edema, contusion, laceration, or necrosis). If there is no diffuse injury, consciousness may be relatively intact even though the child has focal neurologic signs.

The consequences of diffuse trauma include contrecoup effects and diffuse axonal injury. Contrecoup effects reflect the movement of the brain within the skull, with secondary injury on the side of the brain opposite from the site of the initial trauma. Diffuse axonal injury reflects generalized disruption of tissue integrity, particularly in the cerebral white matter. Diffuse injury may cause prolonged impairment of consciousness even in the absence of focal neurologic signs.

Focal brainstem injuries (particularly hemorrhages in the midbrain and pons) result in cranial nerve abnormalities and prolonged unconsciousness. The severity of neurologic dysfunction is typically much greater than one would expect from the extent of brain injury and reflects the critical location of the relatively small area of damage.

CLINICAL ASSESSMENT

Assessment of the head-injured child begins in the field at the scene of the injury and continues in the ambulance and in the emergency department (Jennett and Teasdale, 1981). Initial considerations emphasize assessment of the airway, breathing, and cardiac function. Because of the possibility of critical neck injury as well, the neck must be stabilized until this possibility is excluded (usually by radiograph). Trained professionals should estimate the patient's GCS score on arrival at the scene, again on arrival in the emergency room, and periodically thereafter (Table 27–10). Complete physical examination is necessary to look for evidence of injuries to other organs. Inspection of the body should be conducted to look for bruises and lacerations. Battle sign (ecchymosis behind the ear), blood in the middle ear, or cerebrospinal fluid (CSF) rhinorrhea suggests the presence of a basilar skull fracture. Neurologic examination should be performed to look for signs of focal dysfunction (such as hemiparesis, reflex asymmetry, or Babinski sign) or cranial nerve abnormalities (such as a gaze palsy or pupillary asymmetry). The GCS score is not a substitute for a neurologic examination, since it may fail to detect significant focal findings.

Seizure activity should be noted and described carefully, with attention to evidence of focal seizure activity. Seizures occurring within the first few minutes after the injury ("impact" seizures) should be differentiated from seizures that occur subsequently ("early" seizures). The risk of later epilepsy is thought to be less in children with impact seizures than in those with early seizures.

Neuroimaging (CT or MRI) is indicated in children with moderate and severe head injuries. Contrast studies are usually not necessary in the initial study. CT with "bone window" settings will detect most skull fractures. MRI is better than CT for detecting tissue damage, however. Skull radiographs may be used if neuroimaging is not available, but children with severe head injuries are best managed at facilities that have neuroimaging available. Most clinicians and radiologists agree that skull radiographs are not necessary in many children with mild head injuries. Electroencephalography may be useful acutely to detect subclinical seizures if the patient is sedated or paralyzed. It may be useful later also to help decide whether to continue anticonvulsant drug treatment. Other laboratory studies may be indicated by the nature, extent, and severity of the child's other injuries.

TREATMENT

Children with mild injuries may not need to be admitted to the hospital. Parents can be educated about what to look for at home and instructed about what findings warrant a return to the emergency department. Children with skull fractures or transient neurologic findings whose level of consciousness is normal in the emergency department should probably be admitted for overnight observation. A child with altered consciousness requires frequent, careful observation and should be admitted to an intensive care unit.

Observation in the hospital ("neuro checks") includes assessment of the child's vital signs, arousability, the size and reactivity of the pupils to light, and the extent and symmetry of motor responses. "Neuro checks" are performed every 15 to 30 minutes until the child is alert, then every 1 to 2 hours for 12 hours and every 2 to 4 hours thereafter. Neurologic deterioration may reflect the development of cerebral edema or an expanding epidural or subdural hemorrhage. Repeat neuroimaging is indicated whenever this happens. Intracranial pressure may be increased and need to be treated (see later discussion).

Anticonvulsant drug treatment is indicated if the child has a skull fracture, an intracranial hematoma, or a GCS score of 10 or less on admission. Phenytoin effectively prevents seizures in such patients during the first week after the injury but has no protective effect after that time and should be discontinued (Temkin et al, 1990). If the child has had early seizures or is felt to have a significant risk of seizures because of prolonged coma or severe cerebral injury, it may be helpful to do an EEG at that point. The presence of epileptiform discharges on the EEG would support continuation of anticonvulsant treatment.

INCREASED INTRACRANIAL PRESSURE

Intracranial pressure (ICP) may be increased (greater than 15 mm Hg or 200 mm H_2O) in children with a head injury because of the presence of an intracranial hematoma or because of cerebral edema. Cerebral edema may be either vasogenic or cytotoxic. Vasogenic edema reflects impairment of the blood-brain barrier with leakage of fluid out of blood vessels into the interstitial space and is commonly seen surrounding intracerebral hematomas. Cytotoxic edema reflects neuronal damage with impairment of membrane ion pumping and entry of fluid into the neuron and is commonly seen following diffuse cerebral injury.

In infants with an open fontanel, increased ICP may cause the fontanel to bulge. The cranial sutures will also separate if ICP is raised for a period of time. These mechanisms may relieve ICP to an extent but are inadequate when rapid and severe elevation of ICP occurs. Severe

Table 27–10 • Glasgow Coma Scale

Category	Best Response	Score
Eye opening (E)	Spontaneous	4
	To speech (command)	3
	To pain	2
	None	1
Motor (M)	Obeys (command)	6
	Localizes	5
	Withdraws	4
	Abnormal flexion	3
	Extensor response	2
	None	1
Verbal (V)	Oriented	5
	Confused conversation	4
	Inappropriate words	3
	Incomprehensible sounds	2
	None	1

Total Score = (E + M + V)   Maximum = 15; Minimum = 3

trauma with brain swelling can cause herniation and death even in an infant with an open fontanel.

The best way to detect increased ICP is to measure it directly. When increased ICP is present, continuous ICP monitoring is often desirable to detect changes and to provide treatment promptly. A variety of techniques are available for continuous ICP monitoring, including placement of a catheter, bolt, or pressure transducer into the subdural or subarachnoid space or into the ventricular system. ICP monitoring is indicated in children with persistent unconsciousness. Neurosurgical consultation (if not already obtained) is usually warranted in this situation to place the monitoring device and to assist with treatment.

Treatment of a patient with increased ICP often must be directed toward the underlying etiology (for example, surgical evacuation of a traumatic hematoma) as well as toward the ICP itself. General measures include elevation of the head of the bed to 30 to 45 degrees to facilitate venous return. Fear, anxiety, and agitation may accompany intubation and further increase ICP, so sedation and muscular paralysis should be utilized as necessary. (Sedation should always accompany muscular paralysis.) Hyperventilation to maintain carbon dioxide partial pressure (PCO_2) between 25 and 30 mm Hg effectively reduces ICP. Further reduction below this range provides no additional benefit. If a ventricular catheter is in place, 1 to 2 mL of CSF may be removed to reduce ICP.

Several drugs can be used as needed to reduce ICP. An intravenous injection of a 20% solution of mannitol at a dose of 0.25 to 1.0 mg/kg is effective in many cases and reduces ICP within a few minutes. The effect lasts for 2 to 4 hours and the dose can be repeated for several days. The effect weakens when the serum osmolality is too high, so serum osmolality should be maintained below 310 mOsm by appropriate fluid management. Steroids (dexamethasone 1 mg/kg or its equivalent) may be useful to reduce the vasogenic edema that surrounds a hematoma. High-dose barbiturates can reduce cerebral metabolic activity and thereby reduce cerebral blood flow and consequently ICP as well. A separate neuroprotective effect of barbiturates is often suggested but remains unproven. A short-acting barbiturate like pentobarbital is often used but may cause decreased cardiac function and severe hypotension requiring pressor supports. Phenobarbital (a long-acting barbiturate) is easier to use because it causes less systemic effects and blood levels are readily available, but central nervous system depression is more prolonged (Trauner, 1989; Miller and Ward, 1993).

REHABILITATION AND PROGNOSIS

Many studies of outcome following head injury have used the Glasgow Outcome Scale (Jennett and Teasdale, 1981), which recognizes five classes of outcome: good recovery (no or mild disability), moderate disability, severe disability, persistent vegetative state, and death. One study of children and adolescents with severe head injuries found that recovery was correlated with age, duration of coma, and the presence or absence of focal damage. No child under age 6 and no child in coma for more than a month had a good outcome. A good recovery was observed in 40% of those patients with no focal lesions, compared with only 20% of those with focal lesions (Filley et al, 1987). Another case-control study of children with mild (40), moderate (17), or severe (15) injuries showed that recovery was greatest in the first year after injury and slowed down or plateaued during the next 2 years. Mildly injured children showed minimal deficits, whereas moderately and severely injured children showed academic and cognitive deficits that persisted despite rehabilitation (Jaffe et al, 1995).

The impact of a child's head injury on the family is immense and undoubtedly plays a key role in shaping the outcome for the injured child. Factors include (1) the nature of the child's behavioral disturbances, including impaired social perception, social awareness, and self-control; (2) increased dependency of the child on the family; (3) irritability, anxiety, depression, and other emotional changes; and (4) parental frustration, guilt, social constraints, and financial stress (Lezak, 1988). Preexisting psychiatric problems may be accentuated after a significant head injury and are exacerbated by adverse psychosocial environmental factors (Gerring, 1986). Hyperactivity, conduct disorders, personality changes, mood and affect disorders, behavioral disinhibition, and even organic psychosis can all be seen following head injury and complicate recovery. Methodologic issues need to include consideration of the child's developmental status and potential for growth (Broman and Michel, 1995). A biopsychosocial approach includes psychotherapy, behavioral management, environmental modification, child and family support groups, and judicious use of appropriate psychopharmacology.

Initial rehabilitation following head injury requires a team approach that includes nursing, occupational and physical therapy, speech and language therapy, nutrition, social work, neuropsychology, child life, and appropriate medical, neurologic, and psychiatric therapy (Reilly et al, 1987). Transition and placement into an appropriate educational setting after discharge requires careful planning and coordination. All involved must recognize that the child's performance will be affected initially by fatigue and other medical factors. The child may improve quickly, so classification and placement decisions will need to be re-evaluated periodically (Savage, 1991). The pediatrician and family will need to work closely with the educational team to ensure that the medical and educational intervention is coordinated, comprehensive, and appropriate for the child's needs.

Infectious Diseases

MENINGITIS

Bacterial meningitis remains a frequent cause of neurologic morbidity and mortality in children. Ninety percent of cases are reported in children under 5 years of age, with the highest incidence between 6 and 12 months of age. The most common organisms in newborns are group B streptococci, *Escherichia coli,* and *Listeria monocytogenes.* The most common organisms in older infants and children are *Streptococcus pneumoniae, Haemophilus influenzae* type B, and *Neisseria meningitidis* meningitis. The incidence of *H. influenzae* type B meningitis is decreasing, owing to

Table 27–11 • Typical Cerebrospinal Findings in Infectious Diseases

Test	Bacterial Meningitis	Tuberculous Meningitis	Viral Encephalitis	Aseptic Meningitis
Glucose	Low	Low	Normal	Normal
Protein (mg/dL)	Very high (75–200)	Very high (75–200)	High (50–100)	Normal (15–45)
White blood cell count (cells/mm³)	Very high (300–10,000)	High (100–300)	High (50–1000)	High (10–100)
Cell type	PMN	PMN or lymphocytic	Lymphocytic	Lymphocytic
Red blood cell count	Normal	Normal or high	Normal (high in herpes simplex virus)	Normal
Other	Positive gram stain and culture	Positive acid-fast bacillus stain and culture	Positive titers, polymerase chain reaction, culture (variable)	Positive titers, culture (variable)

PMN = Polymorphonuclear neutrophil leukocytes.

early vaccination against this infection. The mortality rate for bacterial meningitis in children remains 1% to 5% despite modern antibiotics, and the rate of neurologic sequelae may be as high as 40% (Klein, Feigin, and McCracken, 1986). Hearing loss is the most common sequela and may be prevented in some (but not all) instances of *H. influenzae* type B meningitis by early treatment with dexamethasone. Other sequelae include hemiparesis, quadriparesis, ataxia, cognitive disability, and seizures. Some of these sequelae may improve with time (Schrier et al, 1996).

Clinical manifestations include fever, headache, altered mental status, vomiting, and seizures. Patients may complain of neck or back pain and typically resist passive flexion of the neck (nuchal rigidity). Patients may resist knee extension when the hip is flexed 90 degrees (Kernig sign) or may flex the hips and knees involuntarily when the neck is flexed (Brudzinski sign). Increased ICP is present in virtually all patients, and young infants usually have a tense or bulging anterior fontanel. The syndrome of inappropriate (excessive) secretion of antidiuretic hormone is very common and contributes to increased ICP. Focal neurologic signs (deviation of the head or eyes to one side, weakness of the limbs, or reflex asymmetry) occur in 10% to 20% of the infections and often reflect an associated cerebral infarction. Seizures occur in 20% to 30% and are often associated with focal signs. A particularly ominous finding is petechiae or purpura, which may indicate shock due to fulminant meningococcemia.

Young infants may not have many specific clinical signs of meningitis, however, and the absence of these findings cannot be taken as evidence against the presence of meningitis. Thus, the general recommendation is that any febrile infant under 12 to 18 months of age should undergo a lumbar puncture if there are other suspicious signs of cerebral infection such as poor feeding, altered behavior, irritability, lethargy, seizures, or focal neurologic signs. If the child has focal neurologic signs, lumbar puncture may be deferred until after neuroimaging (CT or MRI) has been performed to rule out an abscess. Treatment should not be delayed because of the need for neuroimaging, however. As a rule of thumb, antibiotic treatment should begin within 1 hour of the child's initial presentation to the physician. Antibiotic treatment is a medical emergency and should be initiated whenever bacterial meningitis is suspected, even if the lumbar puncture has been deferred pending neuroimaging.

Cerebrospinal fluid findings may be normal early in the course, but usually there are abnormal findings (Table 27–11). If the clinical and CSF findings are uncertain or atypical, it is usually better to begin treatment with antibiotics and wait for the results of the CSF culture. The CSF culture may not be reliable if the child was treated with antibiotics prior to the lumbar puncture ("partially treated" meningitis), however, and a full course of antibiotics may be necessary even if the CSF culture is negative. Current recommendations for antibiotic treatment are available and should be consulted (Peter, 1997).

Special note should be taken of the diagnostic difficulties in tuberculous meningitis. The course may be more subacute, with initial upper respiratory symptoms followed by headache and altered behavior and consciousness. Results of the tuberculosis skin test may be negative, especially if a control skin test with candida or a similar ubiquitous antigen is also negative (anergy). The CSF findings may not be as dramatic, and the initial stain of the CSF for acid-fast bacilli often shows negative results. The CSF culture may not be positive for mycobacterium tuberculosis until 4 to 6 weeks after lumbar puncture. One of the best indicators of tuberculous meningitis is exposure to or inclusion in a high-risk population, such as recent immigrants from areas of high prevalence of tuberculosis, children who are immunosuppressed due to concomitant steroid treatment, or children with an immunodeficiency syndrome such as HIV-1. To be effective, antibiotic treatment for tuberculous meningitis must be started before the diagnosis is proved. Thus, treatment should be started whenever there is a reasonable clinical suspicion, especially in children at high risk.

ENCEPHALITIS

Encephalitis implies infection of the brain rather than just the meninges. Symptoms and signs usually reflect cerebral involvement and include altered consciousness, seizures, and focal neurologic signs. Some diagnoses of bacterial meningitis as discussed in the previous section are really instances of meningoencephalitis because of the presence of more extensive infection. More typically, encephalitis is caused by viral infection of the brain. The most common sporadic viral encephalitis is caused by herpes simplex virus (HSV). HSV encephalitis can be very acute and fulminant with fever, coma, and seizures, but it can also be subacute or indolent. Focal neurologic signs, focal seizures, evidence on neuroimaging of inflammation of the temporal lobes, or the presence of a high number of red cells in the CSF should suggest the presence of HSV encephalitis. Since HSV is one of the few treatable causes of viral encephalitis, and since treatment is most effective if given early, treatment with acyclovir is recommended whenever HSV encephalitis is suspected (Peter, 1997). Detection of HSV in the CSF may be delayed but can be used for later confirmation of the diagnosis.

Epidemic encephalitis is typically caused by enteroviruses or by arthropod-borne viruses. Most infections occur during the summer and fall. Signs and symptoms are similar as for other instances of encephalitis. Typical CSF findings are shown in Table 27–11. Treatment is predominantly supportive. The prognosis varies with the etiology but can be quite severe (Bale, 1996; Peter, 1997).

ASEPTIC MENINGITIS

The syndrome of aseptic meningitis is very common and fairly distinct. Children present with a fever, headache, and neck stiffness. Typical CSF findings are shown in Table 27–11. Infection is often epidemic and most episodes are caused by one of a variety of enteroviruses. Treatment is generally supportive, but many children are admitted and treated with antibiotics until the CSF culture is negative for bacterial infection. The prognosis is excellent and full recovery can be expected.

REFERENCES

Aicardi J: Epilepsy in Children, 2nd ed. New York, Raven Press, 1994.

Bale JF: Viral infections of the central nervous system. *In* Berg BO (ed): Principles of Child Neurology. New York, McGraw-Hill, 1996, pp 839–858.

Broman SH, Michel ME (eds): Traumatic Head Injury in Children. New York, Oxford, 1995.

Coulter DL: Comprehensive management of epilepsy in persons with mental retardation. Epilepsia 38(Suppl. 4):S24, 1997.

Donat JF, Wright FS: Episodic symptoms mistaken for seizures in the neurologically impaired child. Neurology 40:156, 1990.

Duchowny M: Nonepileptic paroxysmal disorders. *In* Berg BO (ed): Principles of Child Neurology. New York, McGraw-Hill, 1996, pp 285–296.

Filley CM, Cranberg LD, Alexander MP, Hart EJ: Neurobehavioral outcome after closed head injury in childhood and adolescence. Arch Neurol 44:194, 1987.

Freeman JM, Kelly MT, Freeman JB: The Epilepsy Diet Treatment, 2nd ed. New York, Demos Vermande, 1996.

Gerring JP: Psychiatric sequelae of severe closed head injury. Pediatr Rev 8:115, 1986.

Hauser WA, Hesdorffer DC: Epilepsy: Frequency, Causes and Consequences. New York, Demos, 1990.

Holmes GL, McKeever M, Russman BS: Abnormal behavior or epilepsy?

Use of long-term EEG and video monitoring with severely to profoundly mentally retarded patients with seizures. Am J Mental Defic 87:456, 1983.

International League Against Epilepsy: Proposal for classification of epilepsies and epileptic syndromes. Epilepsia 26:268, 1986.

International League Against Epilepsy: Proposal for revised clinical and EEG classification of epileptic seizures. Epilepsia 22:489, 1981.

Jaffe KM, Polissar NL, Fay GC, Liao S: Recovery trends over three years following pediatric traumatic brain injury. Arch Phys Med Rehab 76:17, 1995.

Jennett B, Teasdale G: Management of Head Injury. Philadelphia, FA Davis, 1981.

Klein JO, Feigin RD, McCracken GH: Report of the task force on diagnosis and management of meningitis. Pediatrics 78:959, 1986.

Kraus JF, Fife D, Conroy C: Pediatric brain injuries: The nature, clinical course and early outcomes in a defined United States population. Pediatrics 79:501, 1987.

Levin HS, Eisenberg HM, Benton AL (eds): Mild Head Injury. New York, Oxford University Press, 1989.

Levy RH, Mattson RH, Meldrum BS (eds): Antiepileptic Drugs, 4th ed. New York, Raven Press, 1995.

Lezak MD: Brain damage is a family affair. J Clin Exper Neuropsych 10:111, 1988.

Miller JD, Ward JD: Increased intracranial pressure: theoretical considerations. *In* Pellock JM, Myer EC (eds): Neurological Emergencies in Infancy and Childhood, 2nd ed. Boston, Butterworth-Heinemann, 1993, pp 56–69.

Mizrahi EM, Kellaway P: Characterization and classification of neonatal seizures. Neurology 37:1837, 1987.

Neill JC, Alvarez N: Differential diagnosis of epileptic versus pseudoepileptic seizures in developmentally disabled persons. Appl Res Mental Retard 7:285, 1986.

Nelson KB, Ellenberg JH: Prognosis in children with febrile seizures. Pediatrics 61:720, 1978.

Peter G (ed): 1997 Red Book: Report of the Committee on Infectious Diseases, 24th ed. Elk Grove Village, IL, American Academy of Pediatrics, 1997.

Reilly AN, Lutz MM, Spiegler B, Lynn P: Head trauma in children: the stages to cognitive recovery. Maternal Child Nurs 12:405, 1987.

Roger J, Bureau M, Dravet C, Dreifuss FE, et al: Epileptic Syndromes in Infancy, Childhood and Adolescence, 2nd ed. London, John Libbey, 1992.

Rosman NP, Colton T, Labazzo J, Gilbert PL, Gardella NB, Kaye EM, Van Bennekom C, Winter MR: A controlled trial of diazepam administered during febrile illnesses to prevent recurrence of febrile seizures. N Engl J Med 329:79, 1993.

Savage RC: Identification, classification and placement issues for students with traumatic brain injuries. J Head Trauma Rehab 6:1, 1991.

Schrier LA, Schopps JH, Feigin RD: Bacterial and fungal infections of the central nervous system. *In* Berg BO (ed): Principles of Child Neurology. New York, McGraw-Hill, 1996, pp 749–783.

Temkin NR, Dikmen SS, Wilensky AJ, Keihm J, et al: A randomized, double-blind study of phenytoin for the prevention of post-traumatic seizures. N Engl J Med 323:497, 1990.

Trauner DA: Increased intracranial pressure. *In* Swaiman KF (ed): Pediatric Neurology: Principles and Practice. St. Louis, CV Mosby, 1989, pp 169–175.

Volpe JJ: Neonatal seizures. *In* Volpe JJ: Neurology of the Newborn, 3rd ed. Philadelphia, WB Saunders, 1995, pp 172–207.

Wyllie E (ed): The Treatment of Epilepsy: Principles and Practice. Philadelphia, Lea & Febiger, 1993.

28 Human Immunodeficiency Virus Infection in Children

Allen C. Crocker

 In the United States, the cumulative total for persons with acquired immunodeficiency syndrome reached 612,000 by June 1997 (reporting began in June 1981). The number for children under 13 years of age was 7900, or 1.3% of the total.

It can be stated that the virus is assuredly infectious but not highly contagious; its transmission requires quite specific circumstances of connection.

In the early search for school and other services, young boys with hemophilia (such as Ryan White, the Ray brothers, and Mark Hoyle) made highly effective contributions to public understanding and public policy.

There is now an increased spirit of hopefulness for the situation of children with human immunodeficiency virus infection. Because of improved management in many regards, the disease is becoming a chronic illness with a reasonable short-term prognosis.

The Epidemic

The emergence of *human immunodeficiency virus (HIV)* infection has been a tragic modern development, with critical and widespread effects on civilization. It is generally agreed that HIV infection is the ascendant acute public health dilemma of recent times. Children have been affected directly and indirectly in many ways.

The first identification in the United States of the relevant infection took place in 1981, although retrospective considerations suggest that such a syndrome had been present in this country for several years previously. The disease first appeared to be restricted to men with homosexual practices, especially in San Francisco and New York City. Gradually it was also identified in women who had been using intravenous drugs or had been sexual partners of such men, as well as in persons who received blood transfusions or other blood products. The appearance of infection with similar features in infants and young children was perceived with much difficulty and challenge in Newark, NJ, New York, and Miami in 1983 and 1984 (Shilts, 1987). Demonstration of a specifically involved retrovirus was technically problematic but was finally achieved in both the United States and France.

The epidemic rapidly escalated and broadened in scope. Heterosexual transmission became more prominent, with a gradual rise in the extent of involvement of women (and then, by congenital passage, children). The long latent period between contact and clinical signs of infection, the devastating aspects of disease expression, and the invariable fatal outcome combined to create a plague-like aura about the illness. Needles contaminated with virus produced a strong early link for HIV infection to the drug world; later it was apparent that the use of cocaine and other noninjected drugs led as well to settings of sexual transmission ("intersecting epidemics") (Edlin et al, 1994).

To date, tracking of the epidemic has been achieved principally by required reporting of the presence of *acquired immunodeficiency syndrome (AIDS)*. This refers to the most advanced involvement with the process, including the presence of complicating opportunistic infections, tumors, and serious visceral signs, accompanying HIV isolation or antibodies in the person's blood. These reports are recorded and aggregated by the Centers for Disease Control and Prevention (CDC), with semiannual publication. More people (perhaps three to five times more) have an earlier and milder picture, commonly referred to as *symptomatic HIV infection*. In addition to these individuals, there are many more people carrying the virus who do not yet have identifiable illness. These have positive results on antibody testing, indicating an encounter with the virus. They are said to have *asymptomatic HIV infection,* which can be viewed as being in a latent period. The numbers cannot easily be known (since true surveillance at this level is an exceptional activity), but it is thought that they may be as much as 10 times that for fully expressed AIDS. Included in this category are some infants who are not truly infected but who temporarily demonstrate antibodies that have been passively transferred from their involved mothers ("indeterminate status"). In the United States, the cumulative total for persons with AIDS reached 612,000 by June 1997 (reporting began in June 1981). The number for children under 13 years of age was 7900, or 1.3% of the total. Total deaths at that point had been 375,000, and 4600 for children (CDC, 1997). The number of new cases of AIDS reported, and the number of deaths, dropped slightly in 1996 in the United States, for the first time since the epidemic had begun. These events represented an important recent achievement for prevention efforts and for viral chemotherapy. Regrettably a comparable reduction in incidence rate and survival has not been accomplished in third-world countries.

Acquisition of the Infection

Only blood, semen, vaginal secretions, and human milk have been implicated as a means of transmission of the virus from one person to another. HIV has been documented as being transmitted from an infected person to a noninfected person by three routes: (1) sexual intercourse (either heterosexual or male homosexual); (2) parenteral inoculation of blood (most often among drug users who share syringes and needles for injection; rarely by transfusion, blood products, organ transplantation, or caregiver accidental needle stick); and (3) congenital or perinatal transmission from a woman to her fetus or newborn infant. Although body fluids such as tears, saliva, urine, and stool can contain HIV in low concentration, there is no evidence of real risk of transmission by contact with these fluids (McIntosh, 1994). It can be stated that the virus is assuredly infectious but not highly contagious; its transmission requires quite specific circumstances of connection.

The normal settings of employment, community activities, schools, developmental services such as early intervention or preschools, child care, and medical ambulatory services do not pose consequential risks. In the circumstances of usual family living, including sharing of towels, toothbrushes, clothes, eating utensils, or drinking glasses, there has virtually never been documented transmission. In work with children, particularly those who are not toilet trained or who are rambunctious, concern has been voiced about possible dangers from contact with body fluids or bleeding episodes, but this appears to be unfounded. Numerous lists have been prepared to guide the conduct of human services with mixes of persons including those with HIV infection (American Academy of Pediatrics, Child Welfare League of America, and so on). A common caveat would read, "Improved attention to good hygienic practices is appropriate in all child care activities, including the generous use of hand washing; gloves are not necessary for schoolwork, therapy, feeding, diaper-changing, physical examination, or developmental assessment. Bloody fluids deserve particular respect" (Crocker, 1992).

It is of interest that the existence of the HIV epidemic was needed to cause us to look more thoughtfully at general risks of transmission of common infections within groups of children or adults. The spread of hepatitis B or cytomegalovirus infections is more likely and carries significant personal concern, but the occurrence of these conditions has not been well monitored. In the setting of medical and dental care, child or day care, and even developmental services and classrooms, there is now a widespread use of the general principles of "universal precautions." This has made great contributions to staff peace of mind and a confidence about the admission of infected children. It also guards against complicating illnesses for children with HIV infection, inasmuch as their compromised immunity leaves them susceptible to various viral and bacterial infections.

The route of the original involvement for children with HIV infection is overwhelmingly that of congenital transmission. The CDC surveillance data show that of children currently in the log, including those recently entering, over 90% have an identified maternal infection or risk thereof. Some other children have been involved in transfusion, blood products, or tissue transplant (up to 8% historically). For mothers infecting their babies, the majority are also themselves involved with the use of illicit drugs, or their partners are. The portion of the HIV epidemic that includes women has been growing steadily—from 11.1% of new cases in 1989 and 1990 to 21.3% in 1996 and 1997, with a total for the years since 1981 of 15.7%. The children with infection are 18% white, 23% hispanic, and 58% black (CDC, 1997). There is a strong orientation toward urban settings. Four states account for 57% of the cumulative pediatric AIDS incidence (New York, Florida, New Jersey, and California), and three cities within them (New York, Miami, and Newark, respectively) have national prominence (CDC, 1997). This implies that many of the young children with HIV infection are also involved in urban poverty, drug scenes, and associated disadvantages. There is also a trail of complex suburban lives, with more affluent mothers who have infection, of varying backgrounds, and some others as well from rural settings.

The story of children with hemophilia who became infected with HIV has its own disheartening elements. Infected donors contributed to the pool of blood products used in the treatment of hemophilia, and until 1985 this contamination was not monitored. Eventually 90% of persons with more severe coagulation disorders became HIV positive, adding a maximal new stress to their medical courses (Hall, 1994). The latent period leading to symptomatic infection was often unusually long, but many have died of AIDS, either in childhood or early adult life. Currently more than half of all persons with hemophilia have HIV infection as well. In the early search for access to school and other services, young boys with hemophilia (such as Ryan White, the Ray brothers, and Mark Hoyle) made highly effective contributions to public understanding and public policy. Adolescents with HIV infection understandably may have much difficulty finding effective coping strategies (Brown, Schultz, and Gragg, 1995).

Pregnancy, Newborns, and Infants

It came to be known that between one quarter and one third of the fetuses carried by infected women would themselves become infected, some during various periods of the pregnancy and even more in the delivery process. Anonymous newborn antibody screening served only to provide a measure of the prevalence of ambient maternal infection. A study of seminal importance, with results released in early 1994, showed that zidovudine given orally during pregnancy, intravenously during labor, and then orally to the newborn could reduce the risk of infection by 67% (Connor et al, 1994). This discovery, plus the growing realization of the real potential for prevention of *Pneumocystis carinii* pneumonia by prophylactic chemotherapy, began to relieve much of the threat regarding congenital HIV infection. A new urgency to include HIV serologic testing early in prenatal care, on an informed basis, has yielded much timely diagnosis and allowed intervention. A better understanding of the infant's status is now possible in the early months by improved immunologic testing and culturing, with the setting for prompt and substantial antiretroviral therapy (Scott et al, 1995; Wilfert et al, 1997).

Early clinical manifestations of varying severity appear in most infected infants and may include oral candidiasis, lymphadenopathy, poor weight gain, some developmental delay, recurrent bacterial infections, and lymphoid interstitial pneumonitis. For the infants who have antibodies only by maternal passive transfer, the course is typically unremarkable. By 10 months of age, 50% of the uninfected children revert to seronegativity, and 24 months is the maximum age at which seroreversion usually occurs (Cooper and Pelton, 1996).

Clinical Course

As mentioned in the previous section, there is now an increased spirit of hopefulness for the situation of children with HIV infection. Because of improved management in many regards, the disease is becoming a chronic illness, with a reasonable short-term prognosis. An appreciable number of children have mild symptoms only, involving growth, development, and bacterial and fungal infection. More assertive viral involvement of the organs can include cardiomyopathy, pericardial effusion, acute nephritis, renal tubular dysfunction, pancreatitis, hepatitis, hematologic abnormalities, vomiting, or diarrhea (Cooper and Pelton, 1996). Combinations of antiviral agents are employed, involving reverse transcriptase inhibitors and protease inhibitors; these may be capable of causing a decrease in circulating virus and an increase in CD4 lymphocytes (both are favorable signs).

Infection with HIV in childhood is a multisystem disease that requires comprehensive care by a multidisciplinary team. In such a setting, counseling needs and other supports for the mother and family can be reviewed, with community agency contact as needed. Consideration of nutritional condition will be possible. Child development, both personal and school-related, can be evaluated and assisted. In a shared atmosphere, evaluation of therapy will be much more accurate.

The initial perception of the child's struggle with HIV was that in most instances there was an unalterable progression. Now, assisted by dynamic chemotherapy, the mortality is mild (estimated at 20% in the first 3 years). Various centers report that children surviving beyond the age of 3 years characteristically continue to live on (Meyers, 1994). Barnhart and colleagues (1996) describe a slow evolution of symptomatology. It is clear that a good number of children are getting to the end of childhood or to early adolescence in fair to good condition. Growth may have been poor, developmental achievement less than hoped for, and infections somewhat interfering, but they are active, school-attending young people.

Developmental Outcomes

The encephalopathy resulting from congenital HIV infection has been of central concern. It is part of the qualifying picture for a diagnosis of AIDS, and it has been one of the pervasive and discouraging aspects of HIV infection. For child developmentalists in urban settings, the virus has come to add a new basis for possible troubled progress, with presentations of mental retardation or cerebral palsy or both. The conception of HIV infection as a "disability," identified during the planning process for the Americans with Disabilities Act, drew to some extent on the central nervous system involvement.

It had been the belief, particularly in the United States, that viral effects on the brain are virtually universal in children with HIV infection. Recovery of live virus from the nervous system has been difficult, but related vascular and toxic changes have been implicated. These are well discussed in the remarkable volume *Brain in Pediatric AIDS* (Koslowski et al, 1990). Loss of brain mass, with increasing microcephaly, has been frequent, and calcification of the basal ganglia can be seen on computed tomographic scanning. Serious delays in developmental achievement, with or without regression of previously acquired skills, was commonly seen in the cities, although less often reported from European centers (Diamond and Cohen, 1992; Hittelman, 1990). It was hypothesized that concurrent developmental stresses in our population were accentuating the poorer gains in the cities, such as households having illicit drug use, violence, and parental loss.

Just as the general morbidity and mortality have improved for children with congenital HIV infection now that there is prompt diagnosis and more effective chemotherapy, the cerebral and developmental aspects are also less widespread and severe. There are still important issues, however. A representative and valuable study is the one from Miami that tracks the progress in the first 2 years of life of groups of infected and noninfected Haitian infants with very comparable backgrounds (Gay et al, 1995). Based on Bayley Mental Scale scores at 24 months, 32% of the infected infants had no delay and 21% had severe delay; for the uninfected (seroreverters), these figures were 75% and 1%, respectively. Based on the Performance Scale, 50% of the infected infants were normal and 29% severely delayed; among the uninfected children, 92% were normal and none were severely delayed.

The team from the Rose Kennedy Center in the Bronx, NY, has provided important statistics on the recent capability of school children with HIV infection. These are obviously young people who have passed through the period for early mortality and are on a longer survival course (Papola, Alvarez, and Cohen, 1994). The report describes 90 children from 5 to 14 years of age, most on antiviral therapy and with varying degrees of immunologic failure. Seventy percent of the children had normal intelligence (although many were in the borderline range), 22% had mild mental retardation, 3% had moderate, and 5% had severe retardation, not relating notably to age. About half of the children had significant language impairment, and a quarter had disorders of attention. There were some instances of depression or anxiety disorder, especially in those who were older. In the setting of that time, two thirds of the children were in special education classes, many had counseling, and a few needed habilitative therapies. Now one finds fewer who are requiring special education.

Services in School

A substantial population of children with HIV infection in our country are part of or are awaiting an educational experience. This number is probably about 20,000, skewed toward younger age groups, and potentially relevant to early intervention, child care, Head Start, preschools, and schools (Palfrey et al, 1994). At first, enrollment of these children was contentious and frightening (Kirp, 1989); fortunately the situation has changed.

Program design for very young children (e.g., in Head Start) must capture the principles of the worlds of education, developmental disabilities, and children with special health care needs (Bruder, 1995). These activities must be family-centered, respectful, collaborative, and inclusive and must involve appropriately trained staff.

A survey of the experiences of 84 children with HIV infection attending school in Massachusetts in 1993 to 1994 had favorable conclusions (Cohen et al, 1997). More than half the children had absences of less than 2 weeks during the year; one third had medications administered during the school day. For most of the children, no school personnel had been informed of the HIV infection; among those that were, the school nurses were the most frequent to be notified.

A more extensive survey was made in 1992 of the nation's largest school districts (n = 75) to gather information on local policies (Palfrey et al, 1994). In the process of this work it was possible to note a major transition underway in the nature of the relationship between families and children with HIV infection and the school departments (Lavin et al, 1994). In the 1980s, an authoritarian attitude had prevailed, in which disclosure was expected and there was only "pseudo-confidentiality." There were many restrictive local rules, and universal precautions were rarely used. There was little public support for the children to be in regular classrooms. Staff training was spotty and staff dismay was usual. It was then intriguing to note the fading of use of disclosure by families; by 1994 nondisclosure was the usual behavior, and most school districts had no real idea of how many students with HIV infection were in attendance.

In the previously mentioned (1992) project, an attempt was made to capture the cultural and legal tenets, in addition to consumer hopes, and build a listing of "Best Practices Guidelines" as they are connected to supports for children with HIV infection in school (Crocker et al, 1994). These included a dozen affirmations:

1. An *advisory committee on HIV-related issues* shall be established for the school district and commissioned by the Superintendent.
2. The school district shall adopt *policy statements of relevance to students with HIV infection,* in collaboration with the advisory committee.
3. *Staff education and inservice training* concerning the issues of HIV infection, including transmission, prevention, civil rights, mental health, and death and bereavement, shall be carried out at least annually for all school personnel, including the school board.
4. *Universal precautions relating to blood-borne infections,* as adapted for schools, shall be in effect.

5. The school district shall provide *education relating to the prevention of HIV infection for students in grades K through 12,* within the context of a quality comprehensive school health program.
6. The parent, guardian, or student shall decide *whether or not to inform the school system* about HIV status or other health conditions.
7. Few, if any, personnel in the school or school district shall *receive information about the HIV status* of a student (if disclosed).
8. *Information about a student's HIV status* shall not be included in the educational record, usual school health records, or any other records that are accessible to school staff beyond those whom the parents, guardian, or student has determined should know.
9. The *design of an individual student's program* shall be based on educational needs and not the status regarding HIV infection.
10. *In-school health services* shall be provided as needed, including special regimens required because of HIV infection, but the origin of these programs shall not be identified at the classroom level.
11. School administrators shall provide culturally sensitive information, technical assistance and consultation, and access to resources on HIV issues to the *school's parents and families* through PTAs and other parent organizations.
12. Relevant to existing federal and state statutes, teachers, school health professionals, and other qualified employees shall have the *right to employment and confidentiality* regardless of their own HIV status or other health conditions.

In essence, this will be a situation of universal enrollment, an end of "need to know" rules, presence of student and family autonomy, availability of good information, protection for staff, and support for the public.

Psychosocial Issues

Children with HIV infection have continuing and multifaceted care needs, and their families are challenged on many levels. In the same spirit as was employed for the educational premises, a guide called "Building Quality" has been prepared to consider the dynamics of health care, family support, and community living in the circumstances of children with HIV infection (Boland, Epstein, and Taylor, 1994). Ultimately there may need to be coordination for services in health, mental health, drug rehabilitation, legal issues, public assistance, housing, transportation, support groups, advocacy, and so on. Diverse social work contacts are usual and may be splintered; so-called case management programs are rare but very strategic (Wiener et al, 1992). Many of the mothers are themselves ill and stressed; in some centers as many as half of the children live with extended family, foster parents, or adoptive parents.

Informing a child about his or her HIV infection remains an important but bewildering assignment. There are no uniformly agreed-upon methods for best success, but considerable bias suggests that the process should begin by middle childhood and be carried forward in gradual steps (Funck-Brentano et al, 1997). Ultimate parent leadership is strongly defended by Mary Tasker in her book *How Can I Tell You?* (1992), as she says, "Although in my daily practice and interactions with parents, I frequently raised the topic of telling children the diagnosis, there was never any doubt in my mind that all authority in this decision-making process rested with the parents."

Confidentiality issues are at the core of many conflicts for the clinician and therapist. Terminology in records is a complex assignment if privacy is to be ensured. A particularly unnatural practice is the curtailment of the transfer of information when making referrals to other facilities or consultants whose assistance is desired. Young persons with HIV infection who know their diagnosis must also learn strict rules of discretion; for most of them, their peers are not aware of their secret.

REFERENCES

Barnhart HX, Caldwell MB, Thomas P, et al: Natural history of human immunodeficiency virus disease in perinatally infected children: an analysis from the Pediatric Spectrum of Disease Project. Pediatrics 97:710, 1996.

Boland MG, Epstein SG, Taylor AB: Building Quality: Indicators for Family-Centered Care in HIV Health Services for Children, Youth and Families. Newark, National Pediatric HIV Resource Center, 1994.

Brown LK, Schultz JR, Gragg RA: HIV-infected adolescents with hemophilia: adaptation and coping. Pediatrics 96:459, 1995.

Bruder MB: The challenge of pediatric AIDS: a framework for early childhood special education. Topics Early Child Spec Ed 15(1):83, 1995.

Centers for Disease Control and Prevention: HIV/AIDS Surveillance Report, Midyear Edition. Atlanta, Centers for Disease Control and Prevention, 1997.

Cohen J, Reddington C, Jacobs D, et al: School-related issues among HIV-infected children. Pediatrics 100:e8, 1997.

Connor EM, Sperling RS, Gelber R, et al: Reduction of maternal-infant transmission of human immunodeficiency virus type I with zidovudine treatment. N Engl J Med 331:1173, 1994.

Cooper ER, Pelton SI: Overview of pediatric HIV infection. *In* Libman H, Witzberg RA (eds). HIV Infection. A Primary Care Manual, 3rd ed. Boston, Little, Brown and Co, 1996, pp 631–650.

Crocker AC: Summary of policy recommendations. *In* Crocker AC, Cohen HJ, Kastner TA (eds). HIV Infection and Developmental Disabilities: A Resource for Service Providers. Baltimore, Paul H. Brookes Publishing Co, 1992, pp 247–251.

Crocker AC, Lavin AT, Palfrey JS, et al: Supports for children with HIV infection in school: Best Practice Guidelines. J Sch Health 64:32, 1994.

Diamond GW, Cohen HJ: Developmental disabilities in children with HIV infection. *In* Crocker AC, Cohen HJ, Kastner TA (eds). HIV Infection and Developmental Disabilities: A Resource for Service Providers. Baltimore, Paul H. Brookes Publishing Co, 1992, pp 33–42.

Edlin BR, Irwin KL, Faruque S, et al: Intersecting epidemics—crack cocaine use and HIV infection among inner-city young adults. N Engl J Med 331:1422, 1994.

Funck-Brentano I, Costagliola D, Seibel N, et al: Patterns of disclosure and perceptions of the human immunodeficiency virus in infected elementary school-age children. Arch Pediat Adolesc Med 151:978, 1997.

Gay CL, Armstrong FD, Cohen D, et al: The effects of HIV on cognitive and motor development in children born to HIV-seropositive women with no reported drug use: birth to 24 months. Pediatrics 96:1078, 1995.

Hall CS: The experience of children with hemophilia and HIV infection. J Sch Health 64:16, 1994.

Hittelman J: Neurodevelopmental aspects of HIV infection. *In* Koslowski PB, Snider DA, Vietze PM, Wisniewski HM (eds). Brain in Pediatric AIDS. Basel, Karger, 1990, pp 64–71.

Kirp DL: Learning by Heart: AIDS and Schoolchildren in America's Communities. New Brunswick, NJ, Rutgers University Press, 1989.

Koslowski PB, Snider DA, Vietze PM, Wisniewski HM (eds): Brain in Pediatric AIDS. Basel, Karger, 1990.

Lavin AT, Porter SM, Shaw D, et al: School health services in the age of AIDS. J Sch Health 64:27, 1994.

McIntosh K: Transmissibility of HIV infection: what we know in 1993. J Sch Health 64:14, 1994.

Meyers A: Natural history of congenital HIV infection. J Sch Health 64:9, 1994.

Palfrey JS, Fenton T, Porter SM, et al: Schoolchildren with HIV infection: a survey of the nation's largest school districts. J Sch Health 64:22, 1994.

Papola P, Alvarez M, Cohen HJ: Developmental and service needs of school-age children with human immunodeficiency virus infection: a descriptive study. Pediatrics 94:914, 1994.

Scott GB, Beck DT, Fleischman AR, et al: Perinatal human immunodeficiency virus testing. Pediatrics 95:303, 1995.

Shilts R: And the Band Played On. New York, St. Martin's Press, 1987.

Tasker M: How Can I Tell You? Bethesda, Association for the Care of Children's Health, 1992.

Wiener L, Moss H, Davidson R, et al: Pediatrics: the emerging psychosocial challenges of the AIDS epidemic. Child Adolesc Soc Work J 9:381, 1992.

Wilfert C, Beck DT, Fleischman AR, et al: Evaluation and medical treatment of the HIV-exposed infant. Pediatrics 99:909, 1997.

29 Effects of Nutrition on Development and Behavior

Marion Taylor Baer • Marie Kanne Poulsen •
Roseanne B. Howard-Teplansky •
Anne Bradford Harris

 There has been long-standing interest in the relationship between food intake and later development and behavior. In particular, the effects of malnutrition or undernutrition, have been subjects of in-depth scrutiny. This chapter demonstrates vividly the relevance of nutrition to development and behavior presenting evidence that even mild to moderate deficiencies (e.g., iron deficiency anemia) may have measurable adverse effects on development. This chapter is especially relevant to clinicians who deal with failure to thrive and with programs for early intervention and prevention.

Introduction

Much of what is known about the relationship between nutrition and development and behavior in children is the result of studies of undernourished and poor children in developing countries. In the United States, most of the research relating to failure to thrive has focused on maternal attachment, abuse, and neglect. This reflects a certain complacency surrounding the issue of the nutritional status of children living in the United States, an assumption that most are well nourished, although it is well known that nutrition is basic to growth and development and that optimal nutrition is necessary for optimal growth and development of children. Because of this assumption, measures of infant and child development (e.g., gross and fine motor abilities, language skills, adaptive behaviors, cognitive or achievement scores) rarely include nutritional status, nor do most early intervention programs routinely include a nutrition component. This occurs even though it is clear that malnutrition, even mild to moderate malnutrition, is associated with deficits in growth, development, intellectual function, and behavior patterns, even in the United States (Pollitt, 1994).

Failure to thrive represents approximately 5% of all pediatric admissions in the United States; 10% to 40% of those children, compared to 7% in the general population, had low birth weight, suggesting prenatal origin (Lozoff, 1989). Postnatal nutritional deprivation is implicated as well, by definition, because nutrients for adequate growth have not been offered, accepted, or retained. Failure to thrive is seen much more frequently among low-income children, and in the United States, one of five children is at high psychosocial risk for reasons associated with poverty. One of the latter risk factors is food insecurity (increased likelihood of food inadequacy and hunger at some time during the year), which recently was reported, using US Department of Agriculture data, to affect 12% of households nationwide and up to 17% in some states (Community Nutrition Institute, 1997). Failure to thrive is also more common in children of all income levels at high biological risk (e.g., low birth weight, small for gestational age [SGA], substance exposed) for or with developmental delays or special health care needs (Baer, Farnan, and Mauer, 1990). A recent survey of children with a wide range of special needs in Department of Health and Human Services (DHHS) Region IX indicates that 30% of children younger than 5 years had weights for height below the 5th percentile, 37% had heights for age below the 5th percentile, and nearly 20% had feeding problems (Baer et al, 1997). Because an estimated 35% of families of children with identified disabilities fall below the Census Bureau's threshold for low income (Bowe, 1995) and because two of three children with mild mental retardation have grown up in poverty (Aylward, 1990), many in this group appear to be in double jeopardy.

Research of the past 30 or so years indicates that nutritional status is indeed an important determinant of development and behavior. Adverse effects resulting from generalized undernutrition (both chronic and short-term) and specific nutrient deficiencies in children of all ages, but particularly among the youngest and most vulnerable, can be measured. Recent findings suggest a relationship between undernutrition and the subtle signs of behavioral dysfunction such as sleep disturbance and hyperactivity, which are being seen with ever greater frequency among infants and children. This chapter promotes the integration of nutrition, as one determinant of development and behavior, into the modern complex conceptual framework, illustrating how it interacts with other risk factors, both psychosocial and biological, to affect child outcomes (Fig. 29–1). This chapter outlines the important components of a nutrition and feeding assessment, details some well-established nutrition therapies for the prevention of mental retardation caused by inborn errors of metabolism, and comments on the current status of some controversial dietary interventions proposed to ameliorate behaviors.

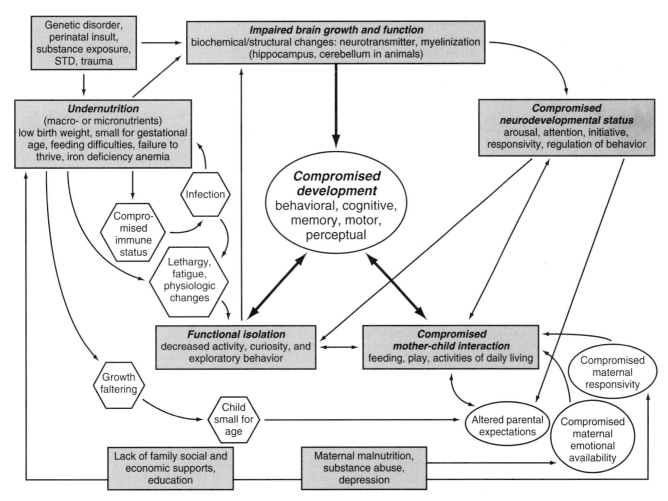

Figure 29–1. The integration of nutrition as one determinant of development and behavior. (Baer MT, Poulsen MK. Used with permission of the Center for Child Development and Developmental Disabilities, University of Southern California University Affiliated Program at Childrens Hospital Los Angeles.)

DEFINITION OF NUTRITIONAL STATUS

Nutritional status can be described as a continuum, from optimal health to death. An individual may, theoretically, fall anywhere along this continuum, depending on past and present nutrient intake. However, obvious malnutrition, defined herein as undernutrition with respect to either energy-providing macronutrients (protein, carbohydrate, fat) or vitamins and minerals (micronutrients), is not apparent clinically until nutrient stores are depleted and there is loss of function. In the case of children, this loss of function is most commonly seen as growth faltering, usually a lack of weight gain (or even weight loss) followed by slowed linear growth as the body conserves energy to preserve metabolic function and muscular activity. Because of the body's ability to adapt to decreased nutrient intake by utilizing the body's stores, much time may pass, depending on the nutrients in question, before clinical malnutrition is recognized.

Nutrition screening can identify risk factors early along the continuum, especially with regard to food intake and feeding skills. Assessment of nutritional status, when indicated, includes not only a complete anthropometric and dietary evaluation but also biochemical analyses to detect depletion of nutrient stores and an evaluation of the child's feeding skills and behaviors (Appendix 29–l). The assessment allows the qualification and quantification of any problems and enables intervention strategies to be designed to ameliorate the child's nutritional status with the goal of preventing the growth faltering that may also signal adverse effects on development.

RELATIONSHIP BETWEEN GROWTH AND DEVELOPMENT

If growth faltering is a functional measure of malnutrition, then to the extent that short stature represents an adaptation to malnutrition in children, it can be used as a proxy for past or chronic undernutrition. This is an important concept, because there are indications that this adaptation may not be a benign reaction to inadequate nutrition, but that it also carries with it certain costs in terms of development in general. For example, Wilson and colleagues (1986) showed a positive association between stature and both intelligence quotient (IQ) and achievement among 14,000 7- to 14-year-old boys surveyed between 1963 and 1970 as a part of the National Health Examination Survey Cycles

II and III in the United States. The relationship between stunting and lowered IQ and/or poor achievement has long been recognized in underdeveloped countries where malnutrition is widespread and often severe. However, the existence of a similarly measurable association between stature and cognitive ability in the United States is somewhat of a revelation.

Genetics plays a role in determining the ultimate size of an individual and has been the common explanation for short stature among populations. The consensus among nutrition professionals is that there is probably no difference in growth potential across ethnic and racial groups, and the use of race-specific growth charts has been rejected. Evidence indicates that where there is dietary improvement as well as other improvements in the environment that affect nutritional and health status in general (e.g., sanitation), there is increased stature from one generation to the next within any given ethnic or racial group until the genetically determined potential is reached. Furthermore, when the mean stature of children from countries as disparate as Nigeria, Guatemala, and India is compared (Johnston and Markowitz, 1993), there is much more similarity between socioeconomic groups across countries than between ethnic groups within countries. The mean stature of the 7-year-old boys from the highest socioeconomic quartile in that study approximated that of 7-year-old boys from the United States, using reference data from the National Center for Health Statistics.

Not only is short stature associated with poverty, but development and achievement scores have also been shown to be associated with poverty. Data from the third National Health and Nutrition Examination Survey (NHANES III), carried out between 1988 and 1994, have shown a relationship between intellectual development as well as academic performance and income level in 2624 children aged 6 to 16 years (Kramer, Allen, and Gergen, 1995). White children from families with incomes at or below the poverty level ($16,050 for a family of four in 1997) scored significantly lower than those from families with incomes three times the poverty level, and similar results were reported for children of other racial groups. Evidence that undernutrition, not necessarily *severe* undernutrition, is one of the mediating environmental factors that explain the associations between poverty, growth, and less than optimal development has been accumulating.

HYPOTHESES TO EXPLAIN THE RELATIONSHIP BETWEEN NUTRITION AND DEVELOPMENT

Historically, there have been two avenues of research attempting to understand the association between nutrition and development and behavior. The first has looked at the effects of undernutrition on brain growth and function; the second has studied its effects on behavior and cognition. Assumptions were made in early studies that demonstrable changes in brain structure and biochemistry were directly related to the alterations in behavior and cognition seen in malnourished children. It was also supposed that the period of vulnerability to nutrition insult was limited to the first 2 years of life while the brain develops rapidly, the so-called critical period. However, it has become clear that the link

between nutrition and behavior is much more complex. Even though structural or biochemical changes in the brain, especially in early life, may have potentially important negative effects, the plasticity of the brain allows for adaptation to environmental influences, and these effects may be overcome to an extent determined largely by the timing, severity, and duration of the insult. It is also believed that the physiologic changes that accompany undernutrition in children and the ones that negatively affect their behavioral repertoire, including the exploratory activity and caregiver-child interaction necessary for optimal development, may be a more important contribution to altered cognitive development and performance. These mechanisms are not unrelated (see Fig. 29–1). The age range of vulnerability to these long-term effects of malnutrition may be much greater than had been suspected, and the minimal amount of nutritional insult necessary to produce them is unknown.

Effects of Undernutrition on Brain Growth and Function

Study of the relationship between malnutrition and cognitive development began with a focus on the effects of inadequate diet on brain structure and function. The fetal brain begins development early in the period of embryogenesis, undergoes a growth spurt during the third trimester (when lipid accretion is the greatest), and continues to develop rapidly during the first 2 to 3 years of extrauterine life, during which it reaches 80% of its adult weight. It has long been known, from work in both animals and humans, that nutritional insults during the period of rapid brain development result in reduced numbers of brain cells, and, because the head grows in response to increased brain size, decreased head circumference. At the micro level, structural and biochemical changes such as modifications in neuronal number, neuronal size, position of neurons in the central nervous system (CNS), development of dendrites and axons, development of synaptic connections, production of neurotransmitters, development of glial cells, and myelination of axons have been observed.

The question remains whether these changes in the brain are permanent and/or related to changes in subsequent cognitive, behavioral or affective development in the child. Studies indicating that onset of growth failure of the head before 26 weeks in infants SGA is associated with lower measures of cognitive ability as well as motor and perceptual scores at 4 to 5 years of age (Vohr, 1991) reinforce the idea that the early and most rapid period of brain growth is the most sensitive to deprivation and suggest that the timing of the insult may be crucial. Animal studies indicate the hippocampus and cerebellum to be the most vulnerable (Strupp and Levitsky, 1995). Permanent alterations remain in these structures whereas others recover, providing clues to potential functional deficits in humans that could be measured. For example, changes in the structure and neurophysiology of the hippocampus might affect short-term memory. Cerebellar changes would be manifested in tests of motor coordination and procedural learning such as reading and writing, skills found to improve with nutritional supplementation (Levitsky and Strupp, 1995).

Neuropharmacologic research in malnourished animals has revealed long-lasting, if not permanent, changes in neurotransmitter activity, which suggests that attentional processes and reaction to stress may be altered. It has even been suggested that cognition per se may not be affected independently, in that deficits in executive function, evidenced by attentional dysfunction and impulsivity, or changes in motivation and/or anxiety can affect every aspect of behavioral function (Levitsky and Strupp, 1995). Previously undernourished animals, for example, seem to be able to perform as well as control subjects in problem-solving situations—at least if the testing conditions do not evoke increased emotionality. Levitsky and Strupp suggest that tests that have been used to determine the effects of undernutrition on development in humans, to the extent that they do not measure affective changes, may have been missing the mark.

Behavioral and Developmental Impact of Undernutrition

PRENATAL NUTRITION

General Undernutrition

The effects of nutrition on development, and the growth of the brain in particular, begin prenatally, because low birth weight is one of the most common risk factors for poor developmental outcome in infants. Undernutrition during pregnancy puts a fetus at risk for intrauterine growth retardation (IUGR) or for being SGA. If a fetus is malnourished throughout pregnancy, the IUGR is described as symmetric, which refers to the fact that both the infant's weight and the head circumference are below the 10th percentile using reference data for intrauterine growth. In asymmetric IUGR, in which the nutritional insult occurs later in the pregnancy, the infant's weight and weight for length are below the 10th percentile but the head circumference is above the 10th percentile. Although there are other reasons for low birth weight (defined as weight less than 2500 g or 5 pounds 5 ounces), maternal nutrition, both before and during pregnancy, is an important determinant of birth weight (Institute of Medicine, 1990); the two variables most consistently associated with low birth weight resulting from IUGR are low maternal prepregnancy weight and low weight gain during pregnancy.

Timing of the prenatal nutritional insult appears to affect outcome. Young Army inductees whose mothers had been exposed during their first trimester to a brief period of famine in Holland during World War II displayed a higher prevalence of conditions antecedent to schizophrenia—in particular schizoid personality (Susser and Stein, 1994). Recently, in the same birth cohorts, aged in their 50s, an association with schizophrenia was demonstrated in both men and women. Exposure in the third trimester had an "unequivocal" effect on birth weight, but not so much on preterm delivery, which points to growth retardation as the underlying process in lowered birth weight. This study, which is ongoing, of children born during the Dutch famine has even affirmed an association between low maternal birth weight and that of the second generation. Because the low birth weights among the mothers in this case were known to be the result of starvation, these data suggest that environmentally induced changes in maternal birth weight may be transmitted to their children.

Other researchers have looked specifically at the relationship between prenatal nutrition and subsequent infant behaviors under conditions of much milder malnutrition. Kirksey and colleagues (1991), for example, have shown, in a semirural Egyptian population, that early maternal pregnancy weight and intake of animal-source foods were significant positive predictors of the newborn's orientation and habituation (a measure of early ability to process information) behaviors.

Micronutrient Deficiencies

Although most reports have related birth weight to the mother's general nutritional status, particularly with respect to energy intake, recent studies have shown maternal riboflavin (Badart-Smook et al, 1997) and other (Doyle et al, 1989) specific micronutrients to be significantly and positively associated with birth weight as well. Prenatal micronutrient deficiencies have also been related to neurologic defects. Iodine deficiency during pregnancy impairs development of the CNS, resulting in cretinism that cannot be fully reversed. Lesser degrees of deficiency have been associated with psychomotor and cognitive deficits that may or may not be reversible. A relative (i.e., subclinical) folate deficiency plays a role in the etiology of neural tube defects and may increase risk of orofacial clefts (Shaw et al, 1995). It has also been suggested that a substantial minority of the general population may have increased folate needs (Molloy et al, 1997).

Some teratogenic drugs, such as valproic acid and carbamazepine, as well as phenytoin and phenobarbital have also been implicated in the etiology of spina bifida and orofacial clefts (King, Lie, and Irgens, 1996). Many of these drugs, as with alcohol, interfere with the metabolism of folate and zinc, another nutrient key to cell multiplication that has been implicated in the etiology of neural tube defects. In addition to acting directly, these teratogens, and other factors in the maternal environment, act indirectly by adversely affecting nutrient intake or metabolism (Williams and Carta, 1997). Smoking, for example, appears to decrease the availability of dietary energy and other nutrients such as folate and zinc while increasing the need for iron (Institute of Medicine, 1990).

INFANT NUTRITION

Feeding and Development

The infant's biological and emotional needs are met through feeding. The infant simultaneously experiences the comfort of a full stomach with solace and communication. Gradually, the physiologic aspect of eating becomes entwined with emotions, as the feeder appeases the infant's hunger and provides interpersonal experience. These feeding interactions promote attachment and have been found to be central to the early relationship of the mother and child. Ainsworth, Bell, and Stayton (1971) found that when there is a high degree of feeding synchrony between the mother and child, the subsequent attachment is strong. The critical elements of maternal caregiving that lead to synchrony include emotional availability; the capacity to read and respond to the infant's cues; expectations that match the child's development, temperament, and neurobehavioral functioning; and the capacity to serve as a buffer from sensory overload (Poulsen, 1993).

Impoverishment, maternal depression, malnutrition, and substance use can interfere with a mother's adeptness at meeting her infant's needs. Impoverished mothers of young children are more vulnerable to depression, apathy, and feelings of hopelessness (Zuckerman and Beardslee, 1987). These depressive symptoms affect parental attention, emotional availability, and infant-parent interactions, their sense of parental empowerment, and capacity to provide appropriate experiential opportunities for their children (see Fig. 29–1).

Lethargy accompanying maternal malnutrition can produce changes in mothers' capacities to initiate interaction with their young and respond to their needs. Mothers who use drugs and alcohol have periods of unavailability and lack facilitating, soothing, and protective parenting strategies that match their infants' developmental and neurobehavioral needs (Poulsen, 1995). In addition, mothers with little education and limited support may have minimal understanding of the role that nutrition plays in infant development and may not make it a priority.

The infant's behavior during feeding also influences the attachment process. At-risk infants may have difficulties with suck-swallow coordination and oral hypersensitivity that interfere with the feeding process. Neurobehavioral dysfunction in alertness, consolability, and depressed interactive behaviors offer misleading feeding cues that disrupt the development of mother-child reciprocity.

An extensive body of child development research has described the influence of the early feeding experience on development. Most theories indicate that feeding plays a role in personality development and interpersonal relationships. Although there are philosophical differences concerning the effect of feeding on development, there is agreement that the more gratifying the feeding experience, the better the effect on development. A gratifying experience involves a successful interaction between the parent and child that is synchronized with the infant's feeding ability, which goes through a marked transition during the 1st year of life as the infant progresses from a totally dependent, somewhat passive feeder to an active participant who increasingly seeks independence. Table 29–1 summarizes the infant's progression in the feeding process. When parents are able to recognize their infants' feeding ability, relinquish control, and allow the infant to progress accordingly, feeding problems are less likely to occur.

Infants at risk for feeding and nutrition problems are those who do not progress appropriately at some stage of feeding development; infants with CNS dysfunction can have feeding problems from birth. Poor sucking ability, prolonged feeding time with small intake, choking, and aspiration are common difficulties. As spoon feeding and solid foods are introduced, problems become more manifest. The persistence of primitive reflexes and abnormal muscle tone are two characteristics of the child with CNS dysfunction that are commonly associated with feeding

problems. The following are often identified as problem areas for which individualized solutions must be found: sitting balance; head and neck control; tongue control; sucking, swallowing, chewing, and drinking; mouth sensation (lack of mouth sensation or hypersensitivity to temperature changes or tactile stimulation); and startle reflex (a common response to a loud noise in children with cerebral palsy). When observed clinically, these organic feeding problems are invariably intermixed with behavioral problems. Because these infants have lost pleasure in the function of eating, possibly because they have been gavage- or force-fed, there can be a conditioned aversion to feeding situations. In addition, families frustrated by the inability to adequately nourish their child and by the amount of time spent attempting to do so may exacerbate the problem as they become more and more stressed (Sechrist-Mertz et al, 1997).

Many factors contribute to the development of a feeding problem, and it is often hard to isolate the organic from the behavioral aspects. Therefore, when there is significant difficulty, an interdisciplinary team evaluation of the infant's oral and fine motor ability, along with an analysis of mother-child interaction during feeding, and a nutrition assessment is needed (see Appendix 29–1). This is especially true for children, including those prenatally exposed to drugs and/or with identified genetic syndromes, who have multifactoral developmental delays. A screening form designed to identify nutrition and feeding problems is especially helpful in determining which children with special health care needs are at risk for feeding and nutrition problems (Baer and Harris, 1997).

A careful review of diet and fluid intake should be made to determine their adequacy, along with determination of the effect of any medications on nutrient absorption and metabolism, taste, appetite, or feeding behavior (e.g., causing drowsiness at mealtime). Children who are nonambulatory, especially if they are undergoing long-term treatment with anticonvulsant agents, should be monitored for vitamin D status (Baer MT, Harris AB, Bujold CR, et al, unpublished data, 1997), as well as for growth and overall dietary adequacy. Determining the status of other nutrients, such as folate, should also be considered in children with seizure disorders.

In the Feeding Development Clinic of the University of Southern California University Affiliated Program at Childrens Hospital, Los Angeles, the feeding team consists of a nutritionist, an occupational therapist, a psychologist, and a consulting pediatrician. The health care team, working together but from different vantage points, can formulate a plan of intervention while considering the total child within the family.

Influence of Breast-Feeding and Preterm Formula on Cognition and Neurobehaviors

Nutritional factors may affect early development even in the absence of undernutrition. There is evidence that infants who are breast-fed have a significant advantage over those who are formula-fed on tests of visual acuity as late as 3 years of age (Uauy and de Andraca, 1995) and cognitive development up to at least 8 years of age (Lucas et al, 1992). In school-aged children, fewer neurologic abnormal-

Table 29–1 • Development of Feeding Skills

Age	Oral and Neuromuscular Development	Feeding Behavior
Birth	Rooting reflex	Turns mouth toward nipple or any object brushing cheek
	Suck-swallow reflex	Initially sucking and swallowing are not differentiated; stimulus introduced into the mouth elicits vigorous sucking followed by a swallow if liquid is present
		Initial swallowing involves the posterior of the tongue; by 9 to 12 weeks, anterior portion is increasingly involved, which facilitates ingestion of semisolid food
		Pushes food out when placed on tongue; strong the first 9 weeks of life
	Bite	Pressure on the gums elicits a phasic bite and release
		Normal occurrence: birth to 3 to 5 months
		Retention produces biting of all objects placed in the mouth
		Interferes with mouthing activities, ingesting food, more mature biting, chewing
		By 6 to 10 weeks recognizes the position in which he or she is fed and begins mouthing and sucking when placed in this position
3 to 6 months	Beginning coordination between eyes and body movements	Explores world with eyes, fingers, hands, and mouth; starts reaching for objects at 4 months but overshoots; hands get in the way during feeding
	Learning to reach mouth with hands at 4 months	Finger sucking—by 6 months all objects go into the mouth
	Able to grasp objects voluntarily at 5 months	May continue to push out food placed on tongue
	Sucking reflex becomes voluntary and lateral motions of the jaw begin	Grasps objects in mitten-like fashion
		Can approximate lips to the rim of cup by 5 months; chewing action begins; by 6 months begins drinking from cup
6 to 12 months	Eyes and hands working together	Brings hand to mouth; at 7 months, able to feed self biscuit
	Sits erect with support at 6 months	Bangs cup and objects on table at 7 months
	Sits erect without support at 9 months	
	Development of grasp (finger to thumb opposition)	Holds own bottle at 9 to 12 months
		Pincer approach to food
		Pokes at food with index finger at 10 months
	Reaches to objects at 10 months	Reaches for food and utensils, including those beyond reach; pushes plate around with spoon; throws eating utensils; insists on holding spoon not to put in mouth but to return to plate or cup
1 to 3 years	Development of manual dexterity	Increased desire to feed self
		15 months—begins to use spoon but turns it before reaching mouth; may hold cup; likely to tilt the cup rather than head, causing spilling
		18 months—eats with spoon, spills frequently, turns spoon in mouth; holds glass with both hands
		2 years—inserts spoon correctly, occasionally with one hand; holds glass; plays with food; distinguishes between food and inedible materials
		2 to 3 years—self-feeding complete with occasional spilling; uses fork; pours from pitcher; obtains drink of water from faucet

Adapted from Getchel E, Howard RB: Nutrition in development. *In* Scipien G, Barnard M (eds): Comprehensive Pediatric Nursing, 2nd ed. New York, McGraw Hill, 1979, p 163, and Fetter L: Feeding the handicapped child. *In* Howard RB, Herbold NH (eds): Nutrition in Clinical Care. New York, McGraw-Hill, 1982, p 613.

ities (Lanting et al, 1994) and better school grades (Rogan and Gladen, 1993) have been reported in those who had been breast-fed. Even though these studies controlled for obvious confounding factors such as maternal education, birth order, and social class, it is clear that differences may remain between mothers who choose to breast-feed and those who use formula. Also, although the act of breast-feeding itself favors the maternal-infant bonding that also positively influences development, the same developmental advantage has been shown in infants fed breast milk by tube (Lucas et al, 1992). The benefits to preterm and infants SGA are greater than to those born at term, suggesting that providing breast milk to the former is even more crucial. Similar developmental advantages have been reported in preterm infants fed an enriched formula (both in protein and micronutrients) either as the sole food or as a supplement to breast milk; again, the effect was especially strik-

ing for infants who were also SGA and, in this case, for males (Lucas et al, 1990).

There are other differences in the composition of breast milk, including hormones and growth factors, which may play a role in nervous system development (Uauy and de Andraca, 1995). However, it is postulated that the beneficial effect of breast milk is due to the presence of long-chain fatty acids, docohexaenoic and arachidonic acids, which make up approximately 30% of brain fatty acid (the lipid content of the brain constitutes about 60% of the total dry weight of the organ), and which are necessary for brain and retinal function as well as psychomotor development. These fatty acids are not included in standard infant formulas in the United States, although their addition is currently being studied by the Food and Drug Administration.

Breast-feeding has also been shown to influence infant electroencephalographic sleep stages and sleep/wake patterns, but little attention has been paid to the role of the composition of the diet in regulating sleep behaviors in infants. It has been demonstrated, however, that changes involving dietary manipulation of nutrients (amino acids), even a single feeding, which influence the synthesis of the neurotransmitter serotonin, can cause a short-term change in newborn sleep behavior (Yogman and Zeisel, 1983).

Impact of Nutrition on Infant Behavioral Regulation and Neurodevelopmental Status

Infants are born with a wide range of temperamental characteristics and regulatory mechanisms that have a neurologic basis. These biologically rooted characteristics influence how the growing infant perceives, initiates, and responds to the persons, objects, and events in his or her world and are the foundation for the development of cognition and social and emotional well-being. Temperamental characteristics and regulatory mechanisms give rise to a spectrum of neurodevelopmental behaviors that account for individual differences in how infants establish feeding and sleeping patterns, learn to control states of

alertness, maintain a balanced sensory threshold, recover from stress, organize behaviors, and, most importantly, develop reciprocal social interactions with the significant persons in their lives.

Neurobehavioral markers refer to the presence of biologically rooted difficulties of self-regulation that are of developmental concern, atypical behaviors that offer suspicion of but not necessarily evidence for neurologic compromise (Neisworth, Bagnato, and Salvia, 1995). These neurobehavioral markers do not directly *cause* behavioral disturbance, cognitive delays, and academic failure, but rather contribute to a state of biological vulnerability that increases the likelihood of negative outcome if they are not adequately addressed in the caregiving process. Table 29–2 describes caregiving strategies that address the neurobehavioral vulnerabilities that affect the feeding process.

Although many biological circumstances can influence the robustness of the child's CNS, poor nutritional status has not yet been well recognized as a risk factor for poor neurobehavioral function and thus has not been adequately addressed by care providers. However, there are indications that undernutrition should also be considered as a cause of neurobehavioral markers. For example, possible

Table 29–2 • Developing Neurobehavioral Competencies Relating to Feeding

	Neurobehavioral Vulnerabilities	Resilience-Building Strategies
Establishment of feeding patterns	Difficulty grasping the nipple Difficulty developing a strong suck Difficulty retaining food Difficulty establishing a feeding pattern	Provide a calm environment for mother and child. Reduce amount of intake with more frequent feedings. Position infant in semisitting flexed position. Burp infant more frequently. Support chin and cheeks to help with suck. Provide frequent rest periods during feeding.
Control over states of alertness	Minimal number of states of alertness Pervasive short duration of alertness Minimal eye engagement	Shield eyes from bright lights. Swaddle infant with arms and knees in flexed position. Sway infant gently to alert. Tickle cheeks to arouse infant. Hold infant upright at shoulder to alert.
Capacity to recover from stress	Prolonged crying even with adult intervention Difficulty in recovering from distress Swift escalation from whimpers to howls	Respond at first whimpers. Place hand firmly across infant's chest. Swaddle infant in flexed position. Provide finger or pacifier. Bathe infant in warm water. Hold infant's folded arms close to infant's chest. Provide skin-to-skin contact. Rock infant vertically and slowly.
Balanced sensory threshold	Overreaction to movement, voice, and lights	Avoid overload to senses (i.e., reduce noise, movement, light touch, and light movement, voice). Sing or speak softly at first. Introduce stimuli gradually. Allow infant to rest when infant averts gaze. Approach infant slowly with warning. Avoid sudden movements when handling infant.
Organization of behavior	Difficulty combining sequences of actions	Protect from intense stimuli. Introduce sensory stimuli incrementally. Introduce multisensory stimuli gradually.
Interactive behaviors	Fewer vocalizations Muted smiles Minimal cuddling Minimal initiation of social contact Diminished eye contact	Position parent's face close for infant touch. Respond to muted infant smiles and glances. Respond to all infant vocalizations. Talk to infant during caregiving activities. Massage and stroke infant with eye engagement or vocalizations. Hold infant in a face-to-face position.

Adapted from Poulsen MK: Building resilience in infants and toddlers at risk. *In* Smith GH, Coles CD, Poulsen MK (eds): Children, Families and Substance Abuse: Challenges for Changing Educational and Social Outcomes. Baltimore, Paul H. Brookes, 1995, p 95.

developmental implications of IUGR (even in children with normal intelligence and no major neurologic problems) include a high rate of the more subtle signs of CNS dysfunction (e.g., speech and language problems, minor neuromotor dysfunction, learning disability, attention deficits, hyperactivity, and behavior problems). Lethargy and difficulties with arousal and in establishing regular sleeping and feeding patterns, identical to those in nutritionally deprived Guatemalan infants, were reported in a group of slightly small for date but clinically normal babies born in Boston (Brazelton et al, 1977). Infants born both preterm and SGA, or those with bronchopulmonary dysplasia, perhaps because of their higher energy requirements (Doyle et al, 1989), are apparently at additional risk for long-term effects compared to preterm infants who are appropriate for gestational age (AGA) (Vohr, 1991). On the other hand, there are opportunities for recovery for the compromised infant, particularly if environmental factors, including nutrition, are positive. Studies of "catch-up growth" in infants SGA suggest that those with optimal nutritional intake postnatally (in this case, those who caught up in weight by 8 months of age) will have increased head size, less neurosensory impairment, and a more optimal developmental outcome than either babies SGA who did not catch up or babies AGA whose growth faltered between term and 8 months (Hack, Klein, and Taylor, 1995).

EARLY CHILDHOOD NUTRITION

Early studies of the links between malnutrition, cognition, and behavior examined the outcomes of very young children who had experienced gross deficiencies of protein, calories, and other nutrients leading to marasmus and found a strong association between early undernutrition and intellectual outcomes. IQ scores for children between the ages of 5 and 11 years who were previously malnourished were consistently lower than their adequately nourished peers. Approximately 50% had IQ scores of 90 or lower, whereas only 17% of the control subjects scored at or below 90 (Galler, 1984). It was hypothesized that this severe malnutrition in the first 2 years of life led to biochemical and structural deficits in brain development, which were reflected in impaired intellectual functioning and behavior patterns. However, it was soon recognized that factors other than nutrition, operant in the environment to which the child was returned after being nutritionally rehabilitated, were playing a role in the poor developmental outcomes measured months, and sometimes years, beyond the severe insult. For example, children who experienced severe short-term malnutrition as a result of illness (such as pyloric stenosis) generally did not show long-term global developmental delays in the absence of socioeconomic deprivation (Lloyd-Still et al, 1974), although some reported significantly lower scores on subscales relating to short-term memory and attention in comparison to siblings and matched control subjects (Klein, Forbes, and Nader, 1975). However, long-term delays remained evident among children undernourished because of poverty (Grantham-McGregor, Schofield, and Powell, 1987). Furthermore, if those undernourished poor children were given developmental stimulation instead of nutritional supplementation, similar beneficial results on development were seen, although the combined interventions were most effective (Walker et al, 1991).

These results suggested that adverse effects of poor nutrition on the developing brain could be largely overcome by environmental enrichment and led to an increased research focus on the effects of nutritional deprivation on behaviors. It was hypothesized that the physiologic changes in the undernourished child influence his or her curiosity, initiative, and motivation to interact with surrounding persons, objects, and events, thus restricting all transactions with the environment that have an energy cost (Pollitt, 1994). The decrease in exploratory activities and spontaneous interactions with the people and objects in the child's world, in turn, changes how caregivers relate and respond to developmental needs. The undernourished child is less active and responsive, has a lower frustration tolerance, is more emotionally unstable, clings more to mother, and initiates less. In return, he or she receives less interpersonal attention from a parent who may perceive and treat a smaller child as a younger child, resulting in "functional isolation" from the interpersonal and exploratory experiences needed to thrive developmentally (see Fig. 29–1).

Thus, poor nutrition and social-environmental deprivation act synergistically to isolate the young child from the experiences necessary for healthy development. The younger the child and the longer the deprivation lasts, the more permanent the adverse effects. The converse is also true. Long-term follow-up to supplementation studies carried out in Guatemala found that children who were exposed to nutrition treatment containing added protein (and energy), as well as the vitamins and minerals given to the low-calorie control group, on a continuous basis beginning prenatally and through the first 2 years of life, performed better at ages 13 to 19 years. After controlling for potentially confounding variables, the group with the greater supplementation scored significantly higher on measures of general intellectual abilities as well as on tests of numeracy, general knowledge, reading, and vocabulary achievement (Pollitt et al, 1995).

These prospective studies confirm the pioneering retrospective studies of young Korean orphans, some of whom had been malnourished during infancy, adopted into middle class American families, which demonstrated that normal academic and behavioral performance can be expected when the malnourished child is provided nutritional (and social-environmental) advantages starting before the age of 3 years (Winick, Meyer, and Harris, 1990). However, within normal limits, significant differences in IQ and school achievement (as well as growth) remained between the malnourished and well-nourished groups of adopted children, demonstrating subtle, but significant, long-term effects of early malnutrition on later intellectual functioning.

Mental abilities test performance is highly contingent on motivational factors, including attention, persistence, and self-confidence. And, as in animal studies, previously malnourished children are more vulnerable to behavioral problems; they have difficulty in maintaining calm, focused attention, concentration, emotional stability, and compliance to classroom expectations (Galler, 1984). Other researchers have noted that adverse behaviors in school-aged children, attributed to early undernutrition, interfere with their capacity to adequately develop early social interaction patterns, particularly with their parents. These vary from aggressive behaviors (Barrett and Radke-Yarrow, 1985) to difficulties in emotional development and social relationships (Rutter, 1979). Thus the poor cognitive performance in previously or chronically undernourished children may be related as much to affective as to intellectual changes. Horowitz (1989) postulates that because the human emotional system is more bound up in the social and cultural environment, it is more vulnerable to nutritional inadequacy than are the motor, language, and cognitive developmental dimensions, which have stronger predetermined courses, allowing them to be achieved under less than ideal interpersonal circumstances.

IMPACT OF POOR NUTRITION AND HUNGER ON SCHOOL PERFORMANCE AND BEHAVIOR

A recent review of literature related to the link between student health risk behaviors and education outcomes in the United States (Symons et al, 1997) includes dietary behaviors as one of the health risk behavioral categories, recognizing the negative impact of poor nutrition. It has been shown that students who participate in school-based breakfast and lunch programs demonstrate greater school attendance, class participation, and academic achievement, better behaviors, and less absenteeism caused by illness.

Studies of the importance of overnight and morning fast (i.e., skipping breakfast) on cognition and school performance, both in the United States and in developing countries, have been recently reviewed (Pollitt, 1995). The author concludes from the data as a whole that brain function, especially with regard to speed and accuracy of information retrieval in working memory (e.g., the Matching Familiar Figure Test), is sensitive to short-term fluctuations in the availability of nutrients, particularly in those children who are nutritionally at risk. In theory, this decrease in performance is due to short-term metabolic and neurohormonal changes in the brain associated with changes in its supply of energy and nutrients.

Cycle of Infection and Malnutrition

Malnutrition is the most common cause of immunodeficiency worldwide. Even moderate protein-energy malnutrition and mild single-nutrient deficiencies alter the immune response. This includes impaired antibody formation, loss of delayed cutaneous hypersensitivity, reduced immunoglobulin concentrations, decreased thymic and splenic lymphocytes, reduced complement formation, reduced secretory immunoglobulin A and interferon, and lower T cells and interleukin-2 receptors. The micronutrients important to these processes include zinc, selenium, iron, copper, magnesium, vitamins A, C, D, E, B_6, and B_{12}, and folic acid (Scrimshaw and SanGiovanni, 1997). Common childhood illness is more abundant in children who are shorter and lighter and who ingest less food than their healthy counterparts (Ballard and Neumann, 1995). Illness also adversely affected cognitive development and behavior; sicker toddlers (18 to 30 months old) performed less well on the Bayley Scales of Infant Development test at 30 months and on other cognitive measures when retested at age 5 years (Neumann et al, 1992).

Conversely, once the child has an infection, the mechanisms that may precipitate malnutrition include anorexia, decreased intestinal absorption, and both catabolic and anabolic losses, even with subclinical infections. Fever and intestinal bleeding in some diseases cause additional losses of energy and, in the latter case, iron. Specific effects on nutrients include protein losses and decreases in serum vitamins A, C, thiamin, niacin, and riboflavin, as well as decreases in copper and zinc (Scrimshaw and SanGiovanni, 1997). Sometimes cultural and therapeutic practices may contribute to the malnutrition (e.g., withdrawal of food from those with fever or diarrhea). It has been suggested that even frequent immunostimulation, by diverting nutrients to support the immune response rather than growth processes, may be an important cause of growth faltering (Solomons et al, 1993).

Effects of Single-Nutrient Deficiencies on Behavior and Development

There are behavioral and developmental effects of specific nutrient deficiencies even in the absence of generalized malnutrition. Work in the 1970s and 1980s revealed a previously unsuspected prevalence of mild to moderate micronutrient deficiencies in humans, especially of trace minerals. Researchers in the area of child nutrition and development had previously been focusing largely on protein-energy malnutrition.

IRON

Since the early 1980s, much attention has been paid to the developmental and behavioral consequences of iron deficiency and iron deficiency anemia (IDA) in infants and children. Of all the micronutrients, iron is the most important determinant of behavior and psychomotor development. Yet IDA is the most common nutritional deficiency worldwide, particularly among the disadvantaged; approximately 25% of the children in the United States living in poverty are anemic. The prevalence is greatest among infants between the ages of 6 and 24 months because of the high demands of rapid growth coupled with frequent dietary inadequacy. This has major significance because the brain is still in its growth spurt at this age and the child is developing rapidly, both in mental and in motor domains.

Recent research indicates that IDA negatively affects an infant's sleep-wake cycles. Anemic infants showed variations in their sleep-wake cycles, including a greater level of variability in respiration during sleep and marked motor activity during the initial periods of sleep, making stabilization more difficult and suggesting less mature motor neurodevelopment. Other researchers have shown longer absolute and interwave latencies and central conduction time in auditory-evoked brainstem potentials (Roncagliolo et al, 1996). These and other indicators of neurologic immaturity, or "soft signs," which have been reported (Walter, 1993), suggest that IDA puts these infants at high risk of lower cognitive development.

Studies evaluating the effects of IDA on infants and toddlers using the Bayley Scales of Infant Development have shown adverse effects on both the psychomotor development indices (PDI) and the indices of mental development (MDI) (de Andraca, Castillo, and Walter, 1997). Most investigators also show differences in the infant behavior record (IBR), as much in emotional tone as in task orientation. The infants are more unhappy and wary of the investigator, at least on initial testing (Lozoff, Abraham, and Jimenez, 1996). Animal studies suggest that the effects may be the result of delayed maturation of the CNS. In addition to its hematologic importance, iron plays an important role in the myelination process and is essential in the metabolism of several neurotransmitters that influence affect and arousal, which may provide a physiologic explanation for observed behavioral effects (Walter, 1993; de Andraca, Castillo, and Jimenez, 1997). For example, iron deficiency appears to lower the activity of brain serotonin, which is thought to help the organism modulate behavior in response to excessive stimuli.

The severity of the iron deficiency is an important variable; several studies show no significant effects on performance and behavior unless the child is overtly anemic. Chronicity of the anemia, which usually co-varies with severity, also plays a role; infants anemic longer than 3 months had lower PDI and MDI scores than those whose anemia developed later (Walter et al, 1989). The reversibility of the adverse effects following oral iron treatment and hematologic response is still in question. Idjradinata and Pollitt (1993) showed a pronounced increase in both mental and motor scores after 4 months of therapy in anemic Indonesian children. On the other hand, Lozoff and colleagues in Costa Rica (1996) were unable to demonstrate improvement in mental or motor functioning after 6 months of treatment, and others have shown adverse effects lasting well into childhood (Walter, 1993). Controlling for environmental factors in the Costa Rican study removed the statistical significance of the iron deficiency as a variable, suggesting that it may serve as a marker for other important nutritional and family variables such as breast-feeding and better-educated mothers.

Studies on the prevention of anemia in high-risk infants in Canada, however, support an independent effect of iron supplementation (Moffatt et al, 1994). Although there were no differences seen in children after 6 months of study, those receiving iron scored significantly higher on the PDI beginning at 9 months, 12 months, and 15 months. There was no anemia, although 4 of 6 measures of iron status were higher in the infants receiving iron beginning at 6 months. In another recent prospective study in Chile, infants who were not anemic at 6 months of age but who became anemic before 12 months of age scored no differently on either MDI or PDI than control subjects who received iron supplementation, suggesting a protective effect of adequate iron intake during the period of most rapid brain growth (de Andraca, Castillo, and Walter, 1997). The importance of nutritional status is underscored by the fact that all the infants in this study weighed more than 3 kg at birth, suggesting adequate iron stores, and had been breast-fed over a prolonged period.

Because the effects of iron deficiency are more apparent during infancy and early childhood, its effects later in childhood are sometimes overlooked or minimized as a risk factor. However, studies of school-aged children in three developing countries (Thailand, Indonesia, and Egypt) suggest that IDA does affect performance on educational achievement tests and that, at least in the case of Indonesian children, iron treatment can improve the scores of the anemic school children (Pollitt, 1997).

ZINC

Zinc is a functionally essential component of more than 200 enzymes that pervade all metabolic pathways, including those of cell replication. In addition to decreased growth velocity, symptoms of human zinc deficiency include slowing and restriction of behavior, lethargy, and apathy. This suggests a possible role for zinc in neurocognitive development; suggested mechanisms include restricted brain growth and delayed neuronal maturation, changes in membrane stability, and altered neurotransmitter and neuromodulator function. Supplementation trials in infants and low-income children in the United States have demonstrated improved growth, especially in boys, indicating suboptimal zinc status, and some researchers have estimated that 50% of US children are at risk of zinc deficiency (Walsh et al, 1994). There have been few studies of the effects of mild zinc deficiency on behavior and development in children, and none in infants or adolescents who are at increased risk because of rapid growth. However, studies of zinc deprivation in immature animals (including monkeys) have shown negative effects on learning, attention, and memory (Golub et al, 1995).

Zinc deficiency is also associated with compromised host-defense mechanisms. Low–birth weight infants have a prolonged impairment of cell-mediated immunity that can be partly restored by providing extra amounts of dietary zinc (Chandra, 1997).

VITAMIN B₆ (PYRIDOXINE)

Vitamin B_6 is an essential cofactor in the developing CNS; deficiencies in animal models appear to alter function of the glutamatergic neurotransmitter system that is thought to play a role in learning and memory. Recent studies of mildly malnourished Egyptian mothers have correlated their B_6 status with scores for infant behavior on the Brazelton Neonatal Assessment Scale. The items related to consolability, rapidity of build-up to the crying stage, and irritability. Poor maternal B_6 status was associated with greater nonresponse to an infant's vocalization, lower response to infant distress, and greater use of sibling caregivers. Vitamin B_6 status also contributed to the prediction of infant vocalization at age 3 to 6 months (McCullough et al, 1990).

LEAD

Although not a nutrient, lead competes with other divalent ions such as calcium, iron, and zinc, which means that a dietary deficiency of any of these elements enhances its absorption. Also, to the extent that iron deficiency is associated with pica, lead in the environment exacerbates the likelihood of lead poisoning, which, because it impairs heme synthesis, compounds the effect of iron deficiency, resulting in a more severe anemia than with iron deficiency alone. Harris, Clark, and Karp (1993) warn of a "veritable epidemic" of low-level lead poisoning in the United States. Based on NHANES II data, DHHS estimated the 1993 numbers of children with serum lead levels of 15 μg/dL or more to be at least 1.2 million, with 400,000 fetuses exposed to maternal levels of 10 μg/dL or more.

Infants exposed to lead levels during gestation (lead crosses the placenta) and early infancy show significant decreases in developmental outcomes and deficits on cognitive, motor, and mental achievement tests. In children, even subclinical lead poisoning has subtle, but permanent, effects on learning and socialization skills and has been associated with school failure, even in children given chelation treatment (Needleman et al, 1990). The current thinking is that *there is no safe blood lead level.*

Nutrition Therapies: Inborn Errors of Amino Acid or Carbohydrate Metabolism

Inborn errors of metabolism originate in the mutations of single genes that are responsible for the synthesis of a specific enzyme. Most inborn errors of metabolism share an autosomal recessive mode of transmission. This either results in a structurally altered enzyme that is incapable of normal catalytic activity or causes an inhibition of enzyme synthesis. The reduced enzymatic function produces a block in the metabolic pathway at a specific point, which, in turn, leads to an abnormal accumulation of substrate before the point at which the block occurs. The level of substrate formed by the subsidiary pathways is increased in the blood, urine, and tissues.

The neurotransmitter system is vulnerable to impeded energy metabolism, abnormal electrolyte metabolism, and alterations of biogenic amine derivatives of amino acids and the catecholamines. Such shifts can affect neurotransmission and behavior. The abnormal biosynthesis of the biogenic amines can be reversed in untreated phenylketonuria by the dietary restriction of phenylalanine. This defect may be a partial explanation for the neuropsychiatric symptoms found in untreated phenylketonuria.

There is a wide range of clinical manifestations in the inborn errors of metabolism. Treatment consists of controlling the substrate accumulation by the restriction or elimination of carbohydrate or protein, or, in certain instances, pharmacologic dosages of vitamins (Table 29–3). Early treatment is essential in preventing the progressive loss of neurologic function, mental retardation, and other serious sequelae of metabolic disorders. For example, treatment for phenylketonuria must be started within the 1st month of life if normal physical and mental development is to occur. There are few reports of improvement in mental development and behavior in individuals with phenylketonuria who undergo treatment in later life (Holmgren, Blomquist, and Samuelson, 1979). To prevent the possible toxic effects on the fetus from elevated blood phenylalanine

levels in pregnant women with phenylketonuria, a phenylalanine-restricted diet begun before conception and continued during pregnancy is used.

Early treatment of inborn metabolic errors has been made possible by newborn screening programs, which can be used to test for more than 20 such syndromes. In the United States, testing for phenylketonuria is commonly mandated by state law. It has been proposed that screening tests for less common disorders can be economically justified when their cost is compared with that incurred when affected infants go undetected. Treatment has been improved by early identification, synthetic formulas, and special dietetic foods. Successful treatment of phenylketonuria is the best example of the prevention of mental retardation through diet.

Nutrition and Behavior: Controversial Therapies

More and more Americans are using unconventional therapies to treat illness. In the case of children with behavior disorders, it is common for parents to be interested in exploring the possibility of using diet (or supplemental nutrient) therapy to improve these behaviors. There are many reasons for this, including the desire to avoid the use of chronic medication, with its possible side effects, and to believe the anecdotal reports and often exaggerated claims of success. Alternative therapies are usually based on overly simplified scientific theories. They may be purported to be effective for a variety of conditions, claiming that most children will respond dramatically, particularly if started early, and to have no side effects. Many are supported by case reports or anecdotal data. Some families may think that they are not included in the process of decision making regarding their child's treatment, whereas the proponents of alternative therapies, including other parents and alternative health practitioners, may be more supportive and allow for more family participation. There are parent support groups organized nationally to provide parents with information, often using newsletters and the World Wide Web (Internet) to disseminate information. However, treatment is sometimes begun with little or no attention to identifying specific objectives or target behaviors (Nickel, 1996). The use of these therapies is widespread, with B_6 with magnesium being the most frequently used controversial therapy (23%) given to children with autism by their parents (Nickel, 1996). The following paragraphs discuss the most prevalent nutritional therapies used to treat autism and attention-deficit hyperactivity disorder.

TREATMENT OF AUTISM

Linus Pauling, the original proponent of orthomolecular psychiatry, defined it as a treatment of mental disorders using optimum concentrations of substances that occur naturally in the body. The theory is that individual needs for these substances, including vitamins and minerals, vary according to that individual's genetic makeup and that disturbances in behavior related to inadequacies of these substances can be ameliorated by providing the substances in optimal amounts. In the case of autism, abnormalities in neurotransmitter metabolism led to the study of vitamin B_6, which is involved in the formation of serotonin, gamma aminobutyric acid, dopamine, norepinephrine, and epinephrine. The early studies, including those of Bernard Rimland and colleagues, had several methodologic flaws that compromised the reportedly positive results. Recently a methodologic analysis of 12 more scientifically valid studies of the effects of vitamin B_6 (usually 30 mg/kg) and magnesium (10 to 15 mg/kg) on behaviors in autistic children was published (Pfeiffer et al, 1995). Behavioral improvements, described as moderate to marked, were reported in 10 of the 12 studies; two reported decreases in autistic behaviors. Although they believed that there were still shortcomings with the research design and interpretation, the authors concluded that the overall results of the studies suggest that treatment with vitamin B_6 and magnesium "may be a promising adjunct" in the treatment of autism, and they recommended that future research explore long-term effectiveness while addressing some of the remaining methodologic weaknesses. The question of dosage is important because the effects are reportedly not seen with doses as low as 3 mg/kg B_6 and 1.4 mg/kg magnesium (Tolbert, 1993). Although there have been no studies of the long-term effects on children, and none of the studies reviewed by Pfeiffer and colleagues (1995) was in that range, chronic use of pyridoxine in high doses (2 to 6 g/day) can cause peripheral neuropathy in adults.

TREATMENT OF ATTENTION-DEFICIT HYPERACTIVITY DISORDER

Although food intolerances and allergies were postulated as having an effect on behavior and learning as long ago as 1922, allergist Benjamin Feingold was the first to implicate diet as the primary cause of hyperactivity, having observed improved behavior in children after they were put on a salicylate-free diet for asthma and chronic urticaria. In 1973, he proposed a diet free of salicylates and artificial flavorings and colorings for the treatment of hyperactivity and reported a 50% improvement rate among his patients. This resulted in great interest among the public, numerous other anecdotal accounts of successful treatment, and a flurry of studies that attempted to replicate his results using controlled and double-blind study designs.

Many years later, the subject remains controversial. Although the findings of some of the studies of the effects of defined diets in the 1970s and early 1980s, which have been recently reviewed (Perry et al, 1996), lend support to his theory, most of those that investigated a single substance or class of substances (e.g., food colorings, food flavors, sugar) failed to demonstrate a decrease in hyperactivity. However, a few more recent, well-designed studies, which have used multiple-elimination diets in addition to food dyes, food flavors, preservatives, monosodium glutamate, and caffeine (or other substances reported by families to affect their particular child), have shown a beneficial response to dietary intervention, particularly among children with allergies.

Although it is clear that a defined diet is not a universal cure for hyperactivity, it appears that for a small subset of children (estimated at about 5%), and perhaps those with allergies, a trial of dietary treatment or continuation of an apparently beneficial diet may be warranted (National Institutes of Health, 1982). As final scientific judgment is awaited, the clinician who may not choose to initiate dietary treatment should respect the experience and desires of families who wish to, working with them to ensure the nutritional adequacy of the diet. There remains a significant number of parents whose beliefs in this treatment are strong and lasting, and these beliefs may, in themselves, lead to a positive placebo effect.

TREATMENT OF MENTAL RETARDATION

Unlike the treatment of hyperactivity and autism, the use of megavitamins to improve cognition and behavior in children with mental retardation, particularly Down syndrome, has never had a solid theoretical foundation. However, when a study published by Harrell and coworkers in 1981 reported dramatic improvement in behavior among a small group of children with mental retardation, increases in IQ scores, and even changes in appearance among those with Down syndrome as a result of treatment with a vitamin and mineral supplement, it spiked great interest among parents of other children with mental retardation and Down syndrome in particular. The Harrell study (Harrell et al, 1981) was plagued with methodologic problems, and subsequent studies, some of which replicated the Harrell design with better methodologies (Pruess, Fewell, and Bennett, 1989), and some of which had better research designs (Kleijnen and Knipschild, 1991), did not find significant effects on cognition or behavior.

Implications for Service Delivery and Policy Development

Evidence is mounting regarding the importance of nutrition to development and behavior in children as methodology becomes more and more sophisticated and knowledge of the underlying biological mechanisms improves. Although further study is needed, it is clear that what used to be considered developmental problems related only to severe malnutrition and extensive environmental deprivation, and therefore of concern mainly in developing countries, are associated with mild undernutrition and even single-nutrient deficiencies as common as IDA, which affects 25% of the poor children in the United States. Also at risk in the United States are children with developmental delays and special health care needs who often have feeding and nutrition problems, many of which begin in infancy when the child is the most vulnerable to lasting nutritional insults. Because the behavioral signs of undernutrition (e.g., emotionality, decreased initiative, responsivity, attention problems) or neurobehavioral markers in infancy (e.g., poor regulation of behaviors, irritability) may closely resemble, or even be causally related to, those of other more commonly recognized risk factors, the clinician who does not consider nutritional etiologies may easily miss a chance to provide the simplest and most basic kind of intervention.

At the same time, many studies have shown the value of early nutrition intervention for children with biological

Table 29–3 • Examples of Inborn Errors of Amino Acid and Carbohydrate Metabolism

Disorder	Incidence	Biochemical Defect	Biochemical Analysis	
			Blood	*Urine*
Amino acids				
Classic phenylketonuria	1 : 10,000	Defective phenylalanine hydroxylase enzyme, which prevents the conversion of phenylalanine, an essential amino acid, to tyrosine, another amino acid	Increased phenylalanine	Increased phenylacids: phenylpyruvic acid, phenylacetic acid, orthohydroxyphenylacetic acid
Classic homocystinuria	1 : 200,000	Defective cystathionine synthase enzyme, which prevents the interaction between an intermediate product of the amino acid methionine with serine to form cystathionine	Increased methionine and homocysteine	Increased homocysteine
Maple syrup urine disease	1 : 200,000	Defective branched chain decarboxylase enzymes Ketoacids of the branch chain amino acids (leucine, valine, and isoleucine) are not converted to fatty acids	Increased leucine, valine, and isoleucine and their ketoacids	Increased leucine, valine, and isoleucine and their ketoacids
Tyrosinemia (Type I)	Not determined	Defect in fumarylacetoacetase enzyme prevents tyrosine metabolites from being converted to fumaric acid	Increased tyrosine and in some cases increased methionine	Succinylacetone present Increased parahydroxy-phenylpyruvic acid; generalized aminoaciduria
Carbohydrates				
Classic galactosemia	1 : 60,000	Defective galactose-1-phosphate uridyl transferase enzyme; galactose, a monosaccharide, is not converted to glucose	Increased galactose and galactose-1-phosphate	Increased galactose; generalized aminoaciduria
Hereditary fructose intolerance	1 : 15,000 to <1 : 100,000	Defect in fructose-1-phosphate aldolase B enzyme; fructose, a monosaccharide, is not converted to glucose	Increased fructose	Increased fructose

Adapted from Howard RB, Herbold NH (eds): Nutrition in Clinical Care. New York, McGraw-Hill, 1982.

Clinical Symptoms	Treatment	Comment
Infant appears normal at birth, followed by hyperactivity, irritability, persistent musty odor, severe mental retardation, decreased pigmentation, and eczema, if untreated	Phenylalanine-restricted diet: no high-quality protein foods (milk, milk products, meat, fish, poultry, eggs, nuts) Controlled amounts of fruits, vegetables, and grain products Special formula, low in phenylalanine, provides protein and is supplemented with vitamins and minerals Treatment monitored with blood phenylalanine levels, growth, and psychological data	Phenylalanine must be provided in amounts sufficient to support growth There are milder forms, which may not require a diet, and there are variant forms that do not respond to treatment
Possible mental retardation; lens dislocation; limb overgrowth; connective tissue defect leading to scoliosis, osteoporosis, vascular thrombosis; fair hair and skin	Methionine-restricted (similar to phenylalanine-restricted) diet, supplemented with cysteine Cysteine, a product of methionine, becomes an essential amino acid when methionine is limited Special low-methionine formula is used, and methionine levels in the blood are monitored, along with growth and psychological functioning	There are other forms of homocystinuria. One is responsive to high doses of pyridoxine (vitamin B_6), a coenzyme of cystathionine synthetase; another is responsive to vitamin B_{12}, a coenzyme in the remethylation reaction of homocysteine to methionine
Infant appears normal at birth, with symptoms showing in the first few days; difficulties with sucking and swallowing, irregular respiration, intermittent rigidity and flaccidity, possible grand mal seizures; urine has the odor of maple syrup; if infant survives, mental retardation is severe if untreated	Diet is restricted in leucine, valine, and isoleucine (similar to phenylalanine-restricted diet) Special formula is used Blood leucine, valine, and isoleucine are monitored, along with growth and psychological functioning	There is a transient form of the disease for which treatment is necessary only during times of illness
Enlargement of liver and spleen noted early in infancy; abdominal distention, liver and renal damage, vitamin D–resistant rickets, possible hypoglycemia; hepatic carcinoma often seen as liver disease progresses	Diet restricted in phenylalanine and tyrosine; the essential amino acid phenylalanine is a precursor of tyrosine Methionine is restricted if blood levels are elevated A special formula is used, and blood levels of phenylalanine, tyrosine, and methionine and growth are monitored Drug NTBC 2-(Nitro-4-trifluoromethylbenzoyl)-1,3-Cyclohexanedione) used to slow the progression of the disease	Dietary treatment can slow the progression of liver disease but does not prevent it; liver transplantation has been successful in a number of children
Infant appears normal at birth with symptoms developing after feedings containing lactose Symptoms include anorexia, vomiting, occasional diarrhea, lethargy, jaundice, hepatomegaly, increased susceptibility to infection; later, cataracts and physical and mental retardation develop	Exclusion of lactose and galactose from the diet; hydrolysis of lactose yields glucose and galactose Diet is milk-free, free of milk products; lactose-free formula is used; if children to not accept formula, diet will need nutrient supplementation Some fruits and vegetables contain free galactose. The clinical implications of galactose-1-phosphate levels are unknown and the need for restriction controversial.	Nonclassic forms include galactokinase and epimerase deficiency; the clinical features are not the same in all three forms Neurological damage and ovarian failure can occur despite dietary treatment
For infants, symptoms include anorexia, vomiting, failure to thrive, hypoglycemic convulsions, dysfunction of the liver and kidney For older children, spontaneous hypoglycemia and vomiting occur after the ingestion of fructose	Elimination of fructose and sucrose from the diet Hydrolysis of sucrose yields glucose and fructose	Differentiate from transient neonatal tyrosinemia

and environmental risk factors that suggest compromised nutritional status such as low birth weight, SGA, substance exposure, and the risks of poverty, especially when nutrition intervention is combined with other forms of environmental stimulation. The finding that ensuring adequate nutrient intake among young disadvantaged children can erase differences in later test scores has enormous public health and policy significance (Pollitt et al, 1995). Of particular note are the apparent developmental advantages (in addition to the already well-recognized health advantages) conferred by breast milk.

Indeed, clinicians in the United States concerned with promoting optimal development in children need to be aware, even vigilant, regarding the possibility of mild to moderate undernutrition, because developmental and behavioral effects can be manifested well before any classic clinical signs of malnutrition such as growth faltering. Care providers should routinely and carefully screen at-risk infants and children for inadequate dietary intake, and they should assess nutritional status, when appropriate, with consistent use of standard and objective measures. All persons who provide pediatric care should also be knowledgeable regarding community resources for nutrition services, including interdisciplinary teams to address feeding problems, and food distribution programs, both public and private (Baer, in press). Nutritional rehabilitation should also be coupled with other social and emotional supports to the family. Finally, there is a need to take an aggressive approach to the primary prevention of growth failure with its attendant risk for suboptimal development, because it is not clear that the deficits can be completely reversed once the undernutrition has occurred.

REFERENCES

Ainsworth M, Bell S, Stayton D: Individual differences in strange-situation behavior of one-year-olds. *In* Schaffer HR (ed): The Origins of Human Social Relations. New York, Academic Press, 1971, p. 17.

Aylward GP: Environmental influences on the developmental outcome of children at risk. Infants and Young Children 2:1, 1990.

Badart-Smook A, van Houwelingen AC, Al MDM, Kester ADM, et al: Fetal growth is associated positively with maternal intake of riboflavin and negatively with maternal intake of linoleic acid. J Am Diet Assoc 97:867, 1997.

Baer MT: Community food and nutrition programs. *In* Kessler DB, Dawson P (eds): Failure to Thrive in Infants and Children: A Transdisciplinary Approach to Nutritional Adequacy in Childhood. Baltimore, Paul H. Brookes, in press.

Baer MT, Farnan S, Mauer AM: Children with special health care needs. *In* Sharbaugh CS (ed): Call to Action: Better Nutrition for Mothers, Children, and Families. Washington, DC, National Center for Education in Maternal and Child Health, 1990.

Baer MT, Harris AB, Bujold CR, et al: Unpublished data, 1997.

Baer MT, Harris AB: Pediatric nutrition assessment: identifying children at risk. J Am Diet Assoc 97:S107, 1997.

Baer MT, Kozlowski BW, Blyler EM, et al: Vitamin D, calcium, and bone status in children with developmental delay in relation to anticonvulsant use and ambulatory status. Am J Clin Nutr 65:1042, 1997.

Ballard TJ, Neumann CG. The effects of malnutrition, parental literacy and household crowding on acute lower respiratory infections in young Kenyan children. J Tropical Pediatr 41:8, 1995.

Barrett D, Radke Yarrow M: Effects of nutritional supplementation on children's responses to novel, frustration and competitive situations. Am J Clin Nutr 42:102, 1985.

Bowe FG: Population estimates: birth-to-5 children with disabilities. J Special Education 20:461, 1995.

Brazelton TB, Tronick T, Lechtig A, et al: The behavior of nutritionally deprived Guatemalan infants. Dev Med Child Neurol 19:364, 1977.

Chandra RK: Nutrition and the immune system: an introduction. Am J Clin Nutr 66:460S, 1997.

Community Nutrition Institute: Nearly fifth of Mississippi homes are food insecure. Nutrition Week 27(43):2, 1997.

de Andraca I, Castillo M, Walter T: Psychomotor development and behavior in iron-deficient anemic infants. Nutr Rev 55:125, 1997.

Doyle W, Crawford MA, Wynn AHA, et al: Maternal nutrient intake and birth weight. J Hum Nutr Diet 2:415, 1989.

Galler JR (ed): Human Nutrition: A Comprehensive Treatise. Nutrition and Behavior, Vol 5. New York, Plenum Press, 1984.

Golub MS, Keen CL, Gershwin ME, et al: Developmental zinc deficiency and behavior. J Nutr 125:2263s, 1995.

Grantham-McGregor S, Schofield W, Powell C: Development of severely malnourished children who received psychosocial stimulation: six year follow-up. Pediatrics 79:247, 1987.

Hack M, Klein NK, Taylor HG: Long-term developmental outcomes of low birth weight infants. *In* Shiono PH, Behrman RE (eds): The Future of Children: Low Birth Weight. Los Altos, CA, Center for the Future of Children, The David and Lucille Packard Foundation, 1995.

Harrell R, Capp R, Davis D, et al: Can nutritional supplements help mentally retarded children? An exploratory study. Proc Nat Acad Sci U S A 78:574, 1981.

Harris P, Clark M, Karp RJ: Prevention and treatment of lead poisoning. *In* Karp RJ (ed): Malnourished Children in the United States: Caught in the Cycle of Poverty. New York, Springer Publishing, 1993.

Holmgren G, Blomquist HK, Samuelson G: Positive effect of a late introduced modified diet in an 8 year old PKU child. Neuropaediatrie 10:10, 1979.

Horowitz FD: Using developmental theory to guide the search for the effects of biological risk factors on the development of children. Am J Clin Nutr 50:589, 1989.

Idjradinata P, Pollitt E: Reversal of developmental delays in iron-deficient anemic infants treated with iron. Lancet 341:1, 1993.

Institute of Medicine Subcommittees on Nutritional Status and Weight Gain During Pregnancy and Dietary Intake and Nutrient Supplements During Pregnancy, Food and Nutrition Board. Nutrition During Pregnancy: Weight Gain; Nutrient Supplements. Washington, DC: National Academy Press, 1990.

Johnston FE, Markowitz D: Do poverty and malnutrition affect children's growth and development: are the data there? *In* Karp RJ (ed): Malnourished Children in the United States: Caught in the Cycle of Poverty. New York, Springer Publishing, 1993.

King PB, Lie RT, Irgens LM. Spina bifida and cleft lip among newborns of Norwegian women with epilepsy; changes related to the use of anticonvulsants. Am J Public Health 86:1454, 1996.

Kirksey A, Rehmanifar A, Wachs TD, et al: Determinants of pregnancy outcome and newborn behavior of a semirural Egyptian population. Am J Clin Nutr 54:657, 1991.

Kleijnen J, Knipschild P: Niacin and vitamin B6 in mental functioning: a review of controlled trails in humans. Biol Psychiatry 29:931, 1991.

Klein P, Forbes G, Nader P: Effects of starvation in infancy (pyloric stenosis) on subsequent learning abilities. J Pediatr 87:8, 1975.

Kramer RA, Allen L, Gergen PJ: Health and social characteristics and children's cognitive functioning: results from a national cohort. Am J Public Health 85:312, 1995.

Lanting CI, Fidler V, Huisman M, et al: Neurological differences between 9-year-old children fed breast-milk or formula-milk as babies. Lancet 344:1319, 1994.

Levitsky DA, Strupp BJ: Malnutrition and the brain: changing concepts, changing concerns. J Nutr 125:2212S, 1995.

Lloyd-Still J, Hurwitz I, Wolff P, et al: Intellectual development after severe malnutrition in infancy. Pediatrics 54:306, 1974.

Lozoff B: Nutrition and behavior. Am Psychologist 4:231, 1989.

Lozoff B, Abraham WW, Jimenez E: Iron-deficiency anemia and infant development: effects of extended oral iron therapy. J Pediatr 129:382, 1996.

Lucas A, Morley R, Cole TJ, et al: Breast milk and subsequent intelligence quotient in children born preterm. Lancet 339:261, 1992.

Lucas A, Morley R, Cole TJ, et al: Early diet in preterm babies and developmental status at 18 months. Lancet 335:1477, 1990.

McCullough AL, Kirksey A, Wachs TD, et al: Vitamin B6 status of Egyptian mothers: relation to infant behavior and maternal-infant interactions. Am J Clin Nutr 51:1067, 1990.

Moffatt MEK, Longstaffe S, Besant J, et al: Prevention of iron deficiency and psychomotor decline in high-risk infants through use of iron-fortified infant formula: a randomized clinical trial. J Pediatr 125:527, 1994.

Molloy AM, Daly S, Mills JL, et al: Thermolabile variant of 5,10-methylenetetrahydrofolate reductase associated with low red-cell folates: implications for folate intake recommendations. Lancet 349:1591, 1997.

National Institutes of Health: Defined diets and childhood hyperactivity. Washington, DC, NIH Consensus Development Conference Statement, January 13–15, 1982.

Needleman HL, Schell A, Bellinger D, et al: Long-term effects of childhood exposure to lead at low dose: an eleven year follow-up report. N Engl J Med 321:83, 1990.

Neisworth JT, Bagnato SJ, Salvia J: Neurobehavioral markers for early regulatory disorders. Infants and Young Children 8:8, 1995.

Neumann C, McDonald MA, Sigman M, et al: Medical illness in school-age Kenyans in relation to nutrition, cognition, and playground behaviors. J Dev Behav Pediatr 13:392, 1992.

Nickel RE: Controversial therapies for young children with developmental disabilities. Infants and Young Children 8:29, 1996.

Perry CA, Dwyer J, Gelfand JA, et al: Health effects of salicylates in foods and drugs. Nutr Rev 54:225, 1996.

Pfeiffer SI, Norton J, Nelson L, et al: Efficacy of vitamin B6 and magnesium in the treatment of autism: a methodology review and summary of outcomes. J Autism Dev Disord 25:481, 1995.

Pollitt E: Iron deficiency and educational deficiency. Nutr Rev 55:133, 1997.

Pollitt E: Does breakfast make a difference in school? J Am Diet Assoc 95:1134, 1995.

Pollitt E: A developmental view of cognition in the undernourished child. Annual Report/Nestle Foundation for the Study of the Problem of Nutrition in the World, Lausanne, Switzerland, 1994 pp. 88–105.

Pollitt E, Gorman KS, Engle PL, et al: The INCAP Follow-up Study: nutrition in early life and the fulfillment of intellectual potential. J Nutr 125:1111S, 1995.

Poulsen MK: Building resilience in infants and toddlers at risk. In Smith GH, Coles CD, Poulsen MK (eds): Children, Families and Substance Abuse: Challenges for Changing Educational and Social Outcomes. Baltimore: Paul H. Brookes, 1995, p. 95.

Poulsen MK: Strategies for building resilience in infants and young children at risk. Infants and Young Children 6:29, 1993.

Pruess JB, Fewell RR, Bennett FC: Vitamin therapy and children with Down syndrome: a review of research. Except Child 55:336, 1989.

Rogan WJ, Gladen BC: Breast-feeding and cognitive development. Early Hum Dev 31:181, 1993.

Roncagliolo M, Garrido M, Williamson A, et al: Delayed maturation of auditory brainstem responses in iron-deficient anemic infants. Pediatr Res 39:20A, 1996.

Rutter M: Protective factors in children's responses to stress and disadvantage. In Kent MW, Rolf JE (eds): Primary Prevention of Psychopathology: Social Competence in Children, Vol 3. Hanover, NH, University Press in New England, 1979, p. 49.

Scrimshaw NS, SanGiovanni JP: Synergism of nutrition, infection, and immunity: an overview. Am J Clin Nutr 66:464S, 1997.

Sechrist-Mertz C, Brotherson MJ, Oakland MJ, et al: Helping families meet the nutritional needs of children with disabilities: an integrated model. Children's Health Care 26:151, 1997.

Shaw GM, Lammer EJ, Wasserman CR, et al: Risks of orofacial clefts in children born to women using multivitamins containing folic acid periconceptionally. Lancet 346:393, 1995.

Solomons NW, Mazariegos M, Brown KH, et al: The underprivileged, developing country child: environmental contamination and growth failure revisited. Nutr Rev 51:327, 1993.

Strupp BJ, Levitsky DA: Enduring cognitive effects of early malnutrition: a theoretical reappraisal. J Nutr 125:2221S, 1995.

Susser M, Stein Z: Timing in prenatal nutrition: a reprise of the Dutch Famine Study. Nutr Rev 52:84, 1994.

Symons CW, Cinelli B, James TC, et al: Bridging student health risks and academic achievement through comprehensive school health programs. J School Health 67:220, 1997.

Tolbert L, Haigler T, Waits MM, et al: Brief report: lack of response in an autistic population to a low dose clinical trial of pyridoxine plus magnesium. J Autism Dev Disord 23:193, 1993.

Uauy R, de Andraca I: Human milk and breast feeding for optimal mental development. J Nutr 125:2278S, 1995.

Vohr BR: Preterm cognitive development: biologic and environmental influences. Infants and Young Children 3:20, 1991.

Walker SP, Powell CA, Grantham-McGregor SM, et al: Nutritional supplementation, psychosocial stimulation, and growth of stunted children: the Jamaican study. Am J Clin Nutr 54:642, 1991.

Walsh CT, Sandstead HH, Prasad AS, et al: Zinc; health effects and research priorities for the 1990s. Environ Health Perspect 102:5, 1994.

Walter T: Review: impact of iron deficiency on cognition in infancy and childhood. Eur J Clin Nutr 47:307, 1993.

Walter T, de Andraca I, Chadud P, et al: Iron deficiency anemia: adverse effects on infant psychomotor development. Pediatrics 84:7, 1989.

Williams RC, Carta JJ: Behavioral outcomes of young children with prenatal exposure to alcohol: review and analysis of experimental literature. Infants and Young Children 8:16, 1997.

Wilson DM, Hammer LD, Duncan PM, et al: Growth and intellectual development. Pediatrics 78:646, 1986.

Winick M, Meyer KK, Harris R: Malnutrition and environmental enrichment by early adoption. Science 19:1173, 1990.

Yogman MW, Zeisel SH: Diet and sleep patterns in newborn infants. N Engl J Med 309:1147, 1983.

Zuckerman B, Beardslee W: Maternal depression: a concern for pediatricians. Pediatrics 79:110, 1987.

Appendix 29–1

Components of a Feeding Evaluation*

Family Story

Child's early feeding experience:

- Feeding abilities
- Medical problems
- History of invasive procedures

Feeding methods used by family:

- Successful
- Unsuccessful

Family goals for feeding

Feeding Environment

- Who feeds the child
- Time of meals
- Seating
- Utensils
- Food preferences (taste, texture, temperature)
- Foods refused

Psychosocial Issues

- Conditioned aversion
- Child's temperament

*From the University of Southern California University Affiliated Program Feeding Development Clinic, Childrens Hospital, Los Angeles, CA.

- Parent-child attachment (eye contact, affection, reciprocity)
- Parent's strengths (flexible schedule, support system, positive attitude, avoidance of overstimulation, firm yet supportive stance, praise and encouragement, follow through with consequences)

Communication

Child

- Communication of pleasure
- Communication of displeasure
- Use of gestures
- Use of verbal language
- Communication of hunger
- Communication of refusal

Parent

- Use of verbal language
- Use of nonverbal communication
- Recognition of child's cues

Parent-Child Dyad

- Mutual understanding of communication
- Match in pace of communication

Position During Feeding

- Head
- Trunk
- Upper extremities
- Lower extremities

Oral-Motor

- Facial muscle tone
- Lip position at rest and during feeding
- Tongue movements
- Jaw movements during chewing
- Jaw stability during biting

Oral Structures

- Palate shape
- Tongue (size in relation to oral cavity, position in the oral cavity)
- Number, position, and condition of teeth
- Gums
- Bite
- Jaw

SENSORY RESPONSIVENESS

	Functional Status	Hyper-sensitivity	Hypo-sensitivity	Comments
Vision				
Hearing				
Touch				
Taste				
Temperature				

Oral Reflexes and Responses to Feeding

- Cough
- Gag

- Bite
- Swallow
- Breathing sounds before, during, and after feeding
- Coordination of breathing and swallowing
- Drooling
- Tongue movements
- Vomiting

FEEDING DEVELOPMENT

	Oral-Motor Pattern	Efficiency
Management of liquids Breast		
Bottle		
Cup		
Straw		
Management of solids Purees		
Lumpy purees		
Chopped table foods		
All table foods		
Prehension Prehension pattern		
Self-feeds by bottle or cup		
Utensils		

Nutrition Intake

- Diet analysis of average 24-hour intake (from dietary recall or 3-day food record)
- Variety of foods, adequate in all food groups
- Nutrient adequacy, energy intake, sources of fiber
- Spacing of meals, snacks
- Developmentally appropriate textures
- Fluid intake
- Contribution of oral versus tube feedings, if applicable

Anthropometric Data

- Weight, height, head circumference
- Arm circumference, triceps and subscapular skinfolds, arm muscle area
- Growth rate (need previous measurements)
- Appropriate reference data (e.g., National Center for Health Statistics [NCHS])
- Energy reserves

Clinical Data

- History of infections, illnesses (recurrent pneumonia)
- Skin integrity
- Previous gastrointestinal workups, findings
- History of reflux, vomiting
- Gastrostomy tube site, if present

Bowel Habits

- Regular
- Constipation
- Diarrhea

Laboratory Findings

- Hemoglobin/hematocrit levels
- Lead levels, if available
- Metabolic indicators, if applicable

Medications

- Types
- Dosage
- Duration
- Time given, with or apart from meals
- Drug/nutrient interactions
- Side effects such as nausea, anorexia, constipation

CASE STUDY

Examination

Tony was born at 35 weeks' gestation with a birth weight of 5 pounds 4 ounces. He was born after premature labor. There were no complications during birth. Tony had a ventricular septal defect (VSD) and pulmonic stenosis. His mother reported that he was having a difficult time feeding by 2 months of age. He was breast-fed for the first 2 months, but it became increasingly difficult for Tony to suck and he became diaphoretic and tachypneic. There was no cyanosis. Tony was hospitalized at 4 months of age for cardiac surgery (after which most babies begin to eat better and have an improved rate of weight gain).

After the surgery, Tony's mother reported that he was not gaining weight, but her pediatrician thought that Tony's failure to gain weight was due to prematurity and there was no intervention. Tony had few periods of the calm, focused alertness that allowed him to engage with his mother. He was lethargic and evidenced developmental delays in all areas.

Finally at age 8 months, at which time Tony had not gained any weight since his surgery, his mother consulted with another pediatrician who referred Tony for admission to the hospital for severe failure to thrive. He was described as marasmic. On admission, his length was 22 inches, weight 7 pounds 10 ounces, and head circumference 41 cm. All were below the 5th percentile for age, even correcting for prematurity. Tony appeared cachectic, in no acute distress, and lying in a fetal position. He had little or no muscular bulk but adequate tone.

Although nurses attempted bottle feeding, it took 30 to 40 minutes to feed 40 mL (a little over 1 ounce). A barium swallow evaluation revealed no swallowing abnormality. An upper gastrointestinal study showed gastroesophageal reflux to the thoracic inlet. Bolus feedings by nasogastric (NG) tube were started. He was first fed by bottle and what was not taken at a feeding was given by tube. He was also started on 30 kcal cardiac formula of Similac with iron, thickened with rice cereal. By day 3, he was calmly alert and somewhat playful. Tony was discharged on day 7 after gaining a total of 240 g (1/2 pound). Feedings were still supplemented by NG tube; mother was trained to insert the tube and check its position in his stomach.

Tony was referred to the University of Southern California University Affiliated Program Feeding Development Clinic for feeding and nutrition follow-up and for developmental and behavioral assistance. At that time he was 9 months old and weighed 8 pounds 3 ounces.

Developmental milestones were delayed: Mental Developmental Index was 82 and Psychomotor Index was 74. Tony had a difficult time, being overly sensitive to being touched and handled. He had short restless periods of sleep and cried excessively. An occupational therapist, nutritionist, and psychologist worked with Tony's mother. The team, with Tony's mother, developed the following plan based on observations of Tony with his mother and mother's report of his special needs.

Mother was advised to give him as much oral feeding as he would take, the rest to be given by NG tube. The bottle would be offered at 3 feedings per day. Tony would have 4 to 5 feedings per day, gradually increasing from 100 to 115 mL per feeding, for a total of 690 kcal per day (about 185 kcal/kg). There was to be weekly monitoring of weight gain and adjustment of intake to promote catch-up growth and establish a normal rate of growth.

Tony's mother would respond to Tony as soon as he began to whimper because he had difficulty calming himself once he started to cry. Tony would be protected from too much noise and sudden bright light. He would be calmed through vertical rocking and ventral pressure. Tony's mother would approach him slowly and speak to him in a soft voice before lifting him so as not to startle him. Mother would respond to all social initiations made by Tony: eye contact, vocalizations, and reaching. Tony would be rocked on a daily basis to provide for vestibular stimulation.

Follow-Up

At 12 months, Tony weighed 14 pounds and measured 24½ inches. Although still small for his age, his weight for height was at the 50th percentile and his head circumference was 45.5 cm, between the 10th and 25th percentiles, showing catch-up growth in all areas.

Developmental milestones were within normal limits with a Mental Developmental Index of 89 and a Psychomotor Index of 85. Even though he was still a sensitive infant, he was able to calm himself and sleep through the night with only one awakening. His neurobehavioral functioning was becoming more robust. He was learning to tolerate transitions and normal household commotion and caregiving. Tony was able to adapt to the give and take of his daily living activities and engaged with his mother with eagerness. Feedings had improved and the NG tube was being used less often.

Long-Term Outcome

Tony continued to show signs of catch-up growth and development. He responded well to early intervention although initially he had delayed milestones in the areas of walking and speech. Tony was placed in a special education program between the ages of 3 and 5, and was fully integrated into a regular first grade by age 6 years, at which time he had achieved low-normal developmental functioning. Compared to his siblings who did not sustain a nutritional insult, Tony's growth and development have been slower. Tony is still small for his age (short stature), although his weight for height and head circumference are at the 50th percentile.

Conclusions/Implications

This child received a severe nutrition insult during the first few months of life, which has permanently affected his overall growth and development. Intensive ongoing interdisciplinary intervention was instrumental in promoting eventual achievement of normal developmental and nutritional status. Although the situation became multifactoral, the insult after the cardiac repair appears to have been primarily nutritional; no other diagnoses have been identified. In other situations, the insult might be less severe and the results less easily detected, especially when the nutritional deprivation occurs in conjunction with other risks for developmental delay. In this case, as in many others, the insult might have been prevented if the nutrition problems had been recognized and treated before they became severe.

30 Toxins

Fred Henretig

 Theories and practical advice on child development rightly point to the importance of the environment, but usually to only the psychosocial part. Not to be forgotten are the various elements of the physical or nonhuman surroundings: natural conditions and disasters, housing, diet, medicines, and physical dangers such as toxins in the air, water, food, and elsewhere. This chapter reviews the hazards for development and behavior of prenatal toxins such as alcohol; breast milk contaminants such as cocaine; postnatal exposures, especially lead and carbon monoxide; and possible unintended effects from standard therapeutic agents such as phenobarbital.

This chapter reviews toxic influences on the central nervous system (CNS) with special reference to those substances that are significant causes of functional brain damage in children. Innumerable neurologic toxins have been described in the toxicology and occupational medicine literature; the focus here is on postnatal exposure to those drugs or toxins with specific pathologic or epidemiologic predilection for cognitive or behavioral effects in young children. Prenatal and perinatal drug or toxin exposures that impact on postnatal cognition and behavior are also addressed briefly. See Chapter 25 for a more focused discussion of teratogenic effects on the CNS, Chapter 29 for a review of dietary and nutritional aspects, and Chapter 50, which focuses on adolescent substance abuse, for further discussions of these additional aspects of neurotoxicity.

General Principles of Neurologic Toxicity

The interaction between various exogenous toxins and the CNS is predictably complex. The CNS tends to be protected from some toxic influences by the blood-brain barrier (Norton, 1985). This barrier is defined conceptually based on observations that many toxins that easily enter cells in other soft tissues, such as muscle or viscera, do not enter the brain. Highly polar compounds tend to be excluded, whereas lipid-soluble, nonpolar compounds tend to cross the barrier easily. The integrity of the barrier varies with age, and the immature brain allows many more substances through. Thus inorganic lead poisoning can cause severe encephalopathy in young children but primarily a peripheral neuropathy in adults. The anatomic substrate of the blood-brain barrier is not yet fully understood, but three major concepts include (1) the function of glial cells wrapped around capillary endothelium, (2) unique properties of the capillary endothelium of the brain, particularly the finding of zonulae occludentes, or structures joining the endothelial cells together into tight junctions, and (3) the extracellular basement membrane between endothelial cells and glia and neurons.

Not all areas of the brain are equally affected by a given toxin, even when it does cross the blood-brain barrier. Variation can result from different vascular patterns and unique sensitivities of different cell types caused by differing neurochemistry. Thus a considerable degree of selectivity occurs in the neuropathologic effects of any given potential neurotoxin.

An additional consideration is the rapid postnatal developmental changes in brain structure, which may be adversely influenced by toxins. At birth, all large neuronal cell bodies are in place in the cerebral cortex and basal ganglia. However, synaptic connections are relatively sparse. Over the first 2 years of life, there is tremendous growth of these connections, such that by age 2 years, synaptic density is almost twice that of adulthood. Over the next few preschool-age years, these synapses are "pruned" selectively, presumably on the basis of sensory and motor stimulation. This process may be altered in the presence of even subtle toxic influences that affect neurotransmitter function, as well as more overt neuronal damage from global insults such as hypoxia or hypoglycemia. Alteration of dendritic architecture may result in difficulties with fine neurocognitive function such as memory, attention, and problem-solving skills. Such a paradigm has been invoked, with experimental evidence in animal models, for the effects of low-level lead toxicity on intellectual function (Goldstein, 1992).

SPECIFIC HAZARDS IN THE PRENATAL AND PERINATAL PERIODS

Many drugs and toxins (e.g., alcohol) exert overt adverse effects on the developing structure and function of the CNS with high-dose exposure in utero. These syndromes (e.g., fetal alcohol syndrome) are described in detail in Chapter 25. Many such agents at lower doses may cause milder effects on postnatal cognitive function without overt structural abnormality (e.g., fetal alcohol effects), and comparable subtle effects may result from maternal exposure to several other substances. Additional perinatal concerns related to drug toxicity include the effects of maternal medications used during parturition and lactation and of those given directly to the newborn (Kulberg and Weisman,

1986). Another important mechanism by which prenatal toxicity can have an impact on postnatal behavior is passive addiction of the fetus to drugs used by the mother.

Prenatal Substance Use and Impact on Postnatal Cognition and Behavior

PRENATAL EXPOSURES

The impact of a given prenatal drug or toxin exposure on the subsequent behavior and development of the exposed child during infancy and childhood is a complex process that involves considerable overlap of prenatal and postnatal influences (Abel and Hannigan, 1995). Many mothers who are chemically dependent, for example, are also of low socioeconomic status, are malnourished, use multiple agents including alcohol and cigarettes, have underlying medical problems (some of which may be secondary to their substance abuse), and may suffer significant emotional disorders and social problems. All these factors may independently impact both prenatal CNS microstructure and function, as well as on the subsequent postnatal maternal-child interaction, and therefore complicate the interpretation of the specific effect of the individual substance, if any, on postnatal behavior and cognition. It is difficult to control for all such factors in clinical studies; in addition, these studies tend to rely on interviewer or questionnaire ascertainment of exposure, which may not be accurate. Animal studies are less useful for observing subtle alterations in behavior and development; even these, as well as in vitro studies, are subject to confounding factors secondary to the occurrence of undernutrition or absence of specific nutritional factors such as vitamins that might attenuate the effect of alcohol in vivo.

The substances most studied in this context include alcohol, cigarettes, cocaine, marijuana, and opiates (Coles and Platzman, 1993). Behavioral effects are described in the neonatal period, infancy, and preschool and school-age years. In general, acute drug effects are often noticeable in the neonatal period and may last several weeks. Aside from neonatal withdrawal syndrome, these are rarely of critical clinical significance. Infants may demonstrate developmental deficits, particularly in motor skills, which become more apparent as they grow older. Information is scarce for older children, and the potential for confounding postnatal influences is almost unavoidable, but evidence suggests that heavy exposures, especially to alcohol, result in specific cognitive deficits and attention disorders (see Chapter 2).

Alcohol

In the absence of frank growth retardation or congenital anomalies (e.g., fetal alcohol syndrome), several studies have found children born to women who drink heavily during pregnancy at increased risk for developmental deficits (American Academy of Pediatrics, 1993b). These have included attention-deficit hyperactivity disorder, fine motor impairment, clumsiness, and subtle speech disorders. This constellation of features is referred to as *fetal alcohol*

effects. It has been difficult to define a precise threshold for toxicity because of the many factors already mentioned. In addition, alcohol consumption has often been characterized as average number of drinks per day, without distinguishing binge drinking (which is more likely to result in higher blood alcohol levels) from daily "social drinking" (e.g., a glass of wine with dinner, which is less likely to result in toxic blood levels). Some authors have cautioned that current dogma proscribing any ingestion of alcohol during pregnancy may be counterproductive, raising unnecessary guilt in otherwise healthy mothers who drink sparingly and failing to focus on the real problem of chronic alcoholism with its attendant comorbidity on the fetus produced by malnutrition, smoking, medical illness, and so on (Alpert and Zuckerman, 1991). Nevertheless, the American Academy of Pediatrics (1993b) recommends that pregnant women and those planning a pregnancy should abstain from alcohol entirely.

Cigarettes

Cigarette smoke contains the toxins nicotine and carbon monoxide, as well as numerous other potentially toxic compounds (e.g., aromatic hydrocarbons). Prenatal exposure to cigarette smoking is believed to result in decreased birth weight, probably because of the vasoconstrictive effect of nicotine on uterine blood flow, and the effect of carbon monoxide on decreasing fetal hemoglobin oxygen-carrying capacity (Byrd and Howard, 1995). Other effects may result from additional toxins, decreased maternal caloric intake, or both. Postnatal effects on behavior and development ascribed to prenatal cigarette exposure include cognitive deficits, decreased attention span, hyperactivity, and increased aggression.

Cocaine

Maternal cocaine use is highly related to numerous catastrophic complications of gestation and the perinatal period (Volpe, 1992). Major CNS anomalies, intracranial hemorrhages, abruptio placentae, and decreased birth weight and head circumference are seen, presumably secondary to the peripheral vasoconstrictive and central monoaminergic effects of this potent drug. Less drastic postnatal effects have also been observed in infants with prenatal exposure. In the neonatal period, some such infants manifest increased tremulousness, poor feeding, irritability, abnormal sleep pattern, and, occasionally, seizures. Older cocaine-exposed infants do not exhibit persistent cognitive deficits using standard tests (e.g., Bayley Scales of Infant Development) in comparison to appropriate control infants.

Marijuana

In general, light to moderate use of marijuana during pregnancy has not been clearly associated with subsequent cognitive deficits. One recent study found an exposure of one or more "joints" per day, but not lesser use, during the third trimester of pregnancy to be associated with a 10-point deficit on Bayley Scales of Infant Development at age 9 months. This effect was no longer apparent at age 19 months (Richardson, Day, and Goldschmidt, 1995).

Opiates

The most profound effect of prenatal opiate exposure is the neonatal withdrawal syndrome (see Neonatal Withdrawal Syndrome). Long-term studies of cognitive function in older children born to heroin-addicted or methadone-maintained mothers are inconsistent in their findings. Perhaps not surprisingly, studies of heroin-exposed children tend to show cognitive deficits, whereas those of children born to mothers provided comprehensive prenatal care in a methadone maintenance clinic do not (Coles and Platzman, 1993).

OBSTETRIC ANESTHESIA

A popular drug for maternal analgesia during labor has been meperidine. However, the slow placental transfer and subsequent metabolism of this compound by the fetus allows considerable accumulation. Thus infants born between 1 and 4 hours after meperidine administration to the mother are likely to experience significant CNS depression. This eventuality can be managed with supportive care and naloxone, 0.01 mg/kg intramuscularly or intravenously.

Both systemic analgesics and regional anesthetic agents have also been shown to have less dramatic but significant effects on newborn behavior. Decreased motor maturity and increased irritability have been noted at 3 days of age after regional anesthesia alone. Systemic agents have been found to affect some variables such as habituation and orientation on the Brazelton Neonatal Behavioral Assessment Scale throughout the 1st month of life. These effects may represent increased pharmacologic action resulting from immaturity of the neonatal blood-brain barrier or metabolic pathways, or both, or they may represent a contribution from interference with normal maternal-infant bonding caused by the combined effects on mother and baby (Lester, Als, and Brazelton, 1982).

OTHER RISKS FOR TOXICITY

A significant iatrogenic source of toxicity in the newborn nursery involves the use of benzyl alcohol as a bacteriostatic agent in frequently used saline "flushes" for intravenous catheters (Gershanik, 1982). Newborns receiving toxic doses after numerous, repetitive flushes experience a syndrome of gasping respirations, CNS depression, metabolic acidosis, hypotension, and renal failure that was occasionally fatal. The affected babies had high blood levels of benzyl alcohol and benzoic acid, presumably reflecting hepatic immaturity in the metabolism of benzoic acid. Thus, seemingly innocuous agents can surface as potential toxins in the context of the metabolically immature neonate.

NEONATAL WITHDRAWAL SYNDROME

A large number of drugs used habitually by pregnant women, including, most notably, opiates, as well as alcohol, barbiturates, benzodiazepines, and several other miscellaneous sedative-hypnotic agents, can cause the neonatal withdrawal syndrome (Volpe, 1987). Many women who are addicted to opiates are polydrug abusers, which complicates the diagnosis and therapy of the clinical withdrawal state in their newborns.

Opiates

Classic features of neonatal opioid withdrawal include wakefulness, jitteriness, irritability that is inconsolable, tremor, hypertonicity and hyperreflexia, vomiting, diarrhea, poor feeding, and failure to thrive. Severe cases can be rarely accompanied by seizures. Most infants of heroin-addicted women display symptoms early, 65% in the first 24 hours of life. Babies born to mothers taking methadone manifest withdrawal slightly later, usually on the 2nd or 3rd day of life, and the duration of their symptoms tends to last longer. Although methadone withdrawal is generally less severe, these infants are more likely to exhibit disturbed feeding patterns and failure to gain weight. Both heroin- and methadone-addicted infants show lower than average gains in development on follow-up testing, although the consensus among researchers is that these differences are probably related more to co-variables, such as poverty and malnutrition, than to drug effects per se. Management of acute neonatal opioid withdrawal, as detailed by Volpe (1995), includes swaddling, hypercaloric diets, and, for severe cases, pharmacologic therapy. Most authorities recommend paregoric, which is effective for both CNS and gastrointestinal symptoms. Generally a starting dose of 3 to 6 drops every 4 to 6 hours is effective. This dosage is continued for several days and is then tapered gradually and discontinued over 2 to 3 weeks. Phenobarbital is also effective for CNS symptoms but not for gastrointestinal symptoms. It can be helpful as an adjunct in severe cases or in situations in which opioid addiction was complicated by barbiturate-sedative-hypnotic abuse. The typical loading dose is 20 mg/kg, followed by 5 mg/kg/day.

Other Drugs

Neonatal withdrawal from short- and long-acting barbiturates, benzodiazepines, tricyclic antidepressants, other sedative-hypnotics, and alcohol is also well described. These syndromes share features of opiate withdrawal and, in particular, can be associated with seizures. Onset varies with the pharmacologic characteristics of the agents (e.g., early for alcohol and short-acting barbiturates; later for phenobarbital). Most such infants can be successfully managed with phenobarbital and supportive care.

Substances in Breast Milk

An additional precaution for the perinatal period is that of illicit drugs or prescribed medications, taken by nursing mothers, that might pass through breast milk. This topic has been summarized by the American Academy of Pediatrics (Committee on Drugs, 1989). General considerations for prescription medications include the necessity of using the medication at all, the possibility of safer alternatives, and the timing of dosing in relation to nursing so that drug transfer is minimized (e.g., just after breast-feeding or just before the baby's longest sleep period).

One area of concern that has surfaced recently is that of subtle developmental effects linked to ethanol exposure of breast-fed infants. Although prenatal toxic effects of alcohol have been recognized for more than a decade, Little and coworkers in 1989 studied postnatal exposure to alcohol through breast-feeding in 400 predominantly middle class women in the Seattle area. After controlling for prenatal alcohol use and many other potentially confounding variables, particularly smoking and other drug use during gestation and the postpartum period, they found a significantly lower score on the Psychomotor Development Index of the Bayley scales in infants regularly exposed to postnatal alcohol, even at levels of one drink daily. Although the amounts of alcohol estimated to be ingested via breast-feeding are small (e.g., a 5-kg infant might receive 3 mL through nursing from a 60-kg woman who had imbibed four drinks), the authors suggested that repetitive doses of alcohol can accumulate in the infant during breast-feeding, as had been shown for other drugs such as caffeine.

The epidemic of illicit cocaine abuse has been the focus of great concern in regard to teratogenic and perinatal morbidity (see Chapter 25). Altered sensorium and seizures have also been observed in infants ingesting cocaine in the perinatal period from breast-feeding (both via milk and from direct contact with cocaine used as a local anesthetic for sore nipples), as well as from environmental acquisition via passive inhalation of ''crack'' smoke, ingestion of crack, or both.

Hazards in Infancy and Childhood

This section highlights significant toxicologic causes of acquired cognitive and behavioral dysfunction in older infants and children. Additionally, adverse cognitive effects of some commonly prescribed therapeutic drugs are discussed.

LEAD

Extent of Problem

The ubiquitous nature of environmental contamination by lead and its documented neurobehavioral toxicity to children should make this hazard one of the most troubling to pediatricians in the 1990s. Lead poisoning (currently defined by blood lead levels in excess of 10 µg/dL by the Centers for Disease Control and Prevention) affects an enormous population of American children. In 1988 to 1991, 8.9% of all preschoolers in the United States were estimated to have lead levels greater than 10 µg/dL (Brody et al, 1994). Recent surveys have found a significant decline in average US lead levels, presumably because of decreased environmental contamination by airborne lead derived from leaded gasoline and decreased use of lead solder in canned foods. Pockets of excessive lead contamination still persist among inner-city, impoverished, minority children. African American inner-city children were estimated to have prevalence rates as high as 36%. In addition, children from ''lower risk'' groups who reside in older homes with deteriorated paint are also found to have elevated lead levels. Thus the number of potential victims of lead-induced effects is staggering. Lead is a modern-day industrial-age nightmare. Sources are numerous, including automobile exhaust emissions, industrial waste, and widespread contamination from deterioration of surfaces painted with lead-based paint Fig. 30–1. This latter phenomenon is not confined to inner-city slums, as previously believed. Many rural and suburban residences date back to the era before lead-containing paint was banned from use for interior surfaces (the 1950s). Thus toddlers in any area in which lead paint exists are potentially at risk. Additional sources include battery casings burned as fuel, dirt and dust in contaminated areas that rest on children's hands and toys, occasional food or water contamination, especially if improperly glazed ceramic cups or plates are used, and lead dust and particles on parental clothing from occupational exposure. Children are more efficient than adults at absorbing ingested lead; this process is further enhanced by concomitant nutritional deficiency, particularly low-iron, high-fat diets, which often coexist with lead paint exposure in low-income families.

Hazards for Development and Behavior

Lead is a typical heavy metal poison, with wide-ranging toxicity on multiple organ systems. Its effects at the subcellular level are probably mediated by affinity for sulfhydryl groups and thereby interference with structural and enzymatic proteins. A commonly observed functional change is in the heme synthesis pathway, in which several key enzymes are interfered with, resulting in measurable increases in delta-aminolevulinic acid and erythrocyte protoporphyrin, as well as decreased heme production with resultant microcytic anemia. Lead effects are also seen in the kidney—acutely with proximal tubular injury and Fanconi syndrome and chronically with interstitial nephritis. However, the most important consequence of lead poisoning, and the focus here, is on the nervous system.

The most dramatic manifestation of lead neurotoxicity in children is acute encephalopathy (Fig. 30–2). Classi-

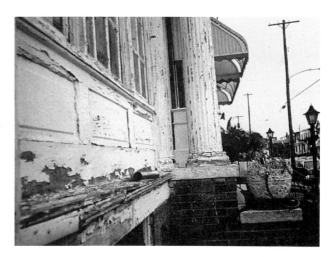

Figure 30–1. A typical inner-city row house with peeling lead paint. (Courtesy of Carla Campbell, MD, and Philadelphia Department of Public Health, Philadelphia, PA.)

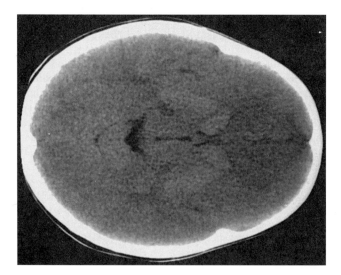

Figure 30–2. Head computed tomography scan of a child with acute lead encephalopathy, demonstrating cerebral edema. (Courtesy of Eric Faerber, MD, and the Department of Radiology, St. Christopher's Hospital for Children, Philadelphia, PA.)

cally seen in the 1- to 3-year-old child, particularly during the summer months, this syndrome is associated with lead levels greater than 100 μg/dL (average 300 μg/dL). Children typically present with stupor or coma and seizures, which are often protracted. The illness can be heralded by days of nausea, vomiting, and irritability or listlessness. It is frequently misdiagnosed as gastroenteritis or a viral syndrome. The pathologic features of acute encephalopathy involve both a vascular lesion with capillary leak and increased intracranial pressure, and direct neuronal damage, particularly in the thalamus, hypothalamus, and basal ganglia (Goyer, 1982). Peripheral neuropathy is also seen occasionally in children, manifested generally by foot drop and generalized weakness. For reasons that are poorly understood, this neuropathy has been observed mainly in children with sickle cell disease. Current government-mandated screening and lead abatement programs have resulted

in a marked decline in the incidence of lead encephalopathy, which has become rare (two patients have been observed in the past 17 years at The Children's Hospital of Philadelphia).

Management considerations for lead encephalopathy include appropriate intensive care with optimal cardiorespiratory support, seizure and intracranial pressure control, close monitoring of fluid provision and urine output to avoid fluid overload but maintain urine flow, and specific chelation therapy (Henretig and Shannon, 1993). Details of chelating medications are outlined in Table 30–1.

The greatest public health concern surrounding childhood lead exposure is related to subencephalopathic effects on the CNS. Numerous studies have attempted to elucidate and quantify cognitive and behavioral deficits in children with "low" lead levels (generally in the 40- to 80-μg/dL range, but recent studies have extended this to levels as low as 10 μg/dL) who were overtly asymptomatic. Many of the early studies were retrospective, and many were poorly controlled. In addition, it is difficult to control for some confounding variables such as innate hyperactivity or learning disability, poor parental supervision, nutritional deficiency, inadequate intellectual stimulation, and low parental intelligence quotient (IQ). Thus, despite the considerable public health consequences of defining asymptomatic lead poisoning as a significant disease with the capacity for intellectual impairment, it has been difficult to demonstrate such causality with precision (Charney, 1982; Pocock, Smith, and Baghurst, 1994).

Studies carried out in the early 1970s demonstrated subtle but statistically significant deficits in cognitive performance in children with elevated lead levels. The findings from most of these studies were suggestive of modest deficits (a reduction of 1 to 5 points on standardized tests of IQ) associated with asymptomatic increased body lead burden in the 40- to 80-μg/dL range and possible impairment at even lower levels. Many of these studies, however, lacked sufficient numbers of patients, adequate markers of lead burden, or proper controls to be fully convincing. The first large, well-controlled study that addressed most methodologic criticisms in detail was reported in 1979 by

Table 30–1 • Chelation Treatment of Lead Poisoning

Clinical Situation	Treatment	Route
I Symptomatic or Pb >70 μg/dL	BAL* 25 mg/kg/day, in every 4-hour doses, for 3–5 days PLUS	Intramuscular
	CaEDTA† 50 mg/kg/day, by continuous infusion over 6 hours for 5 days. (Patients with severe symptoms should be managed in consultation with clinicians experienced in treating symptomatic lead poisoning and pediatric intensive care.)	Intravenous (Intramuscular, rarely, when needed for access or in cases of fluid overload)
II Asymptomatic or Pb >44 and <70 μg/dL	CaEDTA† 25–50 mg/kg/day by continuous infusion or in every 6-hour doses for 5 days OR	Intravenous (Intramuscular)
	Succimer (dimercaptosuccinic acid) 30 mg/kg/day in three doses for 5 days, then 20 mg/kg/day in two doses for 14 days	PO

*Give BAL alone first, then first dose of CaEDTA at least 4 hours later. Usual course for combined therapy is 5 days for encephalopathy. BAL may be discontinued after 3 days in group I patients when Pb level decreases to less than 50 μg/dL.
†CaEDTA for intramuscular use should be mixed with 2% procaine HCl in a ratio of three parts CaEDTA to one part procaine so that final concentration of procaine is 0.5%. When given intravenously, CaEDTA is diluted in dextrose or saline to 500 mg/dL.
BAL = British anti-lewisite (dimercaprol); Pb = lead; CaEDTA = calcium disodium edetate.
Data from American Academy of Pediatrics, Committee on Drugs. Treatment guidelines for lead exposure in children. Pediatrics 96:155–160, 1995.

Needleman and colleagues. These authors compared the neuropsychological performance of 58 children in whom the dentin of shed primary teeth showed a high lead content with that of 100 control children with low dentin lead levels. The children were recruited from first and second grades in the Boston area, and none was identified as having had symptomatic lead poisoning. The high- and low-lead groups were carefully controlled for confounding variables, including medical history, parental education, parental social class and parental IQ, and parental attitudes toward education and school. There was a 4-point deficit in the Wechsler Intelligence Scale for Children (Revised) (WISC [R]) full-scale IQ in the high-lead group (106.6 versus 102.1). In addition, more than 2000 children with known dentin lead levels were evaluated blindly by teacher ratings of classroom behavior. The occurrence of nonadaptive behaviors such as distractibility and impulsiveness was significantly associated in a stepwise dose-related fashion to dentin lead content. The strength of these associations, and the dose-response effect of dentin lead on nonadaptive classroom behavior, was impressive, particularly because the study was a large random sample of an ostensibly normal population of school children. In each group, prior lead levels were known for some children and averaged 23.8 ± 6.0 μg/dL for 23 of 50 in the low-lead group and 35.5 ± 10.1 μg/dL for 58 of 100 in the high-lead group, with both levels being well less than the then-accepted range for significant concern.

Despite these strengths, several criticisms of this Boston study have been noted. The potential issues include lack of concordance on multiple dentin lead analyses from some subjects, a high subject exclusion rate, the focus on WISC(R) score as the primary outcome measure (ignoring differences in tests of academic achievement and perceptual motor skills, presumably because statistical significance was not reached), and the failure to correct for confounding conditions in the analysis of classroom behavior by teachers.

Recent studies have attempted to extend the potential lower limits of both lead burden and critical age by using a longitudinal design, enrolling children at birth or even prenatally. Bellinger and coworkers reported in 1987 on a prospective study of 249 Boston children from birth to 2 years of age. The primary finding was an inverse relationship between prenatal lead exposure and development, with an estimated difference of 4.8 points on the mental scale of the Bayley Scales of Infant Development between the low- and high-exposure groups. Of interest in this longitudinal study, there was no relationship to postnatal blood levels in the range studied, although the differences across the groups between lead levels postnatally were smaller than at birth. Another look at prenatal lead exposure was provided by researchers in Cincinnati (Dietrich et al, 1987). These authors also found an inverse relationship between prenatal and neonatal blood lead and mental scale scores, resulting in a 16- to 22-point mental developmental scale deficit at 6 months of age. These effects were shown to be partly mediated by association with lead-related reductions in gestational age and birth weight. Subsequent follow-up studies of both the Boston and Cincinnati cohorts have found that IQ measured at school entry age is no longer correlated with prenatal lead levels, but rather with peak levels at age 2 years (Pocock, Smith, and Baghurst, 1994).

Postnatal lead exposure was related to effects on development in a longitudinal cohort study from the lead smelter community of Port Pirie in South Australia (McMichael et al, 1988). This study of 537 children found that the blood lead level at each age, particularly at 2 and 3 years, and the integrated average level were inversely related to development, with an estimated deficit of 7.2 points after adjustment for co-variance over a range of lead levels from 10.5 to 31.5 μg/dL. A follow-up on this cohort at age 7 years found a continuation of these cognitive deficits (Baghurst et al, 1992).

Finally, an 11-year follow-up of the 1979 Boston school children study has been published (Needleman et al, 1990). The persistence of dentin lead-associated effects was studied in 132 of 270 young adults originally identified in the 1979 cohort. Among this group, impaired academic status and neurobehavioral function was still found to be related to the lead content of teeth shed 11 years earlier. Measures of cognitive status that correlated with lead burden included failure to graduate high school, frequency of reading disability, and lower high school class rank. Meta-analysis of numerous cross-sectional and prospective studies has estimated that the detrimental effect of doubling blood lead level from 10 to 20 μg/dL is on the order of decreased IQ score of 1 to 2 points. Thus the implications regarding school dysfunction and failure from a public health view are considerable.

Although there may always be some slight doubt regarding the causal relationship between low lead exposure and cognitive effects, the studies of the past decade meet many, if not most, of the usual criteria for relating causality to epidemiologic associations: temporal relationship, strong statistical association, dose-response gradient, control for confounding variables, consistent findings across studies, and biological plausibility. The cumulative weight of these prospective studies adds to the conviction that occult lead poisoning is a potential cause of cognitive deficits.

Pediatric Management

Current recommendations for prevention and screening of children at risk have been recently summarized (American Academy of Pediatrics, 1993a, 1995). Children with a high priority for annual or semiannual screening include those aged 12 to 36 months who reside in older, deteriorated homes; those aged 9 months to 6 years who are siblings or playmates of children with known lead poisoning; children at any age who live in or near older homes undergoing renovation; and any child 9 months to 6 years who lives in older, deteriorated housing or near lead smelters or factories or whose parents work in lead-related jobs or avocations. Additional at-risk groups who are seen for common pediatric problems include children with acute accidental ingestions and those presenting with foreign bodies in the ears, nose, or throat. Intervention should include prompt termination of lead exposure, although this is often difficult to enforce. It is extremely important to remove children from exposure during active lead removal programs.

Recognition and treatment of acute encephalopathy

and symptomatic plumbism have already been discussed and are detailed elsewhere (American Academy of Pediatrics, 1995). The usual chelating medications and treatment regimens are outlined in Table 30–1. Treatment of asymptomatic patients with lead levels greater than 45 μg/dL is generally agreed upon by most authorities; however, the value of chelation therapy to modify the impact on possible neurobehavioral toxicity is unproved. A diagnostic lead mobilization test using one dose of calcium disodium edetate (CaEDTA) for children with blood levels in the 25- to 45-μg/dL range had been recommended in the past, with treatment proposed for those found to have a relatively large, mobilizable pool of lead (American Academy of Pediatrics, 1987); others have argued that such a one-dose or short-course regimen of CaEDTA can actually pose a danger through redistribution of lead to the brain (Chisolm, 1987). The mobilization test is no longer recommended (American Academy of Pediatrics, 1995). The oral chelating agent 2,3-dimercaptosuccinic acid has been used increasingly, with an exceptional safety profile, and this agent is currently the drug of choice for asymptomatic patients with lead levels of 45 to 69 μg/dL (American Academy of Pediatrics, 1995).

MERCURY

Another heavy metal with the potential for significant neurotoxicity and widespread human exposure is mercury. Severe elemental mercury and inorganic mercury salt poisoning (the latter was responsible for pink disease, or acrodynia, from mercurous chloride teething lotions or diaper powder) has become rare. However, a more insidious concern is that of chronic exposure to organic mercurials, particularly methylmercury, resulting from contamination of the food chain. Severe epidemics have occurred in Minamata Bay, Japan, from eating fish contaminated by factory waste discharged into the bay and in Iraq from contaminated bread baked from grain treated with methylmercury as a fungicide. Severe CNS effects occurred in both instances, with a particular susceptibility noted in the fetuses of poisoned pregnant women (almost 30% of children born during the height of the Minamata Bay epidemic had moderate or severe developmental disabilities). The diagnosis of methylmercury poisoning is best confirmed by blood (20 to 50 μg/dL) or hair (50 to 125 μg/g) levels. Treatment is not regularly effective. Currently, dimercaprol for severe cases and D-penicillamine for milder cases have been advocated, although, as for lead poisoning, recent investigations have shown dimercaptosuccinic acid to be promising (Sue, 1994).

OTHER METALS

Aluminum, arsenic, thallium, and manganese are additional unusual causes of neurotoxicity (Ellenhorn and Barceloux, 1988). Aluminum toxicity is manifested primarily as a progressive encephalopathy with dysarthria-apraxia, asterixis, tremor, dementia, and focal seizures. In pediatric patients, the disease is associated primarily with chronic renal failure and long-term hemodialysis or chronic use of aluminum phosphate-binding agents, or both.

Arsenic poisoning still occurs occasionally from pesticides or environmental contamination of well water or food. Chronic exposure is manifested by a classic stocking-glove distribution of sensory neuropathy and encephalopathy. Associated features include alopecia, pruritus, hyperpigmentation and hyperkeratosis; anemia and leukopenia; abdominal pain and diarrhea; and lacrimation, salivation, perspiration, and a garlic-like odor.

Thallium poisoning is uncommon because its use as a pesticide was banned in 1965. Its intoxication was associated with a peripheral neuropathy and encephalopathy and persistent sequelae such as ataxia, tremor, and memory loss. Characteristic accompanying signs include scalp (and facial) hair loss.

Manganese causes a rare CNS disease involving parkinsonian-like features and psychiatric disturbances ("manganese madness"). It is associated primarily with occupational exposure to dust from manganese ore.

These uncommon metal poisonings are reviewed in detail along with specific recommendations for management in reference toxicology texts (Ellenhorn and Barceloux, 1988).

INHALATIONAL TOXINS

Both the accidental or intentional acute exposure to carbon monoxide and the chronic inhalation abuse of various solvents have been associated with CNS syndromes. See Chapter 50 for more detailed discussion of adolescent substance abuse.

Carbon Monoxide

Exposure to carbon monoxide fumes is the most common cause of death from poisoning in the United States, accounting for 3500 to 4000 fatalities per year. Many cases are secondary to smoke inhalation from house fires, although a clinically important and more challenging group to recognize includes individuals with subtle neuropsychiatric or systemic afebrile "flulike" symptoms, or both, resulting from faulty furnaces, automobile exhaust, improperly vented water heaters, kerosene heaters, and so on. One study in The Children's Hospital of Philadelphia emergency department found a surprisingly high incidence (nearly 30%) of carbon monoxide exposure during the winter months in just such a group of 46 patients (Baker, Henretig, and Ludwig, 1988).

Toxicity of carbon monoxide is mediated primarily by cellular hypoxia. It decreases oxygen delivery by binding to hemoglobin to form carboxyhemoglobin and by shifting the oxyhemoglobin dissociation curve to the left; it can also bind to mitochondrial cytochrome oxidase and inhibit cellular respiration as well. As such, carbon monoxide poisoning especially affects organs most susceptible to hypoxia: the heart and brain. In acute, severe exposures, patients may have coma, convulsions, cardiovascular collapse, and respiratory failure. Many survivors (up to 40%) of severe carbon monoxide poisoning have neuropsychiatric sequelae. The effects of severe but nonlethal carbon monoxide exposure on pregnant women can also be manifested as fetal demise or cerebral palsy in the infant. Prolonged low-dose exposure through cigarette smoking (which can produce carboxyhemoglobin levels of 5% to

15%) in pregnancy has been associated with lower birth weights and increased neonatal mortality rates.

Recognition and management of carbon monoxide exposure are detailed elsewhere (Ellenhorn and Barceloux, 1988). The mainstays of treatment are immediate removal from exposure, provision of appropriate supportive care and 100% oxygen, and consideration, if feasible, of the use of hyperbaric oxygen therapy for selected patients. There is some controversy regarding the precise indications for hyperbaric oxygen, but most authorities recommend its use for symptomatic patients with carboxyhemoglobin levels greater than 25% to 40% (or any pregnant patient with levels greater than 15% to 20%), and any patient, regardless of level, who has experienced significant neurologic or cardiac manifestations.

Solvents

The general background for intentional inhalant abuse is discussed in Chapter 50. Several organic solvents have been associated with CNS sequelae, particularly toluene (glue sniffing) and gasoline. The neuropathic effects of toluene include ataxia, tremors, emotional lability, and cognitive effects. Gasoline abuse leads to an encephalopathy characterized by ataxia, tremor, chorea, and myoclonus; there can also be an organic psychosis with hallucinations, paranoia, and violence. The neurologic sequelae of chronic gasoline inhalation are believed to result from tetraethyl lead toxicity, and the diagnosis can be confirmed by finding elevated blood lead levels. There may be some efficacy of standard lead chelation therapy in alleviating the neurologic symptoms of gasoline-related tetraethyl lead toxicity.

Therapeutic Agents

This section discusses observations associating adverse cognitive and behavioral effects with the chronic administration, at therapeutic doses, of therapeutic agents. The focus is on the use of phenobarbital to prevent recurrences of febrile seizures and theophylline for the treatment of bronchial asthma.

Phenobarbital has a long history of relatively safe and effective use as an antiepileptic drug and has been considered the drug of choice for preventing frequent recurrences of febrile seizures in young children. It has been observed for some time, however, that phenobarbital therapy may be associated with behavioral side effects such as moodiness and hyperactivity. Recently there has been some additional concern about the cognitive effects of long-term administration; a study of this agent as used for febrile seizures has reported significant deficits in cognitive performance (Farwell et al, 1990). These investigators followed 217 children who were treated for febrile seizures with phenobarbital or placebo for 2 years and compared IQ as measured by the Stanford-Binet test. They found an 8.4-point deficit in the group randomized to receive phenobarbital; when retested 6 months after phenobarbital had been discontinued, the IQ deficit was 5.2 points. Furthermore, the researchers found no difference in the frequency of recurrent seizures between the two groups. Although earlier studies did not find such cognitive effects in phenobarbital-treated children, Farwell and colleagues' well-controlled study must be considered with concern until further data are available.

Several studies in the 1980s attempted to examine behavioral and cognitive effects of chronic theophylline administration in asthmatic children. Rachelefsky and co-workers reported in 1986 on the effects of a 4-week course of theophylline in children with asymptomatic asthma as compared with placebo administration. Although no effects were found on specific psychological tests or parents' evaluations of symptoms, teachers' ratings of classroom behavior found adverse effects, including deficits in attention and a tendency to become angry easily and fight, for seven of 10 children on theophylline. Similar results were suggested in several other studies of small numbers of children, but these studies were often poorly controlled for confounding variables or lacked follow-up data that would take into account an adaptive effect to the medication, or both. The search for a causal relationship between theophylline and behavioral or cognitive problems has thus far yielded ambiguous and contradictory findings, although there may be a subset of children with heightened sensitivity to this agent for whom treatment choices ought to be appropriately tailored.

Finally, in less rigorously studied therapeutic agents, many practitioners have observed at least temporary behavioral effects from therapeutic courses of antihistamines (drowsiness), decongestants such as pseudoephedrine or phenylpropanolamine (irritability, restlessness), and corticosteroids (emotional lability). The effects of antihistamines and decongestants can be particularly evident in young infants; the therapeutic margin appears low for these agents in some of these patients.

REFERENCES

Abel EL, Hannigan JH: Maternal risk factors in fetal alcohol syndrome: provocative and permissive influences. Neurotoxicol Teratol 17:445–462, 1995.

Alpert JJ, Zuckerman BZ: Alcohol use during pregnancy: what is the risk? Pediatr Rev 12:375–379, 1991.

American Academy of Pediatrics, Committee on Drugs. Treatment guidelines for lead exposure in children. Pediatrics 96:155–160, 1995.

American Academy of Pediatrics, Committee on Drugs: Transfer of drugs and other chemicals into human milk. Pediatrics 84:924, 1989.

American Academy of Pediatrics, Committee on Environmental Hazards; Committee on Accident and Poison Prevention: Statement on childhood lead poisoning. Pediatrics 79:457, 1987.

American Academy of Pediatrics, Committee on Environmental Health. Lead poisoning from screening to primary prevention. Pediatrics 92:176–183, 1993a.

American Academy of Pediatrics, Committee on Substance Abuse and Committee on Children with Disabilities: Fetal alcohol syndrome and fetal alcohol effects. Pediatrics 91:1004–1006, 1993b.

Baghurst PA, McMichael AJ, Wigg NR, et al: Environmental exposure to lead and children's intelligence at the age of seven years. N Engl J Med 327:1279–1284, 1992.

Baker MD, Henretig FM, Ludwig S: Carboxyhemoglobin levels in children with nonspecific flu-like symptoms. J Pediatr 113:501, 1988.

Bellinger D, Leviton A, Waternaux C, et al: Longitudinal analyses of prenatal and postnatal lead exposure and early cognitive development. N Engl J Med 316:1037, 1987.

Brody DJ, Pirkle JL, Kramer RA, et al: Blood lead levels in the US population: phase 1 of the third National Health and Nutrition Examination Survey (NHANES III, 1988 to 1991). JAMA 272:277–283, 1994.

Byrd RS, Howard CR: Children's passive and prenatal exposure to cigarette smoke. Pediatr Ann 24:640–645, 1995.

Charney E: Sub-encephalopathic lead poisoning: central nervous system effects in children. *In* Chisolm JJ Jr, O'Hara DM (eds): Lead Absorption in Children. Baltimore, Urban and Schwarzenberg, 1982, pp 35–42.

Chisolm JJ Jr: Mobilization of lead by calcium disodium edetate: a reappraisal. Am J Dis Child 141:1256, 1987.

Coles CD, Platzman KA. Behavioral development in children prenatally exposed to drugs and alcohol. Int J Addiction 28:1393–1433, 1993.

Dietrich KN, Krafft KM, Bornschein RL, et al: Low-level fetal lead exposure effect on neurobehavioral development in early infancy. Pediatrics 80:721, 1987.

Ellenhorn MJ, Barceloux DG: Metals and related compounds. *In* Medical Toxicology: Diagnosis and Treatment of Human Poisoning. New York, Elsevier, 1988, pp 1007–1066.

Farwell JR, Lee YJ, Hirtz DG, et al: Phenobarbital for febrile seizures—effects on intelligence and on seizure recurrence. N Engl J Med 322:364, 1990.

Gershanik J, Boecler B, Ensley H, et al: The gasping syndrome and benzyl alcohol poisoning. N Engl J Med 307:1384, 1982.

Goldstein GW. Neurologic concepts of lead poisoning in children. Pediatr Ann 21:384–388, 1992.

Goyer RA: Lead toxicity. *In* Chisolm JJ Jr, O'Hara DM (eds): Lead Absorption in Children. Baltimore, Urban and Schwarzenberg, 1982, pp 21–34.

Henretig FM, Shannon M: Toxicologic emergencies. *In* Fleisher GR, Ludwig S (eds): Textbook of Pediatric Emergency Medicine, 3rd ed. Baltimore, Williams & Wilkins, 1993, pp 745–801.

Kulberg HG, Weisman RS: From conception to breastfeeding: toxicologic considerations of pregnancy. *In* Goldfrank LR, Flomenbaum NE, Lewin NA (eds): Toxicologic Emergencies. Norwalk, CT, Appleton-Century-Crofts, 1986, pp 185–197.

Lester BM, Als H, Brazelton TB: Regional obstetric anesthesia and newborn behavior: a reanalysis toward synergistic effects. Child Dev 53:687, 1982.

Little RE, Anderson KW, Ervin CH, et al: Maternal alcohol use during breastfeeding and infant mental and motor development at one year. N Engl J Med 321:425, 1989.

McMichael AJ, Baghurst PA, Wigg NR, et al: Port Pirie Cohort Study: environmental exposure to lead and children's abilities at the age of four years. N Engl J Med 319:468, 1988.

Needleman HL, Gunnoe C, Leviton A, et al: Deficits in psychologic and classroom performance of children with elevated dentine lead levels. N Engl J Med 300:689, 1979.

Needleman HL, Schell A, Bellinger D, et al: The long-term effects of exposure to low doses of lead in childhood—an 11-year follow-up report. N Engl J Med 322:83, 1990.

Norton S: Toxic responses of the central nervous system. *In* Klaassen CD, Amdur MO, Doull J (eds): Toxicology: The Basic Science of Poisons, 3rd ed. New York, Macmillan, 1985, pp 359–386.

Pocock SJ, Smith M, Baghurst P. Environmental lead and children's intelligence: a systematic review of the epidemiologic evidence. BMJ 309:1189–1197, 1994.

Rachelefsky GS, Wo J, Adelson J, et al: Behavior abnormalities and poor school performance due to oral theophylline use. Pediatrics 78:1133, 1986.

Richardson GA, Day NL, Goldschmidt L: Prenatal alcohol, marijuana, and tobacco use: infant mental and motor development. Neurotoxicol Teratol 17:479–487, 1995.

Sue Y-J: Mercury. *In* Goldfrank LR, Flomenbaum NE, Lewin NA (eds): Toxicologic Emergencies. Norwalk, CT, Appleton-Century-Crofts, 1994, pp 1051–1062.

Volpe JJ: Effect of cocaine on the fetus. N Engl J Med 327:399–407, 1992.

Volpe JJ: Teratogenic effects of drugs and passive addiction. *In* Neurology of the Newborn. 3rd ed. Philadelphia, WB Saunders, 1995, pp 834–835.

PART IV

Effects of Medical Illness

31 Acute Minor Illness

William B. Carey

The minor illnesses and injuries of childhood occupy about a half of the time of the average primary care physician, and yet they tend to be regarded as having little or no relevance to the child's development and behavior. This chapter points out the considerable interactions that these universal experiences do have with the child's developmental-behavioral status. The discussion deals both with the dangers of "pediatric pathogenesis" and with the great opportunities for promotion of the child's progress and mental health through skillful handling of these events.

Acute minor illness is defined here as ordinary, brief health problems, such as the common respiratory and gastrointestinal infections and the familiar instances of physical trauma experienced by all children. These are the usual minor complaints that account for almost all the visits to primary health care clinicians because of illness. These illnesses and their management have not generally been considered to be significant factors in the child's development and behavior. However, there is reason to believe that this assumption of their unimportance is incorrect and is attributable to insufficient attention and research. A comprehensive critical review of the meager literature over 25 years ago summarized available data and called for further investigation (Carey and Sibinga, 1972). This chapter draws primarily on that review as to content and organization. Only a little additional material has been published since then (Cunningham, 1989; Richtsmeier and Hatcher, 1994; Schmitt, 1980; Sibinga and Carey, 1976). The recommendations are based more on a pooling of the experience of many pediatricians rather than on extensive formal research findings.

Stresses in the Child and Parents

The child with an acute minor illness experiences the discomfort of the illness and its treatment, the emotional reactions to and fantasies about the illness (such as feelings of guilt, fear, anger, sadness, and apathy), the loss of normal social contacts at school and elsewhere outside the home, the restrictions (such as bedrest and diet), the decreased or altered sensory input, and a change in the relationship with the parents, who may become either more indulgent or more hostile (Freud, 1952).

The parents endure stresses of two sorts: those that arise from the illness itself and its management (such as more responsibility and expense, interference with employ-ment, and less sleep and recreation) and the extraneous factors that complicate the parents' reaction to the illness, such as the parents' personal problems, preexisting physical or behavioral difficulties in the child, and situational pressures, such as unemployment or marital discord. (See also Chapter 16 regarding various forms of family dysfunction.) Another unrelated factor may be the vulnerable child syndrome, in which some parents continue to be inappropriately overconcerned about their children's health long after they have completely recovered from an early health crisis (see Chapter 33). The Family and Medical Leave Act passed by the US Congress in 1993 allows parents leave for the care of their children's major illnesses such as hospitalizations but makes no provision for more common and equally disruptive minor illnesses (Heymann, Earle, and Egleston, 1996).

EFFECTS OF STRESSORS

The effect of acute minor illness on children's behavior, although well known to parents and clinicians, has scarcely been studied. Various possible behavioral reactions such as dependency, withdrawal, irritability, rebelliousness, and feelings of inferiority have been reported, but a comprehensive, systematic delineation of these reactions and their determinants and consequences is still awaited. The child's temperament influences his or her experience of the illness and reactions to it, which are likely to affect the clinical manifestations and outcome (see Chapter 8) (Fig. 31–1).

The parents may also suffer from fears and anxieties, anger, guilt, fatigue, depression, and distortions and misconceptions. They are expected to master these feelings and to adjust sufficiently to meet their child's needs. Ineffective responses may consist of inappropriate feelings or lack of understanding (such as too much or too little anxiety, persistent misconceptions about the illness or its treatment, or an excessive sense of personal injury) or inability to

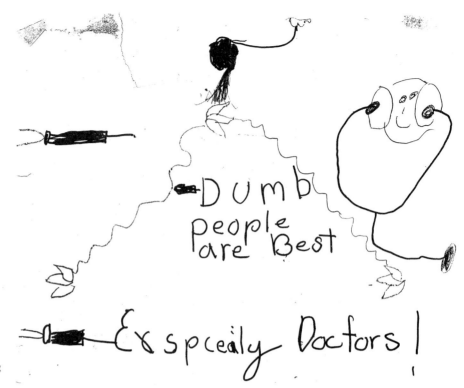

Figure 31–1. A young child's conflicting feelings about her doctor.

muster appropriate behavior to deal with the illness (such as difficulty in carrying out a reasonable share of the treatment process in conjunction with the doctor, as evidenced by noncompliance with the treatment plan).

It seems likely that minor illness and its management account for only a small portion of the more chronic behavioral variations and problems in children, yet these effects are real and must be acknowledged and dealt with. Any experienced pediatrician can think of striking examples of unfavorable outcomes, such as the child who is treated by his parents for years as a semi-invalid because a physician had felt compelled to reveal the existence of a functional heart murmur without considering or assessing the impact of this information on the child and his parents, or the child who is made to feel guilty or inadequate because of recurrent respiratory or urinary infections.

On the other hand, as Parmelee (1997) has observed, it is possible that childhood illnesses "not only *aid* the process of the development of social competence and a healthy personality, but they may be *necessary* for this process. In turn, social competence and a healthy personality provide us the greatest capacity for coping with illness." The recurring experience of minor illnesses furnishes children with a multitude of opportunities to broaden their knowledge of themselves, of their caregivers, and of the relationships between them. Positive outcomes can include enhanced social competence and self-assurance.

Nurturing Sick Children and Supporting Parents

A useful way to describe principles of management of minor illness is in terms of the illness itself, the child, and the parents—how the needs of each are sometimes not met, why this happens, what the consequences may be, and finally how to avoid these complications. Even the best trained, most compassionate physician makes occasional lapses of good judgment in these matters; the objective is to keep "pediatric pathogenesis" to a minimum (Carey and Sibinga, 1972).

TREAT THE ILLNESS

Treatment of illness can go awry in three main ways. Probably the most common error we physicians make in the management of minor illness is in overdiagnosing and overtreating. For example, unnecessary antibiotics are frequently prescribed for viral upper respiratory infections. Insignificant findings such as a functional heart murmur or tibial torsion may be overinterpreted, made into a "pseudo-disease," and managed with greater attention than they deserve. Physicians apparently err in this direction for two principal reasons: problems within the physician himself or herself, such as insufficient training or excessive anxiety, and pressures from the parents, such as their common urging that something decisive be done about recurrent respiratory infections. (See Chapter 16 concerning exaggeration of illness by parents, including Munchausen syndrome by proxy.) Possible consequences of overmanagement include generating fear that the child is sicker than he or she really is, producing harm from unnecessary procedures, and fostering excessive dependence on the physician and his or her treatment.

Undermanagement and mismanagement and their causes and consequences are sufficiently well known to require no further elaboration here.

Obviously, the primary role of the pediatrician or

other clinician is to treat the illness. This means the use of appropriate diagnostic and therapeutic measures with avoidance of the pitfalls already mentioned. In particular, nonillnesses or pseudodiseases should not be treated. Also, reasonable steps should be taken to help the parents and the child prevent recurrences or spread of the illness. Risk-taking behaviors that predispose to illness and injury should be discouraged (see Chapter 51).

NURTURE THE SICK CHILD

Undoubtedly the most common problem in the medical management of the sick child is that the illness itself is treated but the person with the problem is neglected. The clinician may be inadequately sensitive and attentive to the emotional needs of the sick child. The cause is usually a narrowness of interest or a deficiency of empathy. This preoccupation with the illness itself makes it more likely that the experience will be more frightening and stressful for the child than it needs to be.

On the other hand, overattention to the child's feelings, as with our own children or those of our friends or colleagues, with whom we are too closely involved emotionally, may mean that sound professional judgment and proper diagnosis and treatment are in jeopardy.

Third, inappropriate handling of the child—with dishonesty or belittling of his or her concerns for whatever reason—must invariably make the illness experience more hazardous for the child.

Nurturing the sick child means that the physician can reduce the stress of the illness by keeping the discomfort, trauma, and restrictions of the management to a minimum; that he or she can promote the child's adjustment to the illness by listening to the child's concerns and responding to them honestly and supportively; and, at times, that the illness experience can even be an opportunity for psychological growth. By learning about the illness and his or her ability to tolerate discomfort and overcome a problem with the help of the family and physician, the child can gain in self-confidence and avoid developing a sense of physical inferiority or personal inadequacy.

SUPPORT THE PARENTS

Although it may be difficult to define what support for the parents should consist of, there is little problem in identifying unsupportive patterns in the physician-parent relationship. These errors in management are attributable to a variety of professional and personal failings in the physician.

Two common errors are overdomination and oversubmissiveness. The playing of too dominant a role by the physician in the care of minor illness stifles self-reliance in parents, as when the doctor attempts to dictate every detail of the management and leaves nothing to the parents' own resources. Too much submission to the parents' wishes results in abdication of the physician's proper advisory status. Pleasing parents is a reasonable objective but not when it goes, for example, to the extent of allowing parents to change the doctor's mind about use of an antibiotic.

Neglect of the parents entails not giving sufficient attention to their feelings, their need for information, or their help in handling the illness. Insufficient empathy for the parents or being excessively busy are two common sources of this problem. Neglected parents become confused and helpless and are likely to turn elsewhere for assistance.

Inappropriate handling of the parents, such as giving them misinformation about the illness or its management, or doing anything that needlessly upsets them, is, of course, likely to leave them with feelings of incompetence and perhaps with an unwarranted attachment to the doctor through fear or misguided gratitude.

Probably the best way to be supportive to parents with a sick child is to determine their needs and expectations, to help them to deal with the illness and the sick child, to be available in case of further need, and to promote their general self-confidence in handling illness. Following the general guidelines for establishing and maintaining the therapeutic alliance (see Chapters 66 and 76), this process includes listening to the parents' concerns, supplying needed information, helping them use their own ideas and resources as much as possible, giving suggestions about altering potentially dangerous remedies, and providing reassurance. Ineffective but harmless home remedies need not be routinely disapproved. If the parents' fears are disproportionate to the situation, their basis deserves some investigation.

Well-supported, self-reliant parents are more likely to manage well the illness and the child, to relieve the physician of needless repetition of instructions, and to face other aspects of childrearing with greater confidence.

Conclusions

The average American pediatrician spends about half his or her time dealing with minor illnesses, yet problems in development and behavior related to minor illness and its management have been largely ignored. There can be little doubt that the child's developmental and behavioral status affect the experience of and reaction to the illness. The extent of the impact of acute minor illnesses on the child's development and behavior is certainly considerable but demands greater clarification. It remains a major area for expansion of knowledge through research and for enhancement of professional skills.

REFERENCES

Carey WB, Sibinga MS: Avoiding pediatric pathogenesis in the management of acute minor illness. Pediatrics 49:553, 1972.

Cunningham AS: Beware overtreating children. Am J Dis Child 143:786, 1989.

Freud A: The role of bodily illness in the mental life of children. Psychoanal Stud Child 7:69, 1952.

Heymann SJ, Earle A, Egleston B: Parental availability for the care of sick children. Pediatrics 98:226, 1996.

Parmelee AH Jr: Illness and the development of social competence. J Dev Behav Pediatr 18:120, 1997.

Richtsmeier AJ, Hatcher JW: Parental anxiety and minor illness. J Dev Behav Pediatr 15:14, 1994.

Schmitt BD: Fever phobia: misconceptions of parents about fevers. Am J Dis Child 134:176, 1980.

Sibinga MS, Carey WB: Dealing with unnecessary medical trauma to children. Pediatrics 57:800, 1976.

32 Hospitalization, Surgery, and Medical Procedures

Ellen C. Perrin

 A child's developmental-behavioral status can both influence and be influenced by some aspects of medical care, especially the more serious ones described in this chapter: hospitalizations and medical or surgical procedures. Physicians should be aware of the stresses involved in these experiences and the effects they have on children. There are many opportunities for minimizing the stresses on children and for making the experience as positive as possible. Physicians should also be cognizant of the impact that these experiences have on themselves.

Health care professionals have a unique opportunity and therefore a responsibility to help children and their families to minimize the stresses and to capitalize on the opportunities provided by all their health care encounters.

About 5% of children are hospitalized each year in the United States. More and more hospitalizations of children are the result of trauma or are associated with the management of a chronic physical illness. Children with acute illnesses are often cared for outside the hospital, and many elective surgical procedures are performed in day-surgery units. These changes have come about largely as a result of efforts to contain escalating health care costs but also in part because of the recognition among health care professionals and parents that hospitalization itself is associated with extra stresses to children and their families that may be avoided by alternative methods of care.

Major changes in hospital structure, design, and policies have created an environment that is increasingly supportive to children and families and have radically altered the experience of hospitalization over the past 25 years (Thompson, 1986). A great deal of literature has become available for parents and for children to prepare them for hospitalization, and many medical centers provide tours and preparation programs for children anticipating surgery and hospitalization. Wards and patient rooms are designed more appropriately, and play space and appropriate recreation and Child Life programming are often available. Hospital policies generally allow and even encourage siblings and friends to visit and one or both parents to room-in with children (in a few states, such policies are formally legislated).

Sources of Stress

Admission to a hospital is disruptive and bewildering; even after multiple admissions, children report anxiety about and discomfort from the process of entering this strange and frightening world (Table 32–1). The child who is admitted to a hospital is separated from the usual surroundings and routines of his or her everyday life: the support and care of parents, everyday interactions with siblings, school life, and social and sports activities with friends. These interruptions are frequently unplanned, are usually unpleasant, and interfere with children's efforts to maintain autonomy and control. In addition, they generally occur when the child is already anxious and uncomfortable or in pain related to the illness or trauma that precipitated the hospitalization. Even for the few children with severe chronic illnesses who spend many of their days in the hospital, their smoother adjustment to hospital life and routines comes at a cost in disruption of normal social and emotional development.

At the time of hospitalization, children encounter new routines and new adult caretakers and meet other children with a variety of medical problems. They are automatically thrown into a bizarre and unfamiliar environment in which even the most basic functions, such as eating and sleeping, are different from their normal pattern and are under someone else's control. They are introduced to a variety of new technologic equipment and all of the flashing lights and beeps that go with these devices. They may undergo a number of procedures that begin during the process of being admitted to the hospital; these are at the least unfamiliar and often accompanied by discomfort or pain. Almost every child is subjected to poking and

Table 32–1 • Sources of Anxiety Related to Hospitalization

Separation from parents, siblings, friends
New adults and children
Disruption of usual routines
Unfamiliar food, bed, clothes, rules
Interruption of schoolwork
Painful and frightening procedures
Lack of understanding of the experience
Loss of control
Forced dependency
Guilt, shame
Worry about bodily integrity, death
Loss of privacy

pricking, physical restraints, dietary changes, restriction in activity, and perhaps isolation.

In addition to the confusing environment, children often have difficulty understanding what is happening to them, what part they have had in causing or controlling the illness, and why hospitalization and the associated painful procedures are necessary. Young children cannot comprehend the reasons for such traumatic impositions as separation from their parents, being forced to live temporarily in a strange and sterile environment, having to endure painful procedures (sometimes even with the assistance of their parents), and the pain and discomfort that may be associated with the condition itself. Children up to school age may confuse their condition and their hospitalization with some form of immanent justice (e.g., retribution for a rule they have disobeyed or for unacceptable thoughts or activities).

As children get older, their ideas about the causation of illness become more sophisticated, but they do not understand the complexity of the mechanisms of disease and health until well into adolescence (Perrin and Gerrity, 1981). Their limited understanding of illness and its management results in complicated distortions and bizarre notions of their own ability to affect the onset and outcome of the illness (Schonfeld, 1992). Because health care professionals do not necessarily predict accurately how and what children understand about their illness and its treatment, it is helpful to review with children their conceptions and misconceptions in order to avoid maladaptive responses. No matter what else is occurring related to hospitalization, children experience, both in reality and in their fantasy, a frightening loss of control. Much of the time, children feel that they have little control over how and with whom they spend their time and what is happening to them. In that children have a greater belief than do adults in the effectiveness of powerful others (usually adults) in determining their health and well-being, they are especially vulnerable to the ineffectiveness of their own actions and wishes.

Evidence of Effects on Children

Most children who are hospitalized with current hospital procedures are able to cope effectively without any lasting effects on their behavior (Thompson and Vernon, 1992). A few, often those in the most vulnerable age groups, those in whom the preexisting nurturing relationships are tenuous, and those for whom the detrimental or frightening effects of the illness or trauma are overwhelming, cope poorly and require extra attention.

There has been extensive investigation of the psychological impact of hospitalization. The initial work focused primarily on the effects of the separation from parents that accompanied a hospital stay (Douglas, 1975) and began to explore children's fears about their bodily integrity when faced with surgery or extended illness (Davenport and Werry, 1970). Through the 1970s, there were many further elaborations of the vulnerability of children to the many unique stresses of hospitalization and descriptions of the character, extent, and longevity of the behavioral evidence of children's subsequent distress (Gabriel and Danilowicz,

1978; Quinton and Rutter, 1976; Vernon et al, 1975). Since the late 1970s, a large number of interventions have been designed to prevent or ameliorate children's distress (Melamed and Ridley-Johnson, 1988). Most evaluations have concluded that such programs are beneficial, as evidenced by less maladaptive behavior after hospitalization, more rapid physiologic signs of recovery, and growth in both knowledge and understanding (Vernon and Thompson, 1992).

Indications of emotional difficulties are greatest among children between 6 months and 6 years of age and increase markedly if hospitalization is long or frequently recurs. Parents and teachers of children recently hospitalized frequently report behavior problems suggestive of difficulties with separation, fearfulness, and regression (Table 32–2) (Thompson and Vernon, 1992). The number of children who demonstrate behavior problems in this period is greater among children with two or more admissions or who stayed in the hospital more than 2 weeks than among those with a single or a shorter admission. Because children with chronic illnesses are likely to be admitted to hospitals more frequently and to stay longer than generally healthy children, it is possible that these findings are confounded with the known increased prevalence of behavior problems in children with chronic illnesses (Perrin et al, 1993). Davenport and Werry (1970) found no effects of hospitalization 2 weeks after hospital stays of less than 48 hours. A few studies show a direct relationship between difficulties with adjustment after discharge and the amount of visiting the child was allowed (and therefore the amount of separation the child experienced while in the hospital). Studies comparing inpatient treatment with day surgery or outpatient care have demonstrated that although medical outcome was equivalent, hospitalized children displayed higher levels of overall psychological upset than did the group treated as outpatients (Scaife and Campbell, 1988).

Children's prior experience with illness and hospitalization (their own, their peers', or family members') informs their reactions to hospitalization and procedures. It is often helpful to understand children's recent experiences or memories in order to help them separate their current experience from other experiences. Children's intelligence and temperamental style also contribute to their ability to manage and cope with the stresses and threats they confront in hospitalization. Parents can often be helpful in anticipating children's usual reactions to new circumstances, painful or threatening procedures, and separations. Commercially available books and videotapes may guide parents in their support of their children (Association for the Care of Children's Health, 1987).

Parents' attitudes toward the child's illness or condi-

Table 32–2 • Common Behavioral Symptoms After Hospitalization

Regression (thumb-sucking, bed wetting, baby talk)	Sleep disturbances
	Encopresis
Eating disorders	Aggressiveness, acting out
Increased dependency	Fear of doctors and nurses
School phobia	Depression
Decreased attentiveness	Academic underachievement

tion, and their own experiences with hospitalization and illness, may also profoundly influence their child's reaction to hospitalization and his or her ability to cope with it. Parents for whom the illness or trauma and hospitalization generate an apparently excessive amount of anxiety may be helped by learning specific stress management techniques (e.g., hypnosis, deep relaxation, meditation) that may also be helpful for their children. Numerous studies have confirmed that parents can be taught to help their children manage painful procedures by using these techniques. It is important to provide parents with opportunities to get information about their children, to be able to express their concerns and fears to the clinicians working with their children, and, in some cases, to share their emotional reactions and concerns in a caring and safe support group environment. Support groups in the context of children's hospital wards might include such topics as dealing with terminal illness, guilt, financial concerns, working with siblings, and strategies for coping with the subsequent physical and emotional needs of the index child and the rest of the family.

Effects of Children's Serious Illnesses, Pain, and Procedures on Clinicians

It is challenging for nurses, residents, and senior physicians to watch children bewildered, confused, and in pain. Health care providers must understand their own feelings about illness and death, as well as about the necessity for painful procedures, in order to be effective in providing support to children. It is helpful for all members of the health care team to be involved collaboratively with parents in important decisions regarding the care provided to children and families. Conflicts among members of the professional team regarding the division of labor, control of decision making, and responsibility for communication can seriously undermine children's care. Clinicians may identify powerfully with children, or with their parents, and find that such identification interferes with their ability to make dispassionate clinical decisions and to enforce hospital regulations. Past family and personal history with illness, hospitalization, and death may color their ability to deal directly with the powerful affective responses certain children and families may evoke in them. Neither excessive identification nor artificial distancing from children and families is optimally helpful to their patients.

Professionals may have the greatest difficulty in maintaining open communication with children and parents when the child's condition and needed procedures are particularly painful for them. Silence may be interpreted by the child as abandonment or anger as the result of his or her condition and thus may compound the intrinsic difficulty of the circumstance. The death of a child in the hospital is one of the most stressful personal and professional experiences faced by health care providers. It may trigger a grief response similar to that following a personal loss. It is important for health care professionals to have permission and support to discuss these experiences and to have their personal needs met at these times. It is often helpful to encourage some introspection about their own history of losses and a discussion of the impact of their patient's death on their personal and professional lives. Such social institutions as funerals and memorial services can be as helpful to health care providers as they are to families. In some hospital settings, teams of professionals organize support systems to ensure that the expertise and skills of members of multiple related disciplines are available to address these issues. Such support systems often include representatives from the clergy, Child Life, nursing, psychiatry, psychology, and social work.

Opportunities

Children and families can sometimes grow through a hospitalization (Parmelee, 1993; Solnit, 1960) as outlined in Table 32–3. Illness and hospitalization provide opportunities for parents and siblings to care for and nurture the child. The experience provides opportunities for children to increase their understanding of their illness and its care, to increase participation in their own care, and to communicate with health care providers, their parents, and other children about the illness. Hospitalization may be a time when both parents and children can expand their social network, meeting children and families with medical concerns similar to their own. It also provides an opportunity for parents to learn more about their child's illness, gaining both information and skills; to increase their ability to observe their child; and to increase their sense of competence in their ability to care for the child (Fig. 32–1).

Hospitalization also provides special opportunities for health care professionals. The extended period in the hospital allows them to develop or strengthen their alliance with the child and to observe his or her play and interactions with other children, with family members, and with caregiving adults. It allows them to observe the family's strengths and its ongoing needs, the pattern of the child's illness and its response to medications, and the child's response to pain. Pediatricians and other health care professionals can also use the hospital environment to obtain

Table 32–3 • Opportunities Related to Hospitalization

Parents and children have the opportunity to
  Demonstrate/receive nurturing by parents, siblings, friends
  Increase knowledge and skills about the child's illness and its care
  Increase participation in care
  Foster communication with health care professionals
  Develop or enlarge social networks
  Increase available support
  Improve understanding of general mechanisms of health and illness
  Improve confidence and sense of mastery

Health care professionals have the opportunity to
  Develop an alliance with the child
  Observe the child over an extended time (play, interactions with
    peers, family members, adults)
  Assess family's strengths and needs
  Observe pattern of the illness, response to medications
  Provide education, modeling
  Obtain consultations
  Encourage self-care and increase participation and confidence

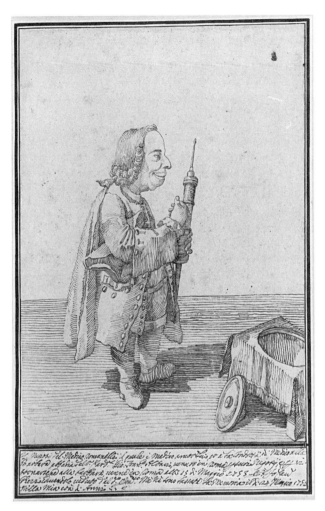

Table 32–4 • Factors Affecting Consequences of Hospitalization

Child's age and development
Whether first or recurrent hospitalization
Length of separation
Previous knowledge or preparation about hospitals, procedures
Child's temperament, personality, and coping style
Characteristics of illness or injury
Family's response to illness or injury
Family cohesiveness and interactions
Procedures/surgery required
Amount of pain and discomfort
Responsiveness of hospital environment
Consistency of hospital personnel

Figure 32–1. Health care professionals can control the nature of the hospital environment to minimize frightening experiences such as this. (Ghezzi, Pierleone: Doctor Holding an Enema Syringe Caricature. Philadelphia Museum of Art: Purchased with funds from the Smithkline Beecham [formerly Beckman] Corporation for the Arts medica Collection.)

cooperative with procedures, to have less resistance to anesthetic induction, to have lower heart rate and blood pressure, to require fewer medications during the recovery period, and to take less time to first voiding and adequate fluid intake after a surgical procedure than children who were not formally prepared before their surgery.

The number of hospital admissions should be kept to a minimum and their length should be limited as much as possible. It is advisable to avoid hospitalization between the ages of 6 months and 4 years. Health professionals should encourage education about health, illness, and hospitals through television and in schools and should facilitate children's hospital tours and meetings with other children and their families who are or who have recently been in the hospital. All children should participate in an organized program preparing them for the experiences associated

consultations, to provide education about the illness and its care, to model appropriate care, and to encourage increased participation in the management of the illness on the part of both the child and the parents, hopefully improving compliance with medical recommendations in the future.

Minimizing Stresses

A number of variables, enumerated in Table 32–4, affect the balance of positive and negative outcomes from a child's hospitalization. What a child and family experience and learn from a hospital stay is strongly influenced by hospital procedures such as those outlined in Table 32–5 and by its health care professionals (Plank, 1971).

Numerous studies have demonstrated unequivocally that systematic preparation for hospitalization or surgery not only reduces children's psychological distress during and after a hospitalization but also results in more adaptive physiologic responses (Melamed and Ridley-Johnson, 1988). Prepared children have been documented to be more

Table 32–5 • Minimization of Stress

Prior preparation
  Television, school, and community programs about illness and hospitals
  Prehospitalization tours
  Systematic preparation for all planned procedures and hospitalizations
  Limited number and length of hospital stays
  Outpatient procedures, evaluation, and treatment whenever possible
  Involvement of parents in decisions about procedures and hospitalizations, their timing, choice of hospitals, and consultants
During hospitalization
  Rooming-in for parents, liberal visiting for others
  Child Life program (recreation and therapeutic play)
  Limited number of nurses and other caregivers
  Child's choice of clothes, food, activities
  Maximal mobility
  Pain control
  Ongoing communication with both children and parents
Procedures
  Limited number
  Preparation of child
  Child's choice of when, where, with whom
  Limited waiting time
  Parents accompany and support child
Hospital structure
  Rooming-in facilities
  Play space
  Waiting space near operating and recovery rooms
  Private rooms for parents
  Cheerful, child-oriented decor
  Single- and double-bed rooms

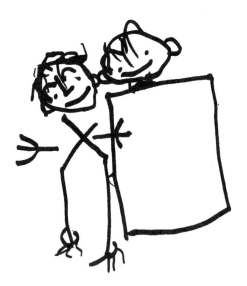

Figure 32–2. Four-year-old child's expression of feeling about the importance of parental presence in the hospital.

with planned surgical or diagnostic procedures (inpatient or outpatient) and hospital stays. Parents should participate in all aspects of planning for and care of children hospitalized or having outpatient procedures.

The factor under the most direct control of health care professionals is the nature of the hospital environment itself and the manner in which surgery and other procedures are carried out. Pediatric hospital units should have a trained staff of Child Life professionals who participate in decisions about the manner and scheduling of children's procedures and who are integrally involved in preparing children for hospitalization, surgery, and procedures. Every pediatric hospital should have a playroom with opportunities for recreation and developmentally appropriate activities to help children deal effectively with their illness, trauma, medical care, and hospitalization. School programs for children of all ages should be integrated into the larger Child Life program to facilitate learning from the child's experiences with illness and hospitalization, as well as from prescribed curricula. Psychologists, social workers, and psychiatrists are often helpful as members of the overall health care team.

Nurses should be assigned in such a way as to minimize the number of different adults caring for a child. Parents should be encouraged to stay with their child as much as possible, and liberal visiting hours should allow friends, teachers, and siblings to visit frequently. Pediatric hospitals can be constructed in such a way that children have opportunities both for being alone or with their family or close friends, and for group activities with their peers. This means that rooms with one or two beds and space for parents to stay are preferable to larger wards. Parents should be encouraged to participate in decision making and care as active members of the health care team (Fig. 32–2).

Procedures, even minor ones such as drawing blood, initiation of intravenous therapy, or radiographic studies, are best limited to those that are absolutely necessary for the child's management. Children should be honestly and appropriately informed about procedures, and, whenever possible, they should be performed at a time, with people, and in a place of the child's choice. Maintaining the child's mobility and autonomy and limiting pain and discomfort are important ways to safeguard the child's security and well-being.

The professionals caring for children in the hospital should be prepared to explain to children and their parents the mechanisms involved in their illness or injury, the plans for its care, and expected outcomes of treatment. They should facilitate and encourage children's taking the maximum possible control of necessary procedures and other aspects of managing their illness both during the hospitalization and after discharge.

It is important that hospital staff be prepared to support parents in their extremely demanding role as children's primary caretakers, both during the hospital stay and afterward. They should encourage participation in resource groups for parents and for older children and should refer parents to the increasing body of literature written for parents and children (Association for the Care of Children's Health, 1987) about surgery, hospitalization, and medical procedures. Health care professionals helping parents and children to cope with these intrusions should refer to the extensive materials available through the Association for the Care of Children's Health,* The Federation for Children with Special Needs,† and many others available commercially.

REFERENCES

Association for the Care of Children's Health (ACCH): Books for Children and Teenagers About Hospitalization, Illness, and Disabling Conditions. Washington, DC, 1987.

Davenport H, Werry J: The effect of general anesthesia, surgery, and hospitalization upon the behavior of children. Am J Orthopsych 40:806–824, 1970.

Douglas J: Early hospital admissions and later disturbances of behavior and learning. Dev Med Child Neurol 17:456–480, 1975.

Gabriel HP, Danilowicz D: Post-operative responses in "prepared" children after cardiac surgery. Br Heart J 40:1046–1051, 1978.

Melamed B, Ridley-Johnson R: Psychological preparation of families for hospitalization. J Dev Behav Pediatr 9:96–102, 1988.

Parmelee AH Jr: Children's illnesses and normal behavioral development: the role of caregivers. Zero to Three 13:4–10, 1993.

Perrin EC, Gerrity PS: There's a demon in your belly: children's understanding of illness. Pediatrics 67:841–849, 1981.

Perrin EC, Newacheck P, Pless IB, et al: Issues involved in the definition and classification of chronic health conditions. Pediatrics 91:787–793, 1993.

Plank E: Working With Children in Hospitals. Cleveland, Case Western Reserve University Press, 1971.

Quinton D, Rutter M: Early hospital admissions and later disturbances of behavior. Dev Med Child Neurol 18:447–459, 1976.

Scaife J, Campbell I: A comparison of the outcome of day care and inpatient treatment of pediatric surgical cases. J Child Psychol Psychiatry 29:185–198, 1988.

Schonfeld, DJ: The child's cognitive understanding of illness. In Lewis M (ed): Child and Adolescent Psychiatry: A Comprehensive Textbook. Baltimore, Williams & Wilkins, 1992.

Solnit AJ: Hospitalization: an aid to physical and psychological health in childhood. Am J Dis Child 99:155–163, 1960.

Thompson R: Where we stand: twenty years of research on pediatric

*3615 Wisconsin Avenue, NW, Washington, DC 20016 (202) 244-1801
†95 Berkeley Street, Boston, MA 02116 (617) 482-2915

hospitalization and health care. Child Health Care 14:200–210, 1986.

Thompson RH, Vernon DT: Research on children's behavior after hospitalization. J Dev Behav Pediatr 14:28–35, 1993.

Vernon D, Foley J, Sipowicz R, Shulman J: The Psychological Responses of Children to Hospitalization and Illness. Springfield, IL, Charles C Thomas, 1975.

Vernon DT, Thompson RH: Research on the effect of experimental interventions on children's behavior after hospitalization. J Dev Behav Pediatr 14:36–44, 1993.

33 Early Health Crises and Vulnerable Children

Brian W. C. Forsyth

 Sometimes in early infancy, transient health problems of varying severity lead to complete recovery in the child but lingering feelings in the parents that the child is sickly and fragile. This "vulnerable child syndrome," with its separation and infantilization interactional issues, has important consequences for the development and behavior of the child. Other factors can precipitate the syndrome, and other outcomes are possible. By contrast, most children and their families respond appropriately to these challenges, and some do so with remarkable resilience.

Green and Solnit (1964) first coined the phrase "the vulnerable child syndrome" in a paper describing children with severe behavioral and learning problems, all of whom had a history of experiencing a serious illness or accident early in life. Although these children had recovered fully from the early life-threatening events, their parents continued to view them as abnormally susceptible to illness or death. These continuing parental fears and the resulting abnormal interactions between the parents and their children were considered responsible for the children's abnormal psychological development. Although this concept had been described previously in the literature, this landmark paper with its use of the term *vulnerable child* brought focus to a psychodynamic process in which the major etiologic factor was the parents' perceptions of vulnerability rather than other factors that might make the child truly vulnerable for adverse outcomes.

Presently, the term *vulnerable child syndrome* is reserved for children who demonstrate all aspects of the syndrome as described by Green and Solnit (Table 33–1), whereas the term *vulnerable child* is commonly used to refer to instances in which parents perceive their children to be abnormally susceptible to illness or death, although the children do not necessarily exhibit the consequences of the parents' abnormal perceptions.

There is a spectrum of vulnerability, with the vulnerable child syndrome representing the extreme end of the spectrum. Both the etiology of vulnerability and the resulting sequelae may be varied; less severe experiences than a near-death experience, such as problems with crying behavior in early infancy, may cause parents to view their child as abnormally vulnerable (Forsyth and Canny, 1991). Similarly, the expression of the disorder might be different; for example, a child who is viewed by parents as vulnerable might be brought to the physician more frequently for minor medical complaints but might not necessarily demonstrate the psychological or behavioral consequences described in the vulnerable child syndrome.

Prevalence of Vulnerability

The true prevalence of perceived vulnerability is difficult to ascertain because it is dependent on the way in which vulnerability is defined. In a community-based study of 1095 children ages 4 to 8 years who were being seen by health care providers, 10% of parents viewed their children as vulnerable using the Child Vulnerability Scale (Forsyth et al, 1996). Twenty-one percent of all mothers reported that they had had prior fears that their child might die. However, using the definitions employed in the study, only 1.8% of children had all three features of the vulnerable child syndrome: (1) prior fears that the child might die, (2) continuing perceptions of vulnerability, and (3) behavior problems (as defined by the Child Behavior Checklist). In another study conducted in medical clinics, 27% of children were described by their parents as vulnerable (i.e., "uniquely threatened by an episode of illness"), although for 40% of these there was no medical basis for concern (Levy, 1980).

Etiologic Factors in the Development of Vulnerability

A number of different types of events and illnesses have been described in the literature as contributing to increased parental perceptions of vulnerability. Examples include

Table 33–1 • Diagnostic Criteria for the Vulnerable Child Syndrome

1. An event early in the child's life that the parent considered to be life-threatening
2. The parent's continuing unrealistic belief that the child is especially susceptible to illness or death
3. The presence of a behavioral or learning problem in the child

From Parker S, Zuckerman B (eds): Developmental and Behavioral Pediatrics. Philadelphia, Lippincott-Raven, 1995.

complications of pregnancy (Burger et al, 1993), premature birth (Perrin, 1989), neonatal jaundice (Kemper, Forsyth, and McCarthy, 1989), hospitalization for infectious illnesses, and problems of feeding and crying behavior in early infancy (Table 33–2) (Forsyth and Canny, 1991). Some of these are truly life-threatening events, whereas others are minor problems that are medically insignificant; it is the parents' understanding and beliefs about the problem that are most important in contributing to perceptions of vulnerability, rather than the reality of the diagnosis as understood by the physician (Carey, 1969). A particular example of this has been referred to in the literature as "nondisease" to describe such entities as innocent cardiac murmurs (Bergman and Stamm, 1967) and sickle cell trait (Hampton et al, 1974), which to the physician are of little consequence but which parents may view with concern and, as a result, treat their child differently.

In general, the earlier in a child's life that an event occurs, the more likely it is to contribute to the parents' perceptions that the child is vulnerable. In some instances, the event that initiates the parents' fears for a child may not be related to a condition of the child but may have occurred before the child's birth, for example, an earlier miscarriage or the experience of the death of a previous child. Also, a crisis that occurred around the time of a mother's pregnancy, such as an illness or death of a close relative, might contribute to irrational fears of death. The newborn period is a time when parents are likely to be particularly anxious about their child's well-being, and medical care that is insensitive to their understanding and concerns might contribute to long-standing perceptions of vulnerability.

In a review of published research related to the vulnerable child syndrome, Thomasgard and Metz (1995) have identified a number of other parental factors that have been associated with vulnerability: for example, perceptions of vulnerability are more prevalent among women who are unmarried, are younger, are less educated, and have lower family incomes. Psychological factors that can contribute to a parent's tendency to view a child as vulnerable include decreased social support and the lack of emotional warmth in relationships, maternal depression particularly in the postpartum period, and a lack of sense of competence as a parent and feeling less in control of one's life (Estroff et al, 1994). Green and Solnit, in their original description of the vulnerable child syndrome, also identified as a predisposing factor a mother's "displacement of unacceptable feelings toward the child or of unacceptable thoughts and reactions associated with the birth of the child." However, it is important to emphasize that the vulnerable child syndrome is a result of the parent's view of the child as somehow defective and is not due to a lack of emotional bonding between the parent and child.

Clinical Presentation of the Vulnerable Child

The vulnerable child may be seen by the clinician with a variety of different types of problems divided by Green and Solnit (1964) into the following major categories:

1. Difficulties with separation. An example of this is a parent's reluctance to leave the child in the care of a baby-sitter. The parent's sense of vulnerability and the resulting abnormality in interactions with the child lead to a decrease in the child's sense of autonomy and independence. Parents may complain of the child's sleep problems, although this may in part be because the child is sleeping in the parents' bed or the parents are regularly checking on the sleeping child to make sure that the child is alive.

2. Symptoms of infantilization. In some cases, the parents are unable to set appropriate disciplinary limits for the child and are overindulgent and excessively protective of the child. The child may become disobedient and argumentative and may refuse to eat. Often the child's episodes of negative behavior disintegrate into physically fighting the parent with hitting and biting, and the parent is unable to handle the behavior appropriately. Even though parental overprotection may be one of the characteristics of the vulnerable child syndrome, there may be other reasons for parental overprotection, for example, young parents with their first child may be overprotective without perceiving their child to be abnormally susceptible to illness or death (see Chapter 16).

3. Overconcern with minor medical problems. A parent who perceives his or her child to be vulnerable is often a frequent visitor to the clinician for what the clinician considers to be only minor medical problems. There is often excessive focus on such things as the regularity of the child's bowel movements and complaints that the child has a sickly appearance or has circles under the eyes. The child may have psychosomatic symptoms such as recurrent abdominal pain or headaches and may have frequent absences from school. Sometimes the Munchausen by proxy syndrome must be considered.

4. School underachievement. Even though school un-

Table 33–2 • Antecedents of the Vulnerable Child

Preexisting
  Death of a relative or previous child early in life
  Prior miscarriage or stillbirth
Pregnancy related
  Pregnancy complications (e.g., vaginal bleeding)
  Abnormal screening results (e.g., abnormal alpha-fetoprotein)
  Delivery complications
Newborn period
  Prematurity
  Neonatal illness or complications
  Congenital abnormalities
  Hyperbilirubinemia
  False positive results of screening (e.g., phenylketonuria)
Early childhood
  Excessive crying, colic, spitting up
  Any serious illness
  Admission to hospital for such things as "to rule out sepsis"
  Self-limited infectious illnesses (e.g., croup, gastroenteritis)

From Parker S, Zuckerman B (eds): Developmental and Behavioral Pediatrics. Philadelphia, Lippincott-Raven, 1995.

derachievement was initially described by Green and Solnit, it is usually not the major presenting problem in the vulnerable child syndrome. The child's school performance may suffer because of distractible, hyperactive behavior in the classroom. The parents' earlier reluctance to separate from the child and the unspoken fear that the child is unsafe out of the parents' presence are transferred to the child. The resulting preoccupation and anxiety interfere with the child's abilities to concentrate and learn.

Making the Diagnosis

Whenever a clinician sees a child with one or more of the aforementioned problems, the possible etiologic role of an earlier event and abnormal parental perceptions of vulnerability should be considered (Fig. 33–1). To make the diagnosis, the clinician must obtain a history that not only identifies the initiating event but also captures the quality of the parents' fears of the risk to the child and provides insight into the abnormal interaction between parent and child. In addition, history taking that is sensitive to the fears of the parent helps to initiate the therapeutic process by conveying to the parent a sense of understanding and empathy.

Often it is necessary to obtain again the child's medical history, beginning from the mother's pregnancy and including history in the family of illness or death. Because parents are truly concerned about their child, they usually welcome the suggestion that a full review of everything that has gone on in the past may shed light on the child's present problems. Whenever the parent reports a prior problem or concern, no matter how minor it was, the details of what the doctor said at the time and what the

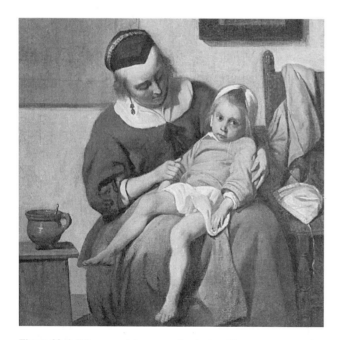

Figure 33–1. When parental concern about minor illness seems excessive, consider the vulnerable child syndrome. (Gabriel Metsu: The Sick Child. With permission from the Rijksmuseum-Stichting Museum, Amsterdam.)

Table 33–3 • Prevention and Management of the Vulnerable Child Syndrome

Prevention at the time of the health crisis
  Understand and discuss parents' beliefs about even minor problems.
  Do not use terms that suggest a diagnostic entity when there is no real evidence supporting it, e.g., "allergy," "colitis."
  Recognize when parents are particularly anxious about an event and specifically deal with their fears.
Management
  After a thorough evaluation, provide a clear statement of the child's physical health.
  Help the parents understand the link between the present problem and their past anxieties regarding their child's health.
  Support and advise parents about interacting with their child in an appropriate manner.
  Make a referral for a psychiatric evaluation and treatment if necessary.

parents understood and feared might be helpful in making the diagnosis. Empathic comments such as "That must have been very frightening to you" and questions such as "Did you at any time fear that he might not make it?" often allow the parents to express their real concerns. If, on the other hand, the event was truly of little concern to the parents, they usually say so. Attention should also be paid to issues of separation both early in the child's life and when the child starts day care or school. Questions should be asked about the parents' level of worry when separated from their child and how comfortable they were leaving the child with a baby-sitter.

Although it is unlikely to be useful in a clinical setting, the Child Vulnerability Scale was developed to be used in research to measure parental perceptions of their children's vulnerability (Forsyth et al, 1996). Both this measure and the adaptation referred to as the Vulnerable Child Scale have been helpful in identifying factors that contribute to vulnerability.

Management

Suggestions for the prevention and management of the vulnerable child syndrome are summarized in Table 33–3.

PREVENTION

Because a parent's understanding of the severity and implications of an illness or event might be very different from reality, it is important that even in minor illnesses the clinician take time to understand parents' beliefs and to discuss them appropriately. For example, a falsely positive screening test for cystic fibrosis might create lingering fears for the parents even after the confirmatory test has proved the initial result to be incorrect. Presenting such findings cannot be done without giving an explanation of the different natures of the two tests (screening versus confirmatory) and making conclusive statements that leave no doubt about the correct diagnosis. Another example is in managing an infant with colic. Suggesting that the infant is allergic to the formula and requires a "special formula" implies to the parents that the child has a medical problem that requires a specific treatment. In contrast, if the clinician describes colic as a self-limited condition affecting normal infants, the risk of parents' perceiving their child as vulnerable can be diminished (see Chapter 37). Some parents may wish to change the formula, but even so, a statement by the clinician ahead of time that the infant can go back to the regular formula within a few weeks serves to emphasize to the parents that this is a self-limited condition without long-lasting effects. Similarly, when discharging a child from the hospital after an acute illness, the clinician should review the diagnosis with the parents, emphasize that recovery is or will be complete, and point out that the child is no more vulnerable to illness than other children.

When a clinician recognizes that a parent is particularly anxious after an illness or other event that could later contribute to perceptions of vulnerability, it may be helpful to ask further questions, such as "Has this brought to mind other things that you've experienced before?" and "Is there anything that you are particularly worried about?" Such questions enable the clinician to deal specifically with the parents' fears and to point out the erroneous links they may have made between two unrelated events. It might also be helpful to question the parents at a later date about an event. Having parents relate their understanding of what went on might help the clinician identify any erroneous beliefs.

APPROACH TO MANAGEMENT

Whenever it is recognized that parental perceptions of vulnerability are affecting or may affect a child's behavior or development, an approach that might be helpful includes the following:

1. The clinician should take an in-depth history and perform a conspicuously meticulous physical examination before giving the parents a clear statement that the child is physically healthy. There should be no equivocal comments, such as "He doesn't look too bad." Conducting laboratory tests just to prove to the parents that there is nothing physically wrong can have the opposite effect of suggesting to them that the clinician is continuing to look for something wrong but has not yet found it.
2. The clinician needs to help the parents understand and accept the notion that the child is considered special by the family and that this derives from their response to earlier events. It is helpful to explain this process as a recognized entity and not something that is particularly unique to them—that there is a way parents who experience the level of anxiety that they have continue to be fearful for their child and that this has an effect on the way they interact with their child, sometimes with a deleterious effect on the child.
3. The parents need to be supported in dealing with the child in a more appropriate manner. Advice should be given on setting consistent limits and discontinuing infantilizing behaviors. Issues of overprotection and problems of separation may need to be examined, and parents may need to be advised on how to respond differently to somatic complaints. In in-

stances when a child probably does have an underlying abnormality (e.g., cerebral palsy following premature birth) but the parents have exaggerated perceptions of their child's vulnerability, the primary care clinician should help the parents distinguish between those issues that are of real concern and those that relate to their past experiences and anxieties. In doing this, the clinician often needs to give parents very specific explanations and advice on how to respond to their child in various circumstances.

4. Although many of these problems can be managed by a primary care clinician, in some instances a referral for psychiatric evaluation and therapy may be necessary. Whether the focus of treatment is primarily on the child or the parents, the importance of the parental perceptions of vulnerability in sustaining the problem needs to remain a central part of the therapy.

In most instances, the time taken by a clinician to establish a diagnosis of vulnerable child syndrome does not necessarily have to be long, particularly if the possibility of the diagnosis is entertained from the beginning and the history is obtained in a systematic fashion, searching for etiologic factors and developing an understanding of the parents' perceptions of the child's vulnerability.

Resiliency

Even though the focus of this chapter is primarily on the adverse psychological effects of early health crises, the concept of resiliency in children is in some respects the other side of the coin from vulnerability and also needs to be considered. The vulnerable child syndrome does not develop in all children who experience a serious life-threatening event, and after an acute, self-limited event, most parents continue to have relatively normal perceptions of their child's vulnerability. The term *resiliency* is most often used to describe the protective processes that result in more positive outcomes for individuals who are at risk because of either adverse social factors (e.g., poverty) or psychological factors (e.g., maternal depression). There is also a body of literature that describes resiliency among children with chronic illnesses or conditions, children who thrive and do well psychologically despite their handicaps.

It is important to recognize that resiliency is not just the result of one or even multiple factors but is a process with many contributing factors. For any individual, the sense of resiliency may change over time and may be influenced by developmental changes (Rutter, 1993). Both preceding and succeeding circumstances may be important. There may, at times, be a turning point in a person's life, when the individual becomes more resilient and less vulnerable, with a resulting change in that person's path in life. From the Kauai Longitudinal Study in which 698 infants were studied into adulthood, Werner (1989) and colleagues identified three different areas that contribute to the development of resiliency: (1) individual factors such as temperament (high activity, sociability, and attention span), cognitive skills, and an internal locus of control, (2) familial factors such as the concern of parents for the well-being of their children despite their own experience of stresses such as poverty or marital discord, and (3) external support factors such as the presence of another caring adult in the life of a child. For children with chronic illness, a number of familial factors that contribute to resiliency have been described. These include the development of good communication within families, the engagement in active coping efforts, the ability to attribute a positive meaning to the situation, and the ability to balance the illness with other family needs (Patterson and Blum, 1996) (see Chapter 34).

There has been little examination of what factors might decrease parental perceptions of vulnerability following an acute, self-limited problem early in a child's life and protect the child from possible adverse psychological consequences. However, it is likely that some of the same individual and familial factors that contribute to the development of resiliency for children with chronic illnesses might also protect a child experiencing an acute health crisis early in infancy. Also, for the child perceived as vulnerable by his or her parents, there is the potential that intervening factors later in development might play a role in contributing to a sense of resiliency rather than vulnerability.

REFERENCES

Bergman AB, Stamm SJ: The morbidity of cardiac nondisease in school-children. N Engl J Med 276:1008–1013, 1967.

Burger J, Horwitz SM, Forsyth BWC, et al: Psychological sequelae of medical complications during pregnancy. Pediatrics 91:566–571, 1993.

Carey WB: Psychologic sequelae of early infancy health crises. Clin Pediatr 8:459–463, 1969.

Estroff DB, Yando R, Burke K, Synder D: Perceptions of preschoolers' vulnerability by mothers who had delivered preterm. J Pediatr Psychol 19:709–721, 1994.

Forsyth BWC, Canny PF: Perceptions of vulnerability 3 1/2 years after problems of feeding and crying behavior in early infancy. Pediatrics 88:757–763, 1991.

Forsyth BWC, Horwitz SM, Leventhal JM, Burger J: The Child Vulnerability Scale: an instrument to measure parental perceptions of child vulnerability. J Pediatr Psychol 21:89–101, 1996.

Green M, Solnit AJ: Reactions to the threatened loss of a child: a vulnerable child syndrome. Pediatrics 34:58–66, 1964.

Hampton ML, Anderson J, Lavizzo BS, Bergman AB: Sickle cell "nondisease": a potentially serious public health problem. Am J Dis Child 128:58–61, 1974.

Kemper K, Forsyth B, McCarthy P: Jaundice, terminating breast-feeding, and the vulnerable child. Pediatrics 84:773–778, 1989.

Levy JC: Vulnerable children: parent's perspectives and the use of medical care. Pediatrics 65:956–963, 1980.

Patterson J, Blum RW: Risk and resilience among children and youth with disabilities. Arch Pediatr Adolesc Med 150:692–698, 1996.

Perrin E, West P, Culley B: Is my child normal yet? Correlates of vulnerability. Pediatrics 83:355–363, 1989.

Rutter M: Resilience: some conceptual considerations. J Adolesc Health 14:626–631, 1993.

Thomasgard M, Metz WP: The vulnerable child syndrome revisited. J Dev Behav Pediatr 16:47–53, 1995.

Werner EE: High risk children in young adulthood: a longitudinal study from birth to 32 years. Am J Orthopsychiatry 59:72–81, 1989.

34 Chronic Illness

James M. Perrin • Ute Thyen

 Chronic illness and disabilities both affect and are affected by the development and behavior of children. Although only a minority of children have serious problems of this sort, the complexity of the diagnosis and management of these children and their families calls for extensive pediatric involvement with much interdisciplinary collaboration and coordination of care. Special pediatric roles other than that of giving medical care include identifying developmental-behavioral consequences, assessing family strengths, educating about illness, and planning for education.

Nature and Extent of Chronic Illness

CHRONIC HEALTH CONDITIONS: A DEFINITION

Chronic illnesses in childhood include a wide variety of health conditions, varying from rare chromosomal disorders to rheumatoid arthritis, epilepsy, asthma, juvenile diabetes, and malignancies. Children and their families face a bewildering number of conditions — most rare, some described in only a handful of cases. Among chronic *physical* conditions, only asthma and recurrent otitis media occur more often than 1 per 100 children. All neurologic diseases (including seizure disorders) taken together approach a prevalence of 1%. Mental health conditions, including those diagnosed as attention-deficit hyperactivity disorder, also occur with relatively high frequency. Other physical conditions are relatively to extremely rare. The experience of child health professionals with chronic conditions differs substantially from that in adult medicine, in which a much higher percentage of patients have a smaller number of relatively common chronic illnesses, such as coronary artery disease, malignancies, adult-onset diabetes, or back pain.

The term *condition* includes both illnesses (diseases) and disabilities. Examples of chronic *illnesses* are asthma, Crohn disease, diabetes, and epilepsy. Disabilities include cerebral palsy, loss of limb function, vision or hearing impairment, or mental retardation. Illness and disability may coexist in the same child and may have different manifestations at changing stages of the illness or the child's growth and development. Children and adolescents with chronic conditions also include those who have no clinical evidence of illness or disability at the time of assessment, for example, symptom-free infants who test positive for human immunodeficiency virus, apparently healthy children on continued replacement therapy or medications, or children during a symptom-free phase of a relapsing condition. The term *handicap* generally describes the social constrictions when the disability creates a barrier to normal participation in social life. Strategies to prevent disease may differ from those to prevent disability or handicap. Any of these levels may also influence behavior and development.

Although the treatment, outcomes, and clinical services for different chronic conditions vary substantially, children with chronic conditions and their families share many common tasks: adaptation to life with a chronic condition, mastering variations in usual developmental transitions, and adjusting to the economic and psychosocial impact of a chronic condition. Many studies of the developmental and behavioral implications of chronic conditions in childhood have examined individual conditions. Nevertheless, an important line of research recognizes the common consequences and service needs of children with a diverse group of conditions, and program organization should reflect these common needs.

General definitions of chronic conditions typically address two main criteria: (1) duration of illness, usually at least 3 to 12 months or the likelihood of permanence (e.g., leukemia, diabetes), and (2) severity, as indicated by limitations in age-appropriate activities, need for long or recurrent hospitalizations, or need for nursing care beyond that generally experienced by healthy children with occasional acute, self-limiting illnesses. This definition of a chronic condition focuses more on the consequences of the conditions than the specific diagnosis.

The use of a generic or category approach to define chronic conditions encourages recognition of the common behavioral and developmental characteristics of all children with these conditions. This approach also allows attention to the characteristics of a condition that may influence behavior and development: duration, age of onset, interference with age-appropriate activities, visibility, expected survival, course (stable versus progressive), level of certainty (episodic versus predictable), mobility, physiologic and sensory impact, impact on cognition and communication, and psychological and social impact (Perrin et al, 1993). These dimensions, which may fluctuate over time, characterize a child's condition more effectively than diagnosis alone and help to frame the impact of the condition on social and psychological growth.

335

EPIDEMIOLOGY OF CHRONIC CONDITIONS IN CHILDHOOD

Although most individual chronic conditions are rare, in the aggregate they cause morbidity for many children and adolescents. Analyses of the 1994 National Health Interview Survey on Disability indicate that 12.9% of children and adolescents have a health-related disability (Harahan et al, 1996). Other studies indicate rates varying from 7% to 31%, depending on the severity of the condition and whether children with mental and development conditions are included along with those with physical conditions. Among conditions that (1) limit the usual daily activities of children, (2) require special therapeutic or diagnostic services, or (3) limit the ability to do regular schoolwork in children older than 6 years, the most frequently reported condition was learning disability (29.5%), followed by speech problems (13.1%), mental retardation (6.8%), asthma (6.4%), and mental or emotional disorders (6.3%) (From the CDC, 1995). These data indicate the higher prevalence of developmental and mental health conditions than physical disorders among chronic problems that affect usual daily activities.

Studies limited to chronic physical disorders generally find that 10% to 20% of children and adolescents have such conditions, although most conditions are mild, and only 2% to 4% of children have severe chronic conditions (Newacheck and Stoddard, 1994; Newacheck and Taylor, 1992). These severe chronic conditions include severe asthma, congenital heart disease, inflammatory bowel disease, arthritis, sickle cell disease, malignancies, and seizure disorders. Severe chronic conditions typically interfere on a daily basis with the child's usual activities and cause major limitations in functioning. These children average 10 days per year in bed and 11 days of school missed annually. They use medical services much more than do other children: 16% are hospitalized each year and they have an average of 16 physician contacts per year.

Boys have higher rates of chronic physical conditions than do females, some because of an X-linked inheritance pattern (e.g., hemophilia, Duchenne muscular dystrophy); in others because male gender is an independent risk factor for adverse outcomes (sequelae of prematurity, childhood accidents and injuries); and in others for unknown reasons. Poor children also have higher rates of chronic conditions and often more severe illness (partially attributable to barriers to care) and higher rates of long-term conditions resulting from low birth weight and/or prematurity or secondary to childhood injury. Specifically, poor children are more likely to develop severe asthma, they run twice the risk of ketoacidosis if diabetic, they have higher rates of severe iron deficiency anemia, and they have two to three times the risk of development of permanent complications from bacterial meningitis (Starfield, 1991).

In years past, many severely ill children died young. Advances in medical and surgical technology and in the delivery of health services over the past quarter century have meant that the large majority (over 90%) of children, even with very severe conditions, survive to young adulthood. Today, almost all children with conditions such as leukemia, cystic fibrosis, or congenital heart diseases survive to young adulthood, although often with significant physical or psychological morbidity. Where long-term planning for many such children appeared to have little purpose before these advances, such planning has taken a central role in child health care.

The epidemiology of chronic conditions in childhood continues to change. New genetic interventions may eradicate some diseases; those relatively rare conditions that continue to have high mortality rates will likely undergo technologic breakthroughs. Nevertheless, given the high levels of survival, aggregate rates of severe chronic conditions in childhood should remain stable. New conditions such as acquired immunodeficiency syndrome in children and adolescents contribute to increases but are offset by the decrease in such conditions as neural tube defects, partly attributable to antenatal screening or folate supplementation during pregnancy. (The incidence in Scotland, for example, which has had the highest incidence of neural tube defects, decreased from 3.0 per 1000 births in the early 1970s to 0.6 in the late 1980s; the US incidence decreased from 1.3 per 1000 to 0.6 during the same time frame and may decrease even further with the folate supplementation of grain supplies.) Antenatal screening for Down syndrome has decreased the prevalence of this condition.

While the overall numbers of children surviving prematurity or low birth weight have increased during the past 3 decades, the incidence of major sequelae has not. Extremely low–birth weight infants have substantial risk of visual and hearing defects, chronic lung disease, cerebral palsy, or mental retardation, but this increase among children who previously would not have survived has been offset by the benefits of modern neonatology for quantitatively larger groups of infants with low birth weight or gestational age of more than 32 weeks who are much more likely to survive with no impairment than in years past.

Impact of Chronic Illness on Development and Behavior

PSYCHOSOCIAL FACTORS AFFECTING CHRONIC CONDITIONS

Most chronic conditions result from a combination of predisposing constitutional factors, often influenced by psychological and environmental factors. The etiology of most diseases is biological (e.g., inborn errors of metabolism or chromosomal abnormalities), although some conditions reflect primarily environmental factors (e.g., lead poisoning) and others mostly social (e.g., head injury secondary to preventable accidents). Thus, social and psychological factors influence the causation of some chronic conditions.

Social and psychological factors also affect the course and severity of chronic illness. Poor children especially lack access to health care, coordination of care, and information and other resources to cope with the illness. Social and community factors can influence the child's or family's ability to normalize life with a chronic illness or disability and thus affect outcomes of chronic conditions, personal aspirations, and preparation for work and independent living. Psychological factors may affect adjustment to the illness and adherence to treatment regimens, perceptions of vulnerability in patients and parents (see Chapter 33), and susceptibility to secondary mental health problems in both the child and the family.

Responses to chronic conditions may be understood by viewing the condition as a chronic stressor. Family members challenged by stress (the affected child as well as parents and siblings) may experience multiple and conflicting emotions and use a wide range of cognitive and behavioral strategies that have both problem-solving and emotion-regulating functions in the process of coping (Lazarus and Folkman, 1984). *Coping* describes a dynamic process in which emotions and appraisal of the stress continually affect and influence each other and change the relationship between the individual and the environment. *Adjustment*, different from coping, describes the outcomes of coping at a specific point in time. Most children and adolescents adhere to certain patterns of coping strategies, dependent on prior experience, learning, beliefs, culture, and environmental influences, although mechanisms change over time and at different stages of development. Although coping mechanisms in children have had less study than in adults, age, gender, and situation appear to predict coping strategy, which is also highly variable among children (Wertlieb, Weigel, and Feldstein, 1987). Children and adults make use of a wide variety of coping patterns. Although problem-focused coping strategies have been associated with more positive emotions in response to stress, different coping strategies may be adaptive depending on the situational circumstances and options available. Clinicians should observe and support the child's preferred coping style rather than change it. A very limited number of coping strategies in an individual should alert the clinician that the coping repertoire may be restricted and adaptive mechanisms poor. Changing clinical practice patterns, which pay more attention to self-help activities, strategies to aid empowerment, sharing of responsibility, and listening to children as they understand their illness and try to cope with it, may benefit children (Perrin, Ayoub, and Willett, 1993). (See also Chapter 8 regarding temperament and coping in children with chronic illnesses and disabilities.)

EFFECTS OF CHRONIC CONDITIONS ON DEVELOPMENT

Adjustment to chronic illness often involves transitions different from those experienced by other children and families, as well as common transitions made more difficult by the presence of a chronic condition. For many families, a key transition takes place at discharge from the hospital, when major responsibility for the child's care transfers from hospital staff to family. Other unusual transitions may include repeat hospitalizations. More typical transitions in a child's life include starting school, the development of autonomy in preadolescents, or initiation of sexual relationships in adolescents, all potentially changed by the presence of a chronic condition. Furthermore, the stage of the child's development at the onset of a chronic condition can affect coping and adjustment. Being born with a chronic illness or congenital abnormality carries with it a different set of coping issues from acquiring the diagnosis of leukemia as a teenager.

In infancy, illness may affect basic growth, cause failure to thrive, and bring about excessive fatigue. The child may be less responsive than other children or may have physical characteristics that interfere with normal nurturing responses of parents. In blind children, for example, normal responsive smiling does not develop, and parents may perceive this phenomenon as indicating an unresponsive, unrewarding infant. Infants with hearing disability show delay in language acquisition, difficulties in communication, and higher rates of behavior problems.

Extensive medical or surgical care during this period often makes the child special and vulnerable in the eyes of parents, and the sense of vulnerability may persist for years, even when medical and surgical care cease.

As toddlers, children should become more independent and explore their environment vigorously. Chronic illness may slow the development of early independence, diminish the child's resilience, and delay the acquisition of normal developmental milestones. It may limit the child's developing sense of competence and task mastery. For school-aged children, frequent absences resulting from illness interfere with learning and usual socialization. Children with visible conditions may feel different or may be subject to teasing. Normal separation from family in early school years may become more difficult because of needs for additional care by parents or increased time at home rather than in school.

Adolescents must develop a new sense of identity, work on their individual identities, develop increasingly adult forms of sexuality, and maintain their educational and vocational development. Many chronic illnesses force continuing dependence on caregivers for medical care or other in-home treatments. Attempts to develop independence in adolescence may lead to rebellion and denial, such as the teenager with diabetes who stops monitoring glucose or diet or who changes insulin dosages whimsically. Sexual development may be affected by disease directly (as with myelomeningocele) or by fears of sexual inadequacy (as in cystic fibrosis). Much of the health care for children and adolescents with chronic illness emphasizes the specific condition they have, neglecting other necessary elements of health supervision and prevention. Teenagers with chronic conditions may require more careful preparation and counseling regarding sexuality than do other children. Chronic illness may affect competitiveness in athletic activities, although health professionals and parents just as commonly underestimate the athletic capabilities of teenagers with chronic illness. Like children without illness, those who are less active in athletics should find other activities that allow them to excel and enhance their self-esteem.

Chronic illness may hamper the development of appropriate individual identity. The development of an appropriate identity emphasizes being a child or adolescent rather than having a disease. Parents, professionals, and adolescents themselves often generalize from their disease to the whole person, labeling the youngster a diabetic or a leukemic, rather than a child or teenager with diabetes. All involved should be encouraged to use "people first" rather than "disease first" language (Table 34–1).

Table 34–1 • Factors That Influence Development and Behavior Among Children With Chronic Health Conditions

Illness or condition characteristics (other than specific diagnosis)
Severity (physiologic or sensory impact)
Duration
Age of onset
Interference with age-appropriate activities
Expected survival
Course (stable versus progressive)
Certainty (predictable versus uncertain)
Impact on mobility
Impact on cognition and communication
Pain
Child factors
Gender
Intelligence and communication skills
Temperament
Coping skills and patterns
Family factors
Family functioning
Parental mental health
Household structure (number of adults and children)
Socioeconomic status
Social factors
Cultural attitudes
Access to health care
Community resources
Geography
School and day care systems

DEVELOPMENT OF CHILDREN'S UNDERSTANDING OF ILLNESS

Children acquire understanding of illness mechanisms in a fashion similar to other areas of cognitive development (Perrin and Gerrity, 1981). Table 34–2 outlines this developmental sequence. Young children of preschool or early school age often associate causation of illness with misbehavior or not following rules. They believe at times that "you get sick by going out in the cold without your coat on." Similarly, getting well is thought to relate to following rules or the doctor's orders. Later, by about age 8 to 11

Table 34–2 • Growth in Understanding of Illness Mechanisms

Typical Age	Level of Understanding
4 to 6 years	Circular, magical, or global responses
6 to 8 years	Concrete, rigid responses with a "parrot-like" quality; little comprehension by the child; enumeration of symptoms, actions, or situations associated with illness
8 to 11 years	Increased generalization, with some indication of child's contribution to the response; quality of invariant causation remains
11 to 13 years	Beginning use of an underlying principle; greater delineation of causal agents of illnesses
Older than 14 years	Organized description of mechanisms underlying illness/recovery; abstract principles

Adapted with permission of Pediatrics from Perrin EC, Gerrity PS: There's a demon in your belly: children's understanding of illness. Pediatrics 67:841, 1981.

years, germ theory becomes prevalent, with the notion that bad germs get into the body and cause disease and that medicines generally help to get rid of germs. It is not until about age 14 years or later that children of average intelligence begin to have a notion of the interaction of host mechanisms and external events in the causation of disease and the role of body functions in recognizing or affecting disease states. It is at this age, too, that children begin to understand the interaction of body parts, that hearts and lungs are not only contiguous but also work together in important ways or that blood vessels interact with bones and joints in arthritis, for example.

Increasing effort goes to educating children about their chronic illnesses; however, few curricular materials that take into account these developmental changes in children's concepts of illness have been developed. Most pamphlets from disease-specific organizations are geared toward children of about the 9- to 11-year-old range, with little available for younger or older children. Recent studies suggest that the acquisition of sophisticated notions of the causation of illness are delayed among children with chronic illnesses compared with apparently healthy children. This finding is unexpected, insofar as a youngster having regular daily experience with illness would be expected to more quickly develop an understanding of the illness. On the other hand, health professionals (physicians, nurses, and developmental psychologists) tend to explain illness to their patients in terminology and concepts appropriate for 9- to 11-year-olds. Enhancing a youngster's understanding of his or her own illness requires developmentally appropriate educational activities.

As children progress from childhood to young adulthood, they should take increasing responsibility for self-management of their chronic condition as part of the usual process of developing independence and autonomy. Application of developmental concepts along with knowledge about how children understand illness and how they use strengths, resources, and skills to cope help clinicians care effectively for children and adolescents with chronic conditions.

BEHAVIORAL IMPACT OF CHRONIC CONDITIONS

Chronic conditions in children increase the risk of associated psychological and behavioral problems. Most larger, community-based studies indicate an approximate doubling of these rates among children with chronic conditions compared with apparently healthy controls. (For a comprehensive review, see Thompson and Gustafson, 1996.) Meta-analyses of behavioral or developmental issues in children with chronic conditions support higher levels of total adjustment problems, with increased rates of both internalizing and externalizing difficulties, and lower self-esteem (Bennett, 1994; Lavigne and Faier-Routman, 1992). Nonetheless, behavioral and psychological differences between apparently healthy children and those with chronic conditions, albeit significant, are generally small, and most children and adolescents with chronic conditions have scores on scales of behavior, mood, or social adaptation within the normal ranges. Of interest is the finding of little variation among different chronic conditions in rates of psychological or behavioral problems. This approximate doubling of risk appears to affect all children with chronic conditions, regardless of the specific diagnosis. The main exception to this rule is that children with chronic conditions affecting the central nervous system directly or indirectly have much higher risk of maladjustment.

Both cognitive impairment and mental health problems may result from the illness directly (e.g., hydrocephalus, brain malformations, head injuries, epilepsy, or encephalitis) or indirectly through the effect of treatments (e.g., neurotoxic medications or radiation therapy in childhood leukemia; theophylline, adrenergics, or steroids for asthma; anticonvulsant medications). For example, the iatrogenic effects of treatment of leukemia have been associated with a mean decline of 10 intelligence quotient points, with attention, concentration, short-term memory, processing speed, sequencing ability, and visual-motor coordination being mostly affected (Cousens et al, 1991). The side effects of phenobarbital for seizure prophylaxis in young children include slowing of cognitive development and at times severe behavioral problems. (See Chapter 30 regarding toxins.)

The mechanisms of increased risk for adjustment problems have not been carefully studied. The increased risk of children with neurologic conditions points to the importance of some condition characteristics or at least the particular impact of central nervous system disease on behavior. Theoretical considerations drawing on knowledge of family development and parent-child interaction indicate parent and family adjustment as powerful mediators of the effect of chronic stress on the child. Maternal self-esteem and depression are highly correlated with child psychological status in many studies, as is high perceived stress in the child and family environment. Psychological difficulties presumably follow from the demands that a chronic condition places upon a child and family beyond the complexities of normal development and psychological growth. Surprisingly, disease severity does not seem to have an impact on child adjustment (Perrin, MacLean, and Perrin, 1989). Although it might be expected that children with the most severe illnesses would have the highest risk of problems in adjustment, few studies have found any association of severity and adjustment. Indeed, some early studies found that children with less severe forms of a condition had greater problems with psychological adjustment than those with more severe forms. These earlier findings do not appear to be supported in more recent studies. Overall, the level of intellectual functioning appears to have an impact on adjustment, with children with lower levels expressing more behavior problems and poorer social functioning. Higher levels of intellectual functioning may protect children with chronic conditions from maladjustment. Whether a condition is congenital or acquired later in childhood or adolescence and the longitudinal effects of course and duration of the condition on behavior have not been well studied.

CHRONIC CONDITIONS: IMPLICATIONS FOR EDUCATION AND WORK

Attending school is important for children's academic, social, and emotional development, yet children with chronic conditions miss a substantial number of school days each year for several reasons: (1) exacerbations of the condition, (2) acute illnesses not related to the chronic condition but likely to have a more protracted course in a child with compromised health status, (3) hospitalizations for treatments, (4) physician or hospital appointments, (5) psychological problems secondary to peer reactions, lack of confidence, or poor academic achievement resulting in school avoidance, and (6) perceptions of vulnerability in parents and inappropriate health beliefs (Weitzman, 1986). Inadequate school nursing care may exclude children who must take medicine, are incontinent or need respiratory therapy, or require parents to come to school. Children with mobility impairments may face barriers to schools or classrooms (Fig. 34–1).

Special education placements are commonly used, despite the fact that most children with mobility problems have no special learning problems that require special education programs. Inadequate school policies may exclude children who must take medicine or require parents to come to school to give medicines. Children who must be at home for extended periods may receive home teaching, especially if the absence is at least for 2 or more consecutive weeks. Yet the child with asthma who has frequent brief absences may find such home services unavailable.

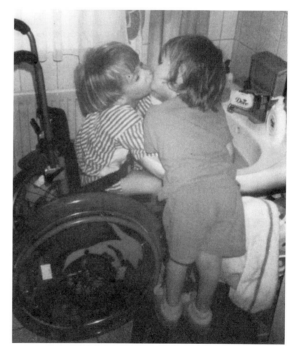

Figure 34–1. Jan (7 years old) and Anna (5 years old) are siblings. Jan has high lumbar spina bifida, bladder and bowel incontinence, and hydrocephalus. He is alert and attends regular classes but also has some special needs. He receives intermittent catheterization four times a day, regular physical therapy to prevent further contractures, and occupational therapy for his sensory motor integration problems. Even though he did walk with braces and mobility aids during preschool years, he has come to depend fully on his wheelchair. Despite the mother's receiving nutritional counseling while pregnant and folate supplementation pregnancy, his younger sister Anna was born with malformation of the sacrum, congenital hip dislocation, and club foot. She needed and still needs intensive orthopedic rehabilitation. She is doing well in kindergarten but has some mild learning difficulties.

Even when available, home teaching typically consists of only a few hours per week and is a poor substitute for the full range of classroom teaching. Furthermore, home teaching cannot replace peer interactions and the socialization that accompanies them. Helping a child maintain active contact with classmates by having them deliver homework and books is one important way of helping to maintain integration.

PROGNOSIS

Psychosocial problems in children and adolescents may persist into young adulthood. Young men who had had chronic physical conditions in childhood or adolescence had significantly higher risks for depression and anxiety, use of mental health specialists, poor educational qualifications, and periods of unemployment. Those with cardiac or respiratory disorders had the highest risks for psychological distress and absence of educational qualifications, those with neurologic and musculoskeletal disorders had highest rates of social isolation, and those with visual or auditory problems had longer spells of unemployment. In contrast, women with a history of childhood chronic conditions had only an elevated risk for having seen a mental health specialist (Pless, Power, and Peckham, 1993). Compared to apparently healthy adults, young adults with a history of chronic physical conditions in childhood are more likely to develop nonspecific psychosomatic complaints (i.e., headaches, back and shoulder pain, dizziness, or palpitations) unrelated to their chronic condition or an overt somatization disorder (Kokkonen and Kokkonen, 1995). The effects of cultural attitudes, which may stigmatize certain diseases, and societal levels of acceptance and tolerance may affect how young people with a chronic condition perceive their quality of life and well-being.

EFFECTS OF CHRONIC CONDITIONS ON THE FAMILY

Each stage of family development is characterized by a set of tasks, for which the family develops its own coping strategies. Societal, historical, cultural, and geographic factors all influence family development and form the context for family beliefs, myths, taboos, expectations, role models, and patterns of adaptation. Developmentally stable (maintenance) periods are interspersed by developmentally less stable (transitional) periods. Normative transitions include the birth of a child, school entry, and onset of adolescence. Unexpected transitions include disruptive life events, such as catastrophic or chronic illness in a family member, or loss and separation.

Families whose child is born with or in whom a chronic condition develops pass through a relatively predictable sequence of emotional reactions similar to those that follow separation and loss: (1) shock (inability to express feelings, communicate, or share feelings), (2) disbelief (denial, wishful thinking), (3) grieving and anger (blaming behavior, lack of control, inappropriate criticism, depression, helplessness, withdrawal behaviors), (4) stabilizing period (demystification, use of cognitive control behavior, adapting to day-to-day routine), and (5) maturation and acceptance (emotional adjustment, feelings of personal development and growth). The different stages are not mutually exclusive, crises may cause setbacks, and different family members typically go through different stages at different times. The onset of chronic conditions varies widely, with some being congenital and others developing and achieving a diagnosis over a long period of time. Similarly, family adjustment varies, reflecting this sequence of response in the context of the family's coping style and strategies.

The resilient family effectively uses resources within and outside the family system to prevent breakdown and promote adaptation to a chronic condition. Parents of children with chronic illness must monitor the child's health, check equipment, administer medications, provide physical therapy, or carry children with mobility impairments, all tasks that go beyond normal parenting. Thus, parents often report feelings of fatigue, depression, and social isolation. The extra burdens of care particularly affect family cohesion, along with less opportunity for social, recreational, and cultural activities in families with a child with a chronic health condition. Overt family dysfunction or family breakdown as a result of a child's chronic illness is uncommon, although families may pay a high price in terms of opportunities, social relationships, career choice, and personal growth to cope with the burden of care. Parents of children with chronic conditions in community-based studies have increased rates of mental health problems, particularly higher rates of depression, but no significant increase in single parenthood, social isolation, alcohol problems, or family dysfunction (Cadman et al, 1991). In contrast, studies of clinical populations indicate more marital discord, dysfunctional family patterns, and overt psychiatric disturbances in families, probably reflecting selection biases in these populations. In families of children with chronic arthritis as an example (Timko, Stovel, and Moos, 1992; Timko et al, 1993), mothers experienced more depressed mood than did fathers but also reported a greater sense of mastery over time. Depressed mood was related to greater functional disability and psychosocial problems in their children and lack of family support. Parental mood and strain also appear to predict child adjustment over time.

Among two-parent families, mothers are significantly less likely to work outside the home if there is a child with a chronic condition than if the family has children without apparent illness. Chronic illness in children has major financial costs as well; the relatively small number of children with severe physical conditions consume at least one third of all child health expenditures. Parents face sizable out-of-pocket expenses, not only for uncompensated health care costs but also for adaptations to the home, transportation, and extra child care. Lost income because a parent quit a job as a result of the child's chronic condition and curtailed career opportunities further increases financial burden.

The multiple demands on the family often leave less parental time for siblings. The few studies of adjustment to a sibling's chronic condition present a mixed picture. Some children find the experience of helping to nurture a sibling with chronic illness one that helps them to develop their own skills, enhances their maturity, and improves their resilience. Others find the parental neglect such a problem that they become depressed, develop aggressive and acting-out behavior, and do poorly in school and are otherwise diminished in their own psychological health. The correlates of adjustment of siblings are not well understood, although parental mental health and the family environment likely play major mediating roles (Dyson, Edgar and Crnic, 1989). (See Chapter 12.)

Families benefit from and contribute to the network of relationships and resources in the community. Effective social support helps families cope better with chronic stress. Self-help and advocacy groups have helped many parents to access information, recruit tangible support, and foster a sense of worth and importance in the work they accomplish.

CHRONIC CONDITIONS IN CHILDHOOD

Asthma

Asthma, the most common chronic illness of childhood and adolescence, has a prevalence of 5% to 10% in North American and European children. Prevalence rates of asthma have increased over the past few decades. Asthma accounts for a large number of school days missed, doctor visits, and hospitalizations. Characteristics of asthma particularly relevant to behavioral consequences include the uncertainty of its diagnosis, the unpredictability of its course, and the effects of medical treatments on behavior. Clinicians vary in their diagnosis of asthma, despite recent efforts to standardize diagnosis and treatment, and there is debate as to when to apply the label "asthma." About half of all children experience at least one episode of wheezing during the first 3 years of life, but, in most, asthma or allergies do not develop later in life. Whereas some clinicians argue that early labeling of a child as having asthma may make parents unnecessarily anxious and increase a sense of vulnerability of the child, others argue that early diagnosis opens access to teaching about the illness, prevention of serious exacerbations, effective medication, and self-management.

The unpredictability of asthma and its exacerbations create particular problems for children and families. Not knowing whether the child's mild wheezing at bedtime will lead to a severe problem in the night or pass quickly and allow the child to attend school in the morning makes planning and care difficult. Having easy access to both medications and treatment as well as to health services when needed acutely substantially improves both children's and parents' sense of well-being. A number of the medications used in the treatment of asthma, especially adrenergics and theophylline preparations, affect cognitive and behavioral functioning (see Chapter 30). The increased use of antiinflammatory medications for asthma will likely decrease the frequency of these consequences. Nonetheless, clinicians and families should be attentive to these issues, with respect to both behavior at home and appropriate planning for educational services. Given the unpredictable nature of exacerbations, children with asthma often need acute access to medications. Both clinicians and families aim toward increasing self-management of asthma; yet, many schools have strong regulations limiting children's access to medication. Timely access may be particularly

difficult for adolescents, because many schools have strong concerns about students' access to any drugs during school hours. Clinicians need to work closely with families and schools to ensure appropriate access in this situation.

Educational programs for school-aged children and adolescents with asthma are widely available and have been shown to increase knowledge and reduce behavioral problems, hospitalizations, and school absenteeism, although little evidence supports their ability to decrease severity or frequency of exacerbations. Effects on long-term morbidity, quality of life, or school performance have not been evaluated. Effective teaching programs typically include developmentally appropriate cognitive strategies to enhance self-management along with emotional and social support to foster self-esteem, social competence, and peer relations. Some programs have added deep relaxation techniques to aid the child's mastery over the signs and symptoms of asthma.

Epilepsy

Epilepsy is the most common neurologic condition in childhood. Although much childhood epilepsy is idiopathic, it occurs in one third of children with cerebral palsy and in 21% of children with mental retardation. Children with epilepsy have a much higher risk of psychological or behavioral problems than other children, with or without other chronic conditions. Although mechanisms have not had adequate study, reasons for these high rates may include (1) the effects of a primary brain disease on other central nervous system functions, (2) the direct mood and behavioral effects of anticonvulsant medications, (3) unpredictability associated with loss of control over one's actions, and (4) continuing social stigma and feelings of shame in the child and the parents. In the Isle of Wight Study, for example, psychiatric disorders were present in 6.6% of the general child population, 11.6% of children with physical disorders not involving the brain, 28.6% of children with uncomplicated epilepsy, and 58.3% of children with complicated epilepsy. In comparison, psychiatric disturbances were present in 37.5% of children with conditions affecting the brain but without seizures (Rutter, Graham, and Yule, 1970). Children with epilepsy show predominantly neurotic or emotional disturbances and less commonly conduct disorders. Parents and teachers regard these children as worried, fearful, miserable, and solitary, rather than acting out, aggressive, or destructive (Hoare and Kerley, 1991). Children with poor seizure control feel helpless, scared, frustrated, and different from others. Two thirds of children with poor seizure control and mental retardation had at least one psychiatric diagnosis in a large Swedish study. Many of the problems had been undiagnosed despite parental concern and conviction that the psychiatric problems were the most burdensome (Steffenburg, Gillberg, and Steffenburg, 1996). As with other chronic conditions, condition-specific factors (type, severity, and anticonvulsant therapy), family stress, and sociodemographic variables contribute to disturbances (Hoare and Kerley, 1991). Behavioral disturbances may improve when seizures are controlled or a specific lesion removed, pointing to an important contribution of the seizures themselves or structural abnormalities of the brain to behavioral or psychological problems.

Parents' anxieties and limited understanding of epilepsy may affect their approach to their children. For example, many parents believe a child may die during a seizure despite the rarity of this occurrence. Overprotection with unnecessary restrictions often results, leading to parenting problems, particularly during adolescence when children strive for more independence. Issues related to driving; cognitive problems such as memory, attention span, and concentration; lack of vocational training or employment; and restrictions related to socializing behavior are major concerns for adolescents and young adults with epilepsy. As for other chronic conditions, educational programs relating to epilepsy have helped parents in raising a child with a seizure disorder (Lewis et al, 1991).

Many children with epilepsy have associated learning disabilities, even if overall intelligence is normal. Early and repeated testing of cognitive functioning should be a standard of care to allow for appropriate school placement and special education when needed. Some children may benefit from speech and language and other therapies, although substantial data supporting their efficacy are lacking. Clinicians and parents face frequent difficult choices in when and whether to use such therapies, especially when they may interfere with normal classroom or social activities for the child.

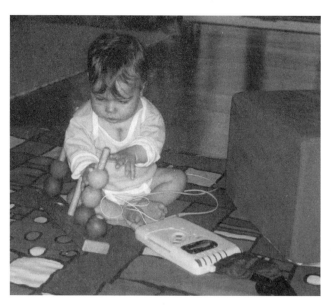

Figure 34–3. One-year-old Finn is on a cardiac monitor. He suffers from complex congenital heart disease (transposition of the great arteries, double inlet left ventricle, mitral valve stenosis and insufficiency, high-grade stenosis of the pulmonary arteries). His first cardiac surgery was at age 4 weeks, and his second operation was at age 10 months after signs of progressive heart failure and congestive liver disease developed. He awaits a third major operation at age 18 months. He has failure to thrive and short stature; however, his cognitive and motor development are somewhat slow but still age appropriate. He is the youngest of three children and hospitalizations at the cardiac surgery center 300 miles from home are a logistic problem, but the family receives social support from grandparents and neighbors.

Children Assisted by Technology

The history of care at home for children assisted by technology dates back to the polio epidemics of the early 1950s, when large numbers of children and young adults dependent on respiratory support required care at home. A second phase of care at home began in the 1980s, when children assisted by other medical devices, especially dialysis, intravenous feeding, enteral alimentation, and mechanical ventilation, were discharged from hospitals. With limited capacities in intensive care units, escalating hospital costs, and improved home equipment, care at home became an accepted alternative. Emerging parent advocacy for their children demanded care at home, pointing to the devastating effects of prolonged hospital admissions and parent-child separation.

Although the number of children assisted by technology at home is small, their numbers have increased substantially since the 1980s. Estimates of US children assisted by technology range up to 100,000 (1.0 per 1000 children). The Office of Technology Assessment defined four categories of technology-assisted children: (1) those who have partial or continuous ventilator assistance, (2) those requiring intravenous administration of nutritional substances or medications, (3) those with daily use of device-based respiratory or nutritional support, and (4) those with daily dependence on other devices that compensate for vital body functions or require daily or near-daily nursing care (Figs. 34–2 through 34–4). Initially developed and administered

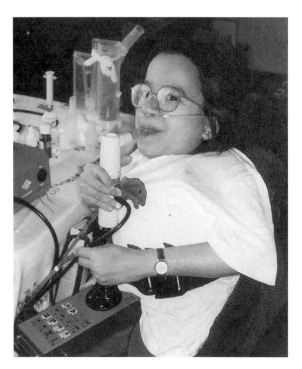

Figure 34–2. Michelle is a 19-year-old woman with osteogenesis imperfecta, restrictive lung disease, cardiomyopathy, intermittent obstructive bowel disease, and frequent fractures. Michelle depends on continuous oxygen, regular respiratory therapy, frequent use of medications per nebulizer, continuous positive airway pressure ventilation at night, and intravenous fluids during episodes of intestinal obstruction. She depends on help in all activities of daily living, with her mother being the main caregiver. She recently finished high school with good reports. She enjoys reading and writing on her personal computer. She is mobile with her electric wheelchair.

in hospitals (mainly large tertiary care centers), these technologies previously required children to have prolonged or frequent hospitalizations. Technologic advances have allowed the transfer of care for children assisted by technology from hospitals back to families and communities. Families have come to provide care for most childhood chronic conditions, relying on hospitals only for acute, life-threatening complications of disease or for review by subspecialists. Providing that care typically requires a broad array of multidisciplinary services that varies substantially according to the health condition and the needs of the child and families. Most families require services well beyond traditional medical and nursing care (Perrin, Shayne, and Bloom, 1993).

Families' experiences with care at home, in particular having substantial hours of nursing in the home, have been ambivalent. Families appreciate having their child home and receiving qualified nursing care. Yet, family privacy, control of parenting and care issues, and independence are in jeopardy. For many families, there may be no guarantee that the services provided at a community level or the hours allotted will be determined with the child's or the family's needs in mind. The training and expertise of nurses may not be sufficient to meet the child's special health care needs.

Management by Clinicians

COORDINATION OF CARE

Children without chronic conditions usually receive all their care close to home from a community-based pediatrician, family physician, or nurse practitioner. Children with chronic conditions receive their care from a multitude of different providers, including the primary care clinician, hospital-based subspecialists, home health agencies, specialized therapists, and sometimes alternative sources of care. Their care may be spread over different sites, sometimes at considerable distance from home, contributing to fragmentation of care. Families with children with chronic conditions may benefit from efforts to coordinate care.

Case management activities have a long history in human services, in which staff from public or voluntary private agencies have helped families, often from economically deprived backgrounds, to determine needs and to gain access to services. As a process, case management is an orderly, planned provision of services intended to facilitate a client's functioning at as normal a level as possible and as economically as possible (Weil and Karls, 1985). The experience with care at home has changed the use and definitions of case management as it applies to children and families (Perrin and Bloom, 1993). The newer and more adequate term *care coordination* places less emphasis on access and management and more on aspects of communication, service delivery, and family support, with the understanding that the professional responsible for coordination works with the family to develop an agenda or a list of short-term and long-term goals and priorities of each family member in close cooperation with the family.

Not all families need care coordination. Family members usually develop increasing competence to direct the management of the child's needs and services provided. Care coordination services may particularly help during the year after the onset of the child's condition, at the time of discharge from hospital, or during difficult transitional periods (e.g., during school entry). Care coordinators come from many different professional disciplines: nurses, social workers, physicians, and educators. Nurses are most commonly employed because of the breadth of their training in health, family, and child development issues. Social workers also frequently provide care coordination because of their expertise in human service programs, access to financial support, and training in working with families and children. Physicians rarely serve as care coordinators, mainly because of lack of training and reimbursement for the time-consuming efforts of care coordination, although they have a central role in coordinating the various aspects of medical and surgical care that a child may need. Increasingly, lay workers and experienced parents from advocacy groups or workers from public health agencies provide care coordination services for families.

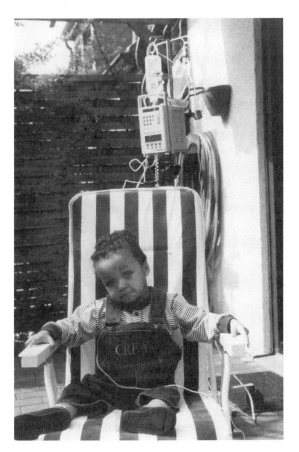

Figure 34–4. Two-year-old Leon has prune belly syndrome with severe obstructive uropathy and inability to have normal bowel movements. The picture shows him with his infusion set for total parenteral nutrition. He depends on parenteral nutrition on a continuous basis (20–24 hours/day) via a broviac catheter, frequent intermittent catherization, nebulizer for intermittent obstructive airway disease, care of his gastrostomy and colostomy, and frequent intravenous antibiotics. He lived in a hospital for the first 1 1/2 years of his life; his mother was single with multiple social problems and was unable to take him home; he lives with foster parents and has made excellent progress developmentally. He walks independently and talks in two-word sentences. He receives intensive early intervention services. However, his health is still fragile and he is frequently hospitalized briefly due to some complications in his management.

The functions of care coordination include teaching families about their child's care, developing a care plan and revising it periodically according to the child's and family's needs, helping the family to access necessary services, communicating effectively with all care providers, including home health services and social and educational services, and helping to resolve conflicts among service providers. Social and emotional support for the family is an important part of the care coordinator's work.

PREVENTION AND MANAGEMENT OF DEVELOPMENTAL AND BEHAVIORAL PROBLEMS

The special needs of families with children who have long-term illnesses require that a wide range of services be available to these families. Pediatricians can help families manage care by ensuring access not only to medical and surgical care but also to a broader array that includes preventive mental health services, appropriate home nursing and educational services, planning and monitoring educational placement, social services, and, at times, other specialized therapies. Furthermore, the pediatric view should include parents and siblings as well as the child with illness (Table 34–3). Modern medical treatments and advanced technology offer great opportunities and many choices for children and adolescents with chronic conditions, both prolonging life and improving quality of life. Families must have good information to help them make sense of medical advice that is often conflicting.

Clinicians working with children with chronic illness should ensure that these children receive all the usual aspects of preventive care and health supervision. Additional pediatric responsibilities include (1) identifying behavioral and developmental consequences of chronic illness for the child, (2) assessing family strengths and coping

Table 34–3 • Areas of Pediatric Evaluation and Intervention

Medical care
   Health maintenance and preventive care
   Acute illness care
   Chronic illness care, collaborating with
      subspecialty health providers
Identification of behavioral and developmental consequences
   Periodic assessment
   Monitoring and referral
Assessment of family strengths
   Knowledge
   Social support
   Coping skills
   Psychological status
Education about illness
   Developmentally appropriate
   Ongoing
   Decision making
Planning for education
   Medication and treatment
   Emergency plans
   Implications of condition for participation in
      classes and outside activities
   Special evaluation or placements

---

skills and identification of family problems (including those of sibling adjustment), (3) educating the child and family about illness, and (4) helping to plan an appropriate educational setting for the child. Given the high cost of many chronic conditions, physicians should also know how to refer families to sources of support, both private and public. (See Bauman et al, 1997, for a recent review.)

Identification of Behavioral/Developmental Consequences

Most children with severe long-term illness are psychologically healthy and without developmental problems. Yet the clinician must be vigilant in developmental and behavioral assessment of children with chronic illnesses and assess both the level at which a child is functioning and the need for referral. Primary care providers apparently recognize adjustment problems in some of their patients with chronic conditions. However, only about half of children with a serious chronic condition and a behavioral or emotional problem receive mental health services (Weiland, Pless, and Roghmann, 1992).

Assessment of Family Strengths

Pediatricians should help families increase the support available to them, become more knowledgeable about their child's health needs, and strengthen their skills both in coping and in nurturing their child. Pediatricians should be particularly sensitive to maternal depression and marital dysfunction, knowing how to identify these problems and where to refer parents when necessary. Although most families need only anticipatory guidance, parent counseling, and empathy, at times a mental health referral is in order (Sabbeth and Stein, 1990).

Education About Illness

Education about illness must take into account the child's developmental level. Explanation of illness and its treatment should be targeted to the child's (and parents') abilities. Education must be a continuing process as the child develops more cognitive sophistication. Periodic review of the child's understanding of illness helps inform the physician of areas needing attention. Pediatricians can help explain the often confusing information that families receive from multiple providers. To do so, they must themselves communicate effectively with specialists and remain current with the main issues of the specific health condition.

Clinicians need to help children and their families make adequate and autonomous decisions. For adults, the principles of informed consent guide clinicians to inform the patient and respect patient decisions. For children and adolescents, the process to achieve informed consent is far more complex. Informed consent requires autonomy and full ability to make judgments, of which children are capable to a limited extent, and should be replaced by a collaborative principle of combined parental permission, child assent, and physician agreement (Fleischman, 1989).

Education of children and families seems necessary but is not sufficient to enhance their self-care skills. Relatively little is known about the exact context of information that families need. Does the child with asthma need to learn about lung physiology, chest anatomy, and the mechanisms of actions of medications and why he or she develops certain kinds of symptoms, where medicines are kept, or how to use them? Much experimentation must continue in this area, and it should take into account the developmental status of the child.

Planning for Education

School is the main workplace of children. Pediatricians should help families work with schools to ensure the best placement for the child. Some children require special education services because of the effect of the illness on their cognitive abilities. Most children with chronic illness can participate in regular education programs, at times requiring modification of the school environment or the school day. Many require planning for dispensing of medication or for emergency care, and school staff need information regarding the illness and its consequences for the child's participation in school. Pediatricians should see that adequate transfer of information occurs and that satisfactory planning occurs for the child.

REFERENCES

Bauman LJ, Drotar D, Leventhal JM, et al: A review of psychosocial interventions for children with chronic health conditions. Pediatrics 100:244–251, 1997.

Bennett DS: Depression among children with chronic medical problems: a meta-analysis. J Pediatr Psychol 19:149–170, 1994.

Cadman D, Rosenbaum P, Boyle M, Offord DR: Children with chronic illness: family and parent demographic characteristics and psychosocial adjustment. Pediatrics 87:884–889, 1991.

Cousens P, Ungerer JA, Crawford JA, Stevens M: Cognitive effects of childhood leukemia therapy: a case of four specific deficits. J Pediatr Psychol 16:475–488, 1991.

Dyson L, Edgar E, Crnic K: Psychological predictors of adjustment by siblings of developmentally disabled children. Am J Ment Retard 94:292–302, 1989.

Fleischman AR: Ethical views and values. In Stein REK (ed): Caring for Children With Chronic Illness: Issues and Strategies. New York, Springer Publishing, 1989, pp 87–100.

From the CDC, JAMA 274:1112–1114, 1995.

Harahan M, Katz R, Miller N, Adler M: Managed care and people with disabilities, conference overview. ALTE/DALTCP Tabulations from the 1994 Disability Phase I Supplement to the National Health Interview Survey. Washington, DC, US Department of Health and Human Services, November, 1996.

Hoare P, Kerley S: Psychosocial adjustment of children with chronic epilepsy and their families. Dev Med Child Neurol 33:201–215, 1991.

Kokkonen J, Kokkonen E-R: Psychological and somatic symptoms in young adults with chronic physical diseases. Psychother Psychosom 64:94–101, 1995.

Lavigne JV, Faier-Routman J: Psychological adjustment to pediatric physical disorders: a meta-analytic review. J Pediatr Psychol 17:133–145, 1992.

Lazarus RS, Folkman SF: Stress, Appraisal, and Coping. New York, Springer Publishing, 1984.

Lewis MA, Hatton CL, Salas I, et al: Impact of the Children's Epilepsy Program on Parents. Epilepsia 32:365–374, 1991.

Newacheck PW, Stoddard JJ: Prevalence and impact of multiple childhood chronic illnesses. J Pediatr 124:40–48, 1994.

Newacheck PW, Taylor WR: Childhood chronic illness: prevalence, severity, and impact. Am J Public Health 82:364–371, 1992.

Perrin EC, Ayoub CC, Willett JB: In the eyes of the beholder: family and maternal influences on perceptions of adjustment of children with a chronic illness. J Dev Behav Pediatr 14:94–105, 1993.

Perrin EC, Gerrity PS: Development of children with chronic illness. Pediatr Clin North Am 31:19–32, 1984.

Perrin EC, Newacheck PW, Pless B, et al: Issues involved in the definition and classification of chronic health conditions. Pediatrics 91:787–793, 1993.

Perrin JM, Bloom SR: Coordination of care for households with children with special health needs. In Wallace HM, Nelson PR, Sweeney PJ (eds): Maternal and Child Health Practices, 4th ed. Oakland, CA, Third Party Publishing, 1993.

Perrin JM, MacLean WE, Perrin EC: Parents' perceptions of health status and psychological adjustment in children with asthma. Pediatrics 83:26–30, 1989.

Perrin JM, Shayne MW, Bloom SR: Home and Community Care for Chronically Ill Children. New York, Oxford University Press, 1993.

Pless IB, Power C, Peckham CS: Long-term psychosocial sequelae of chronic physical disorders in childhood. Pediatrics 91:1131–1136, 1993.

Rutter M, Graham P, Yule W: A Neuropsychiatric Study in Childhood. Philadelphia, JB Lippincott, 1970.

Sabbeth B, Stein REK: Mental health referral: a weak link in comprehensive care of children with chronic physical illness. J Dev Behav Pediatr 11:73–78, 1990.

Starfield B: Childhood morbidity: comparisons, clusters, and trends. Pediatrics 88:519–526, 1991.

Steffenburg S, Gillberg C, Steffenburg U: Psychiatric disorders in children and adolescents with mental retardation and active epilepsy. Arch Neurol 53:904–912, 1996.

Thompson RJ, Gustafson KE: Adaptation to Chronic Childhood Illness. Washington, DC, American Psychological Association, 1996.

Timko C, Baumgartner M, Moos RH, Miller JJ: Parental risk and resistance factors among children with juvenile rheumatic disease: a four year predictive study. J Behav Med 16:571–588, 1993.

Timko C, Stovel KW, Moos RH: Functioning among mothers and fathers of children with juvenile rheumatic disease: a longitudinal study. J Pediatr Psychol 17:705–724, 1992.

Weil M, Karls JM: Historical origins and recent developments. In Weil M, Karls JM (eds): Case Management in Human Service Practice. San Francisco, Jossey-Bass, 1985, pp 1–28.

Weiland SK, Pless IB, Roghmann KJ: Chronic illness and mental health problems in pediatric practice: results from a survey of primary care providers. Pediatrics 89:445–449, 1992.

Weitzman M: School absence rates as outcome measures in studies of children with chronic illness. J Chronic Illness 39:799–808, 1986.

Wertlieb D, Weigel C, Feldstein M: Measuring children's coping. Am J Orthopsychiatry 57:548–559, 1987.

35 Life-Threatening and Terminal Illness

Linda Sayler Gudas • Gerald P. Koocher

 Emotional expression in the infant is primitive and directly linked to impulse and sensation. As the child gets older, mood and reactivity become more stable but fantasies and fears become more important to overall emotional reactivity and adaptation.

Withholding information about the diagnosis and prognosis from the dying child was generally abandoned many years ago.

There is an increasing tendency for families to provide home care for children in the terminal phase of illness.

It would be negligent to stress only the issues of terminal care in this chapter, because the number of long-term survivors grows daily and represents a major challenge for preventive mental health care in pediatrics.

This chapter is intended as a guide to pediatricians and other health care professionals working with children and families who are confronting death. Advances in medical care necessitate considering two aspects of such work. The first involves actual terminal care during an acutely fatal illness. The second and more frequent aspect involves the care of the child with a chronic life-threatening condition, such as cystic fibrosis, cancer, or acquired immunodeficiency syndrome (AIDS). The following pages summarize important treatment approaches related to these distinctions. The development of normal children's views of death are reviewed and linked to the care of seriously ill children. Home care for the dying child and aftercare for the survivors are addressed using a family focus. Finally, issues regarding the effects on the medical provider when caring for such families are explored.

Before the advent of modern chemotherapies in the 1970s, children with acute lymphoblastic leukemia usually died within 6 months of diagnosis. Today acute lymphoblastic leukemia is considered a curable life-threatening illness and children with this illness have a better than 80% chance of surviving 5 or more years in a disease-free state. In the 1950s, most people with cystic fibrosis died in their teens. Today, many people with cystic fibrosis live well into their 30s, with many surviving into their 40s. In the 1990s, medically fragile babies are surviving into childhood and beyond. What of the families and loved ones of such patients? Should they attempt to anticipate the patient's death and accommodate to the loss or attempt to suppress their anxieties about possible death while hoping for the best? Either course can form the basis for a host of psychological stresses. The component of uncertainty clearly cannot be overlooked in considering the adaptation of the child, brothers and sisters, parents, or extended family members.

The psychological stresses associated with the uncertainties of long-term survival among children with life-threatening illness have been described as a *Damocles syndrome* (Koocher and O'Malley, 1981). The quality of life among such patients and their families is often linked to their ability to look beyond uncertainty and adopt an optimistic or hopeful attitude. It would be negligent to stress only the issues of terminal care in this chapter, because the number of long-term survivors grows daily and represents a major challenge for preventive mental health care in pediatrics.

Basic Approaches to Care

The practitioner should strive for awareness of the whole social environment of the patient. A family-based intervention is an absolute necessity if optimal adaptation and support of the patient are the pediatrician's goals. The costs of chronic illness to the patient's family are substantial in both emotional and financial terms. The course of the illness is likely to sap the adaptive capacities of the parents, both as individuals and as a couple. Brothers and sisters are also likely to experience an extra burden of stress. If the patient does die, a family of grief-stricken survivors remains. The practitioner who overlooks the family as part of the "patient care" locus is ultimately likely to compromise care for the ill family member.

In formulating a service plan or clinic structure for children with terminal or life-threatening conditions, teamwork is of critical importance. The most desirable strategy is one that integrates medical and mental health care, along with home care and other associated services, within a single system (Koocher, 1986; Shapiro and Koocher, 1996).

Such a system allows the medical staff to become more familiar with psychosocial issues and allows the psychosocial staff to learn about the medical diagnostic and therapeutic events their patients will be encountering. Patients benefit by virtue of the fact that all caregivers interact closely and more efficiently. Families should not feel that they are singled out as being "crazy" or in need of psychological intervention. Rather, if mental health services are routinely introduced early on as part of the standard care of the illness, no stigma is associated with the service. Integrating medical and mental health services makes using such programs more "normal" for all concerned (Pollin and Kanaan, 1995; Shapiro and Koocher, 1996).

INPATIENT VERSUS OUTPATIENT SETTINGS

Most children with life-threatening illness spend the bulk of their lives outside the hospital. There is also an increasing tendency for families to provide home care for children in the terminal phase of the illness. The psychological issues and needs of pediatric patients and their families are quite different when inpatient care is necessary; it is important for the practitioner to recognize the distinctions.

Outpatient care is generally more reassuring for the child, who will spend more time in the company of familiar caretakers than is the case during an inpatient stay. A degree of normality associated with sleeping in one's own home and returning to the familiar family environment after clinic visits can be supportive and reassuring. However, the stresses on family members can be greater in some instances. Arranging for care of sisters and brothers, missing time at work, managing household chores, and other such disruptions can be quite stressful, depending on the duration of the stay and the treatment required. Some parents are reassured and feel more useful when they are able to care for their child at home, whereas other parents can feel insecure and tense in dealing with the side effects of treatment, administering medication, or other aspects of home care.

During an inpatient stay, a child requires more reassurance and emotional support over a longer period of time than during outpatient visits. Many hospitals now provide rooming-in opportunities and encourage parents or other family members to participate in caring for their child. In some settings or circumstances (e.g., intensive care units) such involvement by family members may be discouraged. Each hospital admission can have a different meaning for the child and family. Some hospital stays can be seen as "routine" therapeutic admissions, while others can generate anxiety, realistic or not, that the illness has worsened.

The important point for health care professionals to remember is that individual family members must be viewed in the context of the current treatment circumstances and the personal meanings of those events. A family who manages well under one set of circumstances can have very different reactions during a subsequent treatment phase. The distinction might well be based on an attribution or perception that is not evident to the physician managing the case. This phenomenon underscores the importance of including mental health professionals on the treatment team.

DEVELOPMENTAL ISSUES

To understand the child's reaction to life-threatening illness, professionals working with ill children must be mindful of important developmental differences among children. Age is only one variable, with emotional, social, and cognitive development each playing its own role in shaping the child's reaction. Experience with loss, separation, and illness also affects the reactions of individual children.

The ability of children to conceptualize the nature and consequences of their illnesses varies dramatically as a function of cognitive development. The infant who is ill probably does not realize that his or her health circumstances could be otherwise and makes little connection of causality with respect to the disease process and the treatment program. As the child becomes a toddler, speech and language development makes it possible to communicate directly about the disease and treatment processes. Magical thinking is active in the preschool years, and the perceived causes of illness-related events can differ radically from reality. By the age of 6 or 7 years, most children have many questions, although they might not always have the vocabulary or feel permission to ask them. A better sense of cause and effect in the illness-treatment process is present. Unlike the situation in younger children, death is now recognized as irreversible rather than as being akin to sleep or other known experiences of the living. With the onset of hypothetical thinking and metacognition in adolescence, alternatives that might not have occurred to the younger child are prevalent (e.g., what will happen if the treatments don't work?). A future orientation becomes meaningful, and the long-range consequences of illness and treatment are now salient for the first time.

Emotional expression in the infant is primitive and directly linked to impulse and sensation. As the child gets older, mood and reactivity become more stable, but fantasies and fears become more important to overall emotional reactivity and adaptation. In the preadolescent years, mastery and competence-building activities help form adaptive mechanisms in the face of emotional stress. Intellectual problem solving becomes useful as a defense mechanism. By adolescence, the child is developing a sense of identity distinct from membership in the family. The teenage years are also ones of self-absorption and narcissism. The ability to cope with pain, body alterations, and similar factors related to life-threatening illness (as well as recognition of the actual threat) varies dramatically as a function of the child's developmental level.

Social issues are also subject to important developmental shifts and have bearing on the steps a pediatrician must take to ensure the best care for the critically ill child. For the infant, separation from loved ones can be akin to abandonment, producing great distress and despair for even the briefest of separations. The toddler might be better able to understand parental separation but can show regressive behavior, such as loss of toilet training or excessive clinging. Whenever possible, parents should be allowed to be present during examinations and procedures of young children. In a clinic or hospital situation, the primary nurse should accompany the child. In such situations, the ability of a small child to hear a caretaker's reassuring voice can be comforting and assist in compliance. Older children with serious illnesses react most severely to perceived threats to their competence, expressing fears of falling behind in school or reacting with marked depression and anxiety to mobility losses. The teenager suffers intense concern with the loss of peer interaction and school activities, since these are the primary delineators of evolving self-esteem in adolescence. The issues of most concern to children are largely linked to their levels of social functioning.

NORMATIVE ADJUSTMENT

Typical or normal behavior in the family of a child with terminal or life-threatening illness is different from the behavior of the same family prior to the diagnosis. This truism is often overlooked by professionals immersed in the process of treating such families or who have known the families for many years. For example, competent, attentive parents talking retrospectively of the day they first learned of their child's diagnosis frequently report, "After the doctor told us our child had leukemia, she said some other things too. . . . I don't remember what they were." The "other things" may have dealt with treatments that were to begin, but the parents, overwhelmed by the threat of a potentially terminal illness, are often too stunned to absorb the information. Such reactions are indeed expected under the circumstances, and the health care team can implement measures to assist such parents. Communication between specialists and the primary care physician should include information important for the parents to absorb (i.e., imminent treatments, side effects of medications). The parents may feel more comfortable communicating with their pediatrician's office for clarification or reassurance. Follow-up phone calls to the family by the physician or nurse should be routine to assess the parents' level of functioning and ability to absorb information. Writing down information or providing written resources allows the parents to have concrete reminders.

Children who are terminally ill or who face an uncertain but potentially fatal outcome from some chronic illness or condition are at substantial risk for emotional problems as a function of stress. Depending on the course and trajectory of the disease process, even children who were asymptomatic prior to becoming ill will predictably experience increased anxiety, loss of appetite, insomnia, social isolation, emotional withdrawal, depression, apathy, and marked ambivalence toward adults who are providing primary care.

These reactions are generally best regarded as responses to acute or chronic stress rather than as evidence of psychopathology. Children or families with preexisting emotional disorders will often experience an exacerbation of symptoms. An important theoretical model for conceptualizing the way in which these reactions occur is best described in the classic work of Seligman (1975) and other writers on the topic of learned helplessness. When individuals believe that the outcome they will confront (i.e., death) is independent of their own behavior, the helplessness syndrome and accompanying emotional stress are dramatic.

Much research has focused on children's awareness of their own fatal illness. Even young children have an awareness of their medical conditions. We know, for example, how anxiety levels in children with leukemia may increase in parallel with increases in the frequency of outpatient clinic visits. This finding is opposite of what is found in youngsters with chronic non–life-threatening illness. Other data demonstrate the increasing sense of isolation dying children tend to experience. One cannot shield sick children from anxiety about their condition.

Even children who otherwise seem to be coping quite well through a prolonged illness can experience specific problems, such as conditioned reflex vomiting, anxiety linked to specific medical procedures, depressive reactions to progressive loss of physical capacities, or family communication inhibitions (Koocher and O'Malley, 1981). Although seemingly a paradoxical reaction to the cessation of a noxious experience, hospitalizations and stressful treatment regimens can become imbued with some protective value.

Children's Perceptions of Death: Developmental Differences

Many misconceptions exist regarding coping with death and loss (Rando, 1993; Worden, 1996; Wortman and Silver, 1989). In addition, there are often-held assumptions regarding children's perceptions of death. First is the assumption that children do not comprehend death. Second is the assumption that adults do comprehend death. Finally, there is an assumption that even if children were able to understand about death, it would be harmful for them to be concerned about it. These assumptions are clearly superficial but did, however, historically provide a basis on which to justify avoiding such discussions with dying children (Evans, 1968). Developmental studies have documented acquisition of the universality and irrevocability of death concepts as well as highlighting children's own awareness of their potential death (Koocher, 1973, 1974).

These studies suggest that egocentrism and magical thinking, which are part of preoperational thought in young children, dominate concerns about death in early childhood. Preschoolers' constructions of reality are based on their physically observable world, limited by their own experiences, and their understanding of death is therefore quite limited. With the beginning of concrete operational thought at about age 6 or 7 years, the child can clearly differentiate between self and others, becomes capable of perspective-taking, and thereby begins to recognize the permanence of death. At this stage, however, the child does not have well-established concepts of cause and effect and can still think of death as something that occurs as a consequence of a specific illness, injury, or action rather than as a biological process. At the time of adolescence, with its accompanying abstract reasoning capability and formal operational thought, a more complete comprehension of death becomes possible. Teenagers also become aware of the complex physiologic systems of the body and comprehend illness and disease in a way younger children cannot. The specific concerns and fantasies expressed by children of different ages with respect to death are reflective of their cognitive understanding about it.

Bowlby's writings (1980) on the theme of attachment and separation demonstrate the importance of social relationships and the consequences of their disruption, especially during the early years of development. It is the interaction of these social relationships and the cognitive accommodation capacities that determine coping abilities in concert with other individual factors. Review of these elements from a child development standpoint can be found in Gudas (1993), Koocher and Gudas (1992), Koocher (1981), and Lonetto (1980).

THE DYING CHILD'S AWARENESS OF DEATH

Withholding information about the diagnosis and prognosis from the dying child was generally abandoned many years ago. The emotions of the pediatricians who must care for terminally ill patients remain an issue, however, at least partially because of a discomfort inherent in the role of working with children who are so gravely ill.

"Protecting" children from the seriousness of their illness does not alleviate their concerns. Reviews of professional opinion and research data have consistently stressed that children as young as 5 or 6 years have a very real understanding of their illness, and still younger children show definite reactions to increased parental stress and other effects of a terminal illness on themselves and their family. Despite this recognition by children of their serious illness, conceptualizations of death and loss do not really differ from the general developmental trends already noted. The predominant modes of response tend to reflect age-related concerns about separation, pain, and disruption of usual life activities. Even among healthy children, there are substantial elements of anxiety with regard to death (Koocher, 1981). It is not surprising, therefore, to find a variety of adverse psychological symptoms and behavioral problems among dying children and members of their families.

The Critically Ill Child: Key Psychological Issues

SEPARATION

Before object constancy develops, the infant who cannot see his or her parent cannot retain the concept that the parent still exists (Piaget, 1960). The infant's reaction of acute distress to the parent's leaving is well recognized (Bowlby, 1980). The infant or toddler in the hospital, an unfamiliar setting with strangers as caregivers, seeks parental reassurance and comfort and finds separation even more anxiety-producing than does the healthy child. Arranging for parents to sleep in the hospital room with their child and to be integrally involved in their child's care is vital at this age. This involvement includes accompanying and comforting the child during medical procedures. At times, the parents' heightened anxiety or withdrawal resulting from anticipatory grief can cause them to defer basic care of their child to the nursing staff. Or, an opposite reaction can be seen where the parent cannot detach from the responsibility of caring for the child and needs permission to be relieved of such care. The pediatrician should assist the parents in openly discussing their emotional reactions

to help them address their personal and family needs and to provide for their child's need for ongoing physical care and comfort.

By approximately 3 years of age, the preschooler can increasingly understand and tolerate parental absence. The presence of a life-threatening illness and the need for prolonged hospitalization, however, can lead to regressive behavior and an increased need for parental reassurance. The preschool-aged child can perceive death as a type of separation or parting from others. Fears and fantasies about illness and dying can be confused with concern about separation. The parents' presence and active involvement remain essential throughout the childhood years.

The adolescent is concerned about potential family withdrawal related to anticipatory grief, the censoring of medical information, and social withdrawal of peers owing to their friends' anxieties about serious illness. Acceptance by peers is very important to the adolescent's sense of identity and self-esteem. Isolation from normal peer activities poses a difficulty for many adolescents.

PAIN MANAGEMENT

The treatment of a life-threatening illness such as cancer, AIDS, or cystic fibrosis requires many painful and noxious procedures and treatments. In addition to the parents' presence, physical comforting, and reassurance, there are other strategies that the treatment team can use to deal with the anxious anticipation of adverse procedures as well as management of pain.

Every child needs preparation for procedures in clear, understandable language. An explanation of the procedure, commensurate with the child's age and ability to comprehend, helps the child anticipate what will transpire and provides an increased sense of control. Play therapy techniques, such as providing children with a stuffed toy animal and asking them to install an intravenous line using actual equipment, provides an opportunity to address emotional concerns and use mastery as a coping strategy prior to the actual procedure. The young child who complains of pain during a procedure can learn distraction techniques, such as deep breathing, squeezing a parent's arm when the pain intensifies, or the use of visual imagery techniques. Allowing the child to maintain some control is also helpful to decrease fear and helplessness. For example, the clinician can suggest that it is okay to cry or to scream during a procedure, as long as the child remains relatively motionless.

Deep muscle relaxation and hypnosis can also be employed with school-aged children and adolescents, both to aid in reducing anxiety and as a strategy to control chronic pain (such as "phantom pain" following amputation or pain from an invasive procedure). Psychotherapy, with the demands of the medical condition framing the goals (Pollin and Kanaan, 1995), can also provide patients with a forum to discuss their emotional reactions and to better understand the psychological context of the pain they are experiencing. The following examples illustrate three approaches specific to pain management.

EXAMPLES

Jill, 4 years of age, had severe distress reactions in response to venipuncture. Play therapy sessions were intro-

duced. These sessions included elaborate preparations for drawing blood from her stuffed toy animal, Snoopy. She was also provided a party blower noisemaker for Snoopy to use during the blood drawing procedure. After a few consultations, she was able to tolerate venipuncture herself, using a party blower without overt signs of distress. The intervention allowed Jill to express herself, gain some mastery over her feelings of anxiety, and learn a distraction technique.

Alan, 9 years of age, had severe phantom limb pain following a leg amputation for osteogenic sarcoma. He was especially fearful of physical therapy. The physical therapist was encouraged to use a Curious George doll at the beginning of each session. Alan would give physical therapy to the doll prior to receiving his own treatment. He was then better able to tolerate the sessions.

George, 15 years of age, complained of chronic pain caused by reflexive sympathetic dystrophy following an orthopedic procedure for severe bone degeneration. A course of training in deep muscle relaxation and guided visual imagery was begun. George learned to induce relaxation and to visualize a pleasant, relaxing scene when he felt the pain becoming intolerable. George found that having this strategy as an alternative to increased levels of pain medication helped him to feel that he had greater control of his pain and his body.

CONTROL

The diagnosis of a life-threatening illness creates an emotional crisis in a family. The loss of control implicit in the diagnosis is one of the most devastating aspects of the crisis. Parents can experience the loss of ability to protect their child from harm and to positively influence their child's future. Their own feelings of loss of control in this situation can generate intensification of their concern and caretaking behavior, thus helping regain a sense of mastery when they feel helpless. Often, however, this behavior can be experienced as infantilizing by the patient.

The preadolescent child, who is seeking achievement in many new areas, can experience the loss of control to plan his or her life. The child might displace anger onto schedules or hospitalizations that interfere with such plans. For example, a 9-year-old child can become furious that chest physical therapy for progressive symptoms of cystic fibrosis interferes with after-school activities. Anger about the diagnosis, per se, might not appear directly.

The preadolescent child might attempt to regain control by testing parental limits. The parents might, in turn, curtail discipline out of guilt or concern for their sick child. Rather than making the child feel special, however, this behavior can make the child feel more out of control.

EXAMPLE

Joey, a 5-year-old boy with AIDS, was permitted by his mother to hit her in the face when he became angry. The mother believed that her son was angry about his illness and its treatments, and she felt guilty for having infected him and was emotionally unable to restrain him in any way. In addition, his mother was worried about Joey's recent weight loss. She therefore offered him multiple choices for each meal. He often made two or three choices and then ate very little. After consulting with the pediatrician and psychologist, the mother was able to talk about her difficulty disciplining Joey. She was encouraged to set firm limits and alternative methods for expressing anger, like hitting a pillow or yelling. Additionally, meals were to include only one choice for the entire family. Two weeks later the parents reported that Joey was less angry and was eating larger meals. The clinic staff also observed that Joey appeared more calm.

Although the loss of control is a salient issue for all patients, it has a heightened impact during adolescence. Adolescents strive for greater autonomy in their environment and increasing independence from parents. These gains are impeded by hospitalizations in which members of the medical staff make decisions that affect the adolescent's health and daily life. Patients often feel bombarded by intrusive medical practices. The hospital experience can foster passivity and regressive dependence that inhibits the adolescent's growing sense of mastery over the environment. The ability to experience competence through school, social experiences, and planning for the future is also seriously disrupted when treatments or symptoms make it difficult for the patient to keep up.

Another adolescent task is developing mastery over one's changing body. Body image issues are directly challenged by the physical changes often accompanying illness. For instance, alopecia, a frequent side effect of chemotherapy, is a visible, inescapable reminder to the patient of the disease, as well as a possible source of embarrassment and diminution of self-esteem. Comfort and confidence in sexual attractiveness are also severely challenged by the effects of both the disease and its treatment.

With children and adolescents, the loss of control accompanying a hospitalization is stressful. The patient's daily schedule is disrupted, and familiar people and activities are absent. Some patients might be especially uncomfortable at some particular time of the day, coinciding with a missed special activity or lonely late-evening hours. Increasing a patient's perception of control can improve the ability to cope with disease (Seligman, 1975). Increasing control can be accomplished by such simple measures as permitting patients to wear their own clothes in the hospital, allowing some choices in time for procedures (e.g., "Should we do this now or after lunch?"), or engaging in other such normalizing activities that offer the child an appropriate degree of control.

HONESTY AND TRUST

Children are aware of the fact they are ill and, sometimes, seem to know innately when they are dying. Children are also often aware of the tendency of parents, loved ones, and medical personnel to withhold or minimize information. The child has many fears and apprehensions about unknown possibilities. Open communication provides an opportunity to dispel them and concentrate on the adjustment required for the realities of treatment. A closed communication style can lead to a sense of isolation for both the child and the parents. Kellerman, Rigler, and Siegal (1977) noted an inverse relationship between a child's open discussion of his or her illness and depression. A child who feels she can ask questions and receive honest answers regarding the disease and treatment will feel more a part of the medical regimen, will trust her caretakers, and will be less anxious regarding her fears and worries. Although such communication may initially be difficult for the clinician, the ultimate gains in compliance and security from such discussions are invaluable.

FAMILY ISSUES

The pediatrician caring for the child with a life-threatening illness comes to recognize that the family, not simply the patient, is the unit of care and attention. A shift in the focus of care—from the patient to the entire family—is especially relevant when issues of home care, respite care, or hospice must be considered (Davies et al, 1995; Jensen and Given, 1991). Studying families is complex, and researchers have too often neglected a family focus in favor of surveying parents only. In coping with life-threatening illness, family members are faced with the problem of managing their own emotions as well as the practical aspects of daily living. Learning to deal with chronic stress, disruption, and uncertainty makes coping a continually trying task. One study summarizes the burdens of coping as "balancing the needs of the patient in the home with those of healthy siblings; fostering the patient's normal social and emotional development while coping with long-term uncertainty; and dealing with unresolved anticipatory grief if the child survives" (Koocher and O'Malley, 1981).

Increased marital stress and financial strain are predictable phenomena. The quality of the marital relationship prior to diagnosis serves as an important predictor of the adequacy of marital coping with the crisis. Differences in parental coping styles, being "out of synch" in the timing of emotional reactions, and differences in managing the family can also exacerbate marital tension (Sourkes, 1977). A decreased sense of parental competence can further impair coping. The survival of a marriage can be linked to survival of the patient, but professional counseling and parent support groups can play important roles in helping to manage parental and marital stress (Koocher and O'Malley, 1981).

The relationship of sisters and brothers to their parents also changes if they experience decreased attention and support. They may feel angry at both the ill child and the parents who have failed to protect them from the consequences of the disease. School and peer relationships can also be adversely affected. School performance can decline in response to family stress. In other instances, brothers and sisters can plunge into academic pursuits as a means of escaping stresses at home or to prove themselves competent in an effort to combat family feelings of hopelessness. Peer relationships can be interrupted for practical reasons, such as school absences to visit the ill child or retreat into the family. Sisters and brothers can also feel alienated from friends who do not understand their irritability and preoccupation. Development of somatic complaints as a means of garnering parental attention or to identify with the ill child has also been observed. Death and mourning for a sibling can raise many issues of vulnerability, anger, misunderstanding, guilt, and confusion (DeMaso, Meyer, and Beasley, 1997).

Open communication between the patient's physician and the siblings, including family counseling sessions, is one very beneficial approach. They may have many questions and fantasies that necessitate clarification but that the parents alone may not be able to answer. Parents' efforts to spend "special time" with their healthy children, to provide consistency, to continue important family routines, and to aid their children in maintaining as normal a life as possible are also important.

COMPLICATIONS FROM TREATMENT

Iatrogenic factors arising from the treatment of the disease can also pose adjustment problems. For example, considerable evidence exists that shows neuropsychological sequelae follow radiation and chemotherapy for cancer patients (Waber, et al, 1990). Although few question the benefit of prophylactic treatment of the central nervous system in terms of greatly sustained remissions in children with leukemia and other cancers, there is argument for more research to ascertain the exact nature, extent, and type of risk factors for such patients.

Psychological iatrogenic factors exist as well. An example involves the patient's development of close ties with other patients and the pain and depression that follows the death of a clinic or hospital friend. This example is especially poignant in cystic fibrosis, when adolescent patients have developed friendships over years or even over a lifetime. The loss of a friend not only precipitates mourning and grief over the death but also forces patients to directly confront their own vulnerability and mortality.

EXAMPLE

Ann, an 18-year-old patient with cystic fibrosis, had known Will, age 19, for several years. They frequently tried to coordinate clinic visits to spend some time together. At one point, they were both hospitalized for "clean-outs" at the same time. As Will's disease progressed, however, and clinic visits and hospitalizations became more frequent and more lengthy, Will became despondent. Witnessing Will's sullen withdrawal, Ann became quite depressed. She worried about the progression of her own disease and experienced refractory psychosomatic abdominal pain.

Another type of complication is functional loss following treatment of a life-threatening illness. The patient with osteogenic sarcoma who must learn to adapt following amputation of a limb illustrates one example of a substantial readjustment problem that is a by-product of treatment. Even patients who are successfully treated can remain at substantial psychological risk as they live with an uncertain future for many years. Evaluating treatment success must include consideration of the whole patient and family, recognizing that predictable serious physical and emotional sequelae can result from treatment.

PLANNING PSYCHOLOGICAL CARE FOR THE CHILD WHO IS DYING

The child who is dying requires and deserves the support, care, and love of family and friends. One of the interdisciplinary team's roles is to encourage and facilitate the family's ability to offer such care. The patient's feeling of being surrounded by a network of understanding people and not being isolated is vital to successful coping with end-stage disease. The knowledge that he or she can openly discuss fears and thoughts about death without being censured is equally important. Knowing that people valued by the patient are available to conduct "unfinished business" is comforting to patients. Clinicians should allow opportunities for interactions such as permitting rival brothers and sisters a time to share their memories and love or helping the parent listen to requests from the patient about managing belongings or the funeral. Consistency in the medical staff who cares for the child (e.g., having a primary nurse, providing the same physical therapist or x-ray technician to do procedures) is also helpful for the child.

THE ROLE OF THE INTERDISCIPLINARY TEAM

Parents and sisters and brothers need consistency and special support as well. Throughout the patient's treatment, the family establishes a network of medical providers whom they come to know and trust. A typical team is composed of the inpatient physician, primary nurse, mental health professional, outpatient pediatrician, and visiting nurse who provide the child and family with clarification of information, assist with practical matters (e.g., tutoring of the child; administration of medications; or in terminal stages, discussing funeral arrangements or wishes for organ donation). Open, frequent communication among team members ensures a uniform approach and underscores the consistent availability of the staff to the patient and family. Liaison with school counselors, teachers, clergy, or other community members is helpful in providing additional support. The designation of an overall team coordinator, who takes responsibility for gathering data and presenting the synthesized information to the family, is crucial for clear communication. This prevents overly anxious parents from "splitting" team members, which can lead to confusing or distorted information. The patient should also be a partner in the treatment team, to the extent that his or her developmental level allows. Rather than diminishing anxiety, exclusion of the patient can exacerbate the sense of loss of control and isolation.

EXAMPLE

Susan, age 9, complained that she was always being treated like a baby. Her physician would often compliment her on her pajamas or ask about her stuffed toy animals, but would not talk with her about what was being decided in his frequent hallway discussions with residents. Susan complained, "I want to know if I need to have another lumbar puncture and when I can go home. I do not care if he likes my teddy bear."

THE ROLE OF THE MENTAL HEALTH PROFESSIONAL

The mental health professional can offer important support to the patient, family, and medical staff by consulting with them on the assessment of the patient's developmental level, the meaning of psychological and psychogenic symptoms, and the care and management of the patient. Indirect consultation can lead to direct patient contact or can allow improved care without such referral. The mental health clinician can also facilitate creation of a forum to discuss team members' emotional reactions to providing care to patients with life-threatening conditions.

The mental health provider can best serve the patient and family when an initial evaluation is made at the time of diagnosis. At this juncture, the psychological consultant can assess the family's functioning and interactional style and make recommendations for managing predictable stresses. This early intervention can help manage predictable reactions and decrease marital tension or sibling problems. Such interventions can also help the family by facilitating clear communication and mutual support. This initial assessment also permits early intervention when one or more family members seem to be at risk.

In responding to the needs of terminal care with a child and family, the mental health professional can provide intervention focused on factors that affect the medical condition and adjustment to those factors. One such approach is described by Pollin (Pollin and Golant, 1994; Pollin and Kanaan, 1995) as medical crisis counseling. Intervention at this time centers on medical issues affecting the family's emotional well-being. The objective of psychological assistance in such medical crises is to help patients and families maintain mental and emotional control, even as they face diminished physical control. "The goal of counseling in respect to death, therefore, is for the patient to focus on living to the fullest extent possible. This is facilitated by grieving losses, finding meaning and joy in the present, coping as effectively as possible with the medical condition, and getting closure whenever possible" (Pollin and Kanaan, 1995, p. 92). Medical and mental health providers can help set reasonable (i.e., concrete, realistic, and focused) goals over which the child and family have some control. For example, alleviation of pain, as discussed earlier in this chapter, is a goal of the child, family, and health care providers and can be obtained only through working collaboratively.

BURNOUT IN PROFESSIONALS CARING FOR TERMINALLY ILL PATIENTS

What of professionals who care for those they cannot cure? In addressing this question, Marquis (1993) states, "Clinical experience and field studies reveal that every form of dying and death places its own distinctive emotional burden on the caretaker" (p. 17). Such an emotional burden can lead to weariness, boredom, progressive loss of interest in work, resentment, frustration, indifference, and eventual exhaustion (Marquis, 1993; Pollin and Kanaan, 1995).

Providers caring for dying children must constantly be aware of their own responses to the vicarious trauma of experiencing repeated death and loss. Physicians must come to terms with being trained (and expected) to heal while facing helplessness and impotence in managing end-stage disease. Advice given to families of terminally ill children applies to providers are well. Most imperative is to seek emotional, social, and professional support. Utilize team members to help confront difficult times or overwhelming defenses. Try to allow a "mourning space" (Marquis, 1993), where feelings and attachments to a deceased patient are addressed before one becomes submerged in the care of yet another dying child. Those who care for others must also learn to care for themselves. To acknowledge and address one's feelings will help prevent the loss of human warmth, compassion, energy, and hope that is necessary to work with terminally ill children and their families.

The Issue of Control in an Inpatient Milieu

There are some critical principles in establishing an environment that enhances the child's perception of control. Such an environment is ideally planned by an interdisciplinary team using a systematic approach to encourage development of the patient's sense of involvement from the time of admission. Continuity of daily life activities is a key issue. Maintaining a social network through visits, phone calls, and letters is encouraged. Making the hospital room a familiar setting by bringing in personal articles from home also promotes continuity and familiarity. Ensuring that the patient continues to be an active, responsible person who makes choices should be the central priority. This active stance is best introduced to patients as a way of helping them cope with disease and hospitalization. Reinforcing messages by pointing out choices in daily hospital life underscores the realistic options. These choices can include activity room programming, academic tutoring, developing a support network by introducing newly diagnosed patients to each other and to "veterans," allowing patients to participate in decisions concerning medical procedures, and soliciting and responding to patient feedback. These components create an atmosphere in which the patient can maintain a sense of dignity and control because he or she knows ways to affect and influence what happens. This type of milieu should have a positive effect on the patient's ability to cope with his or her illness.

Location of Terminal Care

Patients in the terminal stages of disease receive care in a variety of settings. Recent trends in federal and private health care policy have encouraged shortened hospital stays as well as administration of complex medical protocols on an outpatient basis. Such policies have shifted the locus of care of individuals who are terminally ill from the hospital to a home care setting, leaving families to provide the bulk of care (Allen and Fleishman, 1992). Allowing the child to die at home, in hospice, or in a continuing care facility are alternatives that need to be considered by all individuals involved in the care of the child.

Although home- and community-based care is beneficial from many perspectives, such settings carry with them certain costs and potential dangers (Allen and Fleishman, 1992). The anxiety and fatigue generated by being responsible for direct care 24 hours per day; the fear that "something may go wrong" when the medical team is at a distance; and the reality that comprehensive resources necessary to care for the child are scattered, diverse, and complex may prevent families from raising home care alternatives with the physician. If hospice care is a viable option, issues related to competence, reliability, and trust are salient for families. By definition, hospice care implies that the family has acknowledged the terminal nature of the illness, that the patient will not recover, and that the family unit agrees that they can no longer sufficiently care for the child by themselves. The expectation that families can "pull together" to cope with such palliative care decisions may be unrealistic without the support, knowledge, skills, and affirmation of the practitioners involved in the child's care (Davies et al, 1995; Jensen and Given, 1991).

The medical team should discuss location of terminal care with the family and patient at appropriate points in time when the family can plan and have questions thoroughly explored. Mental health and social service clinicians are important consultants for planning at this stage to help the family reach a decision that is personally, financially, and practically reasonable for them. The family needs to be reassured that the entire medical team will support them in whatever decision they reach and that the hospital team will work closely with the home care or hospice team to provide continuity of care. Some families may benefit from meeting a home care or hospice nurse who has a pivotal role in providing medical, emotional, and practical support to the child and family. Davies and colleagues (1995), however, warn the clinician that alternative suggestions for settings can be effective only when the family perceives that the current situation is compounding their stress rather than relieving it.

Theories of Emotional Response to Terminal Illness

Kübler-Ross' (1969) seminal work on stage theory of adjustment to terminal illness stated that people progress through discrete, predictable stages of emotional responses to loss and dying. This theory provided a groundbreaking look at how adults responded to loss at different points in time but oversimplified individual differences in people and situations and did not consider child developmental issues. Two decades following Kübler-Ross' work, other authors questioned whether such theories with intuitive appeal are indeed borne out by empiric research (Stroebe, 1992-93; Wortman and Silver, 1989). Wortman and Silver (1989) noted the relative paucity of controlled studies of such stage theories and concluded that an extreme pattern of variability exists in response to life crises. As is typical of much research, none of the early studies included pediatric patients.

What clinicians and researchers have now begun to document observing in situations of loss and terminal illness is a process of potential reactions that occur, and often recur, over time. Ztalin (1995), for example, refers to two phases of patient response to or understanding of terminal illness. The first phase is one of reaction and questioning, which includes the influence of family and social networks, issues of cause and control, illness severity, and beliefs about world view, and which encompasses reactions in the first four stages of coping described by Kübler-Ross. The second phase is assimilation, in which the patient and family attempt to place the illness within the context of their lives. In response to loss and death, Rando (1993) refers to a schema that divides such responses into three phases (avoidance, confrontation, and accommodation), each of which is characterized by a major response set toward the loss. Researchers studying children's reactions to loss and grief are increasingly referring to psychological tasks rather than stages or phases that children should master in order to cope effectively. Baker, Sedney, and Gross (1992) conceptualize tasks according to early, middle, and late time periods. Early tasks include understanding and self-protection, middle tasks include acceptance and reworking, late tasks pertain to identification and development. Worden (1996) speaks to four tasks necessary for children to grieve and stresses the importance of the child to be able to experience the emotional pain of what is lost.

The crucial point, however, is to recognize the great variability in human response and the nonlinear progression of emotional responsiveness and to conceptualize in terms of reactions rather than lock-step stages. Adjustment to serious illness and loss is not necessarily a continual, orderly, forward movement but is more like the "ebb and flow of tides" (Pollin and Golant, 1994). Wortman and Silver (1989) provide a provocative stance on the variability that exists in response to loss, and they comment that "recognition of this variability is crucial in order that those who experience loss are treated nonjudgementally" and "with the respect, sensitivity, and compassion they deserve." In thinking about adolescents diagnosed with cancer or AIDS, for example, one is likely to see a significant, direct, and continuing expression of anger beyond what early theorists predicted. The adolescent is also much less likely to reach a stage or phase of acceptance of death. Case management must therefore be focused on individual patient responses and needs. The clinician should not fall into the conceptual trap of pondering why a patient has not yet reached a certain stage, phase, or task at an expected juncture nor be concerned that a patient is regressing if he or she seems to be reworking reactions seen at previous points in time.

Another factor impinging upon children's emotional reactivity and ability to cope with illness is their awareness and understanding of what is physiologically happening to them. For example, pediatric patients are aware of when they are feeling energetic or lethargic. A child who is ill and feels weak might be more apt to accept the prognosis than the alert, active child; yet neither child might truly be able to accept his or her fate.

Aftercare Issues

ASSESSING GRIEF REACTIONS

When the patient dies, the pediatrician must consider the needs of surviving family members. Even when the patient was a long-term survivor, the physician must focus special attention on the grief reactions that normally occur. The acute sadness and feelings of unreality or shock that frequently occur immediately after a loss are probably the best recognized manifestations of grief. However, the long-term reactions leading up to a death from chronic illness (often referred to as anticipatory grief) or reactions following the loss by several months create more subtle management problems.

The standard for expression of grief in infancy and toddlerhood is Bowlby's (1980) classic stages of protest, despair, and detachment. Preschoolers and very young children often present as sad, anxious, and scared, which may be related to their concerns about separation (Kranzler et al, 1990). Regression, animistic fantasies, anger, withdrawal, loss of interest in favorite toys or pastimes, and self-blame or guilt over past activities (especially in relation to the deceased) are all common responses. Young children's grief is often less pervasive, more intermittent, and more situation specific than that of older children and adults (Gudas, 1993; Kranzler et al, 1990). School-aged children may develop school and learning difficulties, anger, helplessness, and symptoms that are similar to those of depression. Somatic symptoms are also frequent, and the pediatrician may need to provide great reassurance for these children. Adolescents have been found to experience profound shock and intensity of loss, irritability, anger, sleep disturbances, struggles with being with other people, and intense mood swings (Meshot and Leitner, 1992–93). The adolescent's grief may be expressed in risk-taking behaviors, and caretakers should remain alert if the teenager begins to experiment in dangerous activities.

One key to the diagnostic assessment of childhood grief reactions is the presence or lack of anxiety. The child or adolescent who is in the process of adapting to a family death should be able to verbalize some sadness and related feelings in the course of an interview. Inability to discuss the loss, denial of affect, and anxiety or guilt related to the deceased or surviving family members are all indicators that additional evaluation or psychotherapeutic intervention might be warranted.

Time can also be an important factor in assessing adaptation to loss, but there are no uniform guidelines. Although the intensity of symptoms often abates substantially over a period of months, many precipitants can trigger their return and induce the return of sadness, tension, or stress, along with thoughts of and longing for the deceased person. Rando (1993) discusses a wide variety of such circumstances that can produce subsequent temporary upsurges of grief. Brabant, Forsyth, and McFarlain (1995) refer to the intensity of such periods of grief as similar to aftershocks following an earthquake. Examples of these reactions include realizing the child will never again have Thanksgiving with the family, will not graduate from high school, will not go on a summer picnic, or will no longer sing a favorite song. Some of these reactions are predictable and common (such as sadness around a holiday or anniversary); others may be completely unexpected. Professionals can help the family prepare for when some of these reactions are likely to occur (e.g., Thanksgiving, Christmas, or Hanukah) and also help the family cope with the unpredictable times. Usually these subsequent recurrences of grief are shorter in duration than what occurs during the acute mourning experience. If they persist more than several days following the stimulus events or evoke a heretofore unseen intensity, a psychological assessment is warranted.

The clinician must also be sensitive to the fact that the bereaved child cannot accurately be evaluated outside the family context. Grief reactions in children are subject to both amelioration and exacerbation based on the presence or lack of emotional support within the surviving family. Repeated findings in the literature support that a major factor in how surviving sisters and brothers adjust depends on the functioning of their parents or caregivers and how well those adults are able to provide for the children's needs (Baker, Sedney, and Gross, 1992; Kranzler et al, 1990; Weller et al, 1991; Worden, 1996). Researchers have also found that grieving parents' perceptions of symptoms in their surviving children are different from the children's perceptions and that these parents are often not fully cognizant of their children's depressive symptoms (Hogan and Balk, 1990; Weller et al, 1991). Thus, children should be observed and evaluated directly and clinicians should not merely rely on parent report. Behavioral contagion and social learning also play roles in determining a child's response. Religious rituals and family behavioral patterns provide opportunities for observational learning and imitation that can be either facillitative or inhibitory with respect to the child's adaptation. Children can also react to mourning, depression, or anxiety in their parents or caretakers even though they have had no or minimal contact with the deceased (e.g., a neonatal death or death of a family member who lives far away). The pediatrician must be aware of the parent's grief reaction to consider the family's emotional status as well.

MANAGEMENT OF GRIEF REACTIONS

The emotional care of the bereaved child, whether a surviving brother or sister or another patient, should have two focal points. First is the need to help children differentiate their fate from that of the deceased. Second is the need for children to arrive at a sense of closure with regard to the loss. These areas can involve expressing feelings of guilt or responsibility for the death as well as magical fears about what actually transpired. Both foci are important issues for any child who experiences a loss, although the need is more acute when considerable anxiety or sadness persists.

When another patient known to an ill child dies, the stress can be particularly intense, especially if the surviving child shares the same or similar medical diagnosis. The need to differentiate between the recently deceased and the living is a common cognitive adaptive response among children and adults. Adults are not immune to magical thinking, especially in times of emotional stress, but children have a particular need to distinguish between real and imaginary causes of death. Investigators of cognitive development have long documented the difficulties that children of different ages can have in coping with abstractions. Since death is a one-time-only, final experience for each of us, it qualifies as an abstract experience of individual mastery.

The questions a child might worry about in the after-

math of a death include "Why (i.e., by what means) did that person die?" "Will that happen to me (or someone else I care about)?" "Did I have anything to do with it?" "Who will take care of me now?" (if the deceased was a caretaker). Although these questions might not be specifically articulated by the child, they are almost always part of the underlying anxiety that accompanies a grief reaction. Addressing them must involve both informational and emotional components.

The pediatrician can be extremely helpful to the surviving children and parents immediately following the death. Siblings or peers of the deceased who carry a similar diagnosis need to be reassured in some way how their disease varies from the progression of the child who died. For healthy children, a complete physical examination by the physician (even if their routine check-up was recent) may reaffirm that the child is illness-free. If a surviving child becomes symptomatic (e.g., take on symptoms of the deceased, complain of stomachaches, bad dreams, or difficulty sleeping), the child should be allowed to have contact (even if by telephone) with the primary pediatrician or office nurse to discuss the ailments. Such contact is much more reassuring than being told, "Don't be silly, you're fine" by family members. Additionally, such contact may alleviate any irrational fear of the parents that another child might become ill. The families desperately need the consistent, concerned objectivity that the pediatrician can bring to them in such time of crisis.

In a family context, involvement of surviving brothers and sisters in funerary rituals can also be quite helpful and supportive if such involvement is explained well, if the child is provided with informed choices of activities, and if the activities are consistent with the child's wishes. Vicarious satisfaction of adults' needs during a funeral is not a proper basis for making the decision of whether to involve a child in such activities. Introduction of philosophical or religious concepts solely in a time of intense sadness can tend to confuse and frighten young children, especially without close family support.

FOLLOW-UP VISITS

Inviting the family to return to the hospital or to meet with professionals who helped care for the deceased often can be helpful weeks or months after the death. Some families feel they cannot ask for this contact because the patient is dead and their own needs do not seem a satisfactory basis for "imposing" on the staff. What clinicians need to remember sensitively is that they were a part of the final days of a child's life; and they will forever be indelibly integrated into the family's memories of that experience and incorporated into the meaning of the child's death for the family. To allow parents or brothers and sisters the opportunity to review such events with the medical team is a small but important gesture.

Sometimes an invitation by the staff to discuss autopsy results provides an opportunity for surviving family members to discuss residual emotional issues. A similar opportunity is also frequently welcomed by families who are told that follow-up sessions are "routine." Family members do not want to feel "crazy" or different from other families, and establishing a return visit as "normal" helps accomplish this.

Often friends, neighbors, and relatives do not understand why the immediate family has not "gotten over" or "let go" of the loss after several months. Individuals outside the family can overtly or subtly give messages that they no longer wish to hear about the deceased. Brabant and colleagues (1995) found in a small sample of parents who lost a child that sustained support from extended family was often lacking or short-lived. In such circumstances, those who helped care for the deceased child might offer the only emotional outlet available.

CHILDREN WHO SURVIVE

As noted earlier in this chapter, an ever-increasing number of children with life-threatening medical conditions are becoming long-term survivors. They can live with their disabilities or diseases only to experience complications or relapses after prolonged periods of relatively good health. These patients require special consideration and psychological care as they struggle with the uncertainties of survival beneath a "Damoclean threat" (Koocher, 1984; Koocher and O'Malley, 1981).

The families of such children experience similar stresses with occasional conflicting messages about whether to prepare for a death or hold realistic hope for the child's future. Encouraging such families to make use of psychological services, while offering them appropriate medical information and sensitive follow-up care, is the best intervention strategy. The key issue is not to assume that because the disease is under control, the emotions about the threat of loss are also under control.

A CLOSING NOTE

Many professionals are fearful of working with families of terminally ill children. Most often, they cite their own helplessness or sense of inadequacy in the face of death as a basis for their apprehension. The patients and their families are also afraid but want and need the support of professionals who can provide some encouragement and advice about how to cope with stress and uncertainty. The emotional rewards of working with families during this difficult time are substantial.

REFERENCES

Allen SM, Fleishman J: Problems encountered in home health service delivery to persons with AIDS. Home Health Care Services Q 13:129, 1992.

Baker JE, Sedney MA, Gross E: Psychological tasks for bereaved children. Am J Orthopsychiatry 62:105, 1992.

Bowlby J: Attachment and Loss: Vol. 3. Loss, Sadness and Depression. New York, Basic Books.

Brabant S, Forsyth C, McFarlain G: Life after the death of a child: initial and long term support from others. Omega 31:67, 1995.

Davies B, Reimer J, Brown P, Martens N: Fading Away: The Experience of Transition in Families With Terminal Illness. New York, Baywood Publishing Co, 1995.

DeMaso D, Meyer E, Beasley P: What do I say to my surviving children? J Am Acad Child Adolesc Psychiatry 36:1299, 1997.

Evans AE: If a child must die. N Engl J Med 278:138, 1968.

Gudas L: Concepts of death and loss in childhood and adolescence: a developmental perspective. *In* Saylor CE (ed): Children and Disasters. New York, Plenum Press, 1993, pp 67–84.

Hogan NS, Balk DE: Adolescent reactions to sibling death: perceptions of mothers, fathers, and teenagers. Nurs Res 39:103, 1990.

Jensen S, Given BA: Fatigue affecting family caregivers of cancer patients. Cancer Nurs 14:181, 1991.

Kellerman J, Rigler D, Siegal SE: Psychological effects of isolation in protected environments. Am J Psychiatry 134:563, 1977.

Koocher GP: Psychosocial care of the child during acute cancer treatment. Cancer 58:468, 1986.

Koocher GP: Terminal care and survivorship in pediatric chronic illness. Clin Psychol Rev 4:571, 1984.

Koocher GP: Development of the death concept in childhood. *In* Bibace R, Walsh ME (eds): The Development of Concepts Related to Health: Future Directions in Developmental Psychology. San Francisco, Jossey-Bass, 1981.

Koocher GP: Talking with children about death. Am J Orthopsychiatry 44:571, 1974.

Koocher GP: Childhood, death and cognitive development. Dev Psychol 9:369, 1973.

Koocher GP, Gudas L: Grief and loss in childhood. *In* Walker C, Roberts M (eds): Handbook of Clinical Child Psychology. New York, Wiley & Sons, 1992, pp 1025–1034.

Koocher GP, O'Malley JE: The Damocles Syndrome: Psychosocial Consequences of Surviving Childhood Cancer. New York, McGraw-Hill, 1981.

Kranzler EM, Shaffer MD, Wasserman G, Davies M: Early childhood bereavement. J Am Acad Child Adolesc Psychiatry 29:573, 1990.

Kübler-Ross E: On Death and Dying. New York, MacMillan Publishing, 1969.

Lonetto R: Children's Conceptions of Death. New York, Springer-Verlag, 1980.

Marquis S: Death of the nursed: burnout of the provider. Omega 27:17, 1993.

Meshot CM, Leitner LM: Adolescent mourning and parental death. Omega 26:287, 1992–93.

Piaget J: The Child's Conception of the World. Paterson, NJ: Littlefield, Adams, 1960.

Pollin I, Golant S: Taking Charge. New York, Random House, 1994.

Pollin I, Kanaan SB: Medical Crisis Counseling. New York, W.W. Norton, 1995.

Rando T: Treatment of Complicated Mourning. Champaign, Ill, Research Press, 1993.

Seligman MEP: Helplessness. San Francisco, W.H. Freeman, 1975.

Shapiro DE, Koocher GP: Goals and time considerations in outpatient medical crises intervention. Prof Psychol: Res Pract 27:109, 1996.

Sourkes BM: Facilitating family coping with childhood cancer. J Pediatric Psychol 2:65, 1977.

Stroebe M: Coping with bereavement: a review of the grief work hypothesis. Omega 26:19, 1992–93.

Waber DP, Gioia G, Paccia J, et al: Sex differences in cognitive processing in children treated with CNS prophylaxis for acute lymphoblastic leukemia. J Pediatric Psychol 15:105, 1990.

Weller RA, Weller EB, Fristad MA, Bowes JM: Depression in recently bereaved prepubertal children. Am J Psychiatry 148:1536, 1991.

Worden JW: Children and Grief. New York, Guilford Press, 1996.

Wortman CB, Silver RC: The myths of coping with loss. J Consult Clin Psychol 57:349, 1989.

Ztalin DM: Life themes: a method to understand terminal illness. Omega 31:185, 1995.

36 *Recurrent Pains*

Carolyn H. Frazer • Leonard A. Rappaport

The pains of children have the potential to generate painful experiences for clinicians. These elusive clinical challenges frequently occupy a diagnostic gray zone, a terra incognita somewhere in the borderland between psychological stress and "legitimate" organic illness. The clinician must be vigilant and sensitive while not under- or overreacting to the symptoms presented. In this chapter, some of the common forms of chronic pain are explored in such a way that a practical and systematic approach is presented. Equipped with this knowledge and conceptual framework, the clinician may feel justifiably more confident and find these conditions a bit less of a pain.

Recurrent pains are a common complaint in school-aged children and adolescents. For example, the incidence of recurrent abdominal pain in school-aged children is 10% to 15% (Apley and Hale, 1958; Oster, 1972). When other recurrent pain complaints such as headaches, limb pain, and chest pain are considered as well, pain complaints in children account for many pediatric visits.

Children presenting with recurrent pains are among the most challenging patients encountered in the primary care setting. Much of the difficulty involves the lack of an identified etiology leading to fear of missing a serious or treatable illness, as well as frustration with the chronic nature of the pain complaint on the part of the child, family, and clinician. By using a research-driven model for recurrent pains in childhood to guide the evaluation and management plan, however, most cases of recurrent pains can be managed successfully. In this chapter, we review conceptual models for recurrent pains in childhood, outline a general management approach, and discuss the specific issues of the most common forms of recurrent pain, including abdominal pain, limb and musculoskeletal pains, chest pain, and headache.

Conceptual Model for Recurrent Pains

Western medicine has traditionally used a model for pain that emphasizes a mind-body dichotomy. In other words, pain has been viewed as either "organic," having an identified physical etiology, or "nonorganic," having a psychological origin. Thus the traditional approach to children presenting with pain has involved performing tests to "rule out" an organic etiology and then considering the problem to be psychogenic if no physical disease is identified. More recently, the simultaneous and sequential contributions of

physical, mental, and environmental factors in recurrent pain syndromes have been recognized. Most cases of recurrent pain can be seen to exist on a continuum between organic pain, such as peptic ulcer disease, and psychologically influenced but physiologic pain such as reflex sympathetic dystrophy (Fig. 36–1). Current thinking is that all diseases have organic and psychological components that influence the painful episodes.

In all cases of pain, whether or not an organic basis is identified, there are aspects of physical pain sensation and psychological responses to pain. There is a complex interaction among these forces, the person experiencing pain, and his or her environment, all of which contribute to the pain experience. In a multifactorial model for pain (Fig. 36–2), the child's pain is considered in the context of physical health, temperamental profile, emotional status, family function, and home and school environments. For example, a child's temperamental style may modulate his or her response to pain regardless of the etiology. Similarly, the family dynamics, available supports, and complex interpersonal behavioral patterns may reinforce, modify, or decrease the child's pain experience and complaint.

General Approach to Recurrent Pains (Table 36–1)

SETTING APPROPRIATE EXPECTATIONS

In cases of recurrent pains, setting appropriate expectations initially with the child and family for the evaluation and

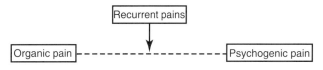

Figure 36–1. Pain spectrum.

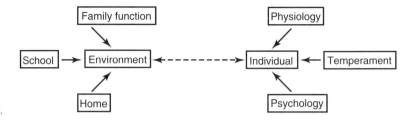

Figure 36–2. Multifactorial system model for pain.

management is crucial. In the majority of children with recurrent pains, a specific cause is never identified. For example, only 10% of recurrent abdominal pain has an identifiable organic etiology (Apley and Hale, 1958). Thus, in the majority of children with recurrent pain complaints, the physician will need to care for the child without ever determining a clear etiology for the pain. If this fact is not shared with the family at initial presentation, they may later feel frustration or fear due to the absence of a diagnosis and pursue further and often unnecessary medical evaluations. Perhaps worse, the child may begin to have the pain intrude upon his or her normal functioning, thus experiencing what Barr has termed an "extended pain syndrome" (Barr, 1983) that affects his or her overall personal life. Families and children need to know that typically a specific treatment will not fully cure recurrent pains. In fact anywhere from one quarter to one half of children with recurrent pains continue to have the same or another type of recurrent pain 3 months later. (Christensen and Mortensen, 1975; Magni et al, 1987). The contribution of physical, psychological, and environmental factors should be considered concurrently, and interventions shown to decrease the pain should be put in place whenever available. If pain relief cannot be achieved, the goal is to support the child to be as functional as possible.

EVALUATION

The first step in the evaluation of recurrent pains is to obtain a careful history and physical examination. The clinician must search for serious disease and treatable conditions. Guided by the literature on the specific recurrent pain complaint, the clinician should gather a review of systems pertinent to the presenting complaint, elicit a family history for similar or related complaints, and perform a thorough physical examination. In addition, a complete

social history including information about the child's temperament, emotional state, current living situation, school history, peer relationships, family function, and any recent or past stressors should be obtained. These factors help provide the context in which the child experiences pain and help assess the supports available for dealing with the pain. Sometimes, this history will provide clues to the etiology for the pain. It is helpful to interview both the parents and the child. With older children, the child should be interviewed separately. Observation of the child's behavior and the interaction between the child and parents provides additional information about the child's response to pain and the family dynamics. Laboratory testing is usually minimal and informed by the results of the history and physical examination. Again, it is important to emphasize from the outset that usually no "cause" is found, so that families are reassured rather than made more anxious if the laboratory test results are normal.

ONGOING MANAGEMENT

Perhaps the most important role for the clinician in the management of recurrent pain complaints is supportive and ongoing care. Establishing appropriate expectations at the first visit allows the clinician to offer support over time. Regular visits will help reassure the family and encourage the child to be as functional as possible, as well as allow for monitoring when the pain complaint or the child's general functioning has altered enough to demand further work-up or intervention. Regular visits also help reassure the clinician that no organic condition requiring treatment is present. Specific recommendations for return visits should be given, including changes in the pain complaint or other concerning signs and symptoms.

Recurrent Abdominal Pain

EXAMPLE

Eva is a 9-year-old girl who is brought to see her primary care physician due to "frequent tummy aches." Eva has previously been healthy. Over the past 3 to 4 months, she has had episodes of severe abdominal pain that come on suddenly and last anywhere from 5 minutes to 1 hour. Sometimes the pain is relieved when her mother rubs her belly. At times she has stayed home from school or been sent home from the nurse's office because of the pain.
There is no association with eating, and other daily activities have not been affected. There is no fever, rash, vomiting, diarrhea, or weight loss. When asked to describe where it hurts, Eva states "kind of all over" and points to

---

Table 36–1 • General Approach to Recurrent Pains

1. Set appropriate expectations at the initial visit.
2. Explain the recurrent and usually benign nature of recurrent pains in childhood.
3. Obtain a thorough history from the parents and child.
4. Perform a complete physical examination.
5. Be alert to "red flags," which indicate a higher likelihood of organic disease.
6. Obtain *limited* laboratory tests guided by the history and physical examination.
7. Discuss the management plan and goal to optimize the child's functioning despite the pain.
8. Review specific criteria for return visits or calls.
9. Provide ongoing and supportive care.

her epigastric area. She is not able to further describe the quality of the pain. Eva's mother reports no changes at home and describes Eva as a "top student" who has many friends.

Recurrent abdominal pain (RAP) is probably the most common recurrent pain syndrome in childhood. Approximately 10% to 15% of all school-aged children will have RAP at some point, with the prevalence being highest in school-aged girls (Apley and Hale, 1958; Oster, 1972). Apley's original description is used to define the syndrome: pain occurring intermittently, at least once a month, for over 3 months, which interferes with a child's home, school, or social functioning.

In most cases the pain is ill-defined and poorly localized. In the majority of cases (90%), the etiology for the pain is unknown. Many cases resolve over time; however, about one third of patients continue to be symptomatic and another third may develop other recurrent complaints, such as irritable bowel syndrome or migraine headaches in adolescence or adulthood. (Christensen and Mortensen, 1975; Magni et al, 1987).

SYMPTOMS

Typically, a child presents with vague abdominal pain that may be dull or crampy, lasts for less than 1 hour, and is poorly localized or periumbilical. There may be associated autonomic symptoms such as palpitations, sweating, or pallor, but results of the physical examination are usually normal. There may be a history of constipation, and in some cases, children will complain of left lower quadrant discomfort during abdominal examination. Growth and development are typically normal, and there are usually no systemic symptoms such as weight loss, fever, rash, joint swelling, or localized gastrointestinal or genitourinary complaints.

SUSPECTED PATHOPHYSIOLOGY

A number of potential mechanisms for RAP have been proposed, including variations in the autonomic nervous system or abnormal responses to gastrointestinal regulatory peptides causing abnormal gut motility, *Helicobacter pylori* infection, vulnerability to lactose intolerance, and constipation. No studies have identified one unifying cause for RAP, however.

DIFFERENTIAL DIAGNOSIS

The differential diagnosis for RAP is broad and includes any pathology of the gastrointestinal or genitourinary systems as well as more systemic conditions such as collagen vascular disease. In the 10% of cases with an identified etiology, there are usually "red flags" on history or physical examination that lead to the diagnosis (Table 36–2). Red flags include an atypical history, systemic symptoms, change in bowel habits, blood in the stool or urine, or pain that is atypical, such as localized, far from the umbilicus, or severe enough to wake the child. Abnormalities in screening laboratory test results are also suggestive of identifiable organic disease.

Table 36–2 • Red Flags: Recurrent Abdominal Pain

Pain farther away from the umbilicus
Pain awakening the child at night
Weight loss
Joint pains or swelling
Fever
Changes in bowel or bladder function
Dysuria
Diarrhea or excessive gas
Anemia
Guaiac-positive stools
Elevated erythrocyte sedimentation rate

WORK-UP

A careful history as outlined in the preceding section should be obtained. Specific details about the pain episodes, duration, frequency, associated symptoms, and exacerbating or relieving factors should be elicited. Physical examination should be complete and include neurologic and rectal examinations. Laboratory investigation should be limited to a screening in the absence of any red flags. The screening may include a complete blood count, erythrocyte sedimentation rate, urinalysis, urine culture in girls, stool guaiac, and stool test for ova and parasites or *Giardia* antigen. In patients in whom a specific etiology is suspected from the history and physical examination, further evaluation is indicated. However, further investigation should be guided only by specific symptoms or findings. For example, in children with diarrhea and bloating, a lactose breath test may be obtained. Abdominal ultrasonography may be useful if there are specific concerns for genitourinary pathology. In children with symptoms of gastritis such as vomiting or epigastric pain, infection with *H. pylori* may be considered.

TREATMENT

Treatment for RAP begins during the initial office visit. It is critical to present a working model of RAP prior to beginning any laboratory investigation. The physician should begin by explaining that abdominal pain of this type is quite common in children. In addition, it should be noted that a pathologic cause is *not* found in most cases of RAP, and the difference between disease and "functional" pain or differences in physiology that can contribute to pain should be explained. The recurrent nature of the syndrome can be discussed; this helps alleviate future frustration when and if symptoms recur. The physician should assure the child and family that he or she understands that the pain is real and should discuss the management plan to screen for any identifiable diseases, provide support and follow-up, and institute specific treatments as indicated. The goal for the physician and family should be to help the child function normally at home, school, and outside the home despite the pain and to work as a team toward that objective.

Specific treatments will be guided by the individual case. If constipation is suspected, the addition of fiber to the diet may improve symptoms. In a random, placebo-controlled study, Feldman and colleagues (1985) documented that 10 g of corn fiber per day produced a significant decrease in pain episodes in unselected children with RAP, so in fact utilizing a fiber intervention may be a good first step in treating RAP and would have no side effects except for inconvenience. In cases in which a specific etiology is identified, such as lactose intolerance or *H. pylori* infection, a dairy-free diet or antibiotic treatment, respectively, may reduce symptoms. Counseling, using a model of cognitive and behavioral family therapy, in conjunction with appropriate medical management, may be beneficial in some cases, particularly to help children and parents develop appropriate coping responses and maximize the child's function (Sanders et al, 1994). Various behavioral therapies including hypnotherapy, relaxation therapy, and biofeedback have helped reduce the pain complaint in children with RAP (Olness, 1989). The most important feature in the treatment of RAP, however, is establishing a supportive working relationship with the family and providing ongoing follow-up and care.

Recurrent Limb Pain

EXAMPLE

John is a 7-year-old boy who is brought to his physician for lower extremity pain. The pain has occurred over the past 3 to 4 months and tends to happen almost exclusively in the early evening and lasts until he falls asleep. There is no swelling or erythema, but the pain does interfere with activity and John tends to want to lie around while he is having the pain. The pain lasts from 3 to 4 hours when John stays up, but when he does finally fall asleep, the pain is always gone when he awakens in the morning. The pain has only rarely awakened him from his sleep. There has been no change in John's activity level, and a complete review of systems finds no abnormalities. The pain is distributed equally on weekdays and on weekends. John has not missed any school because of the pain, since it usually occurs in the evening.

SYMPTOMS

Recurrent limb pains are a common complaint in childhood, occurring slightly less frequently than recurrent abdominal pain but somewhat more commonly than recurrent headaches. The first description of these pains as "growing pains" was by Duchamp in 1823. Since that time, a small series of studies have brought more clarity to the character and cause of this pain complaint, beginning with Hawksley in the 1930s who distinguished these pains from rheumatism, Naish and Apley who provided a population-based study of growing pains in British school children, Brenning from Sweden in the 1960s, Oster from Denmark, and most recently Abu-Arafeh and Russell in a population-based study of children in England (Hawksley, 1938; Naish and Apley, 1951; Brenning, 1960; Abu-Arafeh and Russell, 1996). Abu-Arafeh and Russell were the first to describe the prevalence of various recurrent pain symptoms in childhood as well as their concurrence in the same children.

Generally accepted criteria for recurrent limb pain to be considered as growing pains include the following: the pain most frequently occurs late in the day or awakens the child at night; the pain must be severe enough to interfere with activity; it is not specifically related to the joints; it has been occurring at least monthly for at least 3 months; and it is intermittent, with symptom-free intervals of at least days. In addition, the child must have a normal physical examination.

DIFFERENTIAL DIAGNOSIS

Similar to recurrent abdominal pain, recurrent limb pain can be the presenting symptom of almost any pediatric disorder. The first consideration in the differential diagnosis is whether the child is sick or not sick. The second is to break down the symptoms into joint and nonjoint pain. In both categories, etiologies include infectious, neoplastic, rheumatic, and immune-mediated as well as metabolic disorders. In well children, one should always be especially cognizant of traumatic causes as well as mechanical abnormalities. As with most pain complaints, the physician's first responsibility is to identify children with a recognized organic pathology for their pain complaint with the least invasive and least traumatic work-up that is possible.

EVALUATION

A complete history and physical examination is the first and most important step in the consideration of recurrent limb complaints. If a specific etiology is suggested in the history or physical examination, the evaluation should be directed at confirming or ruling out that specific etiology. For example, if the pain is one-sided and associated with slight swelling of the thigh, a radiograph and perhaps other imaging techniques would be appropriate to rule out a tumor. Searches without leads for the causes of recurrent limb pain, however, can be anxiety-producing for families and traumatic for children. Although recurrent limb pain has not been studied as extensively as recurrent abdominal pain, we suspect that the yield of an undirected work-up will be equally small. While red flags specific for limb pain have not been described, common sense would suggest that utilizing the red flags for abdominal pain with alterations for the obvious area of the body involved would be most reasonable.

TREATMENT

Limb pain from a specific identified etiology should be treated appropriately. To the best of our knowledge, there have been no controlled trials in the treatment of nonspecific limb pain (growing pains). The first step is to reassure the family and child that the pain they describe is common in children, and that it tends to go away over time. The second step is to make sure that the pain symptom is interfering with the child's activity only while the pain is being experienced and that the family has not withdrawn the child from usual childhood activities or social experiences. There is no evidence that limiting activity improves the pain, and withdrawal from activities may cause the child and parent to focus more on the pain. Several interventions (e.g., stretching, warm baths) have been suggested as helpful in growing pains; however, none has been studied in a controlled trial.

Recurrent Headaches

EXAMPLE

Amy is a 12-year-old girl who presents with a month-long history of "daily" headaches. They tend to occur later in the day or during math class and are sometimes associated with feeling tired. The pain occurs "all over" her head and is sometimes relieved with acetaminophen or lying down. There are no associated fevers, weight loss, visual changes, nausea, or vomiting. There is no family history for headaches. Amy did have "stomachaches" from ages 9 to 10 years, which resolved over time.

BACKGROUND

Headaches are another common recurrent pain complaint in childhood. The seminal population survey of 9000 Scandinavian school children by Bille in 1962 demonstrated a prevalence of roughly 15% for frequent recurrent headache and 5% for migraine (Bille, 1962). A more recent study by Abu-Arafeh and Russell showed an incidence of 11% for migraine and 1% for tension headaches in children in Aberdeen, Scotland (Abu-Arafeh and Russell, 1994). The majority of recurrent headaches in childhood are benign—either migraine or "functional" tension headaches. However, potentially lethal causes of headache such as intracerebral hemorrhage or tumor create significant anxiety in parents and clinicians. In addition, many adults are under the impression that children do not get headaches.

SYMPTOMS

Headaches may be categorized by pathophysiology, symptoms, and temporal pattern. With a thorough history and physical examination, it is possible to distinguish between pathologic and functional causes of headache and thus determine an appropriate management plan. The most concerning patterns are acute and progressive. Acute-onset headache may be associated with serious pathology such as infection, head trauma, hypertension, or hemorrhage. There are often associated neurologic or systemic symptoms, and pain is frequently localized. Progressive headaches may indicate increasing intracranial pressure due to hydrocephalus or a mass lesion and thus require further and immediate investigation.

In contrast, recurrent, nonprogressive headaches are much less likely to be associated with serious pathology. Acute recurrent headaches are most commonly migraine, thought to be secondary to paroxysmal constriction and dilation of cerebral blood vessels. Migraine headaches can be unilateral, although in children they tend to be bilateral and may have associated visual, gastrointestinal, sensory, and motor symptoms. They may be preceded by an aura, although children may have a hard time describing the aura since it can be so unusual. In 50% of cases, there is a positive family history for migraine. The headaches may be triggered by stress, certain foods (dairy, chocolate, coffee), and menstruation. Migraines can cause significant discomfort but do not have long-term health sequelae.

Chronic (nonprogressive) recurrent headaches are common in childhood and are also rarely associated with serious pathology. They are often termed "functional" or tension headaches and are characterized by frequent occurrence (often daily), symmetric, poorly defined pain, and few associated symptoms. Occasionally children may present with blurred vision, fatigue, or dizziness. There is sometimes a history of prior episodes of recurrent abdominal or limb pain. Tension headaches are thought to be caused by muscle contraction with resultant ischemia and pain. There are some children who present with a "mixed" pattern, which has elements of both migraine and tension headaches.

DIFFERENTIAL DIAGNOSIS

The differential diagnosis for headache is broad. Pain may be caused by inflammation, traction, or disease in any of the pain-sensitive tissues in the head and skull. Pain in these tissues is mediated by cranial nerves V, VII, IX, and X and upper cervical nerves. The brain itself is not pain sensitive. In the majority of headaches, particularly those that are recurrent and nonprogressive, no significant pathologic etiology is identified. However, in headaches with acute onset or progressive symptoms, more significant etiologies must be considered. These include infection such as sinusitis, otitis, meningitis, and encephalitis; central nervous system tumor with traction on intracerebral tissues and vessels; cerebral or subdural hemorrhage; referred pain from facial or oral structures; inflammation such as arteritis; temporomandibular pain; subtle seizures; head trauma; increased intracranial pressure due to hydrocephalus; visual refractive errors; and use of illicit drugs such as cocaine.

RED FLAGS

Pain that is of acute onset, severe in quality, and very localized is cause for concern. Pain that awakens the child from sleep or occurs early in the morning is more likely due to central nervous system pathology. Pain that is exacerbated by lying down suggests increased intracranial pressure. Localized neurologic findings, papilledema, ataxia, and personality changes are all cause for concern. Seizures, weakness, and visual or gait changes also suggest a pathologic etiology. In addition, systemic symptoms such as fever, joint swelling, fatigue, and weight loss are red flags for a pathologic etiology for headache (Table 36–3).

WORK-UP

The appropriate evaluation for the child presenting with headache begins with a thorough history. The presenting symptoms should be carefully characterized as to onset, duration, severity, temporal pattern, associated symptoms including an aura, and associated factors that exacerbate or relieve the pain. Family history is often positive with migraine headaches. A thorough psychosocial history is also essential to identify any stressors in the child's life that may be contributing to the child's headaches and to determine any impact on the child's function related to the

Table 36–3 • Red Flags: Headache

Acute, severe, and localized
Awakens the child from sleep
Early morning headache
Pain worse when lying down
Vomiting
Papilledema
Focal neurologic findings
Personality change
Seizures
Systemic symptoms (fever, weight loss, joint swelling, fatigue)
Crescendo pattern of pain—worsening with each successive headache

headaches. Recurrent headaches are often associated with school absence, for example. It is important to screen for possible depression, as emotional disorders can potentiate headaches. A complete physical examination is also essential and should include blood pressure measurement, full neurologic examination, fundoscopic examination to rule out papilledema, skin examination for neurocutaneous markings, measurement of head circumference, and auscultation of the head for bruits to rule out an arteriovenous malformation.

Laboratory investigations are rarely indicated and should be guided by specific suspicion based on the history and physical examination. Electroencephalography is rarely helpful except in cases in which the suspicion for a seizure disorder is high. Brain imaging is indicated when there are acute or progressing symptoms or if there are signs or symptoms of increased intracranial pressure.

TREATMENT AND MANAGEMENT

Reassurance and explanation are the most important tools in the management of recurrent headaches. As with all recurrent pain, it is crucial to set the stage from the beginning so that parents and child have appropriate expectations from the clinician. Once serious pathology has been excluded by a careful history and thorough physical examination, the physician should explain to the family that recurrent headaches are quite common in children and not dangerous. There are no long-term sequelae. There are a variety of therapeutic options for treating headaches. School attendance and participation in regular activities is very important, and the main goal is to optimize function at school, at home, and with peers.

Treatment includes pharmacotherapy, counseling, and biofeedback. Analgesics may be very effective, particularly for tension headaches, and have few side effects. Amitriptyline has also been used to treat chronic recurrent headaches, particularly if there are signs of depression (Couch and Hassanein, 1979). For migraines with associated nausea, antiemetics may be helpful. Serotonergic agents and ergotamine compounds act by decreasing vasodilation and can abort a migraine (Rothner, 1989). For migraine prophylaxis, clinicians use a number of medications, including propranolol and cyproheptadine (Bille et al, 1977; Gerber et al, 1995).

Counseling for the child and family may be helpful to develop strategies for coping with the pain and identify

any contributing stressors or triggers and thus reduce episodes and maximize functioning. In some cases, diet modification may be helpful. Relaxation and biofeedback may be beneficial for some patients (McGrath and Masek, 1993). As with any recurrent pain syndrome, regular follow-up and support are the most important elements in clinical management. Families should be given recommendations for when to return or contact the clinician, including a review of potential red flags.

Recurrent Chest Pain

EXAMPLE

Ron is a 9-year-old boy who presented to his pediatrician in an emergency unscheduled visit because of chest pain. He was feeling fine when he experienced severe left-sided pain that worsened with movement but did not go away with staying still. He felt as if the pain was just under his ribs and made it difficult to catch his breath. He had never had the pain before, and by the time he got to the pediatrician's office the pain was gone. His past medical history was unremarkable, he was a good student, and there was no history of early heart disease in his extended family. There was no history of trauma to the area of the pain. On physical examination, his heart sounds had a normal S1 and S2 with no murmur. His chest examination was remarkable for a small bruise above the area where he was having the pain, and the pain was reproducible by pressing on the bruise. When asked about the bruise, Ron recalled that he had fallen on his side when playing football with his friends and landed on a tree branch on the ground. He was reassured that the pain was from the fall and went home with his parents, who had accompanied him, feeling quite relieved.

BACKGROUND

The literature on recurrent chest pain has not been separated into acute and recurrent pain as it has for many other pain symptoms in childhood. It has been noted in several studies however, that in children presenting with chest pain to clinics or to emergency departments, approximately 45% are still experiencing the pain 6 months later, implying that much of what presents as an acute complaint becomes chronic (Leung et al, 1996; Selbst, 1985; Selbst et al, 1990). A unique issue with chest pain is that since in adults this type of pain is frequently associated with life-threatening outcomes, chest pain in children is commonly brought to medical attention almost immediately.

The prevalence of chest pain in children has not been studied to the best of our knowledge; however, the incidence of chest pain in children presenting to an emergency department is approximately 6 per 1000 visits. The male to female ratio is 1:1 and the mean age is 12 years. Young children seem to be more likely to have a cardiorespiratory cause for their chest pain, whereas adolescents are more likely to have a "psychogenic disturbance" (Driscoll et al, 1976; Zavaras-Angelidou et al, 1992). In the literature on chest pain "psychogenic disturbance" is not well defined but loosely means that psychological factors are contribut-

Table 36–4 • Causes of Cardiac-Related Chest Pain

Cardiac Lesion	History or Physical Findings
Severe aortic stenosis	Murmur
Hypertrophic obstructive cardiomyopathy	Autosomal dominant, family history, murmur audible on standing or with Valsalva maneuver
Mitral valve prolapse	Apical midsystolic murmur after a click
Severe pulmonary or aortic stenosis	Diagnosis usually made before pain due to significant murmur and cyanosis (pulmonary stenosis)
Coronary artery disease—post-Kawasaki disease, anomalous coronary arteries	History—no physical findings
Cardiac infection—pericarditis	Fever, sharp stabbing chest pain, respiratory distress, distant heart sounds, friction rub, pulsus paradoxus, pain improves when patient sits up and leans forward
Cardiac infection—myocarditis	Mild pain for several days, fever, vomiting, lightheaded feeling, then more severe pain and respiratory distress; distant heart sounds, gallop rhythm, and orthostatic changes

ing to an overreaction to a normal pain symptom. These factors include a relative who has recently had a significant heart disorder such as a myocardial infarction or a death of a grandparent or friend that makes the adolescent associate mild pain with a frightening outcome. One third of children presenting with chest pain are awakened from sleep by their pain and one third miss school because of the chest pain. After work-up, the chest pain is rarely found to be caused by serious pathology.

The most common sources for chest pain in children are musculoskeletal and pleuritic. In both of these types of pain, it can usually be reproduced by deep breathing, movement, or pressure. Occasionally chest pain can be caused by chest wall abnormalities such as scoliosis or costochondritis.

Chest pain of cardiac origin is unusual in children but obviously of great importance. Ischemic cardiac pain, although quite rare, can result from multiple causes (Table 36–4). Cardiac pain is associated with physical activity and is retrosternal and gripping in character. The pain is typically relieved rapidly by rest. Usually there are hints in the history, such as a past history of Kawasaki disease, or associated findings on physical examination such as the physical stigmata of Marfan syndrome. Children can also experience a cardiac arrhythmia such as supraventricular tachycardia or premature ventricular beats as brief sharp chest pain.

Other causes of chest pain include respiratory disorders such as pneumonia, asthma, pneumothorax, or pneumomediastinum. Rarely children can have pulmonary embolism that causes chest pain, but this is usually associated with specific predisposing conditions such as the use of oral contraceptives, recent severe leg trauma in sports, or abortion. Gastrointestinal problems such as an esophageal foreign body or reflux esophagitis can also present with chest pain. The pain is usually substernal. With a foreign body, the child may or may not experience pain, but the history is very helpful. In esophagitis, the pain is usually burning in character and worsened by lying down or eating spicy food.

EVALUATION

The evaluation of a child or adolescent presenting with chest pain is fully dependent on obtaining a thorough history from the child and parent as well as doing a complete physical examination. Use of the red flags outlined in Table 36–5 plus specific leads from the history and physical examination determine the need for further testing. There are no standard tests that are necessary for a child presenting with chest pain; however, the work-up may be quite extensive if there are worrisome findings in the history or physical examination.

TREATMENT

Although serious pathology is a rare cause of chest pain in childhood, it should be considered and treated appropriately. What a clinician should do with the remainder of children and families who present frightened about chest pain of unclear or benign etiology is another question. Intervention should be directed first at educating the child and family that chest pain is common in children but rarely has a serious etiology or sequelae. Further interventions for chest pain are similar to treatments outlined for chronic pain in the introductory section of this chapter.

Conclusion

Recurrent pains are common in childhood and rarely represent a serious or life-threatening condition. The usually benign outcome of these painful episodes does not diminish the distress experienced by children, their parents, and the clinician. By using an organized approach, however, the majority of children with recurrent pains can be success-

Table 36–5 • Red Flags: Chest Pain

Young age
Worsens with exertion, improves with rest
Awakened from sleep by chest pain
Positive family history of hypertrophic cardiomyopathy, Marfan syndrome, or Ehlers-Danlos syndrome
Pain is crushing in character
Syncope associated with pain
Fever
Signs of chronic disease (weight loss, extreme fatigue)

fully managed in the primary care setting. Appropriate expectations regarding the recurrent nature and usually benign etiology should be discussed with the family at the initial visit. The clinician must identify any potentially serious condition by performing a thorough history and physical examination with attention to red flags. In the absence of serious pathology, the goal is to reassure the family, relieve pain when possible, and promote the child's functioning at home, at school, and with peers. The most important aspect in managing recurrent pain syndromes is to provide supportive and ongoing care to the child and family.

REFERENCES

Abu-Arafeh I, Russell G: Prevalence of headache and migraine in schoolchildren. Br Med J 309:765, 1994.

Abu-Arafeh I, Russell G: Recurrent limb pain in schoolchildren. Arch Dis Child 74:336, 1996.

Apley J, Hale B: Children with recurrent abdominal pains: a field survey of 1000 school children. Arch Dis Child 33:165, 1958.

Barr R: Recurrent abdominal pain. *In* Levine M, Carey W, Crocker A, Gross R (eds): Developmental-Behavioral Pediatrics. Philadelphia, WB Saunders, 1983, pp 521–528.

Bille B: Migraine in school children. Acta Paediatr Scand 51(suppl 136):1, 1962.

Bille B, Ludvigsson J, et al: Prophylaxis of migraine headache in children. Headache 17(2):61, 1977.

Brenning R: Growing pains. Acta Soc Medicor Upsalienis 65:185, 1960.

Christensen M, Mortensen O: Long term prognosis in children with recurrent abdominal pain. Arch Dis Childh 50:1100, 1975.

Couch J, Hassanein R: Amitriptyline in migraine prophylaxis. Arch Neurol 36:695, 1979.

Driscoll D, Glicklick L, et al: Chest pain in children: a prospective study. Pediatrics 57:648, 1976.

Feldman W, McGrath P, et al: The use of dietary fiber in the management of simple, childhood, idiopathic, recurrent, abdominal pain: results in a prospective, double-blind, randomized, controlled trial. Am J Dis Child 139:1216, 1985.

Gerber W, Schellenberg R, et al: Cyclandelate versus propranolol in the prophylaxis of migraine: a double-blind placebo-controlled study. Functional Neurol 10(1):27, 1995.

Hawksley J: The incidence and significance of "growing pains" in children and adolescents. J R Inst Public Health 1:798, 1938.

Leung A, Robson W, et al: Chest pain in children. Can Fam Physician 42:1156, 1996.

Magni G, Pierri M, et al: Recurrent abdominal pain in children: a long term follow-up. Eur J Pediatr 146(1):72, 1987.

McGrath M, Masek B: Biobehavioral treatment of headache. *In* Schechter N, Berde C, Yaster M (eds): Pain in Infants, Children and Adolescents. Baltimore, Williams and Wilkins, 1993, pp 555–560.

Naish J, Apley J: "Growing pains": a clinical study of non-arthritis limb pains in children. Arch Dis Child 26:134, 1951.

Olness K: Hypnotherapy: a cyberphysiologic strategy in pain management. Pediatr Clin North Am 36:873, 1989.

Oster J: Recurrent abdominal pain, headache and limb pain in children and adolescents. Pediatrics 50:429, 1972.

Rothner A: Migraine headaches. *In* Swaiman K (ed): Pediatric Neurology Principles and Practice. St. Louis, CV Mosby Company, 1989, pp 643–648.

Sanders M, Shepherd R, et al: The treatment of recurrent abdominal pain in children: a controlled comparison of cognitive-behavioral family intervention and standard pediatric care. J Consult Clin Psych 62:306, 1994.

Selbst S: Chest pain in children. Pediatrics 75:1068, 1985.

Selbst S, Ruddy R, et al: Chest pain in children: followup of patients previously reported. Clin Pediatr 29:374, 1990.

Zavaras-Angelidou K, Weinhouse E, et al: Review of 180 episodes of chest pain in 134 children. Pediatr Emerg Care 8:189, 1992.

37 "Colic": Prolonged or Excessive Crying in Young Infants

William B. Carey

 Much of the general public and many primary care physicians regard "colic" as an incomprehensible and unmanageable condition that brings great distress to families. Unlike most treatments of this subject, this chapter reports that prolonged crying in young infants is sufficiently understandable in most cases to allow a rational approach that is usually effective. The strategy is to lessen the poorness of fit between the irritable or sensitive behavioral predisposition of the infant and the particular handling techniques of the family.

"Colic" is a poorly defined and incompletely understood state of prolonged or excessive crying seen in young infants who are otherwise well. Although widely regarded by pediatricians and parents as confusing and frustrating, it can usually be successfully improved in a few days.

Definition

There is no standard definition of colic. Pediatric texts and advice books for parents usually (but not always) present a brief section on a phenomenon variously designated by terms such as paroxysmal fussing in infancy, infantile colic, evening colic, or 3-month colic.

Usual descriptions of colic indicate that the condition begins soon after the baby comes home from the newborn nursery and can persist until he or she is 3 or 4 months of age. The crying is characterized as intense, lasting for up to several hours at a time, and usually occurring in the late afternoon and evening. The affected infant is typically pictured as drawing up the knees against the abdomen and expelling much flatus. He or she can appear hungry but is not quieted for long by further feeding or other attempts at soothing. The infant eats well and grows normally, however. The usual explanation offered is that the crying is caused by abdominal pain of intestinal origin.

The standard textbook description in the preceding paragraph is inadequate on several counts:

1. Without a more precise definition of the duration of the crying, it can be extended to apply to almost all young infants at one time or another.
2. Such imprecision makes most studies of the phenomenon of questionable value. Writers on the subject often express strong convictions about favorite theories of cause and management that can be neither refuted nor verified because the infants studied are so poorly identified.
3. Figures relating to the incidence of colic are of little value.
4. Telling parents that their child has colic is at best a confusing message.

The best definition available is still the one used by Wessel and colleagues (1954), that such a young infant is "one who, otherwise healthy and well fed, had paroxysms of irritability, fussing, or crying lasting for a total of more than three hours a day and occurring on more than three days in any one week." Some authors add another criterion of a duration of more than 3 weeks. The prolonged crying is thus identified in terms of total duration but neither as to the frequency of the bouts of crying nor as to its quality. Even this definition, however, is applied with difficulty at times. The term "colic" should ideally be eliminated from clinical use and perhaps restricted to research projects, where it is important to describe accurately the population of subjects.

Any attempt at improving this definition should convey the idea that the child is otherwise well but is crying substantially more than the mean amount for infants of his or her age. The condition might then be better referred to as *prolonged crying* or *primary excessive crying*. The evidence to date does not justify any conclusion that the quality or pitch of the prolonged crying is any different from that of other infants. Most parents do find a high-pitched cry more unpleasant, but it seems to be the quantity that makes them more likely to complain to their child's physician. The flatus might be a consequence rather than the cause of the crying. It is not even certain that such infants are experiencing abdominal pain, as has been commonly assumed. Infants flex their legs in response to a variety of noxious stimuli, such as a pinprick on the foot. It will be difficult to answer with certainty the question of whether such infants are experiencing any kind of pain. Since the crying can generally be markedly diminished within a few days by management techniques that do not reduce pain, it is hard to maintain the view that pain is primarily responsible. The affected infant does not seem to have any disease or malfunction of the bowel or any other organ but differs from the norm only in regard to the amount of crying.

Most studies of prolonged crying have used referred populations, thereby introducing a selection bias. A clearer perspective comes from studies performed in primary care pediatric practices (Carey, 1968, 1972; Taubman, 1988) and from cross-sectional population studies. Such a study of 530 infants in London found that, according to diaries kept by the mothers, 23% of the infants met the Wessel criteria for colic at 6 weeks but that "the overwhelming majority of the crying and associated behavior is unsettled, fussing, and irritable behavior, rather than paroxysmal, abnormally intense or inconsolable crying" (St. James-Roberts, Conroy, and Wilsher, 1995). All infants had periods of inconsolable crying. Those regarded as colicky had more of it but still spent only a small portion of their time in that intense, unsoothable state.

The conclusion to be derived from these and other data is that what is being called "colic" today is the upper end of the normal range of crying rather than a discrete, categorical disorder. Barr (1990) has noted that as the total amount of crying increases or decreases, it is the duration of the bouts that changes rather than the number of separate bouts. Our current understanding of these phenomena is advancing but still far from complete (see recent review of research in Lester and Barr, 1997).

Differential Diagnosis

Since the phenomenon under discussion is prolonged or excessive crying in otherwise well young infants, this condition must be distinguished from two others: normal crying and secondary excessive crying resulting from faulty feeding techniques or physical problems in the infant.

NORMAL CRYING

Brazelton (1962) assessed in detail the crying patterns in a middle class sample of 80 infants. Crying lasted a total of about 2 hours a day at 2 weeks, increased to a peak of almost 3 hours by 6 weeks, and then gradually decreased to about 1 hour by 3 months. The upper quartile of babies were crying 3 1/2 hours per day at 6 weeks. Throughout these 3 months, the principal time for crying for all infants was in the evening. These findings have been supported by similar figures in Canada and England. Pertinence for other populations has yet to be determined.

Several observers have noted that for prematurely born infants, the crying peak occurs at a point 6 weeks after 40 weeks postconceptional age, but this conclusion requires further substantiation. No evidence has been published for gender or birth order differences based on objective data collection.

The amount of parental complaining about crying is not necessarily proportional to the extent of the crying. Some parents are upset about typical periods of fussing, whereas others might not seem disturbed by greater quantities. The first step in the differential diagnosis is to decide whether the crying is merely an ordinary amount that the parents cannot tolerate or is truly longer than average. There seems to be little doubt that parents with greater psychosocial stress are more likely to complain about their infants' crying.

FAULTY FEEDING TECHNIQUES

Underfeeding and overfeeding and inadequate burping or sucking are faulty feeding techniques that should be considered. These possibilities usually can be excluded by a routine history and physical examination. Some have suggested that the type of bottle used or breast- versus formula feeding may affect the amount of crying, but these possibilities are not well supported by current evidence.

PHYSICAL PROBLEMS IN THE BABY

If colic or primary excessive crying in infants is by definition found only in those who are otherwise well, various physical problems in the infant must be excluded before the diagnosis can be applied. Three kinds of problems are usually cited: (1) acute disorders such as otitis media, intestinal cramping with diarrhea, corneal abrasion, a hair tourniquet on a digit, and incarcerated hernia—all of which are relatively easily ruled out by the history and by the examination of the infant—and more chronic conditions such as gastroesophageal reflux; (2) nutritional intolerances such as cow's milk allergy, lactose intolerance, or transmission of irritating substances such as caffeine via breast milk, all of which appear to be relatively insignificant causes of prolonged crying in otherwise well infants; and (3) inadequately defined clinical entities, such as "immaturity" of the central nervous system or of the intestine, which have not been sufficiently studied. Premature infants may be more irritable than full-term ones but are not necessarily colicky.

Despite the widespread opinion that milk allergy can cause excessive crying in otherwise well infants, no study of acceptable design has confirmed this possibility (Carey, 1989). If such a connection should at some point become established in 5% to 10% of prolonged criers, as some believe, the diagnosis of such infants could not be "colic" if that term applies only to infants who are otherwise well. In those infants thought to have lactose intolerance, an elimination of lactose in the diet decreases breath hydrogen but has no effect on the crying.

Contributory Factors in Interaction

If the infant is healthy but is irritable, fussing, and crying substantially more than most, there is usually no single clear-cut explanation for this behavior. The answer appears to lie in the interaction between factors in the infant and the environment. The two principal contributory elements to consider are a physiologic predisposition in the infant and inappropriate handling by the parents, both of which usually appear to be variations of normal rather than abnormalities.

Infants vary considerably in their temperaments or emotional reactivity characteristics (see Chapter 8). The most likely contribution of the infant is a normal predisposition to be more sensitive, more irritable, more intense, less adaptable, or less soothable than average for age. More perceptive infants with low sensory thresholds are prone to increased crying, apparently because they are more vulnerable to disorganization by excessive or inappropriate sensory input from the environment (Carey, 1972, 1984). This relationship between prolonged crying and temperament should become clearer when temperament is studied and clinically assessed before, during, and after the period of excessive crying in the same individuals. So far, such measurements have been attempted only before and after.

Parents may not know at first which methods are most effective for quieting babies in general and theirs in particular. If they cannot understand or tolerate their infant's needs and react to them appropriately, they may engage in unsuitable manipulations that increase rather than decrease the duration of the bouts of crying. Inexperience and anxiety are factors that can make parents even less skillful at responding sensitively. Excessive and inappropriate handling of the infant, such as picking up a fussy, overtired baby, is frequently observed both as a causal factor and as a response to prolonged crying. Prolonged crying probably occurs most typically in the absence of any abnormality in the infant or parent but rather when the parents have not yet learned to interact harmoniously with their infant.

The possible role of psychosocial factors in generating prolonged crying in young infants has been much debated in the literature. An important consideration has been the type of sample used. Infants who are referred to specialty clinics because of the severity of the crying are a selected subgroup of the total population and are probably more likely to demonstrate significant "destabilized maternal functioning" owing to the problems in their lives (Papoušek and von Hofacker, 1995). Primary pediatric care samples and cross-sectional studies, on the other hand, tend to find maternal anxiety and guilt, but it is uncertain how much this differs from what is seen in the general population.

Management

Most advice dealing with the management of prolonged or excessive crying is unreasonably pessimistic about the effectiveness of professional intervention. This defeatism is unjustified; appropriate measures are usually successful in reducing crying to acceptable amounts in 2 to 3 days.

HISTORY

Management begins, as elsewhere, with an adequate history. The first step is to define the symptom: the intensity, duration, and frequency of the crying. Parents often say that the baby is too "gassy" or too hungry, and the clinician must sift the evidence to discover that the crying is the real problem. A good way to make the parents' description of the baby more precise is to ask for a detailed narration of the baby's typical day or for a diary of the crying. Information about the baby's temperamental characteristics can usually be adequately based on brief descriptions of the infant's sensitivity, irritability, intensity, and soothability, but the clinician may choose to use a more detailed questionnaire (see Chapter 67). Having the parents demonstrate their soothing techniques can be helpful in revealing practices that require modification.

The rest of the medical history should be obtained in the usual manner but with an enrichment so as to include parental concern about the pregnancy and the child and anxieties related to their own experience as children or with rearing previous children or to inadequate family support and other stresses. Family psychosocial stressors should be sought and dealt with appropriately, but they will not necessarily be found, and if uncovered, they are not necessarily causative of or resulting from the prolonged crying.

PHYSICAL EXAMINATION

The physical examination seldom reveals anything useful in regard to the diagnosis or management of the crying but is an absolutely necessary part of the procedure. Most parents are doubtful about reassurance that is not preceded by a careful assessment of the infant. For example, a hasty prescription of sedative drops over the telephone is generally not successful.

Laboratory tests, however, are usually not necessary and should not be performed unless specifically indicated by the history and physical examination.

COUNSELING

Counseling has proven to be the most effective method available for helping parents cope successfully with prolonged crying (Carey, 1994). Standard lectures on infant care and simple empathy with the distress of the parents have not been shown to be successful. Counseling should be individualized to the particular situation and should include these main topics:

1. *The infant is not sick.* The physician should reassure the parents that the physical examination has not revealed any problem in the infant's health. The crying may mean distress but is seldom due to pain. Antecedent fears about the infant and anxieties resulting from the crying can be allayed. Counseling about prolonged or excessive crying and its management should avoid "the medical model" that there is probably something, as yet unconfirmed, wrong with the infant's gastrointestinal tract, nervous system, allergic responses, or general viability. Similarly the parents must be unburdened of unjustified worry or guilt about their caregiving abilities. Reassurance about their competence is helpful. Pertinent psychosocial stressors that possibly have contributed to the crying should be discussed.

2. *Education about infant crying.* A comparison of the particular infant's crying with the average for the age should be followed by an educational discussion that includes information such as the following: All young infants are irritable and fussy and cry to some degree, the average in this period being 2 to 3 hours a day. Normal infants vary in how much they cry, how intense the crying is, how sensitive they are to stimuli, and how easily soothed they are. Many parents do not know that fatigue is a common reason why infants cry. Infant crying affects parents' feelings and behavior, such as marital satisfaction and self-esteem. Parents react differently to infant crying,

with varying amounts of guilt, anger, and fear and with stimulation, attempts at soothing, and often overfeeding of the infant. Thus, excessive crying is generally the result of a "poor fit" between the infant's needs and predispositions and the parental response.

3. *The excessive amount of crying can be reduced.* As stated, parental handling of the infant may require alteration. Parents with fussy infants usually are doing too much or doing the right things at the wrong times and they need to shift their tactics. They usually will be successful if they soothe more—as with a pacifier, repetitive sound, and heating pad or hot water bottle—and stimulate less—as with decreasing picking up and feeding the infant in response to every cry. Parents need to learn to be more selective as to when they pick up their crying infant and to refrain from responding to every whimper. A quiet, dimly lit environment with a minimum of unnecessary handling and correction of any faulty feeding techniques without changing the composition of the feedings seem to be helpful. All of these instructions can be given without making the parents feel inadequate.

The essence of this individualized approach is in helping parents to become more skillful at meeting the needs of their infant by observing their infant carefully and interpreting more accurately the behavior their infant displays ("sensitive differential responding"). Perhaps the best way to accomplish this is to watch parent and infant interact during the office visit. Since this is at best a brief episode, however, a more practical method is to ask the parent to relate a typical day, with descriptions of what the infant does, how the parent responds, how the infant in turn reacts, and so on throughout the day. Such observations and descriptions usually reveal ways in which the transactions can be modified to be more soothing for the infant. Such specifically designed behavioral management of the infant has been shown to be more effective in reducing prolonged crying than simply expressing empathy with the parent about the stress of the crying or any other method (Barbero, Rigler, and Rose, 1957; Carey, 1968; McKenzie, 1991; Taubman, 1988; Wolke, Gray, and Meyer, 1994). No study has shown this method to be ineffective when properly applied. These revisions of handling should not be thought of as changing the infants' temperamental predispositions but rather as altering the interaction of the caretakers with them and the resulting output of fussing and crying. The reduction in crying is usually achieved by decreasing the length of the bouts rather than the number of them.

The expression of optimism about the immediate outcome of the foregoing measures is justified and improves chances of success. Although acknowledging with the parents that prolonged crying in young infants is an incompletely understood phenomenon, the clinician is on firm ground in telling parents that if the recommended steps are followed, there is an excellent chance that the crying will diminish considerably in the next 2 or 3 days. This sanguine prophecy is based on experience and is usually correct. On the other hand, telling parents that the

excessive crying will go away by 3 months of age, which may be a condemnation to 2 or more months of further screaming, is not comforting and is likely to be counterproductive.

Close, supportive follow-up of the excessively fussy baby is important. A convenient way to do this is a telephone contact every 2 or 3 days until there is substantial improvement. On rare occasions, it is necessary to reevaluate the child and the situation in a week or so. Referral of the infant or parents for further evaluation and management of physical or psychosocial issues should be pursued if indicated, but it usually is not.

OTHER MEASURES

The use of medication for temporary relief of excessive crying is controversial. Drugs are usually unnecessary. In extreme cases, however, such as with serious sleep deprivation in the parents, medication may have a place in management. The most often recommended drugs are phenobarbital elixir, 10 mg three times daily, or diphenhydramine (Benadryl elixir) 6 mg two to three times a day. Treatment for 1 week is usually sufficient. If excessive crying returns after that, the medication can be given for a second week. There might be some placebo effect in the administration of such substances, but it is likely that there is also a pharmacologic one. The use of a drug alone without the other more important measures, which were mentioned earlier, is only modestly effective. Simethicone has been shown to be of no value (Metcalf et al, 1994). Herbal tea preparations have been thought by some to be helpful in reducing the crying, but their varying constituents make these preparations unacceptable as a general recommendation. Medication, when considered, should be made optional, since some parents want to try first to lessen the crying without it.

Under very extraordinary circumstances and as a last resort, separation of the infant from the parents by a brief period of hospitalization or a stay with a competent relative or friend has been shown to be dramatically effective in reducing the infant's crying. If, however, parental feelings and handling of the infant are not dealt with effectively before the parents are reunited with their infant, the old pattern of interaction and crying is likely to resume (Barbero, Rigler, and Rose, 1957).

Several unsuitable forms of treatment should be mentioned, if only to discourage their use. A change in the composition of feedings, that is from one formula to another, is seldom an appropriate solution. Almost any formula change—in fact, almost any altered procedure done with conviction—is likely to be followed by a temporary reduction in crying because of the placebo effect. But these transient improvements typically wear off in a few days. The lack of support for these techniques has been described elsewhere (Carey, 1989).

Although the use of rectal manipulations and enemas is widely supported by tradition, there is no published evidence to establish their value. Simply carrying the baby for more time each day, regardless of his or her state and needs, has not been demonstrated to be helpful.

Prognosis

Standard pediatric texts and conventional wisdom repeat the notion that colic usually goes away by itself by 3 or 4 months of age and that little can be done to alter that fate. However, clinical experience and reported studies (Barbero, Rigler, and Rose, 1957; Carey, 1968; McKenzie, 1991; Taubman, 1988; Wolke, Gray, and Meyer, 1994) indicate that excessive crying in young infants can be sharply reduced within a few days in most instances if appropriate steps are taken. Some babies and some situations take longer, but virtually all respond to suitable management. Conversely, with inappropriate care, the prolonged crying is likely to continue until 3 or 4 months of age.

Some short-term consequences are commonly seen. A temperamental predisposition to be irritable or sensitive will probably continue to be evident for at least the next few months and probably longer. Parental overattentiveness to the baby or more serious destabilizations of maternal functioning may still be present unless the family and their professional advisors have been able to improve those situations. Both of these factors may have an impact on the infant's subsequent behavior in matters such as night waking in the second 6 months of life. If professional advice has not been sufficiently skillful, the parents may still believe that there is some subtle defect in the child, and a vulnerable child syndrome may have been fostered (see Chapter 33). If the parents' response to the prolonged crying has been too much feeding, the infant may by this time have gained excessive weight.

The long-term prognosis for individuals who as young infants cried more than average has not been sufficiently investigated. Any statement that these infants become more impatient or aggressive as children or adults is pure speculation. Since retrospective data relating to amounts of crying tend to be highly inaccurate, only prospective studies will resolve this issue.

Prevention

No investigation has yet proved that any particular early measures will reduce the subsequent occurrence of colic or excessive crying. Some theoretical possibilities deserve mention.

We do not know how to alter the apparently predisposing temperamental or physiologic factors. We are not even fully certain which are the most important. It may become possible, however, by the use of a measure such as the Brazelton Neonatal Behavioral Assessment Scale or some derivative of it to identify infants in whom excessive crying is particularly likely to develop. So far no such evidence has become available.

It is possible to educate all parents, even starting prenatally, about infant crying and soothing. Some have no idea that even completely normal young infants cry about 2 hours or more a day. Parents often are unaware of the importance of infant fatigue and that a tired baby usually does better if not picked up.

The alert clinician also deals with parental anxieties whenever they are expressed. Concerns revealed prenatally or in the newborn nursery can lead to inappropriate handling of the infant if they are not resolved satisfactorily.

REFERENCES

Barbero GJ, Rigler D, Rose JA: Infantile gastro-intestinal disturbances: a pilot study and design for research. Am J Dis Child 94:532, 1957.

Barr RG: The "colic" enigma: prolonged episodes of a normal predisposition to cry. Infant Mental Health J 11:340, 1990.

Brazelton TB: Crying in infancy. Pediatrics 29:579, 1962.

Carey WB: The effectiveness of parent counseling in the management of colic. Pediatrics 94:333, 1994.

Carey WB: Cow's milk formula and infantile colic [letter to the editor]. Pediatrics 84:1124, 1989.

Carey WB: "Colic": primary excessive crying as an infant-environment interaction. Pediatr Clin North Am 31:993, 1984.

Carey WB: Clinical applications of infant temperament measurements. J Pediatr 81:823, 1972.

Carey WB: Maternal anxiety and infantile colic: is there a relationship? Clin Pediatr 7:590, 1968.

Lester BM, Barr RG (eds): Colic and Excessive Crying. Report of the 105th Ross Conference on Pediatric Research. Columbus, OH, Ross Products Division, Abbott Laboratories, 1997.

McKenzie S: Troublesome crying in infants: effect of advice to reduce stimulation. Arch Dis Childh 66:1416, 1991.

Metcalf TJ, Irons TG, Sher LD, Young PC: Simethicone in the treatment of colic: a randomized, placebo-controlled, multicenter trial. Pediatrics 94:29, 1994.

Papoušek M, von Hofacker N: Persistent crying and parenting: search for a butterfly in a dynamic system. Early Dev Parenting 4:209, 1995.

St. James-Roberts I, Conroy S, Wilsher K: Clinical, developmental, and social aspects of infant crying and colic. Early Dev Parenting 4:107, 1995.

Taubman B: Parental counseling compared with elimination of cow's milk or soy milk protein for treatment of infant colic syndrome: a randomized trial. Pediatrics 81:756, 1988.

Wessel MA, Cobb JC, Jackson EB, et al: Paroxysmal fussing in infancy, sometimes called "colic." Pediatrics 14:421, 1954.

Wolke D, Gray P, Meyer R: Excessive infant crying: a controlled study of mothers helping mothers. Pediatrics 94:322, 1994.

38 Child and Adolescent Obesity

Lawrence D. Hammer • Thomas N. Robinson

 Obesity is one of the greatest developmental-behavioral challenges confronting the primary care physician. It is distressingly common and becoming more so. Medical and psychological sequelae are great. Efforts at prevention and treatment are difficult. This chapter suggests a practical program of diagnosis and management for pediatricians. It is important for patients, their families, and physicians to set realistic goals for success and not expect dramatic results.

A 10-year-old boy was referred to the Obesity Clinic at the Children's Hospital at Stanford for evaluation and management. He had been born at 3.12 kg to a 19-year-old obese woman with a history of gestational diabetes mellitus. His height and weight were at the 95th percentile by the age of 5 years, and, at the time of referral, he was 55% overweight. He had no stigmata of an obesity syndrome or endocrine disorder.

Two years later, the patient developed daytime somnolence, difficulty sleeping at night, enuresis, and encopresis. His weight was 100 kg, 42 kg above the 95th percentile, while his height remained at the 95th percentile. A sleep study revealed evidence of both obstructive and central apnea. After a tonsillectomy and adenoidectomy, a weight loss of 10 kg was associated with improvement in his sleep pattern and a reduction in episodes of obstruction and daytime somnolence.

The following year, the patient's weight had increased to 113 kg, 48 kg above the 95th percentile for a 13-year-old. He had a recurrence of the obstructive sleep apnea syndrome and had a convulsive episode. A sleep study revealed episodes of desaturation at night to levels of 40% to 45%, and echocardiography revealed ventricular hypertrophy. Mask continuous positive airway pressure (CPAP) was initiated, with improvement in his sleep pattern and oxygen saturation during sleep. He was discharged from the hospital and continued to use the mask CPAP apparatus on an outpatient basis.

Slipped capital femoral epiphyses developed in the patient at age 14 years and weight 136 kg. Because of the boy's excessive weight, the orthopedic surgeon was reluctant to operate and recommended an initial period of hospitalization, immobilization, and weight loss. After a 2-week hospitalization and a 3-month period of confinement to bed at home, there was no improvement in his hips, and surgery was undertaken. Postoperatively, type II diabetes mellitus developed. Oral hypoglycemic therapy was initiated, accompanied by weight reduction. The boy's diabetes remained in good control with dietary management and oral hypoglycemic therapy for 6 months, but after an episode of ketoacidosis, the boy was started on insulin therapy.

This patient's medical complications were accompanied by significant psychological distress for both himself and his family. He was subsequently hospitalized twice on an inpatient psychosomatic unit as part of the effort to curb his eating behavior and introduce dietary control.

Prevalence

"Obesity Getting Worse, Especially In Kids," shouted a recent newspaper headline (*USA Today,* March 9, 1997). A consistent trend has been noted, since the first National Health Examination Survey (1960–1962), in the prevalence of overweight and obesity in all age groups. The prevalence of obesity for children and adolescents, using body mass index (BMI) as a criterion, has increased to 14% for children and 12% for adolescents in the most recent cycle of the National Health and Nutrition Examination Survey (NHANES III). Data from NHANES III also indicate that 33% of US men and 36% of US women are overweight and that among women, 34% of non-Hispanic whites, 52% of non-Hispanic African Americans, and 50% of Mexican Americans are overweight (MMWR, 1997). The prevalence of obesity varies with gender, race, and socioeconomic status. Among adolescents, the rates are higher in boys than girls. Low-income children of both sexes tend to be leaner than more affluent children. In general, affluent men are fatter, whereas affluent women and better-educated males are thinner. Within the United States, prevalence of childhood obesity varies geographically, being greatest in the northeast. Obesity is more prevalent during the winter months and in major metropolitan areas than rural areas.

Medical and Psychological Sequelae

Obesity is associated with a variety of medical and psychological sequelae, all of which may begin in childhood. These sequelae include diabetes mellitus, hypertension, and hyperlipoproteinemia. Obesity is the most readily identifiable risk factor for hypertension in childhood. Orthopedic problems, particularly slipped capital femoral epiphyses, may result from the demands of excessive weight on the joints. Acanthosis nigricans occurs in the markedly obese and, in girls, may be associated with the polycystic ovary syndrome. Obese children with histories of snoring or difficulty breathing during sleep have an increased risk of significant sleep-associated breathing disorders, including partial to complete airway obstruction, especially when their obesity is accompanied by adenotonsillar hypertrophy. Many obese children have evidence of the full obesity-hypoventilation syndrome, including hypersomnolence, hypoxemia, hypercarbia, and edema. Obstructive and restrictive abnormalities in lung function have been described in adolescents who are more than 50% overweight, and obesity may result in right and left ventricular dilatation and hypertrophy.

Various endocrine changes occur with increasing adiposity: hyperinsulinemia and insulin resistance, early pubarche, lower serum testosterone, decreased sex hormone–binding globulin, early adrenarche, elevated adrenal androgens and dehydroepiandrosterone, high prolactin at baseline with decreased response to stimulation, and decreased basal and stimulated growth hormone release.

Obesity in adolescence may have long-term consequences on adult health. Must and colleagues (1992) described the association between being overweight in adolescence and later morbidity and mortality in a cohort of 508 persons from the Third Harvard Growth Study. In this 55-year follow-up study, being overweight in adolescence was a significant risk factor for heart disease, gout, colorectal cancer, hip fracture, and arthritis in later adult life. For men, all-cause mortality rate as well as the mortality rates for coronary heart disease, atherosclerotic cerebrovascular disease, and colorectal cancer were significantly increased for those who had been overweight during adolescence.

The social and psychological sequelae of obesity in childhood and adolescence also deserve attention. Poor self-esteem is often accompanied by disturbed body image. The stigma of obesity may lead to difficulty in establishing peer relationships and to social isolation. Obese adolescents are often depressed, dissatisfied with their appearance, and socially inactive. Rejection on the basis of body size and shape begins during the preschool years and can continue throughout life, even leading to discrimination in college acceptance and employment. Rejection by peers at school has been associated with maladjustment during adolescence and adulthood. Obese children are generally judged by peers as less attractive and less active than their classmates. They are accepted less readily by classmates and they are viewed more negatively than classmates of normal weight or children with physical handicaps. Mellbin and Vuille (1989) studied the relationship between an increase in relative weight between 7 and 10 years of age and the development of psychological problems. The highest prevalence of problems was found in the group with most rapid weight gain. The presence of any psychological problems at 7 years of age predicted more rapid weight gain at age 10 years. For both girls and boys, obesity was associated with behavioral and learning problems, and, for girls, obesity was associated with social problems. Boys and girls had almost a threefold increase in risk of rapid weight gain from ages 7 to 10 years if they had a psychological problem rated as "serious."

These social and psychological consequences may also extend into adult life. Gortmaker and colleagues (1993) studied the relationship between being overweight (BMI greater than 95th percentile) and a number of social and psychological variables in a sample of more than 10,000 individuals 16 to 24 years of age, who were assessed on two occasions, 7 years apart. Women who were overweight at the initial assessment were less likely to be married, had lower household incomes, had fewer years of education, and had higher rates of poverty than nonoverweight women, independent of their baseline socioeconomic status. Likewise, men who were overweight at the initial assessment were less likely to be married than the nonoverweight men at baseline. (Their incomes and education were also less, but these differences did not reach statistical significance.)

Psychological problems associated with obesity appear to be more prevalent in clinical samples of children and families seeking obesity treatment. For example, assessment of a group of obese adolescents and their parents before entering into a treatment program revealed clinically significant rates of depression (27%) and low self-esteem (36%) among an initial sample of 58 patients (Mellin L, personal communication, 1994). On the other hand, clinicians should not assume that all obese children have psychological problems. Several studies of population-based, nonclinical samples have found similar prevalences of psychological problems in obese and normal-weight children.

Diagnosis of Obesity

The diagnosis of obesity in childhood and adolescence is usually made on the basis of height and weight. Estimates of body fatness, using techniques such as underwater weighing, potassium counting, or bioelectric impedance, are generally reserved for the research laboratory, whereas skinfold thickness measures can be obtained in the clinician's office. Although clinicians vary in their use of the term *obesity*, it is acceptable to apply the diagnostic label to patients whose body weight is in excess of 20% above that considered appropriate for gender, height, and age.

An alternative approach to the use of height and weight information in the diagnosis of obesity is to use a combination of the two as an index, using the 90th or 95th percentile for age and gender as a criterion (Table 38–1). The BMI, which is calculated using the formula (BMI = weight [kg] divided by height [m] squared), can be plotted on a percentile curve for BMI (Fig. 38–1). Serial measurement of BMI is useful in monitoring a child's obesity over time. Although many clinicians use the ratio of weight to height and curves of weight for height (rather than height squared) in monitoring children over time, this ratio is of more limited utility than the BMI as an index of fatness.

Because weight is composed of lean and fat mass, children who are particularly muscular can be overweight without having excessive fat. In such situations, skinfold thickness measurements are useful in substantiating the diagnosis of obesity. Skinfold thickness in excess of the 85th percentile for age and gender is considered excessive. Table 38–2 lists the 85th percentile values of the triceps skinfold thickness, taken from the National Health and Nutrition Examination Survey (NHANES 1976–1980).

Table 38–1 • Percentile Values of Body Mass Index*

Age	Males			Females		
	50th Percentile	*90th Percentile*	*95th Percentile*	*50th Percentile*	*90th Percentile*	*95th Percentile*
1 year	17.2	19.4	19.9	16.6	18.6	19.3
2 years	16.5	18.4	19.0	16.0	18.0	18.7
3 years	16.0	17.8	18.4	15.6	17.6	18.3
4 years	15.8	17.5	18.1	15.4	17.5	18.2
5 years	15.5	17.3	18.0	15.3	17.5	18.3
6 years	15.4	17.4	18.1	15.3	17.7	18.8
7 years	15.5	17.7	18.9	15.5	18.5	19.7
8 years	15.7	18.4	19.7	16.0	19.4	21.0
9 years	16.0	19.3	20.9	16.6	20.8	22.7
10 years	16.6	20.3	22.2	17.1	21.8	24.2
11 years	17.2	21.3	23.5	17.8	23.0	25.7
12 years	17.8	22.3	24.8	18.3	23.7	26.8
13 years	18.4	23.3	25.8	18.9	24.7	27.9
14 years	19.1	24.4	26.8	19.4	25.3	28.6
15 years	19.7	25.4	27.7	19.9	26.0	29.4
16 years	20.5	26.1	28.4	20.2	26.5	30.0
17 years	21.2	27.0	29.0	20.7	27.1	30.5
18 years	21.9	27.7	29.7	21.1	27.4	31.0
19 years	22.5	28.3	30.1	21.4	27.7	31.3

*Calculated as weight in kilograms divided by the square of height in meters (wt/ht²). Derived from the First National Health and Nutrition Examination Survey, 1971–1974. From Hammer LD, et al: Standardized percentile curves of body mass index for children and adolescents. Am J Dis Child 145:259–263, 1991. Copyright 1991, American Medical Association.

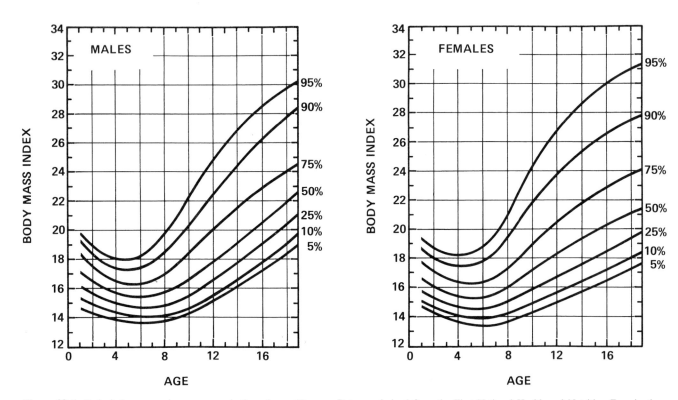

Figure 38–1. Body index curves in young people through age 19 years. Data are derived from the First National Health and Nutrition Examination Survey, 1971–1974. (From Hammer LD, et al. Standardized percentile curves of body mass index for children and adolescents. Am J Dis Child 145:259–263, 1991. Copyright 1991, American Medical Association.)

Table 38–2 • Triceps Skinfold Thickness in Millimeters

Age	Males			Females		
	50th Percentile	*85th Percentile*	*95th Percentile*	*50th Percentile*	*85th Percentile*	*95th Percentile*
6–11 months	10.0	14.0	16.0	10.0	12.5	14.5
1 year	10.0	13.0	15.5	10.5	13.5	16.5
2 years	10.0	13.0	15.0	10.5	13.5	16.0
3 years	9.5	12.5	15.0	10.0	12.5	16.5
4 years	9.0	12.0	15.0	10.0	13.0	15.5
5 years	8.0	11.5	14.5	10.5	14.0	16.0
6 years	8.0	12.0	17.5	10.0	14.5	18.5
7 years	8.5	12.0	17.5	10.5	15.0	20.0
8 years	9.0	16.5	22.0	11.0	16.0	21.0
9 years	9.0	16.0	23.0	13.0	20.0	27.0
10 years	11.0	20.0	26.0	13.5	21.0	24.5
11 years	10.5	22.0	30.0	14.0	21.5	29.5
12 years	11.0	18.0	26.5	13.5	21.5	27.0
13 years	9.0	16.5	22.5	15.0	22.0	30.0
14 years	9.0	15.0	23.0	17.0	25.0	32.0
15 years	7.5	14.5	22.0	16.5	24.5	32.1
16 years	8.0	18.5	25.5	18.0	27.0	33.1
17 years	7.0	12.5	18.0	20.0	26.5	34.5
18 years	9.5	17.5	22.5	18.0	27.0	35.0
19 years	9.0	16.0	23.0	19.0	28.0	33.5

Derived from Najjar MF: Anthropometric reference data and prevalence of overweight, United States, 1976–1980. Vital and Health Statistics, Series II, No. 238, Department of Health and Human Services Publication No. (PHS) 87-1688. Washington, DC, US Government Printing Office, 1987.

Development of Adiposity

Although adiposity may increase at any time, the first 2 years of life and early adolescence are the periods of greatest fat cell proliferation. Even in children of normal weight, fat cells reach adult size by the 2nd year of life. Increases in fat cell number and size are reflected in an increase in subcutaneous fat in the first 1 to 2 years of life, another period of increasing fatness during the school-age years, and continued increase in fatness for adolescent females during and after puberty. Most obese children and adolescents have an increase in both fat cell number and size.

Data concerning the natural history of child and adolescent obesity demonstrate that there is a developmental pattern to the deposition of body fat through childhood and adolescence. Dietz (1994) has suggested that there may be three critical periods in the development of obesity, corresponding to periods of adipose tissue proliferation: gestation and early infancy, ages 5 to 7 years, and adolescence. During the 1st year of life, children tend to accumulate "baby fat," followed by a relative reduction in body fatness over the next several years as the child gains proportionally greater height than weight. Most children again increase their body fat at 5 to 6 years of age. This "rebound" in adiposity continues at a rather steady rate until puberty, after which there is a slower trend toward increasing fat deposition. Investigators have noted that children whose "rebound" in adiposity occurs earlier than the age of 5½ years tend to have a higher likelihood of obesity during adolescence (Rolland-Cachera et al, 1984).

With increasing age, the obese child or adolescent has an increasing likelihood of persistent obesity into adulthood. Serdula and colleagues (1993) reviewed 17 reports of longitudinal studies published between 1970 and 1992 and concluded that less than half of cases of adult obesity can be attributed to child/adolescent obesity. They also concluded that the relative risk for later obesity varied from about 2 for children measured in infancy or early childhood to 6.5 for children assessed at 9 to 13 years of age. Although the risks are markedly elevated compared to the risks among normal-weight children, most longitudinal studies have found that fewer than 50% to 60% of obese children became obese as adults (Robinson, 1993).

Obesity shares a number of characteristics with other chronic conditions. Obesity in adult life generally follows an unremitting course and requires individual and family adaptation. Like hypertension, obesity may have multiple causes and can lead to significant physical and psychological complications. Lifestyle change, including changes in diet and physical activity, often prescribed for non–insulin-dependent diabetes mellitus and hypertension, requires family cooperation and support. Unlike diabetes mellitus or hypertension, no effective pharmacologic interventions are available to provide even symptomatic improvement for the obese individual.

Etiologic Factors

The multifactorial nature of child obesity suggests an important interaction of genetic predisposition, family environment, and personal habits. Whether the origin of obesity is more genetic or behavioral, the clinical approach to evaluating and supporting the treatment of this problem requires that all factors be acknowledged. Dietz and Robinson (1993) suggest that like other diseases that reflect an interaction of host and environment, the most appropriate perspective is that genetics do influence susceptibility to obesity but that the genetic predisposition to obesity can be augmented by environmental factors that increase caloric intake or reduce energy expenditure.

Factors influencing the development of body fatness during childhood and adolescence include caloric intake and energy expenditure. Although differences in caloric intake or energy expenditure might account for differences in body fatness between individuals, it has been generally impossible to demonstrate such differences, even in well-performed naturalistic studies. Numerous studies have reported minimal differences in food intake and physical activity between obese and nonobese children; however, small differences in daily food intake or physical activity, when extended over long periods of time, may account for the excessive weight gain of some children. Nevertheless, the diet history of obese children often reveals either regular or periodic intake of excessive calories and high-fat foods. The intake may be excessive in portion size or in selection of high-calorie foods.

An "obese eating style" has been described in children and adults. This eating style consists of rapid eating, resulting in the rapid consumption of calories. Studies of feeding in infants have revealed a pattern of vigorous feeding, consisting of rapid sucking with higher pressure, resulting in greater caloric intake at a feed, with higher sucking pressure associated with a greater degree of adiposity. This "vigorous suckling style" may represent an early manifestation of the rapid eating style associated with childhood obesity (Agras et al, 1987).

Self-regulation of dietary intake may also be an important factor. Johnson and Birch (1994) studied the relationship of adiposity to children's ability to self-regulate dietary intake. They found that fatter girls were less likely to compensate for intake at a previous meal (regulate their intake) than thinner girls, and that boys with greater lean body mass were better able to regulate their intake. They also found that parents who were more controlling of their children's eating and who were more controlling of their own eating had children with less ability to self-regulate.

Carey and colleagues have proposed a mechanism for inappropriate eating habits and difficulty in maintaining dietary change in some obese children with characteristics of difficult temperament (Carey, Hegvik, and McDevitt, 1988). Using parent questionnaires coded to produce ratings of temperament characteristics, they found that difficult children—those who are low in rhythmicity, approach, and adaptability, high in intensity, and negative in mood—have more rapid weight gain in middle childhood. They speculated that these children may experience more stress in their social interactions and may use eating as a technique for comforting themselves. They also speculated that these children may be less flexible about changing eating patterns when necessary to overcome an established pattern of excessive weight gain. During infancy, these children may also be more irritable, potentially leading to the use of feeding by the parent as a soothing technique (Carey, 1985).

A number of studies have found obese children to be less active than nonobese peers. For example, an analysis of the amount of activity of obese and nonobese participants in a summer camp revealed that despite engaging in similar activities for similar amounts of time, obese campers exhibited significantly less movement than their nonobese counterparts (Bullen, 1964). Because obese children are moving additional mass, however, estimated calorie expenditures of obese and nonobese children have not differed.

Inactivity may also lead to increased weight gain. Excessive television viewing has received increased attention as a potential cause of obesity, although epidemiologic studies have found only weak associations between the two. Evidence from obesity treatment research suggests that interventions to decrease sedentary behaviors, including television viewing, may be effective for increasing physical activity and weight loss (Epstein et al, 1995).

Role of the Primary Care Physician in the Management of Obesity

The primary care physician is often the first medical professional called upon by parents or patients to help understand the problem of obesity in childhood and to offer assistance in its management. Although many others in a child's family or school environment may call attention to the problem, parents often seek guidance first in their pediatrician's office. The primary care physician who has been following a child over an extended period of time is in an excellent position to evaluate the pattern of weight gain and to understand the factors that may be at play in fostering and maintaining the child's obesity. The first concern that most parents raise is that of an underlying endocrine or medical cause of the child's obesity. Except in those situations in which such a cause is likely, referral to a geneticist or endocrinologist is unwarranted. The most important issue that the primary care clinician must raise once the question of etiology has been discussed is the degree of parental and child concern regarding the problem and the extent to which the family may be ready to engage in the difficult tasks of modifying eating and physical activity habits. By and large, the diagnostic evaluation can be undertaken by the primary care physician in the office setting. Depending on the availability of other resources in the community and the needs of the child or family, the physician might consider the additional consultation of a dietitian, psychologist, or family therapist. In addition, for families who might be appropriate for participation in group programs, such programs may be available under the auspices of local clinics, hospitals, school districts, and community organizations, or via the private sector. These programs should contain the elements described below under Behavioral Intervention and should be organized and maintained by appropriately trained professionals, with input from physicians, dietitians, and therapists.

One of the dilemmas for the primary care clinician in the management of child obesity is the time commitment and frequency of office visits involved on an ongoing basis. One of the variables in group programs that predicts success is weekly participation in the group for at least 3 months, and up to 12 months or longer, if possible. Such a frequency of visits to the office may be difficult to achieve as well as costly. A reasonable tradeoff in the office setting is to see the child weekly for 2 to 3 weeks, then monthly once a behavioral program has been established.

Diagnostic Evaluation

HISTORY

Less than 2% of obese children have an underlying endocrinopathy, such as hypothyroidism or Cushing disease, or one of the recognized obesity syndromes, such as the Prader-Willi syndrome, which is notable for its associated history of early hypotonia, feeding difficulty, failure to thrive, and developmental delay, followed by profound hyperphagia, or the Lawrence-Moon-Biedl syndrome, which includes mental retardation, hypogonadism, polydactyly, and eye abnormalities (retinitis pigmentosa, optic atrophy, cataracts, microphthalmia, and colobomata). These diagnoses can almost always be made on the basis of a complete history and physical examination. In general, obese children with normal or above-average height, normal intelligence, and normal gonadal development do not require further medical or laboratory investigation.

A detailed birth and early feeding history should be obtained, and the child's prior growth and development record should be reviewed. The age at which the child was first considered to be overweight and the pattern of weight gain before the evaluation should be noted. A family history of obesity, particularly in one or both parents, or in grandparents, is helpful in supporting the diagnosis of constitutional obesity. The feeding history, beginning in infancy, should be reviewed, with attention given to the current eating habits of the child. Those eating habits might include rapid eating, large portion sizes, multiple frequent meals throughout the day, excessive snacking, bingeing, and nighttime eating. A common pattern seen among older children and adolescents involves skipping breakfast, sometimes skipping lunch, and then having a large dinner, with after-dinner snacking. The child's response to parental limit setting around food should be reviewed and may provide information that is useful during treatment.

The child's past medical history should be reviewed with attention being given to early hypotonia or developmental delay. Current and past medication use, suspected food allergies or intolerance, hospitalizations, and surgeries should also be noted. The review of systems should include attention to excessive daytime sleepiness and snoring, nighttime sleep difficulty, and enuresis, suggesting possible obstructive sleep apnea.

A careful dietary history should be obtained from the child and other family members, preferably after the child or parents have kept diet records at home for 3 to 5 days. These diet records can be combined with a food frequency review to analyze the nutritional composition of the child's diet, and they can be used as a baseline from which the physician or dietitian can probe further for information regarding foods commonly consumed in or out of the household. Diet records from other members of the family provide additional insight into the family's eating patterns. In our experience, a careful diet record, with further probing and interview, has invariably revealed not only excessive dietary intake but also clear opportunities for appropriate dietary modification. Review of the diet record also provides the parent with important objective information concerning the child's dietary habits. In addition to poor food selection, portion sizes may be excessive for the child's age. Mealtime habits, such as "family style" serving, which may promote large portion sizes, should also be noted. A clinical dietitian, particularly one experienced in working with obese patients, can often provide valuable consultation in the evaluation of the child's and family's diet and eating habits.

The child's physical activity should be reviewed, supplemented by a 3- to 5-day physical activity record, to describe the amount and intensity of physical activity. It is also useful to document specific periods of inactivity, including playing video games, viewing television, and using computers, because these are discrete sedentary behaviors that can be targeted for change.

A psychological assessment of the child should be performed by the primary physician or a consultant. The evaluation should focus on ways the child's weight, or that of other family members, might influence the family's functioning, as well as any factors that may influence their eating habits or affect their ability to participate in a treatment program. Ideally, both a family interview and individual interviews with the child and other family members should be included in the evaluation. This is an opportunity to discuss how the child's eating habits or obesity affects the other family members and how the child's obesity may affect peer relationships. The stigma of obesity may be considerable, affecting parents' feelings of competency in their childrearing and promoting parental feelings of guilt for their perceived contributions (genetic or environmental) to the child's obesity. Parental history of obesity or eating disorders should also be ascertained. The presence of significant psychopathology in the child or parents necessitates further psychiatric evaluation and suggests the need for ongoing individual or family therapy as an adjunct to participation in the obesity treatment process. Even the most seemingly well-adjusted child and functional family may find the obesity treatment process arduous and frustrating, and they may benefit from ongoing supportive therapy.

PHYSICAL EXAMINATION

A careful general physical examination should be geared to the identification of underlying endocrine or other syndromes and to the identification of problems that may contribute to, or be a consequence of, the child's obesity. Height and weight should be measured carefully, and skinfold thickness can be measured over the triceps and subscapular areas by an experienced practitioner. Blood pressure should be documented. Examination of the eyes should include fundoscopic evaluation for evidence of retinal or vascular changes. The thyroid should be palpated for presence of enlargement. The heart examination may reveal evidence of cardiac hypertrophy or enlargement. A loud pulmonic second sound suggests an increase in pulmonary vascular resistance, secondary to episodes of obstructive apnea or hypoventilation. The chest examination may reveal evidence of reactive airway disease or restrictive lung disease. The abdomen should be examined for tenderness associated with gallstones or an enlarged fatty liver. Genital examination should be done to rule out hypogonadism and to evaluate pubertal maturation status. The trunk should be observed for evidence of buffalo hump, truncal obesity, and striae. Acanthosis nigricans, or hyperpigmentation and thickening of the skin, particularly in the axillae, around the neck, and in other body folds, is a common physical finding in children with severe persistent obesity. Examination of the hands and feet for evidence of extra digits or particularly small size is important when considering the diagnosis of pseudohypoparathyroidism or Prader-Willi syndrome.

A limited number of characteristics feature prominently in the disorders or dysmorphic syndromes associated with obesity. The presence of mental retardation, short stature, hypogonadism, developmental delay, or other unusual physical stigmata suggests the need for further endocrine or genetic diagnostic evaluation, whereas patients with normal stature, normal cognitive development, and normal gonadal development are unlikely to have a primary diagnosis underlying their obesity.

LABORATORY EVALUATION

Laboratory examination of the obese child is rarely indicated and is used primarily to confirm suspected underlying diagnoses rather than as routine screening. Obese children who are tall, of normal intelligence, and without stigmata of underlying syndromes do not require routine thyroid or other testing. General chemical survey panels and complete blood counts rarely provide useful information in evaluating the obese child. If there is a family history of thyroid or other metabolic disease, parents may be unsatisfied unless such testing is performed. Because hyperlipidemia is more common among obese children and adolescents, measurement of blood lipids is appropriate for these patients.

In patients suspected of having the Prader-Willi syndrome or Turner syndrome, chromosome studies should be undertaken. In addition to chromosome banding studies, fluorescent in-situ hybridization analysis has become the accepted approach to the diagnosis of the Prader-Willi syndrome. Hypothyroidism can be assessed with a serum T_4, T_3 (by radioimmunoassay), and thyroid stimulating hormone assay. In patients with possible Cushing syndrome, cortisol determinations and a dexamethasone suppression test should be obtained.

Radiologic examination should be limited to those patients who complain of hip pain or have limitation of motion at the hip (to rule out slipped capital femoral epiphyses), those with suspected Blount disease (tibia vara), and those suspected of having cardiac or pulmonary disease associated with their excessive weight. Ultrasound examination of the ovaries may be useful for patients with possible polycystic ovary syndrome or symptoms or signs of gallstones. Symptoms of obstructive sleep apnea suggest the need for a sleep study.

PSYCHOLOGICAL ASSESSMENT

A psychological assessment and family assessment can be very helpful in the evaluation of the obese child. This assessment provides important information about the family's concerns and their ability to participate in further evaluation and in treatment. If there is any suspicion of child or family psychopathology, an experienced psychologist or family therapist should be consulted during this process.

During the process of evaluating the obese child and his or her family, it is useful to observe the interaction of family members and to observe their expression of concern, criticism, or support of the child in dealing with this problem. If the opportunity presents itself, it is also useful to note parents' responses to the child's requests for food during the visit. Although overeating may not be the primary factor contributing to the child's obesity, interactions with food are often salient to the evaluation and treatment process.

Treatment

GOALS

The goals of weight reduction are weight loss without adverse health effects, followed by weight maintenance at the reduced weight. The length of time required to achieve ideal weight by weight maintenance can be estimated from the growth chart using the current weight and the weight at the same percentile as height. In order to reach the desired ideal weight, 1 to 2 years of weight maintenance is required for each 20% increment in excess of ideal weight at the time of initiation of treatment.

It is reasonable to establish a target weight for the child. This does not imply that the child must always lose weight. Rather, taking into account appropriate rates of growth, the child's weight should fall into a "healthy range" for height and age. This "healthy weight range" can be defined as 20% above or below the "ideal" weight for height and age, or at a BMI level below the 90th percentile. The process of establishing a goal weight or BMI goal for the child should be reviewed periodically, depending on the child's age and the family's ability to participate in the treatment program. Often, particularly for children who are prepubertal, weight loss may be a less desirable goal than maintenance of weight at a particular level or reduction in the rate of weight gain. Such a goal may be difficult to achieve without periods of weight loss alternating with periods of weight maintenance. Beyond puberty, it may be more appropriate to establish numerical goals for weight loss.

Behavioral treatment should support change in diet and exercise without placing the child at risk for caloric insufficiency. Depending on the age of the child and the severity of obesity, change in behavior may be used to maintain a young child's weight, allowing linear growth to proceed (producing a change toward lower degree of overweight or fatness), or to foster moderate weight loss in the older child (½ to 1 pound per week) or adolescent (1 to 2 pounds per week). By monitoring the child's diet closely and by monitoring rate of weight change and growth in height, nutritional adequacy of the diet can be ascertained. The minimum servings of the US Department of Agriculture food guide pyramid can help families ensure that children and adolescents continue to consume a well-balanced diet during weight loss or maintenance.

In addition to weight loss, it is important to emphasize associated goals of improved fitness, self-esteem, social interaction, and family harmony. All of these outcomes can be achieved without an emphasis on weight loss and may be enhanced by a focus on the development of healthier eating habits and increased physical activity for the whole family. The clinician should be aware of the potential need for family evaluation and support. It is reasonable to include improvement in family relationships and family functioning as a goal of participation in a treatment program for child obesity.

FAMILY INVOLVEMENT

Obesity is often situated within a family context. There are commonly other family members who have struggled with weight and whose experience can be extremely valuable in helping develop a realistic set of goals for the child and family. The tendency for families to feel defeated by obesity comes from their unrealistic expectation of dramatic and continued change.

The family's involvement is critical to the evaluation and management of child obesity. Parents are often confused by what they have read and thought about the origins of their child's obesity. Because obesity has a strong genetic predisposition, parents often feel guilty about their child's obesity and may have already experienced failure in trying to intervene. Because obesity is so resistant to intervention, the family may feel hopeless and at a loss. Efforts to explain the causes of the child's obesity are rarely successful and often lead to confusing or inadequate explanations for the family. Focusing on the impact of the child's obesity on the family and the child and on ways of overcoming the influence of the child's obesity on the family and the child can lead them more directly to effective intervention. For example, rather than using the dietary history as a means of proving the presence of excessive dietary intake, the dietary history should be used as a means of identifying opportunities for dietary change. Likewise, in discussing the child's regular physical activity, it should be possible to identify opportunities for increasing physical activity. Intervention can be approached as a process of gradually modifying the child's eating behavior and physical activity over time, in the context of the whole family. It is critical that the family engage in this process in an active way and agree to initiate and maintain change in the whole family's food and exercise habits.

Intervention for child obesity begins during the evaluation process. Involving the family in the evaluation gives the message that they are part of the solution. In the course of evaluation, if the family appears to be dysfunctional, it is appropriate to delay the implementation of behavioral strategies until the family has had more extensive evaluation and entered into family counseling. Referral to a family therapist, particularly one familiar with many of the issues associated with obesity, can be extremely helpful.

BEHAVIORAL INTERVENTION

For families who appear to be reasonably functional, are interested in supporting the child's efforts, and are able to engage the child in a process of behavior change, the initial strategies are focused on gradual alterations in the child's eating and physical activity. There are a number of behavioral strategies that are useful in the office-based approach to child obesity (Table 38–3). These behavioral strategies include (1) goal setting, (2) self-monitoring, (3) record review, (4) contracting, (5) praise, (6) environmental control, (7) cognitive restructuring, (8) anticipation, (9) periodic reassessment, and (10) maintenance.

Physical activity is an important addition to treatment. Usually insufficient alone to produce adequate negative caloric balance, lifestyle change appears to be more effective than programmed exercise in contributing to weight control. This could include activities such as walking or biking to school, family walks in the afternoon or evening, weekend recreation, or even gardening or yard work that becomes a routine.

Intervention does not require "calorie counting" or

Table 38–3 • Behavioral Treatment Components

Goal setting	Set weekly, achievable goals for change in diet and physical activity.
Self-monitoring	Self-monitoring increases behavioral awareness of behavior change and facilitates reinforcement.
Daily record review	Daily review with a parent helps to provide feedback and reinforcement for behavior change.
Contracting	After setting realistic goals each week, the parent and child contract for agreed-upon behavior change. Rewards should be simple, easy to administer, and inexpensive. Rewards should be deliverable immediately (i.e., weekly or daily).
Praise	Parents can learn to use praise as a powerful tool to reinforce and maintain desired behavior change. Praise should be specific to the behavior. Criticism and punishment are less effective and may be detrimental.
Environmental control	Parents can help by identifying factors within the environment that promote overeating or inactivity. Examples of environmental control include removal of high-fat, high-calorie foods from the household, increasing the availability of cut-up vegetables rather than chips or sweets for snack time, avoidance of television viewing during meal times, reducing the amount of time spent indoors during daylight hours, and increasing the expectation for daily physical activity.
Cognitive restructuring	Parents and children learn alternative ways to think about their beliefs and behaviors in order to reduce the tendency to feel bad about their struggle with weight.
Anticipation	It is important to anticipate obesity-promoting situations and to plan specific strategies for parties, travel, and holidays.
Reassessment	Periodic reassessment enables the child and family to identify lapses in desired behavior change and to reinstitute previously successful strategies before feelings of frustration and failure develop.
Maintenance	There should be ongoing reassessment of goals, strategies, and progress.

a specific calorie intake. An alternative approach is to categorize foods as more or less desirable and to use behavioral techniques that lead to the reduction of less desirable foods and encouragement of more desirable foods. One such system of categorization, the "stoplight diet," categorizes foods as "red light," "yellow light," and "green light" (Epstein and Wing, 1987). By identifying foods in this way, parents can support the child's efforts to reduce intake of "red light" foods and increase intake of foods from the other categories. Gradual reduction in intake of "red light" foods can be rewarded and sustained in association with goals of weight loss or maintenance.

Epstein and colleagues (1990) have reported 5- and 10-year follow-up results of their family-based group treatment program. In their 5-year follow-up, they found that use of conjoint targeting and reinforcement of both child and parent behavior or reciprocal targeting of children and parents yielded better results than a nonspecific control condition in which children were reinforced only for attendance at treatment meetings. Predictors of child success included self-monitoring of weight, changing eating behavior (eating fewer "red light" foods and selecting more low-calorie snacks), parent-reported use of praise, and change in parent percent overweight. Parental outcome was predicted by self-monitoring of weight, baseline parent percent overweight, and participation in fewer subsequent weight control programs. In the 10-year follow-up, results for 158 children who participated in four controlled trials were reported. These children were 6 to 12 years of age when they participated in the family-based behavioral treatment programs. Ten years later, about one third had maintained a greater than or equal to 20% decrease in percent overweight and nearly 30% were no longer obese (Epstein et al, 1994).

In a recent meta-analysis of 41 controlled treatment-outcome studies of child and adolescent obesity, Haddock and colleagues (1994) concluded that three program variables were most consistently related to positive treatment outcome: (1) comprehensive treatment (including a combination of behavioral modification procedures, a special diet, and an exercise program), (2) explicit inclusion of behavior modification techniques, and (3) focus on heavier subjects. Components of the diet that were predictive of better outcome included a simple categorization of foods that was understood easily by children, tailoring of caloric intake to the child's age and metabolic needs, additional focus on fat intake in addition to caloric intake, and supervision by a health professional. In their behavioral treatment studies, Epstein and colleagues (1994) demonstrated greater efficacy from lifestyle change and providing choices for activity than from programmed physical activity.

VERY LOW-CALORIE DIETS

Although widely available for adults, very low-calorie diets (modified fasting, liquid protein diets) should be avoided in children and adolescents, except in appropriate investigational settings. Furthermore, even though they may be effective in promoting initial weight loss, patients who experience severe caloric restriction are likely to regain much of this weight over the subsequent year. Restrictive diets, with close monitoring by an experienced clinician, should be limited to the rare pediatric patient who has a morbid complication of obesity for which rapid weight reduction is necessary (e.g., pseudotumor cerebri, non–insulin-dependent diabetes mellitus, pickwickian syndrome, slipped epiphyses) and must contain sufficient protein, mineral, and vitamin content.

A general word of caution should also be emphasized with regard to the overzealous application of any weight management strategy for the child or adolescent. Significant retardation of growth associated with the dietary treatment of hypercholesterolemia and fear of the development of obesity should be viewed as the unfortunate outcomes of inadequately supervised or misguided attempts at dietary manipulation. In addition, Epstein and colleagues (1994) reported that nearly 20% of 137 patients were treated for psychiatric disorders during the 10-year follow-up. These results suggest that children and adolescents seeking treatment for obesity may be at risk for development of psychiatric problems, particularly eating disorders and depression.

SURGERY

There has been very limited use of surgery (such as reduction of stomach volume) in child obesity, usually only in the presence of severe morbidity or in cases of the Prader-Willi syndrome. Because of the risks of wound infection and dehiscence and because of the limited long-term benefit of surgery in most adults, this approach has not been recommended.

DRUG TREATMENT

Likewise, there is very limited experience with pharmacologic treatments in children and adolescents, including phentermine and fenfluramine (Pondimin), which were recently removed from clinical use due to concern regarding their potential cardiac risk. Other drugs approved for adults include dexfenfluramine (Redux), diethylpropion (Tenuate), mazindol (Sanorex), and phendimetrazine (Bontril). Adults taking these drugs achieve a 5- to 20-pound weight loss in the first 6 months on the drug. Longer use does not seem to be of much added benefit. After discontinuation of drug treatment, patients regain most of the weight they have lost. Frequent side effects include dry mouth, sleep disturbance, polyuria, diarrhea, nervousness, and euphoria. Recently, case-control studies have linked use of these drugs, especially for more than 3 months, with primary pulmonary hypertension. Use of these drugs in children should be considered experimental and done only in a closely monitored clinical trial setting.

FOLLOW-UP

The primary care provider should provide regular follow-up for the child who is involved either in an office-based or in a group treatment program. This follow-up can include periodic monitoring of the child's weight and height and review of the child's self-monitoring records for diet and physical activity. A health professional (physician, nurse, dietitian, or psychologist) should meet with the child and family on a regular basis to review progress, to re-examine the goals of treatment, to assess the extent to which those goals are being achieved, and to begin planning for the posttreatment maintenance period. For the child who is involved in a community-based, school-based, or hospital-based group treatment program, the primary care provider can provide added support, reinforce and encourage the child and family, and help the family monitor their goals and progress along the way. Results from adult weight loss programs indicate that program duration is an important factor in maximizing weight loss and maintenance. Regular follow-up is suggested for at least 1 year and should be longer, if possible.

Prevention

The recent increases in obesity among children and adolescents and the limited long-term effectiveness of most obesity treatments for adults has focused attention on primary prevention of obesity. However, many past approaches to preventing obesity have been disappointing. In general, they have not produced significant changes in adiposity or obesity-related behaviors, and short-term effects consistently decay over time. Several studies are underway to test new approaches to preventing obesity. The current trend is to develop longer-duration prevention programs that address both individual behavior and environmental factors. Many of these programs are based in school settings and include family involvement as well as attempts to influence school meals and physical education. Another approach may be to target the children of obese parents with intensive, family-based behavioral interventions.

REFERENCES

Agras WS, Kraemer HC, Berkowitz RI, et al: Does a vigorous feeding style influence early development of adiposity? J Pediatr 110(5):799–804, 1987.

Bullen BA, Reed RB, Mayer J: Physical activity of obese and nonobese adolescent girls appraised by motion picture sampling. Am J Clin Nutr 14:211, 1964.

Carey WB: Temperament and increased weight gain in infants. J Dev Behav Pediatr 6:128–131, 1985.

Carey WB, Hegvik RL, McDevitt SC: Temperamental factors associated with rapid weight gain and obesity in middle childhood. J Dev Behav Pediatr 9:194–198, 1988.

Dietz WH: Critical periods in childhood for the development of obesity. Am J Clin Nutr 59(5):955–959, 1994.

Dietz WH, Robinson TN: Assessment and treatment of childhood obesity. Pediatr Rev 14(9):337–344, 1993.

Epstein LH, McCurley J, Wing RR, et al: Five year follow-up of family-based behavioral treatments for childhood obesity. J Consult Clin Psychol 58(5):661–664, 1990.

Epstein LH, Valoski AM, Vara LS, et al: Effects of decreasing sedentary behavior and increasing activity on weight change in obese children. Health Psychol 14:109–115, 1995.

Epstein LH, Valoski A, Wing RR, et al: Ten-year outcomes of behavioral family-based treatment for childhood obesity. Health Psychol 13:373–383, 1994.

Epstein LH, Wing RR: Behavioral treatment of childhood obesity. Psychol Bull 101(3):331–342, 1987.

Gortmaker SL, Must A, Perrin JM, et al: Social and economic consequences of overweight in adolescence and young adulthood. N Engl J Med 329:1008–1012, 1993.

Haddock CK, Shadish WR, Klesges RC, et al: Treatments for childhood and adolescent obesity. Ann Behav Med 16:235–244, 1994.

Johnson SL, Birch LL: Parents' and children's adiposity and eating style. Pediatrics 94:653–661, 1994.

Mellbin T, Vuille J-C: Further evidence of an association between psychosocial problems and increase in relative weight between 7 and 10 years of age. Acta Paediat 78:576–580, 1989.

MMWR: Update: prevalence of overweight among children, adolescents, and adults—United States, 1988–1994. MMWR Morb Mortal Wkly Rep 46(9):199–201, 1997.

Must A, Jacques PF, Dallal GE, et al: Long-term morbidity and mortality of overweight adolescents. A follow-up of the Harvard Growth Study of 1922 to 1935. N Engl J Med 327:1350–1355, 1992.

Robinson TN: Defining obesity in children and adolescents: clinical approaches. Crit Rev Food Sci Nutr 33(4-5):313–320, 1993.

Rolland-Cachera M-F, Deheeger M, Bellisle F, et al: Adiposity rebound in children: a simple indicator for predicting obesity. Am J Clin Nutr 39:129–135, 1984.

Serdula MK, Ivery D, Coates RJ, et al: Do obese children become obese adults? A review of the literature. Prev Med 22:167–177, 1993.

RECOMMENDED READING FOR PARENTS AND CHILDREN

Epstein LH, Squires S: The Stoplight Diet for Children: An Eight Week Program for Parents and Children. Boston, Little Brown, 1988.

Satter E: Child of Mine: Feeding With Love and Good Sense. Palo Alto, CA, Bull Publishing, 1991.

Satter E: How to Get Your Kid to Eat but Not Too Much. Palo Alto, CA, Bull Publishing, 1987.

Disordered Eating Behaviors: Anorexia Nervosa, Bulimia Nervosa, Cyclic Vomiting Syndrome, and Rumination Disorder

George D. Comerci

 Each of the various major disturbances in children's eating behavior has complex biopsychosocial origins. Anorexia nervosa involves a distorted body image and self-imposed severe dietary limitation that results in malnutrition. In bulimia nervosa there is binge eating with inappropriate measures taken to avoid weight gain. Cyclic vomiting manifests itself as repeated severe episodes of vomiting in the absence of the usual causes. Rumination disorder entails repeated significant regurgitation of food in infants without any gastrointestinal illness. This chapter defines and clarifies their diagnoses and requirements for management.

Anorexia Nervosa and Bulimia Nervosa

DEFINITIONS AND SUBTYPES

Anorexia, defined as the loss of appetite, is not experienced early in the course of anorexia nervosa, but only later as malnutrition and inanition progress. The diagnostic criteria of *anorexia nervosa* are listed in Table 39–1 (American Psychiatric Association, 1994). The diagnosis is easily made when a hyperactive young woman with unexplained weight loss, cachexia, and amenorrhea claims to be fat and refuses to eat. The patient has an obsessional desire to lose more and more weight, is usually physically hyperactive, and often experiences sleep disturbances. Bizarre eating behaviors are present, as are abnormal attitudes about food, a stubborn denial of illness, and other physical signs of starvation. There is no known physical or other psychiatric illness that can account for the weight loss and other physical and behavioral changes.

Two types of anorexia nervosa are included in the fourth edition of the *Diagnostic and Statistical Manual of Mental Disorders (DSM-IV)* description: the restricting type and binge eating/purging type. In the former there is an absence of binge eating or purging, and in the latter there is self-induced vomiting and laxative, diuretic, and enema use intended to compensate for the increased caloric intake with binge eating. Both types usually involve fasting and inappropriate levels of exercise. Moreover, patients seem to fall into either a water-restricting or water-imbibing category. The above findings constitute the *primary* or *classic* anorexia nervosa syndrome.

Persons who do not meet the official *DSM-IV* criteria for anorexia nervosa or bulimia nervosa (see below) may be considered to have *atypical eating disorders* (Table 39–2). Early in the progression of an eating disorder, many (especially children and preadolescents) may not meet all of the required criteria for a firm diagnosis of anorexia nervosa or bulimia nervosa; they can be considered to have atypical eating disorders, but they still need appropriate treatment (American Psychiatric Association, 1994; Mitrany, 1992). There are other forms of voluntary or psychological undernutrition and food restriction that may be considered atypical and could be referred to as *pseudoanorexia nervosa*. Persons with these variants, or analogues, of anorexia nervosa include obligatory athletes or those motivated by an intense desire to achieve a perfect body

Table 39–1 • Diagnostic Criteria for Anorexia Nervosa

A. Refusal to maintain body weight at or above a minimally normal weight for age and height (e.g., weight loss leading to maintenance of body weight less than 85% of that expected; or failure to make expected weight gain during period of growth, leading to body weight less than 85% of that expected)

B. Intense fear of gaining weight or becoming fat, even though underweight

C. Disturbance in the way in which one's body weight or shape is experienced, undue influence of body weight or shape on self-evaluation, or denial of the seriousness of the current low body weight

D. In postmenarcheal females, amenorrhea, i.e., absence of at least three consecutive menstrual cycles (A woman is considered to have amenorrhea if her periods occur only following hormone, e.g., estrogen, administration.)

Restricting type
During the current episode of anorexia nervosa, the person has not regularly engaged in binge eating or purging behavior (i.e., self-induced vomiting or the misuse of laxatives, diuretics, or enemas).

Binge eating/purging type
During the current episode of anorexia nervosa, the person has regularly engaged in binge eating or purging behaviors (i.e., self-induced vomiting or the misuse of laxatives, diuretics, or enemas).

Adapted from American Psychiatric Association: Diagnostic and Statistical Manual of Mental Disorders, DSM-IV, 4th ed. Washington, DC, American Psychiatric Association, 1994, pp 544–545.

Table 39–2 • Diagnostic Criteria for Atypical Eating Disorders

This category includes those who do not meet the official *DSM IV* criteria for anorexia nervosa and bulimia nervosa:

1. For females: all of the criteria for anorexia nervosa are met except that regular menses are present
2. All of the criteria for anorexia nervosa are met except that, despite significant weight loss, the individual's current weight is in the normal range
3. All of the criteria for bulimia nervosa are met except that the binge eating and inappropriate compensatory mechanisms occur at a frequency of less than twice a week or for a duration of less than 3 months
4. The regular use of inappropriate compensatory behavior by an individual of normal body weight after eating small amounts of food (e.g., self-induced vomiting after the consumption of two cookies)
5. Repeatedly chewing and spitting out, but not swallowing, large amounts of food
6. Binge-eating disorder: recurrent episodes of binge eating in the absence of the regular use of inappropriate compensatory behaviors characteristic of bulimia nervosa

Adapted from American Psychiatric Association: Diagnostic and Statistical Manual of Mental Disorders, DSM-IV, 4th ed. Washington, DC, American Psychiatric Association, 1994, p 550.

suited to a particular body-focused activity. These activities include modeling, ballet and other dance forms, gymnastics, body building, track, and marathon running. Food refusal and restriction associated with schizophrenia, depression, conversion reactions, and other forms of psychogenic undernutrition can be considered *secondary eating disorders*, but they truly are not anorexia or bulimia nervosa. However, psychiatric illness including schizophrenia, conduct disorder, obsessive-compulsive disorder, and personality disorders (borderline, paranoid, or obsessive-compulsive) can be present in some patients with anorexia nervosa or bulimia nervosa as comorbid conditions (Gillberg, Rastam, and Gillberg, 1995; Rastam, Gillberg, and Gillberg, 1995).

Bulimia is defined as a morbid hunger, usually manifested as episodic binge eating or the rapid ingestion of large amounts of food in a relatively short time. *Bulimia nervosa* is a syndrome in which there is binge eating associated with inappropriate compensatory behaviors in attempts to prevent weight gain. The criteria for the diagnosis of bulimia nervosa are listed in Table 39–3 (American Psychiatric Association, 1994). Increased appetite and binge eating usually are not related to increased hunger per se, the exception being when the patient is also involved with prolonged fasting and caloric restriction. The patient also shows frequent weight fluctuations, is dissatisfied with her or his physical shape, and becomes fixated on certain unacceptable body parts. There are depressive symptoms with self-deprecatory thoughts, especially following binge eating. There is no other psychiatric condition or physical abnormality responsible for the symptoms, but it is estimated that up to half of all bulimic patients have another psychiatric disorder such as depression or obsessive-compulsive disorder.

Binge-eating disorder, a proposed diagnostic category in the *DSM-IV*, includes patients who binge eat twice a week or more for 6 months or longer, but do *not* engage in compensatory purging or exercise. Subsequently, these patients are usually overweight. They are difficult to diagnose, show no signs of purging behavior, often refuse to be weighed, and are common among obese populations.

ETIOLOGY

Anorexia nervosa and bulimia nervosa are complex conditions, each having strong biological, psychological, and sociocultural determinants. The eating disorder syndromes are classic examples of biopsychosocial disorders and show the associated developmental and cognitive deficits; they have at their root important psychological and most likely organic determinants (Fig. 39–1). Premorbid conditions of eating disorders and the consequent personality and emotional disorders, family dysfunction, and difficulties with social adaptation interfere with optimal functioning during childhood and adolescence, and for most into adulthood. Most somatic manifestations of eating disorders are the result of semistarvation, purgation, and other inappropriate behaviors; whether all abnormal findings are the result of the eating disorder or a primary biological vulnerability remains to be established (Halmi, 1996; Hartman, 1995; Yates, 1992).

There has been movement away from the concept of eating disorders as being reactive phenomena to an emphasis on developmental, neuroendocrine, and physiologic vulnerabilities, for example, from a focus on the individual's reaction to sociocultural and intrafamilial stressors to a focus on the role of temperament as a predisposing factor and the effect of very early parent-child interactions on personality development. Early separation and emotional

Table 39–3 • Diagnostic Criteria for Bulimia Nervosa

A. Recurrent episodes of binge eating. An episode of binge eating is characterized by both of the following:
1. Eating in a discrete period of time (e.g., within any 2-hour period) an amount of food that is definitely larger than most people would eat during a similar period of time and under similar circumstances
2. A sense of lack of control over eating during the episode (e.g., a feeling that one cannot stop eating or control what or how much one is eating)

B. Recurrent inappropriate compensatory behavior in order to prevent weight gain, such as self-induced vomiting; misuse of laxatives, diuretics, enemas, or other medications; fasting; or excessive exercise

C. Both the binge eating and inappropriate compensatory behaviors occur, on average, at least twice a week for at least 3 months

D. Self-evaluation is unduly influenced by body shape and weight

E. The disturbance does not occur exclusively during episodes of anorexia nervosa

Purging type
During the current episode of bulimia nervosa, the person has regularly engaged in self-induced vomiting or the misuse of laxatives, diuretics, or enemas.

Nonpurging type
During the current episode of bulimia nervosa, the person has used other inappropriate compensatory behaviors, such as fasting or excessive exercise, but has not regularly engaged in self-induced vomiting or the misuse of laxatives, diuretics, or enemas.

Adapted from American Psychiatric Association: Diagnostic and Statistical Manual of Mental Disorders, DSM-IV, 4th ed. Washington, DC, American Psychiatric Association, 1994, pp 549–550.

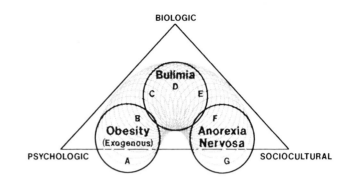

Figure 39–1. Eating disorders. Classic examples of illness with biopsychosocial determinants. Diagram represents reciprocal relationship between obesity, bulimia, and anorexia nervosa, seen along a continuum. (From Comerci GD, Williams RL: Eating disorders in the young. Part 1: Anorexia nervosa and bulimia. Curr Probl Pediatr 15[8]:23, 1985.)

A. Exogenous Obesity
B. Bulimia: Depression/Low Self Esteem
C. Bulimia: Anger (repressed)/Depression
D. Bulimia: Character/Personality Disorder
E. "Atypical" or Secondary Anorexia Nervosa
F. Bulimia Complicating Anorexia Nervosa
G. Classical Anorexia Nervosa

detachment may cause permanent restructuring of neurotransmitter relationships in the young infant with a resultant predisposition to conditions that are associated with eating disorders (Comerci, 1992). The etiologic relationship of conditions such as obsessive-compulsive disorder, depression, avoidant behaviors, shyness, and phobias to eating disorders has been under study (Kasvikis et al, 1986; Wonderlich, 1991). Elevated endogenous opioids and decreased levels of norepinephrine and serotonin may be implicated in the origins and perpetuation of these as well as certain eating disorders. Serotonin and noradrenergic systems are involved with appetite and satiation mechanisms; starvation-induced abnormalities of these transmitter systems have been postulated (Halmi, 1996; Jarry and Vaccarino, 1996; Woodside, 1995). It has been observed that low levels of serotonin in bulimic patients are associated with carbohydrate craving. Because fluoxetine, a serotonin agonist, inhibits the uptake of serotonin, causing higher central nervous system (CNS) levels of this important neurotransmitter, it can be postulated that the higher level of CNS serotonin is at least partially responsible for the success of fluoxetine when used in bulimic patients to reduce bingeing by decreasing carbohydrate craving. Furthermore, cyproheptadine hydrochloride, a serotonin antagonist, may contribute to weight gain when administered to patients with anorexia nervosa by increasing their desire to consume carbohydrates.

The relationship between the neurotransmitters, early parent-infant interactions, and conditions associated with eating disorders, especially depression and obsessive-compulsive traits, is under current study. Yates (1992) gives a review of biological considerations in the etiology of eating disorders.

PSYCHODYNAMICS

In Western society, thinness connotes asceticism and fatness suggests slovenliness and lack of self-discipline and control. Fasting and purging have long been part of a spiritual quest for purity, virtue, and holiness. Through self-sacrifice and denial, the weak become strong, the faint-hearted become brave, and the immoral are cleansed and forgiven. Thus the powerless gain power and by self-control approach a state of godliness and veneration. Whereas affluence and an abundance of food currently seem to be critical environmental factors enhancing the occurrence of eating disorders, in the past, strong religious, family, and cultural forces affected their prevalence (Bell, 1985; Brumberg, 1988). Moreover there is an association between what a society values philosophically and spiritually and how that society defines and seeks physical beauty. It is against this backdrop of fasting, purging, and self-denial as a reciprocal or equivalent of beauty, goodness, and worthiness that eating disorders must be studied. The preoccupation of modern Western culture with physical fitness and thinness, social pressures (including early sexual experimentation), and the recent emphasis on women's achievement and success undoubtedly have played a role in the increase of eating disorders over the past 25 years (Bruch, 1973).

Children in whom anorexia nervosa develops have been described as being obsessive-compulsive, isolated, excessively dependent, and developmentally immature. They are limited in their ability to express emotions, especially anger. Families are described as being overintrusive, overprotective, and skilled at conflict avoidance (Comerci, Kilbourne, and Carroll, 1985). It is believed that the development of symptoms is a way of side-stepping the demands of adolescence and a means of avoiding adulthood.

Patients with bulimia nervosa have many of the same premorbid psychological characteristics as those with anorexia nervosa, but these individuals have greater interpersonal sensitivity and suffer more affective instability.

Indirect evidence exists that biological factors affect the development of anorexia nervosa and bulimia nervosa (see Etiology); there is a higher occurrence of eating disorders in parents and siblings of patients with eating disorders and among twins. It remains unclear whether subtle modifications in the production or metabolism of certain appetite-regulating amines (e.g., cholecystokinen), CNS neurotransmitters, and opioids play a primary role in the initiation and perpetuation of these disorders or whether they are merely associated changes.

INCIDENCE AND MORTALITY

In 1976, it was estimated that there was 1 new case of primary anorexia nervosa each year for every 250 affluent high school girls aged 16 to 18 years (Crisp, Palmer, and Kalucy, 1976). The incidence is believed to be much higher than a generation ago, with a current prevalence rate for white high school girls of 1% to 2% and a female to male ratio of about 10 to 20:1. Two peak times of onset are seen: one around age 14 years and the other at about age 18 years. Although 85% of persons in whom anorexia nervosa develops are between 13 and 20 years of age, 22% are premenarcheal; and approximately 3% of cases begin in childhood (Bryant-Waugh and Lask, 1995). The incidence of anorexia nervosa increases with socioeconomic status and is highest among affluent white females (95%). (See Chapter 17 regarding affluence.) Nevertheless, anorexia nervosa in the United States is being seen in all socioeconomic settings, in patients of all races and ages, and in individuals of varied psychological and social makeup.

Among psychiatric illnesses, anorexia nervosa has one of the higher mortality rates. Anorexia nervosa patients have a fivefold to sixfold increase in mortality rate when compared with the same-sex and same-age general population (Patton, 1985). Reports of mortality rates vary between 5% and 20%, with the American Psychiatric Association, in its *DSM-IV* manual, reporting long-term mortality rates of more than 10% in patients who have been hospitalized. Death is frequently the result of suicide, starvation, and cardiovascular or other complications of starvation and infection. Complications of overly aggressive refeeding regimens are responsible for some deaths. Total parenteral nutrition carries special risks.

Cases of bulimia nervosa increased dramatically during the 1970s and early 1980s. It has come to be considered a major public health problem in the United States, western Europe, Scandinavia, and Australia. With or without associated purging, it probably accounts for the majority of eating disorders in female college students and other young adult women. The prevalence of bulimia nervosa in young women ranges from 2% to 4% (Cooper, Charnock, and Taylor, 1987; Pyle et al, 1983), with 5% of all persons with bulimia being male. Higher reported prevalence rates (up to 19%) may be misleading because many female subjects tend to label the ingestion of a normal meal as bulimic when they feel they have eaten too much. There is a need for more research in this area. The mortality rate for bulimia nervosa is not known but can be considered to be at least as high and probably higher than that for anorexia nervosa. Death may result from severe hypovolemia and electrolyte abnormalities with cardiac dysrhythmias. Suicide is a major cause of death in patients with bulimia nervosa and when bulimia complicates anorexia nervosa. Because the disorder was described relatively recently, there are few or no truly long-term follow-up controlled studies on outcome and mortality rates.

CLINICAL MANIFESTATIONS AND COMPLICATIONS

The usual onset of anorexia nervosa is either in early pubescence or shortly before or after graduation from high school. In boys, the onset is usually earlier, often before pubescence begins. The occurrence of anorexia nervosa seems to coincide with periods of developmental transitions, when the young person is confronted with demands for self-reliance and autonomy and is experiencing the stress of separation from family, as well as other psychosocial pressures. Anorexia nervosa increasingly is occurring in children as young as 9 or 10 years of age and during young and middle adulthood.

The patient's history usually reveals no major illnesses, and the child is described by the parents as having been a "model child" and "no problem at all." The patient is usually a very good student and involved in many activities, such as ballet, other dancing, equestrian sports, and gymnastics. It is less likely that the young person will have been engaged in team sports, more often having excelled at individually focused activities. When rapport and trust are established, the patient may confess to feeling a profound sense of ineffectiveness and low self-esteem, which is likely to be related to a childhood of performing and achieving for the satisfaction and vicarious fulfillment and pleasure of parents, teachers, and others.

The families of patients with anorexia nervosa appear on the surface to be functioning well. With further exploration, however, the marital relationship is found to be lacking (Comerci, 1985; Comerci, Kilbourne, and Carroll, 1985). Fathers are often heavily invested in their work and mothers in their children. As the distance between parents widens, strong intergenerational coalitions, usually between the mother and the affected child, develop. Sometimes with the onset of symptoms, the father becomes more involved in the care of the daughter, and the mother, rebuffed and piqued, withdraws in frustration and anger. With eventual failure to influence the child's behavior, the father in anger and frustration becomes more punitive, and the child stubbornly further isolates herself from friends and family.

Considering the publicity that anorexia nervosa has received in recent years, it is surprising how often there is a long delay by parents in seeking care for their child. The extent of weight loss is well hidden by bulky clothing, and the patient's high degree of physical activity leads parents to believe that all is well. In the early stages, there are few observable signs except for decreased fat tissue, for which the young person often is highly praised. In about one third or more of cases, amenorrhea occurs even before appreciable amounts of weight are lost. It is this symptom that may prompt a mother to finally seek medical consultation. Early on, laboratory tests are normal, which sometimes falsely reassures the physician.

As the condition progresses, physical symptoms and signs appear (Fig. 39–2) and laboratory findings (Tables 39–4 and 39–5) become abnormal. By this time, amenorrhea is an almost universal finding. The skin is dry and has a sallow appearance. The patient still has few complaints and continues to deny there is a problem. However she may complain of loss of scalp hair with shampooing and brushing, the growth of pigmented body hair on the chest and abdomen, and abdominal discomfort and fullness. Appetite decreases, but episodes of severe hunger may disturb sleep with recurrent dreams of eating and food. Constipation is almost always present, but the patient does not complain of it or report it unless asked. Isolating herself from family members and from friends, the patient has little time for socialization and devotes most of her awake hours to exercising, rewriting and perfecting homework

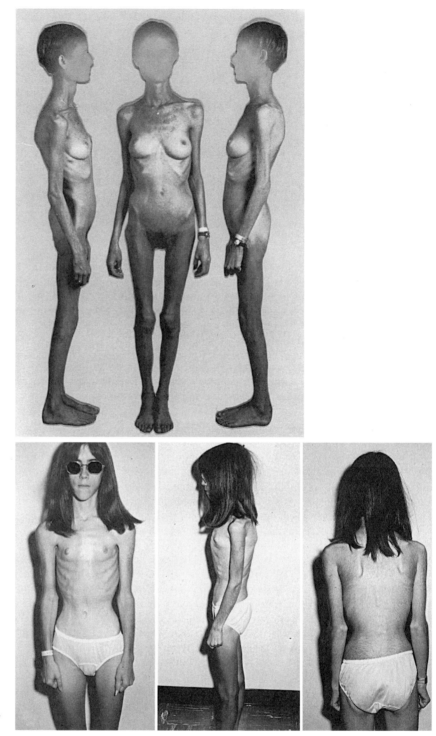

Figure 39–2. Severe emaciation with characteristic physical findings of anorexia nervosa.

assignments, and ruminating and obsessing about food selection, preparation, and avoidance. The young person stays awake studying or exercising past midnight and often awakens before dawn. There is increasing irritability with friends and family and an inability to concentrate. Uncharacteristically, the usually pleasant and compliant adolescent often shows hostility to her friends and impatience with their demands on her time.

With progressive and increasingly severe malnutrition and emaciation, fatigue and muscle weakness occur,

and finally physical activity diminishes. The weakness and fatigue is one of the few symptoms that prompts the young person to seek help or cooperate with parents and physician. With continued weight loss, often greater than 40% of beginning body weight, marked bradycardia (sometimes as low as 25 to 30 beats/minute), hypothermia, and postural hypotension occur (Palla and Litt, 1988). There is increasing weakness and fatigue, leading to depression and apathy. The patient remains at or regresses to a preadolescent or early adolescent stage of cognitive and social development,

Table 39–4 • Physical Symptoms and Signs in Anorexia Nervosa

I. Presenting physical symptoms
  A. Weight loss
  B. Amenorrhea, no cyclic symptoms or physical changes of menstruation (anovulatory)
  C. Hyperactivity (mental and motor)
  D. Aberrant behavior, irritability, isolation-withdrawal, sleep disturbances
  E. Hyperacusis or optic hyperesthesia
  F. May present with depressed mood, feelings of ineffectiveness, and low self-esteem
II. Physical signs
  A. Cachexia, emaciation, debilitation or dehydration, possible signs of shock or impending shock
  B. Covert infectious processes (pneumonia or sepsis; immunologic problems late, anergy-negative skin tests)
  C. Skin changes (dryness, yellowish palms and soles, desquamation, and "dirty" appearance to skin)
  D. Scalp and pubic hair loss, lanugo hair or increased pigmented body hair
  E. Hypothermia (rectal temperature below 96.6°F/36.2°C)
  F. Bradypnea
  G. Bradycardia "quiet" heart (decreased basal metabolic rate)—pulse below 60 beats/minute usual; as low as 25 beats/minute
  H. Hypotension often below 70/50 mm Hg
  I. Heart murmur (infrequent)
  J. Edema of lower extremities
  K. Signs of estrogen deficiency—skin dryness, osteoporosis, small uterus-cervix, vaginal mucosa pink and dry, and gross and microscopic evidence of deficient estrogen
  L. Signs of decreased androgen—no acne, no oily skin

From Comerci GD, Greydanus D: Eating disorders: anorexia nervosa and bulimia. *In* Hofmann AD, Greydanus D (eds): Adolescent Medicine, 3rd ed. Norwalk, CT, Appleton & Lange, 1997.

Table 39–5 • Laboratory Findings in Anorexia Nervosa

I. Chemical
  A. Normal results on most laboratory tests early in process
  B. Elevated blood urea nitrogen (BUN) levels—secondary to dehydration
  C. Hypercarotenemia
  D. Elevated serum cholesterol levels (early—may decrease late)
  E. Decreased transferrin (usually normal protein and albumin to globulin ratio), low complement (C_3), fibrinogen, and prealbumin
  F. Elevated serum lactic dehydrogenase–alkaline phosphatase (possibly related to growth)
  G. Depressed phosphorus level (a late and ominous sign); depressed magnesium and calcium levels (calcium may be elevated)
  H. Possible depression of plasma zinc, urinary zinc, and urinary copper levels
II. Endocrine
  A. Low luteinizing hormone (LH); low or pseudonormal follicle-stimulating hormone (FSH); deficiency of gonadotropin-releasing hormone (GnRH); normal prolactin; low testosterone in males and low estradiol in females
  B. Elevated circulating cortisol (normal production—does not suppress with dexamethasone)
  C. Low normal fasting glucose
  D. Low normal thyroxine (T_4); reduced triiodothyronine (T_3); elevated reverse T_3; normal TSH
  E. Possible elevation of parathyroid hormone (PTH) secondary to hypomagnesemia with resultant hypercalcemia
  F. Elevated resting growth hormone levels
III. Hematological
  A. Leukopenia with relative lymphocytoses (bone marrow hypoplasia), absolute lymphopenia
  B. Thrombocytopenia
  C. Very low erythrocyte sedimentation rate (ESR)—almost always
  D. Anemia late (especially with rehydration)

From Comerci GD, Greydanus D: Eating disorders: anorexia nervosa and bulimia. *In* Hofmann AD, Greydanus D (eds): Adolescent Medicine, 3rd ed. Norwalk, CT, Appleton & Lange, 1997.

and sexual development and interest cease. Certain clinical findings are observed in voluntary starvation, which might help distinguish anorexia nervosa from involuntary malnutrition (Table 39–6).

Bulimia nervosa is difficult to diagnose by physical examination alone because bulimic persons, unless engaging in a high level of inappropriate compensatory behaviors (purgation, exercising, and fasting), often exhibit no signs of illness and usually are of normal weight. They may be underweight but are less likely to be cachectic. When the condition is complicated by caloric and fluid restriction, signs of dehydration and electrolyte disturbance are seen. There is hypovolemia with postural hypotension and tachycardia. The parotid and submandibular glands can become enlarged, presumably as a result of excessive reflex stimulation or reflux into salivary ducts. Abdominal tenderness can simply result from straining with retching and vomiting or, if severe, can be due to pancreatitis. Esophagitis and mucosal tears can occur. The physical symptoms and signs and laboratory findings of bulimia nervosa are listed in Tables 39–7 and 39–8.

DIFFERENTIAL DIAGNOSIS AND EVALUATION

Early recognition of eating disorders and prompt intervention is associated with improved outcome, but common

adolescent preoccupation with dieting and unusual eating attitudes should not be prematurely attributed to an eating disorder. Distinguishing between anorexia nervosa and bulimia nervosa and a normal variation in eating and eating attitudes is a challenge that must be met if inappropriate labeling is to be avoided (Maloney et al, 1989).

Table 39–6 • Voluntary Starvation of Anorexia Nervosa and Involuntary Starvation

	Starvation	
Clinical Finding	*Voluntary*	*Involuntary*
Vitamin deficiencies	Rare	Frequent
Serum cholesterol	Elevated	Decreased
Serum carotene	Elevated	Elevated
Serum albumin	Normal	Decreased in kwashiorkor
Anemia	Infrequent	Common
Lymphocytes	Normal	Increased T cells, increased null cells
Humoral immunity	Unimpaired	Impaired
Skin testing	Moderately impaired	Significantly impaired
Breast tissue	Maintained	Atrophied
Muscle weakness	Less pronounced	More pronounced
Activity level	Often increased	Decreased

From Comerci GD, Kilbourne KA, Carroll AE: Eating disorders in the young: anorexia nervosa and bulimia, Part 2. Curr Probl Pediatr 15(9):1–59, 1985.

Table 39–7 • Physical Symptoms
and Signs in Bulimia Nervosa

I. Presenting physical symptoms
  A. Weight may be normal, overweight, or underweight
  B. Complaints of bloating, diarrhea, swelling
  C. Hyperactivity (mental and motor)—exceptions common
  D. Constant or extreme thirst and increased urination (hypokalemic nephropathy-hypovolemia)
  E. May present with depression, anxiety, despair, and suicidal ideation
II. Physical signs
  A. Usually well groomed and good hygiene; definite exceptions, especially patients with a severe character disorder or chronic addictive conditions
  B. Usually normal weight or mild to moderate obesity (exception: food restrictors or anorexia nervosa patients with associated bulimia–vomiting-purging)
  C. Generalized or localized edema of lower extremities (compensatory renal retention of sodium and water, i.e., hypovolemia with secondary hyperaldosteronism or pseudo-Bartter syndrome)
  D. Physical findings of extreme weight loss (self-starvation) if bulimia–vomiting-purging is complication of anorexia nervosa or food restriction; loss of scalp hair, skin changes of anorexia
  E. Swelling of parotid and other salivary glands
  F. Dental enamel dysplasia and discoloration due to gastric juices (vomiting)
  G. Bruises and lacerations of palate and posterior pharynx; lesions of fingernails, fingers, and dorsum of hand(s) (due to self-induced vomiting)
  H. Pyorrhea and other gum disorders
  I. Diminished reflexes, muscle weakness, paralysis, and, infrequently, peripheral neuropathy with muscle weakness and paralysis
  J. Muscle cramping (with induced hypoxia or positive Trousseau sign)
  K. Signs of hypokalemia: cardiac dysrhythmias, hypotension, decreased cardiac output, weak pulse, and poor quality heart sounds; abdominal distention, ileus, acute gastric dilatation; and myopathy. Shortness of breath, depression, and mental clouding

From Comerci GD, Greydanus D: Eating disorders: anorexia nervosa and bulimia. *In* Hofmann HD, Greydanus D (eds): Adolescent Medicine, 3rd ed. Norwalk, CT, Appleton & Lange, 1997.

As part of the initial evaluation of patients with eating disorders, the differential diagnoses of anorexia nervosa and bulimia nervosa must be considered. Other psychiatric and organic conditions can closely simulate anorexia nervosa. Schizophrenia, obsessive-compulsive disorder, bipolar or depressive disorders, conversion reactions, and psychophysiologic disorders must be considered. Other mental health disorders that should be considered, especially in bulimic patients, include personality disorders (borderline, paranoid, obsessive-compulsive) and conduct disorder (Gillberg, Rastam, and Gillberg, 1995; Rastam, Gillberg, and Gillberg, 1995). Approximately 30% of patients with anorexia nervosa also have recurrent affective disorders, and suicide occurs in 2% to 5%. Anxiety disorders (e.g., obsessive-compulsive disorder, social phobia, or body dysmorphic disorder) may have some elements similar to aspects of anorexia nervosa (American Psychiatric Association, 1994).

Organic conditions to be considered by the pediatrician include malignancies (especially CNS and gastrointestinal), Addison or hypopituitary disease, hypothyroidism, chronic infection (including with cytomegalovirus, Epstein-Barr virus, and human immunodeficiency virus), chronic lung disease (including undiagnosed cystic fibrosis), ulcer disease, chronic inflammatory bowel disease (regional enteritis or Crohn disease), diabetes mellitus and diabetes insipidus, immunologic, renal, and collagen vascular disease, and drug use (especially cocaine and other stimulants). When patients with weight loss and vomiting complain of dysphagia and firmly deny self-induced vomiting, upper gastrointestinal obstruction such as achalasia must be considered.

In bulimia nervosa, the presence of hyponatremia and hypovolemia associated with marked weakness and fatigue may lead to the suspicion of Addison disease, kidney disease, or diuretic abuse. Patients with bulimia nervosa commonly have difficulty with fluid retention, which in older patients may closely mimic idiopathic edema or the premenstrual syndrome. A more complete review of the medical complications of eating disorders is available (Comerci and Greydanus, 1997; Fisher, 1992; Kreipe, 1995a; Kreipe and Harris, 1992).

MANAGEMENT

Management of an eating disorder is a complex process and a challenge to even the most skilled and experienced practitioner. Although an organized approach to care and a protocol for treatment is essential, each patient must be considered unique and deserving of individual care. There are four general principles of care that should be followed: (1) establishment of rapport and trust, (2) restoration of nutritional and metabolic state to normal, (3) involvement of the family, and (4) implementation of a team approach. A number of excellent reviews are available (Comerci and Greydanus, 1997; Halmi, 1996; Herzog and Beresin, 1997; Kreipe, 1995b).

Once the primary care physician is confident of the diagnosis, there are a number of screening laboratory and psychological tests that are helpful (Fig. 39–3). To better delineate underlying psychopathology, some patients require not only a test to identify abnormal eating attitudes

Table 39–8 • Laboratory Findings in
Bulimia Nervosa–Vomiting-Purging

A. Bulimia alone: no abnormalities reported—possible alterations in glucose metabolism
B. Bulimia with vomiting:
  1. Metabolic alkalosis with hypochloremia, elevated serum bicarbonate levels
  2. Hypokalemia (secondary to number 1 above)
  3. Hypovolemia with secondary hyperaldosteronism (also contributes to hypokalemia) (pseudo-Bartter syndrome)
C. Bulimia with vomiting and laxative-diuretic abuse:
  1. All findings in A and B (above)
  2. Decreased body potassium due to small bowel (diarrhea) and renal losses
  3. Metabolic acidosis with spurious normal serum potassium levels
  4. Hypokalemic nephropathy with a urine-concentrating deficit
  5. Hypokalemic myopathy (including heart)
  6. Hypocalcemia or hypercalcemia, hypomagnesemia, hypophosphatemia

From Comerci GD, Greydanus D: Eating disorders: anorexia nervosa and bulimia. *In* Hofmann AD, Greydanus D (eds): Adolescent Medicine, 3rd ed. Norwalk, CT, Appleton & Lange, 1997.

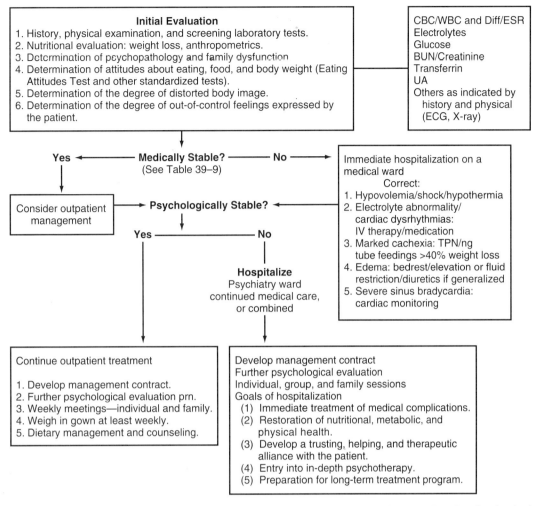

Figure 39–3. Initial evaluation and management of the eating disorder patient. (Adapted from Comerci GD, et al: Eating disorders in the young. Part 2: Anorexia nervosa and bulimia. Curr Probl Pediatr 15[9]:7–16, 1985.)

(Eating Disorders Inventory) (Garner, Olmsted, and Polivy, 1983) but also formal psychometric tests such as the Minnesota Multiphasic Personality Profile.

After malnutrition is corrected, treatment should be directed to the resolution of disturbed family interactions and individual psychotherapy. This phase of treatment almost always requires referral to a team of professionals who are experienced in the care of eating disorder patients. Psychological treatment is critical to the overall success of management. It is estimated that of the patients with anorexia and bulimia who recover, 80% do so through formal treatment. Focus of therapy is on the psychological underpinnings of these disorders: low self-esteem; depression; difficulty identifying, expressing, and tolerating strong feelings; constant thoughts of helplessness; sense of ineffectiveness; distorted body image; and family of origin issues. These young women usually are ambitious and shy, do very well academically or in their careers, and are reasonably well adjusted socially. Many, however, despite their distress and desire to gain control over their bulimia and purging behaviors, require intensive individual, family, and group therapy; the use of antidepressants or anxiolytics may be pivotal.

Primary care physicians should consult a psychiatrist before administering psychotropic medications in adolescents with eating disorders. Caution should be exercised to avoid prescribing such medications to adolescents who are using alcohol and other drugs. There should be careful discussion with the patient and parents regarding the side effects, benefits, and risks of such medications. Permission should be obtained from the parents. The use of fluoxetine (Prozac), a selective serotonin reuptake inhibitor, has been found to be beneficial, especially in bulimic patients. In general, medication is less effective in anorexia nervosa. When an affective disorder is present, antidepressant medication may help, but, if possible, prescribing should be delayed until the patient is medically stable or a stable weight gain has been achieved. Obtaining an electrocardiogram (ECG) before prescribing medication is recommended. Cyproheptadine (Periactin) may help some patients with nonpurging anorexia nervosa by reducing anxiety and increasing appetite.

Outpatient therapy can be attempted by the primary care physician if the duration of the illness is less than 2 to 4 months, there are no severe purgative behaviors, there is a low level of family dysfunction, and the family fully supports the treatment program. Indications for immediate hospitalization include (1) hypovolemia and impending shock, (2) electrolyte imbalance including hypokalemia, hypomagnesemia, and hypophosphatemia, (3) uncompensated metabolic alkalosis or acidosis, (4) marked cachexia, especially if weight loss is 40% or more from appropriate or beginning weight, (5) generalized edema or congestive heart failure, (6) marked bradycardia and ECG abnormalities, and (7) hypothermia (see Fig. 39–3 and Table 39–9).

The primary goal of early inpatient treatment is to save life by restoration of body weight and physiologic homeostasis. Secondary goals include (1) the development of trust by the patient in the physician and other members of the eating disorder team, (2) a time out (isolation) from a self-perpetuating disturbed home environment, (3) patient education regarding nutrition and eating habits, and (4) the provision of structure, giving the patient an opportunity to establish realistic priorities and to achieve a feeling of being safe and in control.

PROGNOSIS AND OUTCOME

Controlled studies of effective therapy for eating disorders are lacking. Because starvation causes major psychological as well as physiologic deviations from normal, psychological approaches alone will fail if malnutrition and physiological abnormalities are not first corrected. Conversely, a simplistic approach to weight gain and control of vomiting and purgation as a cure in itself will have only short-term success. About 70% of all patients with eating disorders show short-term recovery with current treatment methods,

but the long-term prognosis is uncertain. Studies with adequate follow-up find that more than 40% of patients recover, 30% improve, 20% do not improve and are chronically affected, and 9% die as a result of the illness (Garfinkel and Garner, 1982; Herzog and Beresin, 1997). In general, males have a less favorable prognosis. Early motivation for change and early intervention are believed to be a good prognostic sign. Anorexic patients with late onset of illness, extreme weight loss, and long duration of symptoms and multiple hospitalizations carry a poor prognosis, as do patients with bulimic components to their illness (especially laxative abusers), persistent distorted body image, and severe personality disorders or major family pathology. Whether treatment has an effect on the ultimate long-term course of eating disorders remains controversial.

There are few long-term follow-up studies of bulimia nervosa, because the identification of bulimia as a distinct disorder has occurred only in the recent past. Serious medical complications, including death, can occur in purging bulimic patients because of electrolyte imbalance and hypovolemia. It is estimated, however, that only 40% to 50% of treated patients can be completely "cured" to the point of being no more preoccupied with body weight and food than their unaffected peers and having comparable feelings of being in control. Some clinicians speculate that "cure" may not be a realistic goal for persons with bulimia (or anorexia), but rather long-term maintenance is preferred, as often is described with a chronic disorder. Anorexia nervosa and bulimia nervosa are chronic disorders and, as such, can be expected to have relapses and remissions, making evaluation of treatment programs difficult.

PREVENTION

Eating disorders are complex biopsychosocial conditions and their cause is indefinite and multifactorial. Risk factors are difficult to know with full confidence; therefore preventive measures are uncertain.

Pediatricians should suggest guidelines to parents and intervene when childrearing methods appear to be detrimental to the child's development. Parents should be encouraged to provide nurturing without being overprotective or overinvolved. They should be alert to the needs of the child and avoid putting their own vicarious pleasure from the child's accomplishments over the inner joy felt by the child. The parents should encourage autonomy and independence but not as a justification for neglect or preoccupation with their own needs and activities. Children should be made to feel wanted, loved, and valued but not possessed, overprized, or indulged.

Mealtimes should be regular and relaxed. Parents should not totally avoid conflict. Children should be encouraged to express differing opinions. Avoidance of conflict by parents can reflect an underlying insecurity on their part regarding their child's love.

Primary care physicians should use moderation in their advice to parents and children regarding the need for fat restriction, avoidance of obesity, and the need for exercise. The media are very effective in this regard—indeed, too effective. Physicians should be alert to inappropriate media messages that generate anxiety about body shape,

---

Table 39–9 • Parameters for Inpatient Management of Anorexia Nervosa

1. Unstable vital signs, such as pulse under 45 beats/minute (BPM), blood pressure under 90 mm Hg systolic, or such orthostatic changes as pulse change over 35 BPM or systolic blood pressure change over 10 mm Hg; also temperature instability: less than 36.2°C or more than 38.0°C
2. Severe electrolyte abnormalities (as potassium less than 3.0 mEq/L, sodium less than 130 mEq/L, or phosphorus less than 2.0 mg/dL)
3. Cardiac dysrhythmias
4. Inability to drink or eat
5. Inability to stop the binge-emesis-food restriction cycles
6. Critically low weight: over 40% loss of body weight, 25%–30% loss in less than 3 months, or under 70% of ideal body weight
7. Arrested growth and development
8. Acute medical emergencies
   A. Gastric perforation
   B. Cardiac failure
   C. Emetine (Ipecac) overdose
   D. Postbinge pancreatitis
   E. Severe hematemesis
   F. Mallory-Weiss syndrome (laceration of the lower end of the esophagus associated with bleeding or mediastinal penetration and resultant mediastinitis)
   G. Boerhaave syndrome (spontaneous rupture of lower esophagus; variant of Mallory-Weiss syndrome)
   H. Aspiration pneumonia
9. Psychiatric emergencies
10. Failure to respond to outpatient management.

Adapted from Comerci GD, Greydanus D: Eating disorders: anorexia nervosa and bulimia. *In* Hofmann A, Greydanus D (eds): Adolescent Medicine, 3rd ed. Norwalk, CT, Appleton & Lange, 1997.

appearance, and physical fitness. Exercise should be reasonable and have an appropriate, but not all-consuming, place in the lives of adults (who serve as models of behavior for children) and the lives of children.

Cyclic Vomiting Syndrome

Described as early as 1882, cyclic vomiting syndrome (CVS) has been variably referred to as cyclic, periodic, or recurrent vomiting of childhood. The cause is not definitively known but has been suspected to be a form of epilepsy or a seizure equivalent, an allergic manifestation, or a psychogenic condition. It has long been an enigma to clinicians faced with symptoms suggestive of serious organic pathology, and only recently has there been a somewhat better understanding of the cause and prevention of this condition. Credence has been given to migraine as the cause of this perplexing syndrome.

CLINICAL MANIFESTATIONS

CVS is characterized by repeated episodes of vomiting, often occurring in clusters, and severe enough to cause ketosis, hypochloremic alkalosis, and dehydration. Episodes may be separated by variable intervals of 2 or usually more weeks, during which the child or adolescent appears to be entirely well. During attacks lasting 6 to 48 hours, patients have uncontrollable vomiting or violent retching, often associated with nausea, abdominal pain, and sometimes photophobia, retrosternal burning, and motion sickness. The vomitus may be mildly blood stained. There may be facial flushing, marked salivation, and drooling. Frequently the patient experiences intense thirst and headache. Withdrawal, lethargy, and somnolence often follow the episodes of vomiting. The severity of the initial episode necessitates consideration of CNS, gastrointestinal, or other pathologic condition; the physical examination, neurologic evaluation (except occasional electroencephalographic variations), and radiographic studies are normal.

PREVALENCE

The prevalence of CVS is unknown and there are few data regarding its frequency (Fleisher and Matar, 1993). It is estimated that at a busy US children's hospital, the condition might be seen five or six times a year (Pfau et al, 1992). Recently, a study from Scotland using stringent diagnostic criteria found a prevalence rate of 1.9% (Abu-Arafeh and Russell, 1995). In that study, children with CVS had a mean age of onset of 5.3 years and an overall sex ratio of 1:1. The clinical features overlapped to a large extent with those of migraine. Other researchers have found CVS to be more common in preschool boys and 6- to 7-year-old girls.

ETIOLOGY

The overlap in the features of CVS with those of childhood migraine supports the prevailing theory that the condition is a migraine variant or equivalent. There is a higher prevalence of migraine in children with CVS, and con-versely, more children with migraine have CVS. There are common clinical features of CVS and childhood migraine: (1) there is an episodic and stereotypic mode of presentation for each patient, (2) episodes are often triggered by travel, stress, or excitement and are relieved by sleep and darkness, (3) there are associated gastrointestinal and sensory symptoms (irritable bowel syndrome and motion sickness), (4) similar vasomotor changes occur during the attacks, (5) there is a significantly higher prevalence of migraine among first-degree relatives of children with CVS, and (6) there is a good response to migraine pharmacotherapy. Nevertheless, CVS remains a poorly understood syndrome, a disorder defined by its clinical pattern and likely to have multiple etiologies.

DIFFERENTIAL DIAGNOSIS

The nature of CVS, with its alarming paroxysms of severe vomiting, often with sudden onset during the night, headache, abdominal pain, pallor, and eventual dehydration requiring intravenous fluids, demands that the physician consider each episode as a possible life-threatening illness. The possibility of a supervening or previously overlooked organic disease is always a challenge to the physician. Brain tumors, especially brainstem gliomas, may make magnetic resonance imaging necessary. Urinary tract disease, including hydronephrosis, appendicitis, and intermittent small bowel obstruction, must be considered.

MANAGEMENT

Intravenous glucose and fluids continue to be the mainstay of treatment for episodes lasting more than a day. Esophagitis should be treated and electrolyte deficits, especially hypokalemia, corrected. The use of intravenous benzodiazepines (lorazepam) to sedate, reduce anxiety, and induce sleep may shorten attacks. Ondansetron, a serotonin antagonist, has been used as an antiemetic and has advantages over phenothiazine and metoclopramide (Reglan), both of which may cause extrapyramidal reactions. Erythromycin, a prokinetic agent, may be useful as well.

CVS, like migraine, may be a reaction to psychological stress. It is important that the clinician address such issues when discussing with patient and family the cause and management of vomiting episodes. CVS may be a manifestation of individual or familial psychopathology, in which case a mental health referral is in order. The episodes of vomiting are frightening to parents and sometimes generate a fair amount of anger because of the expense and inconvenience of repeated episodes. Moreover, when patients are seen by medical personnel unfamiliar with CVS in urgent care and emergency departments, a good deal of resentment because of unnecessary studies and inappropriate treatment recommendations can result. Primary care physicians may want to prepare the family of such patients to deal with covering physicians and emergency room situations.

PREVENTION

The more the patient and family are aware of the precipitating factors associated with CVS, and the more knowledge and understanding they have of what is thought to be its cause, the more likely future episodes can be avoided. When there is significant family psychopathology, it is important that it be addressed. Insight by the child and the parents into their interpersonal and familial relationships may diminish occurrences.

With the emphasis on CVS being a migraine equivalent or an early manifestation of migraine, preventive measures have included medications such as propranolol, amitriptyline, and cyproheptadine. Results of a study of children and adolescents unresponsive to various interventions showed good results to both amitriptyline and cyproheptadine prophylaxis (Andersen et al, 1996). Effective doses of cyproheptadine were similar to those published for migraine prophylaxis. The effective dose of amitriptyline varied widely; most responded to doses for migraine prophylaxis. Although no therapy has been shown to abort an acute attack, such medications are promising.

As the child grows older, the attacks may subside and evolve into "typical" migraine attacks.

Rumination Disorder

Included in *DSM-IV* as an eating disorder, rumination disorder (RD) is a potentially fatal condition characterized by repeated regurgitation of ingested food without nausea or associated gastrointestinal illness. Before the diagnosis is made, congenital anomalies that affect the gastrointestinal system should be ruled out. There are two types of merycism or rumination disorder: psychogenic and self-stimulating. *Psychogenic* rumination is rare and occurs primarily in young male infants between 3 and 14 months of age. Development is otherwise normal; the behavior with resultant weight loss and failure to thrive is believed to result from a seriously disturbed parent-child relationship. Mortality rate is reported to be as high as 25%. *Self-stimulatory* rumination is not uncommon, is seen in mentally retarded individuals of any age, and occurs even when parents are very nurturing and attentive.

CLINICAL MANIFESTATIONS

Young affected infants are often found lying in a small pool of regurgitated liquid. They are observed to actively gag themselves either by manipulation of the tongue or with their pacifier or fingers. Chewing movements and finger mouthing often precede or accompany the regurgitation. The amount of food regurgitated appears small but may result in significant nutrient loss. Repetitive regurgitation and reswallowing of ingested liquids and solids, gagging, mouthing, constant head movement, and failure to thrive are the hallmarks of the condition.

PREVALENCE

Psychogenic rumination disorder is relatively rare, but the self-stimulatory type in developmentally compromised or disabled individuals (e.g., autism, pervasive developmental disorders, mental retardation, cerebral palsy) is encountered in pediatric practice. Rumination in adolescents and adults of normal intelligence is underdiagnosed in general, but

particularly in those suffering from anorexia and bulimia nervosa (O'Brien, Bruce, Camilleri, 1995). Features in the O'Brien study included daily, effortless regurgitation of undigested food starting within minutes of meals. Weight loss was substantial. Manometry confirmed the diagnosis in 33% but was otherwise normal in all subjects. Seventeen percent of female patients had a history of bulimia.

ETIOLOGY

The etiology of RD is unclear. Self-stimulation in those who are mentally or visually impaired, abnormal or altered interpersonal interactions with caretakers and the environment, and prolonged lack of stimulation in newborn intensive care units have been associated with the condition and are considered to be possible etiologic factors. An association with anorexia nervosa and bulimia nervosa has been described (Parry-Jones, 1994). Neurologically impaired infants and children are at high risk for both gastroesophageal reflux (GER) and RD, but the two conditions should be separated. GER can be diagnosed with the use of pH monitoring and treated, but psychosocial factors are often not pursued; more overlap than has been documented may exist between GER and RD.

Self-limited rumination as a reaction to situational stress (maladaptation to a new school situation or to being adopted) has been described in two mentally and developmentally normal 6-year-old children (Reis, 1994). The author describes these cases as "distinctly different" from that defined in the DSM. RD has been described in adolescents and adults of normal intelligence (O'Brien, Bruce, and Camilleri, 1995).

DIFFERENTIAL DIAGNOSIS

A barium swallow roentgenogram should demonstrate a hiatal hernia, esophageal atresia malformations, stricture, achalasia, or chalasia. An upper gastrointestinal series and small bowel follow-through may be necessary to diagnose other intestinal lesions, including duodenal ulcer. Upper gastrointestinal manometry reportedly confirms the diagnosis of RD. Manometry or endoscopy is seldom indicated when the clinical picture is typical of rumination. The 24-hour esophageal pH monitor is most helpful in ruling out GER. Esophagitis and severe dental caries are common manifestations of GER and self-induced vomiting associated with eating disorders and may occur in RD. Endoscopy and cultures for *Helicobacter pylori* may be indicated.

Rumination may be associated with Sandifer syndrome in which there is reflux, esophagitis, iron deficiency anemia, vomiting, and characteristic posturing of the head, neck, and shoulders. Premalignant changes of the epithelium (Barrett's epithelium or esophagus) may develop in patients with long-standing reflux esophagitis and may occur with chronic rumination.

MANAGEMENT

A comprehensive evaluation of family dynamics and the relationship between the primary caretaker and infant (or older patient) should be undertaken. Exploration for hidden underlying conflicts should be incorporated into counseling. Enhanced mothering, intense family therapy and counseling, and environmental manipulation are required if intervention is to succeed. Psychotherapy should be combined with behavioral modification. Behavioral treatment is especially indicated in the self-stimulating type of rumination most often encountered in developmentally disabled children and adolescents. Positive reinforcement for desired eating behaviors and adverse conditioning for rumination and undesirable behaviors should be implemented. Parents and family should be helped, through education and training, to use appropriate approaches to the child, to the child's feeding, and to changing the child's social and physical environment as indicated.

Caloric deprivation should be corrected. Recurrent bronchitis or pneumonia, reflex laryngospasm, bronchospasm, and asthma caused by repeated pulmonary aspiration of gastric fluid may, as with GER, complicate the condition. Medical treatment, similar to that appropriate for GER, may be indicated. In children not responding to intensive medical, psychiatric, and behavioral therapy, an antireflux surgical procedure (gastroesophageal fundoplication) may be considered. It may stop regurgitation, but it does not eliminate the underlying problem nor improve other associated symptoms.

PREVENTION

Prevention of psychogenic rumination requires identification of high-risk maternal-infant relationships and sources of stress on the infant-mother dyad and the family. Psychosocial factors that may be contributing to early feeding difficulties should be explored and addressed. In situations of extreme neglect or maternal deprivation, the infant should be removed and hospitalized or provided a nurturing caretaker. Sources of major stress should be explored when confronted with an older child or adolescent who is "spitting up" or holding saliva. The possibility of rumination in patients with anorexia or bulimia nervosa should be considered.

Developmentally disabled individuals and those with sensory deprivation (vision, hearing) or severe emotional problems should be considered at high risk for development of RD. With early signs of rumination, attempts should be made to identify and address any underlying psychopathology, and, when indicated, to work with the parents to increase stimulation of the child, modify rumination behaviors, and otherwise change existing circumstances and factors contributing to the problem.

REFERENCES

Abu-Arafeh I, Russell G: Cyclical vomiting syndrome in children: a population-based study. J Pediatr Gastroenterol Nutr 21:454–458, 1995.

American Psychiatric Association: Diagnostic and Statistical Manual of Mental Disorders, DSM-IV, 4th ed. Washington, DC, American Psychiatric Association, 1994, p. 544.

Andersen J, Lockhart J, Sugerman K, Weinberg W: Effective prophylactic therapy for cyclic vomiting syndrome in children using amitriptyline (Elavil) or cyproheptadine (Periactin). North American Society for Pediatric GI and Nutrition Annual Meeting (abstract), 1996.

Bell RM: Holy Anorexia. Chicago, University of Chicago Press, 1985.

Bruch H: Eating Disorders: Obesity, Anorexia Nervosa, and the Person Within. New York, Basic Books, 1973.

Brumberg JJ: Fasting Girls: The Emergence of Anorexia Nervosa as a Modern Disease. Cambridge, MA, Harvard University Press, 1988.

Bryant-Waugh R, Lask B: Eating disorders in children. J Child Psychol Psychiatr 36:191–202, 1995.

Comerci GD: Eating disorders: evolving, controvertible, and irresolute issues. Pediatr Ann 21:711–715, 1992.

Comerci GD: Eating disorders in the young: a new plague. In Green M (ed): The Psychosocial Aspects of the Family: The New Pediatrics. Lexington, MA, Lexington Books, 1985.

Comerci GD, Greydanus D: Eating disorders: anorexia nervosa and bulimia. In Hofmann A, Greydanus D (eds): Adolescent Medicine, 3rd ed. Norwalk, CT, Appleton & Lange, 1997.

Comerci GD, Kilbourne KA, Carroll AE: Eating disorders in the young: anorexia nervosa and bulimia, Part 2. Curr Probl Pediatr 15:26, 1985.

Cooper PJ, Charnock DJ, Taylor MJ: The prevalence of bulimia nervosa: a replication study. Br J Psychiatry 151:684, 1987.

Crisp AH, Palmer RL, Kalucy RS: How common is anorexia nervosa? A prevalence study. Br J Psychol 128:549–554, 1976.

Fisher M: Medical complications of anorexia and bulimia nervosa. State of the art reviews. Adolesc Med 3(3):487–502, 1992.

Fleisher DR, Matar M: The cyclic vomiting syndrome: a report of 71 cases and literature review. J Pediatr Gastroenterol Nutr 17(4):361–369, 1993.

Garfinkel PE, Garner DM: Anorexia nervosa: a multidimensional perspective. New York, Brunner/Mazel, 1982, p 103.

Garner DM, Olmsted MP, Polivy J: Development and validation of a multidimensional eating disorder inventory for anorexia nervosa and bulimia. Int J Eat Disorder 2:15, 1983.

Gillberg IC, Rastam M, Gillberg C: Anorexia nervosa 6 years after onset: Part I: personality disorders. Compr Psychiatr 36:61–69, 1995.

Halmi KA: Eating disorder research in the past decade. Ann N Y Acad Sci 78:67, 1996.

Hartman D: Anorexia nervosa—diagnosis, aetiology and treatment. Postgrad Med J 71:712, 1995.

Herzog DB, Beresin EV: Anorexia nervosa. In Textbook of Child and Adolescent Psychiatry, 2nd ed. Washington, DC, American Psychiatric Press, 1997, pp 543–562.

Jarry JL, Vaccarino FJ: Eating disorder and obsessive-compulsive disorder: neurochemical and phenomenological commonalities. J Psychiatr Neurosci 21:36, 1996.

Kasvikis YG, Tsakiris F, Marks IM, et al: Past history of anorexia nervosa in women with obsessive-compulsive disorders. Int J Eat Disorder 5:1069–1075, 1986.

Kreipe RE: Bone mineral density in adolescents. Pediatr Ann 24:308–315, 1995a.

Kreipe RE: Eating disorders among children and adolescents. Pediatr Rev 16:370–379, 1995b.

Kreipe RE, Harris JP: Myocardial impairment resulting from eating disorders. Pediatr Ann 21:760–768, 1992.

Maloney MJ, McGuire J, Daniels SR, et al: Dieting behavior and eating attitudes in children. Pediatrics 85:482, 1989.

Mitrany E: Atypical eating disorders. J Adolesc Health 13(3):400–443, 1992.

O'Brien MD, Bruce BK, Camilleri M: The rumination syndrome: clinical features rather than manometric diagnosis. Gastroenterology 108:1024–1029, 1995.

Palla B, Litt IF: Medical complications of eating disorders in adolescents. Pediatrics 81:613, 1988.

Parry-Jones B: Merycism or rumination disorder. A historical investigation and current assessment. Br J Psychiatry 165:303–314, 1994.

Patton GC: Mortality in eating disorders. Psychol Med 18(4):947, 1985.

Pfau BT, Li BUK, Murray RD, et al: Cyclic vomiting in children: a migraine equivalent? Gastroenterology 102:A23, 1992.

Pyle RL, Halvorson PA, Neuman PA, et al: The increasing prevalence of bulimia in freshman college students. Int J Eat Disorder 5(4):631, 1983.

Rastam M, Gillberg IC, Gillberg C: Anorexia nervosa 6 years after onset: Part II: comorbid psychiatric problems. Compr Psychiatry 36:70–76, 1995.

Reis S: Rumination in two developmentally normal children: case report and review of the literature. J Fam Pract 38(5):521–523, 1994.

Wonderlich S: Comorbidity of personality disorders and eating disorders: five year follow-up. Presented at North American Scientific Symposium on Eating Disorders in Adolescence, Seattle, WA, December 6, 1991.

Woodside DB: A review of anorexia nervosa and bulimia nervosa. Curr Probl Pediatr 25:67–89, 1995.

Yates A: Biologic considerations in the etiology of eating disorders. Pediatr Ann 21:739–744, 1992.

40 *Common Issues in Feeding*

Martin T. Stein

The feeding of infants and children by their caregivers is a primary focus of their interactions, which is affected by many factors including the cultural setting, parental experience, the child's developmental level, and temperament. Parents experience a variety of satisfactions and worries and frequently turn to their medical caregivers for help. Concerns about the content and amount of the food consumed are frequent and include issues such as rate of weight gain, spitting up, fussiness, food dislikes, and pica. Opportunities for anticipatory guidance and prevention of behavior problems are numerous.

Feeding: A Major Event

Feeding infants and young children is a behavioral event. Beyond the need for adequate nutrients to ensure physical growth, the process of feeding is important to the emotional and social development of the child. The sheer time spent feeding consumes an enormous part of an infant's life. Beyond the consumption of nutrients for growth, feeding represents the earliest opportunity for an infant to experience novel social interactions.

The interplay between the child, parent, and environment begins during fetal life and accelerates immediately after birth. A prolonged gestation in humans provides time for the development of an intense attachment to the fetus that prepares a mother for the nurturing behaviors needed after birth. When the nursing infant sucks and swallows, the infant visually locks into the mother's face, hears her voice, and feels her skin. Nursing infants exhibit behaviors associated with specific tastes from foods consumed by the mother (Mannella and Beauchamp, 1991). These sensory stimuli are experienced by the infant, who has a relatively mature neurologic system ready to interact with the immediate environment. The range of emotional responses experienced by the baby and the mother is broad. The feeding dyad is built on these reciprocal and contingent behaviors of an infant and mother.

An individual child's temperament, state regulation, physiologic variables, and behavioral organization contribute to the interactional process. The mother's or caretaker's unique characteristics also make an important contribution. The mother's psychological health, concepts of parenting, social support, and, in the newborn period, recovery after delivery are important variables. To encourage a pleasurable experience associated with feeding, the child-parent dyad must find a common ground to maintain a nurturing encounter.

Individual variation in both child and parent temperaments guides the feeding interaction. Early in a child's life, effective parents learn to respond to subtle feeding cues that reflect hunger, satiety, and the desire to feed slower or faster. Infants and children often develop predictable patterns of feeding behavior, and parents participate by developing good observation skills and reading the infant's cues accurately. Whereas many parents naturally learn the value of monitoring and responding to behavioral cues, others benefit from a supportive family member or health care professional who can guide the process (Satter, 1990).

Multiple events in early childhood ensure the development of a sense of "basic trust." The achievement of this psychological task requires predictable, pleasurable, and secure feelings as the child experiences other caregivers in the first few years of life. At around 3 months of age, the child learns to anticipate feeding routines and is more interested in the feeding activities of others. The enormous pleasure derived from sucking when fed by a responsive caregiver and the self-satisfaction that comes later with independent feeding fuel the development of basic trust.

The introduction of solid foods between 4 and 6 months of age is a nutritional and social landmark. Solid foods provide the infant with an opportunity to explore new textures, smells, colors, and tastes of foods. Other than the requirement for additional iron found in some solids, nutrients in breast milk alone are adequate for the first 12 months. Solids, however, promote development by encouraging the use of new motor skills, visual milestones, and social behaviors. At around 6 months of age, tongue-thrusting behavior decreases, head and trunk control allow the infant to sit upright, and the ability to reach for and grasp objects develops in association with hand-eye coordination skills. Steady sitting is associated with readiness for the use of a cup. A pincer grasp and effective hand-eye coordination are requirements for eating finger foods. The infant has more control over choice of food type and amount as he or she experiments and explores.

Similar to play in late infancy and among toddlers, feeding explorations are often accompanied by messy tables and messy kids. Self-discovery and mastery of individual tasks inevitably require a messy environment (Fig. 40–1). Parental response to the events modulates the child's experience—with exploration in general and with feeding specifically. Parents should be encouraged to respect the child's quest for autonomy and mastery over feeding. Parents can be advised that although new foods tend to be

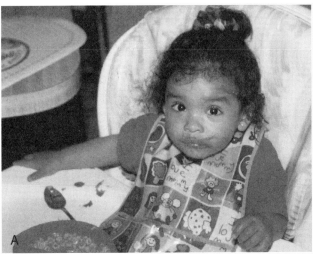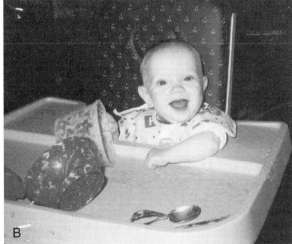

Figure 40–1. Typical toddler messiness.

rejected initially, preference for novel foods increases with repeated exposure (Sullivan and Birch, 1994). Clinicians should be sensitive to temperament differences that may guide a child's interest, tempo, and responses to new foods.

Feeding is central to the development of autonomy in the 2nd and 3rd years of life. Motor skills (to independently discover, prepare, and pick up food), language skills (to express desires for food now!), and psychological development (to convey needs through strong feelings, to be aggressive and egocentric) come together in the toddler to make feeding, at times, a dramatic family event. Independent feeding at this age can be viewed as one component of a child's journey toward self-regulation, self-determination (including sleeping, playing, verbal expression, and toilet training), and psychological separation. As with all these emerging skills, learning about feeding occurs at different rates, and setbacks (or regression) may occur following intercurrent events in the family (Hammer, 1992).

Parents are most responsive to guidance around nutritional concerns when they can be framed in the context of developmental skills (Dixon, 1992). This approach to anticipatory guidance (and feeding problems) encourages parents to respond to a child's cues and needs at a particular developmental age. As illustrated in Table 40–1, the most significant changes and challenges to feeding occur in the first 3 years when the ground rules for feeding change frequently with emerging neurodevelopmental milestones.

Feeding in the Context of Culture

Culture dominates feeding practices and styles (see Chapter 10). There are many examples in both developed and developing countries. Breast-feeding was universal until dairy and biochemical technologies produced infant formulas. That single innovation dramatically changed infant feeding. Among ancient hunter-gatherer societies, babies were fed frequent, small feedings while being carried constantly, meaning that babies were in continuous skin contact with their mothers and were fed at the slightest clue of hunger for most of human history. Children slept with parents and siblings in close proximity (co-sleeping), which allowed for frequent nighttime feeds. Currently, as many as 50% of African American young children co-sleep with their mothers (Lozoff, Wolf, and Davis, 1984). This same practice is found in Southeast Asian families and in other cultures.

Weaning is another feeding practice that varies significantly among cultures. In developing countries, weaning is delayed because breast-feeding remains the cheapest, most nutritious form of sustenance, serves as a form of birth control, and encourages survival of the child. Co-sleeping, traditionally discouraged in Western countries as a disincentive to mastering independence and self-regulation of sleep, has been shown recently to encourage prolonged breast-feeding (McKenna, Mosko, and Richard, 1997). In Western countries, early weaning from breast milk or formula to a cup has been viewed by many clinicians in the context of a toddler's quest for autonomy. If the breast or artificial nipple is an infantile symbol, the cup represents independence and encourages self-regulation. Yet there are no data that support a developmental advantage in children weaned at 12 months compared with those weaned at 24 months.

Clinicians should practice tolerance for the wide variety of early childhood feeding practices. Unless a particular practice is shown to affect adversely either the nutritional intake or the developmental progress of a child, culturally dependent feeding patterns should be encouraged, monitored for effects, and used by the clinician as a potential source of clinical insight.

A recent cultural change with an impact on feeding patterns in developed countries has been the trend for mothers of infants and toddlers to work outside the home. The increased use of day care has been associated with earlier weaning from breast to formula as well as a social change in the feeding environment. Young children in day care are fed by individuals other than parents or family, and by age 1 year, they experience feeding in groups. Neither developmental disadvantage nor clear advantages have been shown to come from these changes in feeding patterns.

Table 40–1 • Behavioral and Developmental Abilities Related to Feeding

Age	Behavioral/Developmental Abilities
Newborn–2 months	Primitive reflexes (rooting, sucking, swallowing) facilitate feeding and quickly become organized into a whole pattern of behavior; hunger cry initiates feeding interaction; minimal vocal, visual, or motor activity during feeding
2–4 months	More alert and interactive during feeding; explosive cough to protect self from aspiration; beginning ability to wait for food; associates mother's smell, voice, and cradling with feeding; hand-to-mouth behavior quiets infant, increases interest in mouthing activities
4–6 months	Readiness for solids; excellent head and trunk control; reaching for objects; raking grasp; increased hand-to-mouth facility; loss of extrusion reflex of the tongue; may purposefully spit out food as part of food exploration; adaptation to introduction to solids may be affected by infant's temperament
6–8 months	Sits alone with a steady head during sitting feedings; chewing mechanism developed; holds bottle; vocal eagerness during meal preparation; much more motor activity during feeding
8–10 months	Finger food readiness; thumb-forefinger grasp (i.e., inferior pincer); grasps spoon but cannot use it effectively; feeds self crackers and so on; enjoys new textures, tastes; emerging independence
10–12 months	Increasing determination to feed self; neat pincer grasp; drops food off highchair onto floor to see where it goes; holds cup but frequently spills it; more verbal and motor behavior during feeding
12–15 months	Demands to feed self without help; decreased appetite and nutritional requirements; improved cup use (both hands); uses spoon, fills poorly, turns at mouth; can use spoon as extension of hand; messy play
15–18 months	Eats rapidly, short feeding sessions; wants to be motorically active (too busy to eat); fairly good use of spoon and cup; enhanced ability to wait for food; plays with/throws food to elicit response from parent
18–24 months	Feeds self, using combination of utensils and fingers; verbalizes "eat, all gone"; asks for food; negativism emerges, says no when really wanting offered food; wants control of feeding situation
2–3 years	Uses fork; ritualistic, repetitive at mealtimes; food jags, all one food at a time; dawdles; likes to help set/clear table; may begin to help self to refrigerator contents
3–4 years	Spills little; uses utensils well; washes hands with minimal help; likes food preparation; reasonable table manners when eating out
4–5 years	Serves self; choosy about food; resists some textures; begins to request foods seen on television ads (especially junk food); makes menu suggestions; likes to assist in washing dishes; helps in food preparation
5–6 years	Uses knife; assists in preparing and packing own box lunch; can be responsible for setting/clearing table; aids younger siblings' request for food or drink
6–8 years	Does dishes independently and willingly; increases pressure to buy junk food; interested in, often critical of, and attempts to negotiate about daily menu; manages money for school meal ticket
8–10 years	Enjoys planning and preparing simple family meals; wants supplemental spending money to buy snacks when away from home; more reticent to trying new foods; resists kitchen chores

Adapted from Dixon S, Stein M (eds): Encounters With Children: Pediatric Behavior and Development, 2nd ed. St. Louis: Mosby-Year Book, 1992.

Opportunities for Preventing Feeding Problems

Primary prevention through anticipatory guidance can limit or eliminate many common feeding problems. Education about early infant feeding can begin at the prenatal visit and newborn examination. Plans for feeding should be explored, and breast-feeding should be encouraged by emphasizing nutritional, immunologic, and psychological benefits. Realistic expectation for nursing and instructions to ensure proper latching on and effective sucking by the infant should be reviewed before mother and infant are discharged home. A follow-up office visit within 1 week should be encouraged for first-time nursing mothers. Lactation counseling by the baby's clinician or another person assists many mothers and prevents early discontinuation of breast-feeding (Powers and Slusser, 1997).

Clinicians can assist parents to prepare for each stage in feeding by reviewing anticipated milestones that change a feeding pattern (see Table 40–1). Temperament variations and cultural differences should be evaluated and incorporated into recommendations.

When talking directly to school-aged children and adolescents, nutritional counselors should take into consideration cognitive stages of development in terms of the child's ability to understand cause and effect (concrete operations) and to hypothesize an outcome (formal operations) (see Chapters 5 and 6).

Parental Concerns About Feeding

"My child is not gaining enough weight."

Standard growth measurements and monitoring practices during health supervision visits allow tracking of growth on height and weight charts. When a concern about growth is expressed by the parent of a child who is growing at an expected rate, the visual image of growth illustrated by a chart is often therapeutic. It is also useful to ask the parent to describe a meal in terms of the child's behavior and the immediate environment. Curious and active children may show so much interest in the surrounding environment during feeding that they may only appear to be undereating. Parental expectations may be a clue to developmentally inappropriate goals. Concerns about too-frequent meals, picky eating patterns, spitting up, and food preferences or aversions may provide an opening to discuss behaviors that impact on broader aspects of the child's development (Birch and Martin, 1982).

Failure to thrive (FTT), defined as weight loss that crosses at least two major percentile lines on a standard growth chart or weight lower than the 5th percentile, is discussed elsewhere (see Chapter 41). Milder forms of weight loss secondary to *underfeeding* are frequent in the first 3 years of life. A pediatric approach to a mild form of FTT requires a comprehensive medical and psychosocial evaluation. Caution should be taken in assuming that a behavioral or interactional problem is the cause for underfeeding. A common form of mild FTT can be seen in infants and toddlers who exhibit a transient but dramatic weight loss following a series of common intercurrent infections. These frequent febrile illnesses may be associated with irritability, painful oral lesions, sore bottoms, and anorexia. Even though the infant or toddler may recover quickly from the illness, feeding patterns may not rebound as efficiently, especially when a parent perceives the child as vulnerable or fragile. A parent at risk for depression, substance abuse, or other significant psychosocial stress may not adapt effectively to the child's changing feeding behaviors. Attentive observations of parent-child interactions in the office, a 2-day nutritional diary, and a clear explanation of the effect of illness on appetite and temporary weight loss begin the evaluation and treatment process.

"My baby is spitting up all the time."

Spitting up (or regurgitation) is common during infancy. In the absence of projectile vomiting and poor weight gain, it usually is a result of *gastroesophageal reflux* (GER). When infants regurgitate with every feeding, a parent is usually concerned about a serious disease. In a thriving infant with a normal physical examination, GER is the likely cause. A simple diagram that illustrates the course of a meal from the mouth to the stomach allows the clinician to illustrate the anatomy and function of the gastroesophageal sphincter and its predictable maturation during infancy. Smaller, more frequent feeds, holding the infant's head well above his or her abdomen during feeding, and (in formula-fed babies) thickening the milk with rice cereal diminishes spitting up in most infants. Cisapride, a prokinetic drug that promotes gastric emptying, is prescribed occasionally, but only in the most severe case. GER is an example of a common developmental problem with a physiologic cause that may be associated with significant parental concerns and anxiety. This is especially true when more severe reflux causes peptic esophagitis, "heartburn," and dramatic arching of the trunk and neck (Sandifer syndrome).

A related problem is the excessive air swallowed (*aerophagia*) by some infants during feeding. Fussiness, abdominal distention, and regurgitation may result from an overly distended stomach. Attention to the infant's latching on to the nipple during nursing, proper holding, feeding in a calm environment, and adequate burping are beneficial. When regurgitation or aerophagia does not respond to these techniques or when the feeding interaction is chaotic and stressful, an examination of maternal-child interactions and stresses in the family is usually helpful.

Regurgitation may also be a sign of *overfeeding*. At other times, the only clinical clue may be excessive weight gain. Caution in infancy is recommended because many breast-fed infants are chubby in the 1st year. Bottle-fed infants who gain more than 1 ounce each day or who consume greater than 35 ounces of formula each day may be overfeeding. In early childhood, overfeeding is usually responsive to education of parents about appropriate weight gain and alternative ways to comfort and soothe. A similar approach is appropriate for older children after an evaluation of family mealtime behaviors, food quantities and types available to the child, and the child's functional psychosocial status (see Chapter 38).

"My baby is so fussy. The formula isn't satisfying him."

Some parents may interpret prolonged periods of fussiness in a healthy infant as an expression of hunger. Even though this may be true in some infants, episodic fussiness in early infancy is more commonly a reflection of a child's inborn temperament (see Chapter 37). Frequent feeding that may lead to excessive weight gain is not in the best interest of the child.

"I know she's growing; you've shown me her growth chart. But she only eats a few preferred foods and refuses most of the foods we serve. It's very frustrating."

The time and emotional energy spent feeding an infant during the 1st year of life changes dramatically when toddlers and preschool children make choices about content, amount, and timing of meals. For some parents, it is a difficult transition. In other families, mealtime is so central to family life that performance expectations are set high. Most parents find reassurance in a few important facts. First, when offered nutritional foods, without sweets, and an appropriate level of fat content, children select a balanced diet over a period of a few weeks (Pilner and Pelchat, 1986; Story and Brown, 1987). Second, growth rates for height and weight are expected to decrease after 1 year of age. Many children normally develop a leaner body at this time as activity level and energy output increase. Third, no parent has ever won "a battle" over food intake or preferences. By encouraging choice in the diet, parents promote autonomy, mastery, and self-esteem. Keeping healthy foods in the home for meals and snack time, limiting junk food for special occasions, and reviewing food choices among adults in the home promote adequate nutrition habits.

Less common than food fussiness are *food phobias*, in which a child experiences a severe emotional anxiety or a tantrum related to a particular food. Avoidance of the food that elicits the phobic response is usually sufficient unless the phobia is associated with other psychological problems. For most children without a suspicion of disease after a complete medical history and physical examination, a parent's concern about a picky eating pattern or limited food preferences is a behavioral problem that should focus on developmental expectations and parent-child interactions. It should be seen as an opportunity for a behavioral intervention through education.

Parents can be advised not to use food as a reward for behavior and not to reward a child for finishing a meal (Finney, 1986). Most children respond when they see other children eating foods they have avoided (Davis, 1938). Meals including a variety of foods, served in a family setting, without television or video watching and without forcing, promote healthy eating habits.

"My child will always choose junk foods over good foods."

Food preference is a learned behavior. The preferences of children (and adults) reflect their exposure to foods at mealtime and snack time and their exposure to food advertising. To prevent preferences for foods with excessive sugar and fat content, early counseling of parents about nutrition is appropriate in the 1st year of life and periodically after that during health supervision visits (American Academy of Pediatrics, 1997). Office wall posters and literature for parents may be informative. When parents watch television with their children or see an advertisement for junk food in a magazine or on a billboard, they can be advised to comment and engage their child in a conversation about appropriate nutrition and health. Role modeling of parental snacking habits at home—especially eating high-fat, sweet, or salty foods while watching television—should be reviewed.

When junk food intake is frequent and excessive, it may be helpful to review the parents' goals for nutrition and patterns of mealtime behaviors and snacking at home and away from home. Eliminating junk foods in the home is a good start. Encouraging fruit and vegetable sticks for snacks is helpful. For older children, a reward program of self-directed healthy eating can be initiated. Realistic counseling goals inform parents that they can control the availability of food in the home and give their child appropriate nutrition information. Eating behaviors outside the home may be influenced, but not entirely controlled, by parental guidance.

Pica is seen in children who frequently ingest non-food substances. It is found in all children in the first 2 years as a reflection of normative hand-to-mouth exploratory behavior. When pica occurs persistently, beyond age 2 years, or involves dangerous substances, it is a medical and behavioral problem. Children with mental retardation, significant psychological disorders, autism, and sensory impairment may exhibit pica extensively. Children with insufficient emotional or intellectual stimulation ingest nonfood substances as well. This practice may be harmful when it involves lead in peeling paint, dirt, or other toxic substances.

Alternative Diets—Nutritional and Behavioral Considerations

For a variety of reasons, some parents and older children choose to consume foods in a pattern outside the cultural mainstream. These alternative diets are embraced by a subset of the population, either temporarily or long term. Religious, ethical, and cultural contexts often guide the choice for these diets. Other parents and older children may sublimate a desire to gain control over their lives through a commitment to an alternative nutrition system. Concern for environmental pollution in the food chain or water supply initiates the decision for others. Even though most of the diets are not harmful, pediatric clinicians should be aware that specific nutrient deficiencies can occur with some alternative diets. A lacto-ovo vegetarian diet (which includes dairy and egg consumption) may be iron deficient. Vegans (no animal products at all) benefit from iron and vitamin B_{12} supplements. Megavitamin diets may cause vitamin D toxicity, decrease vitamin B_{12} absorption (ascorbic acid excess), and decrease breast milk production (pyridoxine excess). A macrobiotic diet may be deficient in calories, protein, and some minerals and vitamins (Forbes, 1980).

Food fads are common beginning at the age of puberty. The decision to break away from family tradition and begin some form of a vegetarian diet is linked closely with an age-appropriate quest for independence. Pediatricians can support the adolescent at the time of this decision, as well as reassure parents, by reviewing both the benefits and the potential nutritional deficiencies in the diet. The most frequent choice, a lacto-ovo vegetarian diet, is healthful and without risk except for the need for a supplemental iron source. A pure vegetarian diet (vegan) requires more nutritional knowledge to ensure adequate protein and caloric intake for the growing body. A diet diary for a few days may be useful when there is concern about excessive restrictiveness of essential nutrients. Self-imposed limits on caloric intake may be an early sign of anorexia nervosa (see Chapter 39).

REFERENCES

American Academy of Pediatrics: Guidelines for Health Supervision Visits, III. Elk Grove Village, IL, American Academy of Pediatrics, 1997.
Birch LL, Martin DW: I don't like it; I never tried it: efforts of exposure on two-year-old children's food preferences. Appetite 3:353, 1982.
Davis CM: Self-selection of diet experiment: its significance for feeding in the home. Ohio State Med J 34:862, 1938.
Dixon SD: Nine to ten months: active exploration in a safe environment. *In* Dixon SD, Stein MT (eds): Encounters With Children: Pediatric Behavior and Development, 2nd ed. St. Louis, Mosby-Year Book, 1992.
Finney JW: Preventing common feeding problems in infants and young children. Pediatr Clin North Am 33:775–788, 1986.
Forbes GB: Food fads: safe feeding of children. Pediatr Rev 1:207, 1980.
Hammer LD: The development of eating behavior in childhood. Pediatr Clin North Am 39:379–394, 1992.
Lozoff B, Wolf AW, Davis NS: Co-sleeping in urban families with young children in the United States. Pediatrics 74:171–182, 1984.
Mannella JA, Beauchamp GK: Maternal diet alters the sensory qualities of human milk and nursling's behavior. Pediatrics 88:737–744, 1991.
McKenna J, Mosko S, Richard C: Bed sharing promotes breastfeeding. Pediatrics 100:214–219, 1997.
Pilner P, Pelchat ML: Similarities in food preferences between children and their siblings and parents. Appetite 7:333, 1986.
Powers NG, Slusser W: Breastfeeding update 2: clinical lactation management. Pediatr Rev 18:147–161, 1997.
Satter EM: The feeding relationship: problems and interventions. J Pediatr 117:S181–S189, 1990.
Story M, Brown JE: Do young children instinctively know what to eat? The studies of Clara Davis revisited. N Engl J Med 316:103, 1987.
Sullivan SA, Birch LL: Infant dietary experience and acceptance of solid foods. Pediatrics 93:271–277, 1994.

41 Failure to Thrive

Patrick H. Casey

 Young children sometimes fail to grow at the expected rate for reasons other than inadequate diet and physical disease. Various factors in the child, parents, and environment influence the mother-child interaction in ways that result in insufficient provision of nutrition. The differing clinical presentations require a comprehensive diagnostic evaluation including growth, physical status, development, behavior, the psychosocial setting, and the parent-child interaction. Management calls for attention to the nutritional state and to all the factors that contributed to the problem. The diverse outcomes depend on the gravity of the precipitating factors and the effectiveness of the intervention.

Failure to thrive (FTT) is a descriptive term for a condition in infants and toddlers who do not grow at the expected rate for children of that age and gender. This clinical problem, which usually comes first to the attention of primary care pediatricians and family physicians, is a diagnostic and therapeutic challenge because of the broad array of medical and environmental causes. The current incidence of this condition is difficult to ascertain. Although population-based data are not available for the United States, recent community population-based studies in England and Israel found a prevalence of 3% to 4% in the 1st year of life (Skuse et al, 1994). FTT occurs frequently, with an estimated 10% prevalence in rural and urban outpatient settings (Altemeier et al, 1985; Mitchell, Gorrel, and Greenberg, 1980). Certain clinical populations, for example, low–birth weight preterm infants, have a higher incidence, as much as 21% (Kelleher et al, 1993). Whereas older publications suggest that FTT accounted for 3% to 5% of admissions to academic hospitals (Berwick, 1980), a recent publication documented that 34.9% of hospitalized children younger than age 2 years demonstrated some degree of malnutrition (Hendriks et al, 1995).

Definition

The term *failure to thrive* is generally used to describe a condition in infants or toddlers whose weight is abnormally 2 standard deviations less than the mean (i.e., less than the 5th percentile) for gestation-corrected age and sex or whose weight crosses two major percentiles downward on a standardized growth grid. Height, head circumference, and developmental skills can also be affected, depending on severity, duration, age of onset, and cause of the clinical condition.

All children who fit these criteria, whether because of organic or nonorganic causes, are considered to have FTT. The term *abnormal* in the foregoing definition has two implications. Children who are genetically short because they have small parents are often *normal*, although they are less than 2 standard deviations from the average

for gender and age. Also, infants whose growth is retarded at birth may never rebound to normal for population. The definition suggests the importance of correcting for the degree of prematurity when plotting on a growth grid. This procedure should be followed at least to 18 months of chronologic age for most infants born prematurely and probably longer for extremely low–birth weight infants. Finally this definition of FTT suggests that the *rate,* or velocity, of growth of the child is not adequate. Reference to percentile lines on the growth grid (90%, 75%, 50%, 25%, 10%, and 5%) is suggested to monitor rate of growth, because there are no objective data and no unanimous opinion regarding how long a growth concern should exist before a child meets criteria for FTT. An overweight infant might cross percentile lines as a normal growth pattern during a process of trimming weight.

In summary, FTT implies an abnormal velocity of weight growth that is disproportionate to height growth, taking into account genetic growth potential and appropriateness of size and degree of prematurity at birth. Figure 41–1 displays a typical pattern of growth in an infant with FTT, compared with the growth pattern of a premature infant and an infant with an endocrinopathy.

Etiology

Inadequate nutrition has come to be recognized as the central cause of FTT (Wright, Ashenbury, and Whitaker, 1994). All children with FTT suffer the biological insult of calorie deprivation, because inadequate calories are delivered or more than normal calories are required. Whether or not a biological disease is present, most children with FTT demonstrate catch-up growth when adequate calories are provided (Bell and Woolston, 1985; Bithoney et al, 1989). Many biochemical, endocrinologic, immunologic, and neurobehavioral consequences of malnutrition have an impact on the development, course, and prognosis of FTT (Bithoney and Dubowitz, 1985).

CLINICAL CATEGORIES

Pediatricians have historically dichotomized the etiology of FTT into organic or nonorganic causes. Organic FTT

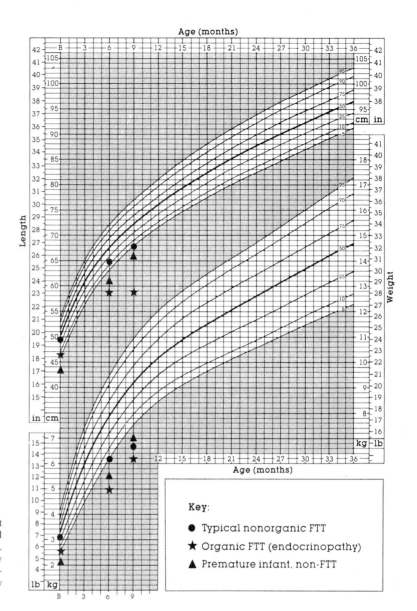

Figure 41–1. Failure to thrive versus premature infant growth curves. (Adapted from Hamill PVV, et al: Physical growth: National Center for Health Statistics percentiles. Copyright Am J Clin Nutr 30:607, 1979, American Society for Clinical Nutrition. Data from the Fels Research Institute. Wright State University School of Medicine. Yellow Springs, Ohio.)

includes any biomedical condition that is severe enough to result independently in the growth problem. Disease in any organ system can cause FTT. Pediatricians typically attribute the child's FTT to nonorganic causes when problems in the child's environment are judged to be the primary cause of FTT, in the presence or absence of medical disease. A third category of mixed-cause FTT has been described for children whose FTT results from a combination of organic and environmental causes (Homer and Ludwig, 1981). Most children with FTT suffer from nonorganic FTT (Berwick, 1980). No more than 30% of children with FTT suffer from organic causes alone. Of 131 children seen in a referral clinic, 17% had organic disease only, 45% had nonorganic FTT, 35% had a mixed cause, and 3% had FTT of unknown cause (Casey, Wortham, and Nelson, 1984). These percentages are likely to vary depending on how a sample is identified. Compared to children in a community setting, children diagnosed and treated in a clinical or hospital sample are more likely to have physical or psychological-emotional pathology.

The exclusionary diagnostic approach presents several problems. The symptoms of the child with FTT at presentation, such as persistent vomiting or diarrhea, are often not clearly caused by either organic or nonorganic problems, and concerns persist regarding the cause of the FTT. In addition, few features of the family other than overt parental poverty or emotional instability are used to make a positive diagnosis of nonorganic FTT. Although significant weight gain during a hospital stay is often the most positive clinical feature used to diagnose nonorganic FTT, this approach is subject to error. Some children with nonorganic FTT require weeks to gain weight. Likewise some children with growth problems resulting from physical disease can demonstrate rapid growth when hospitalized (Bell and Woolston, 1985). Even the "mixed cause" terminology is problematic, because it suggests only a "blending" of biomedical and environmental psychosocial causes.

Psychiatrists, on the other hand, have developed specific diagnoses in the fourth edition of the *Diagnostic and Statistical Manual of Mental Disorders* (*DSM-IV*) that may be used in children with FTT. *DSM-IV* criteria for the diagnosis of feeding disorder of infancy or early childhood include (1) feeding disturbance manifested by persistent failure to eat adequately with significant failure to gain weight or significant weight loss over at least 1 month, (2) manifestations that are *not* due to associated gastrointestinal or other medical conditions, (3) manifestations that are *not* better accounted for by another mental disorder or lack of food, and (4) onset before 6 years of age. This diagnosis would be given to many children for whom pediatricians would consider nonorganic FTT, but the feeding disorder diagnosis is rarely used by pediatricians. FTT was one of the defining features of another diagnosis, *reactive attachment disorder,* in the 1980 third edition of the *Diagnostic and Statistical Manual of Mental Disorders* (*DSM-III*). This disorder of attachment, as currently described in *DSM-IV,* results in developmentally inappropriate social relatedness and has its onset during preschool years; it results from grossly pathologic caregiving that fails to meet the children's emotional or physical needs. This diagnosis may be associated with FTT in some cases, but in *DSM-IV,* FTT is no longer described as a defining feature of reactive attachment disorder (Richters and Volkmar, 1994).

INTERACTIONAL MODEL

The term *maternal deprivation* was used by many clinicians almost interchangeably with FTT decades ago, but research and experience have subsequently demonstrated that overt neglect of the infant is infrequently associated with FTT, and the use of that term is not appropriate. Clinicians and theoreticians are increasingly using an interactional-transactional model of the causation of FTT, except in those infants with overt organic or nonorganic causes (Bithoney and Dubowitz, 1985; Casey, 1989; Frank and Zeisel, 1988).

The model in Figure 41–2 conceptualizes interaction at several levels. The central cause of FTT is viewed as a breakdown in the parent-infant interaction (the mother is usually the involved parent). The parent does not "read" or respond to the infant appropriately, and the infant has difficulty in eliciting attention and appropriate care from the parent. This bidirectional problem ultimately results in nutritional and nurturing deficiencies that then result in FTT. Certain extreme physical, emotional, or social problems in the parent cause unidirectional effects that would result in FTT in any child. This parent-to-child effect has dominated the literature on nonorganic FTT. More commonly, minor or subtle abnormalities in physical, temperamental, or emotional aspects of the parent, or all of these factors, combine with real or perceived similar abnormalities in the infant to result in interactional FTT. For example, infants who are difficult to care for, such as in feeding or soothing, place stress on the parent-infant interaction. Infants who are unpredictable and have difficulty signaling their needs can also impede a mutually rewarding relationship. Such problems occur more commonly in premature infants, infants born small for gestational age, drug-exposed infants, children with difficult or placid, easy temperaments, and children with neurologic dysfunction. Undernutrition in infants has an independent detrimental effect on parent-infant interaction as early as the first 6 months of life (Lozoff, 1989).

Finally the interaction between the parent-child pair is viewed in the context of their microenvironment and macroenvironment. Physical aspects of the home provide the milieu in which the parent-infant interaction occurs. The number of people present in the home, the adequacy of the physical house, the organization of the home, and the availability of support all affect parent-infant interaction and the parent's ability to meet the infant's needs. Strengths (supports) and weaknesses (stressors) in the home, marital relationship, extended family, neighborhood, and workplace enhance or impede the quality of parent-child interaction and can have a direct impact on the development of FTT (Casey, 1989).

This interactional model of FTT implies a multifacto-

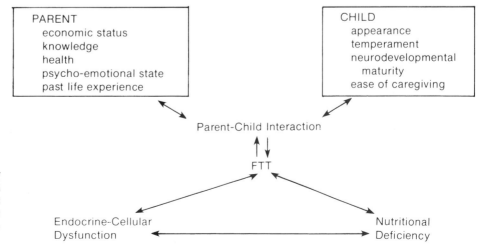

HOME AND SOCIETAL ENVIRONMENT

Figure 41–2. Interactional model of failure to thrive. (From Casey PH: The family system and failure to thrive. *In* Ramsey CN [ed]: Family Systems in Medicine. New York, Guilford Press, 1989, p 348.)

rial causation mediated by the maladapted parent-infant interaction. The maladapted interaction results in nutritional and, ultimately, endocrine-cellular abnormalities, which, in turn, lead to FTT. This clinical model supersedes the organic versus nonorganic diagnostic dichotomy.

Clinical Presentations

NEURODEVELOPMENTAL

Differentiating the age of onset, severity, and duration of FTT is clinically important from a neurodevelopmental perspective. Detrimental effects of undernutrition on brain size, structure, and function are most likely to occur during rapid brain growth from midgestation to the toddler years, particularly in the 1st year of life. Neuronal and glial cell differentiation and growth, myelination, formation of synapses, dendritic arborization, and cellular metabolism can all be affected by undernutrition (Frank and Zeisel, 1988). Thus an infant in whom FTT develops in the 1st year of life, particularly if it is of significant duration and degree, is more likely to suffer irreversible neuropathophysiologic effects, with a subsequent negative impact on developmental and behavioral course, than is a child who is older with a milder degree of FTT (Skuse et al, 1994).

SOCIOEMOTIONAL

Other researchers have described subtypes of FTT from a socioemotional developmental perspective. This perspective generally divides the first 8 months of life into *neurophysiologic stabilization* in the first 3 months and the subsequent development of the *attachment relationship* based on the quality of mother-child interaction in the following 5 months. Infants older than 8 months of age enter a phase referred to as *separation and individuation*. In this phase, FTT often results when control of the feeding process, with resultant refusal of food, becomes a focus of a more global struggle for independence from the parent (Chatoor et al, 1984). This problem often relates to the introduction of solid foods and the process of becoming an independent eater. Clinical manifestations of FTT in this situation usually occur in the 2nd year of life and are associated with mealtime behavioral problems (e.g., spitting, throwing), multiple food dislikes, and atypical eating habits (e.g., nibbling all day rather than eating at structured mealtimes).

There are thus two "typical" clinical presentations of children with FTT. The first involves infants who are first seen with FTT at younger than 8 to 10 months of age. Such infants are more likely to have a presenting symptom such as vomiting or diarrhea and are more likely to have an organic cause for their FTT such as gastroesophageal reflux or oral-motor feeding problem. They are more likely to be developmentally delayed. Most of these infants, however, feed well and grow rapidly in a controlled environment, such as a hospital. Conversely, parents of infants older than 10 to 12 months of age often complain that they "have no appetite" or they "just will not eat." Such children often never learned to eat a normal range of foods at typical mealtimes and often nibble at inappropriate foods

or drinks throughout the day. Most of these infants are normal in developmental status but, as already suggested, have a range of behavioral problems that can come into focus at mealtime.

Diagnostic Evaluation

The diagnostic approach to a child with FTT requires a thoughtful medical, developmental-behavioral, nutritional, and social evaluation in order to understand etiology, develop a treatment plan, and understand prognosis. Data collection in all of these areas should occur simultaneously, if possible, in order to develop a comprehensive interactional-transactional perspective based on positive findings, rather than undertaking a medical exclusionary diagnostic approach. Almost all of the initial data can be collected in the pediatrician's office (Table 41–1).

MEDICAL EVALUATION

Growth Status

First the presence of FTT is documented by obtaining accurate measurements of height, weight, and head circumference. Using standard collection techniques is critical. Measurements of midarm circumference and triceps skinfold thickness are not necessary for clinical purposes, unless weight is confounded by edema of protein malnutrition. Growth charts developed by the National Center for Health Statistics are recommended for reference, because they include the most recent standard growth data from a representative national sample of children. Growth grids for use with low–birth weight preterm children based on a longitudinal sample are available to provide reference data for such children younger than 3 years of age (Casey et al, 1991). The infant's height, weight, and head circumference are plotted to determine the percentile for age (corrected for gestational age if necessary) and the percentile for weight for height. Weight for age less than the 5th percentile suggests undernutrition. A weight to height ratio that plots at less than the 5th percentile, even in a short child, suggests acute recent malnutrition. Crossing percentile lines on the growth grid suggests a growth velocity problem. Velocity growth curves are available for use in as-

Table 41–1 • Diagnostic Evaluation

Growth assessment: confirm the diagnosis with height and weight—present and past

History—predisposing factors?

Physical examination—significant findings other than malnutrition?

Developmental-behavioral assessment—delayed development? behavioral abnormality?

Laboratory—variable requirements, stepwise approach

Nutritional and feeding evaluation—content and mealtime structure, technique of feeding; nutritionist can be helpful

Social history—liabilities and assets; social worker can be helpful

Parent-child interaction—especially in feeding; social worker can be helpful

Psychiatric evaluation—when caregivers' emotional problems (e.g., depression) negatively affect parent-child interaction or their ability to meet child's needs

sessing weight and length gain over time at various ages for infants younger than 2 years of age (Guo et al, 1991).

The weight percentile usually decreases before a change in the length or head circumference percentile in a child with FTT. The length and ultimately head circumference percentiles also decrease if the problem is sufficiently severe and chronic. Some term infants with weight, length, or head circumference less than normal at birth (small for gestational age) demonstrate a stable rate of growth, with normal weight for length, but remain at less than the 5th percentile for age. Often these children have had a problem in utero that precludes normal growth; these children do not have FTT. On occasion a child demonstrates a normal weight to height ratio but a progressive deterioration of length percentile. This situation suggests an endocrinopathy or constitutional short stature. Some children whose weight and height percentiles at birth are greater than their ultimate growth potential cross growth curve percentiles downward between the ages of 6 and 24 months as a normal growth pattern. It is thus critical to take into account the heights of both parents in assessing normal growth expectations.

History

The medical history and physical examination should identify any condition or cluster of symptoms that negatively affect the infant's growth potential (such as in utero growth retardation), increase the child's basic caloric requirement (such as chronic infection), decrease the availability or utilization of calories (such as malabsorption), negatively affect the child's ability or willingness to feed (such as gastroesophageal reflux [Rudolph, 1994]), or negatively influence the parents' ability to meet nutritional needs. The medical history begins with the description of the development of the growth problem. How do the parents perceive the problem and its cause, and if both parents are present, how do they relate in describing this problem? How old was the infant at the beginning of the problem and what medical conditions and symptoms were present? Were problematic feeding or behavioral styles present? A complete review of systems elicits information about recurring symptoms that might have been omitted from the general history. Organic problems that most likely result in FTT are recurring diarrhea and vomiting, neurologic disease (particularly early cerebral palsy), and chronic upper airway disease (otitis media) and obstruction (Bithoney and Newberger, 1987; Fleisher, 1994; Sills, 1978).

A thorough past medical history is established. Some past conditions (e.g., gastroesophageal reflux) may result in ongoing food aversion, even if the condition is not active. Even children with nonorganic FTT tend to have been smaller at birth and to have had more illness than children who grow normally (Altemeir et al, 1985). Birth weight, gestational age, and complications in the prenatal, perinatal, and postnatal periods are noted. In utero toxin exposure (e.g., alcohol, tobacco, cocaine) and infection (e.g., acquired immunodeficiency syndrome, cytomegalovirus infection) are increasingly common causes of FTT. Such conditions also increase the burden of caring for the infant, which stresses the parents' ability to provide. For example, some premature infants or infants who have been exposed to toxins can be hyperirritable and demonstrate

deficient responses to visual, auditory, or tactile stimuli. Their unpredictable behavior, difficulty in signaling needs, and problems in coordinating sucking and swallowing interfere with parent-child interaction and the feeding event.

The child's developmental milestones and progress are substantiated. Children with FTT commonly demonstrate developmental delays and subtle deviations from normal behavior (Powell, Low, and Speers, 1987). A description of the child's temperament and eating ability and the presence of problems such as "colic" are solicited. Normal children might have temperamental traits that stress parents beyond their ability to cope (Bithoney and Newberger, 1987). They might feed with difficulty, be poorly able to modulate their moods, whine or show other evidence of irritability, and be excessively clinging. In contrast, some children described as "good" babies might actually be withdrawn, depressed, or unable to place normal demands on their environment.

Finally a family history is obtained to detect inherited problems such as cystic fibrosis, sickle cell disease, diabetes mellitus, or other endocrine, metabolic, neurologic, or gastrointestinal diseases that can affect ultimate growth. The physical size of the parents, siblings, uncles, aunts, and grandparents assists in predicting growth prognosis.

Physical Examination

Careful evaluation for minor dysmorphic features can suggest syndromes associated with short stature such as fetal alcohol syndrome or Russell-Silver syndrome. Head size; configuration of eyes, ears, and mouth; proportion of trunk to extremities; and abnormalities of digits and extremities require particular attention. Specific organ diseases are sought, particularly those that can be asymptomatic, such as chronic serous otitis media, congenital heart disease, or abdominal masses. A neurologic examination evaluates the child for cranial nerve or motor tract dysfunction, particularly abnormalities of muscle tone and peripheral reflexes. Cranial nerve dysfunction associated with difficulty in swallowing can result in FTT. Hypertonicity and hyperreflexia, sometimes prematurely diagnosed as cerebral palsy, can actually result from progressive undernutrition in infancy. Finally the child is evaluated for evidence of abuse, such as unexplained burns or skin lesions, fractures, or retinal hemorrhages (Fig. 41–3).

DEVELOPMENTAL AND BEHAVIORAL ASSESSMENT

The Denver Developmental Screening Test continues to be the best standardized and most easily administered and interpreted instrument for screening developmental status in a pediatric office (see Chapter 68). Referral to a pediatric psychologist to document developmental status with a more comprehensive standardized technique, such as the Bayley Scale of Infant Development, may be useful. Assessment of oral-motor function, including lip and tongue coordination and swallowing, can yield relevant data, particularly in infants (Ramsey, Gisel, and Boutry, 1993). An array of atypical behaviors seen in infants with nonorganic FTT has been described, including general inactivity, flexed hips and knees, expressionless face, gaze aversion, and lack of

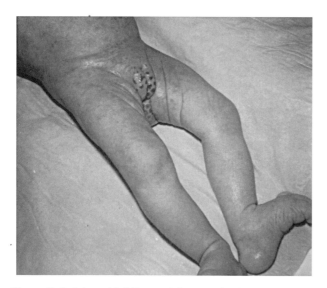

Figure 41–3. Infant with failure to thrive assuming hypertonic posture. (Courtesy of Drs. S. Ludwig and A. Rostain, The Children's Hospital of Philadelphia, Philadelphia, PA.)

motor activity in response to stimulus. These behaviors differentiate children with FTT from children without FTT (Powell, Low, and Speers, 1987). Finally behavior at mealtime and general behavioral style is of particular importance to the assessment of the child with the onset of FTT in the 2nd year of life. Observation of behavior at mealtimes to assess problems such as food refusal, spitting, throwing, and oral retention may be useful in this diagnosis.

LABORATORY ANALYSIS

The results of the history and physical examination guide the laboratory evaluation. When no significant symptoms or physical findings are present, a stepwise laboratory approach is recommended. A thorough history and physical evaluation detect most organic causes of FTT, and laboratory tests almost never contribute to the diagnosis independently (Homer and Ludwig, 1981; Sills, 1978). Some conditions, for example, lead poisoning, tuberculosis, and giardiasis, can be endemic in certain geographic areas and require routine laboratory assessments. Laboratory evaluation can also be useful to document nutritional status. The albumin level is used to assess protein status in severe FTT. Deficiency in minerals, particularly iron and zinc, can have an independent detrimental effect on the development of FTT (Lozoff, 1989). Interpretation of growth patterns on growth grids can assist in decisions regarding laboratory evaluation. A child with a decreasing height growth velocity with a symmetric weight to height ratio might require bone age and thyroid studies and perhaps growth hormone evaluation. Conversely these endocrine studies are not warranted in a typical FTT growth pattern.

NUTRITIONAL AND FEEDING EVALUATION

A nutritional and feeding history assesses the calorie, protein, and micronutrient intake; the quality and appropriate-

ness of food for age; and the social nature of the feeding event. A first-level evaluation in these areas can be performed by a pediatrician or nurse. Children with FTT have a lower intake of calories, protein, and certain vitamins and minerals than do normal children. The average daily requirement for infants younger than 6 months of age is 100 to 120 kcal/kg/day; for children 6 through 12 months of age, this amount decreases to about 105 kcal/kg/day, and it is somewhat less for children older than 1 year of age. It is helpful to use a 24-hour diet recall for infants. For infants younger than 6 months of age who receive formula or breast milk, the frequency and amount of feedings are recorded, along with how the formula was prepared (i.e., too dilute or concentrated) and delivered (propped or not), the infant's skill in sucking and swallowing, and whether the feedings are retained. Observation of bottle feeding is useful to assess the parents' style. How long did the feeding take and how much did the infant consume? Was there a good suck without vomiting? Was the social interaction (i.e., eye and body contact) good? Was the parent excessively stimulating, withdrawn, or disruptive?

A 3-day diet recall is used to ascertain intake for older children who are eating solid foods. Some children are described as good eaters who eat "all the time." Children who demonstrate this "grazing" pattern might nibble on nonnutritious foods throughout the day but fail to meet daily requirements. Drinking an excessive amount of fruit juices and other sweet liquids may be particularly problematic. One should inquire about the feeding event for the toddler taking solid foods. Are three meals provided per day? Are they eaten in a highchair or in a chair at the table, and are they supervised by an adult? Children with FTT often suffer in these contextual aspects of the feeding event.

The parents' understanding and attitude toward normal nutrition and feeding is ascertained. Some families adhere to atypical feeding practices because of lack of knowledge or experience, but in some cases it is because of excessively zealous application of breast-feeding, vegetarian diets, diets to prevent obesity or cardiovascular disease, or medical regimens to treat diarrhea or suspected food allergies (Frank and Zeisel, 1988).

SOCIAL HISTORY

There are few specific socioenvironmental causes of FTT (e.g., extreme poverty, parent with mental retardation or psychosis), and there is no single set of factors that routinely results in FTT. Most controlled research has found no difference between families with children with FTT and control subjects in maternal age, marital status, knowledge, stress, mental health, number of family members, birth order of index child, or number of rooms in the household (Casey, 1989). However, mothers who have children with FTT reported more negative perceptions of their own childhood and of their relationship with the child's father (e.g., arguments and separations) (Altemeir et al, 1985), and they demonstrated more disorganized homes (Casey, 1989), more neglectful and less nurturant styles (Black et al, 1994), and more social isolation and less support from families and neighbors (Bithoney and Newberger, 1987; Bithoney et al, 1995).

The comprehensive social status interview, which is usually performed by a clinician trained in the collection of such data, solicits information regarding the parents, family, and their environment, which may potentiate (vulnerability factors) or compensate (protector factors) the development of FTT. Historical features of specific importance are maternal and paternal education; household income and income per capita; availability of adequate food in the house; marital status; the number of people and rooms in the child's home; the presence of parental psychoemotional dysfunction or habit disorders (e.g., alcohol or drug use); history of neglect or abuse with the parents' other children; the history of parental abuse as a child; history of major stress to the parents such as spousal abuse, loss of job, or recent death; atypical family feeding and cultural practices; problems in family routines and organization; and the presence of emotional, financial, and physical support available to the primary provider. Children with FTT are often raised primarily by day care providers, relatives, or neighbors, and the primary problem might lie outside the immediate household. The clinician interprets the interaction of the relative strengths and weaknesses in these various areas in determining their contribution to the development of FTT. Psychiatric referral and evaluation can be helpful when concerns arise regarding the psychoemotional stability (e.g., depression, psychoses) of a primary caregiver, particularly when it results in distortions in the quality of the parent-child interaction.

PARENT-CHILD INTERACTION ASSESSMENT

There is no generally accepted clinical approach to assess the quality of parent-child interaction, despite its theoretical and practical value. Such an assessment can occur at home or in a clinical setting, by a pediatrician, nurse, social worker or psychiatrist, in a feeding event or nonstructured situation, with a standardized instrument or global clinical judgment. In general, the clinician attempts to assess the appropriateness, warmth, sensitivity, and responsiveness of the interaction between parent and child. There is no substitute for a home visit to observe the child and parent in the context of their own environment. The HOME inventory is the most commonly used standardized instrument for assessing the quality of home environment and parent-child interaction during a home visit. A questionnaire for assessing a child's physical and social environment for use by pediatricians in clinical settings, derived from the HOME inventory, has been shown to predict child development status (Casey et al, 1993). Attention to the parent-child interaction during a feeding event is of particular relevance in FTT.

Management

NEED TO HOSPITALIZE

The first decision after the initial outpatient evaluation is whether to hospitalize the child to initiate management.

Successful outpatient management of most children with FTT has been demonstrated in settings with multidisciplinary groups (Bithoney et al, 1989; Casey, Wortham, and Nelson, 1984). Physicians with access to social workers and nutritionists can attempt to manage in outpatient settings children who are mildly to moderately underweight (greater than 60% average weight for age) and mildly wasted (greater than 80% average weight for height), who constitute the majority of all FTT children (Wright, Ashenburg, and Whitaker, 1994). This outpatient intervention has the advantage of being less costly, of working with the family in the reality of their own environment, and of keeping the parent and child together as the focus of the intervention. Hospitalization is required for the following: (1) to protect the child from abuse when evidence of nonaccidental trauma is found at the time of initial evaluation, (2) to protect a severely malnourished child from the sequelae of further starvation, (3) in extremely problematic parent-child interaction, particularly toddlers with feeding behavior problems, (4) when practicality of distance and transportation preclude outpatient management, and (5) after failure of an adequate attempt at outpatient management. Inpatient care allows completion of the medical evaluation, observation of the child's spontaneous feeding ability and style, more detailed observation of parent-child interaction and parenting style, and the development of a realistic nutritional plan based on these observations. These goals require the presence of the parent during the hospitalization. Involving the parents in the development of the treatment plan and educating them regarding the details of this plan are more likely to ensure cooperation and follow-through on discharge. On occasion it is necessary, however, to excuse the parents from part of the hospitalization if their presence disrupts the successful achievement of nutritional rehabilitation.

NUTRITIONAL REHABILITATION

Nutritional rehabilitation is at the core of the management of FTT, whether it is inpatient or outpatient management (Table 41–2) (Maggioni and Lifshitz, 1995). To allow growth to compensate toward normal, one to two times the normally expected caloric intake for age should be given. Mathematic formulas are available to calculate this nutritional goal (Frank and Zeisel, 1988). Enriched formulas (24 to 30 calories per ounce) using carbohydrate, triglyceride, or dried milk added to normal formula are used for infants younger than 12 to 15 months of age. A specific plan of quantity and frequency to achieve the nutritional goal is suggested as a minimum. Formula beyond this goal,

Table 41–2 • Management of Failure to Thrive

Nutritional rehabilitation—establishing appropriate intake, restoration, and maintenance
Improved parent-child interaction
Special stimulation of infant in some cases
Management of organic disease
Amelioration of social-family problems
Mental health support for parents when indicated
Regular follow-up

and solid food if needed, are encouraged. Vitamin and mineral deficiencies, such as that of iron or zinc, can negatively affect behavior, appetite, and growth, and supplementation might be required (Lozoff, 1989). A randomized controlled study of zinc supplementation in children with FTT demonstrated a significant increase in weight gain in the zinc-supplemented children (Walvarens, Hambridge, and Koepfer, 1989).

Attention must be given to the environmental context of feeding. Some infants and toddlers require a quiet setting with little distraction, and some toddlers need to be restrained in a highchair. Anorexic infants or toddlers with feeding and behavioral problems present particular challenges in nutritional rehabilitation. Elimination of nonnutritious intake (e.g., colas, sweetened drinks, sweets) and structuring the timing and environment are first steps. Strict behavioral protocols to modify mealtime behavior and the use of nasogastric feeding tubes to expand intake are occasionally required (Rudolph, 1994).

Monitoring daily weight gain during hospitalization or during a 1- to 3-week follow-up visit in the outpatient setting allows determination of the success of this nutritional protocol. Although catch-up growth can occur rapidly, up to 2 weeks can pass before growth occurs in the child with more involved FTT. Children with FTT, like malnourished children from third-world countries, can demonstrate weight gains three to four times the daily amount expected during this rapid catch-up phase.

OTHER MANAGEMENT NEEDS

Other aspects of the management plan are based on the problems identified in the initial evaluation. The goals of treatment are to improve parent understanding of child care, nutrition, and the health and development of their child, and to minimize stressors and stabilize the home environment, all with the focus of improving parent-child interaction. For example, helping the parent understand, tolerate, and manage better any contributory temperament traits may be helpful. Aggressive management of organic diseases associated with FTT is warranted. For example, placement of ventilation tubes in a child with recurrent otitis media might result in a striking return of appetite. A hospital-based social worker or nurse, or both, often in conjunction with community social workers or public health nurses, can work with the family for ongoing education and support and to stabilize the home environment. Use of an array of appropriate community resources (e.g., community financial supports; the Women, Infant, Children [WIC] program; housing authority; homemaker assistance) is required in most cases. Referral for mental health support might be necessary for some parents. Therapy focused on improving parent-child interaction is available in some settings. The child might benefit from out-of-home care at a developmental stimulation program.

Recent controlled research with home-based intervention and center-based educational stimulation has resulted in more nurturing home environments and improved developmental status in children with FTT (Black et al, 1995; Casey et al, 1994).

FOLLOW-UP

All of the aforementioned steps, along with ongoing monitoring in the clinical setting, serve to provide the family with an anchor to the world to minimize their social isolation. The relationship of the physician and other health care workers to the family during this monitoring process is a supportive one, which increases the likelihood of compliance with the management plan and clinical follow-up. The frequency of follow-up is based on the course of the child's and the family's responses to the plan. All aspects of the management plan are modified based on course.

Prognosis

The outcome of children with FTT is predictably variable, given the broad range of severity, age of onset, and etiology. Even in the absence of diagnosable disease, children with FTT vary considerably in degree of malnutrition, subtle neurodevelopmental abnormality, and quality of nurturance and stimulation of their home environments, all of which independently contribute to ultimate outcomes in growth, development, and behavior.

Most controlled and noncontrolled follow-up studies of children with FTT in the United States and undernourished children in developing countries generally document negative long-term effects on growth, development, and behavior (Black and Dubowitz, 1991; Casey et al, 1994). In many of these reports, children with FTT functioned in the lower range of normal in outcome measures, although lower than the control groups (Kelleher et al, 1993; Sturm and Drotar, 1989). Long-term outcomes may be affected positively by treatment (Casey et al, 1994). Several randomized controlled interventions have been performed with malnourished children in developing countries, using nutrition or psychosocial stimulation (Black and Dubowitz, 1991). In general, these studies yielded beneficial effects on growth, development, and behavior. For example, 129 growth-retarded children in Jamaica were randomly assigned to four groups: control, nutritional supplementation, psychosocial stimulation, or both treatments. Developmental stimulation and nutritional supplementation had significant independent beneficial effects on 2-year developmental status. The treatment effects were additive, and the combined interventions were more effective than either alone (Grantham-McGregor et al, 1991).

In summary, most children with FTT can be expected to achieve normal growth and developmental status. In contrast, many children remain small and continue to be at risk for long-term negative developmental and behavioral sequelae. Because of the variation in clinical subtypes and etiologic contributors on the transactional spectrum, no generalization regarding prognosis is adequate for an individual child. Nutritional, family support, and childhood stimulation intervention will likely improve outcomes of children with FTT.

Advocacy

Many advocacy roles exist for the physician who manages children with FTT. Although these children usually do not have organic disease, their illness carries unacceptable prognosis without concerted action. The first advocacy role relates to early identification, because chronicity of the problem correlates with poor outcome. Beyond vigilance for high-risk clinical situations and careful monitoring of growth, physicians can assist in early identification by educating community providers such as public health nurses, social workers, and nutritionists regarding FTT. Next, management requires communication and cooperative interaction with many community organizations. The advocate physician can expend significant effort to develop an adequately coordinated management and monitoring plan. Finally and perhaps most difficult is the need to advocate for the child against the family in the juvenile court system when the management plan fails despite the clinical team's best efforts in working with the family. There is some suggestion that foster care placement can have a beneficial impact on the course of FTT in certain circumstances.

REFERENCES

Altemeir WA, O'Connor SM, Sherrod KB, et al: Prospective study of antecedents for nonorganic failure to thrive. J Pediatr 106:360, 1985.

Bell LS, Woolston JL: The relationship of weight gain and caloric intake in infants with organic and nonorganic failure to thrive syndrome. J Am Acad Child Psychiatry 24:447, 1985.

Berwick DM: Nonorganic failure to thrive. Pediatr Rev 1:265, 1980.

Bithoney WG, Dubowitz H: Organic concomitants of nonorganic failure to thrive. In Drotar D (ed): New Directions in Failure to Thrive: Implications for Research and Practice. New York, Plenum Press, 1985, p 47.

Bithoney WG, Newberger EH: Child and family attributes of failure to thrive. J Dev Behav Pediatr 8:32, 1987.

Bithoney WG, McJunkin J, Michalek J, et al: Prospective evaluation of weight gain in both nonorganic and organic failure to thrive children: an outpatient trial of a multidisciplinary team intervention strategy. J Dev Behav Pediatr 10:27, 1989.

Bithoney WG, Van Sciver MM, Foster S, et al: Parental stress and growth outcomes in growth-deficient children. Pediatrics 96:707, 1995.

Black M, Dubowitz H: Failure to thrive: lessons from animal models and developing countries. J Dev Behav Pediatr 12:259, 1991.

Black MM, Dubowitz H, Hutcheson J, et al: A randomized clinical trial of home intervention for children with failure to thrive. Pediatrics 95:807, 1995.

Black MM, Hutcheson JJ, Dubowitz H, Berenson-Howard J: Parenting styles and development status among children with non-organic failure to thrive. J Pediatr Psychiatry 6:689, 1994.

Casey PH: The family system and failure to thrive. In Ramsey CN (ed): Family Systems in Medicine. New York, Guilford Press, 1989, p 348.

Casey PH, Wortham B, Nelson JY: Management of children with failure to thrive in a rural ambulatory setting. Clin Pediatr 23:325, 1984.

Casey PH, Kraemer HC, Bernbaum J, et al: Growth status and growth rates of a large varied sample of low birth weight, preterm infants: a longitudinal cohort from birth to age three. J Pediatr 119:599, 1991.

Casey PH, Barrett KW, Bradley RH, et al: Pediatric clinical assessment of mother-infant interaction: concurrent and predictive validity. J Dev Behav Pediatr 14:313, 1993.

Casey PH, Kelleher KJ, Bradley RH, et al: A multifaceted intervention for infants with failure to thrive: a prospective study. Arch Pediatr Adolesc Med 148:1071, 1994.

Chatoor I, Schaefer S, Dickson L, et al: Nonorganic failure to thrive: a developmental perspective. Pediatr Ann 13(11):829, 1984.

Fleisher DR: Functional vomiting disorders in infancy: innocent vomiting, nervous vomiting, and infant rumination syndrome. J Pediatr 123(6):S84, 1994.

Frank DA, Zeisel SH: Failure to thrive. Pediatr Clin North Am 35(6):1187, 1988.

Grantham-McGregor SM, Powell CA, Walker SP, et al: Nutritional supplementation, psychosocial stimulation, and mental development of stunted children: the Jamaican study. Lancet 338:1, 1991.

Guo S, Roche AF, Fomon SJ, et al: Reference data on gains in weight and length during the first two years of life. J Pediatr 119:355, 1991.

Hendricks KM, Duggan C, Gallagher L, et al: Malnutrition in hospitalized pediatric patients. Arch Pediatr Adolesc Med 149:1118, 1995.

Homer C, Ludwig S: Categorization of etiology of failure to thrive. Am J Dis Child 135:848, 1981.

Kelleher K, Casey PH, Bradley RH, et al: Risk factors and outcomes for failure to thrive in low birthweight preterm infants. Pediatrics 91:941, 1993.

Lozoff B: Nutrition and behavior. Am Psychol 44:231, 1989.

Maggioni A, Lifshitz F: Nutritional management of failure to thrive. Pediatr Clin North Am 42(4):791, 1995.

Mitchell WG, Gorrell RW, Greenberg RA: Failure to thrive: a study in a primary care setting. Epidemiology and follow-up. Pediatrics 65:961, 1980.

Powell GF, Low JF, Speers MA: Behavior as a diagnostic aid in failure to thrive. J Dev Behav Pediatr 8:18, 1987.

Ramsay M, Gisel EG, Boutry M: Non-organic failure to thrive secondary to feeding skills disorder. Dev Med Child Neurol 35:285, 1993.

Richters MM, Volkmar FR: Reactive attachment disorder of infancy or early childhood. J Am Acad Child Adolesc Psychiatry 33:328, 1994.

Rudolph DC: Feeding disorders in infants and children. J Pediatr 125:5116, 1994.

Sills RH: Failure to thrive: the role of clinical and laboratory evaluation. Am J Dis Child 132:967, 1978.

Skuse D, Pickles A, Wolke D, Reilly S: Postnatal growth and maternal deprivation: Evidence for a "sensitive period." J Child Psychol Psychiatr 35(3):521, 1994.

Sturm L, Drotar D: Prediction of weight for height following intervention in three-year-old children with early histories of nonorganic failure to thrive. Child Abuse Negl 13:19, 1989.

Walvarens PA, Hambridge KM, Koepfer DM: Zinc supplementation in infants with a nutritional pattern of failure to thrive: a double-blind, controlled study. Pediatrics 83:532, 1989.

Wright JA, Ashenburg CA, Whitaker RC: Comparison of methods to categorize undernutrition in children. J Pediatr 145:944, 1994.

42 *Enuresis*

Michael E. K. Moffatt

To awaken each morning immersed, if not submersed, in a lagoon of urine must be one of the more humiliating ways to launch a day. Children with enuresis lack a primitive form of control and, in many cases, feel this shortcoming with deep pain. Their parents are apt to be exasperated by this unrelenting nuisance. In this chapter, the author examines the range of mechanisms that can underlie this chronic developmental-behavioral problem. He offers excellent suggestions for a systematic approach to successful and minimally traumatic management.

Types of Enuresis

Enuresis, or urinary incontinence beyond an age when a child should be developmentally capable of continence, is one of the most common developmental problems. It can be a source of embarrassment for the child and a source of frustration for parents.

There are two common ways to classify enuresis, and each has some clinical merit. The first way is based on relationship to sleep. *Nocturnal enuresis* occurs only while sleeping (afternoon naps included), whereas *diurnal enuresis* occurs when the child is awake. There seems to be a continuum between these two types of enuresis. The child with monosymptomatic nocturnal enuresis has achieved daytime continence at a normal age, has excellent daytime control, does not have frequency, urgency, hesitancy, or dysuria, and has a normal bladder capacity. Further along the continuum is the child who has only nocturnal wetting but some bladder symptoms. Next are children who have the aforementioned manifestations plus an occasional episode of daytime wetting. At the far end of the spectrum is the child who has both regular day and night wetting and bladder symptoms. Bladder capacity in these children is often well below expected values (capacity = age in years + 2 = ounces of bladder capacity) (Koff, 1983).

The second way of classifying enuresis is into primary and secondary types. The child with *primary* nocturnal enuresis has never been consistently dry, whereas the child with *secondary* enuresis has had at least 6 months of consecutive dryness. The child with secondary bed-wetting is somewhat more likely to have psychological factors as an etiologic basis (Feehan et al, 1990). Organic causes, such as recent onset of diabetes mellitus, must also be considered.

Epidemiology

The prevalence of nocturnal enuresis is estimated at approximately 7% of 8-year-olds, with a subsequent decrease of 1 percentage point per year. Boys outnumber girls by a

ratio of 1.4:1. A Swedish study (Hellstrom, Hanson, and Hansson, 1990) has confirmed the ratio of boys to girls for 7-year-old school entrants and has provided information on the frequency of other symptoms. Bed-wetting was monosymptomatic in 39% of girls and 59% of boys. Day wetting of volumes greater than 1 mL at least once per week was found in 3.1% of girls and 2.1% of boys. In the group with socially significant enuresis, 61% wet only at night, 17% wet both day and night, and 22% wet only during the day.

Etiologic Factors

Enuresis is not a disease. Rather, it is a symptom that may have multiple etiologic factors. Some of the more well-established factors are genetics, psychological and social factors, sleep state, large urine volume, small bladder capacity, prematurity, and constipation.

GENETICS

Numerous studies (Bakwin, 1973; Hallgren, 1956; Kaffman and Elizur, 1977) have documented a strong familial tendency for nocturnal enuresis. Some authors have hypothesized that there is a dominant gene with variable penetrance for the most common presentation of nocturnal enuresis. Recently, Danish researchers identified a dominant gene on chromosome 13 (Eiberg, Berendt, and Mohr, 1995). Replication of this finding and identification of the gene product holds the potential to give new insights into the problem of enuresis.

PSYCHOLOGICAL AND SOCIAL FACTORS

Children from lower socioeconomic circumstances, broken or stressed homes, and institutions are more likely to have problems with enuresis. This is particularly true for secondary nocturnal enuresis, which may have its onset after the birth of a sibling, a death in the family, or a separation of parents (Feehan et al, 1990). A chaotic social situation may also contribute to the development of poor voiding habits, which may lead to problems with daytime control. There is little or no support for the once-common notion that nocturnal enuresis is a psychiatric problem. Most children with enuresis have normal psychological profiles or minor increases in behavior symptoms (Moffatt, 1989).

SLEEP

The exact role of sleep and arousal remains elusive. Parents consistently report that nocturnal enuretic children are deep sleepers who are difficult to arouse compared with their siblings who do not have enuresis. Although differences in the electroencephalographic sleep pattern have not been found and nocturnal wetting episodes have been shown to occur randomly throughout the sleep stages, recent evidence does point to some difficulty in arousal for these children (Wille, 1994). Even though the hypothesis is unproven, many researchers believe the reason that children outgrow their enuresis is that there is a maturation in sleep pattern that allows the child to recognize and respond to a full bladder while asleep.

URINE VOLUME AND ANTIDIURETIC HORMONE

Children with nocturnal enuresis may produce large volumes of dilute urine. Danish studies (Djurhuus, Norgaard, and Rittig, 1992) have shown that many children do not have the diurnal variation in arginine vasopressin that non-wetting children have. Whether this finding applies to all children with nocturnal enuresis is unclear, but it seems to be present in at least some of those with monosymptomatic bed-wetting.

BLADDER CAPACITY

Bed-wetting occurs when functional bladder capacity is reached (Djurhuus, Norgaard, and Rittig, 1992). There is considerable variation in bladder capacity of children, and enuretic children have consistently been shown to have smaller bladder capacities than their dry counterparts (Zaleski, Gerrard, and Shokier, 1973).

PREMATURITY (MINOR NEUROLOGIC DAMAGE)

Epidemiologic evidence (Kass, Diokno, and Montealegre, 1979) has distinguished prematurity as one of the most significant risk factors for children at the end of the spectrum with daytime symptoms. These children were also likely to have a comorbid condition, such as attention-deficit hyperactivity disorder. Jarvelin and associates (1988) hypothesize that minor neurologic damage may be the linking factor.

CONSTIPATION

It is common to find bowel elimination problems in children with enuresis, particularly those with daytime symptoms. This may be simply comorbidity, but one study (O'Reagan et al, 1986) suggested it might also be an etiologic factor. Encopresis (see Chapter 43) is usually due to obstipation, and it is plausible that a dilated rectum could impinge on the bladder, making bladder control more difficult.

Evaluation of Child and Family

The evaluation is an opportunity to gain the trust of the child and the child's family. Thus it is a part of the therapeutic process and should be given adequate consideration.

HISTORY

Careful history-taking is the main element of the evaluation.

Reason for Consultation

The reason and timing for consulting a physician about the problem often give considerable insight into the family dynamics.

Pattern of Enuresis

The onset, pattern, and severity of the wetting must be established. Is it primary or secondary and does it ever occur during the day? Are the volumes large or small? Does the child seem to wet more than once per night? It is helpful to have a calendar mailed to the family several weeks before the consultation so that wetting events can be prospectively recorded.

Psychosocial History

How does the child feel about the problem (Fig. 42–1)? It is common for children to be embarrassed or to cry, necessitating sensitivity on the part of the clinician. Who is most distressed by the wetting—the child, the mother, or the father? Have the parents ever punished the child for wetting? Is there a difference in approach between the parents? Is the child motivated for treatment? Are there recent or current emotional stresses within the family? What effect is the problem having on the child's life? Is the child missing out on sleepovers, summer camp, trips with the baseball or hockey team, or any other important social development activities? How much do the parents know about enuresis? Are their expectations realistic? Do they blame the child?

Family History

Family history is best obtained by mailing out a questionnaire in advance. Because enuresis is still largely secret, families do not discuss it and are often unaware of the family history.

Previous Treatments

The date, intensity, duration, and success of all previous treatments, both medical and alternative, give some insight into the family and what is likely to be effective. Often treatments have not been optimally applied.

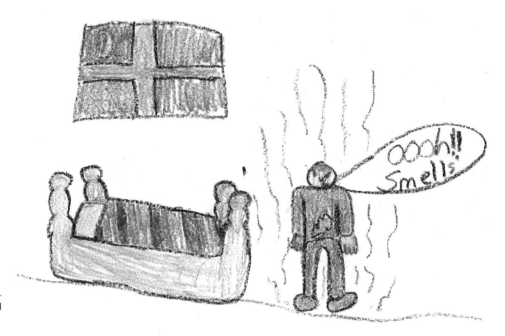

Figure 42–1. A 9-year-old boy illustrates how he feels about nocturnal enuresis.

Voiding History

Voiding history is the basis on which a decision is made about the likelihood of urinary tract pathology and the need for further investigations. Inquiry should be made about frequency (more than six voids during the waking day), urgency, intermittent or weak stream, staccato stream, squatting (usually in girls), or posturing (in both sexes). Infrequent voiding (e.g., in the child who gets up in the morning and does not have to void and may void only a couple of times during the day) may also be an indicator of bladder pathology, as is a history of urinary tract infection.

Stool Pattern

Stool pattern should be recorded. Soiling, very large or painful bowel movements, or a history of 3 or more days between bowel movements may all be indications of constipation.

Miscellaneous

Sleep pattern and ease of arousal may be helpful in planning therapeutic approaches. Food allergies have been associated with enuresis. Sleep apnea has also been associated in a few case reports. Thirst and fluid consumption may help identify children with diabetes or difficulty with urine concentration.

PHYSICAL EXAMINATION

The physical examination should be directed to the abdomen, the genitals, perineal sensation and anal wink reflex, the lower spine (for sacral dimple or cutaneous abnormality), and the neurologic system. If a voiding problem is suspected, it is worthwhile to observe the child void. Results of the physical examination are normal in most enuretic children.

LABORATORY INVESTIGATION

The only routine tests recommended are a careful urinalysis to look for signs of infection, chronic renal disease, and diabetes mellitus and a culture to rule out infection. Other tests such as sickle cell prep and tests of urinary concentrating ability are indicated only if history specifically points to a suspicion. Radiography of the genitourinary system is invasive, costly, and, for most children with nocturnal enuresis, unrewarding. The following section presents some guidelines as to when it might be indicated.

Uncomplicated Versus Complicated Enuresis

Most cases of enuresis are uncomplicated. The investigative scheme put forward in Figure 42–2 (Rushton, 1989) is an appropriate approach with one proviso: because encopresis often occurs in the absence of organic pathology (see Chapter 43), unless there are clear indicators of neurologic or urinary tract pathology, it seems reasonable to try treatment for constipation before embarking on invasive tests. Rushton (1989) suggests that complicated enuresis is seen in children with neurologic abnormality, current or past urinary tract infection, and symptoms suggestive of urinary tract pathology—either severe frequency and persistent regular daytime incontinence associated with poor urinary stream and/or encopresis or the child with very infrequent voiding. These children should undergo renal sonograms and vesicourogram (VCUG). If vesicoureteral reflux, hydronephrosis, a thickened unstable bladder, or posterior urethral valves are found, the patient requires further urologic evaluation. It may, at times, seem like the physician is walking a fine line in making the decision about who to recommend for further investigation. A recent Swedish study (Hellstrom, Hanson, and Hansson, 1990) supports a conservative approach. Of 3556 7-year-old school entrants, the researchers found 173 who had some day wetting, and none of these were identified as having organic pathology.

Management

RATIONALE

The first principle of management is to provide support and education to the family and the child. In some cases, this is all that is required. Because enuresis is not a disease and the symptom nearly always disappears with time, the decision to treat rests on several considerations. There is a cost to the family for persistent enuresis. A recent estimate (Norgaard and Andersen, 1993) put the annual figure at $1000. More important are the stress factors, which vary greatly from family to family. When the stress level is high, it reflects negatively on the child. The most important factor is how the child feels about wetting and about himself or herself. Young children are often not bothered by enuresis and it has little effect on their social development unless the family environment is hostile. Although it has not been demonstrated that enuretic children have lower than normal self-esteem, it has been shown that scores on self-concept tests improve after treatment (Moffatt, Kato, and Pless, 1987). This constitutes a strong rationale for offering treatment. Standard treatments are less effective with very young children. Treatment should be considered at around 7 years of age, although for mature children with high motivation, success is possible a little earlier.

EDUCATION AND DEMYSTIFICATION

Parents are frequently ignorant of the incidence of enuresis, are unaware that other families have the problem, and blame the child or consider the child to be lazy. The first step is to uncover such misconceptions and attitudes and provide information on the epidemiology, physiology, etiologic factors, and natural history of enuresis. For children old enough to understand, it is helpful, with the aid of diagrams or models, to explain how urine is produced, what the bladder is for, and how the bladder is connected to the brain and nervous system. Nocturnal enuresis can be presented as arising from two factors: (1) a full bladder and (2) the inability to sense that full bladder when sleeping. The full bladder may be due to large amounts of urine or a small bladder capacity. Daytime enuresis when there is no suspicion of organic pathology may be explained to the child (taking into account the child's developmental level and ability to integrate the facts) as a small bladder that is hyperresponsive and, when full, does not give enough warning before it overcomes sphincter resistance.

TREATMENT FOR NOCTURNAL ENURESIS

Conditioning

The conditioning alarm, first developed nearly a century ago, is by far the best method of treating night wetting. A recent systematic review (Houts, 1995; Houts, Berman, and Abramson, 1994) has confirmed an overall success rate of 66% and a 1-year success rate of 51%. When several other behavioral interventions are added in conjunction with conditioning, the 1-year success rate increases to more than 60%. How conditioning actually works is a mystery. The simplest explanation is that it is operant conditioning with the alarm acting as an aversive stimulus. The conditioned stimulus is probably pelvic floor or sphincter contraction. When the alarm sounds consistently every time the bladder reaches the point that it is contracting, the child learns to respond in anticipation. The result is that most children successfully treated with this method end up sleeping through the night and holding a larger volume of urine. Conditioning is no "quick fix." It takes a minimum of 3 to 5 months to complete, and the family must be patient and supportive. Nevertheless, if the method is explained in a positive fashion, most parents are willing to try it.

Conditioning alarms are inexpensive and uncomplicated. They are attached to the child and a probe is placed in front of the urethra. Two of the earliest available and most commonly used alarms in North America are the Nytone (worn on the wrist with a probe that is clipped onto a layer of cloth from the underwear) and the Palco (attached to the shoulder by a Velcro band with a flat probe that fits into a Velcro pocket, which is sewn onto the crotch of the underwear). These devices and many other brands (choice is largely personal preference, because results are similar with all standard alarms) are widely available, but a local supplier must be sought. This may be a medical

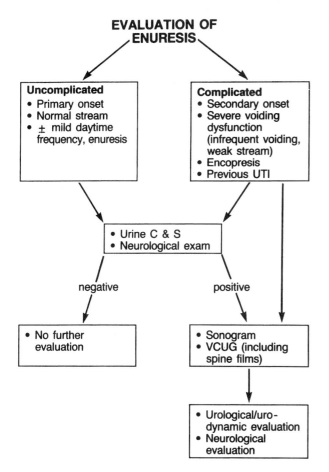

Figure 42–2. Flow chart for evaluation of uncomplicated and complicated enuresis. C & S, culture and sensitivity testing; UTI, urinary tract infection; VCUG, voiding cystourethrogram. (From Rushton HG: Nocturnal enuresis: epidemiology, evaluation, and currently available treatment options. J Pediatr 114[suppl 4 part 2]:692, 1989.)

supply company, pharmacy, or department store. Because urine is a saline solution, it conducts electricity. The first drops of urine complete the circuit and the alarm sounds. The child is instructed to arouse, get up, remove the probe, and go to the bathroom to finish voiding. The alarm should then be reconnected on a dry pair of underwear in case there is a subsequent wetting. Children younger than 10 years often do not hear the alarm. Conditioning still works, however, if the parent gets up and awakens the child. Over time, a motivated child begins to hear the alarm. A daily record should be kept of the number of alarms that are activated and the size of the wet spot in the child's underwear. This record should be brought to each follow-up visit where the therapist can point out the signs of improvement. Reinforcing arousal has been shown to correlate with success. Decreasing size of the wet spots is another sign of success, usually occurring before the dry nights increase. For children who wet more than one time per night (often something the parents are unaware of before the alarm is used), a decrease in the number of wets per night is also a positive sign. Finally, there is an increase in the number of dry nights (no alarm response and not even a wet spot). The initial target is 14 dry nights in a row. When this is achieved, the next phase should be overlearning or over-conditioning. Extra fluids are taken before bed—usually 16 to 32 ounces. This often results in the resumption of wetting, but studies have shown that overlearning reduces the relapse rate, which otherwise can be as high as 40% (Morgan, 1978). The wetting usually disappears after a few weeks and the child can remain dry again. When the child goes 14 consecutive nights without wetting in this overlearning stage, it is possible to stop the drinking and the alarm, and the relapse rate will be reduced to 10% or 15%. In children who have daytime symptoms and a small bladder capacity, it may be wise to gradually increase the fluid by increments of 60 mL (Houts, Peterson, and Whelan, 1986).

EXAMPLE: MONOSYMPTOMATIC PRIMARY NOCTURNAL ENURESIS RESPONSIVE TO CONDITIONING

Eleven-year-old Patricia had primary nocturnal enuresis and was highly embarrassed about it. She had no bladder symptoms but the family history was positive—both her grandmothers had wet until age 9 and her brother until age 8. When Patricia was 8 years old she underwent a 6-week trial with an enuresis alarm, but she and her parents had given up in frustration because she failed to awaken when the alarm sounded (which was every night). The parents had not been instructed to assist her. Another trial of the alarm with parental input was suggested. During the first 2 weeks, there was a decrease in the size of the wet spots in her underwear, but she had only sporadic dry nights. When she had achieved 14 consecutive dry nights, she was started on overlearning, beginning with drinking one 8-ounce glass of water before bedtime. When she was dry again for 3 nights in a row, the fluid was increased to 16 ounces and by successive increments of 8 ounces up to 32 ounces per night. By 11 weeks after starting the alarm, Patricia had completed 14 consecutive dry nights on full overlearning. She was able to stop the alarm and the fluid load and she has remained dry.

Conditioning is most effective when the wetting intensity is lowest, but this also appears to be true of pharmacotherapy. It is least likely to work when there are major family problems, the child has significant behavior problems, or the family has used punishment for bed-wetting. Conditioning requires a positive presentation and considerable patience. The therapist does not have to be a physician or a psychologist but may be a nurse or other trained health care worker.

Pharmacotherapy

Two types of pharmaceutical agents shown to be effective in treating nocturnal enuresis are tricyclic antidepressants and desmopressin (DDAVP).

Tricyclic Antidepressants

For more than 3 decades it has been known that tricyclic antidepressants reduce the frequency of nighttime wetting (Blackwell and Currah, 1973). The most common theory about how they work is that they lighten sleep enough to allow bladder filling to be detected. They also have an anticholinergic effect, but because anticholinergic drugs alone have no effect on bed-wetting, the latter is an unlikely explanation. Imipramine is the most studied and the least expensive. The dosage required is usually in the range of 1 to 1.5 mg/kg given within 1 hour before bedtime. Imipramine has side effects in some children, usually insomnia and behavior and mood change. Significant side effects necessitate discontinuation. The biggest danger is overdose, which can be fatal as a result of cardiac arrhythmia. The drug should never be prescribed in unstable family situations, and only small quantities should be dispensed at a time.

A meta-analysis (Houts, Berman, and Abramson, 1994) estimated that 43% of children became dry on imipramine, but this is likely an underestimate because the study included many trials in which the dosage was probably too low. As with all pharmacotherapy, the effects are symptomatic and not curative. Relapse is the rule once the drug is stopped. Nevertheless, when a child responds, it is worth continuing it for 6 months and then tapering it slowly. A few children remain dry. It can also be used as an intermittent treatment for special occasions in which wetting would be an embarrassment (e.g., at sleepovers). Sometimes it is important to gain a few dry nights in an older child who has never been dry in order to improve confidence and motivation. Because of its anticholinergic effect, it may be a useful symptomatic treatment for children with small bladder capacities.

Desmopressin Acetate (DDAVP)

The rationale for the use of DDAVP is the absent circadian rhythm for arginine vasopressin. A systematic review (Moffatt et al, 1993) found clear evidence of efficacy in reducing wet nights, but less optimism about the production of complete dryness, which appeared to be only about 25%. The presumed mechanism of effect is decreased urine volume. Dosage is usually gradually increased from 10 to

40 µg before bed. Experience has shown little evidence of serious side effects. Minor side effects include headaches, nasal stuffiness, and abdominal pain. The most feared side effect is water intoxication, but relatively few cases have been reported and most have been in children with metabolic or neurologic disorders for whom the drug is inappropriate. It is important to explain this risk to the child and family and stress the importance of not drinking anything after the drug has been taken. Like imipramine, DDAVP is not a cure, but it provides symptomatic relief. Some investigators have found that it can be used without problems for periods longer than 1 year. A major drawback is its cost, which ranges from $50 to $200 per month depending on dose.

EXAMPLE: MONOSYMPTOMATIC NOCTURNAL ENURESIS RESPONDING TO DDAVP

Donald was 13 years old when he was seen at the enuresis clinic with a lifetime history of night wetting five to seven times per week. There was no day wetting and no daytime symptoms. His social history indicated neglect and he had spent 6 years in foster care, but he was currently living with his natural mother and a foster father. Evidence evolved later that Donald pretty much took care of himself. A trial of an enuresis alarm failed because he did not wake up and got little help from his parents. A trial of DDAVP was initiated at a dose of 30 µg at bedtime. Donald became dry. He was so pleased with his dryness that he regulated the medication himself. Trials of stopping DDAVP at 3-monthly intervals consistently resulted in prompt relapse. After 3 years of continuing on DDAVP 30 µg, Donald was still pleased to be dry and reported no side effects. The cost of the DDAVP was supported by a social assistance program.

Other Therapies

Hypnotherapy

Hypnotherapy is a nondrug therapy that holds promise. After 9 months of a nonrandomized trial (Bannerjee, Srivastav, and Palan, 1993), 68% of a hypnotherapy group were dry compared with 24% in an imipramine group. Hypnotherapy is child-centered therapy in which the physiology of bladder-brain connections are explained to the child and the child is taught self-hypnosis and visual imaging to assist in responding to a full bladder while sleeping. Proper randomized controlled trials are needed to determine the true efficacy of this therapy. Therapists interested in using this method should be properly trained and certified by an appropriate body such as the American Society for Clinical Hypnosis.

Treatment of Constipation

Where encopresis or severe constipation is present, catharsis should be tried. It has its greatest effect on daytime symptoms.

Dietary Therapy

Dietary therapy may be worth exploring if the child has a clear history of allergy to foods such as milk, chocolate, or citrus fruits (Egger et al, 1992), but it requires the assistance of a dietitian. Evidence that dietary therapy is effective treatment for enuresis is weak, and it is not advocated as standard treatment.

TREATMENT FOR DIURNAL ENURESIS

Most children with day wetting also have night wetting. The results of treatment for nocturnal enuresis are not very good for those children who have regular day wetting or urgency and small bladder capacity. It is essential to approach the day wetting first. Children who fit the criteria for complicated enuresis and are found to have abnormalities on sonogram or VCUG are appropriately referred to urologic specialists. Those with mild day wetting and those who were screened as complicated but have normal imaging may be divided into those with bladder dysfunction and those with lazy bladder (urgency but infrequent voids). For both groups, the removal of constipation, when present, is a first step. Children with small bladder capacity may respond to bladder stretching exercises, which include stopping and starting urine flow and holding urine for as long as possible to increase bladder capacity. Baseline measurements of bladder capacity may be obtained by having the child distracted by some pleasant activity and holding the urine as long as possible before voiding in a measuring container. Usually several measurements are obtained over a period of time, and the largest volume is taken as a measure of capacity. Thereafter the child is asked to hold his or her urine as long as possible at least one time per day and to record the volume on a chart. A reward system can be set up for modest (5%–10%) increases in bladder capacity. These children also may respond to anticholinergic drugs. Most commonly used is oxybutynin in doses of 5 mg three times per day, which can be used in conjunction with exercises. Usually the drug is used for 2 or 3 months and then withdrawn slowly.

Children with lazy bladder are more responsive to timed voiding every 90 to 120 minutes to avoid urgency.

Nighttime wetting in all children with diurnal enuresis can be treated with conditioning or pharmacotherapy, but initial improvement in bladder capacity is advised.

There have been very few comparative studies of different methods of managing children with diurnal enuresis; this is an area that requires further research.

EXAMPLE: COMPLICATED NOCTURNAL AND DIURNAL ENURESIS

Nine-year-old James was referred to enuresis clinic for day and night wetting. He had a long history of cyclic episodes of both. He had urgency and frequency (urinating more than eight times a day). There was also a history of constipation and soiling. He had had two past documented urinary tract infections. Trials of imipramine and DDAVP had been given by his family physician with no success. He had also been placed on oxybutynin with a minor improvement in his daytime symptoms. An earlier VCUG had shown grade 1 reflux. Physical examination did not reveal spinal, neurologic, or urologic problems. The boy was referred to a urologist, and a repeat VCUG was ordered. Treatment of his constipation resulted in some improvement of his daytime wetting and a disappearance of his soiling. He continues to be followed up by both urologists and pediatricians.

Conclusion

Children who have success with any method of treating enuresis often show a more outgoing positive attitude as treatment progresses. Both children and their families are extremely grateful for clear explanations and successful treatments, making this developmental symptom one of the most rewarding to manage.

REFERENCES

Bakwin H: The genetics of enuresis. *In* Kolvin I, MacKeith RC, Meadow SR (eds): Bladder Control and Enuresis. London, William Heinemann, 1973, pp 73–77.

Bannerjee S, Srivastav A, Palan BM: Hypnosis and self-hypnosis in the management of nocturnal enuresis: a comparative study with imipramine therapy. Am J Clin Hypn 36:113, 1993.

Blackwell B, Currah J: The Psychopharmacoloy of nocturnal enuresis. *In* Kolvin I, MacKeith RC, Meadow SR (eds): Bladder Control and Enuresis. London, William Heinemann, 1973, pp 231–257.

Djurhuus JC, Norgaard JP, Rittig S: Monosymptomatic bedwetting. Scand J Urol Nephrol Suppl 141:7, 1992.

Egger J, Carter CH, Soothill JF, Wilson J: Effect of diet treatment on enuresis in children with migraine or hyperkinetic behavior. Clin Pediatr 302, 1992.

Eiberg H, Berendt I, Mohr J: Assignment of dominant inherited nocturnal enuresis (ENUR1) to chromosome 13q. Nat Genet 10:354, 1995.

Feehan M, McGee R, Sranton W, Silva PA: A 6 year follow-up of childhood enuresis: prevalence in adolescence and consequences for mental health. J Paediatr Child Health 26:75, 1990.

Hallgren B: Enuresis I. A study with reference to the morbidity risk and symptomatology. Acta Psychiatr Neurol Scand 31:379, 1956.

Hellstrom AL, Hanson E, Hansson S: Micturition habits and incontinence in 7-year-old Swedish school entrants. Eur J Pediatr 149:434, 1990.

Houts AC: Behavioural treatment for enuresis. Scand J Urol Nephrol Suppl 173:83, 1995.

Houts AC, Berman JS, Abramson H: Effectiveness of psychological and pharmacological treatments for nocturnal enuresis. J Consult Clin Psychol 62:737, 1994.

Houts AC, Peterson JK, Whelan JP: Prevention of relapse in full-spectrum home training for primary enuresis: a component analysis. Behav Ther 17:462, 1986.

Jarvelin MR, Vikerainen-Tervoven L, Moulainen I, Huttenen N-P: Enuresis in seven-year-old children. Acta Paediatr Scand 77:148–153, 1988.

Kaffman M, Elizur E: Infants who become enuretics: a longitudinal study of 161 kibbutz children. Monogr Soc Res Child Dev 42(2 serial no. 170):1, 1977.

Kass KJ, Diokno AC, Montealegre A: Enuresis: principles of management and results of treatment. J Urol 121:794, 1979.

Koff S: Estimating bladder capacity in children. Urology 21:218, 1983.

Moffatt MEK: Nocturnal enuresis: psychological implications of treatment and nontreatment. J Pediatr 114:697, 1989.

Moffatt MEK, Harlos S, Kirshen AJ, Burd L: Desmopressin acetate and nocturnal enuresis: how much do we know? Pediatrics 92:420, 1993.

Moffatt MEK, Kato C, Pless IB: Improvements in self-concept after treatment of nocturnal enuresis: a randomized controlled trial. J Pediatr 110:647, 1987.

Morgan RTT: Relapse and therapeutic response in the conditioning treatment of enuresis: a review of recent findings on intermittent reinforcement, overlearning and stimulus intensity. Behav Res Ther 16:273, 1978.

Norgaard JP, Andersen TM: Nocturnal enuresis—a burden on the family economy. Scand J Urol Suppl 163:49, 1993.

O'Reagan S, Yazbeck S, Hamberger B, Schick E: Constipation: a commonly unrecognized cause of enuresis. Am J Dis Child 140:260, 1986.

Rushton HG: Nocturnal enuresis: epidemiology, evaluation, and currently available treatment options. J Pediatr 114(suppl): 691, 1989.

Wille S: Nocturnal enuresis: sleep disturbance and behavioural patterns. Acta Paediatr 83:772, 1994.

Zaleski A, Gerrard JW, Shokier MHK: (1973). Nocturnal enuresis: the importance of small bladder capacity. *In* Kolvin I, MacKeith RC, Meadow SR (eds): Bladder Control and Enuresis. London, William Heinemann, 1973, pp 95–109.

43 Encopresis

Randal Rockney

Involuntary defecation can be a perplexing and treatment-resistant condition, a plight whose victims feel helpless and totally diminished. In most cases, this disorder is neither a traditional organic disease nor a purely psychogenic condition. It is likely to be the end product of multiple predisposing factors and underlying mechanisms. These pathways are explored in this chapter. Additionally, the author provides guidelines to the management of this sometimes therapy-defying disorder of development and behavior. Probably no patient is more grateful than a successful graduate of an encopresis treatment protocol.

EXAMPLE

A 13-year-old boy is suspended from school because neither his teachers nor his classmates can stand being around him. There are concerns as well about his mental health because much of his conversation refers to life in a distant galaxy, Bright Star, the subject of a novel he is writing, which he brings to the clinic. In the clinic waiting room, other families give him and his mother plenty of space. In the closed confines of the examination room, the smell is nearly overwhelming. Later, when the boy and his mother have left, a delegation of clinic nurses and secretaries march into the examination room and demand that the patient never be allowed to return. What is going on?

This unfortunate youth had long-standing, untreated encopresis. His near-constant state of fecal soiling accompanied by a perhaps acquired near-total neglect of personal hygiene in general caused him to become a pariah in the eyes (and noses) of his teachers and classmates. His sense of alienation from others had advanced to such a degree that his thought processes bordered on the delusional, no doubt an accommodation to and a defense against personal isolation.

While the circumstances of an encopretic child are not always as dramatic as in this case, a child with encopresis and his or her family can often feel isolated and hopeless as a result of the problem. Toileting in general and defecation in particular are sensitive subjects about which people do not like to converse. The secrecy and shame often attendant upon these subjects is immense when the function is disordered or out of control.

Statement of Problem

Encopresis, or fecal soiling, is a distressing and surprisingly common disorder of children. The reported prevalence of encopresis among 7- and 8-year-old children is 2.3% for boys and 1.3% for girls (Bellman, 1966), and among 10- to 12-year-olds it is 1.3% and 0.3%, respectively (Rutter, 1975). The male to female ratio for encopresis ranges from 2.5:1 to 6:1. In two studies, encopresis accounted for 3%

of visits to a general pediatric outpatient clinic (Levine, 1975; Loening-Baucke, 1995). Functional fecal retention, often accompanied by fecal soiling, accounts for 25% of all children referred to a pediatric gastroenterologist. These prevalence figures are higher than most families and even clinicians are aware of. Many researchers and clinicians believe that the problem is probably more common than the literature might indicate. Both children and parents often feel hopeless and ashamed about the problem and try to keep it a secret, even from the doctor. That there is so much secrecy attendant upon the symptom should not be unexpected, as lack of control of bowel function is perceived as shameful and disgusting by many in society. To quote Levine (1992), who has written extensively on the subject, "In appreciating the tragedy of encopresis, one must conceptualize a human condition in which a child is ridiculed, shamed, or blamed (by himself and others) for something he did not cause and over which he has had little, if any, actual control."

Definition and Classification

According to *Diagnostic and Statistical Manual of Mental Disorders,* fourth edition *(DSM-IV)* (American Psychiatric Association, 1997), the criteria for the diagnosis of encopresis are as follows:

1. Repeated passage of feces into inappropriate places (e.g., clothing or floor), whether involuntary or intentional.
2. At least one such event a month for at least 3 months.
3. Chronologic age is at least 4 years (or equivalent developmental level).
4. The behavior is not due exclusively to the direct physiologic effects of a substance (e.g., laxatives) or a general medical condition except through a mechanism involving constipation.

That same manual goes on to code the disorder differentially as "with constipation and overflow incontinence" and "without constipation and overflow incontinence." This differentiation has important etiologic and therapeutic implications, as will be seen. Another means of classifying encopresis is *primary* (or continuous) and *secondary* (or discontinuous) subtypes. The former is often described by parents as the situation in which, in their eyes, the child has never successfully mastered toilet training; whereas the latter is the circumstance in which the child has had a significant period, 6 months or a year, of continuous bowel continence prior to the development of the symptom of bowel incontinence.

Pathogenesis: Vulnerable Stages and Symptom Potentiation

In discussing the pathogenesis of encopresis, it is helpful to paraphrase Shakespeare: Some children are born encopretic; some children achieve encopresis; and some children have encopresis thrust upon them. Ninety-five percent of children with fecal incontinence have encopresis in association with functional constipation. Constipation alone, however, is not the sole risk factor present for most children with encopresis; but it is, probably, the most powerful predisposing condition.

Levine (1992) describes a useful framework for thinking about the development of fecal soiling (Table 43–1), in which he describes critical stages in the potentiation of encopresis as a function of age and developmental level. In most children with encopresis, more than one of these potentiating factors can be recognized as having played a role in the pathogenesis of the problem.

Defining the exact etiology in any given child may be less important than recognizing potential contributing factors in young children and providing intervention and anticipatory guidance with the goal of preventing the occurrence of the problem later on.

Table 43–1 • Critical Stages in the Potentiation of Encopresis*

Stage I potentiators (infancy and toddler years)
Simple constipation
Early colonic inertia
Congenital anorectal problems
Other anorectal conditions
Parental overreaction
Coercive medical interventions
Stage II potentiators (training and autonomy—3 to 5 years)
Psychosocial stresses during training period
Coercive or extremely permissive training
Idiosyncratic toilet fears
Painful or difficult defecation
Stage III potentiators (extramural function—early school years)
Avoidance of school bathrooms
Prolonged or acute gastroenteritis
Attention deficits with task impersistence
Possibly food intolerance, including lactase deficiency
Frenetic lifestyles
Psychosocial stress

*Children who ultimately develop encopresis are likely to have accumulated multiple risk factors on this list.

STAGE I: EARLY EXPERIENCE AND CONSTITUTIONAL PREDISPOSITION

Infants and toddlers born with a tendency toward constipation, whether on a genetic basis or in response to other factors such as changes in the type of milk they are consuming, are at risk for the later development of encopresis. Aggressive management of constipation in the first few years of life can often prevent the eventual development of encopresis (Loening-Baucke, 1993). Constipated infants and toddlers have an increased vulnerability for the development of encopresis, because of both their tendency toward "colonic inertia" and the secondary effects of chronic constipation: large or hard stools that cause pain when they are passed. Infants and toddlers, like people at any age of life, desire the avoidance of pain and learn how to withhold bowel movements to avoid pain. Later, this learned ability to avoid the passage of stools can be recognized by parents who witness the children stiffening and hyperextending their bodies in an effort to prevent the passage of stools. Because these events often occur simultaneously with a soiling episode, parents often interpret them as the child's deliberate act of defecation into the clothes, sometimes increasing the intrafamilial tension surrounding the soiling.

STAGE II: TRAINING AND EARLY AUTONOMY

Under the best of circumstances, the toilet training process can be difficult or confusing to a child. Successful toilet training represents the mastery of a number of complex skills, skills that must be employed under the proper circumstances and in the correct order to allow for the accomplishment of the task at hand (see box). There are inevitable false starts, and progress does not usually proceed in a series of steady advances, but rather with advances and setbacks. These developmental skills take years to master.

> An infant (without constipation) has no difficulty passing stools because she makes no attempt to exercise control over this function. In contrast, a 5-year-old child is able to perceive the urge to defecate, suppress the impulse to pass stool immediately, leave off from whatever activity, such as play, in which she is engaged, find a bathroom, make sure she has privacy (this need may vary from child to child), loosen or take off her clothes, sit down on the toilet, initiate the passage of stool, recognize when finished, get off the toilet, wipe herself (a developmental skill little remarked upon, with a likely wide age range for developmental attainment), refasten or put on her clothes once more, wash her hands, open the door (if it is closed), and be prepared to resume her previous activity.

Any intercurrent stresses during the toilet training process can prove distracting to the child or the parent, or both. Common sources of distraction are the birth of a new sibling, the mother's returning to work, parents' marital discord, or combinations of these and other factors. If parental expectations are too high or tolerance for uneven progress is too low, anxiety and confusion can be the result for the child. Oftentimes this confusion manifests as fecal withholding: the child is unsure what to do but senses that there is something wrong with allowing the passage of stool. Any tendency toward fecal withholding, whether as the result of constipation or deliberate withholding, can then compound the difficulty by leading to painful stools, which further condition the child to withhold stool.

STAGE III: EXTRAMURAL FUNCTION

As one author (Anthony, 1957) observed over 40 years ago, "The battle of the bowel seemingly won in the nursery is destined to be lost on the playing field at school." These are the children who have constipation thrust upon them and often present as secondary encopretics.

Children who have successfully mastered toilet training at home have their normal routine interrupted by their attendance at school. Instead of the safe, familiar environment, including bathroom, at home, they are faced with the choice of accommodating their biological rhythms to a new routine and using the school bathroom or withholding stool until they return home. The former option is often unappealing for a variety of reasons. Children may be reluctant to call attention to their need to have a bowel movement by asking to be excused from class to use the bathroom. The bathrooms themselves may prove to be powerful disincentives for their use. As stated by Levine (1992), "A child who used to defecate each morning at 11 AM at home may discover that there are no doors in front of the toilets or that the school lavatory is a well-publicized amphitheater with a varied program of humiliating scenarios."

A very potent contributing factor, which probably plays a role at any age but is most easily identified in school-aged children, is concomitant attention-deficit disorder with its attendant task impersistence. Children with attention problems often have a difficult time sitting still to complete any activity, including passing stool. In addition, the urge to defecate may pass through their minds but be supplanted by other thoughts before the child takes the time to act on that urge. If these events happen often, which is likely, the end result is chronic fecal retention and ultimate loss of the ability to completely sense the urge to have a bowel movement.

Busy schedules—school, music lessons, soccer practice, the parents' agenda—and inadequate availability of bathrooms at home or at school can also contribute to a child's withholding of stool. Also, psychosocial stresses, as at early ages, can prove sufficiently distracting to prevent a child's paying full attention to an urge to defecate. Stressors such as physical or sexual abuse can also play a role. In both instances, the distraction created by the powerful emotional disturbance is more commonly responsible for the fecal soiling than the direct physical effect of the particular abusive behaviors, including sodomy. The urge, if not acted upon, will go away, but the increasing amount of stool in the rectum will not.

Other potentiating factors include prolonged illnesses, especially ones involving the gastrointestinal tract, or injuries that result in prolonged inactivity, which can alter bowel function, again producing fecal retention.

Etiology

In most cases, regardless of the specific pathogenetic factors involved, fecal retention and the consequent loss of sensation of rectal distention and overflow incontinence are the final common pathway in the development of encopresis (Fig. 43–1). Chronic fecal retention, stool withholding, and incomplete defecation result in an overdistended rectum. The normal mechanism by which the child senses rectal fullness is subverted. Instead, the rectal walls are chronically stretched and the tissue architecture itself thereby distorted such that the child's awareness of rectal distention is dulled. Although the child may not sense rectal fullness and therefore does not know when to leave off from the activity in which she is engaged, stool nonetheless is produced and continues to fill and distend the rectum. Fecal incontinence comes about in one of two ways. Either new, liquid stool from the proximal colon leaks around and through the interstices created by the obstructing fecal mass in the distal colon and rectum; or, when a critical mass of stool accumulates in the rectum, a

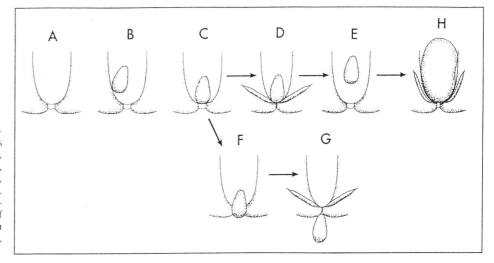

Figure 43–1. Diagrammatic representation of the sequence of events during defecation, fecal continence, and chronic fecal retention. A, B, C, F, G: Normal defecation. A, B, C, D, E, H: Pathway of fecal retention. (Reprinted from Fleisher DR: Diagnosis and treatment of disorders of defecation in children. Pediatr Ann 5:701, 1976; SLACK Incorporated, Thorofare, NJ.)

Table 43–2 • Disorders of Defecation

Soiling Without Retention		Retention With or Without Soiling	
Organic	*Functional*	*Organic*	*Functional*

Diarrheal diseases
Rectal pull-through surgery (without stenosis)
Occult spinal dysraphism
	Functional nonretentive fecal soiling
	Spock-Bergen syndrome
	Prolonged use of diapers for defecation
		Motility failures
		  Hirschsprung disease
		  Pseudoobstruction
		  MEN III
		Impaired Valsalva maneuver
		Pharmacologic and endocrinologic causes of fecal stasis
			Functional fecal retention syndrome caused by physically and/or emotionally difficult bowel movements

MEN = multiple endocrine neoplasia.
From Hyman PE, Fleischer DR: A classification of disorders of defecation in infants and children. Semin Gastrointest Dis 5:20, 1994.

process akin to the calving of a glacier occurs and stool falls out into the child's clothing. The latter process seems to be more common.

Other Causes of Fecal Incontinence

When a child presents with fecal soiling, it is important to bear in mind other causes for the symptom (Table 43–2). It is helpful to distinguish whether the soiling is or is not accompanied by fecal retention.

Organic causes of soiling in the absence of fecal retention include diarrheal diseases like giardiasis, which may exhaust the pelvic floor muscles' ability to maintain continence. Children born with imperforate anus may have fecal incontinence because of misplacement of the rectum or damage to the levator muscles during surgery. Impairment of corticospinal pathways or the cauda equina because of occult or obvious spinal dysraphism also may produce fecal incontinence.

Functional disorders causing fecal soiling in the absence of fecal retention are behavioral in origin. Most children who soil in the absence of fecal retention are young, and their soiling represents incomplete or disordered toilet training. Some preschool-aged or early school-aged children use the toilet appropriately for urination but insist on the use of a diaper for defecation. Alternatively, they refuse to use the toilet for bowel movements during the day but will pass stool into a diaper while asleep at night. This behavior probably represents overanxiousness on the part of the child who is reluctant to try something new, that is, passing stool on the toilet. This problem can be complicated by overly coercive interventions by the parents or physician, which can cause fecal retention where none had existed. In those instances, it is important to encourage bowel regularity first, and defecating in the toilet only after the child has overcome his anxiety about using the toilet. Another functional cause of delayed toileting skills, again uncommon, is the Spock-Bergen syndrome. Fecal incontinence results from parental ambivalence regarding toilet training, an apparent result of excessive fears regarding the risk of causing emotional trauma to the child undergoing toilet training.

There are children who soil more or less deliberately and probably out of anger, the result of a disordered parent-child relationship. It should be emphasized that such children make up a tiny fraction of children who present with fecal incontinence and can probably be recognized both by the absence of fecal retention and by the presence of other irritating behaviors and psychiatric symptoms.

Organic causes of fecal soiling that may present with or without fecal retention include motility disorders of the colon, the most important of which is Hirschsprung disease (congenital aganglionic megacolon) (Table 43–3). Hirschsprung disease is rare, the incidence being approximately 1 in 5000 births. The child with encopresis usually appears healthy and well-nourished, whereas the child with Hirschsprung disease is likely to look wasted and chronically ill and to have had intermittent obstructive symptoms. Most often, the bowel symptoms of children with Hirschsprung disease present early in infancy, whereas symptoms of encopresis present later in childhood. Also, children with encopresis often have a history of producing large-caliber

Table 43–3 • Encopresis and Hirschsprung Disease

	Encopresis	Hirschsprung Disease
Stool incontinence	Always	Rare
Constipation	Common, may be intermittent	Always present
Symptoms as newborn	Rare	Almost always
Infant constipation	Sometimes	Common
Late onset (after age 3 years)	Common	Rare
Problem in bowel training	Common	Rare
Avoidance of toilet	Common	Rare
Failure to thrive	Rare	Common
Anemia	None	Common
Obstructive symptoms	Rare	Common
Stool in ampulla	Common	Rare
Loose or tight sphincter tone	Rare	Common
Large-caliber stool	Common	Never
Preponderance of males	86%	90%
Incidence	1.5% at age 7 or 8	1 in 25,000 births
Anal manometry	Sometimes abnormal	Always abnormal

stools, while those with Hirschsprung disease are more likely to produce thin, ribbony stools.

Evaluation

HISTORY

It is important to openly discuss the presenting symptoms and associated findings commonly present in children with fecal soiling, with both the parent and the child. This can serve both a diagnostic and a therapeutic function. There are many clinical manifestations common to most children with encopresis. Questioning the child and his or her parent about the presence of these common features can be reassuring because of the implicit acknowledgment of how frequently the disorder is encountered. Also, asking the child and parent these questions provides a natural lead-in to a discussion of the many day-to-day issues that encopretic children and their parents grapple with.

Particular attention should be paid to the child's past and current habits with regard to bowel movements during infancy, the toilet training process, and enrollment in day care or school. A thorough discussion of the possible staged potentiators previously discussed is important to elucidate how the particular child became encopretic; an explanation is often sought by the parents. Also, any ongoing factors responsible for the encopresis need to be addressed to prevent perpetuation of the problem.

Most children soil between 3 and 7 PM, that is, after school, commonly on the way home from school. Soiling at school is usually a marker of a more severe problem. Very rarely do children soil during sleep. Soiling frequency varies from several times per day to less often, with severity most often reflected by frequency. Many parents (but not all) perceive that encopretic children pass large-caliber stools and sometimes even clog the toilet with feces when they defecate in the toilet. It is surprising how often parents respond with a "how did you know?" when asked if they keep a broomstick in the bathroom to break up their child's feces before attempting to flush them down. Absence of a report of large-caliber stools is not always reliable, however, as objective standards for stool caliber do not exist and many parents do not look at their child's stools anyway.

It is important to elicit and discuss three historical features that are frequently the source of conflict between encopretic children and their parents. The children often hide their soiled underwear, an expression of denial and shame, which usually only serves to increase the parents' aggravation. Parents can be lulled into a false sense of complacency because they see fewer soiled underpants, only to be disappointed when either the child has no more underwear or the cache of soiled underpants is discovered by the family dog. Also, most children with encopresis have lost the ability to sense rectal fullness. This is a difficult point to elicit because the child will often say he does feel the urge when he really does not, or the parent cannot believe that the child cannot appreciate the need to pass stool. Children with encopresis often become inured to the fecal odor that accompanies them. These are difficult points for parents to grasp and common sources of aggravation.

It is important to ask about previous efforts to deal with the problem. Parents often attribute their child's symptom to laziness. Punishment is often employed because of the parents' perception that the soiling is a willful behavior. The frequent history of retentive posturing, often witnessed but misinterpreted by the parents, in which the child desperately attempts to preserve continence by intentionally contracting the gluteal and pelvic floor muscles, may contribute to that perception. Children have often had some form of medical intervention in the past, with or without successful outcomes. Oftentimes the earlier intervention did not succeed because it was limited or there was inadequate follow-up. In some studies, a lot of earlier medical intervention is a poor prognostic feature, either because previously treated children represent more difficult cases or because failed treatment is a marker for inadequate compliance.

Associated symptoms often include constipation, abdominal pain, decreased appetite, daytime urinary incontinence, nocturnal enuresis, and recurrent urinary tract infections. Constipation is here defined as stools less often than every other day or the passage of painful stools because of large size or hard consistency. Some parents of children with encopresis do not perceive their children to be constipated because the child has daily bowel movements, in which case it is helpful to point out that the child may be having a daily bowel movement that is incomplete, that is, the child is not effectively emptying his or her rectum. Abdominal pain, a complaint in 50% to 60% of cases, is especially prominent in those instances that constipation is severe. The parents often report the complaint of abdominal pain with a long interval between bowel movements. Abdominal distention follows a similar pattern. Appetite suppression is often noted in retrospect, when the appetite improves after the child is successfully treated. Urinary incontinence during the day has been reported in 27% of children with encopresis. The urinary incontinence can often be attributed to crowding within the abdomen brought about by the fecal retention (Fig. 43–2). It often resolves when the fecal retention is relieved. Nocturnal enuresis is present in 30% to 40% of children with encopresis but is less likely to resolve with treatment of the fecal retention (Loening-Baucke, 1995). A common and little discussed syndrome occurs in girls who have encopresis, urinary incontinence, and recurrent urinary tract infections. Treatment of the encopresis often brings dramatic relief of the other symptoms (O'Regan, Yazbeck, and Schick, 1985).

PHYSICAL EXAMINATION AND OTHER STUDIES

Evaluation of the problem of fecal soiling should include a complete physical examination. Special attention should be directed to the child's general appearance, including an assessment of personal hygiene, growth percentiles, and abdominal, rectal, and neurologic examinations. Children with encopresis are usually otherwise healthy and do not have a sickly appearance.

Abdominal examination may reveal distention and a nontender, sausage-shaped mass, most often in the left lower quadrant. The absence of such a mass, however, does not rule out fecal retention because some children

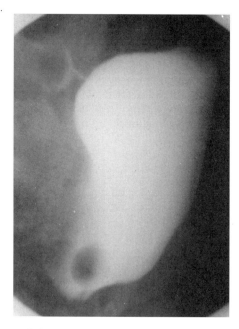

Figure 43–2. Voiding cystourethrogram in a constipated child.

are obese or excessively ticklish, causing this part of the examination to be less reliable.

It is important to inspect the anus, paying particular attention to the presence or absence of soiling and whether the anus is patulous. Evidence of scarring or other signs of trauma such as anal fissures should be noted. Anterior displacement of the anus, the mildest form of the anal atresia spectrum, can be ruled out by noting its relation to the posterior fourchette of the vagina in girls and the base of the scrotum in boys. In girls, the distance between the posterior fourchette and the anus should be at least one third the distance between the posterior fourchette and coccyx, while in boys the scrotoanal distance should be half the scrotococcygeal distance (Reisner et al, 1984). Anal sensation and the anal wink reflex can be assessed by light touch of the anus.

Digital rectal examination should be done to determine sphincter tone and the contents of the rectum. A large amount of stool in the rectum has a high positive predictive value for the presence of fecal retention, although no stool in the rectum has a low negative predictive value for fecal retention (Rockney, McQuade, and Days, 1995). In the latter case, a plain abdominal radiograph can be obtained to look for evidence of fecal retention (Barr et al, 1979) (Fig. 43–3). Use of the rectal examination to determine the presence of fecal retention is quicker and cheaper and does not expose the child to radiation. The abdominal radiograph may be preferred in situations in which the child is not willing to allow a rectal examination or if that examination is best deferred because of concern that the examination itself may be traumatic, such as when the child has suffered sexual abuse. A plain abdominal radiograph may also help to demystify the problem or educate the patient and his or her family about the underlying pathophysiology of the condition.

Neurologic examination should include assessment of deep tendon reflexes and gait. Visual inspection of the back should be carried out to look for evidence of occult spinal dysraphism.

In cases in which Hirschsprung disease is suspected, a barium enema examination can be useful. Such an examination can also be useful if a child has had surgery for anal atresia or Hirschsprung disease at a younger age but has persistent fecal incontinence. In both instances, a transition zone between aganglionic and ganglionic segments of the colon may be visualized, indicating the need for surgical intervention.

Anorectal manometry, if available, can be used to distinguish Hirschsprung disease from constipation with encopresis. Demonstration of internal anal sphincter relaxation with rectal balloon distention makes Hirschsprung disease unlikely. Use of biofeedback in conjunction with anorectal manometry has demonstrated improved short-term outcome from encopresis but has not increased long-term recovery above the conventional treatment as described subsequently (Loening-Baucke, 1995).

Management

Encopresis is an interesting clinical problem in that it presents a useful paradigm for the management of a behavioral pediatric disorder: behavioral and emotional issues are interwoven with actual physiologic derangement, and solution of the problem requires an integrated behavioral and medical approach. A very important part of treatment involves education about encopresis, which should include a description of its etiology and pathophysiology. Visual aids such as drawings, diagrams, and radiographs can help children and parents understand both the origin of the problem and the rationale for treatment (Fig. 43–4).

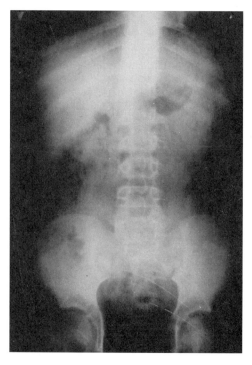

Figure 43–3. Plain abdominal radiograph.

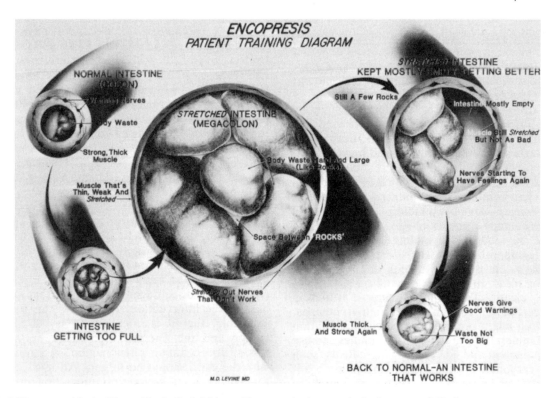

Figure 43–4. Diagram used in the "demystification" of children with encopresis. A poster-sized enlargement of this diagram serves to represent normal intestinal musculature, its distention with "rocks" of body waste, the development of a megacolon with stretched-out, thin muscles and nerves, the beginning resolution of the problem, and ultimately the restoration of normal function. This teaching aid can help the clinician during initial counseling of the child and parents. An enlarged reproduction of this diagram can be obtained by writing to Dr. Melvin D. Levine.

There is no universal agreement on the best approach to management of encopresis. Most approaches, however, involve a combination of bowel catharsis and behavior modification. Children without underlying fecal retention, if absence of fecal retention can be determined with certainty, should not undergo a bowel catharsis regimen. Instead, therapy should be focused on behavioral changes, especially bowel and diet habits, as described subsequently.

Because of the complex nature of the problem and the need for a long-term approach to therapy, it is rational to use a two-stage approach to treatment. At the first visit, after establishing a diagnosis of underlying fecal retention, some means of effecting bowel catharsis should be proposed. In almost all cases, the bowel catharsis procedure can be carried out at home. One approach is to employ a 2-week bowel catharsis regimen that consists of four consecutive 3-day cycles of treatment, each cycle consisting of an enema (day 1), a suppository (day 2), and a laxative tablet (day 3) (Table 43–4). Alternatives to this approach include daily enemas for 3 to 7 days depending on the output of feces, or high-dose mineral oil, up to 1 ounce per year of age, twice a day (Davidson, Kugler, and Bauer, 1963). The mineral oil treatment, which was the first method of achieving bowel catharsis to appear in the pediatric literature, is difficult because of children's lack of enthusiasm for consuming mineral oil, especially in high doses.

It is important to tell parents that successful completion of the bowel catharsis regimen does not guarantee a cure and that more and different therapy will be necessary

following its completion. There are instances when the response to the bowel catharsis program is so dramatically positive that the family does not comply with the follow-up appointment, only to have the child present several months later with a relapse of the encopresis.

In the rare instance in which the child and family have difficulty complying with a bowel catharsis regimen on their own, a visiting nurse service can be helpful. In very difficult-to-treat cases that have failed multiple attempts at outpatient management, bowel catharsis can be achieved in an inpatient setting. Because of third-party payor restrictions on hospital lengths of stay, bowel catharsis must be achieved more rapidly. Instead of one intervention per day, two (an enema and a suppository) may be necessary. Another approach in the inpatient setting is to use a balanced electrolyte solution (GoLYTELY) to flush

Table 43–4 • Encopresis Cleanout Regimen

Day 1	Fleet* enema (adult size)	Day 8	Dulcolax suppository
Day 2	Dulcolax† suppository	Day 9	Dulcolax tablet
Day 3	Dulcolax tablet	Day 10	Fleet enema
Day 4	Fleet enema	Day 11	Dulcolax suppository
Day 5	Dulcolax suppository	Day 12	Dulcolax tablet
Day 6	Dulcolax tablet	Day 13	Dulcolax tablet
Day 7	Fleet enema	Return to clinic	

*Monobasic sodium phosphate and dibasic sodium phosphate.
†Bisacodyl.

Table 43–5 • Bowel Continence Maintenance Program

1. Stool softener, e.g., mineral oil, at a starting dose of 2 tablespoons twice a day. Dose to be titrated to facilitate regular soft stools and avoid mineral oil leakage.
2. Daily multivitamin to guard against possibility of mineral oil interference with absorption of fat-soluble vitamins.
3. Other laxatives or stool softeners may be substituted for mineral oil (see Table 43–6).
4. Toilet sitting for 10 minutes each time at least twice a day at times child is most likely to have a bowel movement (upon awakening, after school, or after meals).
5. Encourage increased activity, increased fluids (other than milk, e.g., water and juices) and a high-fiber diet (25–35 g per day).

out the colon from above (Ingebo and Heyman, 1988). Because large volumes of fluid are necessary to clean out the colon (up to 40 mL/kg/hr), use of GoLYTELY most often necessitates placement of a nasogastric tube. Children brought into the hospital for bowel catharsis often require desensitization before invasive procedures such as enemas and nasogastric tube placement can be undertaken. Mental health professionals can often provide assistance in preparing these children to undergo such procedures.

It is important to assess the response to the bowel catharsis regimen as soon as possible upon its completion.

Over 30% of children still have fecal retention after a bowel catharsis regimen. This is especially likely if there has been poor or incomplete compliance with the suggested interventions. If compliance or response is poor, more education about the problem and suggested interventions and 1 to 2 more weeks of similar treatment are often necessary. Some children will require enemas in the clinic or office setting.

When bowel catharsis has been satisfactorily achieved, usually by parental report of abundant fecal production and decreased episodes of soiling, it is important to initiate a bowel continence maintenance program. The goals of this program are (1) no soiling; (2) regular (at least every other day) soft bowel movements; and (3) improvement in the ability to sense the urge to have a bowel movement. To achieve these goals, a list of suggestions (Table 43–5) should be given to families to help their child acquire bowel control. The main determinants of long-term bowel continence are good bowel habits and a diet conducive to fecal regularity. Subsequent follow-up visits are necessary to monitor and encourage progress and to individualize the specific interventions that are most helpful and acceptable to the child and parent.

There are many stool softeners and laxatives that can be used to encourage "hyper-regularity," that is, the production of frequent, soft bowel movements, to keep the

Table 43–6 • Medications for Constipation and Impaction

Medication	Dosage	Comments
Stool softeners		
Mineral oil	1–2 mL/kg/dose bid Adolescents: 60 mL/dose (max 8 oz/d)	Do not use in children with gastroesophageal reflux, vomiting, or who are not yet walking Emulsified types (Petrogalar, plain Agoral, Kondremul) taste better
Lactulose	0.5–1.0 mL/kg/dose bid Adolescents: 15 mL bid (max 3 oz/d)	This is a prescription item
Laxatives		
(Listed in order of increasing potency)		
Phillips' Milk of Magnesia (MOM) or Haley's M-O (75% MOM, 25% mineral oil)	1 mL/kg/dose bid Adolescents: 60 mL bid	1 tablet MOM = 2.5 mL liquid
Senokot	<5 yr: 1–2 tsp syrup >5 yr: 2–3 tsp syrup Adolescents: 1 tbsp (max 2.5 tbsp or 8 tablets)	1 tablet = 3 mL granules = 5 mL syrup
Fletcher's Castoria	<5 yr: 1–2 tsp >5 yr: 2–3 tsp Adolescents: 2 tbsp max	
Dulcolax, 5-mg tablet	>5 yr: 5 mg >12 yr: 10 mg (2 tablets) Adolescents: 4 tablets max	No liquid form
Phenolphthalein		Do not use because of prolonged gastrointestinal irritation
Rectal suppositories		
Glycerin suppository		
Dulcolax, 10-mg	>2 yr: 1 suppository	
Enemas		
Mineral oil enema	1–2 oz/20 lb of weight Adolescents: 4 oz	Squeeze bottle size: 4.5 oz
Sodium phosphate enema (Fleet)	1 oz/20 lb of weight Adolescents: 4 oz (max 8 oz)	Squeeze bottle size: 2.25 oz children, 4.5 oz adult

From Schmitt BD, Mauro RO: Twenty common errors in treating encopresis. Contemp Pediatrics May, pp 47–65, 1992. © 1992 by Medical Economics Company.

rectum relatively empty to allow for its attainment of a more normal configuration (Table 43–6). It is important that children with encopresis be maintained on at least one of these compounds for an extended length of time, anywhere from months to a year.

Prognosis

Outcome studies using the approach just described indicate a reasonably good prognosis 1 year after presentation and initiation of therapy, with 63% to 94% of cases showing improvement of symptoms (Bulut and Tekant, 1991; Gleghorn, Heyman, and Rudolph, 1991; Levine and Bakow, 1976; Nolan et al, 1991; Stark et al, 1990; Wakefield et al, 1984). In the only prospective clinical trial to document the benefit of laxative therapy in the management of encopresis, Nolan and colleagues (1991) showed 63% of encopretic patients to be in partial (noticeably improved since presentation) or complete (no soiling episodes for at least 1 month) remission. There are few long-term studies of outcome after treatment for encopresis (Davidson, Kugler, and Bauer, 1963; Loening-Baucke, 1995; Rockney et al, 1996). These studies indicate that achievement of remission becomes more likely as more time elapses between presentation and outcome assessment, indicating an unknown rate of spontaneous resolution of the symptom. There has never been (and probably never will be) a study to assess the rate of spontaneous remission from encopresis analogous to Forsythe and Redmond's study (1974) of the natural history of enuresis.

Encopresis is a chronic problem that is difficult to treat and prone to frequent relapses of symptoms. A significant number of encopretic children, 23% to 37%, do not respond to the treatment outlined earlier. Treatment failure can often be attributed to inadequate compliance or associated behavior problems that make good compliance less likely.

A more rigorous behavioral approach using group therapy can often be effective for the difficult-to-treat patients (Stark et al, 1990). The group therapy approach emphasizes education about encopresis and the integration of behavioral parenting procedures, specifically appropriate toileting habits and high fiber consumption, with medical management.

In the case presented at the beginning of the chapter, the boy responded well to the bowel catharsis regimen. At follow-up, he had regained control of his personal hygiene and he did not smell bad. His conversation focused on sports and girls rather than a distant galaxy.

REFERENCES

American Psychiatric Association: Diagnostic and Statistical Manual of Mental Disorders, 4th ed. Washington, DC, American Psychiatric Association, 1997.

Anthony EJ: An experimental approach to the psychopathology of childhood: Encopresis. Br J Med Psychol 30:146, 1957.

Barr RG, Levine MD, Wilkinson RH, Mulvihill D: Chronic and occult stool retention: a clinical tool for its evaluation in school-aged children. Clin Pediatr 18:674, 1979.

Bellman M: Studies on encopresis. Acta Pediatr Scan 170 (suppl):1, 1966.

Bulut M, Tekant G: Encopretic children: experience with fifty cases. Turk J Pediatr 33:167, 1991.

Davidson M, Kugler MM, Bauer CH: Diagnosis and management in children with severe and protracted constipation and obstipation. J Pediatr 62:261, 1963.

Forsythe WI, Redmond A: Enuresis and spontaneous cure rate: study of 1129 enuretics. Arch Dis Child 49:259, 1974.

Gleghorn EE, Heyman MB, Rudolph CD: No-enema therapy for idiopathic constipation and encopresis. Clin Pediatr 30:669, 1991.

Ingebo KB, Heyman MB: Polyethylene glycol-electrolyte solution for intestinal clearance in children with refractory encopresis. Am J Dis Child 142:340, 1988.

Levine MD: Children with encopresis: a descriptive analysis. Pediatrics 56:412, 1975.

Levine MD: Encopresis. *In* Levine MD, Cary WB, Crocker AC (eds): Developmental-Behavioral Pediatrics, 2nd ed. Philadelphia, WB Saunders, 1992, p 390.

Levine MD, Bakow H: Children with encopresis: a study of treatment outcome. Pediatrics 58:845, 1976.

Loening-Baucke V: Biofeedback treatment for chronic constipation and encopresis in childhood: long-term outcome. Pediatrics 96:105, 1995.

Loening-Baucke V: Constipation in early childhood: patient characteristics, treatment, and longterm follow up. Gut 34:1400, 1993.

Nolan T, Debelle G, Oberklaid F, Coffey C: Randomized trial of laxatives in the treatment of childhood encopresis. Lancet 338:523, 1991.

O'Regan S, Yazbeck S, Schick E: Constipation, bladder instability, urinary tract infection syndrome. Clin Nephrol 23:152, 1985.

Reisner SH, Sivan Y, Nitzan M, Merlob P: Determination of anterior displacement of the anus in newborn infants and children. Pediatrics 73:216, 1984.

Rockney RM, McQuade WH, Days AL: The plain abdominal radiograph in the management of encopresis. Arch Pediatr Adolesc Med 149:623, 1995.

Rockney RM, McQuade WH, Days AL, et al: Encopresis treatment outcome: long-term follow-up of 45 cases. J Dev Behav Pediatr 17:380, 1996.

Rutter M: Helping Troubled Children. Harmonds-Worth, England, Penguin Education, 1975.

Stark LJ, Owens-Stively J, Spirito A, et al: Group behavioral treatment of retentive encopresis. J Pediatr Psychol 15:659, 1990.

Wakefield MA, Woodbridge C, Steward J, et al: A treatment programme for faecal incontinence. Dev Med Child Neurol 26:6134, 1984.

44 Sleep Disorders

Henry L. Shapiro

 Children who fail at sleeping cause their parents and sometimes their pediatricians to endure sleepless lives themselves. A child's sleep deprivation can interfere with daytime function while creating high levels of anxiety for all concerned. Fortunately, our growing knowledge regarding the mechanisms underlying normal and perturbed sleep patterns contributes significantly to the intervention repertoire available to these children. In this chapter, the mechanisms are tied to a number of effective and practical therapeutic options.

The drive to sleep ranks with breathing, drinking, and eating in its intensity. Sleep problems are among the most common behavioral complaints in pediatric populations. Most sleep problems can be diagnosed and managed clinically even though special studies in the sleep laboratory may be necessary in some cases. This chapter reviews relevant aspects of normal sleep, common variations, classification of sleep problems in children, and current approaches to evaluation and treatment.

Normal Sleep and Its Variations

Sleep is a highly organized physiologic process with strong social and cultural influences. In this section, sleep stages, sleep rhythms, and developmental aspects of sleep are discussed. Sleep is a primordial biological rhythm (Webb, 1994). The concept of sleep stages was derived from relatively recent understanding of this complex rhythm. There are cyclic changes in arousability to sensory stimuli, electroencephalographic (EEG) waves, motor activity, and autonomic function.

SLEEP STAGES

From the standpoint of the EEG, sleep can be divided into (1) a "quiet" phase of low-voltage, increasingly synchronized activity and (2) an "active" rapid eye movement (REM) phase in which the pattern is more like a waking rhythm. After infancy, quiet sleep is divided into four stages of non-REM (NREM) sleep. Stages I and II are transitional stages, marked by characteristic EEG patterns that include K-complexes and sleep spindles, and have a relatively low threshold for arousal. Stages III and IV are defined by synchronized EEG activity referred to as slow-wave sleep (SWS). A very high-sensory threshold of arousal characterizes this "deep" phase of sleep. REM sleep is characterized by a low threshold to nonmeaningful stimuli, rapid eye movements, dreaming, central skeletal muscle paralysis, and increased autonomic variability. In REM sleep, meaningful environmental stimuli are often incorporated into dream content instead of causing arousal. Normal individuals experience recurring cycles of stages I

through IV, followed by a period of REM sleep. There are normal periods of wakefulness (arousal) between each sleep cycle (stages I through IV plus REM). The sleeper usually forgets these arousals because of anterograde and retrograde amnesia that occurs after sleep onset. The relative "volume" of each of these stages varies both by age and over the course of each night. SWS predominates during the first few cycles, and REM predominates during the final cycles during the night.

There is a physiologic need for both REM and SWS. Individuals who are deprived of these stages tend to make them up on subsequent nights. This is true both for total sleep-deprived individuals (both adults and children) and for individuals selectively deprived of specific stages. The increasing "pressure" for REM and SWS can be relieved only by sleep. "Sleep intrusions" in the form of microsleep, characterized by EEG-identifiable sleep lasting as short as 30 seconds, are inevitable with sleep deprivation.

SLEEP LATENCY

Sleep latency is the time between the attempts to sleep and EEG-identifiable sleep. In the laboratory, this can be measured by the Multiple Sleep Latency Test (MSLT), which consists of five attempted daytime naps taken every 2 hours. Normal sleep latency varies from 7 to 20 minutes and follows a characteristic circasemidian (12-hour) rhythm and is at its nadir in the middle of the sleep period and 12 hours later. The greatest sleep latency (resistance to sleep) occurs in between these nadirs. "Night owls" and "larks" represent the temperamental extremes in the timing of the sleep phase.

Sleep rhythms come in multiples of the Basic Rest Activity Cycle, the circa 90-minute cycle described by Kleitman and his followers (Webb, 1994). This "ultradian" rhythm is present in many animal species, including birds and mammals, and persists through both sleep and wakefulness. In addition to this 90-minute cycle, there is the well-known daily (circadian) cycle as well as a clear-cut 12-hour (circasemidian) rhythms.

These rhythms are normally in phase with the solar day because of physiologic entrainment of intrinsic pacemakers such as the circadian clock. Environmental cues or "Zeitgebers" can reset (entrain) the pacemakers. The strongest of these cues is the light-dark cycle, which is responsible for setting the biological clock on a daily basis. Zeitgebers include social routines such as working, eating, bathing, and travel. Without these external cues, rhythms become free-running, usually with a time period slightly longer than the 24-hour solar day. Totally blind individuals who are otherwise neurologically normal often have a great deal of difficulty maintaining a normal 24-hour schedule, and their free-running rhythms often lead to fragmented or disrupted sleep patterns. Developmentally disabled individuals may have difficulty regulating their sleep patterns and often require highly predictable and structured environments. Melatonin, a serotonin derivative produced by the pineal gland, is one of the primary neurochemicals involved with sleep regulation. Its secretion is strongly inhibited by light. Exogenous melatonin may be helpful in entraining sleep rhythms in blind and severely disabled children (Jan, Espezel, and Appleton, 1994).

DEVELOPMENTAL ASPECTS (SLEEP ONTOGENY)

Newborn infants sleep for 16 to 18 hours a day and spend the majority of their time in REM sleep. As children get older, this time is broken up with periods of wakefulness and frequent naps. Consolidation of these cycles (sleeping through the night) varies greatly and may not occur until the end of the 1st year of life in many children. Because of the well-known pattern of separation-related sleep problems that occur as object permanence develops, some normal children do not sleep through the night until well into their 2nd year. Napping also follows a well-described developmental pattern (Weissbluth, 1995). In nonsiesta cultures, naps are probably abandoned almost universally by middle childhood. By age 7 years, total sleep time is approximately 10 hours. For adolescents, total sleep requirements are similar to adults', 7 to 9 hours, but there is a well-recognized delay in sleep phase, leading to later bedtimes and more difficulty waking in the morning (Carskadon, Vieira, and Acebo, 1993).

SLEEP AND COGNITION

Dahl (1996) has reviewed the work in the area of cognitive and behavioral effects of sleep loss. Much of the information regarding attention, memory, executive functioning, and cognition comes from studies of sleep deprivation in normal adult volunteers. There are only a few studies involving children. Both experimental and observational studies suggest that there are a variety of specific problems that appear to be related to sleep restriction. These include deficits of focused attention, motivation, and effort; emotional self-regulation; short-term memory; and memory consolidation. Children with sleep restriction share many characteristics of children diagnosed with attention-deficit hyperactivity disorder, although previously normal children may show these symptoms when acutely or chronically deprived of sleep.

Limited data suggest that treatment of the sleep problem may resolve many of the cognitive and behavioral problems attributed to the sleep restriction. The associations of sleep problems in children who have developmental variations of attention, higher-order cognitive executive functions, memory, and self-regulation are less well understood. Sleep disorders, like environmental factors and general medical conditions, should be considered in the differential diagnosis of learning and behavioral problems.

Sleep Problems

Herein, the term *problem* is used interchangeably with the term *disorder*, recognizing the difficulty of making a distinction. Temperamental differences become problems when they lead to sleep loss and difficulty with daytime functioning. This discussion generally follows the 1990 nosology of sleep (Table 44–1), which includes problems seen in childhood but is primarily derived from the study of adults (Thorpy, 1994).

GENERAL CLINICAL APPROACHES

The sleep history is the most important part of diagnosing the sleep problem (Table 44–2). Obtaining the history takes about an hour and is often made more efficient by having parents fill out questionnaires before the child is seen by the clinician. Areas that are often overlooked include identifying barriers to therapy and a detailed physical description of the sleep environment. Having parents complete a 2-week sleep log before the first visit is often instructive. An example is available at the author's World Wide Web site, http://www.dbpeds.org.

A general physical and neurologic examination is indicated in all children. A more extensive neurodevelopmental examination is indicated when there are associated

---

Table 44–1 • Summary Classification of Pediatric Sleep Disorders

Dyssomnias
  Intrinsic sleep disorders (e.g., obstructive sleep apnea, narcolepsy, restless legs syndrome)
  Extrinsic sleep disorders (e.g., limit-setting disorder)
  Circadian rhythm sleep disorders (e.g., delayed or advanced sleep phase)
Parasomnias
  Arousal disorders (e.g., sleepwalking, sleep terrors)
  Sleep-wake transition disorders (e.g., head banging, sleep talking)
  REM parasomnias (e.g., nightmares, sleep paralysis)
  Other parasomnias (e.g., bruxism, enuresis, sudden infant death syndrome)
Medical-psychiatric sleep disorders
  Associated with other mental disorders (e.g., psychoses, mood and anxiety disorders)
  Associated with neurologic disorders (e.g., headache, epilepsy, degenerative disorders)
  Associated with other medical disorders (e.g., asthma, gastroesophageal reflux, pain)
Proposed sleep disorders (e.g., short sleeper, menstrual-associated sleep disorder)

Adapted from Thorpy MJ: Classification of sleep disorders. *In* Kryger MH, et al (eds): Principles and Practice of Sleep Medicine. Philadelphia, WB Saunders, 1994, pp 426–436. Copyright 1990, International Classification of Sleep Disorders, American Sleep Disorders Association, reprinted by permission.

Table 44–2 • Sleep History

Description of problem	Otitis media
Duration	Chronic pain (e.g. arthritis)
Impact on family	Reflux esophagitis
Associated problems	Hypothalamic/pituitary
Description of sleep behavior	dysfunction
Sleep routines and	Medications
associations	Neurologic disorders
Sleep environment	Other symptoms
Bed partners	Daytime sleepiness
Snoring	Cataplexy
Sleep position	Sleep paralysis
Description/video of	School failure
behaviors	Hyperactivity and irritability
Two-week sleep log	Depression
Developmental and behavioral	Interventions tried
history	Medications
Birth factors	Changes in sleep environment
Temperament	Sleep associations and rituals
Development	Cautions and warning signs
Behavior	Seizure symptoms
Learning	High-risk social situation
Emotional	Potential barriers to therapy
Sexual abuse and trauma	Attitudes and beliefs
Medical and family history	Lack of resources and support
Asthma and allergy	Parental secondary gain

developmental concerns. The clinical approach varies according to the setting of the practitioner. Laboratory investigations such as polysomnography can be helpful but are not needed in most cases.

Sleep is a window into an individual's social, emotional, and family functioning. Psychiatric, neurologic, and general medical conditions can disrupt sleep, leading to both nighttime and daytime symptoms. Medications and other substances have an impact on sleep as well. Ferber (1995) writes that 23% to 33% of 1- and 2-year-olds exhibit enough night-waking to worry their parents and that up to one third of preschoolers exhibit night-wakings.

Cultural differences have a large impact on many sleep practices. Co-sleeping is a good example. The current medical opinion against co-sleeping with infants and young children needs to be re-evaluated because there is evidence from multicultural studies (Lozoff, Askew, and Wolf, 1996) that co-sleeping has benefits and is more "normal" from the standpoint of evolution (McKenna and Mosko, 1994). It is important for the clinician to avoid labeling a cultural preference as a problem in the absence of parental concerns.

SLEEPLESSNESS

Refusal to go to bed or nap, sleep onset problems, and sleep maintenance problems are common in young children, and they are rarely due to an intrinsic disorder of sleep. It is helpful to distinguish between a disorder of initiating and maintaining sleep as a result of medical factors and the wide variety of environmental, behavioral, and social factors that lead to the complaint of sleeplessness. It is rare for younger children to become sleep deprived because they tend to make up the sleep on their own. Parents, however, can rarely recover their lost sleep. Sleepy parents show performance deficits, leading to further impairment in their ability to set limits, maintain consistent rules, and be patient.

Ferber (1995) points out the need to divide the phenomenon of sleeplessness into categories by age and mechanism. Fragmentation of sleep and frequent night-wakings are normal in infants and toddlers and may persist in up to 33% of 1- and 2-year olds. Nighttime feedings may contribute to this problem, especially because increased fluid intake leads to increased urination. The colic syndrome is associated with night-wakings in infants. Conditions such as otitis media, gastroesophageal reflux, and possibly food allergy have been implicated as medical causes of sleep disturbance in infants and toddlers. Preschool and school-aged children have more complicated causes of sleeplessness.

Older children often fight or stall sleep. Even though this is often referred to as a limit-setting disorder, this appears to be an oversimplification of complex interactional problems. Children vary in their ability to self-soothe and their tendency to signal when distressed. It is important to explore parental beliefs, temperamental issues, and the family context before simply instructing parents to "set limits and be consistent," even though this is certainly good advice in otherwise well-functioning families.

Treatment of behavioral sleep disorders relies on a cognitive behavioral framework, consisting of teaching the patient and family about the relevant aspects of sleep physiology, describing a step-by-step behavior plan, and monitoring and supporting the implementation of the plan. The most effective approaches to bedtime tantrums and night-wakings are based on changing sleep associations by extinction and reinforcement of other behaviors. Ferber (1986) made a great contribution by describing and popularizing approaches to these common problems.

Simple ignoring ("let them cry it out") is effective, but unpopular with parents (and children). Variations of ignoring, such as graduated extinction, are effective, as is introducing positive bedtime routines (Adams and Rickert, 1989). Both procedures begin with putting the child to bed around the child's usual sleep time, which is often considerably later than the child's bedtime. Time in bed should be limited to the typical sleep duration (determined by history and review of the sleep log).

In *graduated extinction*, parents are trained to ignore the protests for short time periods determined by the child's age and the parents' estimate of how long they could ignore the behavior. Parents are allowed to check or comfort their child between intervals for 15 seconds but otherwise are to firmly return the child to bed. The intervals are lengthened on a weekly basis.

Positive routines consist of quiet activities that the child is trained to do by himself or herself at bedtime. These routines should last no longer than 20 minutes. If children protest or have a tantrum after the routines are over, the child is firmly redirected to bed. Children should initially be put to bed close to the actual time they fall asleep, even if it is later than the desired bedtime. Parents should be told to expect a treatment period of 6 to 8 weeks, after which the bedtime can be gradually adjusted to an earlier time. If problems re-emerge, parents should be praised for their attempts and instructed to restart at an earlier part of the sequence.

EXAMPLE: 30-MONTH-OLD WITH BEDTIME STRUGGLES

History: A 30-month-old child had persistent bedtime struggles for 3 months and the problem was thought to be severe. The child's mother reported nearly falling asleep while driving on two occasions, and the father reported that his job performance was suffering. A sleep log showed that the problem occurred almost every weeknight and occasionally on weekends. The total sleep time was about 11 hours because of daytime naps. The problem started with frequent episodes of the child calling out for the parents, requesting a drink, or coming to the parents' bed. When ignored, the child became increasingly irritable and started having nightly temper tantrums when put to bed. The parents were up nightly with the child to avoid these tantrums. There were no signs of daytime emotional or behavioral problems, and medical and neurodevelopmental examinations were normal.

Diagnosis: Limit-setting disorder in a "signaler" with secondary parental sleep deprivation without significant comorbid family dysfunction or attachment problems.

Intervention: The parents were counseled about normal sleep function and sleep hygiene and were given different options of treatment including a checking routine and positive routines. They agreed on a realistic goal of reducing the behavior. The parents chose a hybrid approach with frequent checking and reassurance after establishing a brief bedtime ritual for about 2 weeks. Each parent was assigned a night, or portion of the night, to be responsible for this routine. A simple calendar was made to monitor the therapy. The parents were warned about the possibility of an "extinction burst," but they were counseled that this is actually a sign that their strategy was likely to be effective. The problem was largely resolved at the 2-week follow-up visit.

SLEEP PHASE PROBLEMS

Delayed sleep phase syndrome is frequent enough in adolescents to be considered a normal variation. Beyond the normal variation of morning or evening preferences, some children experience significant delays or advances in sleep phase, leading to complaints of evening or morning insomnia, respectively. There are also individuals who seem to be short sleepers on a constitutional basis. They wake up refreshed and function well despite shorter than normal sleep times.

Adolescents typically exhibit a normal, physiologic delay in sleep phase, resulting in late hours, reduced sleep on school days, and weekend recovery sleep (Dahl and Carskadon, 1995). Adolescents complain of inadequate sleep and sleep onset insomnia, often staying up more than 2 hours beyond their desired bedtime. Social and emotional issues, substance abuse, medication use, and environmental factors are increasingly present in this age group and should be ruled out. Adolescents may also "voluntarily" stay up and develop irregular sleep patterns. Habits formed in adolescence may persist into adulthood, leading to a more chronic sleep disorder. Because parents are less affected by the adolescent's sleep problem (in that their own sleep may not be disrupted), the physician may not become aware of adolescent sleep dysfunction except in extreme cases.

Treatment of delayed sleep phase problems relies on sleep hygiene (Table 44–3) and schedule manipulation. In addition to sleep hygiene measures, manipulation of the sleep schedule is often necessary to get adequate sleep time during the school week. Weekend replacement sleep may be essential for sleep-deprived adolescents. Later school starting times would be a possible solution, but in my experience, educators are not receptive to this idea because of school transportation issues. In a recent review, Regestein and Monk (1995) discuss different clinical approaches to this problem. Very gradual adjustments to an earlier bedtime (15 minutes a week) may work. It is sometimes possible to readjust the adolescent's sleep schedule by having him or her go to bed progressively later until the desired bedtime is achieved, with the adolescent being up at night and sleeping during the day for a period of time. This may take a few months and normally has to be done during an extended vacation. Delayed and advanced phase disorders may respond to morning or evening bright light exposure to force a shift in the circadian phase. Adolescents with phase delay should be encouraged to avoid bright lights in the evening and to get early morning bright light exposure. The opposite approach is effective for early morning insomnia.

SLEEPINESS

Excessive daytime sleepiness in middle childhood is always a cause for concern. Usually this is caused by sleep restriction, from either decreased total sleep time or disruptions in sleep. Voluntary sleep restriction also results in daytime sleepiness. Excessively sleepy children often fall asleep in the car, but they may fall asleep in other locations, such as school or church, or while reading if their sleepiness is more severe.

Narcolepsy is a serious, chronic cause of excessive daytime sleepiness that is being recognized more frequently in children and adolescents. It is rare, with a prevalence in the range of 0.04% to 0.1% (Dahl, Holttum, and Trubnick, 1994). The classic tetrad of narcolepsy consists of (1) irresistible attacks of daytime sleepiness in the setting of normal total sleep time, (2) cataplexy (loss of muscle tone during strong emotions leading to drop-attacks), (3) sleep-onset REM associated with hypnagogic hallucinations, and (4) sleep paralysis. Narcolepsy can be familial, and there

Table 44–3 • Sleep Hygiene

Provide quiet, dark, cool environment.
Keep bedtime ritual simple and reproducible by child.
Limit time in bed.
Limit nighttime feeding.
Use bedroom for sleeping only (e.g., not for homework, punishment)
Avoid medications.
Consider allergy prevention.
Consider effect of sleep partners (including pets).
Remove distractions (e.g., televisions, telephones, video games).
Maintain consistent 7-day schedule.
Avoid naps but allow for replacement sleep (e.g., in adolescents).

is an association with HLA types DR2 and DQw1, although HLA typing is not useful as a diagnostic test. Diagnosis of narcolepsy is by history, polysomnography, and formal evaluation of sleep latency, usually with the MSLT done in the sleep laboratory. Narcolepsy may present like an attention-deficit hyperactivity disorder in younger children or like a neurologic or psychiatric disorder.

Treatment of narcolepsy consists of scheduled naps and pharmacologic intervention, especially psychostimulants in relatively large doses. Patients benefit from support groups, because there may be significant occupational and social problems associated with narcolepsy.

There are some rare causes of hypersomnia such as the Kleine-Levin syndrome (hypersomnia, excessive eating or sexuality, and emotional disturbance) and menstrual-associated periodic hypersomnia (Brown and Billiard, 1995).

SLEEP-RELATED BREATHING DISORDERS

Sleep-related breathing problems (e.g., apnea) often escape evaluation and diagnosis. They can have a dramatic impact on daytime function (Carroll and Loughlin, 1995). Sleep apnea consists of an absence of effective ventilation during sleep and may result from complete or partial airway obstruction, from loss of normal central respiratory control, or as a mixed phenomenon. Future studies may provide better age-specific criteria, but currently *apnea* is defined as lack of oronasal airflow lasting more than 10 seconds. *Hypopnea* is a less severe form of hypoventilation, which may result in frequent arousals or insufficient oxygenation. These episodes are defined by more than 50% obstruction of airflow and are associated with capillary oxygen desaturation and increased end-tidal carbon dioxide levels. The apnea index is a measure of the mean number of apnea episodes per hour. In adults, more than five such episodes or 10 hypopneas per hour during sleep is considered abnormal. Carroll and Loughlin (1995) argue that these criteria are too stringent in children and that children experience oxygen desaturation more readily than adults.

Sleep apnea is often suspected because of loud snoring or observed pauses in breathing. Sometimes it is discovered as part of an evaluation for excessive daytime sleepiness and less often as a result of daytime or nighttime behavior disturbance. Sleep apnea and hypopnea may be major causes of daytime learning and behavior problems, although there is little population-based data to indicate the prevalence or severity of this problem. It is probably more frequent than the 1% to 2% prevalence reported in adults. Children with craniofacial abnormalities, including Down syndrome, as well as children with cerebral palsy or hydrocephalus are known to be at increased risk of sleep apnea. The same is true for children with degenerative or neuromuscular disorders. Obesity is a common contributor to sleep apnea. Other sleep-related breathing problems include alveolar hypoventilation (pickwickian syndrome) and central hypoventilation.

Treatment of obstructive sleep apnea and hypopnea can be complex but rarely requires extreme measures such as tracheotomy. Tonsillectomy and adenoidectomy can often be curative in obstructive sleep apnea associated with tissue hypertrophy. Carroll and Loughlin (1995) state that polysomnography should be performed on children with suspected sleep apnea even if tonsillectomy is already being considered in order to distinguish apnea from benign primary snoring. Other procedures, such as continuous or bilevel positive airway pressure devices, positioning, dental devices, or other surgeries, can be effective in selected cases.

PARASOMNIAS AND ABNORMAL AROUSALS

Children frequently exhibit disturbing behavior at night, including common parasomnias such as sleepwalking and sleep terrors, and more rare phenomena (in children) such as periodic limb movement disorder (e.g., restless legs syndrome). They can be distinguished based on historical and behavioral features (Table 44–4). Evaluation of parasomnias consists of a good sleep history and review of other information such as videotapes obtained by parents. Sleep studies should be done mainly to rule out other suspected conditions (Table 44–5).

Nightmares

Common nightmares occur during REM sleep and are classified as *dream anxiety attacks*. Their etiology appears to be identical to other anxiety-related phenomena. Children and adolescents are usually able to report the content of the nightmare, at least immediately afterward. For occasional nightmares, reassurance and attention to transitory stressors should be enough. It is easy to underestimate children's ability to imagine and worry about the future,

Table 44–4 • Common Parasomnias

Head banging: Rhythmic banging of head against soft or hard object during sleep
  Age: 9 months to 12 years
  Sleep stage: Sleep onset, stages 1 and 2
  Comments: Head banging is common and persistent. Medications have limited utility. Behavior modification has been shown to be effective. Benzodiazepines and levodopa have been reported to be effective in case studies.
Sleepwalking: Walking or running during partial arousals from sleep
  Age: 3 to 10 years
  Sleep stage: Slow-wave sleep (3 to 4), more during first third of night
  Comments: Safety is primary concern.
Bruxism: Grinding or clenching teeth during sleep
  Age: Any
  Sleep stage: Any, perhaps more during early part of night
  Comments: Dental appliances may be indicated if dental damage is present.
Nightmares: Frightening dreams associated with sleep disturbance
  Age: Any
  Sleep stage: Rapid eye movement
  Comments: Children are awake and can report their experience. Nightmares should be treated like daytime fears or anxiety; it should be distinguished from posttraumatic stress disorder by history.
Sleep terrors: Sudden disturbance of sleep associated with screaming and autonomic discharge
  Age: After 18 months
  Sleep stage: Slow-wave sleep (stages 3 and 4), first one third of night
  Comments: Occurrences may be persistent but they are benign.

Table 44–5 • Selected Indications for Polysomnography

Excessive daytime sleepiness
Periodic leg movements (restless legs)
Behavioral disturbance in high-risk individuals
   Craniofacial abnormalities
   Tonsillar hypertrophy
   Obesity
Suspected sleep apnea
   Loud snoring
   Observed respiratory pauses in sleep
   Neuromuscular disorders
   Cor pulmonale
   Hypertension
Assess effectiveness of intervention
   Continuous positive airwavy pressure/bilevel positive airway pressure
   Tonsillectomy
   Antiepileptic drugs
Atypical or severe parasomnias to rule out epilepsy
   Bruxism (also to rule out dyskinesia or dystonia)
   Sleepwalking with automatisms
   Multiple or frequent sleep terrors
   Excessive sleepiness in epilepsy patient

death, and the multitude of anxiety-provoking events. If nightmares become severe or frequent and interfere with family life or daytime functioning, mental health referral is warranted.

Posttraumatic stress disorder is an important pattern to recognize. In addition to frequent nightmares, often with repetitive content, children may show symptoms of re-experiencing their trauma ("like a movie"), episodes of numbing, reenacting events, or irrational fear of specific objects. On rare occasions, prescription medication (e.g., alpha-2 agonists, beta-blockers, and L-dopa) may cause nightmares (Hartmann, 1994).

Arousal Disorders

Even though arousals usually occur at the end of a complete sleep cycle, they may completely or partially interrupt normal sleep. Arousal disorders, such as sleep terrors (parvor nocturnus), sleepwalking (somnambulism), and confusional arousals, occur more often in the first 1 to 3 hours after sleep onset because of their association with SWS (Anders and Eiben, 1997). Proportionately more time is spent in SWS during the first one third of the night, and this is when parents may be awake to notice the behavior. Arousal disorders usually occur just once during the sleep period but can be multiple and take place during other sleep stages. Physiologically, these partial arousals occur in transition from SWS and may be precipitated by sleep deprivation, changes in sleep schedule, illness, or stress.

Sleepwalking may be calm or agitated and has been reported to occur in 40% of children age 6 to 12 years, with an annual prevalence of 6% to 17%. It may persist for 5 years in 33% of children and for more than 10 years in 12% (Rosen, Mahowald, and Ferber, 1995). Only 2% to 3% of children sleepwalk more than once a month. Quiet sleepwalkers get out of bed and may walk around in their room and even negotiate stairs, although they do have an increased risk of injury. They may engage in semipurposeful activity and even return to their bed with no signs of

having left it. In some cases, they may become agitated, cry out, run around, or respond defensively if interfered with.

Confusional arousals are often upsetting to parents because children may appear frightened or disturbed, and even cry out, but do not respond to attempts to wake them. These episodes may be brief or last up to 45 minutes, with a typical duration of 5 to 15 minutes (Rosen, Mahowald, and Ferber, 1995). Sleep terrors are a more disturbing phenomenon, although they are benign and rarely cause excessive daytime sleepiness. Formerly referred to as night terrors, sleep terrors can be very dramatic. The child often sits up and emits a blood-curdling scream, thrashing around aimlessly or even getting out of bed and running around. This is associated with autonomic overflow such as sweating and tachycardia. Sleep terrors occur suddenly and without warning, more often during the first half of the night (with the highest percentage of SWS). The child falls back asleep without memory of the incident (although this is not true for parents!).

Treatment of sleep terrors, sleep walking, and confusional arousals is often disappointing. If the episodes occur at predictable times, scheduled wakings about 15 minutes before the expected episode can be effective. It is also important to consider daytime stressors, medications, and sleep deprivation as precipitating factors. Drug therapy is not a good long-term solution, given the persistence of sleep terrors (Rosen, Mahowald, and Ferber, 1995), although clonazepam and tricyclic antidepressants have been suggested. Excessive parental intervention during arousal disorders may result in unintended conditioning of night-waking, especially if parents set up sleep associations that interfere with normal transition back to sleep. Safety measures for sleepwalking include installing gates and door alarms. Parents should quietly redirect sleepwalkers back to bed rather than try to wake them.

Rhythmic Movement Disorders

A number of movement disorders are associated with transition to sleep, including head banging, body rocking, limb slamming, and restless leg movements. Anders and Eiben (1997) quote Klackenberg as saying that rhythmic movement disorders affect up to 58% of 9-month-old children, decreasing to about 22% at age 2 years. While these disorders are self-limited problems and not a serious cause of pathology in most cases, they can be persistent.

Head banging is a common, persistent, but usually benign problem that occurs during transition to sleep. Bruises or calluses on the forehead develop in some children from head banging. It is reasonable to provide extra padding in the sleep environment, but helmets are rarely necessary except in children with more severe development disabilities. Interrupting the head banging and reinforcing an alternative, interfering behavior (such as squeezing a pillow) is a reasonable approach. Drug therapy is not usually indicated, although, as with many parasomnias, clonazepam may be effective.

Bruxism is characterized by grinding or clenching of the teeth during any stage of sleep. This is rarely a serious problem, but it does have some potential to cause dental injury. It is a common symptom in children and can be present in adults. Dental devices may prevent damage to teeth and may be helpful. Mahowald and Thorpy (1995) identify some rare etiologies of bruxism such as orofacial dyskinesia, mandibular dystonia, and tremor.

Nocturnal Enuresis

Nocturnal enuresis (bed-wetting) is another common concern (see Chapter 42). It is divided into primary nocturnal enuresis (no period of nighttime dryness more than 6 months) and secondary nocturnal enuresis. Medical causes such as neurogenic bladder and anatomic abnormalities can be ruled out if the child is dry during the day. Secondary enuresis may signal concern for psychosocial or emotional problems as well as neurologic disorders (e.g., tethered cord and other spinal lesions), but the distinction between primary and secondary nocturnal enuresis is somewhat arbitrary. History and urinalysis can rule out diabetes mellitus and urinary tract infections, and neurologic examination looking for lower spinal reflexes (anal wink) is important.

Parents often report that bed-wetting occurs when the child is in deep sleep because they are more likely to check the bed and try to wake the child in the first half of the night, when there is a higher probability of the child's being in a deep sleep stage. There is no correlation between sleep stage and nocturnal enuresis when the time spent in each stage is controlled for (Anders and Eiben, 1997).

Bed-wetting alarms are highly effective for school-aged children who are motivated to stop wetting the bed. It is important for the child and parents to form an alliance, because it is essential to wake the child completely when the alarm goes off, followed by a trip to the bathroom to empty the bladder. Because the child is not always woken by the alarm, parents usually have to be involved in this process regardless of the child's age. After dryness has been accomplished, a period of overtraining with increased water consumption before bedtime can improve long-term results. Bladder training exercises may help by improving bladder capacity. Hypnotherapy may also be effective. Children at any age can be given a positive role in removing wet bedsheets and helping with laundry. Treatment of encopresis or chronic constipation, if present, can help greatly. Pharmacologic agents such as desmopressin (DDAVP) and imipramine provide short-term relief of symptoms but have not been shown to "cure" bed-wetting and have potential for low-frequency but potentially serious complications, such as hyponatremia and seizures.

GENERAL MEDICAL DISORDERS AFFECTING SLEEP

Chronic pain, asthma, gastroesophageal reflux, infection, and inflammatory disorders have all been shown to disturb sleep, leading to excessive daytime sleepiness or masquerading as parasomnias and even seizures. Migraine and cluster headache may occur at night and disturb sleep. Many medications can affect sleep. All stimulants, including medications such as methylphenidate and dextroamphetamine, as well as commonly used asthma medications and over-the-counter decongestants can interfere with sleep onset. Dietary stimulants such as caffeine and chocolate can have similar effects. Both sedative and paradoxical effects can be seen with most antihistamines. Most antiepi-leptic drugs have sedative effects but usually do not affect sleep per se. A number of drugs affect REM sleep and may be associated with nightmares.

It is important for the pediatrician to ask about sleep in their patients with chronic health problems, as both an indicator of the status of their illness and an important social and emotional consideration. After making appropriate efforts to treat the underlying problem and making adjustments and substitutions in treatment when possible, the clinician needs to teach the principles of good sleep hygiene (see Table 44-3). Medications to induce sleep continue to have major negative side effects, including rapid tolerance, dependence, and impairment of performance, and they are rarely indicated except for short-term use.

NEUROLOGIC AND PSYCHIATRIC DISORDERS

Epilepsy

Epilepsy is an infrequent cause of sleep disturbance, although several forms of epilepsy occur at night and may be confused with parasomnias. Often the timing of the event, the age of onset, and associated neurologic or developmental findings allow the clinician to make an appropriate differential diagnosis (see Table 44-4). In difficult cases, many sleep laboratories can combine polysomnography with an extended EEG montage as a screen for epilepsy. Rhythmic movement disorders appear to raise the most concern about epilepsy. However, they are usually characteristic in terms of age of onset, duration, and relationship to sleep stage. There would be more concern about a new paroxysmal sleep event that occurred sporadically, during adolescence or adulthood, especially if associated with daytime sleepiness, performance, or behavior problems.

In juvenile myoclonic epilepsy, myoclonic and/or generalized tonic-clonic seizures occur at sleep onset or on waking, but not during sleep. Children with infantile spasms or Lennox-Gastaut syndrome exhibit seizures during sleep that are said to be more frequent in REM sleep. Children with complex partial seizures and rolandic epilepsy also experience seizures during sleep, which might reduce their volume of REM sleep (Bourgeois, 1996). Most of these seizure types can be readily distinguished from parasomnias. Because associated daytime symptoms can overlap (daytime performance problems, excessive daytime sleepiness, school failure, behavior disturbances), epilepsy needs to be considered carefully during an evaluation of a child for sleep problems. The relative frequency of these problems should be kept in mind, because certain parasomnias may be 30 to 60 times more common than epilepsy, and they may coexist in the same individual.

Psychiatric Disorders

Many major psychiatric disorders can have associated sleep problems, including depression, mania, anxiety, and psychoses. In addition, different psychiatric drugs can induce sleep maintenance or insomnia, most notably selective serotonin-reuptake inhibitors such as fluoxetine, sertraline, and paroxetine. Tricyclic antidepressants suppress REM sleep. Psychostimulants can also cause sleep-onset insomnia. Drugs of abuse can disturb sleep as well. In particular, tobacco and caffeine can contribute to insomnia, and alcohol can lead to sleep fragmentation. Posttraumatic stress disorder, child sexual abuse, and substance abuse need to be considered in children with recurrent nightmares or recent onset of their sleep problem.

Conclusion

Sleep problems are common in children but are often misdiagnosed. Different problems appear at characteristic ages and at characteristic times during the sleep-wake cycle. Sleep appears to have an important function in attention, memory, learning, and behavior. Problems require a detailed biopsychosocial approach to diagnosis and treatment. Developmental-behavioral pediatricians are in a unique position to manage many sleep problems, but they may need to rely on other consultants when it comes to neurologic and breathing disorders. The most effective approaches to sleep problems include education about basic processes related to sleep, improvement in sleep hygiene, and behavioral management aimed at developing appropriate sleep associations.

REFERENCES

Adams LA, Rickert VI: Reducing bedtime tantrums: comparison between positive routines and graduated extinction. Pediatrics 84:756–761, 1989.

Anders TF, Eiben LA: Pediatric sleep disorders: a review of the past 10 years. J Am Acad Child Adolesc Psychiatry 36:9–20, 1997.

Bourgeois B: The relationship between sleep and epilepsy in children. Semin Pediatr Neurol 3:29–35, 1996.

Brown LW, Billiard M: Narcolepsy, Kleine-Levin syndrome, and other causes of sleepiness in children. *In* Ferber R, Kryger M (eds): Principles and Practice of Sleep Medicine in the Child. Philadelphia, WB Saunders, 1995, pp 125–134.

Carroll JL, Loughlin GM: Obstructive sleep apnea syndrome in infants and children: diagnosis and management. *In* Ferber R, Kryger M (eds): Principles and Practice of Sleep Medicine in the Child. Philadelphia, WB Saunders, 1995, pp 193–216.

Carskadon MA, Roth T: Sleep restriction. *In* Monk TH (ed): Sleep, Sleepiness, and Performance. New York, John Wiley & Sons, 1991, pp 155–167.

Carskadon MA, Vieira C, Acebo C: Association between puberty and delayed phase preference. Sleep 16:258–262, 1993.

Dahl RE: The impact of inadequate sleep on children's daytime cognitive function. Semin Pediatr Neurol 3:44–50, 1996.

Dahl RE, Carskadon MA: Sleep and its disorders in adolescence. *In* Ferber R, Kryger M (eds): Principles and Practice of Sleep Medicine in the Child. Philadelphia, WB Saunders, 1995, pp 19–28.

Dahl RE, Holttum J, Trubnick L: A clinical picture of child and adolescent narcolepsy. J Am Academy Child Adolesc Psychiatry 33:834–841, 1994.

Ferber R: Sleeplessness in children. *In* Ferber R, Kryger M (eds): Principles and Practice of Sleep Medicine in the Child. Philadelphia, WB Saunders, 1995, pp 79–89.

Ferber R: Solve Your Child's Sleep Problem. New York, Simon and Schuster, 1986.

Hartmann E: Nightmares and other dreams. *In* Kryger MH, Roth T, Dement WC (eds): Principles and Practice of Sleep Medicine. Philadelphia, WB Saunders, 1994, pp 407–410.

Jan JE, Espezel H, Appleton RE: The treatment of sleep disorders with melatonin. Dev Med Child Neurol 36:97–107, 1994.

Lozoff B, Askew GL, Wolf AQ: Cosleeping and early childhood sleep problems: effects of ethnicity and socioeconomic status. J Dev Behav Pediatr 17:9–15, 1996.

Mahowald MW, Thorpy M: Nonarousal parasomnias in the child. *In* Ferber R, Kryger M (eds): Principles and Practice of Sleep Medicine in the Child. Philadelphia, WB Saunders, 1995, pp 115–123.

McKenna JJ, Mosko SS: Sleep and arousal, synchrony and independence, among mothers and infants sleeping apart and together (same bed): an experiment in evolutionary medicine. Acta Paediatr Suppl 397:94–102, 1994.

Regestein QR, Monk TH: Delayed sleep phase syndrome: a review of its clinical aspects. Am J Psychiatry 152:602–608, 1995.

Rosen G, Mahowald MW, Ferber R: Sleepwalking, confusional arousals, and sleep terrors in the child. *In* Ferber R, Kryger M (eds): Principles and Practice of Sleep Medicine in the Child. Philadelphia, WB Saunders, 1995, pp 99–113.

Thorpy MJ: Classification of sleep disorders. *In* Kryger MH, Roth T, Dement WC (eds): Principles and Practice of Sleep Medicine. Philadelphia, WB Saunders, 1994, pp 426–436.

Webb WB: Sleep as a biologic rhythm: a historical review. Sleep 17:188–194, 1994.

Weissbluth M: Naps in children 6 months–7 years. Sleep 18:82–87, 1995.

45 Repetitive Behaviors

Nathan J. Blum

 A wide variety of repetitive behaviors are common during childhood. Generally they are normal variations such as thumb-sucking and nail-biting, requiring only reassurance or minimal management. Sometimes they become problematic because they cause stigmatization, subjective distress, or tissue damage, which necessitate more help. In some children they are a signal that a child is experiencing significant stress, making better management of that stress a vital part of the plan. Consideration must also be given to the possibility that they are accompanied by developmental or neurologic problems such as retardation, autism, or sensory impairment. This chapter clarifies the broad range of causes, manifestations, and treatments of repetitive behaviors.

Repetitive or stereotypic behaviors are common during childhood. They are usually defined as repeated purposeless actions that are often rhythmic. Repetitive behaviors frequently occur in normally developing children and are benign and self-limited. However, children with repetitive behaviors deserve careful consideration because such behaviors occur with increased frequency in children with developmental, emotional, or physical disorders. Furthermore, the behaviors themselves may be problematic in that they may cause tissue damage, may be socially undesirable, or may cause subjective distress to the individual. This chapter discusses the etiology of repetitive behaviors and the current method of classification for them. Information on the evaluation and treatment of specific repetitive behaviors and repetitive behavior syndromes is also presented.

Etiology

Investigations into the etiology of repetitive behaviors have found that both biological and environmental factors are important in causing or maintaining these behaviors. Studies of infants have found that repetitive behaviors are nearly universal phenomena that occur with a distinctive developmental progression (Table 45–1). In typically developing infants, hand sucking occurs in 89% within 2 hours of birth; foot kicking begins between 2 and 3 months of age; object banging and body rocking begin at approximately 6 months of age; and hand clapping begins at 7 to 8 months of age (Kravitz and Boehm, 1971; Thelen, 1979). The nearly universal occurrence of these behaviors in the 1st year of life and the distinctive developmental progression have led to the theory that they represent intrinsic movement patterns generated by the developing nervous system (Thelen, 1979). Repetitive behaviors may serve as a transition between uncoordinated movements and more mature goal-directed behaviors.

Other evidence for the importance of biological factors in the etiology of repetitive behaviors comes from pharmacologic and neuroanatomic studies. These studies have implicated the basal ganglia, frontal lobes, and dopamine neurotransmitter systems in the etiology of at least some of these behaviors. Large doses of amphetamines administered to a variety of laboratory animals have been shown to induce repetitive behaviors (Ridley, 1994), and treatment of humans with stimulant medications produces tics or repetitive picking behaviors in some individuals. Infusion of dopamine into the caudate nucleus in rats also produces stereotyped oral behaviors (Fog and Pakkenberg, 1971). Ablations of the frontal lobe in laboratory animals and neurologic disorders associated with degeneration of the frontal lobes in humans have also been reported to cause repetitive behaviors (Ames et al, 1994; Ridley, 1994). The fact that a variety of brain injuries and alterations in neurotransmitters produce repetitive behaviors may be explained by linkages between these systems. For example, the frontal lobes have a modulating effect on the activation of motor movements by the basal ganglia, and dopamine is a regulatory neurotransmitter within the basal ganglia.

Although there is strong evidence that biologic factors play a role in the etiology of repetitive behaviors, there is also strong evidence that environmental factors play an important role in determining their frequency. Both high and low levels of arousal may increase the frequency of repetitive behaviors. Conditions of severe sensory deprivation have been shown to produce these behaviors in both laboratory animals and humans. Programs to enrich environmental stimulation have been shown to decrease repetitive behavior in institutionalized children with mental retardation. Thelen (1981) found that in the 1st year of life, most repetitive behaviors could be associated with either a change in stimuli (e.g., appearance of a caretaker, presentation of a toy) or a nonalert (usually fussy) state. In older children, repetitive behaviors are reported to occur most frequently either during periods of low arousal such as when tired, bored, or distracted by other stimuli (e.g., reading, television) or during periods of high arousal such as when concentrating, angry, or frustrated (Sallustro and Atwell, 1978; Troster, 1994).

Repetitive behaviors may also be maintained by their

Table 45–1 • Onset and Prevalence of Some Repetitive Behaviors in Early Childhood

Repetitive Behavior	Mean Age of Onset (months)	Percent of Children Exhibiting the Behavior			Comments	Reference
		0–1 yr	*1–2 yr*	*2–6 yr*		
Hand, finger, thumb-sucking	Birth	100%	40%–50%	14%–19% at 5 yr	In the United States; in other cultures, reported prevalence ranges from 0% to more than 50%.	Kravitz and Boehm (1971); Mahalski and Stanton (1992)
Lip biting or sucking	4–5	93%		1%–10%		Kravitz and Boehm (1971); Troster (1994)
Foot kicking	2–3	99%			May continue as leg swinging in older children.	Kravitz and Boehm, (1971)
Body rocking	6	91%	9%–30%	3%		Kravitz and Boehm (1971)
Head banging	8–9	7%	5%–19%	1%–3%	Male to female ratio of 3:1; 9% of those with head banging at age 3 years had persistent banging at age 7 years.	Abe et al (1984); Kravitz and Boehm (1971); Sallustro and Atwell (1978).

effects on the environment. This has been demonstrated most frequently in individuals with disabilities in which repetitive behaviors (especially those causing self-injury) are often found to be reinforced by caretakers who respond to the behaviors by providing attention to the individual, by allowing the individual access to tangible reinforcers, or by allowing the individual to avoid undesired activities (Guess and Carr, 1991). In toddlers, similar factors may reinforce head banging, leading to increased rates of head banging during tantrums. In an experimental situation, Rovee and Rovee (1969) demonstrated that when a string is attached between a mobile and the leg of a 2- to 3-month-old infant, the infant engages in an increased rate of leg kicking when compared with control infants whose mobile moved noncontingently. Thus, in both normally developing children and those with disabilities, environmental variables play an important role in determining the rate at which repetitive behaviors occur.

Classification

The classification system for repetitive behaviors used in the fourth edition of *The Diagnostic and Statistical Manual of Mental Disorders* (DSM-IV) (American Psychiatric Association, 1994) and *The Classification of Child and Adolescent Mental Diagnoses in Primary Care: Diagnostic and Statistical Manual for Primary Care (DSM-PC) Child and Adolescent Version* (Wolraich et al, 1996) is shown in Table 45–2. Repetitive behaviors may be classified as normal variations, as problems, or as specific disorders based primarily on the degree of dysfunction or stigmatization that is associated with the behaviors. In addition, repetitive behaviors may occur as part of a general medical or neurologic condition, in response to some medications, or as part of a developmental disorder, sensory impairment, or psychiatric disorder. In these cases, it is important to recognize the underlying condition. In some cases, the underlying condition may preclude the diagnosis of a separate repetitive behavior disorder. This is the case when the repetitive behaviors that cause dysfunction are thought to be part of the underlying condition, such as in the pervasive developmental disorders or obsessive-compulsive disorder, and when the repetitive behaviors occur in response to a medication or other substance. In individuals with mental retardation or sensory impairments, repetitive behaviors are recognized to occur more frequently than in the general population, but they are not usually associated with significant functional impairment. In these cases, when significant functional impairment does exist, the diagnosis of a separate repetitive behavior disorder should be considered.

Repetitive Behaviors

SUCKING

Sucking of the hand, fingers, or thumb has been observed in utero as early as 29 weeks of gestation and is a nearly universal phenomenon in healthy neonates within hours after birth (Kravitz and Boehm, 1971). Sucking is viewed as a biologically driven behavior that develops into a habit in some children. The habit may be adaptive for many infants and toddlers in that it may provide stimulation to delay the onset of boredom during periods of low stimulation and it may help soothe the child when he or she is tired, sick, or upset.

Thumb- or digit-sucking is usually a harmless behavior in infants and young children, but it has been associated with a number of sequelae when it persists, especially at high frequency or intensity, beyond age 4 to 6 years. Some of the most frequent sequelae involve dental problems such as an anterior open bite, decreased alveolar bone growth, mucosal trauma, and even altered growth of the facial bones. Thumb- or digit-sucking is a common cause of paronychia in children and it may be associated with an

Table 45–2 • Classification of Repetitive Behaviors

Repetitive behaviors—variation (V65.49)
  Sporadic repetitive movements are of limited duration, cause no physical harm, and do not impair normal development or activities.
Repetitive behaviors—problem (V40.3)
  Repetitive behaviors cause some social disruption and/or dysfunction that results from the behavior itself and from the response of others to that behavior, but is not sufficiently intense to qualify for a diagnosis of a repetitive behavior disorder.
Repetitive behaviors—disorders
  Stereotypic movement disorder (SMD; 307.3)
    Motor behavior that is repetitive, often seemingly driven, and nonfunctional. The behaviors are clearly associated with social dysfunction and stigmatization.
  Trichotillomania (312.39)
    Recurrent pulling out of one's hair, resulting in noticeable hair loss. Associated with tension before hair pulling and gratification or relief after pulling.
  Transient tic disorder (307.21)
    Single or multiple motor and/or vocal tics that occur many times a day, nearly every day, for at least 4 weeks, but for no longer than 12 consecutive months.
  Chronic motor or vocal tic disorder (307.22)
    Single or multiple motor or vocal tics, but not both, have been present at some time during the illness. The tics occur many times a day nearly every day or intermittently throughout a period of more than 1 year. The disturbance causes marked distress or significant impairment in social and academic functioning.
  Tourette syndrome (307.23)
    Similar to chronic motor or vocal tic disorder except that both multiple motor and one or more vocal tics have to be present at some time during the illness.
Repetitive behaviors associated with general medical conditions
  Examples: Multiple sclerosis, postviral encephalitis, head injury, Sydenham chorea, Huntington chorea, Lesch-Nyhan syndrome
Repetitive behaviors associated with sensory impairments
  Examples: Repetitive behaviors occur with increased frequency in children with hearing impairment and children with visual impairment
Repetitive behaviors associated with substances
  Examples: Stimulants, seizure medications, hypnotics, anxiolytics
Repetitive behaviors associated with developmental disorders
  Examples: Mental retardation, pervasive developmental disorder
Repetitive behaviors associated with psychiatric disorders
  Examples: Obsessive-compulsive disorder, schizophrenia

Data from Wolraich ML et al (eds): The Classification of Child and Adolescent Mental Diagnoses in Primary Care: Diagnostic and Statistical Manual for Primary Care (DSM-PC), Child and Adolescent Version. Elk Grove Village, IL, American Academy of Pediatrics, 1996, and American Psychiatric Association: DSM-IV, Diagnostic and Statistical Manual of Mental Disorders, 4th ed. Washington, DC, American Psychiatric Association, 1994.

increased incidence of accidental ingestion. Deformities of the fingers and thumb may occur. Finally, thumb- or digit-sucking may have psychological sequelae. It has been shown that when 1st grade children are asked to rate pictures of peers who are thumb-sucking and pictures of the same peers when they are not thumb-sucking, they rate the children pictured while thumb-sucking as less intelligent, happy, attractive, likable, and fun, as well as less desirable as a friend or playmate (Friman et al, 1993). Children who suck their thumbs may also be exposed to frequent reprimands or nagging from parents, which may lead to unhappiness or insecurity.

There has been some controversy as to whether thumb-sucking is a marker for underlying emotional stress, anxiety, or other behavior problems. When groups of children who suck their thumbs are compared with groups of children who do not suck their thumbs, some studies have found increased behavior problems in the group with thumb-sucking, whereas others have not (Mahalski and Stanton, 1992). Reports of an increased prevalence of specific behavior problems in children with thumb-sucking have not been consistent between studies. Within an individual child, the events that occur around the time of thumb-sucking should be evaluated to determine whether the thumb-sucking seems to be related to emotional stress or anxiety, but the presence of thumb-sucking alone does not necessarily indicate that the child is experiencing emotional stress or anxiety.

Treatment of thumb-sucking is rarely indicated in children younger than age 4 years. In older children, if thumb-sucking occurs infrequently (e.g., only at night) or only as a temporary response to a significant stressor, then treatment is not usually indicated. Treatment is indicated if thumb-sucking causes dental problems (a dental evaluation may be necessary to ascertain this), digital malformations, or distress to the child. Children older than age 4 years who suck their thumb or fingers in multiple settings or both during the day and at night are at increased risk for medical and psychologic sequelae, and treatment should be considered.

A variety of successful treatments for thumb-sucking have been described. If thumb-sucking has resulted in significant negative reactions from the parents, a moratorium on parental comments on the thumb-sucking should precede any other treatment. This reduces tension between the parent and child and may decrease the thumb-sucking if it had been reinforced by parental attention. If other sources of stress or anxiety are thought to be related to the thumb-sucking, a plan to manage these stressors should be developed.

Treatment for thumb-sucking usually involves some combination of reinforcement (praise and sometimes tangible rewards) for not thumb-sucking, application of an aversive taste substance to the thumbnail, or physical barriers (gloves, hand socks, thumb splints) to thumb-sucking. Friman and Leibowitz (1990) combined a reward system with an aversive taste treatment. The child's thumbnail was coated with Stop-Zit (Purepac Pharmaceutical Co.), an aversive taste substance, in the morning, before bed, and any time the child was observed sucking his or her thumb. Small tangible rewards were offered if the child went without thumb-sucking for specified intervals. The researchers report that this treatment resulted in cessation of thumb-sucking in 12 of 22 subjects within 3 months and 20 of 22 subjects within 1 year. Intraoral dental appliances that serve as a reminder not to suck and/or that interfere with the seal that sucking creates are effective treatments when needed.

BANGING

Rhythmic banging behaviors such as the banging of one's hand or an object against a surface occurs commonly during infancy. Thelen (1981) observed this behavior in all of the 20 infants she followed during the 1st year of life. Head banging, however, is the most dramatic banging behavior and the one that is most likely to elicit concern from parents.

Head banging involves the rhythmic hitting of the head against a solid surface, often the crib mattress, but sometimes harder surfaces. While head banging, the child is usually quiet and relaxed. Head banging occurs in 5% to 19% of children during the infancy and toddler years. It occurs most frequently when children are tired or at bedtime, but it may also occur when the child is alone or upset (Sallustro and Atwell, 1978). Many children who bang their heads have had other rhythmic behaviors, often body rocking or head rolling, earlier in infancy. Each episode of head banging usually lasts for less than 15 minutes, but episodes lasting a few hours may occur. Although the frequency of head banging declines rapidly after 18 months of age, 1% to 3% of children continue the behavior after age 3 years. Nine percent of children who bang their head at age 3 years are still head banging at age 7 years (Abe, Oda, and Amatoni, 1984).

Although most children who bang their heads do not have physical illness, in some cases, the onset of head banging has been associated with episodes of otitis media and with teething (Kravitz and Boehm, 1971). In these cases, head banging has been postulated to serve as a pain-relieving function.

Parents are often concerned that head banging will result in brain injury and that it is indicative of a developmental or emotional disorder. However, studies suggest that infants who bang their head may actually reach certain gross motor milestones earlier than children who do not (Sallustro and Atwell, 1978). In one study, children with persistent head banging at age 3 years were found to be more moody and restless when followed up at 8 years of age (Abe, Oda, and Amatoni, 1984), but in most children head banging is not a sign of an emotional disorder. Head banging can result in callus formation at the site of the banging, abrasions, and contusions; however, with the possible exception of children with severe developmental disabilities (most commonly autism) or bleeding disorders, head banging does not result in intracranial injury.

Treatment primarily involves reassurance of the parents that head banging alone is not a sign of emotional disturbance or developmental disability and that injury is unlikely. If the child is banging against a hard surface, padding the surface decreases the chance of abrasions or contusions. In most cases, parents should be counseled to ignore the behavior while it is occurring. This is especially true for head banging that occurs during tantrums. Attention in the form of concern or punishment for the behavior may inadvertently reinforce the behavior. Similarly, when head banging is occurring primarily during temper tantrums, one must investigate whether the head banging is being reinforced by helping the child gain access to desired items or helping the child avoid undesired parental demands. In children with developmental disabilities, severe and persistent head banging may necessitate the use of helmets and pharmacologic treatment in some cases (see section on repetitive behaviors in children with developmental disorders in this chapter and also Chapter 62.

ROCKING

Body rocking occurs in most infants during the 1st year of life. It usually begins around 6 months of age and has been reported to occur most frequently when infants are listening to music or are alone in their cribs (Sallustro and Atwell, 1978). It usually involves a rhythmic forward and backward swaying of the trunk at the hips that occurs most frequently in a sitting position, but also in the quadruped position. It can be gentle or violent enough to shake or even move a crib. The peak prevalence has been variably reported to be between 6 and 18 months of age, with a rapid decline in the prevalence of the behavior after 18 months of age. Most episodes of uninterrupted body rocking last for less than 15 minutes, but Sallustro and Atwell (1978) found that 12% of parents reported that their children had episodes lasting 15 to 30 minutes.

Body rocking may persist beyond age 2 years in approximately 3% of typically developing children. A variety of functions of rocking behaviors have been proposed, including self-stimulation and tension reduction. In children with developmental disorders and children with visual impairments, body rocking has been associated with a lack of environmental stimulation.

In most cases, body rocking does not cause significant functional impairment or stigmatization. However, cases in which rocking occurs throughout most of the day, interfering with functional activities and causing significant impairment or stigmatization, have been described in children, adolescents, and adults (Castellanos et al, 1996). These cases meet criteria for stereotypic movement disorder.

BREATH-HOLDING SPELLS

Breath-holding spells are not typically thought of as a repetitive behavior, but they do have some similarities to repetitive behaviors in their management.

Breath-holding spells are reflexive events in which the child becomes apneic at end expiration. Typically there is a provoking event that causes anger, fear, frustration, or minor injury and results in the child's beginning to cry. The crying may be brief or may be prolonged and gradually intensifying. In either case, the crying stops at full expiration when the child becomes apneic and cyanotic or pale.

In some cases, the spell resolves at this point as the child takes a deep breath (simple breath-holding spells), whereas in other cases the event continues and the child may lose consciousness and muscle tone and fall to the ground. Occasionally the child may have a brief seizure. After the event, there may be a period of drowsiness.

Breath-holding spells are generally reported to occur in 4% to 5% of the pediatric population. They may begin as early as 2 months of age, but most frequently begin between 6 and 18 months of age. It is unusual for the spells to last beyond 6 to 7 years of age (Dimario, 1992).

Breath-holding spells may be divided into cyanotic spells or pallid spells based on the child's color during the event. Cyanotic spells are more common and are thought to be related to an abnormality in respiratory regulation that leads to prolonged expiratory apnea. Pallid spells are thought to be related to an overactive vagal response leading to bradycardia or asystole.

The differential diagnosis for breath-holding spells includes seizures, cardiac arrhythmias, or a brainstem tumor or malformation (e.g., Arnold Chiari malformation). Anemia may increase the frequency of breath-holding spells, and treatment with ferrous sulfate (5 mg/kg/day) has been reported to decrease the frequency of the spells (Daoud et al, 1997). Breath-holding spells have also been reported to occur with increased frequency in children with familial dysautonomia and Rett syndrome, but they would not be the sole manifestation of these disorders. Usually the history of a provoking event and the presence of color change before the loss of consciousness allow one to distinguish breath-holding spells from seizures on clinical grounds, but occasionally an electroencephalogram is helpful. If a child has pallid spells, one should consider obtaining an electrocardiogram to evaluate the child for conditions associated with cardiac arrhythmias such as long QT syndrome.

Breath-holding spells are frightening to parents. Treatment primarily involves reassurance that the spells will not harm the child and demystification of the events leading to the loss of consciousness. Parents should understand that if the child does lose consciousness, he or she will begin breathing at that time. In cases of very frequent and severe (i.e., associated with seizures) pallid breath-holding spells, treatment with atropine has been shown to decrease the frequency of the seizures (McWilliam and Stephenson, 1984).

Treatment with iron is indicated in children who are anemic, but the role of iron for children with breath-holding spells who are not anemic is less clear. Daoud and colleagues (1997) found that iron was effective in decreasing breath-holding spells even in some children who were not iron deficient. The mechanism by which iron decreases breath-holding spells is not known.

The response of parents to the breath-holding spells should also be investigated. Parents who remain fearful of the events may try to prevent the child from experiencing pain, fear, minor injury, anger, or frustration. In trying to prevent these events, the parents may unnecessarily restrict some activities, may have difficulty setting consistent limits when the child has tantrums, or may provide attention in response to tantrums. In these cases, the parents' behavior may reinforce the tantrums, and the child may learn to trigger the breath-holding spells during tantrums in order to get the desired response from his or her parents. In these situations, if demystification and reassurance do not change the parents' behavior, referral to a mental health professional is indicated.

NAIL-BITING

Nail-biting is uncommon in preschool children but is common in school-aged children, occurring in 30% to 60% of children at age 10 years. The incidence then decreases to about 20% during adolescence and about 10% during adulthood (Leung and Robson, 1990). During childhood, the incidence of nail-biting is similar in boys and girls, but during adolescence and adulthood, more boys than girls bite their nails. Nail-biting is often thought to be an indication of tension or anxiety. In some cases, the habit itself may be the source of tension within the family. Bakwin and Bakwin (1972) reported that monozygotic twins show concordance for the habit about twice as frequently as dizygotic twins, suggesting a possible genetic contribution.

Nail-biting is usually confined to the fingernails, and most individuals bite all 10 nails equally. Occasionally specific fingernails are bitten (or avoided) selectively, and some individuals bite toenails. The bitten nails are short and irregular. Sometimes the skin margins of the nail bed or the cuticle are bitten. This may result in paronychia or, in cases of oral herpes, development of herpetic whitlow on the bitten finger. In severe cases, nail-biting may be harmful to dentition, resulting in apical root resorption, fractures in the edges of the incisors, and gingivitis.

When specific stressors related to nail-biting can be identified, treatment should be directed at helping the child to cope with these stressors. Efforts should be made to be supportive of the child because punishments, nagging, or ridicule related to the nail-biting are likely to worsen the behavior or create other difficulties in the parent-child relationship. Good nail hygiene is recommended because the rough nail edges may be irritating and worsen the behavior. In adolescents and adults, the habit reversal procedure (see Habit Reversal) has been effective in reducing nail-biting (Fig. 45–1) (Azrin, Nunn, and Frantz, 1980a).

BRUXISM

Bruxism refers to the grinding and clenching of teeth. It is common in both children and adults. In children, the incidence of bruxism has been reported to vary between 7% and 88%, with most studies reporting an incidence between 15% and 30% (Cash, 1988). During childhood, bruxism increases in frequency, reaching a peak between ages 7 and 10 years and then decreasing after that. The peak at 7 to 10 years has been postulated to be related to the mixture of deciduous and permanent teeth that are present at this age.

Diurnal (daytime) bruxism should be distinguished from *nocturnal bruxism.* Nocturnal bruxism is associated with both grinding and clenching of the teeth and generates tremendous forces that produce audible grinding sounds. In general, each episode of nocturnal bruxism is brief, lasting 8 to 9 seconds, and during a night of sleep, an average of 42 seconds of bruxing occurs (Attanasio, 1991). In contrast to nocturnal bruxism, diurnal bruxism usually

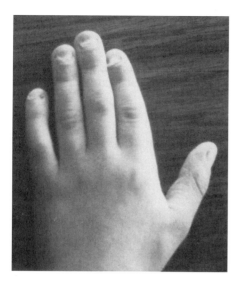

Figure 45–1. Severe destruction of the fingernails caused by biting and picking.

does not produce grinding sounds (except in individuals with central nervous system dysfunction) because it is associated primarily with clenching of the teeth and the forces generated are less than those produced during nocturnal bruxism. Diurnal bruxism is thought to be related to other oral habits such as nail-biting or lip-biting and chewing on objects, because these behaviors tend to occur in similar settings.

Symptoms from bruxism are less common in children than in adults. In children, the most common symptom is pain on palpation over the muscles of mastication (Cash, 1988). Other symptoms such as dysfunction of the temporomandibular joint, recurrent headaches, and thermal hypersensitivity of the teeth may be related to bruxism in some cases. The most common sign of bruxism is abnormal wearing of the teeth. Hypermobility of the teeth, injury to the periodontium, fractured teeth, and pulpitis may also occur.

Investigations of bruxism have not identified clear etiologic factors, and it is likely that its cause is multifactorial in most cases. Studies have centered on dental occlusion problems and psychological factors. The role of dental occlusal discrepancies in bruxism remains controversial. Whereas some studies have suggested that the creation of occlusal discrepancies in laboratory animals and in humans may lead to bruxism, many studies have failed to identify a direct relationship between nocturnal bruxism and an individual's dental occlusion. Nonetheless, evaluation of dental occlusion in individuals with bruxism is important because the occlusion affects the distribution of the forces generated by the bruxism.

Many psychological factors have been thought to be related to the occurrence of bruxism. Most frequently, bruxism is associated with emotional stress such as frustration, anger, anxiety, or fear. Vanderas (1995) demonstrated that children aged 6 to 10 years who had experienced unpleasant life events were more likely to have bruxism than control subjects who had not experienced one of the unpleasant life events. However, this and other studies that

have reported a relationship between bruxism and emotional stressors have failed to distinguish between nocturnal and diurnal bruxism. When studies are limited to individuals with nocturnal bruxism, the finding of a relationship between nocturnal bruxism and emotional stressors is less consistent (Cash, 1988).

Treatment of bruxism in children needs to be considered carefully, because bruxism is often transient and children are less likely to have symptoms than adults. Thus reassurance is often the only treatment that is needed. If the child is having significant symptoms, a thorough medical and dental evaluation should occur before treatment. If treatment is indicated, the options include occlusal adjustment of the dentition, interocclusal dental appliances, psychological therapies, physical therapy, or pharmacologic treatment.

Occlusal adjustment involves altering the teeth and is permanent. It should be considered only when there is an obvious interference with occlusion. A variety of interocclusal devices worn over the surface of the teeth have been developed. They have been reported to decrease bruxism in about 50% of individuals but to reduce symptoms of bruxism in an even greater number of individuals. In these latter cases, it may be the redistribution of masticatory forces that is responsible for the benefit (Attanasio, 1991).

Psychological treatments aimed at decreasing stress or teaching the individual to manage stress are helpful in some cases. Nocturnal alarms that arouse the individual during bruxing events have been shown to decrease the frequency and duration of bruxing during treatment, but the gains may not be maintained after treatment. Relaxation training and biofeedback have also been reported to have at least short-term benefit in adults, but they have not been studied in children.

Exercises, heat applications, ultrasound, and transcutaneous electric stimulation are treatments that may be used by physical therapists to help manage pain associated with bruxism. Nonsteroidal antiinflammatory agents may also be helpful for pain management. Muscle relaxants may decrease bruxism, but they have significant side effects and are not a long-term solution.

COUGH

Habit or "psychogenic" cough has been described in children, in adolescents, and rarely in adults. Usually the cough begins after a minor upper respiratory infection associated with a cough, but the cough persists long after the other respiratory symptoms resolve. The cough is often described as a harsh nonproductive barking. It may occur multiple times per minute and can be very disruptive in a classroom.

Individuals with a habit cough are often misdiagnosed as having asthma, and a number of patients have received treatment with daily bronchodilators and even daily steroids. In contrast to those with many other causes of a chronic cough, those with a habit cough do not cough while asleep and are likely to have a decrease in the frequency of the cough when distracted by vigorous physical exertion.

Habit cough is occasionally associated with other behavioral or emotional problems. The most common are school problems. In these cases, school absenteeism resulting from the cough may serve to reinforce the cough. However, many children with a habit cough do not have other behavioral or emotional disorders.

If habit cough is associated with school avoidance, school problems, or other emotional or behavioral problems, a comprehensive plan to treat these problems should be developed. A number of treatments for the habit cough have been described. Lokshin and colleagues (1991) successfully treated nine children and adolescents using brief suggestive therapy. They described to the patient that the cough is related to a cycle in which coughing leads to bronchial irritation, which leads to further coughing. They provide the patient a distractor to "help decrease the irritation" (e.g., breathing nebulized medicine, sipping warm water). The patient is encouraged and praised for resisting the urge to cough and told that each second of delay makes further inhibition easier. When some ability to suppress the cough is noted, which usually takes about 10 minutes, they are asked, "You are beginning to feel that you can resist the urge to cough, aren't you?" When the patient goes for 5 minutes without a cough, he or she is asked, "Do you feel you can resist the urge to cough on your own?" When the patient answers this question affirmatively, the session ends and the patient is advised to repeat the procedure for any recurrence of the cough. All patients had a significant decrease in symptoms 1 week after treatment and at follow-up a median of 3.4 years after treatment.

Lavigne and colleagues (1991) described an alternative behavioral treatment for habit cough. Parents were instructed to monitor the frequency of the symptom during a 30-minute period of the evening. Goals were then set for a 10% reduction in the frequency of the coughing with further 10% reductions occurring when the child met the goal for 3 days. In some cases, parental praise for reaching the goal was the only reinforcer needed, whereas in other cases tangible rewards were offered for reaching the goal. The decrease in coughing generalized to other times of the day in all four patients in the study.

PICKING

Repetitive picking behavior may involve picking at the skin or nose. There has been little systematic study regarding nose picking, although one survey study found that 91% of adults answering the survey reported current nose picking and 8% reported eating what they picked (Jefferson and Thompson, 1995). Similar data are not available for children, but these behaviors are commonly observed in children. Young children often pick their noses in public, whereas older children are more likely to do so when they are alone or when they feel protected from public view. Nose picking may begin in association with rhinorrhea resulting from colds or allergies or may begin in association with nasal irritation or itchiness. The most common complication of nose picking is epistaxis, and recurrent epistaxis in children is often attributed to nose picking. Other complications such as infections or perforation of the nasal septum are much less common but can occur. When nose picking is associated with allergic symptoms or rhinorrhea resulting from a cold, treatment with antihistamines or decongestants may be helpful. Despite the emotional re-

sponse that nose picking often elicits from parents, specific treatments are rarely indicated in young children because the behavior tends to decrease (or at least occur predominantly in private) as children get older and develop more social consciousness. Repeated attention to the behavior in the form of reprimands or punishments is not usually helpful and, in some cases, may serve to inadvertently reinforce the behavior.

Individuals may also pick at their skin or at scabs, resulting in excoriations, which at times may become infected. The cause of skin picking has not been well investigated, but it is often thought that stress and anxiety play a role. In adolescents, skin picking may occur in response to an imagined or slight defect in the appearance of the body or skin (body dysmorphic disorder) (see Chapter 46). In some cases, skin picking may occur in response to or be exacerbated by treatment with stimulant medications. Skin picking occurs relatively commonly in adolescents and adults with Prader-Willi syndrome.

Little systematic information on the treatment of skin picking is available. Good skin care to prevent infection and blocking access to the picked site until it heals are sufficient in some children. In more difficult cases, behavioral treatment using the habit reversal procedure (see Habit Reversal) could be attempted. There are case reports of adolescents and adults (including individuals with Prader-Willi syndrome) whose skin picking has improved on the serotonin-reuptake inhibitor fluoxetine (Warnock and Kestenbaum, 1992).

TRICHOTILLOMANIA

Trichotillomania is a disorder characterized by recurrent pulling of one's own hair, resulting in alopecia. Typically hair is pulled from the scalp, eyebrows, or eyelashes, but hair pulling can involve any site in which hair grows, including axillary and pubic hair. Occasionally hair may be pulled from dolls, pets, or other materials. The *DSM-IV* diagnostic criteria for trichotillomania require that individuals experience an increasing sense of tension before pulling out their hair and a sense of gratification or relief when pulling out their hair. However, many individuals who pull out their hair do not report this sense of tension and gratification. Thus, the prevalence of trichotillomania depends on the criteria used to make the diagnosis. Using *DSM-IV* criteria, Christenson and colleagues (1991) found a lifetime prevalence of trichotillomania of 0.6% in college freshman. However, hair pulling resulting in alopecia is more common, occurring in 1% to 2% of individuals (Christenson et al, 1991), and hair pulling that does not result in alopecia may occur at some point during childhood or adolescence in 10% or more of the population.

The diagnosis of trichotillomania can be difficult. It is not unusual for individuals with trichotillomania to deny hair pulling and to engage in the behavior surreptitiously. Trichotillomania must be distinguished from other causes of alopecia in children, most commonly tinea capitis or alopecia areata. In both trichotillomania and tinea capitis, the hair loss is usually patchy, but tinea capitis is usually associated with scaling of the scalp and broken hairs at the scalp. In alopecia areata, the hair loss is usually complete in the affected area, whereas in trichotillomania the hair loss is usually incomplete and hairs of various length are present in the area of alopecia. General thinning of the hair may occur in response to severe stressors, hypothyroidism, hyperthyroidism, and certain medications.

Clinical reports suggest that at least two subtypes of trichotillomania may exist. One form that tends to begin in younger children (usually younger than 6 years of age) is viewed as a benign habit that is self-limited or easily treated with behavior modification or counseling (Swedo and Rapoport, 1991). In these cases, the behavior often occurs in association with thumb-sucking and may be most frequent during periods of low stimulation such as at nap time or bedtime. When trichotillomania begins in older children and adolescents, it appears more likely to become a chronic condition and more likely to be associated with an anxiety disorder or depression (Reeve, Bernstein, and Christenson, 1992). Most adults with trichotillomania describe its onset during childhood or adolescence. In all cases, the clinician should inquire about trichophagia, because treatment is more urgent in children who are eating their hair, in order to prevent formation of a trichobezoar.

A variety of treatments for trichotillomania have been described. Behavioral treatments have the best demonstrated efficacy. In young children who suck their thumb while pulling their hair, treatment of the thumb-sucking often stops the hair pulling (Friman, 1990). For others, behavioral treatments using a habit reversal procedure (see Habit Reversal) or modifications of the habit reversal procedure have been successful in decreasing or eliminating hair pulling (Azrin, Nunn, and Frantz, 1980b; Blum, Barone, and Friman, 1993). Effective treatment with hypnosis has also been described (Kohen, 1996).

Recently there has been a lot of interest in the use of the serotonin-reuptake inhibitors, particularly fluoxetine and clomipramine, in the treatment of trichotillomania. These studies have predominantly occurred in adults. Even though many studies that have not used placebo-controlled designs suggest that these medications are helpful, studies using experimental designs have produced mixed results for clomipramine and generally negative results for fluoxetine (Jaspers, 1996). In those who initially benefit from the medication, a relapse in symptoms may occur during treatment.

HYPERVENTILATION

Hyperventilation syndrome describes a group of symptoms that may be caused by overbreathing. These symptoms include dizziness, paresthesias, blurred vision, chest pain, dry mouth, muscle spasms, headache, confusion, hallucinations, and feelings of impending doom (Evans, 1995; Herman, Stickler, and Lucas, 1981). A number of physiologic alterations brought about by hyperventilation are thought to account for these symptoms. Specifically, hyperventilation is known to decrease cerebral blood flow, which may account for the dizziness, visual changes, headache, and confusion. Alterations in electrolytes (e.g., calcium or phosphorus) may account for the paresthesias and muscle spasms.

The diagnosis of hyperventilation syndrome is not difficult when the patient's symptoms are associated with a rapid respiratory rate. However, in most cases of hyperventilation syndrome, the hyperventilation is not grossly visible. Small changes in tidal volume with a normal respiratory rate can significantly alter arterial carbon dioxide pressure, leading to symptoms. Reproduction of the symptoms on voluntary overbreathing can be helpful in making the diagnosis. This may be done by asking the patient to take deep breaths at a rate comfortable for the patient for 3 minutes. Dizziness and blurred vision may begin within 20 to 30 seconds, whereas paresthesias take longer to develop. Chest pains are reproduced in only about 50% of individuals in the 3 minutes (Lum, 1987). The differential diagnosis of hyperventilation syndrome includes disorders such as asthma, thyrotoxicosis, salicylate ingestion, pneumothorax, metabolic abnormality, cardiac arrhythmia, or neurologic disorder.

Hyperventilation syndrome is often associated with symptoms of anxiety, panic, phobias, or depression. In a follow-up study of 30 children at 2 to 28 years after the diagnosis of hyperventilation syndrome, Herman and colleagues (1981) found that more than 50% reported problems with anxiety and more than 33% reported problems with depression. Forty percent were still having episodes of hyperventilation.

Reassurance and education are vital components of the treatment of hyperventilation syndrome. When significant symptoms of anxiety, fear, stress, or depression are present, the patient should receive appropriate psychological and, if necessary, pharmacologic treatment. A number of possible interventions have been suggested when patients begin to experience symptoms. The most common is to have individuals hold their breath, count to 10, and then slowly breathe out. Breathing in and out of a paper bag has also been suggested on the principle that this leads to restoration of a normal arterial carbon dioxide pressure. However, the distraction provided by the paper bag and the suggestion that it is helpful may also be important factors that contribute to the efficacy of this approach. Other treatments include breathing retraining (Tweeddale, Rowbottom, and McHardy, 1994), biofeedback, and hypnosis.

Tics and Tourette Syndrome

Tics are involuntary, brief, rapid, repetitive, nonrhythmic movements or vocalizations. Individual tics are usually classified as motor or vocal (if they involve the movement of air through the mouth or nose) and as simple or complex. Simple motor tics are those that involve an individual muscle group and include blinking, shoulder shrugging, squinting, and lip licking. Complex motor tics involve either a cluster of simple tics or a more coordinated pattern of movements such as touching, jumping, manipulating clothing, or facial grimacing. Simple vocal tics involve making sounds such as grunting, sniffing, and throat clearing. Complex vocal tics involve saying words, parts of words, or phrases, palilalia (repeating one's own words), or echolalia (repeating other's words).

Recently, there has been a lot of interest in sensory phenomena that often precede tics. Many individuals with Tourette syndrome have an unpleasant feeling that may be described as a pressure, urge, or itch that becomes progressively more bothersome until they perform the tic. Premonitory sensations most often involve the shoulders, palms of the hands, abdomen, and throat, and tics in these areas seem more likely to be associated with them than tics that involve the eyes, face, and head (Scahill, Leckman, and Marek, 1995). However, there is not always correspondence between the location of the premonitory sensation and the site to the tic.

Individuals with tics may be further classified as having one of three tic disorders (see Table 45–2) based on both the duration and type of tics that are present. *Transient tic disorder* requires that single or multiple motor or vocal tics be present for less than 1 year. Because there is no accurate way to predict whether tics will resolve or become chronic, the diagnosis of transient tic disorder can only be made in retrospect. Nonetheless, transient tic disorder is the most common tic disorder, occurring in 5% to 24% of school-aged children (Singer, 1993). *Chronic tic disorder* is diagnosed when single or multiple tics, which are only motor or less commonly only vocal, occur for more than 1 year. Chronic tic disorder occurs in 1% to 2% of the school-aged population. *Tourette syndrome* is diagnosed when both motor and vocal tics occur and tics have been present for more than 1 year. Tourette syndrome occurs in 1 to 8 of every 1000 boys and in 0.1 to 4 of every 1000 girls (Peterson, 1996). A substantial amount of evidence from genetic studies suggests that chronic tic disorder and Tourette syndrome are part of the same spectrum of tic disorders, whereas questions remain as to whether transient tic disorders represent the mildest end of the Tourette syndrome spectrum or an unrelated tic disorder (Lombroso et al, 1995).

The modal age for the onset of motor tics is 7 years old and for vocal tics is 9 years old, but tics may occur as early as 2 years of age, and in rare cases, the new onset of tics has been described as late as the early 20s. Usually Tourette syndrome has a gradual onset with one or more episodes of transient tics followed by more persistent motor and vocal tics. The tics usually have a waxing and waning course and may be exacerbated by anxiety, stress, excitement, or fatigue. Over time, new tics may replace old tics or be added to the preexisting repertoire of tics. Even within the group of children who meet the diagnostic criteria for Tourette syndrome, there is a lot of variability in the severity of the tics. In some, the tics may be of low frequency and intensity, whereas in others the tics may be of such high frequency and intensity that they cause significant subjective distress to the individual and interfere with interpersonal relationships and classroom or other activities. Occasionally, complex tics involve obscene gestures (copropraxia) or obscene words (coprolalia). Even though copropraxia and coprolalia are often emphasized in descriptions of Tourette syndrome, they are not required for the diagnosis and occur in less than 10% of individuals with Tourette syndrome.

Tourette syndrome is often associated with other behavioral or learning problems. Obsessive-compulsive behaviors have been described in as many as 90% of affected individuals, and 40% to 50% meet criteria for obsessive-compulsive disorder (Como, 1995; Singer, 1993). Genetic studies have also pointed to a relationship with obsessive-compulsive disorder, which occurs at a 9 to 13 times higher frequency in first-degree relatives of individuals with Tourette syndrome than in the general population. Furthermore, data are consistent, with Tourette syndrome being transmitted in an autosomal dominant manner with obsessive-compulsive disorder being an alternative expression of the Tourette syndrome gene (Como, 1995). In these studies, males are more likely to have Tourette syndrome and females are more likely to have obsessive-compulsive disorder without tics.

Other disorders have also been described as occurring frequently in individuals with Tourette syndrome. Attention-deficit hyperactivity disorder (ADHD) is diagnosed in approximately 50% of affected individuals, and the ADHD symptoms often predate the onset of the tics. Anxiety disorders and depression have been described in 25% to 50% of individuals with this condition (Lombroso et al, 1995) and learning disabilities occur in about 25%.

Treatment of children with Tourette syndrome must focus on determining the impact of the tics as well as on the impact of comorbid conditions on the child's functioning. Often the comorbid conditions have a greater impact on the child's functioning than the tics, and treatment should focus on the management of the identified comorbid conditions (management of the various comorbid conditions is discussed elsewhere in this book, especially Chapter 64).

The presence of tics alone is not a reason for treatment. However, when the tics cause significant disruption in motor or speech functions or are interfering with the child's social or emotional development or interpersonal relationships, then treatment is indicated. Thus, even in a referred population of children, only about 60% of the children with Tourette syndrome receive pharmacologic treatment for the tics (Singer, 1993).

Pharmacologic treatments for tics (Table 45–3) have the best documented efficacy. (See Chapter 82 regarding drugs and doses). Neuroleptic medications such as risperidone, haloperidol, pimozide, and fluphenazine are the most effective for suppressing tics, but side effects such as sedation, weight gain, dysphoria, anxiety (including school phobia), cognitive dulling, and extrapyramidal effects often limit the dose that can be administered or compliance with the treatment. In addition, the risk of tardive dyskinesia restricts the use of these medications to children with the most severe symptoms. When neuroleptics are used, they should be started at a low dose, which can be increased on a weekly basis until the lowest effective amount is identified. Although doses higher than those listed in Table 45–3 are sometimes used, it is unusual to have a dramatic decrease in tics at higher levels. When the treatment efficacy is not dramatic, it can be difficult to distinguish between a response to medication and the natural waxing and waning that occurs with tics.

The alpha-2 adrenergic agonists clonidine and guanfacine are less effective than neuroleptics in suppressing tics but still may be used as the first-line medication because they have fewer side effects and do not have the long-term risk of tardive dyskinesia. In addition, these medications may help decrease hyperactivity and are often used in children with ADHD and a tic disorder. Maximum efficacy of these medications may not be seen for 3 to 4 weeks, but even at this point 50% to 75% of individuals

Table 45–3 • Medications Used in the Treatment of Tics

Medications: Generic Name (Brand Name)	Usual Dose Range* (mg/day)	Schedule (doses/day)	Potential Adverse Effects
Neuroleptics			
Haloperidol (Haldol)	0.5–3.0	1–2	Acute dystonia, extrapyramidal symptoms, tardive dyskinesia, akathesia, fatigue, weight gain, cognitive blunting, neuroleptic malignant syndrome
Pimozide (Orap)	1.0–6.0	1–2	Same as Haldol and long QT interval, monitor EKG
Fluphenazine (Prolixin)	0.5–3.0	1–2	Same as Haldol
Atypical neuroleptics			
Risperidone (Risperdal)	0.5–4.0	1–2	Similar to Haldol, but fewer extrapyramidal symptoms and more postural hypotension
Alpha-2 adrenergic agonists			
Clonidine (Catapres)	0.05–0.5 0.003–0.01 mg/kg/day	3–4	Sedation, dry mouth, constipation, irritability, sleep disturbance, nightmares, hypotension, anxiety, depression, hallucinations (rare), rebound hypertension if stopped suddenly
Guanfacine (Tenex)	0.5–4.0 0.015–0.05 mg/kg/day	2–4	Similar to clonidine, possibly with less sedation

*Doses above these ranges are often accompanied by significant side effects.

report little or no improvement in tic symptoms (Peterson, 1996). The most common side effect of these medications is sedation, which, although it tends to decrease over the first 3 to 4 weeks of treatment, still limits the use of the medication in some children. Rapid discontinuation of these medications can produce rebound hypertension as well as worsening of the tics, and thus the medications should be tapered before they are discontinued.

Nonpharmacologic treatments for tics, including habit reversal (see Habit Reversal), relaxation training, biofeedback, and hypnosis, have been reported to decrease the frequency of tics in some individuals. However, the generalizability (especially to children) of reports of effective treatments using these procedures is not clear, and further research is needed before they can be widely recommended.

Habit Reversal

The original habit reversal procedure was described by Azrin and Nunn (1973). It is a multicomponent behavioral treatment (Table 45–4) that has been demonstrated to be effective for a wide variety of repetitive behaviors including thumb-sucking, nail biting, hair pulling, and tics (Woods and Miltenberger, 1995). The components of the treatment are designed to accomplish three goals: (1) increase the individual's awareness of the habit, (2) teach the individual a competing response to engage in when they feel as if they are about to engage in the habit, and (3) help sustain compliance and facilitate generalization of the response. When habit reversal has been compared with other behavioral treatments for repetitive behaviors, habit reversal has generally been found to be more effective in suppressing them (Azrin, Nunn, and Frantz, 1980a, 1980b; Peterson and Azrin, 1992).

Since the original description of the habit reversal procedure, effective treatments that have used modifications of the procedure have been described. Studies that have removed components of the original procedure suggest that the training to increase awareness of the habit and the use of the competing response are the most important components of the treatment, although it has been hypothesized that the social support procedure may have increased importance in children (Woods and Miltenberger, 1995). Other studies have added components to the habit reversal procedure that include progressive muscle relaxation, relaxed breathing, and visual imagery.

Although the habit reversal procedure has the best documented efficacy for the behavioral treatment of repetitive behaviors, most group studies have occurred in adolescents and adults. Use of this procedure in children often requires simplification of the procedures, motivation on the child's part to change the behavior, and a high level of cooperation between the child and parents. If the child is not motivated to change the behavior or if the repetitive behavior is resulting in significant conflict between the parent and child, these issues need to be managed before implementing the habit reversal procedure. Teaching patients the habit reversal procedures takes some time and experience. Most often, patients are taught the habit reversal procedure by a behavioral psychologist, but other clinicians interested in treating habits can learn to use the procedure effectively.

Repetitive Behaviors in Children With Developmental Disorders

Individuals with developmental disorders such as autism, mental retardation, and severe visual impairments have higher rates of repetitive behaviors than are found in the general population. These behaviors may be of concern because they are stigmatizing, because they occur to the exclusion of more adaptive behaviors, or because they result in self-injury. Self-injury is the most severe form of repetitive behavior and is the focus of this section.

Self-injurious behaviors include a wide range of behaviors such as repeated wetting and rubbing of the hands in the mouth, causing maceration of the skin; biting or

Table 45–4 • Components of Habit Reversal Procedure

I. Increase individual's awareness of habit
    A. Response description—have individual describe behavior to therapist in detail while reenacting the behavior and looking in a mirror.
    B. Response detection—inform individual of each occurrence of the behavior until each occurrence is detected without assistance.
    C. Early warning—have individual practice identifying earliest signs of the target behavior.
    D. Situation awareness—have individual describe all situations in which the target behavior is likely to occur.
II. Teach competing response to habit
    The competing response must result in isometric contraction of muscles involved in the habit, be capable of being maintained for 3 minutes, and be socially inconspicuous and compatible with normal ongoing activities, but incompatible with the habit (e.g., clenching one's fist, grasping and clenching an object).
III. Sustain compliance and facilitate generalization
    A. Habit inconvenience review—have individual review in detail all problems associated with target behavior.
    B. Social support procedure—family members and friends provide high levels of praise when a habit-free period is noted.
    C. Public display—individual demonstrates to others that he or she can control the target behavior.
    D. Symbolic rehearsal procedure—for each situation identified in situation awareness procedure, individual imagines himself or herself beginning the target behavior, but stopping and engaging in the competing response.

picking skin, resulting in open lesions that may become infected; and violent banging of the head or other body parts against hard surfaces, which may result in fractures, retinal detachments, intracranial hemorrhages, and even death. Self-injury is a major reason for intensive special education programming and hospitalization, thus greatly increasing the costs associated with an individual's care (Fig. 45–2).

Environmental and biological factors are associated with repetitive behaviors in general and self-injurious behaviors in particular. Increases in repetitive behaviors have been shown to be a response to the level of environmental stimulation. Prolonged institutionalization, especially when associated with low levels of stimulation or confinement of the individual, has been shown to increase repetitive

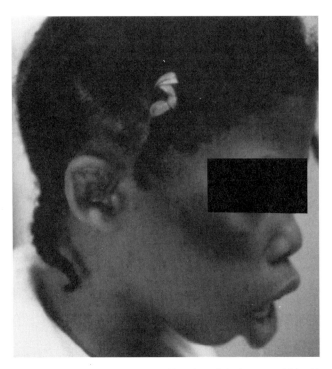

Figure 45–2. Scarring of the ear and bruising of the face caused by self-injurious behavior in a child with severe mental retardation.

behaviors, which may be fulfilling a self-stimulatory function. For example, visually impaired individuals may compress the optic globe (which may result in injury to the eye), because such an action stimulates the retina. In this type of situation, increasing environmental stimulation may decrease the repetitive behaviors (Guess and Carr, 1991). On the other hand, high levels of stimulation that produce anxiety, stress, or frustration may also increase repetitive behaviors. Individuals with severe disabilities may have limited abilities to describe their experiences, requiring clinicians and caretakers to observe carefully and describe the individual and situations that elicit the repetitive behaviors.

Studies of self-injurious behavior have demonstrated that the predictable reactions of caretakers to the behavior often reinforce the self-injurious behaviors. For example, this may occur when self-injury results in care providers' giving attention to the individual or when caregivers respond to the behavior by allowing the individual access to materials or activities that may be otherwise restricted (e.g., food, going on a walk). Self-injurious behavior may also be reinforced when it causes care providers to remove task demands (Mace and Mauk, 1995). In these cases, the repetitive self-injurious behaviors are best viewed as learned behaviors that serve as a form of nonverbal communication.

Biological factors are also important in the occurrence of self-injurious behavior. Alterations in neuro-transmitter systems are thought to contribute to some self-injurious behaviors. Dopamine deficiency early in development is thought to cause the nearly universal occurrence of self-biting in individuals with Lesch-Nyhan syndrome (Breese et al, 1995). It has been hypothesized that in some cases, the ability of self-injurious behavior to release endogenous opiates may maintain the behavior, and effective treatment with the opiate antagonist naltrexone has been described. Other biological variables may affect the likelihood that an individual will engage in self-injurious behavior. Increased rates of self-injurious behavior have been suggested to occur in association with menstruation, physical conditions such as otitis media, fatigue, and allergies. Although it is unlikely that these factors directly cause self-injury, they could certainly decrease one's tolerance for task demands or frustration and thus alter the likelihood of a specific event triggering self-injurious behavior.

For a review of the assessment and treatment of self-injurious behavior, see Mace and Mauk (1995) and Steege and colleagues (1989). Briefly, the treatment plan must first protect the individual from significant injury. In some cases, this may involve the use of helmets or even restraints, but these devices limit adaptive functioning and thus are best used as temporary measures to protect the individual until an assessment is completed and an effective treatment plan is implemented.

An assessment must include an evaluation of the potential communicative role for the behaviors. Although in some cases the communicative role of the behaviors may be clear to care providers, in many cases it is not. A functional analysis of the behavior conducted by a behavior analyst (Steege et al, 1989) may be necessary to identify the communicative function of the behavior. When a communicative function is identified, treatment should focus on training the individual to use more adaptive means for communicating his or her needs.

Occasionally a communicative function for the self-injurious behaviors is not identified or the self-injury is so severe that pharmacologic intervention is required. Neuroleptic medications are the most frequently used medication in this situation, and these medications seem to be most helpful when the behavior occurs in a very stereotyped manner. However, neuroleptics must be used with caution both because of their sedating effects, which may decrease adaptive functioning, and because of their potential for other severe side effects. Research into the use of other medications, such as opiate antagonists, serotonin-reuptake inhibitors, and beta-blockers, may allow more targeted pharmacologic treatment for self-injury (Mace and Mauk, 1995).

ACKNOWLEDGMENT

I would like to thank Drs. Patrick Friman and Marianne Mercugliano for their review and helpful comments on an earlier version of this chapter.

REFERENCES

Abe K, Oda N, Amatoni M: Natural history and predictive significance of head-banging, head-rolling and breath-holding spells. Dev Med Child Neurol 26:644–648, 1984.

American Psychiatric Association: DSM-IV, Diagnostic and Statistical Manual of Mental Disorders, 4th ed. Washington, DC, American Psychiatric Association, 1994.

Ames D, Cummings JL, Wirshing WC, et al: Repetitive and compulsive behavior in frontal lobe degenerations. J Neuropsychiatry Clin Neurosci 6:100–113, 1994.

Attanasio R: Nocturnal bruxism and its clinical management. Dent Clin North Am 35:245–252, 1991.

Azrin NH, Nunn RG: Habit reversal: a method of eliminating nervous habits and tics. Behav Res Ther 11:619–628, 1973.

Azrin NH, Nunn RG, Frantz SE: Habit reversal vs. negative practice treatment of nailbiting. Behav Res Ther 18:281–285, 1980a.

Azrin NH, Nunn RG, Frantz SE: Treatment of hairpulling (trichotillomania): a comparative study of habit reversal and negative practice training. J Behav Ther Exp Psychiatry 11:13–20, 1980b.

Bakwin H, Bakwin RM. Behavior Disorders in Children. Philadelphia, WB Saunders, 1972, pp 505–516.

Blum NJ, Barone VJ, Friman PC: A simplified behavioral treatment for trichotillomania: report of two cases. Pediatrics 91:993–995, 1993.

Breese GR, Criswell HE, Duncan GE, et al: Model for reduced dopamine in Lesch-Nyhan syndrome and the mentally retarded: neurobiology of neonatal-6-hydroxydopamine lesioned rats. MRDD Res Rev 1:111–119, 1995.

Cash RG: Bruxism in children: review of the literature. J Pedodontics 12:107127, 1988.

Castellanos FX, Ritchie GF, Marsh WL, et al: DSM-IV Stereotypic movement disorder: persistence of stereotypies of infancy in intellectually normal adolescents and adults. J Clin Psychiatry 57(3):116–122, 1996.

Christenson GA, Pyle RL, Mitchell JE: Estimated lifetime prevalence of trichotillomania in college students. J Clin Psychiatry 52:415–417, 1991.

Como PG: Obsessive-compulsive disorder in Tourette's syndrome. Adv Neurol 65:281–291, 1995.

Daoud AS, Batieha A, Al-Sheyyab M, et al: Effectiveness of iron therapy on breath-holding spells. J Pediatr 130(4):547–550, 1997.

Dimario FJ: Breath-holding spells in childhood. Am J Dis Child 146:125–131, 1992.

Evans RW: Neurologic aspects of hyperventilation syndrome. Semin Neurol 15(2):115–125, 1995.

Fog R, Pakkenberg H: Behavioural effects of dopamine and p-hydroxyamphetamine injected into the corpus striatum of rats. Exp Neurol 31:75–86, 1971.

Friman PC: Concurrent habits: what would Linus do with his blanket if his thumb-sucking were treated? Am J Dis Child 144:1316–1318, 1990.

Friman PC, Leibowitz J: An effective and acceptable treatment alternative for chronic thumb and finger sucking. J Pediatr Psychol 15(1):57–62, 1990.

Friman PC, McPherson KM, Warzak WJ, et al: Influence of thumb sucking on peer social acceptance in first-grade children. Pediatrics 91(4):784–786, 1993.

Guess D, Carr E: Emergence and maintenance of stereotypy and self-injury. Am J Ment Retard 96(3):299–319, 1991.

Herman SP, Stickler GB, Lucas AR: Hyperventilation syndrome in children and adolescents: long-tem follow-up. Pediatrics 67(2):183–187, 1981.

Jaspers JPC: The diagnosis and psychopharmacological treatment of trichotillomania: a review. Pharmacopsychiatry 29:115–120, 1996.

Jefferson JW, Thompson TD: Rhinotillexomania: psychiatric disorder or habit. J Clin Psychiatry 56(2):56–59, 1995.

Kohen DP: Hypnotherapeutic management of pediatric and adolescent trichotillomania. J Dev Behav Pediatr 17(5):328–334, 1996.

Kravitz H, Boehm JJ: Rhythmic habit patterns in infancy: their sequence, age of onset, and frequency. Child Dev 42:399–413, 1971.

Lavigne JV, Davis AT, Fauber R: Behavioral management of psychogenic cough: alternative to the "bedsheet" and other aversive techniques. Pediatrics 87(4):532–537, 1991.

Leung AKC, Robson LM: Nailbiting. Clin Pediatr 1990; 29(12):690–692.

Lokshin B, Lindgren S, Weinberger M, et al: Outcome of habit cough in children treated with a brief session of suggestion therapy. Ann Allergy 67:579–582, 1991.

Lombroso PJ, Scahill LD, Chappell PB, et al: Tourette's syndrome: a multigenerational neuropsychiatric disorder. Adv Neurol 65:305–318, 1995.

Lum LC: Hyperventilation syndromes in medicine and psychiatry: a review. J R Soc Med 80:229–231, 1987.

Mace FC, Mauk JE: Bio-behavioral diagnosis and treatment of self-injury. MRDD Res Rev 1:104–110, 1995.

Mahalski PA, Stanton WR: The relationship between digit sucking and behaviour problems: a longitudinal study over 10 years. J Child Psychol Psychiatry 33(5):913–923, 1992.

McWilliam RC, Stephenson JBP: Atropine treatment of reflex anoxic seizures. Arch Dis Child 59:473–485, 1984.

Peterson AL, Azrin NH: An evaluation of behavioral treatments for Tourette syndrome. Behav Res Ther 30:167–174, 1992.

Peterson BS: Considerations of natural history and pathophysiology in the psychopharmacology of Tourette's syndrome. J Clin Psychiatry 57(suppl 9):24–34, 1996.

Reeve EA, Bernstein GA, Christenson GA: Clinical characteristics and psychiatric comorbidity in children with trichotillomania. J Am Child Adolesc Psychiatry 31(1):132–138, 1992.

Ridley RM: The psychology of perseverative and stereotyped behaviour. Prog Neurobiol 44:221–231, 1994.

Rovee CK, Rovee DT: Conjugate reinforcement of infant exploratory behavior. J Exp Child Psychol 8:33–39, 1969.

Sallustro MA, Atwell CW: Body rocking, head banging, and head rolling in normal children. J Pediatr 93(4):704–708, 1978.

Scahill LD, Leckman JF, Marek KL: Sensory phenomena in Tourette's syndrome. Adv Neurol 65:273–280, 1995.

Singer HS: Tic disorders. Pediatr Ann 23(1):22–29, 1993.

Steege MW, Wacker DP, Berg WK, et al: The use of behavioral assessment to prescribe and evaluate treatments for severely handicapped children. J Appl Behav Anal 22:22–23, 1989.

Swedo SE, Rapoport JL: Annotation: trichotillomania. J Child Psychol Psychiat 32(3):401–409, 1991.

Thelen E: Rhythmical behavior in infancy: an ethological perspective. Develop Psychol 17(3):237–257, 1981.

Thelen E: Rhythmical stereotypes in normal human infants. Anim Behav 27:699–715, 1979.

Troster H: Prevalence and functions of stereotyped behaviors in nonhandicapped children in residential care. J Abnorm Child Psychol 22(1):79–97, 1994.

Tweeddale PM, Rowbottom I, McHardy GJR: Breathing retraining: effect on anxiety and depression scores in behavioral breathlessness. J Psychosom Res 38:11–21, 1994.

Vanderas AP: Relationship between craniomandibular dysfunction and oral parafunctions in caucasian children with and without unpleasant life events. J Oral Rehab 22:289–294, 1995.

Warnock JK, Kestenbaum T: Pharmacologic treatment of severe skin picking behaviors in Prader-Willi syndrome: two case reports. Arch Dermatol 128(12):1623–1625, 1992.

Wolraich ML, Felice ME, Drotar D (eds): The Classification of Child and Adolescent Mental Diagnoses in Primary Care: Diagnostic and Statistical Manual for Primary Care (DSM-PC) Child and Adolescent Version. Elk Grove Village, IL, American Academy of Pediatrics, 1996.

Woods DW, Miltenberger R: Habit reversal: a review of applications and variations. J Behav Ther Exp Psychiatry 26(2):123–131, 1995.

46 Body Image: Development and Distortion

Myron L. Belfer

 The body image that the individual knows is not the reflection of the body as it is, but an interpretation of it.

Despite demonstrated competence in social, intellectual, and vocational skills, children with manifest deformities are often stereotyped in disadvantaged ways.

The child who is less verbal or is reticent in his or her answers may be approached by being asked to draw a picture of a person, followed by the request to draw a picture of himself or herself. The usefulness of the data obtained increases with the age of the child.

The term *body image* encompasses a complex psychological concept related to the mental representation of the self and is not merely a function of objective appearance. The development of one's body image is an intricate evolutionary process with multiple determinants. The growth of normal body image is influenced by biological, psychological, social, and cultural inputs. Understanding the creation and meaning of body image is necessary to appreciate certain developmental hurdles for children with more subtle deficits in motor function, unobservable abnormalities, and metabolic disease. Distortions of body image may arise with genetic syndromes, congenital illnesses, alterations in body morphology, and trauma (Anthony, 1968; Belfer, Harrison, and Murray, 1979; Belfer, Harrison, and Pillemar, 1982; Green and Levitt, 1962; Kaufman, 1972; Kaufman and Hersher; 1971). In the past decade, complex disorders involving body image, such as eating disorders and body dysmorphic disorder, have occupied the attention of clinicians.

The main objective of this chapter is to delineate the trajectory of normal body image development and to identify potential concerns for physicians responsible for the continuing medical care of children who might have problems with their body image that affect self-esteem and psychological functioning. Although the concluding section addresses specific psychological and treatment considerations, recommendations for the management of children with body image disturbances are interspersed throughout.

Body Image Development

Body image is defined as that aspect of the self-concept that begins to develop in the earliest stages of awareness of self. It has the physical body as a focus, and other aspects of self-concept are elaborated around it. Kaufman and Hersher (1971) make the important distinction between the body as a physical object and "the mental representation of the body which is a psychological construct." The body image that the individual knows is not the reflection of the body as it is, but an interpretation of it. This interpretation, which is affectively charged, is influenced by individual factors and contextual ones, such as the meanings and values that the culture confers on the masculine and feminine bodies (Rodriquez-Tome, Bariaud, and Cohen Zardin, 1990; Bruchon-Schweitzer, 1990).

Normal Early Development

At the earliest stages of development, children gain an appreciation of their own bodies and their environment by often delicate sensory input, and they obtain feelings of mastery through an increasing sense of competence in their manipulative functions, whether of the hands, feet, tongue, or other body parts. Infants are capable of integrating multiple perceptions. For example, in the feeding and sucking process, the mouth is the first area to be stimulated. As the child's capacity to explore the environment grows, primary kinesthetic and tactile sensations form the foundation upon which the beginnings of self-awareness and individuality are built (Kolb, 1959).

Similar to the progressive development of a child's perceptual capacities, the development of cognitive functions influences the perception of his or her body and defines the limits of body image development (Goodenough, 1926; Katz and Zigler, 1967; Shapiro and Stine, 1965). Developmentally, children learn about the body and its parts in a sequential fashion that coincides with a progressive increase in cognitive functioning. The development of a coherent and constant body image occurs during Piaget's preoperational subperiod, between the ages of approximately 2 and 7 years. This aspect of self-experience consolidates between the ages of 5 and 7 years. Children with low intellectual potential can be limited in their perceptions of their body, and younger children, because of their immature cognition, perceive their bodies in different ways than do older children. Mental retardation can significantly limit the development of a child's body image because of the inability both to form abstract concepts of bodily functions and to relate self-perceptions to the bodies of others. In those youngsters, there is a persistent emphasis on the function of body parts, more so than on aesthetic considerations.

All children, regardless of their physical normalcy, experience a sense of "like" and "not like." They compare their bodies with those of parents, brothers and sisters, and peers and later with those that are presented by the culture as a whole. During this process a child becomes aware of similarities and differences. How a child reacts to inherent differences between self and others depends not only on the objective nature of the difference, but also on the interaction of the child with the significant persons in the environment who place a value on certain attributes, as well as on cultural values that are conveyed to the child in a variety of ways.

There is evidence that children as young as 6 years already understand the importance of looking good and being thin (Flannery-Schroeder and Chrisler, 1996). Further, children of this age associate "bad" adjectives with endomorphic body types (Brenner and Hinsdale, 1978). Thus, for instance, stigmatization of obese individuals is established in early childhood (Goldfield and Chrisler, 1995).

In many cultures children with obvious physical differences are viewed with disapproval, revulsion, and rejection. Such attitudes have both psychological and social meaning. The etiology of these attitudes may reside in the individuals offering the criticism, whose body image may be inadequate. These individuals project their inadequacies onto those they feel may be more vulnerable and who have more obvious differences. This accounts for the verbal assault experienced by some children with more obvious bodily differences.

PARENTAL ROLE

The parents' perceptions of their child as having positive bodily attributes gives the child permission to appreciate himself or herself and his or her body, to gain self-esteem, and to become comfortable with himself or herself. Early in the child's life, parental attitudes, feelings, and behavior in regard to a deformity influence the child's ability to relate positively to his or her body. Social learning theory proposes that parents are important agents of socialization who, through modeling, feedback, and instruction, influence their children's body image (Striegel-Moore and Kearney-Cooke, 1994). It is normative for parents to view their children as physically attractive. Parents tend to focus on the body's physical appearance in girls but emphasize physical function in boys (Rodin, Silberstein, and Striegel-Moore, 1985). Acculturative effects on body image perception remain largely unexplored in the literature (Pate et al, 1992).

The capacity for a satisfying adaptation among children with deficits in bodily development is dependent more on parental, family, and cultural attitudes toward the body structure than on the presence of a specific bodily difference. A child who is normal but who does not fulfill expectations for athletic prowess might be viewed as defective. When family and cultural attitudes toward the difference are constructive and supportive, the child has a greater possibility for successful compensatory development without the development of a host of complex psychological defenses that may distort healthy development.

Early Deformity

Failure to gain feelings of mastery and competence and the inability to appreciate subtle nuances of stimuli deprive children with birth defects or acquired differences of a sense of wholeness and satisfaction that other children obtain. The lack of mastery of basic bodily kinesthetic and tactile sensations has a negative influence on the development of a child's body image and self-concept. In the child with a congenital abnormality, a sense of bodily incompetence can develop when the abnormality is associated with a functional impairment. For example, the child with syndactyly may fail to gain tactile satisfaction, or the patient with a cleft palate may have impaired oral perception and difficulty with nasal secretions (Tisza et al, 1958).

The child with a deformity who looks dull or retarded tends to be considered so regardless of his or her true intellectual capacity. When a youngster has a congenital deformity based on some definable genetic diathesis, such as trisomy or a diffuse craniofacial abnormality, the child's appearance can contribute to the impression that he or she has an intellectual deficit greater than that present and may, in fact, mask a normal intellectual potential. An example of this phenomenon is seen most dramatically in children with Apert and Crouzon syndromes, in which, despite frequent misconception, there is a broad range of intellectual functioning, including totally normal levels of verbal and performance intelligence. Wright (1964) noted that this phenomenon occurs with respect to self-perceptions as well. Cohen and Yasuna (1978), studying children with Apert and Crouzon syndromes, showed that the fears of children with facial disfigurements that they were mentally retarded stemmed in part from concerns about their facial structures. Children with congenital or acquired deformities internalize a sense of impaired cognitive ability that can then inhibit normal cognitive development because of the occurrence of self-defeating defenses. It must be remembered that the child's internal sense of self does not reflect reality; rather it reflects what is psychologically important to him or her (Kaufman, 1972). A child who incorporates a sense of distorted bodily function, and in particular a perceived sense of deficit, can internalize this as a sense of "badness."

PARENTAL ROLE

The negative effects on social interaction for a child with a congenital or acquired defect are most strongly felt in the child's encounters with the parents. Bowlby (1969) suggests that the infant emits biologically programmed responses that "trigger" nurturing behavior on the part of the mother. Two important elicitors of maternal behavior are smiling and vocalization. A structural abnormality around the mouth could interfere with recognizable smile responses or vocalization. Thus, the physical deficit may lead to complex problems in bonding and psychological development.

Parents are challenged to understand and relate to the child who is born not meeting their expectations. The mother and father are faced with the task of adapting to meet the needs of the child while working through their issues of what led to the birth of the child with the developmental problem. In this era, parents are inevitably concerned with the genetics of the observable problem, which parent's genes might be responsible, what the implications are for having other children, and at a deeper level a sense of personal responsibility, guilt, or blame directed at others, including the other parent. The latter is a demonstrable stress that is now well recognized and in more dramatic situations requires counseling to avoid the all-too-common consequence of marital discord and disruption.

It is to be expected that parents will experience a sadness that should resolve with time. Failure of this grief response to resolve may be an indication for counseling. Failure to resolve some of the conflicts noted can have an adverse effect on how parents later see their child. It must be borne in mind that it is the parental perception of the child's problem that is most important and that this may not fit with the objective appearance of the child. The child may appear far better to the professional than to the parent who has a predetermined set of expectations. Support groups for parents are available, some addressing specific syndromes related to aspects of the body. (See listing of selected support groups at the end of the chapter.)

Denial of the reality of a child's deformity and "undoing" the defect by referring to it as "cute" are common defense mechanisms used by parents whose child has a congenital or acquired deformity. In the extreme, some parents seek through reconstructive or cosmetic surgery to "undo" or deny the congenital deformity or the stigmata associated with certain chromosomal abnormalities, such as trisomy 21. The pediatrician needs to be aware that the notion of such reconstruction has its ardent proponents as well as its detractors. Some parents and clinicians believe that the surgical intervention frees the child to pursue a more "normal" life. Others see the surgery as an effort to deny reality.

In another scenario, a sense of "specialness" can be attributed to the child with a congenital deformity that impedes reality development and the evaluation of a child's capacities. There is an important difference between supporting a youngster's strengths and helping him or her to gain particular skills or talents, and identifying the child as "special" in the sense that he or she is endowed with special attributes of a spiritual nature. The latter does not equip the child with the means for successful later coping in situations where peers and others will not accept the premise for this more abstract "specialness."

In some instances parents may respond to a child's differentness through reaction formation or emotional withdrawal. These defenses are particularly damaging to the child for two reasons. First, children tend to emulate their parents' methods of coping with anger, loss, and disappointment and employ similar defensive styles. Second, these defenses can lead to an impairment of reality testing in the child so that an unrealistic sense of self, owing to the differentness, is formed. Although some psychological defenses are necessary in order for both parents and child to cope, the degree and intensity to which they are maintained should be taken into consideration.

EXAMPLE

Javier is a child who grew up with hemifacial microsomia. Valued for his pleasant personality and friendliness, he was expected to never be angry with his younger siblings, parents, or other adults in his environment. When surgery was being considered to reconstruct his outer ear and improve the appearance of his face, it was not possible to get Javier to express realistic anxiety about the pending procedure. Further, in therapeutic work he was unable to express normal feelings of anger that would have helped him to achieve more independence in his life. These inabilities to express feelings can be traced back to Javier's incorporation of his caregivers' need to deny his differentness and overemphasize his extraordinary reaction formation.

With a younger child, the physician can gain information about the child's coping mechanisms through discussion with the parents. Parents who have resolved their personal conflicts tend to speak about the child's disorder rationally and realistically. They also tend to accept and follow through on offers of help, whether the offer of aid is physical or psychological. A certain degree of denial may be healthy and sustain positive functioning. It is not helpful to confront either the parent or the child with a harsh reality; rather it is preferable to support denial to the extent that it preserves a functioning family unit and then proceed to work on lessening the denial over time as one sees the child and family through evolving developmental phases.

In the situation of an older child, the physician would do well to investigate the child's capacity to deal verbally with the consequences of the disorder without interfering too greatly with the youngster's adaptive defenses. Again, one should not abruptly take away denial that facilitates coping.

The father has a special influence on body image development, for he is a potential source of support for the mother and can offer valued acceptance and support to the child. If the father is seen by the mother as sympathetic and positive, many of her attitudes of guilt, humiliation, or depression can be alleviated. In addition, the mother is often less anxious over the birth of a child with a deformity if the father expresses his distress over the event, perceiving that she is not alone with her feelings. As with other significant persons, such as friends and relatives, the father can either support the mother's adaptation to their child or increase the difficulties she might experience. Matters are made more complex when the child has a deformity that is similar to a parental deformity, and thus various parental issues are aroused, including a pathologic identity, increased guilt, and blame by others.

Observation of both the verbal and nonverbal communications between parents, as well as those between parent and child, is one source of data that permits the physician to measure the quality of the marital relationship and the degree of parent-child attachment. Parents who belittle or blame each other, be it subtly or overtly, constitute a source of conflict that can affect the overall psychological development of the child, as well as the child's sense of body image.

Brothers and sisters further contribute to the development of body image in siblings, both indirectly in terms of comparison and directly in terms of the nature of their responses toward the child with differentness. In some cases brothers and sisters reinforce whatever messages the child receives from the parents. In other instances, depending on the developmental stage of the sibling, vulnerability may lead to a negative focus on the affected child manifested by jealousy or devaluation.

Following the responses of parents and siblings are those of the child's peers, teachers, and the culture as a whole. Developmentally, responses from an increasing number of persons occur when the child reaches the age at which he or she is eligible for organized day care or school. Extensive research exists on the manner in which children with physical disabilities are responded to in settings such as schools and camps and by peer groups (Dion and Berscheid, 1974; Lerner and Lerner, 1977).

Later Changes in Body Image

Development of a healthy body image can be disrupted by trauma or surgery. Children who acquire a deformity as a result of illness, trauma, or surgical procedures are more likely to receive sympathetic acceptance from both parents and society. Moreover, children with acquired deformities have had the opportunity to begin the process of normal body image development prior to the trauma.

The age at which the deformity occurs has an impact on parental attitudes toward the child, thereby influencing the child's developing body image. Children born with congenital deformities appear to suffer more from social stigma as well as from a mother's sense of "punishment" than do children with later distortions, such as obesity. Pierce and Wardle (1993) showed that parental perceptions of a child's being overweight is associated with lower self-esteem in girls. This, coupled with social pressures for thinness, are held responsible for affecting the psychological functioning of young girls.

Comparisons of same-age children, who are themselves in the process of change, occupy an important place in the social context that influences the adolescent in his or her self-perception. The peer group provides the adolescent with comparison references, sends back images of himself or herself, and enables him or her to experience new forms of friendship and interaction (Coleman and Hendry, 1990; Rodriquez-Tome, Bariaud, and Cohen Zardi, 1993). Roles become increasingly sex-typed with sexual maturation of the body, which occurs at puberty, and sexual differences become more significant and pervasive in social situations.

Early puberty in girls has been negatively associated with body satisfaction and self-esteem (Slap et al, 1994). Blyth and colleagues (1985) reported that early-maturing girls in the sixth grade had more difficulty with body image and with the transition to middle school than did girls who matured at a more normal age. The association with the rate of breast development versus degree of breast development and body image was strong and independent of other potential events. In adolescent boys, the more they develop (pubertal level) or the earlier they develop (pubertal timing), the more they are satisfied with their physical appearance (Rodriquez-Tome, Bariaud, and Cohen Zardir, 1993).

Short stature can have profound psychological consequences for a developing child (Frankel, 1996). Short stature is not necessarily pathogenic (Vance, Ingersoll, and Golden, 1994), however, and need not lead to manifest psychopathology (Frankel, 1996). The etiology of the short stature appears to affect the ultimate psychological functioning of the child, although this remains an area of controversy. Children who are dependent on growth hormones who are medically treated appear to do better psychologically than do children with constitutionally short stature or those with a constitutional delay in growth (Drotar, Owens, and Gotthold, 1980; Gordon et al, 1982). All categories of child appear to do better with advancing age (Stabler et al, 1994). Adjustment of children with short-stature appears to be a function of socioeconomic status, growth hormone treatment, and the availability of psychotherapy at an early age. For those who are symptomatic, there are long-term difficulties in social and vocational adjustment and marriage. Traditional wisdom and some studies support these findings, but the reported experience of Little People of America, a group representing many people with dwarfism including those with achondroplasia, suggests that with support, pride can be a dominant outcome.

Adaptation to Distortions and Alterations in Body Image

Reconstructive surgery must be viewed as a concrete intervention occurring at one point in time in an otherwise long developmental course (MacGregor et al, 1953). It is an intervention capable of provoking the most dramatic of changes. These changes have been documented to be substantially positive, with enhanced ability to interact with peers, documented alterations in body image, and improved social relations and academic performance (Belfer, Harrison, and Murray, 1982; Phillips and Whitaker, 1979). More recent studies by Pillemer and Cook (1989) suggest that longer term residual difficulties in adjustment can be expected in some youngsters. The precise determinants of psychosocial outcome remain to be determined. It has been emphasized in past studies that supportive but not overly protective families, absence of family conflict, adequate cognitive functioning, good adjustment before the surgery, and peer support enhance adaptation. Ironically, children with adequate parental, peer, and societal support will adapt to their facial difference or other difference to such an extent that change brought about through surgery may lead them to question their identity and worry about the preservation of friends established prior to the surgery. The following story illustrates the complexity of postsurgical adaptation:

EXAMPLE

John was a 17-year-old with Crouzon syndrome who underwent a one-stage procedure to advance the midface and otherwise remove the facial stigmata. Upon the successful completion of the surgery and for approximately 1 year during the postoperative period, John deliberately attempted to determine whether friends would recognize him, tried to provoke situations to determine whether he would be treated as he had been prior to surgery, and attempted a number of "personality changes." With time, John adjusted to his new image, maintaining the essential peer relationships of the past and no longer engaging in provocative behavior.

Despite demonstrated competence in social, intellectual, and vocational skills, children with manifest differences or failure to achieve full development are often stereotyped in disadvantageous ways. Children's concerns with negative stereotyping may be based on reality. Children with manifest "differentness" are often the subject of humiliating, rejecting, and hostile responses by parents, peers, and society at large.

ATTITUDINAL ISSUES

Clifford and Walster (1973) studied the effects of attractiveness on teachers' expectations of pupil performance. The same report card was distributed to a large group of teachers with varying photographs of children attached. The attractive child was rated significantly higher on intelligence, educational attainment, educational potential, and social potential. Barocas and Black (1974), reviewing referrals for "remedial" versus "control" problems, speculated that attractive children were more likely to receive teachers' attention and help. Teachers' negative expectations for unattractive children can have important consequences. The effects of teacher expectations on student performance are well documented (Rosenthal and Jacobson, 1968). It might be that teachers' negative expectations for these children actually help to "produce" the expected intellectual and social deficits.

The child's responses to such attitudes depends upon his or her adaptation to the differentness. Children who refuse to look in the mirror or who refuse to go to school appear to have difficulty in integrating their differentness into a healthy sense of self. Such behavior should alert the physician to possible body image disturbances. The physician's contribution, whether directly or indirectly, can greatly facilitate a child's adjustment to a real or perceived deficit in body image by helping the child gain an enhanced understanding of the meaning and etiology of the deformity. Children can be helped by their parents or pediatricians to adapt, by modeling responses to provocative questions from peers or adults. Giving a child a simple explanation of their deformity to give to others, such as, "I was born that way, that's all!," can alleviate anxiety. Learning these easier ways of responding lessens the likelihood of morbid obsessing or getting into complex, equally stigmatizing discussions, such as might be encountered with a discussion of genetic etiology. The following illustrates both a potential problem and a most satisfactory response.

EXAMPLE

Sally is a 6-year-old child who entered 1st grade after partial reconstructive surgery for hemifacial microsomia.

Her mother actively involved her in a broad range of activities, and Sally was described as more social and assertive than her older sister. In the dance class, another mother informed her daughter that she should not attend a class with a child who looked like Sally. That mother then urged the teacher to remove Sally from the class. Sally, aware of the comments, expressed a desire to remain in class, and her mother was supported by other parents and the teacher.

In the current era, groups of youngsters with similar differentness have formed support networks. Through these networks, which may involve group discussions, common activities, and education, affected individuals gain an enhanced sense of self. They may feel empowered to see their differentness as positive and to capitalize on it, as has been noted earlier in relation to people with dwarfism.

Children without manifest body deformities can suffer the effects of body image disturbance more than those with obvious body disorders. Many apparently normal children have body image disturbances resulting from constitutional predisposition and life experience. Children who are subjected to physical abuse or who as infants exhibited a failure to thrive are examples of situations of possible body image disturbances in which there is no manifest deformity. Since their bodies appear intact, disturbances of body image can go unnoticed by the physician caring for such children, unless one observes or seeks out the symptoms that would reveal such a disturbance. For instance, cryptorchism and nevi in covered places can negatively influence a child's body image. Hidden deformities carry with them the added burden that feelings or worries about the differentness may go undiscussed. Children with hypospadias or cryptorchism, as they mature, may well be more concerned about their reproductive function than the precise correctness or manifest function of their body. Reassurance may not be sufficient, and detailed explanations of the capacity for normal function or limitations may be in order. Parents cannot be relied on as sources of this information but need to be included in the overall effort by professionals.

Children do better when they have an opportunity to speak with parents, siblings, and peers about the observable differences in their appearance. Offered the possibility, young children and even older adolescents may need encouragement over a period of time to share their concerns. Rarely will one office visit suffice to address a body-image issue. Children who are able to speak about their sense of differentness, or their efforts at adaptation, are in a better position to manage the inevitable assaults on self-esteem, real or imagined, that all children and adolescents are vulnerable to as they mature. When parents can join in the dialogue, or when counselors, as an adjunct, encourage the dialogue, the youth gains added support.

With older children, manifest disturbances of affect, notably dysphoria, may be apparent. This may result from the negative evaluation of personal attractiveness (McCabe and Marwit, 1993). Dysphoric children see themselves as less attractive than their peers. Attractiveness is the most salient body image dimension implicated in dysphoria with children (McCabe and Marwit, 1993). The depression of childhood, the sense of alienation, and lowered self-esteem are not self-limited; rather they can become significant personality characteristics with lifelong implications for a disordered personality.

Assessment of Body Image Development

The complexity of body image development and disturbance can often make the assessment of such disturbances difficult. There are a number of reliable indicators of possible body image disturbance, however. Perhaps the simplest indicators are observations of the parent-child dyad, interactions between parents, and the functioning of the family as a unit. Children with manifest body deformities are different, and familial and social responses to a child's "differentness" are good measurements of possible body image disturbance. The previously noted observations of extreme denial, overemphasis on specialness, discrepant views of the parents, or lack of engagement of the youngster are all possible indicators that the child may be at risk for distortions of body image development.

With children who are preverbal or who lack the motor capacity for more sophisticated assessment techniques, the physician must depend solely on observation. The child with syndactyly who hides his or her hands, or the child who refuses to undress, may have a body image problem. Further, the quality of responses to any child's body can provide information concerning later body image disturbances in the context of psychosomatic conditions, such as anorexia nervosa and bulimia, or somatoform disorders, such as hypochondriasis and conversion reactions. A focus on issues such as the need for thinness or muscle building can provide clues.

There are a number of procedures that allow the physician to assess body image disturbance. These procedures complement the information acquired through observation of the child in his or her environment. The choice of assessment technique varies according to the age of the child.

When a concern about body image exists, a simple psychological examination in the context of a physical examination will yield useful results (Levy, 1929). The physician follows the physical examination by asking the child to comment on what he or she notices about the various parts of the body, and how he or she would like to see his or her body parts at maturity. If the child cooperates with this procedure, the physician makes further inquiry regarding ideas and feelings about the importance or lack of importance of characteristics such as height, weight, strength, and appearance.

Using this method, the child who spontaneously and comfortably responds to such questions indicates a degree of acceptance of the body or adaptation to deformity. Children who tend to hide their bodies or who are reluctant or embarrassed to speak about their feelings toward body parts or functioning may have a body image disturbance. It should be noted, however, that the quality of the relationship between the child and the physician, as well as the length of time during which a relationship with a child is developed, also influence the child's responses to intimate questions.

The child who is less verbal or is reticent in his or her answers may be approached by being asked to draw a picture of a person, followed by the request to draw a picture of himself or herself. This is the clinical application of the Draw-a-Person test (Machover, 1949), which can be used with children approximately 3 years old and older. The usefulness of the data obtained increases with the age of the child. The test is a projective technique devised to elicit unconscious attitudes and perceptions of body image. The usefulness of the Draw-a-Person test as an office technique is underscored by the drawings shown in Figures 46–1 and 46–2, which demonstrate the picture of a child with typical lowered self-esteem and body distortion, respectively.

Although it is easier to see the impact of life-threatening and chronic diseases on body image, less well defined and less apparent afflictions can be equally devastating. Hemangiomas, eczema, and gross motor dysfunction impose the same burden as more life-threatening illnesses. The pediatrician needs to be mindful of the impact of these types of diseases or disturbances on the development of a sense of bodily competence. Acknowledging with the patient the impact of eczema, for example, can provide the opportunity for the youngster to vent feelings of disgust, guilt, and failure. Discussing these issues with a helping individual can relieve the youngster. If the concerns are significant and are broached with a sense of helpfulness, the caregiver will have the opportunity to offer therapeutic support.

The issue of compliance is covered elsewhere in this text, but in illnesses such as diabetes, a contributor to noncompliance is a failure to value one's own body. Thus, children with diabetes who sense a defective body require help to invest in themselves. That self-investment, and

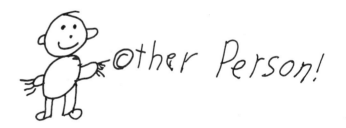

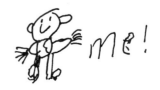

Figure 46–1. Drawing by a child with low self-esteem.

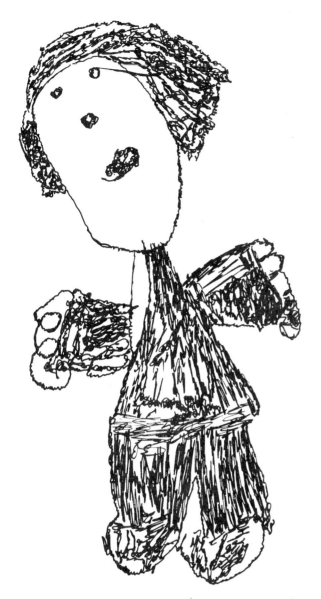

Figure 46–2. Drawing by a child with cystic hygroma and obesity.

realistic understanding of the disorder, are essential to support compliance.

The child who experiences trauma, such as the traumatic amputation of a limb, and who had normal body image development can be expected to go through a grief response. There is the shock with disbelief and anger followed by an appraisal of the functional deficit and the cosmetic impact. This process of appraisal is in itself prolonged and should not be foreshortened. The initial self-assessment can be grossly exaggerated or can embody massive denial. Only after an appropriate period of mourning the loss of limb or function can the child and the parent achieve a sense of realistic deficit. Therapeutically, children should be followed closely and involved actively in appropriate rehabilitation programs at the earliest possible time.

Therapeutic Considerations

As in other areas, the best treatment for disturbance of body image is the prevention of body image distortion when possible. The issues related to the parental role in prevention have been discussed previously. The pediatrician, working with the child, parents, and teachers, can further facilitate the development of a normal body image in vulnerable children through a variety of means. Alertness to specific vulnerabilities of certain children and the emphasis on compensatory strengths are vital to this strategy.

The role of the physician is critical at the birth of a child with a deformity. Parental education as to the nature and consequences of the malformation can be helpful but must be repeated more than once because of the parents' inability to deal with information at a time of acute stress. Referral to a professional for a specific psychotherapeutic intervention for parental or family support at the time of birth can assist in parental adjustment and minimize potential body image disturbance in the child when it is believed that the parent's response is pathologic or when unusual vulnerability is noted. However, it is most important that any referral not be made at the first instant, but should come only after the pediatrician feels that he or she has adequately attempted to educate and reassure the parents but has not had the desired effect.

Preventive measures designed to aid parents in coping successfully with a child born with a birth defect should be considered the preferred choice of treatment, and therefore referral to parent groups such as those for the parents of children with cleft palate can be helpful. Both local and national organizations can provide resource directories or resources specific to a multitude of disorders or for the provision of general support. (See listing of resources.)

In children without specific deformities but with other conditions that may be associated with a poor body image, working with the parents to help them modify their expectations can be of great usefulness. This approach is applicable to a wide range of conditions associated with vulnerability in the intellectual, physical, or aesthetic spheres. Regular supportive visits with a child and the parents, when possible, enhances this approach. The caring relationship with the pediatrician can be valuable and sustaining. For instance, with the child who is clumsy, it is rewarding to see such a youngster gain self-esteem from participation in chess, cross-country running, and other activities that can accentuate a child's strengths but not emphasize fine motor coordination. Story-telling or citing models of alternative forms of prowess to support or encourage the child's ability in areas that de-emphasize athletic prowess is appropriate.

Environmental manipulation, that is, altering a child's experience through directed activities or changes in environment such as school or camp, is an effective therapeutic technique. Examples of such manipulations include encouraging the parents to place their child in a summer camp that will emphasize supportive activities, to enroll an artistically gifted child in art classes, or to enroll a child who has difficulty with competition in a supportive, small-group athletic program. Guidance for the parents in relation to this type of manipulation can be constructive.

Coupled with the preceding therapeutic approaches, it can be useful to systematically employ behavioral reinforcement, essentially to give positive reinforcement to activities, actions, and statements that imply or corroborate competence and mastery. It is important, at times, for the pediatrician to be a parent and patient ally when approaching the school system and classroom teacher to provide consistency in this type of positive behavioral reinforcement.

When the supportive interventions fail to bring about a positive change in a child as manifested by an improved sense of self-esteem, the pediatrician, the family, and the patient need to consider psychotherapeutic approaches. Unfortunate consequences of a failure to gain a sense of completeness, mastery, or competence are depression, anger, alienation, and a sense of lowered self-esteem. Individual or group psychotherapy addressing depression and anger at an early stage can facilitate resolution of underlying conflicts and, coupled with the approaches already discussed, can bring a child back along a path of healthy psychological development.

In special instances, additional therapeutic approaches can be employed to help a child gain a better sense of mastery. For instance, groups for youth with eating disorders are an important part of any treatment regimen. The child who is hospitalized following trauma or surgery or the child with a chronic, debilitating illness can benefit from a Child Life activities–based program. Because children who have body image problems can hold back from participation in these programs, the pediatrician needs to give active encouragement and support for participation.

The development of a realistic and satisfying body image is complex. The complexity is more apparent as children and families cope with differentness. The efforts to help youth achieve a positive body image rely on the given propensity of children toward healthy psychological development, support of the parent and child, and appropriate therapeutic intervention when indicated. Perfection should never be the goal, but the achievement of reasonable self-satisfaction recognizing the importance of differentness in our society.

. . . soul is the same thing in all living creatures, although the body of each is different.

—HIPPOCRATES, REGIMEN, BOOK I, SECTION 28.

REFERENCES

Anthony EJ: The child's discovery of his body. Phys Ther 48:1103, 1968.

Barocas R, Black H: Referral rate and physical attractiveness in third grade children. Perceptual Motor Skills 39:731, 1974.

Belfer ML, Harrison AM, Murray JE: Body image and the process of reconstructive surgery. Am J Dis Child 133:532–535, 1979.

Belfer ML, Harrison AM, Pillemer FG, et al: Appearance and the influence of reconstructive surgery on body image. Clin Plast Surg 9:307, 1982.

Blyth DA, Simmons RG, Zakin DF: Satisfaction with body image for early adolescent females: the impact of pubertal timing within different school environments. J Youth Adolesc 14:207, 1985.

Bowlby J: Attachment. New York, Basic Books, 1969.

Brenner D, Hinsdale G: Body build stereotypes and self-identification in three age groups of females. Adolescence 13:551, 1978.

Bruchon-Schweitzer M: Une Psychologie du Corps. Paris, Presses Universitaires de France, 1990.

Clifford M, Walster E: The effect of physical attractiveness on teacher expectations. Sociol Educ 46:248, 1973.

Cohen F, Yasuna A: Cognitive and psychological assessment of the child with craniofacial abnormalities. Presented at Symposium on a Comprehensive Approach to Craniofacial Deformity. Boston, 1978.

Coleman JC, Hendry L: The Nature of Adolescence, 2nd ed. London, Routledge, 1990.

Dion K, Berscheid E: Physical attractiveness: perception among children. Sociometry 37:1, 1974.

Drotar D, Owens R, Gotthold J: Personality adjustment of children and adolescents with hypopituitarism. Child Psychiat Hum Dev 11:59, 1980.

Flannery-Schroeder EC, Chrisler JC: Body esteem, eating attitudes, and gender-role orientation in three age groups of children. Curr Psychol 15:235–248, 1996.

Frankel SA: Psychological complications of short stature in childhood: some implications of the role of visual comparisons in normal and pathological development. Psychoanal Study Child 51:455, 1996.

Goodenough F: Measurement of Intelligence by Drawings. Yonkers, New York, World Book, 1926.

Gordon M, Crouthamel D, Post E, Richman F: Psychosocial aspects of constitutional short stature: social competence, behavior problems, and family functioning. J Pediatrics 101:477, 1982.

Green M, Levitt EE: Constriction of body image in children with congenital heart disease. Pediatrics 29:438, 1962.

Katz P, Zigler E: Self-image disparity: a developmental approach. J Pers Soc Psychol 5:186, 1967.

Kaufman RV: Body image changes in physically ill teen-agers. J Am Acad Child Psychiatry 11:157, 1972.

Kaufman RV, Hersher BA: Body image changes in teenage diabetics. Pediatrics 48:123, 1971.

Kolb LC: Disturbances of the body-image. In Arieti S (ed): American Handbook of Psychiatry, Vol 1. New York, Basic Books, 1959.

Lerner RM, Lerner J: Effects of age, sex and physical attractiveness on a child-peer relative, academic performance, and elementary school adjustment. Dev Psychol 13:585, 1977.

Levy DM: Method of integrating physical and psychiatric examination with special studies of body interest, overt protection, response to growth and sex difference. Am J Psychiatry 9:121, 1929.

MacGregor FC, Abel TM, Bryt A, et al: Facial Deformities and Plastic Surgery. Springfield, IL, Charles C Thomas, 1953.

Machover JA: Personality Projection in the Drawing of the Human Figure. Springfield, IL, Charles C Thomas, 1949.

McCabe M, Marwit SJ: Depressive symptomatology, perceptions of attractiveness, and body image in children. J Child Psychol Psychiatry 34(7):1117, 1993.

Pate JE, Pumariega AK, Hester C, Garner DM: Cross-cultural patterns in eating disorders: a review. J Am Acad Child Adolesc Psychiatry 31:802–809, 1992.

Phillips J, Whitaker LA: The social effects of craniofacial deformity and its correction. Cleft Palate J 16(1):7, 1979.

Pierce JW, Wardle J: Self-esteem, parental approval, and body size in children. J Child Psychol Psychiatry 34:1125–1136, 1993.

Pillemer FG, Cook KV: The psychological adjustment of pediatric craniofacial patients after surgery. Cleft Palate J 26(3):201, 1989.

Rodin J, Silberstein LR, Striegel-Moore RH: Women and weight: a normative discontent. In Sonderegger TB (ed): Nebraska Symposium on Motivation. Lincoln, University of Nebraska, 1985, pp 267–308.

Rodriquez-Tome H, Bariaud F, Cohen Zardi MF: The effects of pubertal changes on body image and relations with peers of the opposite sex in adolescence. J Adolescence 16:421, 1993.

Rosenthal R, Jacobson L: Pygmalion in the Classroom. New York, Holt, Rinehart and Winston, 1968.

Shapiro T, Stine J: The figure drawings of three-year-old children. Psychoanal Study Child 20:298, 1965.

Slap GB, Khalid N, Paikoff RL, et al: Evolving self-image, pubertal manifestations, and pubertal hormones: preliminary findings in young adolescent girls. J Adolescent Health 15:327, 1994.

Stabler B, Tancer M, Ranc J, Underwood I: Psychiatric symptoms in young adults treated for growth hormone deficiency in childhood. In Stabler B, Underwood I (eds): Growth, Stature, and Adaptation: Behavioral, Social, and Cognitive Aspects of Growth Delay. Chapel Hill, University of North Carolina Press, 1994, pp 99–106.

Striegel-Moore RH, Kearney-Cooke A: Exploring parents' attitudes and behaviors about their children's physical appearance. Int J Eating Disorders 15(4):377, 1994.

Tisza VB, Silverstone B, Rosenblum O, et al: Psychiatric observations of children with cleft palate. Am J Orthopsychiatry 28:416, 1958.

Vance M, Ingersoll G, Golden M: Short stature in a nonclinical sample: not a big problem. In B Stabler, L Underwood (eds): Growth, Stature and Adaptation: Behavioral, Social, and Cognitive Aspects of Growth Delay. Chapel Hill, University of North Carolina Press, 1994, pp 35–46.

Wright BA: Spread in adjustment to disability. Bull Menninger Clin 28:198, 1964.

RESOURCES

Alliance of Genetic Support Groups, 35 Wisconsin Circle, Suite 440, Chevy Chase, MD 20815

Children's Craniofacial Association, 9441 LBJ Freeway, Suite 115, LB 46, Dallas, TX 75243

Let's Face It, Box 711, Concord, MA 01742-0711 [Can provide a listing of resources for individuals with a broad range of facial and physical differences.]

Little People of America, Inc., 7238 Piedmont Drive, Dallas, TX 75227-9324

March of Dimes, 1-888-663-4637 (MODIMES)

National Organization for Rare Disorders, Inc., P.O. Box 8923, New Fairfield, CT 06812-8923

National Self-Help Clearinghouse, Room 620, 25 West 43rd Street, New York, NY 10036

Support Organization for Trisomy 18, 13 and Related Disorders, 2982 S. Union Street, Rochester, NY 14624-1926

47 Gross Motor Dysfunction: Its Evaluation and Management

Lynn Mowbray Wegner

Clumsy children often have to endure profound feelings of inadequacy at the same time that they withstand a recurring series of humiliating life events. Often these children develop an inadequate body image and self-concept. Additionally, they are likely to be deprived of the special gratification that comes with motor mastery. In this chapter, various forms of gross motor dysfunction are described, along with an approach to their systematic assessment and management. Through understanding of a child's patterns of gross motor performance, a pediatrician can play a valuable role in finding motor success for all patients. It has been said that "any kid can hit a home run if the bat is wide enough!"

Gross motor activity allows children to explore their environments, interact with others, form friendships, gain self-confidence, and learn about themselves. Most children develop gross motor skills through a series of seamless transitions from one developmental level to the next. Children with gross motor dysfunction lack this ability to make the transition with proficiency. For example, they may not be able to jump rope without tripping, ride a bicycle quickly and confidently, or catch a ball without dropping it. Gross motor dysfunction may be a child's only developmental variation; however, comorbidity with other developmental differences is more common. For example, gross motor dysfunction may be an accompaniment of impaired language and speech, reading disorders, or attention deficits (Taft, 1989). Other associated findings may include perceptual disorders, incomplete cerebral dominance, and lack of experience or opportunity. Emotional disturbances may occur as a primary or secondary finding. The term *nonpathologic gross motor dysfunction* presupposes normal anatomy, strength, and sensation and a central nervous system without focal asymmetry.

Normal Gross Motor Function

Gross motor development is a continuous, orderly process of accreting skills. Optimal gross motor function reflects the orchestration of visual-motor abilities, dexterity, balance, coordination, reaction time, and rate of movement. Neural control affects motor behavior. Additional biological factors and influences, including visual acuity, hearing sensitivity, proprioception, vestibular integration, strength, and overall health and fitness, directly shape skill attainment. Environmental factors such as opportunity for practice and encouragement of the child's efforts can affect the level of skill development, motivation, and degree of perseverance. Movement quality directly reflects the integration of these factors involved in motor learning and movement control.

The development of neuromuscular control in infancy follows a cephalocaudal, proximal-distal direction (Fig. 47–1) (Sturner, personal communication, 1997). Initial gross control subsequently refines to increasingly more precise control. For example, the 1- or 2-month-old infant moves his arms in a flailing pattern, but by his 4th month he can control the movement and bring his hands together in the midline of his body. Although the sequence of motor skill development is predictably similar for all children, these skills develop at varying rates among children. Accelerated rate of skill acquisition at one childhood stage may not be repeated and, in fact, may be followed by a slower rate of skill attainment. Furthermore, there are stages in a child's life when the motor imprecision is expected. The imperfect balance of the 4- to 6-year-old with rapidly

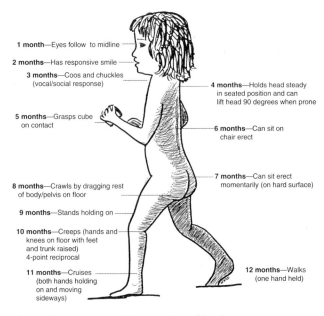

1 month—Eyes follow to midline

2 months—Has responsive smile

3 months—Coos and chuckles (vocal/social response)

4 months—Holds head steady in seated position and can lift head 90 degrees when prone

5 months—Grasps cube on contact

6 months—Can sit on chair erect

7 months—Can sit erect momentarily (on hard surface)

8 months—Crawls by dragging rest of body/pelvis on floor

9 months—Stands holding on

10 months—Creeps (hands and knees on floor with feet and trunk raised) 4-point reciprocal

11 months—Cruises (both hands holding on and moving sideways)

12 months—Walks (one hand held)

Figure 47–1. Cephalocaudal progression of development.

changing visual motor abilities and the awkward coordination of the early adolescent whose body possesses a discrepant ratio of upper to lower body segment size are not surprising when they occur.

Gross Motor Dysfunction

EXAMPLE

Ten-year-old Alex was brought to his pediatrician's office for an evaluation of his awkward motor skills. Alex had achieved his developmental milestones at the appropriate times and was very active as a younger child. Although he had been receiving extra help for poor handwriting, his parents reported his written output was "slow and messy." He was slow in running, watched his feet when he walked up stairs, often tripped when he ran, and could not throw a ball at a target with any power or accuracy. His parents thought a community youth soccer team would help Alex improve his skills; however, he had not been chosen to play in any games and recently he had begun complaining of intense stomach pains before practices.

Prevalence rates of gross motor dysfunction range from 5% to 8% (Denckla, 1984). Incidence is not related to the child's educational level or socioeconomic status, and the label is usually applied after the age of 4 or 5 years, with peak age range for identification being between 6 and 12 years.

As most children develop and grow, they perform motor activities with increasing ease. Despite the predictable uneven gross motor development in younger children, children entering the years of middle childhood are expected to perform motor tasks with more rigid age-equivalent abilities. Children having qualitative gross motor skill differences show immature and substandard performance in motor skills relative to their same aged peers. The child does not progress to the next performance level.

Gross motor dysfunction encompasses a wide spectrum of motor behaviors, and there is no agreed upon physical sign representing motor awkwardness. Descriptive criteria have been established in *The Diagnostic and Statistical Manual for Primary Care (DSM-PC) Child and Adolescent Version* for several conditions divided as a variation, problem, or disorder of developmental coordination (Wolraich et al, 1997).

Evaluation

The primary care health provider is an initial professional resource for the assessment of a child's gross motor dysfunction. The evaluation heavily depends on a detailed history and careful physical examination. The assessment of younger children focuses on the sequence and integration of skills: "Is this child's motor development commensurate with the age equivalence of his other developmental domains?"

QUESTIONNAIRES

A brief screening of motor development can be obtained in a time-efficient manner through parent reports such as the Denver II Pre-Screening Questionnaire for children up to 60 months old (Frankenburg and Dodds, 1995). The ANSER Questionnaires (Levine, 1996), elicits detailed information about the parents' perceptions of 3- to 18-year-old children's interest and ability in various motor activities. Noting the amount of time spent in motor activities and the forms of participation is also important.

HISTORY

The child may be interviewed in the company of his or her parents or individually for older children and adolescents, with the interviewer identifying the gross motor areas perceived as difficult or for which the child has experienced embarrassment. These interviews may be poignant with memories of humiliation and failure.

Either the child or parents may report activities or observations that are relevant to the etiology of the gross motor dysfunction (e.g., frequent play on a trampoline with skull contact, use of the head in soccer, or decreased exercise tolerance).

The family history should focus on other members who did not have proficiency in motor skills. A graphic pedigree may be drawn if there are neurologic conditions (e.g., neuromuscular disease) in any family members. Additional significant family history might include associated learning or attention differences, or childhood or early adulthood demise with signs of physical "wasting," unexpected death, or limited physical endurance.

Observations commonly made about children with gross motor dysfunction are shown in Table 47–1.

Table 47–1 • Observations Indicating
Gross Motor Dysfunction

Home environment
   When given a choice, these children avoid physical activity in which definite skills are used (e.g., neighborhood softball, street hockey, jumping rope, roller skating).
   These children prefer to play with younger children whom they can dominate and with whom their physical coordination may be more compatible.
   They may shy away from events or opportunities that have an athletic component, such as summer camp or Scouting.
Classroom
   These children bump into classmates, desks, and chairs.
   These children collide with objects or drop them.
   Boys especially may adopt the "class clown or bully" identity to compensate for motor ineptness.
   These children may avoid friendships with peers who like sports.
Physical education class
   These children may require many demonstrations of a motor skill, even having another person physically touch their bodies to help them move in the appropriate manner.
   They may show a relatively short span of focused attention, and often the focus may not be on the sport but on extraneous details in the environment (watching the clouds in the sky instead of looking for the path of a ball).
   When these children play actively with peers, they usually lose a contest.
   These children are usually the last ones chosen for competitive games.
   They may display signs of anxiety or "act up." This naughty behavior may be somewhat adaptive if the teacher sends them out of the class.

PHYSICAL AND NEUROLOGIC EXAMINATION AND RELATED TESTING

Watching a child demonstrate motor skills during a physical examination provides corroborating information about milestone achievement in the younger child and qualitative proficiency in the older child. Extra time may be needed for the neurologic examination because repeated maneuvers are sometimes necessary to elicit subtle findings, suggesting a specific etiology for the dysfunctions. As an example, exertional weakness as a finding in mitochondrial disease may be demonstrated only after a period of activity lasting several minutes. Running up and down a hallway in the health care provider's office may not be strenuous enough to create sufficient fatigue. Pertinent physical findings and their implications are summarized in Table 47–2, and additional description of the neurologic examination is found in Kandt (1984).

Associated movements are extra actions that represent the child's inability to inhibit motor movements not associated with the required task. For example, mirror movements reflect this weakness of motor inhibition. These are thought to represent neurologic immaturity or "soft" signs of neurologic difference (Hoekelman, 1997). These perceptual, behavioral, and motor "soft signs" of nervous system dysfunction have not been accompanied by measurable laboratory abnormalities; however, recent advances in nuclear imaging of the central nervous system have revealed structural differences in some of these children (Lyon and Rumsey, 1996).

The standard neurologic examination should also include several additional maneuvers that are helpful in assessing integrated physical performance. The tasks described in Table 47–3 also permit the observer additional

Table 47–2 • Physical Examination Signs Frequently Accompanying Gross Motor Dysfunction

Anthropometric measurements: Skeletal abnormalities, including leg length discrepancies, circumferential measurements of the midcalf and midthigh regions, head circumference (megalocephaly)
Skin markings: Hyperpigmented macules (neurofibromatosis); asymmetry of thumbnails (associated with growth disturbance, such as mild hemiparesis)
Neurologic examination:
  Cranial nerves: II: Vision screening indicating farsightedness
  Motor system: Muscle strength is grossly ascertained by having the child walk, run, skip, hop, arise from sitting on the floor, and walk up and down steps. Menkes (1990) suggests the pronator sign maneuver as a sensitive test for upper extremity weakness. With the child's arms raised above his or her head, the hand on the hypotonic side hyperpronates to palm outward and the ipsalateral elbow may flex.
  Coordination: Finger-to-nose and heel-to-shin: Accentuation of tremor as the finger or heel approaches the target strongly suggests cerebellar dysfunction. Rapidly alternating movements with attention to rate, tremors and/or choreiform movements, Gower maneuver
  Sensory: Primarily position maneuvers to assess intact posterior column
  Reflexes: Focal increases or asymmetry
  Accessory movements and "soft signs": Choreiform rotatory movements of the fingers or tongue, spooning (dorsal concavity) of fingers, choreiform twitches of tongue or fingers, synkinesia (mirror movements), and motor overflow

Table 47–3 • Gross Motor Tasks and Their Underlying Neurodevelopmental Functions

Rapid alternating movement: The child may demonstrate dysdiadichokinesis by quickly alternating pronation and supination of the hand or by grasping a small object, like a ping pong or squash ball, and holding it above the head with the arm fully extended, and quickly rotating the wrist. Children should be able to inhibit proximal muscle groups while facilitating distal groups. Motor coordination is dependent on this balanced motor facilitation and inhibition. Other functions assessed include motor planning and sequencing and maintenance of a rhythm.
Sustained motor stance: Asking the child to stand erect for 15 seconds with arms and fingers extended, feet together, eyes closed, and tongue protruding beyond the lips may reveal problems with motor inhibition. Balance, somesthetic input, and vestibular function contribute as well.
Tandem balance: In this task, which requires maintenance of a static posture without visual monitoring, the instructions are identical for the sustained motor stance except the child is requested to put one foot directly in line in front of the other ("like on a tightrope"). This task allows assessment of motor monitoring, self-righting skills, vestibular function, somesthetic input, balance, body position sense, selective motor inhibition, and motor persistence.
Hopping in place: The child is asked to hop in place on one foot in the following sequences: right—two times, left—two times; right—two times, left—three times; right—three times; left—two times. Each alternating sequence is performed three cycles. Some children cannot hop at all. These children may be requested to perform the same alternating sequences by patting their laps or a table surface. This task entails the integration of auditory input and gross motor output. Motor planning, motor sequencing, short-term motor memory, motor inhibition, and the ability to establish and maintain a rhythmic pattern are all involved. Children who cannot perform this task standing may have lower extremity weakness or the problem may be with lower extremity coordination.
Catch a ball: This can be assessed in two ways. If the child is younger than 10 years, or if the child is with historical evidence of very poor motor skills, tossing a tennis or squash ball back and forth between the examiner and the child 7 to 10 times provides information about eye-arm coordination, motor planning, and balance. An older, more physically adept child may be given a squash ball and a lightweight cup just slightly larger than the diameter of the ball and be requested to toss the ball above the child's head and catch the ball in the cup. Interpretation of visual-spatial input, development of a consistent motor pattern, strategy formation, and bimanual coordination are important functions assessed during this task.

Adapted from Levine MD: The Pediatric Examination of Educational Readiness at Middle Childhood (PEERAMID 2). Cambridge, MA, Educators Publishing Service, Inc., 1996:

opportunity to evaluate the child's ability to translate verbal instructions into an effective motor plan, emotional response to imperfect performance, social interaction skills, and further emergence of associated movements. The neurodevelopmental functions are described with each task.

LABORATORY AND IMAGING STUDIES

Radiographic studies, including computerized tomography and magnetic resonance imaging, are seldom necessary in this evaluation unless there are specific signs indicating upper motor neuron dysfunction or a history of acute changes in gross motor skills. If the child shows signs of poor muscle mass or limited physical exertion, preliminary laboratory values of lactic dehydrogenase and creatine kinase may indicate possible muscle deterioration or specific illness. Progressive and nonprogressive disorders influencing gross motor function are listed in Table 47–4. Some of

Table 47–4 • Medical Causes of Childhood Gross Motor Dysfunction

Progressive
Tumors: Frontal, parietal, cerebellar, spinal cord
Metabolic: Poisoning, drug toxicity, aminoacidurias, leukodystrophies, lipid storage diseases, Wilson disease, hepatic precoma
Degenerative: Spinocerebellar degenerations, extrapyramidal syndromes, spinal disorders, brainstem disorders, cerebellar disorders
Neuromuscular disease: Kugelberg-Welander syndrome, acquired and hereditary neuropathy, muscular dystrophy polymyositis, mitochondrial disease, myotonia congenita, myasthenia gravis
Hydrocephalus
Myoclonic epilepsy
Acute cerebellar ataxia
Nonprogressive
Congenital encephalopathies
Acquired brain injury sequelae: Posttraumatic, postmeningitic, postencephalitic, vascular accidents, anoxia, hypoglycemia
Tic disorders
Mental retardation
Visual deficits: Poor vision (specifically relative farsightedness), congenital nystagmus
Arthropathies: Traumatic, rheumatoid, arthrogryposis
Orthopedic impairments
Vertigo: Meniere disease
Connective tissue disorders
Chronic medical conditions: Anemia, endocrinopathies, cardiac, pulmonary, renal, diseases, obesity

From Levine MD: Developmental Variation and Learning Disorders. Cambridge, MA, Educators Publishing Service, Inc., 1987.

these disorders show signs beginning in infancy whereas others emerge in later childhood stages.

Management

The first step in management begins with an explanation to the child and the child's family relating his or her motor problems to the particular profile of neurodevelopmental strengths and weaknesses. For example, a child who is significantly affected by a slower rate of motor production might have this identified along with excellent hand-eye coordination and balance skills. The child as well as the adults see the child as having strengths on which to build while trying to increase the child's motor rate.

The second step in management is the selection of appropriate physical venues for the child. Children who have weaknesses in their gross motor function often avoid physical activities—much to the chagrin of their parents. Parents often believe the treatment for poor gross motor abilities is to be more aggressive in participation. This approach frequently results in many opportunities for failure, humiliation, and consistent erosion of the child's self-esteem. The following questions are helpful in selecting appropriate activities:

1. Does the child want to participate in this activity?
2. Is the environment safe for the activities and developmental levels of the children?
3. Are children grouped by age or developmental skill level?
4. If children are grouped by developmental skill level, are younger, and possibly smaller, children, in a situation devoid of intimidation from larger children and

are the activities not infantilizing for the older children?
5. Does the leader understand the developmental tasks as the children progress through childhood? Do activities in the class reflect developing selective attention abilities, variability in sequencing skills, and variations in learning styles (visual, auditory, kinesthetic input as the primary input modality for acquisition of new information)?
6. Does the atmosphere of the class reflect the leader's acceptance and encouragement of individualism, curiosity, sensitivity, willingness to try the unknown, and even diversity?
7. Does the leader demonstrate an approach of describing the child's endeavors without the use of qualitative labels? Labeling movements as "good," "artistic," or "nice" may subtly encourage imitation or restrict expressions to those conforming to the leader's expectations.

The identification of specific strengths is helpful to make suggestions of activities in which the child may have a reasonable chance of success. Common activities and their emphasized neurodevelopmental strengths are listed in Table 47–5.

For more extensively affected children, direct therapy is helpful. Children with a primary nervous system or musculoskeletal disorder can be eligible for therapeutic resources in the public school setting. Consultation with the adaptive physical education specialist in the school system enables a child with motor dysfunction to participate in organized physical recreation class as much as possible. These accommodations are made under Title 504 "Other Health Impaired" classification. Other management measures can include referral to a local occupational therapy professional. Many occupational therapy centers offer group sessions in which children of similar motor patterns learn skills transferable to sport situations. Receiving remediation in a setting with peers who share similar motor proficiency profiles is effective and enhances the child's sense of self-esteem.

Prognosis

The few outcome studies of children with gross motor dysfunction attributed to unspecified, nonprogressive causes indicate a relatively favorable outcome if the initial motor dysfunction is not severe (Knuckey, 1983). As these

Table 47–5 • Physical Activities to Develop Gross Motor Function

Running: Balance, rate
Bicycling: Balance, depth perception, hand-eye coordination
Swimming: Endurance, coordination of upper and lower body segment actions
Tennis/badminton/squash: Hand-eye coordination, balance, rate
Diving: Balance, motor memory, rate, flexibility, sequential processing
Soccer: Rate, temporal and sequential processing, depth perception
Softball/baseball: Hand-eye coordination, balance, rate
Field events (shot put, discus): Upper torso strength, balance

children mature, their gross motor function usually improves. Children who are more extensively affected may not show significant improvement in their motor function, however (Losse et al, 1991). Many of the children develop other recreational interests, allowing them successful experiences to offset the minimal gratification they receive from physical activities. If these children can be guided into movement areas that emphasize their motor skill strengths and minimize their weaknesses, they will not be unduly at risk for the health concerns that accompany inactivity.

REFERENCES

Denckla MB: Developmental dyspraxia: the clumsy child. *In* Levine MD, Satz P (eds): Middle Childhood: Development and Dysfunction. Baltimore, University Park Press, 1984, p 246.

Frankenburg WK, Dodds JB: Denver Developmental Screening Questionnaire. Denver, Denver Developmental Materials, Inc., 1990.

Hoekelman RA (ed): Primary Pediatric Care, 3rd ed. St. Louis, Mosby-Year Book, 1997, p 675.

Kandt RS: Neurologic examination of children with learning disorders. Pediatr Clin North Am 31:296–314, 1984.

Knuckey NW, Gubbay S: Clumsy children: a prognostic study. Aust Paediatr J 19:9–13, 1983.

Levine MD: The ANSER System Follow-up Questionnaires. Cambridge, MA, Educators Publishing Service, 1996.

Losse A, Henderson SE, Elliman D, et al: Clumsiness in children—do they grow out of it? A 10-year follow-up study. Dev Med Child Neurol 33:55–68, 1991.

Lyon GR, Rumsey JM (eds): Neuroimaging. Baltimore, Paul H. Brooks, 1996. p 39.

Menkes JH: Textbook of Child Neurology. Philadelphia, Lea and Febiger, 1990.

Taft LT: Clumsy child. Pediatr Rev 10:247–253, 1989.

Wolraich M (ed): The Classification of Child and Adolescent Mental Diagnoses in Primary Care: Diagnostic and Statistical Manual for Primary Care (DSM-PC) Child and Adolescent Version. Elk Grove Village, IL, The American Academy of Pediatrics, 1996.

SUGGESTED READINGS FOR PROFESSIONALS AND PARENTS

American Academy of Pediatrics: Committees on Sports Medicine and School Health. Organized athletics for preadolescent children. Pediatrics 84:583–584, 1989.

American Academy of Pediatrics: Infant exercise programs. Pediatrics 82:800, 1988.

American Academy of Pediatrics: Physical fitness and the schools. Pediatrics 80:449–450, 1987.

American Academy of Pediatrics: School-aged children with motor disabilities. Pediatrics 76:648–649, 1985.

Burnett DJ: Youth, Sports, and Self Esteem. Indianapolis, IN, Masters Publishing Press, 1993.

   (To order: 1-800-722-2677. This publisher has a series of books about children and specific sports: The Spaulding Youth Series)

Cratty BJ: Clumsy Child Syndromes. Langhorn, PA, Harwood Academic Publishers, 1994.

Ehrlich MG, Hulstyn M, d'Amato C: Sports injuries in children and the clumsy child. Pediatr Clin North Am 39:433, 1992.

Jacobs AG (ed): Basketball Rules in Pictures. New York, Putnam Publishing Group, 1993.

   The line drawings in this guide may be easier for a child to interpret than a photograph.

National Youth Sports Coaches Association: Basic Level Member's Handbook. West Palm Beach, FL, National Youth Sports Coaches Association, National Alliance for Youth Sports.

   The National Clearinghouse for Youth Sports Information provides parents and professionals with access to a variety of resource information and materials pertaining to youth sports. Its resource library includes academic research, books, pamphlets, instructional videos, and other assorted publications and information. Information is available from National Youth Sports Coaches Association, National Alliance for Youth Sports, 2050 Vista Parkway, FL, 33411 at 1-800-729-2057.

Schmidt RA: Motor Control and Learning, 2nd ed. Champaign, IL, Human Kinetics, 1988.

48 Development of Sexuality and Its Problems

Iris F. Litt • John A. Martin

 Issues of the development of sexuality arise throughout the pediatric years, as biological and psychosocial factors interact in the maturing individual. Children and their caregivers are often confused and concerned by questions about matters such as masturbation, initiation of sexual intercourse, and feelings and behaviors that do not fit with the prevailing sexual stereotypes. Pediatricians have a unique opportunity to promote appropriate education about sexuality and to provide specific advice about worries or problems before or after they arise.

Infancy and Early Childhood

The development of sexuality is often considered a task of adolescence. The reality, however, is that sexuality begins to develop from the time of conception and often continues throughout life. Sexuality represents an amalgam of gender role, gender identity, physical characteristics, hormonal influences, society's expectations, peer and parental influences, and cognitive, psychological, and moral development superimposed on actual experiences. When it is viewed in this way, descriptive terms such as *sexually active* are rendered meaningless, as every growing child has a sex life. Development of gender is discussed in Chapter 9. This chapter concentrates on the psychosocial, biological, and behavioral aspects of the development of sexuality throughout childhood and adolescence.

FREUD'S THEORY OF SEXUAL DEVELOPMENT

Freud built a complex and convincing argument for the existence of sexuality in infants and saw the infant's orientation toward humans growing directly out of its need to discharge sexual tensions (Freud, 1964a, 1964b).

Freud argued that sexual impulses in the neonate are identical in kind to the adult sexual response; sexual behavior involves an interplay between excitation and satisfaction. Excitation for the newborn occurs primarily in terms of instinctual needs, the most pressing of which, according to Freud, is the need for nourishment. The satisfaction of the need for nourishment comes from feeding.

The notion of the anaclitic—which is similar to the idea of conditioned reinforcers—was invoked by Freud to explain the relationship between the satisfaction of the need for food and a more generalized notion of "pleasure." The satisfactions of feeding generalize to satisfactions associated with the process of sucking. Thus sucking for nourishment in effect becomes sucking for pleasure. In this sense the child's first sexual object is the mother's breast, which both nourishes and gives pleasure.

Although Freud failed to distinguish between the nature of the satisfactions associated with nourishment and sucking for its own sake, it is clear that both forms of pleasure are part of the same phylogenetic system, one of which has specific survival value, whereas the other serves simply to reinforce that value. The basic survival value of feeding and the taking in of nourishment is the force behind infantile sexual gratification.

Freud's major contribution to the study of sexual development, then, was his idea that sexual behavior—originally considered to be associated exclusively with adolescence and adulthood—in fact begins, though in an immature form, in newborn infants. The specific manifestations of sexuality undergo developmental transformations throughout the life cycle, like other behavioral systems, but Freud argued that there are continuities between the manifestations of sexuality in infancy and adulthood. His ideas paved the way for clinicians and researchers to focus on sexual behavior in infancy and early childhood.

SEXUAL AROUSAL IN INFANCY AND EARLY CHILDHOOD

A number of investigators have observed spontaneous erection in infant boys as young as 2 days old. Erection tends to be associated with various forms of arousal, specifically with restlessness, stretching, limb rigidity, crying, fretting, and thumb-sucking. Erection is also associated with fullness of the bladder and bowels and frequently follows voiding. In addition there has been some suggestion that the period between voidings of the bladder or bowels is elongated when interposed by erections. Spontaneous erections are quite common during sleep in infant boys—much more common, according to some investigators, than is spontaneous erection in adult men. There is lack of agreement regarding the stage of sleep during which erection is most common. When erection occurs during rapid eye movement (REM) sleep, it is typically accompanied by smiling and rhythmical mouthing or tonguing.

Stimulation of the genitals in infants of both sexes has been shown to lead to arousal. Genital stimulation of boys frequently results in penile erection; in older infants such stimulation also leads to smiling and cooing. It has further been suggested that most infants, both boys and girls, have orgastic capacity by age 3 to 4 years but have few opportunities to "test" this capacity. In young boys, orgasm tends to occur very quickly, followed by a brief refractory period, often only several seconds in length. In girls, orgastic capacity also occurs very early in life but is less common than in boys.

Thus it appears that physical and psychological response to sexual stimulation begins very early in life and that orgasm is possible at all ages, for both males and females.

MASTURBATION IN INFANCY AND CHILDHOOD

Given that sexual arousal occurs early in life and that there are some indications that this arousal is associated with pleasure, it comes as no surprise that masturbation is a common occurrence in both boys and girls.

Masturbation probably occurs accidentally in infancy during the natural process of bodily exploration. When the genitals are discovered and randomly fingered, the infant discovers the relationship between this behavior and arousal and pleasure. Therefore the infant is motivated to repeat the activity. Some writers have suggested that by age 5 to 6 years, masturbation is universal, systematic, and intentional in children of both sexes.

Alternatively it has been suggested that masturbatory activity often begins with some physiologic discomfort in the genital area. Diaper rash, urethral infection, and bladder distention are frequently cited as drawing attention to the genital area.

The repression of masturbation is common in many cultures. In the past, Western child guidance experts suggested a variety of severe "treatments" for masturbation, ranging from the suggestion that parents refrain from allowing their infants and young children to be alone in bed while still awake to the shackling of arms or legs and the use of tranquilizers. More recently clinicians have more commonly counseled parents that masturbation is normal and harmless.

A variety of interpretations have been made of the psychological meaning of masturbation. Some psychoanalytical writers have described masturbation as serving as a precursor to the oral-genital shift, whereas others have gone so far as to argue that it involves an anxiety-ridden identification with the opposite sex and a desire to become a member of the opposite sex. It has also been argued, however, that masturbation in infancy and early childhood might be an entirely different phenomenon from masturbation in young and later adulthood, although the specific form of the behavior can be quite similar. Kleeman (1975), while acknowledging the frequency of masturbatory behavior among young infants, observed that emotional excitement is rarely associated with the behavior, at least through 2 years of age. Spitz (1949) and Kinsey and colleagues (1948) de-emphasized the importance of childhood masturbation: "It is still to be shown that these elemental tactile experiences have anything to do with the development of the sexual behavior of the adult." Thus although there is ample evidence that self-manipulation is common among

even very young infants, and that parents and physicians are sharply aware of these episodes when they occur, there is yet some question about the significance of the experiences for the child.

SOCIOSEXUAL BEHAVIOR IN EARLY CHILDHOOD

Ample evidence exists that sociosexual experiences occur very early in a child's life, in some studies as early as 5 years of age. The question has been raised repeatedly, by both parents and clinicians, whether such experiences have deleterious effects on the child's development in general or in particular. Martinson (1973), in an extensive literature review, concluded that there is little or no evidence of long-term consequences—either positive or negative—from early sexual experiences. The amount of arousal associated with early childhood sex play is minimal.

Regarding the origins of interpersonal sex play in children, Broderick (1968) favored a modeling explanation. In his review of cross-cultural materials, he found that interpersonal sex play among children, especially oral-genital contact and copulatory attempts, were most common in cultures in which children were permitted to watch adult love making. Thus interpersonal sex play among children is common. Its form can be influenced by various social factors, but there is little evidence that such childhood experiences have any adverse developmental effects.

THE PARENTS' ROLE IN SEXUAL DEVELOPMENT

As with other forms of social development, parents exert direct socialization pressure on their children with respect to the development of sexual behavior. Both because sex is such a strong driving force in childhood behavior and because our culture has strong and rather explicit rules about "acceptable" sexual behavior, we might expect parents to be quite consistently nonpermissive about sexuality in their children. In fact, however, there appears to be considerable variability in parents' attitudes toward sexual behavior.

Research on the impact of differences in these attitudes has been striking in its consistency. In general, permissiveness toward sexual behavior is related to parental warmth, supportiveness, and nonpunitiveness, all of which appear to promote sexual adjustment later in life. The problem with this research, however, is that most of the information about parents comes from the retrospective reports of adults identified as sexually adjusted or maladjusted. Moreover parents who are permissive about sexual issues tend to be warmer, more supportive, and less punitive than parents who are not permissive, so it is difficult to know, on the basis of existing information, whether it is the permissiveness or the quality of the parent-child relationship, or both, that is implicated in the development of "healthy" sexuality.

Clinicians and researchers in child development have given divergent sorts of advice to parents about various topics relevant to sexual socialization. The advice has ranged from the very general, such as Ellis's (1938) caveat that parents ought not to assist in rendering the unconscious erotic impulses of their children conscious, to the very specific, such as Finch's (1969) suggestion that to avoid early incestuous relations, parents ought not to let opposite-sex siblings share the same bedroom. Some of the advice offered to parents seems to be in accordance with existing knowledge and theories about the effect of socialization practices on sexual development; sometimes, however, the advice has been rather counterintuitive, such as Ellis's (1938) suggestion that mothers avoid excessive tenderness and warmth (lest their sons become sexually excited). There seems to be overwhelming agreement that any socialization of sexual behavior that does seem necessary should be performed with as little fanfare as possible. Finch (1969), for example, stated: "Parents should be aware that sex play may occur and should discourage it when it is observed, but without harsh scoldings and punishment." Likewise Burch (1952) reassured parents that sex play is normal, and that "sudden scolding or a terrifying scene will do more harm than good." Ausubel (1958) cautioned that "making a scene" can be counterproductive; he noted that children quickly learn that sexual behavior is likely to elicit a response from their parents, and thus might use their sexuality as "a weapon with which to shock adult sensibilities and express defiance of adult authority." A dramatic negative response on the part of the parent, in this context, might therefore serve to reinforce the child's behavior.

Adolescence

PSYCHOLOGICAL DETERMINANTS OF ADOLESCENT SEXUALITY

Organization of the adolescent's experience of sexuality has been viewed from four major vantage points—psychoanalytical, psychosocial, cognitive developmental, and learning theory (Table 48–1).

Psychoanalytic theory, best articulated by Freud, sees adolescence as the time when instinctual sexuality is re-awakened under the influence of surging hormones. The repression of the ego, which characterizes the antecedent latency stage, is no longer tenable, and the major task of the adolescent becomes that of fulfilling the internally driven sexual mandate within the confines imposed by the ego and the id. "In the Freudian view, the individual enters adolescence possessing a fully articulated set of erotic meanings that seek appropriate objects and behavior. . . . Adolescence is the beginning of a quest for an appropriate interpersonal sexual script to articulate with a largely formed intrapsychic script" (Miller and Simon, 1980).

In contrast to Freud, Erikson (1950) sees adolescence as a change in social rather than biological status. Adolescent sexuality is viewed on the continuum of identity development. Sexual identity is developed during adolescence in the context of mastering the capacity for trust, intimacy among peers, and autonomy from parents. Preparation for heterosexual selection of a mate by confirmation of a heterosexual commitment signifies successful progress in the Eriksonian view.

While concurring with Erikson in rejecting the Freudian position of sexuality as an innate drive that must be controlled, Gagnon (1972) is in disagreement with him on the matter of continuity with earlier stages. In his view, early adolescence represents a break with the past, and the continuity of socialization exists not in the sexual but in the nonsexual, specifically in gender role training. The major task of the early adolescent is the integration of new definitions of a potentially sexual self with prior gender role training. Gagnon believes that the physical changes of puberty provide a signal to adults, who then attribute new sexual meanings to the adolescent's behavior and react to

Table 48–1 • Development of Sexuality

Age	Biological Development	Cognitive Stages (Piaget)	Social Development	Psychosexual Stages (Freud)	Psychosocial Crises (Erikson)
0	Chromosomal sex Genital dimorphism	↑	Gender assignment	Oral	(1) Trust versus mistrust
1	Capacity for orgasm	Sensory motor	Self-exploration		
2	Growth in size		Mutual exploration	Anal	(2) Autonomy versus shame and doubt
3		Preoperational		Phallic	(3) Initiative versus guilt
4					
5			Genital play	Latency	(4) Industry versus inferiority
6					
7		Concrete operational			
8					
9					
10					
11					
Adolescence	Puberty Secondary sex characteristics	Formal	Dating Petting	Genital	(5) Identity versus role diffusion
Young adulthood	Menarche Ejaculation		Coitus		(6) Intimacy versus isolation

early adolescents as being more sexual than they really are (Gagnon, 1972).

The third organizing factor of adolescents' sexuality, proposed by Piaget (1948) and Kohlberg (1972), is cognitive development. The capacity for formal operations develops during adolescence in most but not all youths. This capacity enables the adolescent to transform erotic objects and thoughts into symbolic abstractions, which can then be explored rationally. Conflict resolution is then possible without the necessity for actually acting out the potentially conflicting scenarios (Kohlberg, 1972; Piaget, 1948).

Finally, learning theory has been invoked to explain the development of adolescent sexual behavior. According to such theory, pleasurable acts are reinforced and tend to be repeated because they are pleasurable. Kinsey is the major proponent of this view. He argues, for example, that homosexual acts in adolescence are largely rooted in the gratification experienced during previous same-sex experimentation (Kinsey, Pomeroy, and Martin, 1948). This theory addresses only the perpetuation rather than elucidating the initiation of behavior.

It is important to remember that these sometimes disparate views of adolescent sexual development are based largely on theoretical models, which are yet to be validated. The limited body of empirical data relating to adolescent sexuality suffers from sampling bias and other methodologic limitations. The difficulty in obtaining systematic prospective data is addressed by Money (1976): ". . . childhood sexuality remains a research frontier, unopened to empirical and operational study. Any attempt to cross the frontier is subject to condemnation, as if juvenile sexology constituted a branch of pornography which, in turn, is stigmatized as illicit and immoral." A case in point is the experience of Sorensen (1973), who in an effort to maximize parental acceptance so that they would allow their adolescents to participate in his study of adolescent sexuality, struck from the final draft of his questionnaire exceptionally sensitive questions dealing with oral sex, anal sex, and intercourse with animals. As a result there are no data relating to these behavioral patterns.

The theories of intrapsychic determinants of adolescent sexuality thus far discussed fail to address differences between the sexes. Gagnon (1965), however, attributes adolescent sex differences in masturbatory activity, sexual fantasies, and sexual intercourse to differences in earlier gender role training. For example, the central themes for female socialization involve a commitment to future marriage and to the rhetoric of romantic love, whereas for adolescent males, whose sexual activity of all types is more frequent, these acts often suggest themes of achievement and mastery. Social class differences in motivations for sexual behavior are also described, especially among young adolescent boys. He ascribes the lower incidence of masturbatory behavior among working class males to both a less complex fantasy life and their view of this behavior as being unmanly, and, to a lesser extent, to the earlier onset of intercourse in this group.

BIOLOGICAL DETERMINANTS OF ADOLESCENT SEXUALITY

All the hypothalamic and pituitary-gonadal structures necessary for pubertal onset appear to be present from the

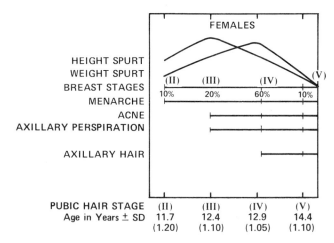

Figure 48–1. Females: Interrelationship of secondary sex characteristics during puberty.

time of birth. The reasons for their dormancy until the 2nd decade of life remain enigmatic. It appears, however, that a feedback system exists so that gonadotropin-releasing hormone stimulates gonadotropin, which, in turn, causes release of sex steroids from the gonads. These, in turn, inhibit further release of gonadotropin-releasing hormone until sex steroid levels again fall below a threshold level, at which time the cycle repeats itself.

Shortly before any structural changes of puberty emerge, a shift occurs in the anterior pituitary gland from a consistent pattern of secretion of low levels of gonadotropins (3 to 4 mIU/mL), which characterizes childhood, to one in which surges of up to 10 mIU/mL of these hormones are secreted coincident with each 90-minute sleep cycle. Sex steroid concentrations fluctuate in synchrony with the gonadotropins, coincidentally for testosterone, and following a 10- to 12-hour delay for estrogens. The daytime secretory patterns remain unchanged from the prepubertal state.

The interrelationships of the changes that characterize

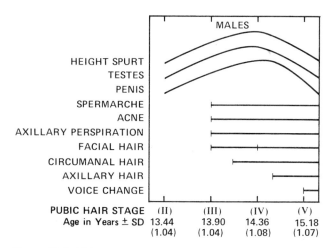

Figure 48–2. Males: Interrelationship of secondary sex characteristics during puberty.

Table 48–2 • Development of Primary and Secondary Sex Characteristics, Both Sexes

Sex Maturity Rating	Endocrine	Pubic Hair
II (Boys = 10.5–14.5 years; Girls = 10.4–12.9 years)	Gonadotropins—sleep augmentation Growth hormone—elevated	Midline Long, downy, and silky
III (Boys = 11.8–14.9 years; Girls = 11.1–13.4 years)	Gonadotropin—peaks higher Growth hormone—detectable in daytime	Spreads laterally, lightly pigmented, few longer and coarser
IV (Boys = 12.8–15.4 years; Girls = 11.8–14.3 years)	Continuation of preceding pattern Growth hormone—highest peaks	Covers entire mons, coarse and curly
V (Boys = 13.8–16.3 years; Girls = 13.2–17.1 years)	Adult pattern and range No sleep augmentation	Extends to medial thighs

the development of the secondary sex characteristics of puberty are diagrammed in Figures 48–1 and 48–2, and the timing of various stages is shown in Tables 48–2 through 48–4.

THE INTERFACE OF BIOLOGY AND BEHAVIOR

The relationship of sexual behavior to hormonal states has long been of interest to researchers. Studies of pubertal male primates have demonstrated a correlation between increasing sexual behavior and serum testosterone levels. The effect of the social setting also has been found to exert an influence, both testosterone levels and sexual behavior being decreased when adult males were present in the social group.

Attempts to replicate these findings in humans have been inconclusive, undoubtedly owing to the greater complexity of determinants of sexual drive and interest in humans. Studies by Bancroft (1986) of hypogonadal men have shown that although they experience impaired nocturnal penile tumescence, which is reversible with androgen administration, they are able to have erections in response to erotic movies, suggesting that some but not all elements of sexual arousal are androgen-dependent. Variations in

androgen levels among normal adult men do not correlate with differences in coital frequency, sexual excitement, or desire (Persky, 1983).

Even less is known about the role of estrogens in human female sexual behavior. Studies by Persky and colleagues (1978) found no relationship between plasma estradiol levels and sexual arousal, frequency of intercourse, or sexual gratification. Conflicting results have been found in studies of the role of progesterone in affecting sexual desire. More consistent, although not conclusive, are findings of studies implicating testosterone as contributing to the level of arousal and sexual desire in females (Gray and Gorzalka, 1980; Sherwin, Gelfand, and Brender, 1985).

The implications of the dramatic changes in physical appearance at puberty for the development of sexuality are myriad. It has been postulated that the primary evolutionary significance of pubic and axillary hair might have been to act as wicks for the dissemination of the odor of secretions produced by the apocrine and sebaceous glands. In lower primates, body hair and odors of sexual maturity serve as sexual attractants, territorial markers, and determinants of social hierarchy. The advanced state of socialization of the human race has reduced the sexual significance of these dermatologic appendages, but across cultures and at various periods within our own history, one or another secondary

Table 48–3 • Development of Primary and Secondary Sex Characteristics, Boys

Sex Maturity Rating	Testes	Scrotum	Accessory Structures	Penis
II 10.5–14.5 years	Seminiferous tubules—↑ size Leydig and Sertoli cells—↑ number Greater than 3 mL total volume	Thinning Hypervascularity	↑ Size epididymis ↑ Size seminal vesicles ↑ Size prostate	Elongation begins
III 11.8–14.9 years	Continued growth of above	Continued	Continued	Continued elongation
IV 12.8–15.4 years	Spermatogenesis	Pigmented	—	Growth of corpora cavernosa → widening of shaft
V 13.8–16.3 years	Adult size ~ 2.5 cm	—	Adult size	Adult length and width

↑ = increased; → = leads to.

Table 48–4 • Development of Primary and Secondary Sex Characteristics, Girls

Sex Maturity Rating	Breasts	Vaginal Mucosa	Labia Majora	Ovaries	Uterus
II 10.4–12.9 years	Budding	Thinning	Vascularization and wrinkling	Enlarge greater than 3 g	Corpus equal in size to cervix
III 11.1–13.4 years	Separation of areolar and breast tissue	Watery, mucoid discharge	—	Continued growth	Cervix longer than corpus
IV 11.8–14.3 years	—	Folds become more prominent and develop ciliated epithelial lining, pH is acid	—	Average, 6 g	Menarche in 90% by this stage
V 13.2–17.1 years	Adult configuration	—	—	Ovulatory cycles more frequent than anovulatory	—

sex characteristic (typically the female breasts or buttocks) gains ascendance in the scale of social desirability.

Breasts are considered to be normal sequelae of puberty in girls, yet our society stigmatizes gynecomastia, which develops in one third to one half of healthy young adolescent boys. Embarrassment, doubts about masculinity, and withdrawal from social interactions, and often from the school locker room, can result from this normal phenomenon.

The more visible of the secondary sex characteristics, particularly the breasts, are important signals to parents and peer groups that childhood has passed and that sexuality, as adults know it, becomes a possibility. The timing of appearance of these characteristics in relationship to the peer group has an impact on the young adolescent female's self-image, which can indirectly affect peer interaction. The social behavior of dating might be one such example. In some circumstances, however, societal expectations might be geared more to the age than to the adolescent's stage of physical maturation. In a large study in the United States in the late 1960s, "individual differences in sexual development seem not to have a strong influence on dating, which is commonly thought of as reflecting the development of biological drives.... . Social pressures appear to overwhelm the individual whose rate of biological development deviates from the norm" (Dornbusch, Carlsmith, and Gross, 1981).

There are other sequelae of pubertal development that affect appearance and hence sexual attractiveness in the eyes of adolescents. The increased production of dihydrotestosterone in both sexes stimulates the size and secretions of sebaceous follicles, often resulting in the production of acne. Frequent requests for comedo extraction or lancing of cysts prior to an important social event remind us that it is of small comfort to the adolescent to know that acne signifies normal pubertal development. Another effect of the pubertal growth spurt is to cause elongation of the optic globe and hence myopia in the genetically predisposed. The appearance of a bespectacled Playboy centerfold notwithstanding, most adolescents feel that

glasses detract from their sexual attractiveness. Similarly it is socially unfortunate that completion of pubertal growth is also the time preferred by orthodontists for affixing braces. In addition, in late adolescence, in 10% of sexually mature males, wedge-shaped indentations over each lateral frontal region of the forehead result in receding of the hairline.

SEXUAL BEHAVIOR IN ADOLESCENCE

Male Orgasm

Postpubertal orgasm in boys is accompanied by ejaculation, the discharge of semen or spermarche, which usually begins approximately 1 year after the onset of testicular growth. In Kinsey's sample, 90% experienced ejaculation between the ages of 11 and 15 years, with 1 year's difference in the mean age between the socioeconomically deprived and the advantaged (14.6 versus 13.6 years, respectively). In the majority of the sample, the first nocturnal emission occurred almost 1 year following achievement of ejaculatory ability (Kinsey, Pomeroy, and Martin, 1948).

Kinsey used the phrase "total outlet" to describe the total number of orgasms achieved in a typical week through any form of sexual stimulation (masturbation, sex dreams, petting, coitus, or homosexual or animal contacts). He found the highest frequency of total outlet in the youngest group, consisting of males 15 years of age and younger (but all pubertal) with a mean of 2.9 orgasms per week. These observations run contrary to the popular notion that sexuality is awakened during adolescence, gradually reaches its peak during early adulthood, and then wanes.

In the Kinsey sample, the most frequent source of orgasm for the more highly educated youth was masturbation, followed by nocturnal emissions, in contrast to intercourse for the less-educated group. Comparable figures for the present are not yet available.

Female Orgasm

Kinsey found that sexual behavior less frequently culminates in orgasm for women. There were also marked differences between males and females in the age distribution of orgasmic behavior, with girls 15 years or younger averaging one orgasm every 3 weeks, and the peak of activity reached and maintained in women between 30 and 40 years of age. The source of orgasm for females was reported not on the basis of educational status, as with the males, but rather on the basis of marital status at the time of the survey. In the unmarried group, masturbation provided the most frequent source (84%), whereas marital coitus did so for the married group.

Masturbation resulted in orgasm for 71% of female adolescents surveyed by Sorensen (1973). More than half the adolescent females with intercourse experience reported that they had an orgasm during sex "rarely or never." Only one third of this group believed it important to reach orgasm during sex, compared with more than two thirds of those who actually experienced orgasms.

Dating and Petting

The onset of dating signifies one of the few, albeit unofficial, rites of passage in our society. It characteristically begins in the adolescent age period. Accordingly it represents an early social decision-making point, which often creates tension between parents and their teenaged children. As such, it can serve as a battleground for the struggle for independence. The conflict can be in response to the teenager's desire to date and the parents' opposition, or vice versa. Parental opposition is often based on the nonspoken fear that early dating might increase the risk of sexual experience and pregnancy. Rather than discussing these concerns with their offspring, parents might respond by imposing stringent restrictions about curfew, chaperones, and modes of travel. Adolescents might react by rebelling—through sexual acting out or other mechanisms designed to test injunctions of control—rather than out of desire for the sexual act itself. Available data suggest, however, that pregnancy is unlikely, for sexual intercourse is a rare event during the early adolescent dating experience.

Unchaperoned dating was a post–World War I development, whereas the custom of "going steady" in high school became popular about the time of World War II. Dating appears not to be a single behavior but rather one that undergoes its own developmental sequence. Adolescents move from having friends of the same sex, to having friends of both sexes, to dating, to having the desire for having a steady date, to actual steady dating, and lastly to having sexual intercourse (Chess, Thomas, and Cameron, 1976). Even within a steady dating relationship, a spectrum of behavior is experienced. Schofield (1965) describes five stages, which occurred in a fairly predictable sequence, at least among the 15- to 19-year-old British youths he studied in the early 1960s. Stage 1, in which there is little heterosexual contact, is limited to kissing and the rare dates that are devoid of kissing. In stage 2, sexual contact is limited to kissing and stimulation of breasts while fully clothed. Stage 3 involves "sexual intimacies which fall short of intercourse" and might include breast stimulation under clothes, genital stimulation, or apposition. Stage 4 involves sexual intercourse with a single partner, and in stage 5 there might be intercourse with more than one partner.

Sorensen (1973), in studying a cross section of American youth a decade later, found a similar pattern. He reported that in 22% of American adolescents aged 13 to 15 years (20% of boys, 25% of girls), there was a total lack of any sexual contact, other than kissing, that either aimed at or resulted in pleasurable physical reactions. Another 17% (14% of boys, 19% of girls) were virgins who had participated in beginning sexual activities (kissing, touching, exposing one's body to another for sexual pleasure) but had not yet had sexual intercourse. The duration of this phase could not be judged because of the cross-sectional nature of his data. That limitation notwithstanding, the degree of satisfaction expressed by this group, both with the amount of sexual gratification and with peer and parental relationship, suggests that these activities might represent more than just foreplay. Petting appears to be pivotal in initiating heterosexual psychosocial encounters. In addition to providing a bridge to adult heterosexual intercourse, it teaches adolescents about each other's bodies, emotional and sexual responses, notions of masculinity and femininity, and social rules and customs of sexual behavior and thus allows for beginning consolidation of the disparate components of sexual identity.

Chilman (1979) notes that male writers are frequently puzzled by the apparent contentment of young women to restrict themselves to heavy petting without moving on to intercourse. There are a number of possible practical reasons for this behavior: It greatly reduces the chance of becoming pregnant, females might be more readily orgasmic through direct clitoral stimulation brought about by petting, and withholding full intercourse from the male until marriage is thought to increase his desire for this commitment.

In contrast to those parents who oppose their adolescents' initiation into dating, others encourage it to the point of creating intergenerational conflict over the issue. "Says 15-year-old Marilyn, 'I would rather spend an evening with my girlfriends than with a boy I do not like. But my parents push me into dating. They think I don't go out enough. They are angry when I turn down a date. 'You don't have to like the boy to have fun,' they say. I feel it is dishonest to let a boy spend money on me when I have no feelings for him' " (Ginott, 1969). In Sorensen's study, 19% responded in the affirmative to the statement, "Ever since I was 12 or 13 years old, my parents have encouraged me to go out on dates." Perhaps some of these parents place a premium on the youngster's popularity, either to enhance their own social image or out of a genuine conviction that such popularity will increase the adolescent's happiness, whereas others might live out their sexual fantasies vicariously through their children.

The determinants of adolescent dating behavior have attracted research interest. The question posed is whether the age of onset of dating is biologically or socially determined. Data from a cross-sectional study of a large national probability sample of 12- to 17-year-olds were used to explore the correlates of dating. Assessing the stage of sexual maturation by Tanner staging, it was found that dating in girls was more closely linked to progression through age grades than to sexual maturation (Dornbusch, Carlsmith, and Gross, 1981). Using a longitudinal sample and defining sexual maturation on the basis of attainment of menarche for girls and of peak velocity of growth in height for boys, another group found a dominant role for biological factors in determining dating behavior. Females with early onset of pubertal development dated more in middle school than those who were later maturers (Blyth, Bulcroft, and Simmons, 1981).

The consequences of dating have been variously perceived. One group demonstrated a detrimental effect of dating on self-esteem among white girls in the seventh grade. This finding was compounded for those who were early maturers and had entered junior high school during that grade. Moreover they reported that girls who dated early were more likely to score low in achievement tests and to have lower grade point averages than did those who had not yet dated (Simmons et al, 1979).

Sorensen's survey also suggested better school performance, as well as greater religiosity, among adolescents who did not yet date. Is it that better students and those who are more religious refrain from interactions with the opposite sex or, conversely, that lack of dating allows for pursuit of scholastic and religious interests? The direction of the relationships between these variables is difficult to ascertain.

Chess and associates (1976) found physical attractiveness to affect the relationships among adolescents; the less attractive the adolescent, the less likely was she or he to have a steady date. Obesity was a strong deterrent.

Gagnon (1972) believes that early dating is advantageous, especially for middle class boys. "These steady dating experiences may well serve to increase the young male's investment in the rhetoric of love and emotional commitment which seem so necessary a part of the marriage pattern of this society."

Sexual Intercourse

There are gender and ethnic differences in the age of onset of sexual intercourse among American adolescents, with boys and African Americans generally initiating this behavior earlier than girls and whites, respectively. The gap between African American and white girls appears to be narrowing recently, however. Data for other ethnic groups have not been systematically collected. Approximately 5% of 13-year-old, 30% of 16-year-old, and 60% of 19-year-old girls report sexual intercourse compared with 20%, 45%, and 80% of boys at these ages. Over the course of the 1970s, there was a 66% increase in sexual activity among unmarried girls 15 to 19 years of age, most of which was accounted for by whites. During the decade of the 1980s, the average age of onset of intercourse decreased for girls. In 1988, 51.5% of 15- to 19-year-old girls had premarital intercourse (US Dept. of Health and Human Services, 1991).

In Sorensen's study, 71% of the boys had had intercourse by age 15 years, and only 5% waited until 18 years of age. He believed that the age of onset of intercourse might predict subsequent sexual behavior, in that 60% of the sexual adventurers (those with multiple sexual partners) had had intercourse by 14 years of age, compared with 26% of the monogamists (those with a single sexual partner). Jessor and Jessor (1975), in a large sample (1126 subjects) followed prospectively for 4 years after junior high school, from 1969, found 75% of tenth grade and 51% of twelfth grade boys to be virgins.

In the Sorensen study, one quarter of the boys first had intercourse with a casual acquaintance, whereas one third of girls did so with a boy they intended to marry. The first instance of intercourse occurred in the home of one of the adolescents in 40% of the cases and in automobiles half as often as that.

The transition from virginity to sexual intercourse was studied by Jessor and Jessor. Characterizing nonvirginity in secondary school as a manifestation of "transition proneness," they were able to predict which students would lose their virginity in the next year. This group valued independence more and achievement less than the virgin group, and appeared to be more influenced by the views of friends than those of parents. In a cross-sectional study, Sorensen reported similar differences between virginal adolescents and those who had experienced intercourse. Both studies reported greater religiosity, less tolerance for drug usage, and higher scholastic achievement among the virgins.

First intercourse experiences among young adolescents are characterized by the lack of use of effective contraception. Only 32% of sexually active adolescents did anything to reduce the chance of pregnancy at the time of first intercourse, condom and withdrawal (18% each) being the most commonly used methods. In a 1971 study, it was found that 50% used birth control at last intercourse, whereas in 1979 the use of contraception by the same group increased to 70% (Zelnik and Kantner, 1980). A careful perusal of the data, however, reveals that the increase is based almost entirely on greater dependence on totally ineffective methods, such as withdrawal, and that use of reliable methods, such as orally administered contraceptives, IUDs, or combinational barrier methods actually decreased. Earlier studies demonstrated a lag period of approximately 1 year between initiation of intercourse behavior and seeking of a birth control method by adolescent girls. In the 1979 study, only 34% of sexually active adolescents stated that they consistently practiced contraception.

Once the adolescent actually obtains an effective birth control method, there is no guarantee that he or she will continue to use it. In a study of compliance with birth control, it was found that only 45% of female adolescents continued to use the prescribed method for longer than 4 months following its receipt. The noncompliers were the younger adolescents, those experiencing infrequent intercourse, those with a sexual relationship of short duration (less than 6 months), and those who had not taken the initiative for their medical visit (Litt, Cuskey, and Rudd, 1980). A variety of explanations has been offered for nonuse of contraception by this age group. In a large study, the majority of the two thirds of sexually active adolescents who had never practiced contraception thought that they could not become pregnant because of the erroneous impression that it was the wrong time of the month (41%). Sixteen percent did not use contraception because they had not expected to have intercourse, and 8% did not know how to obtain contraception. Only 9% were actually trying to become pregnant (Alan Guttmacher Institute, 1981).

An unfortunate result of nonuse of contraception by this age group has been an increase in pregnancy. Within the first month after initiation of intercourse, one fifth of the first pregnancies among adolescents occur, and within the first 6 months, 50% of the first pregnancies occur. In 1990 there were 835,000 pregnancies among adolescents (Centers for Disease Control and Prevention, 1995). Approximately 33% were terminated by induced abortion and about 15% by spontaneous abortion. Forty-nine percent resulted in live births, half of which were to unmarried female adolescents. Whereas the pregnancy rate among older adolescents has decreased over the past decade, that for girls under 15 years of age has held constant at about 30,000 per year.

The sequelae of young adolescent pregnancy are myriad. They include a higher incidence of obstetric complications, such as toxemia (15% higher), anemia (92% higher), and postpartum hemorrhage and infection, as well as neonatal problems such as prematurity and small for date status. The infant death risk is two times greater among babies born to adolescents than to women older than 20 years of age. The relative contribution of poor obstetric care is unclear owing to delay in presentation and physiologic factors in the pathogenesis of these problems. The negative educational, social, and economic consequences to the adolescent and her baby have been described. They include an increased risk of cognitive deficits, poorer school performance, and more behavior problems than among children born to older women (US Congress OTA, 1991). Follow-up of a large sample of children born to poor African American adolescents in the 1960s suggests that they continue to be disadvantaged into adolescence, having a higher frequency of delinquency, school failure, and emotional difficulties, as well as their increased risk of adolescent pregnancy themselves (Furstenberg, Levine, and Brooks-Gunn, 1990).

Another adverse consequence of sexual intercourse in adolescents is the possibility of contracting a sexually transmitted disease. Adolescents lead the United States in the actual rate of gonorrheal, chlamydial, and human papillomavirus infections, as well as in the rate of rise of these infections over the last 15 years. Prevalence ratios for acquired immunodeficiency syndrome (AIDS) are also increasing rapidly for this age group (see Chapter 28). Youth and multiple sexual partners are two factors that correlate with the increased risk of pelvic inflammatory disease. The explanation for the increased risk of infection based on chronologic age is not clear. Although the number of AIDS cases among adolescents presently is small, it is likely that a large number of 20- to 24-year-olds contracted HIV during adolescence. The increase in intercourse behavior among adolescents has been accompanied by increased use of condoms (estimated to be about two- to threefold in the last 2 decades).

Effeminate Behavior and Homosexuality

A pediatrician is often consulted, directly or obliquely, by worried parents of a young boy who dresses in female clothing or enjoys playing with dolls or girls. They are concerned about the relationship of this behavior to adult homosexuality. As adolescence approaches, the gentle stu-

dious young man with a slight build might cause his former football star father to question his son's masculinity. A visit to the pediatrician for the purpose of "giving him something to help him grow" can result. The teenaged boy might seek counsel himself when faced with the appearance of gynecomastia. Alternatively he may choose not to discuss it at all but rather to ask the doctor for an excuse from gym class for his "painful ankle" rather than suffer the embarrassment of undressing in the locker room. These young men are well served by pediatricians who prepare them in advance for this, or reassure them once the gynecomastia develop.

To be in a position to deal with these common situations, the clinician needs information about the development of sexual preference choices and the significance of cross dressing in childhood and same-sex sexual experiences in adolescence.

Unfortunately there has been little definitive research in this vital area. The majority of studies have dealt with adults whose retrospective recall of childhood events and feelings is obviously colored by their present sexual orientation. In the few prospective studies of male children with effeminate qualities, the question of self-fulfilling prophecy must be raised as a methodologic limitation. What is the parent's or child's understanding of why they were selected for participation in the study, and how might this affect subsequent social interactions? Another major problem with the existing body of information about homosexuality is that it has been derived from studies on select samples, for example, prisoners, patients undergoing psychotherapy and, more recently, members of homophile organizations. It is reasonable to question how easy it is to generalize about the information gathered from these potentially biased samples. Finally, the existing literature, until recently, has addressed itself only to male homosexuality, so that even less is understood about sexual preference among females. Keeping in mind these major limitations, we review some of the existing body of knowledge.

Issue 1: Is homosexuality determined from early childhood, or is sexual object preference variable and not determined until late adolescence?

Bieber and colleagues (1962) support the position that there is the "prehomosexual" child and that one feature distinguishing him from his peers is his early childhood sexual feelings toward males. This position is supported by Manosevitz (1972), who compared two adult samples, one homosexual and the other heterosexual, on the basis of responses to personality tests and to a specially designed life history questionnaire. Although he found no significant differences in early parental treatment in relation to sex play, early sexual or dating experiences with girls or boys, or the age of first ejaculation between the groups, he reports other areas in which major differences were found. The homosexuals recalled more frequent and stronger sexual attractions to one or more males, including adult males, than did the heterosexual group. Fewer of the latter group admitted having had childhood sexual activity with another male. As regards masturbation, more of the homosexuals acknowledged masturbation prior to 13 years of age, and more reported fantasizing about other males while engaging in masturbatory activity. Of interest was the notation that only 9 of the 25 subjects in the homosexual group agreed with the statement that they had been "born homosexual." On the basis of these data, Manosevitz concluded that one major distinguishing feature of the prehomosexual male child when compared with the preheterosexual male child is his bidirectional sexual orientation.

There is variability in the recall of the heterosexual, bisexual, and homosexual men with regard to their gender-conforming (masculine) behaviors during childhood. For example, almost the same percentage of homosexual men had gender-conforming as had gender-nonconforming memories in a study by Phillips and Over (1992).

Green (1986) reports one of the few prospective studies of childhood antecedents of adult homosexuality. In his 15-year follow-up he found that 75% of boys considered to be effeminate in childhood reported themselves to be homosexual or bisexual as adults, compared with less than 1% among control subjects who did not manifest effeminate behavior as children.

A different view is proposed by Glasser (1977), who is of the opinion that homosexual behavior can occur at successive developmental stages during adolescence, a period characterized by "change and flux." Accordingly its significance must be viewed against a background of other components of the developmental process. In early adolescence (puberty to 15 years), for example, the boy is involved in gradual withdrawal from dependent emotional involvement with his parents, while still acknowledging their authority. During this process the youngster becomes narcissistically self-absorbed and selects friends who possess characteristics he would like to possess and whom he loves as he would like to be loved. In this context, mutual masturbation is viewed as a means of self-exploration and experimentation, comparison, and reassurance. Glasser notes a similar phenomenon in adolescent girls, although the manifestations are more emotional than physical. He compared this "normal" homosexual activity among adolescent boys with that found in those destined to be homosexuals. The former group always had a strong heterosexual interest, and the activity never occurred with an adult man.

In middle adolescence (15 to 17 or 18 years), the youth rejects parental ideals, values, and authority, develops his own code of ethics and morals, and turns to his peer group for support and approval. In working toward the establishment of such an identity, the adolescent, according to Glasser, is driven toward a final confrontation with his revived oedipal conflicts. How he resolves them will determine his future functioning. In his view, castration anxiety at this age can lead the young adolescent to deny the existence of people without penises or to adopt a passive and submissive posture because of fear of authority figures, either of which might drive him to homosexuality. Glasser also applies this Freudian interpretation of homosexual orientation to females and asserts that they arrive at their lesbian sexual orientation as a result of the persistence of the attempt to deny what they believe to be their anatomic inferiority. He believes that resolution of anxieties and guilt during middle adolescence will result in a heterosexual orientation, but that by late adolescence (18 to 21 years), homosexuality is established. This view of adolescent homosexual development remains untested, being based in psychoanalytical theory and supported only by anecdotal material.

A study of female homosexual college students explores their perceptions of their parents. In a study of 34 lesbians and an equal number of control subjects, using the adjective checklist of human behavior and the Liphe test of parent-child relationships, Neel and Martin (1981) found that the lesbians viewed their fathers as being less nurturing, more aggressive, less heterosexual, and more self-abasing, and as having less interest in and less respect for their daughters compared with the control subjects.

Issue 2: The significance of homosexual acts during adolescence.

As reported by Glasser, heterosexual males might engage in sexual activity with other males during adolescence. Sorensen's study (1973) also found that 11% of the males and 6% of the females surveyed had had at least one homosexual experience. In the majority of the boys, the first of these experiences occurred at 11 or 12 years of age, whereas in the majority of the girls it occurred at 6 to 10 years of age. In approximately one third, the experience was with someone older, but in only 12% of the males, and in none of the females, was the partner an adult. Continuing homosexual activity among this adolescent group was minimal. Only 2% of the boys and none of the girls had a homosexual experience within the month prior to the survey. The weight of the present evidence is that homosexual experiences during adolescence are not uncommon, nor do they predict later homosexuality; conversely, however, most homosexuals report having had homosexual experiences during adolescence.

Issue 3: Is there a physical basis for homosexuality?

Following the report of Kolodny and colleagues (1971) of low testosterone and high luteinizing hormone levels in the serum of homosexual adult men, a number of other researchers have attempted to confirm this finding. Using different techniques and sampling schedules, others have found higher but normal levels of male hormones in homosexual males, compared with heterosexual males, as well as elevated plasma estradiol levels in the homosexuals.

The only endocrine study of adolescents was carried out by Parks and associates (1974). In their study of six homosexual and six heterosexual boys (age 17.8 ± 1.1 years) over 28 consecutive days of sampling, follicle stimulating hormone, luteinizing hormone, and testosterone levels were found to be comparable for the two groups and appropriate for maturational age.

From these data, sexual preference cannot be explained on the basis of hormonal differences during adolescence or adulthood. It remains possible, however, that differences can be found in prenatal or neonatal hormone levels.

Issue 4: Implications of cross dressing.

During childhood, occasional cross dressing and other effeminate behavioral patterns among boys have no implications for later sex role choices (Bakwin, 1968).

Adolescent cross dressing, or more specifically, boys dressing in female clothing, however, signifies the existence of transsexualism, transvestism, or effeminate homosexuality. The differences among these three conditions, although not always clear-cut, relate to the function of the clothing, the sexual object choice, and the role of the penis

Table 48–5 • Categorization of Male Gender Identity Variants

	Transsexuals	Effeminate Homosexuals	Transvestites
Core gender identity	Female	Male	Male
Cross dressing	To fulfill feminine role	To attract partner	Fetishistic
Desired sex partner	Heterosexual male	Homosexual male	Heterosexual female
View of penis	Abhorrent	Source of gratification	Source of gratification

in sexual gratification (Table 48–5). Transsexuals cross dress because they truly view themselves as females and recall that their first cross dressing experience made them feel secure and warm. In contrast, transvestites use women's clothing fetishistically to augment or stimulate sexual arousal, whereas for effeminate homosexuals, being "in drag" serves to attract sexual partners and often has a flamboyant quality. The desired sexual partner for a transsexual is typically a heterosexual male; for a transvestite, a heterosexual female; and for an effeminate homosexual, a homosexual male. The penis is abhorred by the transsexual and is never the source of sexual gratification, in contrast to the transvestite and effeminate homosexual, both of whom derive pleasure from the genital organ.

Sexual Learning and Sex Education

The notion that teaching about sex will stimulate children to engage in sexual experimentation cannot be supported. In fact, all existing evidence indicates that it is ignorance about sex that is more likely to result in sexual experimentation.

Given that children should be provided with sexual information, there remain a number of issues relevant to the implementation of sex education. When should it be taught? What should be taught? Who should do the teaching, and how is it best taught? These questions are obviously interrelated, but we attempt to review them separately.

WHEN SHOULD SEXUAL INFORMATION BE PROVIDED?

To decide when to initiate sex education, it is important to relate the issue to the development of cognitive function throughout childhood and adolescence. The studies by Bernstein and Cowan (1975) of children from 3 to 12 years of age indicate that sex information is not simply taken in but is transformed to the child's present cognitive level. In response to the question, "How does the baby happen to be inside the mother's body?" the youngest children (3 to 4 years old), paralleling Piagetian levels, are preformist and believe that a baby who now exists has always existed. At level II, children begin to attribute causality to the existence of babies, but they do so in the context of the manufacture of inanimate objects. By level III, children in transition from preoperations to concrete operations, although aware of the three major ingredients in the creation of babies (social relationship, the external mechanics of sexual intercourse, and the fusion of biological-genetic materials), are unable to coordinate any of the variables in

a coherent system. By the stage of concrete operations (level IV), a coordinated system of biological causality, the union of sperm and egg, is espoused without any attempt to explain why it must be so. Children at level V envision one gamete uniting with the other and releasing the preformed embryo as a result. By 11 to 12 years of age, on the average, children have reached level VI and recognize that the equal contribution of genetic material from both parents results in formation of the embryo.

In addition to understanding how children process information about sexuality at various ages, it is important to recognize that their social experiences will result in the acquisition of certain information regardless of whether it is taught intentionally. Kleeman (1975) found that by the second year of life, boys have knowledge about their genitals. Between the ages of 4 and 5 1/2 years, 98% of the 185 boys studied by Kreitler and Kreitler (1966) knew that their genitals were different from those of girls. By 9 to 11 years of age, more than 15% had extensive knowledge of genital function during coitus, according to Conn and Kanner (1947); by the age of 12 years, more than 50% of Ramsey's (1943) sample knew about ejaculation, the origin of babies, nocturnal emissions, contraception, masturbation, intercourse, and prostitution. By 14 years of age, more than half the boys had knowledge of venereal disease. It is important to note that the Ramsey and the Conn and Kanner studies were done prior to the advent of television as a major source of education, in 1940 and 1947, respectively.

Addressing the question of when to teach, Gagnon and Simon (1969) state: "If information is given too soon, it may be meaningless, or worse, anxiety provoking. If given too late, the young think we are slightly hypocritical. In the absence of highly individualized teaching in which a young person can seek information as he needs it from a responsive and caring adult, it might be best to opt for being slightly late." Conversely, in providing information about certain topics, such as birth control to the sexually active, one does not have the luxury of being "slightly late."

WHO SHOULD TEACH ABOUT SEX?

The recent literature suggests that parents are attempting to provide some sex education for their children but that in so doing they have a number of barriers to overcome. Most significant among them is a feeling among parents of inadequacy. This concern appears to be realistic, as in one study only 45% of the mothers had correct information concerning the time of the month when pregnancy was most likely to occur (Alan Guttmacher Institute, 1981). More than half of university students whose parents indicated that they had discussed sex with them reported that the talks had not been meaningful (King and Lorasso, 1997). Many parents are of the belief that children do not want to talk with their parents about sex. The reality is, however, that most youngsters express the desire to do so. In Sorensen's study, for example, 50% of the adolescent males and 63% of the females stated that they wanted to be able to talk to their parents about sex. In surveys in Arizona and New Zealand, parents and the schools were the youths' preferred sources of sex education.

It may be that little sex information comes from the home at least in part because many parents fail to provide unambiguous and direct answers to their children's questions. Conn and Kanner (1947) found that between the ages of 4 and 12 years of age, an average child asks only two questions of parents about sex-related matters. This might be, they suggest, because the parents fail to answer their children's questions adequately, and the children therefore do not bother to ask further questions in this apparently sensitive area. Since parents seem willing to answer other sorts of questions, sex often stands out for young children as a peculiar topic, leading to heightened curiosity. Parents should be counseled that children are generally ready to accept correct information about any topic for which they seek information, and that they should be answered directly, honestly, and simply. Parents should stop wondering whether they should reveal basic information about sex to their children and ask, rather, when and how this information should be transmitted to be most effective and useful for the child (Broderick, 1968).

Yet as Gagnon noted, the prevailing attitude of parents toward sexual socialization of their children seems to be that the best sexual teaching is that which teaches without provoking further questions or overt behavior. Three main types of information control seem to characterize parental attitudes toward their children's sex education. The first is called unambiguous labeling: Parents call attention to some behavior and label that behavior as "wrong." Generally they do so unambiguously and without explanation. A second type of information control, called nonlabeling by Gagnon, involves an attempt to avoid the issue. A third type is called mislabeling: In this case negative sanctions are interpreted to be outside the area of sex. For example, masturbation might be warned against because of the danger of the child's "getting germs." Likewise, interpersonal sex play might be mislabeled by parents as aggression and punished as such (Gagnon, 1965). Another type of mislabeling involves avoiding labels altogether. Most commonly masturbation and the genitals are given amorphous names, if any names at all, by parents who wish to avoid sexual labels (Sears, Maccoby, and Levin, 1957).

Information control of this kind can have deleterious effects on sexual development. The parental negative sanctions associated with unambiguous labeling and mislabeling can be well learned so that the negative, "dirty" interpretations of sexual behavior might never be revised. Likewise mislabeling can result in spillage from nonsexual areas to sexual ones, for example, if interpersonal sex play is mislabeled as aggression, a child's growing sense of social attitudes about aggression might translate into inferred attitudes about sexual behavior. Sears similarly suggested that mislabeling leads to misunderstandings about sex and inappropriately long persistence of the belief system that results from the mislabeling. Gagnon cautioned that punishment for mislabeled sexual behavior can cause a variety of problems for a growing child. With mislabeling it is unlikely that the child will understand why he or she is being punished, since it seems that the punishment is nonspecific to the behavior. Thus such punishment is likely to have few inhibitory effects. In contrast, punishment for mislabeled behavior can result in generalized anxiety about the behavior.

Nevertheless information control can have its payoffs (Gagnon, 1965). Nonlabeling can serve to protect a child against the parents' anxieties. Given that most adults in our culture have some anxieties about their own attitudes toward sex, it is difficult for them to be totally open with their children about sex.

Children and adolescents apparently learn early which topics might be acceptable to discuss with parents and others that are taboo. In families in which mothers and daughters communicated about sex, the daughters were more likely to initiate discussions about dating, boyfriends, and menstruation, whereas mothers were more apt to raise issues of sexual morality, intercourse, and birth control (Fox and Inazu, 1980). The type of issue raised by youngsters varies with their age. Preadolescents present more sexual situations to parents than do adolescent children, and the former are more likely to involve the topics of genitals, intercourse, in utero development and birth, female development and menstruation, and modesty and nudity, whereas adolescents raise issues of petting and premarital sex, dirty words and jokes, and abortion (Gilbert and Bailis, 1980).

This developmental sequence in parent-child communication about sex was confirmed by Chess and coworkers (1976). In the only prospective longitudinal study of the subject, they found that "by the time youths are 16, sex is a closed topic between themselves and their parents. The adolescents guard their privacy . . . and, for the most part, parents respect that privacy." Avoidance of discussions of sex reflects both the adolescent's effort to establish independence and the desire to avoid the conflict and tension that such discussions might precipitate. This notwithstanding, Fox and Inazu (1980) reported later ages of onset of coitus and more effective use of contraception among those who received information about sex within the family context.

The most common source of sex information seems to be same-sex peers. When teachers or siblings were reported as the primary source of information, accuracy scores were highest (Ansuini, Fiddler-Woite, and Woite, 1996).

WHAT AND HOW TO TEACH

Against this background of limited communication between parents and their children about sexual matters came reports of the increasing rate of venereal disease and pregnancy among young people in the late 1960s. Just as our society responded to Sputnik by demanding more mathematics and science in the schools, these developments placed new demands on the formal education system to provide sex education. Over the ensuing years, programs in family life education were introduced into the curriculum in most school districts; yet in reality, by 1980 no more than 10% of the students had received comprehensive sex education in school. In most programs, the curriculum consists of the presentation of basic biological factors about reproduction and less often includes attitudes, clarification of values, and decision making. Much has been written about how to set up programs, although evaluations of their efficacy are rare. When evaluations are performed, the outcome variables are typically cognitive, centering on the acquisition of factual knowledge, rather than attitudinal or behavioral outcomes. For a more complete review of the subject of program evaluation, the reader is referred to the article by Parcel and Luttman (1981).

Gordon (1975) emphasizes the importance of each school's examining its own atmosphere critically before deciding on curriculum content. If the environment is one in which student trust is lacking, attempts at teaching sexual values and attitudes will fail. In such settings he suggests a simple presentation of factual information. In recognition of the power of the peer group in the sex education process, an alternative to formal classroom teaching might be afterschool programs that use peer counselors for sessions in the clarification of values and responsibility for sexual activity. Physicians can provide valuable help in either of these contexts. In one community, for example, a pediatrician worked effectively with the Parent-Teacher Association to organize and teach a program in pubertal development for parents and their seventh grade children.

In addition to the role of consultant responding to requests for educational input, the physician should stimulate creation of educational opportunities within schools and families for youngsters with disabilities. The needs of such young people for sexual information often go unrecognized by those most closely involved with their care.

The observation that children with certain disabilities, such as blindness or meningomyelocele, tend to have earlier menarche than normal suggests their need for earlier education about reproduction and the prevention of pregnancy. In one study of parents of children with meningomyelocele, however, more than one third had the erroneous belief that their disabled children would be incapable of reproduction. Another implication of the disabled state is the fact that these individuals cannot avail themselves of the informal educational opportunities for sexual exploration and transfer of information among peers that are available to normal children. In a study of adolescents with meningomyelocele, three fourths had less than the average knowledge of sex, as compared with only one quarter of age-matched control subjects (Hayden, Davenport, and Campell, 1979).

Conclusion

Every stage of development in childhood and adolescence is equally important in the development of sexuality.

Parents, as the major agents of socialization, can contribute most significantly to this process by teaching modesty, by serving as role models for mutual respect and nonexploitation between the sexes, and by providing factual information and a yardstick against which children

and adolescents can measure their own behavior. Peers undoubtedly contribute heavily during adolescence by providing the most information about sex as well as an arena for sexual experimentation. Physical development, though not the primary stimulus for this experimentation, undoubtedly forces confrontation with new issues and choices during puberty. The physician, through contact with parents and the developing child throughout this period, is in a unique position to serve as a resource person to both and, in so doing, potentially to reduce the anxiety that often surrounds the issue of sexuality. Sexual development should be made a routine part of the curriculum of anticipatory guidance sessions provided with each well-baby, well-child, or well-adolescent visit. Rather than waiting for questions to be asked, the physician should take the opportunity at each such visit to indicate the sexual behavioral patterns normally engaged in at the youngster's level of development and those to be expected in the interval before the next visit. Once adolescence is reached, a similar approach should be taken with the patient and parent individually. Since the adolescent is faced with a number of options in terms of the wide range of sexual behavioral patterns, it is appropriate to use these sessions to help explore the basis for decision making, as well as to discuss possible sequelae of a decision to engage in intercourse, with the goal of preventing those that are undesirable, such as pregnancy and sexually transmitted diseases.

REFERENCES

Alan Guttmacher Institute: Teenage Pregnancy: The Problem That Hasn't Gone Away. New York, Alan Guttmacher Institute, 1981.

Ansuini CG, Fiddler-Woite J, Woite RS: The source, accuracy, and impact of initial sexuality information on lifetime wellness. Adolescence 31:283, 1996.

Ausubel DP: Theory and Problems of Child Development. New York, Grune & Stratton, 1958.

Bakwin H: Deviant gender-role behavior in children: relation to homosexuality. Pediatrics 41:620, 1968.

Bancroft J: The role of hormones in female sexuality. Proceedings of the Eighth International Congress of Psychosomatic Obstetrics and Gynecology. Amsterdam, Excerpta Medica, 1986.

Bernstein AC, Cowan PA: Children's concepts of how people get babies. Child Dev 46:77, 1975.

Bieber I, et al: Homosexuality: A Psychoanalytic Study. New York, Basic Books, 1962.

Blyth DA, Bulcroft R, Simmons RG: The impact of puberty on adolescents: a longitudinal study. Presented at Annual Meeting of the American Psychological Association, Los Angeles, August 26, 1981.

Broderick CB: Preadolescent sexual behavior. Med Aspects Hum Sexuality 2:20, 1968.

Burch B: Sex and the young child. Parents Magazine 27:36, 1952.

Centers for Disease Control and Prevention: State-specific pregnancy and birth rates among teenagers—United States 1991–1992. MMWR 44:677, 1995.

Chess S, Thomas A, Cameron M: Sexual attitudes and behavior patterns in a middle-class adolescent population. Am J Orthopsychiatry 46:689, 1976.

Chilman CS: Adolescent Sexuality in a Changing American Society: Social and Psychological Perspectives. DHEW Publication (NIH) 79–1426. Washington, DC, Department of Health, Education, and Welfare, 1979.

Conn JH, Kanner L: Children's awareness of sex differences. J Child Psychiatry 1:3, 1947.

Dornbusch SH, Carlsmith JM, Gross RT: Sexual development, age and dating: a comparison of biological and social influences upon one set of behaviors. Child Dev 52:179, 1981.

Ellis H: Psychology of Sex. New York, Emerson Books, 1938.

Erikson GH: Childhood and Society. New York, WW Norton, 1950.

Finch SM: Sex play among boys and girls. Med Aspects Hum Sexuality 3:58, 1969.

Fox GL, Inazu JK: Mother-daughter communication about sex. Family Relations 29:347, 1980.

Freud S: Three essays on the theory of sexuality. *In* Strachey J (ed and translator): The Standard Edition of the Complete Psychological Works of Sigmund Freud, Vol 7. London, Hogarth Press, 1964a.

Freud S: Lecture 20 of the introductory lectures on psycho-analysis. The sexual life of man. *In* Strachey J (ed and translator): The Standard Edition of the Complete Psychological Works of Sigmund Freud, Vol 16. London, Hogarth Press, 1964b.

Furstenberg FF, Levine JA, Brooks-Gunn J: The children of teenage mothers: patterns of early childbearing in two generations. Fam Plann Perspect 22:54, 1990.

Gagnon JH: Sexuality and sexual learning in the child. Psychiatry 28:212, 1965.

Gagnon JH: The creation of the sexual in early adolescence. *In* Kagan J, Coles L (eds): 12 to 16: Early Adolescence. New York, WW Norton, 1972, pp 231–257.

Gagnon JH, Simon W: Sex education and human development. *In* Fink PJ, Hammett UBO (eds): Sexual Function and Dysfunction. Philadelphia, FA Davis, 1969.

Gilbert FS, Bailis KL: Sex education in the home: an empirical task analysis. J Sex Res 16:148, 1980.

Ginott HG: Between Parent and Teenager. Avon Books, 1969, p 142.

Glasser M: Homosexuality in adolescence. Br J Med Psychol 50:217, 1977.

Gordon S: What place does sex education have in the schools? J School Health 44:186, 1975.

Gray DS, Gorzalka BB: Adrenal steroid interactions in female sexual behavior: a review. Psychoneuroendocrinology 5:157, 1980.

Green R: The Sissy-boy Syndrome and the Development of Homosexuality: A 15-year Prospective Study. New Haven, Yale University Press, 1986.

Hayden PW, Davenport SLH, Campbell MM: Adolescents with myelodysplasia: impact of physical disability on emotional maturation. Pediatrics 64:53, 1979.

Jessor SL, Jessor R: Transition from virginity to nonvirginity among youth: a socio-psychological study over time. Dev Psychol 11:473, 1975.

King BM, Lorasso J: Discussions in the home about sex: different recollections by parents and children. J Sex Marital Ther 23:52, 1997.

Kinsey AC, Pomeroy WB, Martin CE: Sexual Behavior in the Human Male. Philadelphia, WB Saunders, 1948.

Kleeman JA: Genital self-stimulation in infants and toddler girls. *In* Marcus IM, Francis JJ (eds): Masturbation: From Infancy to Senescence. New York, International Universities Press, 1975.

Kohlberg L: The adolescent as a philosopher. *In* Kagan J, Coles L (eds): 12 to 16: Early Adolescence. New York, WW Norton, 1972, pp 144–175.

Kolodny RC, Masters WH, Hendryx BS, et al: Plasma testosterone and semen analysis in male homosexuals. N Engl J Med 285:1170, 1971.

Kreitler H, Kreitler S: Children's concepts of sexuality and birth. Child Dev 37:363, 1966.

Litt IF, Cuskey WR, Rudd S: Identifying adolescents at risk for noncompliance with contraceptive therapy. J Pediatr 96:742, 1980.

Manosevitz M: The development of male homosexuality. J Sex Res 8:31, 1972.

Martinson FM: Infant and Child Sexuality: A Sociological Perspective. St. Peter, Minnesota, Book Mark, 1973.

Miller PY, Simon W: The development of sexuality in adolescence. *In* Adelson J (ed): Handbook of Adolescent Psychology. New York, John Wiley & Sons, 1980.

Money J: Childhood: The last frontier in sex research. The Sciences, 16:12, 27, 1976.

Parcel GS, Luttmann D: Evaluation in sex education: evaluation research for sex education applied to program planning. J Sch Health 51:278, 1981.

Parks GA, Karth-Schütz S, Penny R, et al: Variation in pituitary-gonadal function in adolescent homosexuals and heterosexuals. J Clin Endocrinol Metab 39:796, 1974.

Peck MW, Wells FL: On the psychosexuality of college graduate men. Ment Hyg 7:697, 1923.

Persky H: Psychosexual effects of hormones. Med Aspects Hum Sexuality 17:74, 1983.

Persky H, Charney N, Lief HT, et al: The relationship of plasma estradiol level to sexual behavior in young women. Psychosom Med 40:523, 1978.

Phillips G, Over R: Adult sexual orientation in relationship to memories of childhood gender conforming and gender nonconforming behaviors. Arch Sex Behav 21:543, 1992.

Piaget J: The Moral Judgment of the Child. Glencoe, Illinois, Free Press, 1948.

Ramsey GV: The sex information of younger boys. Am J Orthopsychiatry 13:347, 1943.

Schofield CBS: The Sexual Behavior of Young People. Boston, Little, Brown, 1965.

Sears RR, Maccoby EE, Levin H: Patterns of Child Rearing. Evanston, Illinois, Row, Peterson, 1957.

Sherwin B, Gelfand M, Brender W: Androgen enhances sexual motivation in females: a prospective crossover study in steroid administration in surgical menopause. Psychosom Med 47:339, 1985.

Simmons RG, Blyth DA, Van Cleave EF, et al: Entry into early adolescence: the impact of school structure, puberty, and early dating on self-esteem. Am Sociol Rev 44:948, 1979.

Sorensen RC: Adolescent Sexuality in Contemporary America. Mountain View, CA, World Publications, 1973.

Spitz RA: Autoeroticism: some empirical findings and hypotheses on three of its manifestations in the first year of life. Psychoanal Study Child 3–4:85, 1949.

US Congress, Office of Technology Assessment (OTA): Adolescent Health. Vol. II: Background and the Effectiveness of Selected Prevention and Treatment Services. OTA-H-466. Washington, DC, US Government Printing Office, 1991.

US Department of Health and Human Services, PHJ, CDC: Premarital sexual intercourse among adolescent women: United States, 1970–1988. Mortal Morbidity Weekly Report 39:929, 1991.

Zelnik M, Kantner JF: Sexual activity, contraceptive use and pregnancy among metropolitan area teenagers, 1971–1979. Fam Plann Perspect 12:230, 1980.

49 Aggressive Behavior and Delinquency

W. S. Yancy

Aggressive children are at risk to become tomorrow's violent adolescents. Understanding the roots of acting-out behaviors therefore comprises a critical component of preventive developmental-behavioral pediatrics. In this chapter, the author goes beyond the reductionist notion of "conduct disorder" to examine in detail the underpinnings of previolent and violent activity. This chapter makes it clear that the prevention and early detection of aggression needs to be an important role of the primary care clinician. Suggestions for the management of these maladaptive behaviors also need to be included in the treatment plans of these potentially destructive and self-destructive youngsters.

Aggressive Behaviors

EXAMPLE

A distraught Mrs. Jones is observed in the examining room struggling to keep her 20-month-old son from jumping out of her lap. Almost in tears, she exclaims, "Johnny is just impossible. His second day care center is threatening to expel him. He can't sit still and bites the other children. His older sister was never like this. What can I do?"

By definition, aggression is a hostile attack and is often considered a negative trait. But, in animals and early humans, aggression may have been necessary in the "survival of the fittest." In modern times, aggression may be seen as beneficial in the classroom, on the sporting field, and in the business world. Aggressiveness may be viewed as assertiveness. It may be acceptable, even encouraged, at the appropriate time and place. When it is not excessive, aggression may be beneficial to the individual. But when is aggression too much? When does teasing become malicious? When does enthusiastic ambition lead to lying and cheating? When does forceful play become "win at all costs?" When does assertive salesmanship lead to misrepresentation and dishonesty? Does aggressive behavior in the toddler lead to violent behavior and delinquency in the adolescent?

Information regarding these questions is scarce. Aggressive behavior that is mild and intermittent is thought to be common among young children. In a study of 8- and 11-year-old boys and girls, 51% reported having had at least one aggressive fight during the previous year (Boulton, 1993). Other studies have shown that children who initially display high rates of antisocial behavior are more likely to persist in this behavior than children who initially show lower rates of antisocial behavior (Loeber, 1982). Of 97 delinquent males evaluated 9 years after discharge from a correctional institution, all but six had adult criminal records, most for violent crimes (Lewis et al, 1994). These studies suggest that aggressive behavior is stable over time, but it cannot be concluded that all aggression progresses to problem behavior.

The Diagnostic and Statistical Manual for Primary Care (DSM-PC) Child and Adolescent Version (Wolraich, 1996) presents criteria for the diagnoses of aggression problems ranging from aggressive/oppositional variations through oppositional defiant disorders to conduct disorders. Figure 49–1 demonstrates the format of this manual, which provides common developmental presentations from infancy to adolescence. This manual is also helpful in providing criteria and codes for variations and problems that do not meet the criteria for more classic disorders. Mild biting, kicking, and verbal abuse may not arouse much concern but may require considerable discussion and anticipatory guidance to avoid escalation of the problem. Oppositional defiant disorder implies hostile behavior toward others that persists for at least 6 months. The behavior must occur frequently and cause clinically significant impairment in social and academic functioning. The diagnosis of conduct disorders (Fig. 49–2) is applied to those with repetitive, persistent behavior that violates the rights of others or disregards age-appropriate societal norms or rules. These patients may be cruel to people and animals, initiate physical fights, and use weapons. They may engage in firesetting and other property destruction. Lying and stealing are not uncommon, and such children are often truant from school and run away from home.

CAUSES

As a basic character trait, aggression may be beneficial if channeled appropriately, but the cause of excessive aggression is often not clear. In young children it may be due to frustration, retaliation, or attention-seeking behavior. In a study of 8-year-old girls and boys, aggressive fighting was observed to be due to retaliation to playful assault 15.4% of the time and to disputes over space 13.5% of the time (Boulton, 1993). In 43.3% of the fights observed, no obvious immediate cause could be detected. Family adversity and poor parenting are often cited as causes of negative behaviors. In such a setting, the child who behaves well may receive little attention but be quickly scolded when he or she acts out. Thus, a pattern of aggressive behavior may be established because the child prefers negative attention

PROBLEM	COMMON DEVELOPMENTAL PRESENTATIONS
V71.02 Aggressive/ Oppositional Problem **Aggression** When levels of aggression and hostility interfere with family routines, begin to engender negative responses from peers or teachers, and/or cause disruption at school, problematic status is evident. The negative impact is moderate. People change routines; property begins to be more seriously damaged. The child will display some of the symptoms listed for conduct disorder but not enough to warrant the diagnosis of the disorder. However, the behaviors are not sufficiently intense to qualify for a behavioral disorder.	**Infancy** The infant bites, kicks, cries, and pulls hair fairly frequently. **Early Childhood** The child frequently grabs others' toys, shouts, hits or punches siblings and others, and is verbally abusive. **Middle Childhood** The child gets into fights intermittently in school or in the neighborhood, swears or uses bad language sometimes in inappropriate settings, hits or otherwise hurts self when angry or frustrated. **Adolescence** The adolescent intermittently hits others, uses bad language, is verbally abusive, may display some inappropriate suggestive sexual behaviors.
	SPECIAL INFORMATION
	Problem levels of aggressive behavior may run in families. When marked aggression is present, the assessor must examine the family system, the types of behaviors modeled, and the possibility of abusive interactions.

DISORDER	COMMON DEVELOPMENTAL PRESENTATIONS
313.81 Oppositional Defiant Disorder Hostile, defiant behavior towards others of at least 6 months' duration that is developmentally inappropriate. • often loses temper • often argues with adults • often actively defies or refuses to comply with adults' requests or rules • often deliberately annoys people • often blames others for his or her mistakes or misbehavior • is often touchy or easily annoyed by others • is often angry and resentful • is often spiteful or vindictive (see *DSM-IV* Criteria Appendix)	**Infancy** It is not possible to make the diagnosis. **Early Childhood** The child is extremely defiant, refuses to do as asked, mouths off, throws tantrums. **Middle Childhood** The child is very rebellious, refusing to comply with reasonable requests, argues often, and annoys other people on purpose. **Adolescence** The adolescent is frequently rebellious, has severe arguments, follows parents around while arguing, is defiant, has negative attitudes, is unwilling to compromise, and may precociously use alcohol, tobacco, or illicit drugs.

Figure 49–1. Aggressive/oppositional problem: oppositional defiant disorder. (From American Academy of Pediatrics: Diagnostic and Statistical manual for Primary Care [DSM-PC] Child and Adolescent Version. Elk Grove Village, IL, American Academy of Pediatrics, 1996, p 123.)

to no attention. Although data relative to the long-term effects of corporal punishment, such as spanking, are as yet inconclusive, Straus (1994, 1996) has shown that teenagers who were hit by their parents are more likely to steal and assault someone else physically. It has also been shown that the more spanking used by parents attempting to correct misbehavior, the worse the child's antisocial behavior was 2 years later (Straus, Sugarman, and Giles-Sims, 1997). Certainly, physical or sexual abuse and family violence are correlated with subsequent antisocial behavior.

Oppositional defiant disorders, especially when associated with aggressive behavior, may be an antecedent to conduct disorders (Loeber et al, 1995). This study also found that low socioeconomic status of parents and parental substance abuse were highly predictive of the development of conduct disorder in adolescents.

The relationship between attention-deficit hyperactivity disorders (ADHD) and the development of conduct disorders is described in a longitudinal study by Gittelman (1985). Antisocial behavior is reported to be six times more frequent in youth whose ADHD symptoms persist through adolescence. Adolescents whose ADHD symptoms had remitted were no different than control subjects. Conduct disorders are more likely to develop in children with ADHD plus aggressive behavior, but even in a group of pure ADHD children, without aggression symptoms, conduct disorder developed in 20%.

The frequency of violence in movies and on television has been widely documented. Music videos are tremendously popular with youth and they have also been reported to have high rates of violence (DuRant et al, 1997). Although still a controversial conclusion, 3 decades

DISORDER	COMMON DEVELOPMENTAL PRESENTATION
312.81 Conduct Disorder Childhood Onset **312.82 Conduct Disorder Adolescent Onset** A repetitive and persistent pattern of behavior in which the basic rights of others or major age-appropriate societal norms or rules are violated. Onset may occur as early as age 5 to 6 years, but is usually in late childhood or early adolescence. The behaviors harm others and break societal rules including stealing, fighting, destroying property, lying, truancy, and running away from home. (see *DSM-IV* Criteria Appendix) **309.3 Adjustment Disorder With Disturbance of Conduct** (see *DSM-IV* Criteria Appendix) **312.9 Disruptive Behavior Disorder, NOS** (see *DSM-IV* Criteria Appendix)	**Infancy** It is not possible to make the diagnosis. **Early Childhood** Symptoms are rarely of such a quality or intensity to be able to diagnose the disorder. **Middle Childhood** The child often may exhibit some of the following behaviors: lies, steals, fights with peers with and without weapons, is cruel to people or animals, may display some inappropriate sexual activity, bullies, engages in destructive acts, violates rules, acts deceitful, is truant from school, and has academic difficulties. **Adolescence** The adolescent displays delinquent, aggressive behavior, harms people and property more often than in middle childhood, exhibits deviant sexual behavior, uses illegal drugs, is suspended/expelled from school, has difficulties with the law, acts reckless, runs away from home, is destructive, violates rules, has problems adjusting at work, and has academic difficulties.
	SPECIAL INFORMATION
	The best predictor of aggression that will reach the level of a disorder is a diversity of antisocial behaviors exhibited at an early age; clinicians should be alert to this factor. Oppositional defiant disorder usually becomes evident before age 8 years and usually not later than early adolescence. Oppositional defiant disorder is more prevalent in males than in females before puberty, but rates are probably equal after puberty. The occurrence of the following negative environmental factors may increase the likelihood, severity, and negative prognosis of conduct disorder: parental rejection and neglect, inconsistent management with harsh discipline, physical or sexual child abuse, lack of supervision, early institutional living, frequent changes of caregivers, and association with delinquent peer group. Suicidal ideation, suicide attempts, and completed suicide occur at a higher than expected rate. If the criteria are met for both oppositional defiant disorder and conduct disorder, only code conduct disorder.

Figure 49–2. Conduct disorder. (From American Academy of Pediatrics: Diagnostic and Statistical manual for Primary Care [DSM-PC] Child and Adolescent Version. Elk Grove Village, IL, American Academy of Pediatrics, 1996, p 124.)

of research would suggest that there is a causal link between exposure to television violence and the development of aggressive behavior (Sege and Dietz, 1994).

Biogenetic causes for aggressive behavior have recently received increased attention. The children of parents with criminal records have been shown to have high rates of criminal behavior, even when raised in adoptive noncriminal families. Concordance studies of twins born to criminal parents but who were raised in different families also show an increased likelihood of antisocial behavior in the children. Use of a genetic loading technique and comparison of the frequency of symptoms in relatives has demonstrated the important role of genetic factors in oppositional defiant disorder and conduct disorder (Comings, 1995). Emerging data regarding the role of neurotransmitters in the development of aggressive behavior have concentrated on serotonin, but evidence of abnormali-

ties in catecholaminergic and peptidergic systems is also available. These studies involve cerebral spinal fluid serotonin, platelet-receptor binding, and psychopharmacologic challenge tests. The finding of decreased numbers of serotonin transporter sites on the platelets of patients with aggressive conduct disorder may provide a biological marker for some patients with this diagnosis (Birmaher et al, 1990; Stoff et al, 1987). The report by Halperin et al (1994) of differences in the fenfluramine challenge responses in aggressive ADHD patients compared with nonaggressive control subjects also provides evidence to implicate an abnormality in the serotonin system.

Specific food allergies, adverse reactions to sugar, and sensitivity to food additives have all been implicated as a cause of aggressive behavior and hyperactivity. Although numerous studies have reported no evidence in support of these claims, they are mentioned herein to discourage dietary interventions that are not effective and may not be benign.

PREVENTION AND TREATMENT

Treatment approaches to aggression in children and youth depend on the frequency, duration, and intensity of the aggressive behavior and whether there is an underlying or associated emotional disorder. Parents must avoid corporal punishment and learn positive methods of discipline. They can be taught the developmental aspects of aggression and can learn how to channel it into positive acts. Because behavior does not persist or recur if it is not reinforced, "time out" techniques have been frequently recommended to parents and teachers. This may be all that is necessary to help the young child with mild aggressive behavior. However, because the only sure way to avoid reinforcing a behavior is not to be around it, the parent or teacher must remove the child from sight. Simply placing the child in a corner where he or she can still receive attention from classmates or from siblings is not effective. It is also important to recognize the benefit of rewarding nonaggressive behavior. *Parent Effectiveness Training* (Gordon, 1975) and *Defiant Children* (Barkley, 1997) present two programs that have been successful in teaching parents problem-solving skills, negotiation techniques, and methods of rewarding desirable behavior. More disordered behaviors may require referral to a physician with developmental-behavioral training or to other mental health professionals. These specialists may use individual or group therapy, family therapy, parent training, or peer group counseling.

Pharmacologic therapy for aggressive behavior may be beneficial in conjunction with behavioral, educational, or community program interventions. However, it is not clear whether medication can decrease aggression when it occurs independently of a comorbid psychiatric disorder, such as ADHD or conduct disorder (Connor and Steingard, 1996). Methylphenidate and dextroamphetamine have been shown to reduce aggression in ADHD children by teacher and parent reports and by direct observation studies. When buspirone is given in conjunction with stimulants, additional improvement is noted. Clonidine has been shown to be of benefit to aggressive patients with conduct disorder and/or ADHD. Further studies of the serotonin system may identify antiaggression-specific medications.

Outside of the family, programs for the prevention of aggressive behavior have focused on the schools and communities. Outcome evaluations of these programs are limited, but in a randomized trial of second- and third-grade children, a curriculum teaching social skills related to anger management, impulse control, and empathy demonstrated an overall decrease in physical aggression and an increase in prosocial behavior in the study group compared with a control group (Grossman et al, 1997). Most effects were noted to persist 6 months later. Another study demonstrated that a behavioral treatment classroom program was effective in reducing children's hyperactive, impulsive, and aggressive behaviors and in improving their self-control and social skills (Barkley et al, 1996). Children in the study group were also found to have fewer symptoms of a conduct disorder.

Delinquency

EXAMPLE

John, a 13-year-old youth, is brought to the office because he ran away from home. He has been taking Ritalin (methylphenidate) for 4 years and initially responded quite well. However, during the past year he has been frequently truant from school and is currently on probation for vandalism and disorderly conduct. His mother wants to know why his medicine is no longer working.

Delinquency is more a legal term than a medical term. A youth is considered to be a delinquent if he or she commits an act that violates the law and the violation comes to the attention of the police or the court system. Usually youth are tried in juvenile courts, but at adjudication they may be determined to be delinquents, status offenders, or persons in need of supervision, or they may be waved to criminal court for processing as an adult. A "status offense" is an act that is illegal when committed by a juvenile and one that can only be tried in a juvenile court. For example, truancy, disobedience to parents, or running away from home would not be considered a crime if committed by an adult. "Index offenses" are acts such as homicide, burglary, auto theft, prostitution, and disorderly conduct that would be considered criminal acts at any age. The extent of delinquent behavior is enormous, and the increasing rate of violent behavior is staggering. In 1995 there were 2,084,428 arrests among persons younger than 18 years and 711,348 arrests in the age group younger than 15 years (Federal Bureau of Investigation, 1996). From 1986 to 1995, the overall arrest rate of male youth increased 24.4%, with arrests for murder and aggravated assault increasing by 91.9% and 69.2%, respectively. Arrests for other assaults increased by 97.8%. The overall arrest rate for girls younger than 18 years increased 50.1%, with arrests for murder and aggravated assault increasing by 62.4% and 128.1%, respectively. Other assaults committed by girls increased by 154%. These figures reflect the increased rate of violence among all age groups in the United States. These figures report only those youth who have come to the attention of the court system. Data from nationwide self-report surveys of high school students indicate that more than 90% of these youth engaged in at least one delinquent act that, if detected, would have resulted in juvenile court involvement. Using The National Youth Risk Behavior Survey, Sosin and colleagues (1995) reported that 8% of high school students had been in a fight during the 30 days prior to the survey and 26% had carried a firearm. Of all students, the fighters accounted for 49% of those carrying a firearm.

CAUSES

In the legal system, all of the 15 criteria for conduct disorder in *The Diagnostic and Statistical Manual of Mental Disorders (DSM-IV)* would at least be status offenses and seven of the 15 would be index offenses. For this reason, the aforementioned causes for conduct disorder would also apply to most delinquents.

Much attention has been paid to social and environmental determinants in the families of delinquents. Delinquent behavior is common in children belonging to highly stressed families of low economic status. Parents may have marital discord, have psychopathologic behavior, abuse alcohol and other drugs, be unemployed, and/or abuse their spouses or children. In a prospective study, 49% of the childhood victims of abuse had criminal records as young adults and were twice as likely as unabused control subjects to have been arrested for a violent crime (Maxfield and Widom, 1996). Poor role models and poor monitoring and disciplinary efforts by parents are correlated significantly with police contacts and self-reported delinquency by children. However, not all delinquent youth are raised in low-income, stressful, neglectful situations. Youth from middle-income families may be less likely to commit violent crimes, but their rates of status offenses and minor delinquent acts are equal to those of youth in low-income families. Delinquents report poor self-esteem and perceive themselves as more socially inadequate, more alienated, and more isolated than do nondelinquents. These characteristics may be fostered unknowingly by parental permissiveness or ambivalent communication from parents who are unable to cope with their own antisocial traits. Even when parents are not violent to each other, the more corporal punishment they inflict on their children, the greater the chances of delinquency (Straus, 1994).

Poor school performance, learning disabilities, and ADHD have been frequently reported in association with delinquent behavior. Studies have reported up to 70% of delinquent youth to have learning disabilities, especially reading problems. A review of boys with ADHD found that 50% had conduct disorders, and they were reported to have five times the number of arrests and 25 times the number of incarcerations compared with normal control subjects (Klein and Mannuzza, 1991). Children with a learning disability or ADHD are likely to become frustrated and have low self-esteem because of their inability to perform up to the scholastic standards of their classmates and because their impulsive, hyperactive behavior creates disruption in the classroom. These behaviors may cause teachers and parents to view such children as oppositional or difficult, causing further alienation and reduced self-esteem. This may lead to aggressive, delinquent behavior.

Biogenetic factors in the development of delinquency are similar to those related to conduct disorder development. With delinquents, especially violent offenders, it is the serotonin system that is most frequently implicated. Linnoila and colleagues (1983) reported lower spinal fluid serotonin in impulsive violent offenders compared to violent offenders who acted with premeditation, which suggests that it is the impulsive aggression in these former individuals that correlates with reduced central serotonin levels. Alm and associates (1994) suggest that low platelet monoamine oxidase (MAO) activity in young delinquents may predict an increased risk for continued criminal behavior. They found significantly lower platelet MAO activity in subjects with early and late criminal behavior compared to subjects who had early but not late criminal records. There was no significant difference between control subjects and the early delinquents who had no late criminality.

Nutritional concerns, especially about sucrose, as a cause for delinquent behavior have received so much publicity that some juvenile detention centers eliminate or reduce sugar in their institutional diets with the objective of preventing undesirable behavior. This practice has persisted despite studies that demonstrate no significant negative effects of a sucrose challenge. Bachorowski and associates (1990) found that delinquents who were asked to perform a series of tasks that were relevant to delinquency actually had improved performance after sucrose ingestion.

PREVENTION AND TREATMENT

The approach to prevention and treatment for delinquency is similar to that for conduct disorders and it begins with the family. Good role models, open communication, appropriate supervision, avoidance of punitive disciplinary practices, promotion of education, reinforcement of positive behavior, and cultivation of good self-esteem are all beneficial characteristics of an environment that reduces the potential for delinquent behavior. Comprehensive family support and early education in parenting skills have a positive effect in the reduction of risk factors for delinquency and may reduce the incidence of subsequent delinquent behavior (Yoshikawa, 1994).

Pharmacologic therapy may be of some benefit, especially for delinquents with comorbid psychological diagnoses and in the reduction of violent behavior. However, multimodality treatment (MMT), which combines drug therapy with individual or group therapy, social skills training, and parent skills training, has been shown to be much more effective than drug treatment alone. Satterfield, Satterfield, and Schell (1987) followed two groups of hyperactive boys for 9 years. The MMT group had one third the arrest rate for felony crimes as the group treated with methylphenidate alone. Institutionalization occurred in 22% of the drug-only group but in only 8% of the MMT group. For boys receiving MMT for longer than 2 years, no institutionalization occurred. Two other programs, one in a school setting (O'Donnell et al, 1995) and one in a community setting (Jones and Offord, 1989), documented equally promising long-term results among children from low-income families. These studies reported reduced antisocial behaviors and substance abuse and increased social and school work skills.

Physician Involvement

Physicians who provide health care for children and youth have the opportunity and the responsibility to help them avoid the development of aggressive, delinquent behaviors. Screening questions on violence and anticipatory guidance for violence prevention should be a part of every well-child examination. Parents need to be reminded about the promotion of self-esteem, the monitoring of television viewing habits, the effects of corporal punishment, and the value of appropriate supervision for their children. They can be taught good communication skills, constructive disciplinary techniques, and the benefits of compromise in conflict resolution approaches. They can learn how to establish rules and to reinforce appropriate behavior. To know when intervention is indicated, the physician must be familiar with risk factors such as parents' marital discord, punitive disciplinary practices, ADHD, and poor school performance. Warning signs such as biting, lying, petty stealing, cruelty to animals, and aggressive, oppositional behavior are cues for early intervention. Physicians are often asked to help youth who have committed delinquent acts but have not come in contact with the court system or who have not yet been incarcerated. To provide optimal care for these youth, the physician needs to be familiar with community agencies and programs that can provide family support, educational assistance, vocational training, substance abuse counseling, and group or family therapy.

The most important role of the physician is as an advocate for school and community programs that promote the learning of social skills, problem-solving skills, and nonviolent approaches to conflict resolution. Physicians can encourage local governments and school boards to develop programs such as the ones described by Barkley and colleagues (1996), O'Donnell and associates (1995), or Jones and Offord (1989). The expense of institutionalization, property damage, and theft and the increased cost of police, fire, and court services far exceed the cost of these preventive programs. The personal cost to the individual and the family and the loss of educational achievement and career productivity cannot be measured. Physicians have a responsibility to their patients and to their communities to recognize these problems and to help develop and implement appropriate solutions to them.

REFERENCES

Alm PO, Alm M, Humble K, et al: Criminality and platelet monoamine oxidase activity in former juvenile delinquents as adults. Acta Psychiatr Scand 89(1):41, 1994.

Bachorowski J, Newman JP, Nichols SL, et al: Sucrose and delinquency: behavioral assessment. Pediatrics 86(2):244, 1990.

Barkley RA: Defiant Children, 2nd ed. New York, Guilford Press, 1997.

Barkley RA, Shelton TL, Crosswait C, et al: Preliminary findings of an early intervention program with aggressive hyperactive children. Ann N Y Acad Sci 794:277, 1996.

Birmaher B, Stanley M, Greenhill L, et al: Platelet imipramine binding in children and adolescents with impulsive behavior. J Am Acad Child Adolesc Psychiatry 29:914, 1990.

Boulton MJ: Proximate causes of aggressive fighting in middle school children. Br J Educ Psychol 63(2):231, 1993.

Comings DE: The role of genetic factors in conduct disorder based on studies of Tourette syndrome and attention-deficit hyperactivity disorder probands and their relatives. J Dev Behav Pediatrics 16(3):142, 1995.

Connor DF, Steingard RJ: A clinical approach to the pharmacotherapy of aggression in children and adolescents. Ann N Y Acad Sci 794:290, 1996.

DuRant RH, Rich M, Emans SJ, et al: Violence and weapon carrying in music videos. Arch Pediatr Adolesc Med 151:443, 1997.

Federal Bureau of Investigation: Uniform crime reports for the United States—1995. Washington, DC, US Government Printing Office, 1996.

Gittelman R, Mannuzza S, Shenker R, et al: Hyperactive boys almost grown up. Arch Gen Psychiatry 42:937, 1985.

Gordon T: Parent Effectiveness Training. New York, New American Library, 1975.

Grossman DC, Neckerman HJ, Koepsell TD, et al: Effectiveness of a violence prevention curriculum among children in elementary school. JAMA 277(20):1605, 1997.

Halperin JM, Sharma V, Siever LJ, et al: Serotonergic function in aggressive and nonaggressive boys with attention deficit hyperactivity disorder. Am J Psychiatry 151:243, 1994.

Jones MB, Offord DR: Reduction of antisocial behavior in poor children by nonschool skill-development. J Child Psychol Psychiatry 30(5):737, 1989.

Klein RG, Mannuzza S: Long-term outcome of hyperactive children: a review. J Am Acad Child Adolesc Psychiatry 30:383, 1991.

Lewis DO, Yeager CA, Lovely R, et al: A clinical follow-up of delinquent males: ignored vulnerabilities, unmet needs and the perpetuation of violence. J Am Acad Child Adolesc Psychiatry 33(4):518, 1994.

Linnoila M, Virkkunen M, Scheinin M, et al: Low cerebrospinal fluid 5-HIAA concentration differentiates impulsive from nonimpulsive violent behavior. Life Sci 33:2609, 1983.

Loeber R: The stability of antisocial and delinquent child behavior: a review. Child Dev 53(6):1431, 1982.

Loeber R, Green SM, Keenan K, et al: Which boys will fare worse? Early predictors of the onset of conduct disorder in a six-year longitudinal study. J Am Acad Child Adolesc Psychiatry 34(4):499, 1995.

Maxfield MG, Widom CS: The cycle of violence. Revisited 6 years later. Arch Pediatr Adolesc Med 150(4):390, 1996.

O'Donnell J, Hawkins JD, Catalano RF, et al: Preventing school failure, drug use and delinquency among low-income children: long-term intervention in elementary schools. Am J Orthopsychiatry 65(1):87, 1995.

Satterfield JH, Satterfield BT, Schell AM: Therapeutic interventions to prevent delinquency in hyperactive boys. J Am Acad Child Adolesc Psychiatry 26(1):56, 1987.

Sege R, Dietz W: Television viewing and violence in children: the pediatrician as agent for change. Pediatrics 94(4):600, 1994.

Sosin DM, Koepsell TD, Rivara FP, et al: Fighting as a marker for multiple problem behaviors in adolescents. J Adolesc Health 16:209, 1995.

Stoff DM, Pollock L, Vitiello B, et al: Reduction of (3H)-imipramine binding sites on platelets of conduct-disordered children. Neuropsychopharmacology 1(1):55, 1987.

Straus MA: Spanking and the making of a violent society. Pediatrics 98(4):837; 1996.

Straus MA: Beating the Devil Out of Them—Corporal Punishment in American Families. New York, Lexington Books, 1994, pp 106, 108.

Straus MA, Sugarman DB, Giles-Sims J: Spanking by parents and subsequent antisocial behavior of children. Arch Pediatr Adolesc Med 151:761, 1997.

Wolraich ML (ed): Diagnostic and Statistical Manual for Primary Care (DSM-PC) Child and Adolescent Version. Elk Grove Village, IL, American Academy of Pediatrics, 1996.

Yoshikawa H: Prevention as cumulative protection: effects of early family support and education on chronic delinquency and its risks. Psychol Bulletin 115(1):28, 1994.

50 *Substance Use, Abuse, and Dependence*

John R. Knight

 The most commonly used substances are tobacco, alcohol, and marijuana. Although the prevalence of tobacco and alcohol use among teenagers has remained fairly stable during the 1990s, marijuana use has increased. There has also been a rise in the use of volatile inhalants, stimulants, LSD, and other hallucinogens.

The developmental stages of adolescent drug and alcohol use can include abstinence, experimental use, regular use, problem use, abuse, and dependency.

The most effective method of screening is a good history, taken without parents present in the room. Teenagers will reliably report use of alcohol and drugs if they are assured of confidentiality.

Use and abuse of psychoactive substances is a major national problem, and one of great concern to pediatricians. Treatment of medical problems related to the use of tobacco, alcohol, and other drugs places a considerable drain on time and other health care resources. Even more important is the cost in human pain and suffering to individual abusers and their family members. Physicians can make a difference by recognizing substance use early on and intervening before serious harm results. This chapter presents an overview of the problem and describes methods for screening, assessment, office intervention, and referral to treatment programs. Because this problem often affects families, the chapter ends with a discussion of substance abuse by parents.

Adolescent Development

Puberty refers to the physiologic changes that occur between late childhood (8–10 years of age) and young adulthood (16–18 years). These include acceleration in linear growth, gametogenesis, and development of secondary sexual characteristics. *Adolescence* describes the accompanying psychosocial changes that occur as individuals leave childhood and develop into independent, contributing members of adult society. To accomplish this change, a number of strategies may be employed, including experimentation, exploration, risk taking, limit testing, and questioning of established rules and authority. While these strategies are often functional, they can also lead to serious injury and illness in the context of alcohol or drug use. Simple warnings about risks may be insufficient to bring about change in behavior, as teenagers tend to see themselves as invulnerable. All too often, warnings elicit the classic response, "Don't worry, that can never happen to me," (Elkind, 1992). On the more positive side, research on adolescent development indicates this is not a tumultuous period of emotional lability and suicidality (Offer and Schonert-Reichl, 1992). In fact, it is a very positive period, when interpersonal relationships are transformed and new cognitive abilities emerge. In social relationships, there is

movement from predominant family influence (preconformist), to peer influence (conformist), to independent thinking (postconformist) (Peterson and Leffert, 1995). Cognitively, the development of formal operations leads to the ability to think in the abstract (Piaget, 1962). This allows for the use of propositional logic, that is, the formation of a hypothesis and consideration of possible solutions. Adolescents also develop metacognition, or the ability to think about the thought process itself. These abilities are essential for the establishment of therapeutic doctor-patient relationships and for cognitive-behavioral interventions such as resistance planning.

Risk and Problem Behaviors

Problem-behavior theory and social cognitive theory provide a conceptual framework for understanding risk behaviors during the adolescent period. Problem-behavior theory defines *risk behavior* as anything that can interfere with successful psychosocial development; and *problem behavior* as risk behaviors that elicit either formal or informal social responses designed to control them (Jessor and Jessor, 1977). These may cluster to form a *risk behavior syndrome* when they serve a common social or psychological developmental function (e.g., affirming individuation from parents, helping to achieve adult status, gaining acceptance from peers). These behaviors may also help the adolescent cope with failure, boredom, social anxiety, unhappiness, rejection, social isolation, low self-esteem, or a lack of self-efficacy. For example, adolescents who are poor students may use drugs as a way of achieving social status among their peers.

Social cognitive theory explains human functioning in terms of *triadic reciprocal causation,* in which behavior, personal determinants, and environmental influences all interact to determine behavior (Bandura, 1977). According to this theory, individuals learn how to behave through a process of modeling and reinforcement, imitating behaviors observed in others that are perceived to have positive consequences. Therefore, exposure to successful, high-status role models who use drugs will likely influence adolescents. According to this theory, health risk and problem behaviors are both purposeful and functional. Peer influences may suggest to adolescents that drug use and sexual behaviors will help one to become popular, cool, sexy, grown-up, sophisticated, macho, or tough.

Epidemiology

The federal government has commissioned several longitudinal studies of alcohol and drug use, including the *National Household Survey on Drug Abuse* and the *Monitoring the Future Study* (formerly knows as the *High School Senior Survey*) (SAMHSA, 1996; NIDA, 1995). These studies have followed patterns of use over the past 20 years and found that while prevalence of use of individual psychoactive substances may wax and wane, it does not disappear. Data released in 1996 indicate that drug use among youth is on the rise, and initiation of use is occurring at younger ages. In addition, the perceived risk-of-harm has decreased while the perceived availability of drugs has increased. The most commonly used substances are tobacco, alcohol, and marijuana. Although the prevalence of tobacco and alcohol use among teenagers has remained fairly stable during the 1990s, marijuana use has increased. There has also been a rise in the use of volatile inhalants, stimulants, LSD, and other hallucinogens.

TOBACCO

There have been a number of positive developments regarding tobacco use over recent years. The acceptability of cigarette smoking in public places has declined, and there is a widespread perception that tobacco use is hazardous to health. There has also been an increase in the number of laws restricting tobacco use, and better enforcement of laws prohibiting sale of tobacco products to minors. Despite these advances, prevalence of tobacco use among high school students has remained essentially unchanged, with just under 20% of seniors reporting daily smoking (NIDA, 1995). This makes cigarettes the drug most commonly used on a daily basis among high school students. These data have great significance in that tobacco is a "gateway" drug for youth, and cigarette smokers are more likely to be heavy drinkers and to use illicit drugs (Epps, Manley, and Glynn, 1995).

ALCOHOL

Despite the fact that alcohol is an illegal substance for teenagers, the overwhelming majority of them have tried it. Although there has been an overall decline in teenager's use of alcohol over recent years, over half of eighth-graders and 80% of twelfth-graders have had a drink (SAMHSA, 1996). The average first-time drinker is 12 to 13 years old. Of greatest concern is the prevalence of binge drinking, defined as having five or more drinks in a row. The prevalence of this behavior is reported at 15%, 24%, and 28% among eighth-, tenth-, and twelfth-graders, respectively. It is more common among males than females and often occurs in cars or at parties from which young people drive

home. Accidents are the leading cause of death among young people in the United States, and 45% of motor vehicle fatalities are directly related to alcohol consumption (CDC, 1991; NHTSA, 1991). Even though most teenagers report that they are aware that driving after drinking is dangerous, almost one third have accepted a ride from a driver who had been drinking, and almost half of the students who drink have taken this risk (OIG, 1991).

ILLICIT DRUGS

More than 40% of twelfth-graders have tried some kind of illicit drug. The most commonly used substances are marijuana, volatile inhalants, and stimulants. Marijuana use rose sharply between 1991 and 1994. Thirty-eight percent of high school seniors have tried it, 19% have used it within the past month, and 3.6% use it daily (NIDA, 1995). Frequent marijuana use is particularly problematic for students, as it can result in suppression of motivation and lead to a downward spiral of worsening academic performance and increased use. The potency of this drug has increased dramatically over the past 30 years, making the marijuana used currently more hazardous than that smoked during the 1960s by present-day parents of teenaged children. Inhalants are another class of drugs whose use is on the rise. These are defined as fumes or gases that produce euphoria when inhaled and include solvents, glues, aerosols, and butane. These chemicals are found in many common household products and thus are readily available to young people. Inhalants may be brought into school as small bottles of typewriter correction fluid. This is the only class of drug whose use is highest among eighth-graders, the youngest group surveyed (NIDA, 1995). Approximately 20% of eighth-graders have tried some form of inhalant. Other illicit drugs such as cocaine and heroin are more likely to be used by older teenagers and young adults. Although the use of heroin is relatively uncommon, its popularity in some US cities is currently on the rise.

PRESCRIPTION DRUGS

Over recent years, there has been an increased public awareness of attention-deficit hyperactivity disorder (ADHD), and more children are being treated with stimulant medications (Safer, Zito, and Fine, 1996). This, in turn, has been associated with an increase in the diversion, sale, and abuse of stimulants. Methylphenidate can be ground up with a mortar and pestle and then self-administered by nasal insufflation ("snorting"). As with cocaine, this can potentially lead to sudden cardiac arrhythmia and death. As there is significant comorbidity of ADHD and substance abuse, clinicians should carefully consider this risk and recommend adult supervision of stimulant medication storage and administration when treating high-risk youth. Since for some teenagers drug use is considered "cool" and appealing, over-the-counter stimulant medications (e.g., "stay-awake" pills or "diet pills") may also be abused.

Risk Factors

Multiple factors have been found to influence the development and manifestation of substance use problems in young people. These include genetic, familial, social, environmental, and characterologic factors. Genetic predictors have been found in both twin and adoption studies. This suggests that alcohol abuse and dependency disorders are at least mildly inheritable, particularly from fathers to sons (Murray and Clifford, 1983). Other family factors have been implicated in the development of substance abuse problems, such as parental use of alcohol or drugs or permissive attitudes regarding substance use (Patton, 1995). Socially, having substance-abusing friends is associated with increased likelihood of initiating substance use (Freeland and Campbell, 1973). This may be due both to peer pressure and to availability of supply. Peer influences, however, do not predict the development of substance use problems or disorders (Patton, 1995). In fact, adolescents who use for social reasons are more likely to stop than those who use for psychological reasons (Kandel and Raveis, 1989). Environmental risk factors include deprivation and low socioeconomic status (Dusenbury, Khuri, and Millman, 1992). Personality characteristics associated with substance abuse problems include low assertiveness, low self-esteem, low self-efficacy, low self-confidence, low social confidence, and external locus of control (Dusenbury, Khuri, and Millman, 1992). Substance users also tend to have lower religiosity, higher identification with counterculture, higher impulsivity, higher anxiety, and a stronger need for peer approval (Newcomb and Felix-Ortiz, 1992).

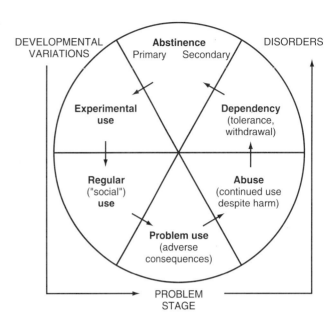

Figure 50–1. Adolescent drug and alcohol use: a developmental view. (Data from Knight JR: Adolescent substance use: screening, assessment, and intervention in medical office practice. Contemp Pediatrics 14[4]:45, 1997; and Wolraich ML [ed]: The Classification of Child and Adolescent Mental Diagnoses in Primary Care. Elk Grove Village, IL, American Academy of Pediatrics, 1996.)

Associated Problems

Significant comorbidity exists between substance abuse and depression, bipolar disorder, ADHD, and antisocial behavior disorders (Bukstein, Brent, and Kaminer, 1989). The use of alcohol and drugs is also associated with truancy, juvenile delinquency, and early sexual experimentation (Jessor and Jessor, 1977, Jessor, 1991). This last association is an important factor in the present epidemic of human immunodeficiency virus (HIV) and acquired immunodeficiency syndrome (AIDS). The Centers for Disease Control and Prevention (CDC) report that as of December 30, 1993, there were 1554 cases of AIDS in the 13- to 19-year-old age group, and AIDS was the sixth leading cause of death among persons 15 to 24 years of age (CDC, 1993a, 1993b). Behavior-related exposures continue to account for the majority of adolescent HIV and AIDS cases. Use of drugs increases the risk of HIV exposure by impairing judgment, increasing the likelihood of participating in sexual behavior, and reducing the likelihood of condom use (Friedman, Stunin, and Hingson, 1993; Hingson et al, 1990).

Stages of Use

According to the new *Diagnostic and Statistical Manual for Primary Care (DSM-PC) Child and Adolescent Version,* substance use occurs on a continuum from the "developmental variation" of experimentation, through "substance use problems," to the disorders of abuse and dependency (Wolraich, 1996). One way of conceptualizing this (Knight, 1997) is described subsequently and illustrated in Figure 50–1.

Abstinence is the stage at which adolescents have not yet begun to use any psychoactive substances.

An initial trial of tobacco, alcohol, or other drugs defines the stage of *experimental use.* It is characterized by using substances that are usually obtained from and used with friends. At this stage, intoxicants produce a mild euphoria with a return to baseline mood and feeling. The teenager thus experiences a good feeling without serious adverse consequences. Experimentation can still be a hazardous activity for teenagers, however. They have insufficient experience to know their own limits or safe "doses" of alcohol and drugs. Urged on by their peers, they may rapidly consume toxic quantities without realizing the potential danger. Or they may put themselves and others at risk by participating in hazardous activities like operation of a motor vehicle. Some individuals may not like the results of their experimentation and go back to abstinence for at least a time.

In other cases, the experience is viewed positively and the behavior is repeated. This latter activity defines the stage of *regular use,* characterized by the intermittent, occasional, continuing use of alcohol or drugs. In adults, this may be referred to as *social use.* This term is misleading if applied to teenage drinking, however, as the typical "social" pattern is *binge drinking* (defined as five or more drinks in a row). In addition to alcohol, regular users tend to use marijuana, inhalants, and stimulants.

Problem use is said to occur when adverse consequences develop as a result of use, even though the individual may not realize or acknowledge that there is any cause-and-effect relationship. School failure, family stress, fights, accidents, and legal problems may appear at this stage. These are often accompanied by significant changes in dress, behavior, and peer group. Health care providers should therefore ask every adolescent patient about school failure, detentions, suspensions, problems with parent or peer relationships, motor vehicle accidents, emergency room visits, and physical or sexual assaults. At the problem use stage, alcohol- or drug-induced euphoria may or may not be followed by return to baseline mood and feeling. There may be associated anxiety, discomfort, and guilt feelings and changes in both quantitative and qualitative aspects of the use of the substance, such as increased amounts, increased frequency, and increase in variety of substances used (beyond tobacco, alcohol, and marijuana). At this stage, some individuals are still able to cut back or eliminate their use with minimal intervention. Others seem to have crossed over an "invisible line" and progressed to the disorders of abuse and dependency. These require more intensive intervention and treatment.

Substance abuse is a disorder characterized by loss of control over use. To paraphrase *DSM-IV,* substance abuse is a maladaptive pattern of substance use that causes impairment in social or school functioning, recurrent physical risk or legal problems, and continued use despite harm occurring over a 12-month period (APA, 1994). Individuals at this stage no longer have a return to baseline mood after using. Alcohol and drug use often become a coping mechanism for dealing with negative feelings. Thus, despite major consequences and losses, there is a *need* for continued use of the substance. Feelings of powerlessness and inadequacy emerge.

Dependency is a disorder characterized by a maladaptive pattern of use, negative consequences, preoccupation with use, and tolerance or withdrawal. *Tolerance* is the need to use more and more to get the usual effect. *Withdrawal* is feeling ill when substance use is stopped. Tolerance and withdrawal symptoms can be physiologic, psychological, or both. Dependency is true addiction, characterized by constant use of substances when available, disrupted family ties, and loss of outside supports. Addicts often become solitary users. They increase risk-taking and self-destructive behaviors. Significant medical and psychiatric problems develop, including hepatic dysfunction, infectious diseases, overdoses, blackouts, depression, and paranoia. Referral to a formal treatment program is required. *Secondary abstinence* becomes the goal of treatment, as control over use is almost impossible to reestablish once it is lost.

All of these stages may or may not be progressive. Although appropriate diagnosis is always important, the disorders of abuse and dependency are relatively easier to recognize and more difficult to treat. Pediatricians should therefore try to identify as early as possible the high prevalence–low severity behaviors of experimentation, regular use, and problem use and intervene before serious harm results (Knight, 1997).

Screening and Assessment

Screening is the process of identifying individuals with a high likelihood of having a problem, while *assessment* is the process of determining the magnitude of the problem and the best type of treatment. Thus, screening is applied to a population at large, while assessment is reserved for individuals who have already screened positive. When it comes to psychoactive substance use, all adolescents should be screened. The American Academy of Pediatrics supports this by saying, "Inquiry regarding the extent of tobacco, alcohol, and other drug use, as well as sexual activities, should be part of the routine history of every teenager presenting for periodic health care" (AAP, 1989). Beyond routine screening, pediatric clinicians should have a high index of suspicion when any adolescent presents with behavioral problems, school failure, or emotional distress. In any case, the most effective method of screening is a good history, taken without parents present in the room. Teenagers will reliably report use of alcohol and drugs if they are assured of confidentiality (Brener et al, 1995; Knight et al, in press). They should be told straight away that "anything you tell me will be kept confidential unless I think there is a risk to your safety, or some else's safety. Should that happen, I promise to let you know, and you and I together will figure out how to tell your parents. I will never pass on information to someone else behind your back." The interview should begin with general questions about health and then progress to psychosocial functioning. The HEADS FIRST mnemonic (Fig. 50–2) summarizes the areas that should be covered in all adolescent interviews (Fuller and Cavanaugh, 1995; Goldenring and Cohen, 1988).

Some clinicians may prefer to use a questionnaire for screening purposes. One that has received considerable attention recently is the Problem Oriented Screening Instrument for Teenagers (POSIT), developed by the National Institute on Drug Abuse. (Rahdert, 1991). This is a 139-item yes/no questionnaire, written at a sixth-grade reading level, that includes 10 scales: alcohol and drug use, physical health, mental health, family relations, peer relations, educational status, vocational status, social skills, leisure/recreation, and aggressive behavior/delinquency. The POSIT has been found to have good reliability among adolescents in a medical office setting (Knight, in press).

When taking a substance use history, a "transitional" strategy in information gathering works best (Adger and Werner, 1996). The clinician should begin with questions about the use of legitimate substances (i.e., prescribed and over-the-counter medications), then progress to asking about those substance that are socially tolerated (tobacco,

H HOME: Separation, support, "space to grow"
E EDUCATION: Expectations, study habits, achievement
A ABUSE: Emotional, verbal, physical, sexual
D DRUGS: Tobacco, alcohol, marijuana, others
S SAFETY: Hazardous activities, seatbelts, helmets

F FRIENDS: Confidant, peer pressure, interaction
I IMAGE: Self-esteem, looks, appearance
R RECREATION: Exercise, relaxation, TV, video games
S SEXUALITY: changes, feelings, experiences, identity
T THREATS: Harm to self or others, running away

Figure 50–2. HEADS FIRST mnemonic. (HEADS mnemonic invented by Goldenring JM, Cohen G: Getting into adolescent heads. Contemp Pediatrics 5:75, 1988; FIRST mnemonic added by Fuller PG, Cavanaugh RM: Basic assessment and screening for substance abuse in the pediatrician's office. Ped Clin North Am 42[2]:295–307, 1995.)

alcohol), and finally to those that are socially disapproved of (marijuana) and to those that are frankly illegal and socially proscribed (cocaine, heroin). With younger adolescents, a second transitional strategy involves moving from a general statement about use, to a question about use among school peers, to a question about friends' use, to a question about personal use. "I know that kids your age are often curious about cigarettes. Has anyone in your school tried smoking? How about any of your friends? Have you thought about it at all? Have you ever tried smoking? The style of the interview should be one of alliance and mutual discovery (the "Lt. Colombo" method) using open-ended questions and concentrating on what have been the *effects* on the teenager of his or her alcohol or drug use. This is contrasted to the potentially alienating interrogative style (the "Sgt. Friday" method), which uses closed-ended questions on amount, frequency, and types of substances used.

There are several alcohol brief screening tools that have been validated in adults, of which the CAGE questions are certainly most popular (Bush et al, 1987; Ewing, 1984). The RAFFT questions were developed specifically for adolescent alcohol and drug use, but no studies on their psychometric properties have yet been published (Riggs and Alario, 1987). In one study of another instrument, the Drug and Alcohol Problem Quickscreen (DAP), four questions were found to have good ability to discriminate between high-risk and low-risk alcohol and drug use (Klitzner et al, 1987; Schwartz and Wirtz, 1990). These questions asked about cigarette smoking, school suspension, suspicion by others, and driving while intoxicated or riding in a car with an intoxicated driver. I suggest melding together items from all of these screening tools. The result, known by the mnemonic CRAFFT, is shown in Figure 50–3.

The last CRAFFT question should be broken into several parts: "Have you gotten into any trouble recently?", and if the answer is yes, "Were you using alcohol or drugs at the time?", and if the answer is yes again, "Do you think there could be a link between your alcohol/drug use and getting into that trouble?" Adolescents may not have yet made this association. Asking these questions in serial fashion elicits more information, and also begins the process of intervention by increasing the adolescent's awareness of problems.

EXAMPLE, PART 1

Brittany is a 15-year-old girl who has just been suspended from school. Because of concern about alcohol and drug use, her principal has insisted she be evaluated by a physician before returning to school. Her parents tell you that Brittany is currently in the ninth grade. Since she moved up to the high school, she has become friendly with a group who her parents say "dress and act like punk rockers." Her grades have fallen, and she seems more moody and distant at home. They also tell you they know she has been drinking alcohol because they smelled it on her breath when she returned from a party 3 weeks ago. They are also worried that her present "crowd" may be using marijuana or other drugs.

You interview Brittany alone and use a transitional strategy to ask about things at home, at school, and her goals and leisure activities. You then take a substance use history. Brittany tells you that she has tried cigarettes but does not smoke regularly. She began drinking alcohol during the summer break, and now likes to "party on weekends" with her friends. She occasionally smokes "herb" after school, but denies trying other drugs. When asked the CRAFFT questions (see Fig. 50–3), Brittany answers "no" to the Alone and Forget questions. She answers "yes" to the Car and Relax questions, and "probably, why else would I be here?" to the question about having a family member who thinks she should cut down.

You then ask, "Have you gotten into any trouble recently?"

"Well, I did get suspended from school."

"How did that happen?" you ask.

"I threw a beer bottle at the side of the school, and it hit the window accidentally."

"So were you drinking at the time this happened?"

"Oh, yeah. We all were," Brittany replies.

"Have you ever considered that if you hadn't been drinking, you might not have gotten suspended?"

Appearing reflective and mildly surprised, Brittany answers, "I never really thought about it that way."

The parent interview is an important part of screening and assessment. Clinicians may gain valuable additional information. The CRAFFT questions can be easily modified for a "third person" history, for example, "Has your son/daughter ever ridden in a car driven by someone (including themselves) who was 'high' or had been using alcohol or drugs?"

A complete physical examination should be performed, including a full set of vital signs. When performing the eye examination, be sure to note pupil size. Nasal mucosa should be examined for inflammation or erosion characteristic of drug insufflation ("snorting"). Liver and spleen should be carefully palpated. A skin examination may reveal needle marks, although this finding is quite rare in adolescents presenting for regular medical care. Abnormal breath sounds (e.g., wheezing) may be found in patients who are smoking tobacco, marijuana, cocaine, or

C Have you ever ridden in a **CAR** driven by someone (including yourself) who was "high" or had been using alcohol or drugs?
R Do you ever use alcohol or drugs to **RELAX,** feel better about yourself, or fit in?
A Do you ever use alcohol or drugs while you are by yourself **ALONE**?
F Do your **FAMILY** or **FRIENDS** ever tell you that you should cut down on your drinking or drug use?
F Do you ever **FORGET** things you did while using alcohol or drugs?
T Have you ever gotten into **TROUBLE** while you were using alcohol or drugs?

Figure 50–3. CRAFFT questions. Two or more "yes" answers indicate a need for further assessment and/or referral to specialty treatment. (Adapted from Knight JR, Shrier LA, Bravender TD, et al: CRAFFT: A new brief screen for adolescent substance abuse. Abstract presented at Ambulatory Pediatric Association meeting, New Orleans, 1998.)

heroin. Urine and serum toxicologic examination are of limited usefulness and are generally less sensitive than a good history. Except in cases of a true emergency, they should not be performed without the knowledge and consent of the patient (AAP, 1996). Pediatric clinicians should avoid performing drug screens at the request of parents or legal authorities. They may order drug tests as an adjunct to outpatient treatment, when the results will be available only to the patient and treatment team. Results must always be interpreted with caution, and clinicians must be familiar with sensitivity and specificity (threshold values) for specific drugs and methods of testing. Urine specific gravity should always be obtained, as urine concentration directly affects the sensitivity of the screening test. All positive results should be confirmed by gas chromatography and mass spectrometry. In general, serum half-lives of drugs of abuse are brief, and urine testing reflects drug use only within the last 24 hours. The exception to this rule is marijuana, because its active ingredient, tetrahydrocannabinol (THC), may be detected in the urine for several weeks after discontinuation of use (Woolf and Shannon, 1995). Therefore, when drug testing for THC is being done as part of a treatment program, serial urine specimens must be sent out for *quantitative* THC and creatinine (as a measure of urine concentration or dilution). Abstinence is supported by a finding of serial decreases in the ratio of THC to creatinine.

Adolescent patients may present with symptoms of acute or pathologic intoxication. Table 50–1 lists the signs and symptoms of intoxication and withdrawal and the treatment options for common drugs of abuse.

Following the screening process, pediatric clinicians must make an initial assessment of problem severity and the need for treatment (Fig. 50–4).

Individuals who are experimental users or regular users do not necessarily need to be referred to mental health specialists. They are amenable to brief office interventions as described in the next section. On the other hand, teenagers who seem likely to have a disorder (abuse or dependency) should be referred to specialized treatment right away. Clinicians should also refer those who have signs or symptoms of a comorbid mental disorder such as major depression, bipolar disorder, bulimia, or ADHD. In all instances, the most important assessment has to do with the immediate safety of the patient. If it is at all in jeopardy, admission to a hospital should be arranged.

Brief Office Intervention

Brief interventions should involve less time than is usually associated with formal treatment programs, be delivered by nonspecialists, emphasize self-help and self-management, reach large numbers of patients, and be considerably less expensive than conventional treatment (Heather, 1989). To be effective, an intervention statement must be appropriate to the stage of use the young person is at. For "abstinence," practitioners should offer positive reinforcement by, for example, making a statement such as, "I think it's great that you have decided to stay away from trying cigarettes, alcohol, or other drugs. That's a very intelligent and courageous choice. I'm really proud of you! I also want you to know that I understand how tempting it can be for teens to try them, and so I still plan to ask you about this again on your next visit. If things ever change, I hope you'll trust me enough to talk about it. My only concern is for your health." For the stages of "experimentation" and "regular use," the intervention should be aimed at reducing risk. For example, most teenagers drink in cars or at parties (and then get into cars). Therefore, an effective intervention strategy is the development of a "rescue plan" (Knight, 1997). The health care provider assists in the development of a contract with the parents or another adult that promises a ride home, no questions asked, any time the adolescent calls and asks for one. When this is not feasible, an alternative plan might involve having the teenager carry emergency taxi or public transit fare. Adolescents who have progressed to the stages of problem use, abuse, or dependency require office interventions that move them toward total abstinence from alcohol and drug use or formal treatment programs. For most individuals, this kind of significant behavior change will be a process rather than an event. A useful model for understanding behavior change is illustrated in Figure 50–5 (Prochaska, 1994; Prochaska and Diclemene, 1982, 1983; Prochaska et al, 1994).

Precontemplation is a precursor to the process of change. The individual at this stage has not yet begun to consider change as an option. His or her problems are attributed to misfortune, misunderstanding, or other external forces. Defensive thinking is prominent and may be manifested as denial, minimization, projection, rationalization, justification, or blaming of others. *Contemplation,* on the other hand, is heralded by consideration on the part of the individual that he or she may indeed have a problem. The pros and cons of changing behavior are being weighed. Individuals at this stage are ambivalent about changing problem behaviors. *Determination* is characterized by making a clear decision to change. At this stage, the mind has changed but the behavior has not. A quit date may be set, or a plan made to get help (e.g., enter a treatment program).

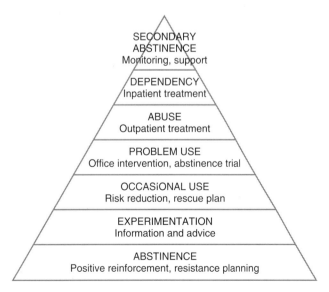

Figure 50–4. The Substance Use Intervention pyramid.

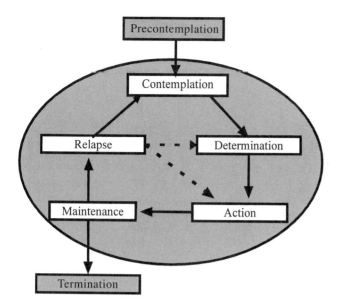

Figure 50–5. Stages of change. (Data from Prochaska JO: Strong and weak principles for progressing from precontemplation to action on the basis of 12 problem behaviors. Health Psych 13:47, 1994; Prochaska JO, DiClemente CC: Stages and processes of self-change of smoking: toward an integrative model of change. J Consult Psych 51:390, 1983; Prochaska JO, DiClemente CC: Transtheoretical therapy: toward a more integrative model of change. Psychotherapy 19:276, 1982; and Prochaska JO, Velicer WF, Rossi JS, Goldstein MG, Marcus BH, Rakowski W, Fiore C, Harlow LL, Redding CA, Rosenblum D, Rossi SR: Stages of change and decisional balance for 12 problem behaviors. Health Psych 13:39, 1994.)

Action is defined by evidence of actual change in behavior. It takes a while, however, for the individual to feel comfortable with the new behavior. He or she may struggle with urges to resume the use of alcohol or drugs. When the new behavior becomes learned enough to be automatic, the individual is said to be in *maintenance*. Maintenance may lead to either a permanent exit (*termination*) from the change cycle, or *relapse* and entry into another cycle. Practitioners must remember that relapse is part of the early recovery process, and patients should not be stigmatized or abandoned when one occurs. The relapse should be viewed as a learning experience. Supports and treatments should be reviewed and increased.

According to this theory, the goal of any single patient encounter is to facilitate movement of the patient from any one stage of change to the next. (Miller and Rollnick, 1991; Rollnick, Heather, and Bell, 1992). For individuals at the precontemplation stage, the clinician should try to raise doubt and increase the awareness of risks and problems. This may be done by skillful questioning ("Have you ever considered that you might not have gotten suspended from school if you hadn't been smoking pot?") or by simple delivery of information ("Are you aware that car accidents, particularly those caused by drinking, are the number one cause of death for young people your age?"). For those in contemplation, the clinician should acknowledge their ambivalence ("So it sounds like part of you wants to stop and part of you wants to keep on drinking . . ."), try to evoke reasons to change, and then tip the balance in favor of change. Once determination is reached, the goal of the intervention is to help the

adolescent find the best course of action. This is done by listing treatment options, making an appropriate referral, and following up. During maintenance, the clinician should offer positive reinforcement and discuss relapse prevention strategies. The content of an effective brief intervention statement is summarized in the FRAMES mnemonic, illustrated in Figure 50–6 (Miller and Sanchez, 1994).

The clinician should begin with feedback concerning problem or risk behavior by listing the facts, stated in the patient's own words. Facts are less likely to lead to arguments than are interpretations or diagnoses. After listing the pertinent facts, emphasize that the patient is the one who is responsible for changing his or her behavior. Advice should be clear, with an emphasis on stopping completely. In those cases in which the teenager is unwilling to stop, a further menu of options, including cutting down and risk reduction, should be offered. Further choices involve options for formal treatment, including referral to counseling, 12-step support groups, or more intensive treatment programs. The clinician must project an attitude of empathy and faith in the patient's ability to make the necessary change (self-efficacy). During the course of the intervention, clinicians should avoid attempts to pressure the patient, as this may only lead to increased resistance to change. It is better to try to elicit self-motivational statements from the adolescent ("How might you imagine your life could improve if you gave up using drugs?"), and then summarize and support those statements that favor change. Most importantly, the clinician must establish and maintain a supportive relationship with the adolescent (Schonberg, 1988). The relationship needs to be firm, consistent, and nonrejecting. A written behavior change contract is a useful adjunct to office intervention (NIAAA, 1994). One example is the "Change Plan Worksheet" illustrated in Figure 50–7. In the example shown, the young person has contracted to stop using alcohol and drugs and to enter a formal treatment program if she is unable to follow through on her plan.

EXAMPLE, PART 2

Following the history, you assess that Brittany is most likely in the problem use category, and you make an interventional statement using the FRAMES format:

"I want to thank you, Brittany, for being honest with me today. I have to tell you, though, that I've heard a few things that have me concerned. You told me that you have accepted a ride home from a driver who had been drinking. I know from national statistics that many

Text continued on page 488

F	**FEEDBACK** on personal risk or impairment
R	Emphasis on personal **RESPONSIBILITY** for change
A	Clear **ADVICE** to change
M	A **MENU** of alternative change options
E	Therapist **EMPATHY**
S	Facilitation of client **SELF-EFFICACY** or optimism

Figure 50–6. The FRAMES mnemonic. (Data from Miller WR, Rollnick S: Motivational Interviewing. Guilford Press, New York, 1991; and Miller WR, Sanchez VC: Motivating young adults for treatment and lifestyle change. *In* Howard G, Nathan P [eds]: Issues in Alcohol Use and Misuse by Young Adults. Notre Dame, IN, University of Notre Dame Press, 1994, pp 51–81.)

Table 50–1 • Medical Management of Drug Intoxication and Withdrawal

Names/Preparations	Intoxication		Withdrawal	
	Signs and Symptoms	Treatment	Signs and Symptoms	Treatment
A. Alcohol				
Beer Wine Hard liquor	*Mild-moderate:* ↓ level of consciousness, poor coordination, ataxia, nystagmus, conjunctival injection, slurred speech, stupor, gastrointestinal bleed, orthostatic hypotension	Observation and supportive care, protect airway, position on side to avoid aspiration	*Mild-moderate:* restlessness, agitation, coarse tremor, ↑ sensitivity to sensory input, nausea, vomiting, anorexia, autonomic hyperactivity (tachycardia, hypertension, hyperthermia), anxiety/depression, headache, insomnia	Thiamine 100 mg IM, benzodiazepine taper (chlordiazepoxide 25–50 mg q6h × 24 hrs, then 25 mg q6h × 48 hrs; or diazepam, clonazepam, oxazepam), multivitamins
	Severe: Respiratory depression, coma, death. (*Chronic:* pancreatitis, cirrhosis, are rare in adolescents)	Ventilatory support, intensive care	*Severe:* seizures, hallucinations, delirium, death	Seizures: benzodiazepines (diazepam 0.2–0.5 mg/kg/dose IV, maximum dose = 10 mg, or 0.5 mg/kg/dose PR) Hallucinations: haloperidol
	Pathologic: belligerent, excited, combative, psychotic state (even after small amount in susceptible person)	Physical restraint, low-dose benzodiazepine (lorazepam 1–5 mg PO as needed), or haloperidol 1–5 mg q4–8 hrs IM or 1–15 mg/dose PO		

Miscellaneous information: Alcohol is highly addictive, and withdrawal from it is associated with serious, potentially lethal side effects that begin 6–24 hours after the last drink. Alcohol dependency is rare in adolescents, however, but alcohol-related deaths are not. Adolescents tend to be binge drinkers and are at high risk for alcohol-related accidents and acute alcohol poisoning.

Names/Preparations	Signs and Symptoms	Treatment	Signs and Symptoms	Treatment
B. Cannabis				
Marijuana *Pot, herb, grass, weed, reefer, dope, buds, sinsemilla, Thai sticks* THC capsules Hashish Hashish oil	*Acute:* Euphoria, sensory stimulation, pupillary constriction, conjunctival injection, photophobia, nystagmus, diplopia, ↑ appetite, autonomic dysfunction (tachycardia, hypertension, orthostatic hypotension), temporary bronchodilatation	Reassurance and observation	*Chronic users:* mild irritability, agitation, insomnia, electroencephalographic changes	Reassurance; symptoms disappear in 3–4 days
	Chronic: gynecomastia, reactive airway disease, ↓ sperm count, weight gain, lethargy, amotivational syndrome	Discontinuation of use, symptomatic treatment/care (bronchodilators for wheezing) Psychosis: neuroleptic medication		
	Pathologic: panic, delirium, psychosis, flashbacks			

Miscellaneous information: Cannabis derivatives have relatively low addictive potential. These drugs are commonly used by adolescents, however, and are associated with adverse psychologic effects. The potency of marijuana has tripled over the past 25 years.

C. Hallucinogens

Drug	Effects	Treatment	Dependence
Phencyclidine (PCP) *Angel dust, super grass, peace weed* Lysergic acid diethylamide (LSD) *Acid, blotters, orange sunshine, blue heaven, microdot, sugar cubes* Mescaline *Mesc* Peyote *Buttons, cactus* Psilocybin *Magic mushrooms, shrooms* Jimson weed *Locoweed* Nightshade	*Acute:* Perceptual (visual, auditory) distortion and hallucinations, nystagmus, feelings of depersonalization, mild nausea, tremors, tachycardia, hypertension, hyperreflexia *Chronic:* flashbacks *Pathologic:* panic, paranoia, psychosis	Reassurance and observation (for anticholinergics, e.g., Jimson weed, nightshade, symptoms are more severe and may require gastric lavage, benzodiazepine sedation and hospitalization) Discontinuation of use Psychosis: close observation in a quiet room, benzodiazepines (lorazepam 1–5 mg PO); use of neuroleptic medication is controversial	Psychologic	Reassurance

Miscellaneous information: PCP may be sprinkled on marijuana and smoked. Exposure can thus occur without the user's knowledge.

D. Inhalants

Drug	Effects	Treatment	Dependence
Nitrous oxide *Laughing gas, whippets* Amyl nitrite *Poppers, snappers* Butyl nitrate *Rush, bullet, climax* Chlorohydrocarbons *Aerosol spray cans* Hydrocarbons *Gasoline, glue, solvents, typewriter correction fluid*	*Acute:* euphoria, disorientation, sedation, conjunctival injection, acute toxicity to CNS, liver, kidneys Nitrates: sudden hypoxemia, hypotension *Chronic:* peripheral nerve, CNS, liver, and kidney damage Leaded gasoline (not in US): plumbism *Pathologic:* cardiac arrhythmia and arrest	Symptomatic medical treatments Discontinuation of use, supportive therapies (dialysis, etc) Plumbism: chelation therapy Resuscitation, hospitalization	Psychologic Physiologic—unknown	Reassurance, support

Miscellaneous information: Nitrous oxide is sometimes sold at rock concerts inside balloons. Nitrate compounds have been most popular among gay men, alledgedly to enhance sexual experiences. The volatile hydrocarbon compounds are favored by younger adolescents and popular in some Latin-American countries, on Native American reservations, and in Latino communities within the United States.

Table continued on following page

Table 50–1 • Medical Management of Drug Intoxication and Withdrawal (*Continued*)

Names/Preparations	Intoxication		Withdrawal	
	Signs and Symptoms	*Treatment*	*Signs and Symptoms*	*Treatment*
E. Stimulants				
Cocaine *Coke, snow, flake, blow, nose candy* Crack *Freebase, rocks* Amphetamines *Speed, black beauties* Methamphetamine *Crank, crystal meth, ice* Methylphenidate Ritalin Pemoline Cylert Rx Diet Pills Didrex, Tenuate, Ionamin, Sanorex, etc. "Legal speed" *OTC diet or stay-awake pills*	*Acute:* exhilaration, euphoria, restlessness, irritability, insomnia, pupillary dilatation, tachycardia, arrhythmia, chest pain, hypertension, anorexia, hyperpyrexia, hyperreflexia *Chronic:* (if snorting: inflamed nasal mucosa, septal erosion or perforation) confusion, sensory hallucinations, paranoia, depression *Pathologic:* sudden cardiac arrest, hypertensive crisis, seizures	Reassurance and observation Symptomatic care Agitation: high-dose benzodiazepines (diazepam 10–25 mg) Tachycardia hypertension: (controversial, see below) Hyperthermia: external cooling Discontinuation of use, symptomatic treatment/care Psychosis: neuroleptic medication Resuscitation, hospitalization Hypertensive crisis: beta-blockers, phentolamine, nitroprusside Seizures: IV diazepam (see alcohol section above), or phenytoin 15–20 mg/kg slow IV push with cardiac monitor	*Chronic users:* severe depression with suicidal/homicidal ideation, exhaustion, prolonged sleep, voracious appetite	Close observation, reassurance; symptoms disappear in 3–4 days

Miscellaneous information: While use of cocaine and crack has declined somewhat in recent years, amphetamines have become more popular. Methamphetamine is more commonly available in California, the West, and the Southwest. With the increased public awareness of ADHD and the popularity of stimulant medications to treat it, Ritalin has now become a drug of abuse among some adolescents. It can be ground up and "snorted," and has been implicated in several reports of sudden cardiac arrest and death. So-called "legal speed," OTC preparations that are available in pharmacies and through mail order houses, can cause toxicity similar to more potent stimulants when taken in high doses.

Names/Preparations	Intoxication		Withdrawal	
	Signs and Symptoms	*Treatment*	*Signs and Symptoms*	*Treatment*
F. Depressants				
Benzodiapines Valium, *V's*, Librium, Serax, Klonopin, Tranxene, Xanax, Halcion, Rohypnol, *ruffies* Barbiturates Nembutal, Seconal, Amytal, Tuinal, *downers, barbs, blue devils, red devils, yellows, yellow jackets* Methaqualone Quaaludes, *ludes, sopors*	*Mild-moderate:* CNS sedation, pupillary constriction, disorientation, slurred speech, staggering gait *Severe:* Respiratory depression, hypothermia, coma, death *Pathologic:* paradoxical disinhibition, hyperexcitability	Observation and supportive care, protect airway, position on side to avoid aspiration Acute overdose: Gastric lavage Supportive: ventilator, warming blanket, ICU care Symptoms pass in a matter of hours; physical restraint, low-dose benzodiazepine rarely needed	*Mild-moderate:* restlessness, anxiety, agitation, tremor, abdominal cramps, nausea, vomiting hyperreflexia, hypertension, headache, insomnia *Severe:* seizures, delirium, hyperpyrexia, hallucinations, death	Gradual reduction of the drug of dependency, or phenobarbital substitution (calculate phenobarbital equivalent of daily dose, or give 3–4 mg/kg/day ÷ q8h) with gradual taper, or change short-acting benzodiazepine to longer-acting benzodiazepine and then taper Seizures: diazepam Hallucinations: haloperidol (see alcohol section above for doses)

Miscellaneous information: These compounds are all similar to alcohol in effect and highly addictive. Withdrawal symptoms are severe and may begin 12–16 hours after last dose, or may be delayed for up to a week.

G. Narcotics

Drug	Clinical effects	Treatment	Detoxification
Heroin *Smack, horse, junk, brown sugar, big H, mud* Opium	*Acute:* Euphoria, pupillary constriction, depression of respirations and gag reflex, bradycardia, hypotension, constipation	Airway protection, judicious use of naloxone	*Acute detoxification:* Methadone (PO) Children: 0.7 mg/kg/day ÷ q4–6 hrs, or adult 30–40 mg/day in 3–4 divided doses, with 5 mg/day taper Clonidine (PO) Children: 5–7 µg/kg/day ÷ q6–12 hrs (max = 0.9 mg/day) Adult: 0.1 mg test dose, check postural blood pressure; if stable, 0.1–0.2 mg PO q4–6 hrs *Long-term treatment:* Long-term therapeutic support; methadone or LAAM maintenance (specialized clinics only)
Rx narcotics Morphine, meperidine, fentanyl, oxycodone, hydrocodone, codeine, Darvon, etc.	*Chronic:* complications of IV use include hepatitis B, HIV/AIDS, SBE, brain abscesses *Pathologic:* acute overdose may cause respiratory arrest and death	Discontinuation of use, targeted medical care for infectious complications Intubation and ventilation, naloxone (IV, IM, SC, ETT): children <20 kg: 0.1 mg/kg; dose q2–3 hrs; children >20 kg: 2–5 mg/dose	*Chronic users:* restlessness, lacrimation, yawning, pupillary dilatation, rhinorrhea, sniffing, sneezing, sweating, flushing, tachycardia, hypertension, muscle cramps, abdominal cramps, nausea, vomiting, diarrhea

Miscellaneous information: Individuals who abuse narcotics seldom seek treatment for intoxication. They are more often found semi-comatose and brought to the hospital by friends or the EMS for treatment. When treating an overdose, remember that naloxone has a shorter duration of action than most narcotic drugs, and doses therefore need to be repeated at fairly frequent intervals. These patients require lengthy (12–24 hr) periods of observation in hospital.

H. Designer Drugs

Drug	Clinical effects	Treatment
Fentanyl analogues Synthetic heroin, *China White*	Similar to narcotics (above)	Similar to narcotics (above)
Meperidine analogues *MPPP, MPTP*	Similar to narcotics (above)	Similar to narcotics (above)
Amphetamine analogues *MDMA, Ecstasy, Adam, EVE, STP, PMA, TMA, DOM, DOB,* etc.	Similar to amphetamines (above)	Similar to amphetamines (above)
PCP analogues *PCPy; PCE*	Similar to PCP (above)	Similar to PCP (above)

Miscellaneous information: More popular on the West Coast, designer drugs can be both stronger and cheaper than the parent compound. Quality is not controlled during illicit manufacturing, posing great danger to users. For example: MPTP, a contaminant of the meperidine analogue MPPP, causes irreversible Parkinson disease.

AIDS = acquired immunodeficiency syndrome; CNS = central nervous system; EMS = emergency medical response system; ETT = via endotracheal tube; HIV = human immunodeficiency virus; ICU = intensive care unit; IM = intramuscularly; IV = intravenously; LAAM = levo-alpha acetyl methadol; OTC = over-the-counter; PO = orally; PR = rectally; q = every; Rx = prescription; SBE = subacute bacterial endocarditis; SC = subcutaneously; THC = tetrahydrocannabinol; ↓ = decreased; ↑ = increased.

Acknowledgment: Michael Shannon, MD, MPH (Toxicology Program), and Brigid Vaughan, MD (Department of Psychiatry), at Children's Hospital, Boston assisted with the preparation of this table.

Data from Barone MA (ed): The Harriet Lane Handbook. 14th ed. St. Louis, Mosby, 1996; Chang G, Kosten TR: Emergency management of acute drug intoxication. *In* Lowinson JH, Ruiz P, Millman RB (eds): Substance Abuse: A Comprehensive Textbook. Baltimore, Williams & Wilkins, 1992; Schonberg SK (ed): Guidelines for the Treatment of Alcohol- and Other Drug-Abusing Adolescents. Treatment Improvement Protocol (TIP) Series 4. CSAT, USDHHS 93-2010, Washington DC, US Government Printing Office, 1993. Wesson D (ed): Detoxification for Alcohol and Other Drugs. Treatment Improvement Protocol (TIP) Series 19. CSAT, USDHHS 93-2010, Washington, DC, US Government Printing Office, 1995.

1.   **The change(s) I want to make are:**

     Stop drinking alcohol

     No smoking herb

2.   **The most important reasons for changing are:**

     I don't want to drink right now

     Smoking is unhealthy

     To get my parents off my back

     I get in trouble when I drink

3.   **The steps I plan to take in changing are:**

     To not put myself in bad situations where others
     are using herb or drinking

     To go to one AA meeting and check it out

4.   **The ways other people can help me are:**
     Person   Possible ways to help

     Parents   pick me up anytime I call

     David   stop drinking at least around me

     Dr. Jones check in with me in 3 weeks

5.   **I will know that my plan is working if:**

     I do not use alcohol or drugs

     I stay out of trouble

6.   **Some things that could interfere with my plan are:**

     Hanging out with my friends who use

     Fights with my parents

7.   **If my plan doesn't work, I will:**

     Go to AA 3 times a week

     Go to family counseling

     Brittany Smith   *11/21/97*
     Signature   **Date**

Figure 50–7. Change plan worksheet.

young people have died as a result of this. You also told me that using alcohol and drugs helps you to relax, and that your parents have become worried about you. And then you told me about being suspended from school, and that this could be related to your drinking. All of these things together could indicate that alcohol and drugs are becoming a problem for you. I wonder if you would be willing to stop for a while. I'd like to see if you are able to do this. If you are, we will at least know that you haven't lost control completely. If you can't stop, we should see about getting you some additional help. I also want to suggest that you try going to a meeting of Alcoholics Anonymous just to hear some of the stories. You might learn something about how alcohol problems de-

velop in people. In any case, I want to work with you on this and would like to see you again in a few weeks. What do you think? Will you give this a try?"

Brittany agrees to a trial of abstinence. You ask her to fill out a Change Plan Worksheet (see Fig. 50–7), review it with her before she leaves, and arrange for a follow-up appointment.

Treatment

Pediatric clinicians should be familiar with treatment resources in their own communities. Programs vary in both intensity and philosophy, but complete abstinence from alcohol and drugs is the primary goal. In general, treatment programs fall into one of the following categories: detoxification, methadone maintenance, inpatient treatment, therapeutic communities, and outpatient treatment (Dusenbury, Khuri, and Millman, 1992). Detoxification programs are relatively short-term inpatient programs whose goal is medical management of physiologic withdrawal symptoms, although outpatient detoxification is now more widely available. Traditionally, these programs have concentrated on alcohol dependency, as withdrawal symptoms can be life-threatening. Detoxification is also appropriate for individuals who are addicted to sedatives, barbiturates, heroin, and other opioids. Most teenagers do not require detoxification, as physiologic dependence is relatively uncommon in this age group. In those cases in which it is necessary, detoxification should be viewed as a first step in treatment and always followed by long-term counseling and support. Methadone maintenance originated, and continues to be, the treatment of choice for narcotics (e.g., heroin) addiction. Methadone is a synthetic opioid drug that does not induce euphoria in therapeutic doses and blocks the euphoric effect of other narcotics. Methadone treatment is usually combined with outpatient counseling, group therapy, educational and vocational assistance, and psychosocial support. Inpatient programs, usually hospital based, saw a rapid rise in popularity during the 1970s and 1980s. They were intensive, highly structured, month-long programs run by medical providers, counselors, psychologists, and family therapists. In recent years, many of these programs have closed as managed care entities have become reluctant to fund this relatively expensive form of treatment. There are few remaining inpatient programs for adolescents. Therapeutic communities originated largely for treatment of heroin addiction but have expanded to include alcohol, marijuana, and polydrug abuse. These programs tend to be long-term (6–12 months), highly structured, founded on self-help or 12-step principles, and often staffed by recovering addicts. A present-day example of this type of treatment is Phoenix House, including programs in New York, California, and Texas. There are other residential programs designed to remove the adolescent substance abuser from his or her environment (e.g., wilderness programs). All of these residential treatment programs are best reserved for those teenagers who have failed outpatient treatment or who have a high degree of antisocial behavior associated with their substance use. Outpatient treatment is a useful first option. The vast majority of adolescents who receive substance abuse treatment receive it in an outpatient

setting. Treatment settings can vary from structured hospital-based day treatment, to varying combinations of individual counseling, family therapy, group therapy, cognitive-behavioral therapy, hypnosis, biofeedback, acupuncture, random drug testing, and self-help groups. Whatever the level of intensity, teenagers should be referred to programs that specialize in people their own age. Group therapy is a component of virtually all treatment programs, and adolescents do not relate well to groups of older adults. For those adolescents at the problem use–abuse end of the spectrum, simple outpatient counseling by a mental health professional specially trained in adolescent substance use may be sufficient. Referral to 12-step support groups, like Alcoholics Anonymous or Narcotics Anonymous, may also be useful. Clinicians should obtain a "meeting list" from one or both of these fellowships and become familiar with its use. Contact can be made with recovering volunteers from these organizations by calling the number listed in the telephone directory. These volunteers are usually happy to recommend specific meetings in the local area that are appropriate for young people and may often volunteer to bring the patient to a meeting and introduce him or her to the group. Twelve-step groups are developmentally challenging for adolescents and will often not work without an interested recovering person who acts as an initial liaison or "temporary sponsor." The clinician must continue to support adolescents who are in treatment. Follow-up visits should be scheduled at regular intervals. The clinician should find out what the components of treatment are, or what goes on in 12-step groups, then check with the adolescent at each visit to see how things are going and offer encouragement and support. (*"So tell me, have you joined an AA group? Have you found a sponsor yet? Which of the 12 steps are you working on now?"*) A clinician should never hesitate to tell recovering adolescents how proud he is of them. The process of recovery is a difficult one for all individuals and poses special challenges (e.g., changing friends, accepting that they have a "chronic" disease) during the teenage years.

Family members should be encouraged to participate in treatment with their child. They may need to receive counseling themselves and may also benefit from self-help groups like Alanon. While parents should not become overly restrictive, they must be encouraged to adopt a firm yet reasonable stance. In the most severe cases, they may need the support of the clinician in taking a very difficult position, such as informing a teenager who continues to use that he or she must either go into treatment or find another place to live. Occasionally, clinicians will encounter parents who are either unwilling or unable to assist in treatment. For example, they may refuse to eliminate alcohol or other drugs from the house, often because they have a substance use problem of their own.

Substance-Abusing Parents

Current estimates are that there are 11 million children and adolescents in the United States who have an alcoholic parent, or one out of every eight children (Macdonald and Blume, 1986). Clinicians should be aware that the problem is not uncommon and should routinely ask about parental use of alcohol and drugs during office visits. Particular

C   Have you ever felt that you should **CUT DOWN** on your drinking?
A   Have people **ANNOYED** you by criticizing your drinking?
G   Have you ever felt bad or **GUILTY** about your drinking?
E   Have you ever had a drink first thing in the morning to steady your nerves or get rid of a hangover (**EYE-OPENER**)?

Figure 50–8. The CAGE questions. (Data from Bush B, Shaw S, Cleary P, DelBlanco TL, Aronson MD: Screening for alcohol abuse using the CAGE questionnaire. Am J Med 82:231, 1987; and Ewing JA: Detecting alcoholism: the CAGE questionnaire. JAMA 252(14):1905, 1984. The CAGE mnemonic was invented by JA Ewing.)

vigilance is called for when seeing children in the medical clinic with chronic vague complaints, or when they present to school function clinics or mental health programs. In recent years, there has been a growing awareness of the problem, and there is now a body of scientific research on the special problems and challenges of these children. Children of alcoholics have long been known to be at risk for serious medical problems such as fetal alcohol syndrome and fetal alcohol effect (Jones et al, 1973). More recent research indicates that having an alcoholic parent is associated with higher health care costs and a host of medical problems, including sleep disturbance, gastrointestinal problems, musculoskeletal complaints, vascular and migraine headaches, chronic fatigue, and decreased appetite (Emshoff and Price, 1997). Having an alcoholic parent also places children at higher risk for becoming substance abusers themselves (Smart and Fejer, 1972). It is also associated with mental health problems such as ADHD, anxiety disorder, depression, and conduct disorder (Earls et al, 1988). School problems are also common among children of alcoholics. They are more likely to have language-based learning difficulties, poor attention, behavioral problems, suspensions, truancy, absenteeism, and grade retention; and yet they are less likely to receive special educational services than other children with special needs (Emshoff and Price, 1997). Within the family, parental abuse of alcohol is associated with increased family violence, separation and divorce, parental absence, poverty, and child abuse and neglect (Johnson and Leff, 1997). In addition, children of drug-addicted parents are susceptible to special problems, which include passive exposure to smoked drugs and the more severe problem of congenital HIV or AIDS. Children of drug abusers also are exposed to more chaos within the home, often due to illegal activity surrounding the acquisition, sale, and use of illicit substances. Despite all these risks, studies have been inconsistent in identifying personality characteristics of children from substance abusing families (Johnson and Leff, 1997). They are not a homogeneous group and do not have a defined profile of psychopathology. Clinicians should avoid labeling them and should always consider relative strengths and weaknesses within the child and the home.

The CAGE questions, shown in Figure 50–8, are a useful screening tool. A "yes" answer to two or more questions is highly predictive of a diagnosis of alcohol abuse or dependency (Bush et al, 1987).

When a parent has a positive CAGE, the pediatric clinician should explain the result, share his or her concern, and suggest that the parent go for a formal substance abuse evaluation. In those instances in which a child is at significant risk, clinicians must do more than suggest an evaluation; they must insist on it. Figure 50–9 lists the essential components of a formal intervention with parents. Following such an intervention, clinicians must not avoid future contact with the parent, remembering instead that parents so affected are sick people rather than bad people. When at all possible, this view should be communicated to the child. The child should also be told that the parent's disease is not the fault of the child, and its "cure" is not the child's responsibility. Individual and family counseling is needed, and a referral to child-centered support groups (e.g., Alateen, Alatot) may be helpful.

Conclusion

Substance use and abuse is a leading cause of morbidity and mortality for adolescents in the United States. Pediatric clinicians should routinely screen all teenagers and view the use of alcohol and drugs on a spectrum from the high-prevalence–low-severity phenomenon of experimentation, through the low-prevalence–high-severity disorders of abuse and dependency. On the low-severity side of the continuum, brief office interventions are most appropriate. Once a teenager has progressed to abuse or dependency, however, referral to specialty treatment is needed. Clinicians should be familiar with treatment resources in the local community and provide follow-up during the process of recovery. More research is needed on what constitutes effective treatment. All health care providers should also be aware that children may be affected by substance use and abuse on the part of their parents. Questions about parental use of alcohol and drugs should be part of a

F   Give parents a listing of the **FACTS** that have led to your concern.
R   Explain that you are legally **REQUIRED TO REPORT**.
A   Have **ANOTHER PERSON** present. There is strength in numbers, and this will help avoid later confusion about exactly what was said or recommended.
M   The intervention should be a series of **MONOLOGUES**, not a discussion or debate. If interrupted, ask the parent to please let you finish; you will then be happy to listen to him or her without interrupting.
E   Referring the parent(s) for formal **EVALUATION** is the goal of the intervention. Avoid giving a diagnosis of substance use/abuse, as this will lead to arguments.
R   If the individual is acutely intoxicated, arrange for a **RIDE**. Do not allow him or her to drive. Insist that you receive a **REPORT BACK** from the evaluation. This will let you know it has been done, and help you better care for the child.

Figure 50–9. Principles of effective intervention with parents. The FRAMER mnemonic. (Data from Knight JR, Vandeven A: Substance Abusing Parents: A Guide to Brief Interventions in Pediatric Practice. Workshop presented at Ambulatory Pediatric Association Meeting, Washington, DC, 1997.)

standard family screening. When problems are identified, clinicians should refer parents to adult mental health professionals for formal evaluation and treatment and insist on being a part of continuing family health care.

REFERENCES

Adger H, Werner MJ: The pediatrician. *In* Identification and Treatment of Substance Abuse in Primary Care Settings supplement. Am J Addictions 5(4):s20, 1996.

American Academy of Pediatrics (AAP) Committee on Adolescence, Committee on Bioethics, and Provisional Committee on Substance Abuse: Screening for drugs of abuse in children and adolescents. Pediatrics 84(2):396, 1989.

American Academy of Pediatrics (AAP) Committee on Substance Abuse: Testing for drugs of abuse in children and adolescents. Pediatrics 98(2):305, 1996.

American Psychiatric Association (APA): Diagnostic and Statistical Manual of Mental Disorders, 4th ed. Washington, DC, American Psychiatric Association, 1994.

Bandura A: Social Learning Theory. Englewood Cliffs, NJ, Prentice Hall, 1977.

Barone MA (ed): The Harriet Lane Handbook, 14th ed. St. Louis, Mosby, 1996.

Brener ND, Collins JL, Kann L, et al: Reliability of the youth risk behavior survey questionnaire. Am J Epidemiol 141(6):575, 1995.

Bukstein OG, Brent DA, Kaminer Y: Comorbidity of substance abuse and other psychiatric disorders in adolescents. Am J Psychiatry 146(9):1131, 1989.

Bush B, Shaw S, Cleary P, et al: Screening for alcohol abuse using the CAGE questionnaire. Am J Med 82:231, 1987.

Centers for Disease Control and Prevention (CDC): Alcohol and other drug use among high school students: United States, 1990. MMWR 40:776, 1991.

Centers for Disease Control and Prevention (CDC): HIV/AIDS Surveillance Report. Year-end Edition 5:5, 1993a.

Centers for Disease Control and Prevention (CDC): Mortality trends and leading causes of death among adolescents and young adults: United States, 1979–1988. Morbid Mortal Wkly Rep 42:459, 1993b.

Chang G, Kosten TR: Emergency management of acute drug intoxication. *In* Lowinson JH, Ruiz P, Millman RB (eds): Substance Abuse: A Comprehensive Textbook. Baltimore, Williams & Wilkins, 1992.

Dusenbury L, Khuri E, Millman RB: Adolescent substance abuse: a sociodevelopmental perspective. *In* Lowinson JH, Ruiz P, Millman RB (eds): Substance Abuse: A Comprehensive Textbook. Baltimore, Williams & Wilkins, 1992.

Earls F, Reich W, Jung KG, Cloninger CR: Psychopathology in children of alcoholic and antisocial parents. Alcoholism Clin Exper Res 12(4):481, 1988.

Elkind D: Cognitive development. *In* Friedman SB, Fisher M, Schonberg SK (eds): Comprehensive Adolescent Health Care. St. Louis, Quality Medical Publishing, 1992.

Emshoff JG, Price AW: Prevention and Intervention Options for Children of Alcoholics. Monograph presented at meeting on Core Competencies for Involvement of Health Care Professionals in the Care of Children and Adolescents in Families Affected by Substance Abuse, Office of National Drug Control Policy, Washington DC, 1997.

Epps RP, Manley MW, Glynn TJ: Tobacco use among adolescents. Ped Clin North Am 42(2):389, 1995.

Ewing JA: Detecting alcoholism: the CAGE questionnaire. JAMA 252(14):1905, 1984.

Freeland JB, Cambell RS: The social context of first marijuana use. Int J Addict 8:317, 1973.

Friedman LS, Stunin L, Hingson R: A survey of attitudes, beliefs, behaviors and knowledge about AIDS and HIV testing by adolescents and young adults enrolled in alcohol and drug treatment. J Adol Health 14(6):442, 1993.

Fuller PG, Cavanaugh RM: Basic assessment and screening for substance abuse in the pediatrician's office. Ped Clin North Am 42(2):295, 1995.

Goldenring JM, Cohen G: Getting into adolescent heads. Contemp Pediatrics 5(7):75, 1988.

Heather N: Psychology and brief interventions. Br J Addict 84:357, 1989.

Hingson RW, Strunin L, Berlin B, et al: Beliefs about AIDS, use of alcohol and drugs and unprotected sex among Massachusetts adolescents. Am J Public Health 80:1, 1990.

Jessor R, Jessor SL: Problem Behavior and Psychosocial Development: A Longitudinal Study of Youth. New York, Academic Press, 1977.

Jessor R: Risk behavior in adolescence: a psychosocial framework for understanding and action. J Adolescent Health 12:597, 1991.

Johnson JL, Leff M: Overview of the Research on Children of Substance Abusers. Monograph presented at meeting on Core Competencies for Involvement of Health Care Professionals in the Care of Children and Adolescents in Families Affected by Substance Abuse, Office of National Drug Control Policy, Washington DC, 1997.

Jones KL, Smith DW, Ulleland CN, et al: Pattern of malformation in offspring of chronic alcoholic mothers. Lancet 1(815):1267, 1973.

Kandel DB, Raveis VH: Cessation of illicit drug use in young adulthood. Arch Gen Psychiatry 46:109, 1989.

Klitzner M, Schwartz RH, Gruenwald P, Blasinsky M: Screening for risk factors for adolescent alcohol and drug use. Am J Dis Child 141:45, 1987.

Knight JR: Adolescent substance use: screening, assessment, and intervention in medical office practice. Contemp Pediatrics 14(4):45, 1997.

Knight JR, Goodman E, Pulerwitz T, DuRant RH: Reliability of the Problem Oriented Screening Instrument for Teenagers (POSIT) in an adolescent medicine clinic population. Substance Use and Misuse, in press.

Knight JR, Vandeven A: Substance Abusing Parents: A Guide to Brief Interventions in Pediatric Practice. Workshop presented at Ambulatory Pediatric Association Meeting, Washington, DC, 1997.

MacDonald DI, Blume SB: Children of alcoholics. Am J Dis Child 140(8):750, 1986.

Miller WR, Rollnick S: Motivational Interviewing. Guilford Press, New York, 1991.

Miller WR, Sanchez VC: Motivating young adults for treatment and lifestyle change. *In* Howard G, Nathan P (eds): Issues in Alcohol Use and Misuse by Young Adults. Notre Dame, IN, University of Notre Dame Press, 1994, pp 51–81.

Murray RM, Clifford H: Twin and adoption studies: how good is the evidence for a genetic role? *In* Galanter M (ed): Recent Development in Alcoholism, Vol I. New York, Plenum Press, 1983.

Newcomb MD, Felix-Ortiz M: Multiple protective and risk factors for drug use and abuse: cross-sectional and prospective findings. J Person Soc Psychol 63(2):280, 1992.

National Highway Traffic and Safety Administration (NHTSA), US Department of Transportation: Fatal Accident Reporting System: 1989 Annual Report. DOTHS07693, Washington, DC, US Government Printing Office, 1991.

National Institute on Alcohol Abuse and Alcoholism (NIAAA), US Department of Health and Human Services: Motivational Enhancement Therapy Manual. USDHHS 94-3723, Washington, DC, US Government Printing Office, 1994.

National Institute on Drug Abuse (NIDA), U.S. Department of Health and Human Services: National Survey Results on Drug Use From the Monitoring the Future Study, 1975–1994. Rockville MD, NIDA, 1995.

Offer D, Schonert-Reichl KA: Debunking the myths of adolescence: findings from recent research. J Am Acad Child Adolesc Psychiatry 31(6):1003, 1992.

Office of the Inspector General (OIG): General reports on youth and alcohol. DHHS-RPO799, Washington, DC, US Government Printing Office, 1991.

Patton LH: Adolescent substance abuse: risk factors and protective factors. Ped Clin North Am 42(2):283, 1995.

Petersen AC, Leffert N: Developmental issues influencing guidelines for adolescent health research: a review. J Adolesc Health 17:298, 1995.

Piaget J: The Moral Judgment of the Child. New York, Collier, 1962.

Prochaska JO: Strong and weak principles for progressing from precontemplation to action on the basis of twelve problem behaviors. Health Psych 13:47, 1994.

Prochaska JO, DiClemente CC: Stages and processes of self-change of smoking: toward an integrative model of change. J Consult Psych 51:390, 1983.

Prochaska JO, DiClemente CC: Transtheoretical therapy: toward a more integrative model of change. Psychotherapy: Theory, Research and Practice 19(3):276, 1982.

Prochaska JO, Velicer WF, Rossi JS, Goldstein MG, Marcus BH, Rakowski W, Fiore C, Harlow LL, Redding CA, Rosenblum D, Rossi SR: Stages of change and decisional balance for 12 problem behaviors. Health Psych 13:39, 1994.

Rahdert ER (ed): The Adolescent Assessment/Referral System Manual. USDHHS (ADM)91-1735, Washington, DC, US Government Printing Office, 1991.

Riggs SR, Alario A: RAFFT questions. Project ADEPT Manual. Brown University, Providence, RI, 1987.

Rollnick S, Heather N, Bell A: Negotiating behavior change in medical settings: the development of brief motivational interviewing. J Ment Health 1:25, 1992.

Safer DJ, Zito JM, Fine EM: Increased methylphenidate usage for attention deficit disorder in the 1990s. Pediatrics 98(6):1084, 1996.

Schonberg SK (ed): Guidelines for the Treatment of Alcohol- and Other Drug-Abusing Adolescents. Treatment Improvement Protocol (TIP) Series 4. Center for Substance Abuse Treatment, USDHHS 93-2010, Washington, DC, US Government Printing Office, 1993.

Schonberg SK (ed): Substance Abuse: A Guide for Health Professionals. Elk Grove Village, IL, American Academy of Pediatrics, 1988.

Schwartz RH, Wirtz PW: Potential substance abuse: detection among adolescent patients. Clin Pediatrics 29(1):38, 1990.

Smart RG, Fejer D: Drug use among adolescents and their parents: closing the generation gap in mood modification. J Abnormal Psychiatry 79:153, 1972.

Substance Abuse and Mental Health Service Administration (SAMHSA), US Department of Health and Human Services: Preliminary Estimates from the 1995 National Household Survey on Drug Abuse. Rockville MD, Office of Applied Studies, 1996.

Wesson D (ed): Detoxification for Alcohol and Other Drugs. Treatment Improvement Protocol (TIP) Series 19. CSAT, USDHHS 93-2010, Washington, DC, US Government Printing Office, 1995.

Wolraich ML (ed): The Classification of Child and Adolescent Mental Diagnoses in Primary Care. Elk Grove Village, IL, American Academy of Pediatrics, 1996.

Woolf AD, Shannon MW: Clinical toxicology for the pediatrician. Ped Clin North Am 42(2):317, 1995.

51 Developmental Implications of Violence in Youth

Joy D. Osofsky • Howard J. Osofsky

In one moderate-sized city, 51% of the fifth-graders had been direct victims of violence. Ninety-one percent had personally witnessed some type of violence.

Reports based on clinical experience with the Boston Medical Center's Child Witness to Violence Project emphasize that domestic violence can be particularly damaging for young children when they see assaults between people to whom they are emotionally attached.

Exposure to trauma can interfere with normal development of trust and later emergence of autonomy through exploration.

Other risk factors include (1) the ready availability of guns; (2) youth involvement in drugs, both as consumers and in other aspects of the drug economy; (3) peer pressures; and (4) fragmented, and at times inadequate, family, school, and community supports.

Violence and children's witnessing of violence have been characterized as a "public health epidemic" in the United States. Violence among youth ages 11 to 17 years, including murder, rape, robbery, and aggravated assault, has increased 25% in the last decade (Fingerhut and Kleinman, 1990). Homicide ranks as the second leading cause of death among males between 15 and 24 years of age, and the rate has more than doubled since 1950 (reported by the Federal Bureau of Investigation [Centers for Disease Control and Prevention, 1994; Jenkins and Bell, 1997] in 1991 as 37 per 100,000). For African American males between 15 and 24 years of age, the rate is much higher, reported in 1991 as 159 per 100,000. A recent survey at a public hospital–based pediatric clinic in a major US city found that 1 of every 10 children under the age of 6 reported having observed a shooting or stabbing (Groves et al, 1993). Half of these incidents occurred at home and half on the streets. Only in some developing countries is there a higher incidence of violence than in the United States.

It is important to understand the *meaning* that an experience of violence may have for a child. This meaning will be influenced by the nature of the threat and the damage, the child's relationship with the victim or perpetrator, the severity and duration of the violence, and its proximity to the child. While consistent prospective data are not yet available, it is likely that different types of violence have different effects on children and families. In predicting negative developmental effects it seems probable that witnessing domestic violence among people whom the child knows, as well as exposure to chronic violence, will have the most significant consequences in children.

Recent data obtained from approximately 300 children between 6 and 12 years of age indicate that school-aged children are victims of and witnesses to significant amounts of violence. In one moderate-sized city, 51% of the fifth-graders had been direct victims of violence. Ninety-one percent had personally witnessed some type of violence. Children's reports of distress symptoms indicated a significant relation to a violent event. Parents reported concerns about being safe and about protecting their children in neighborhoods where violence occurs frequently (Osofsky et al, 1993). Very early in their lives, many children must learn to deal with loss and to cope with grieving for family members and friends who have been killed. Parents often feel helpless and hopeless as they try to deal with the trauma that children experience.

Parallels have been drawn between children growing up in inner cities in the United States and those living in war zones (Garbarino et al, 1992). In many urban areas, children commonly tell pediatric health care providers that they hear gunshots outside their homes, have viewed shootings on playgrounds and in their neighborhoods, and have a family member or relative who has been a victim or perpetrator of violence.

The effect of contact with domestic violence on children is receiving increasing attention from health care providers, mental health professionals, law enforcement, and the judicial system related to the recent work of advocates and policy makers (Groves et al, 1993; National Research Council, 1997; Osofsky, 1997). At least 3.3 million children see domestic violence each year, which includes a range of attacks from hitting and slapping to fatal assaults with guns or knives. Despite the presumed underreporting of family violence, it is likely that 30% of young adult women in the United States (perhaps as many as 15 million) have experienced at least one episode of physical

---

This paper has been modified from an earlier chapter written by the first author for *Rudolph's Pediatrics,* J. Shonkoff and T. Boyce, eds. Stamford, CT, Appleton & Lange, 1994.

abuse by a male intimate. In many such instances, there are not just adult victims but also child witnesses.

Estimates vary on the number of children who witness one parent abusing another. It is estimated that at least 3.3 million children yearly are at risk of being exposed to parental violence (Jaffe, Wolfe, and Wilson, 1990). It is likely that this estimate is low, however, since it includes only proximity with serious violence, and the study on which it was based (Straus, Gelles, and Steinmetz, 1980) excluded families with children under 3 years of age and families in which parents were separated or divorced. Figures from a program in Miami providing court-referred interventions estimated that approximately 75% of children from violent homes are spectators of their fathers battering their mothers (Farr, personal communication, 1997). Several informal reports have indicated that children are present in approximately half of the homes where police intervene because of domestic violence. The effects on children who witness such violence manifest as psychological, behavioral, affective, and somatic symptoms similar to those of children who are abused and neglected. In addition, between 50% and 75% of men who abuse their partners also abuse their children (McKibben, DeVos, and Newberger, 1989; Straus, Gelles, and Steinmetz, 1980). Further, a child's response to the father's abusing the mother is one of the strongest risk factors for transmitting violence from one generation to another (Table 51–1).

Recent studies of television and movies indicate that children of all ages also are exposed to a great deal of media-based violence that has a demonstrable effect on the development of aggressive behaviors as well as attitudes toward violence (Huesmann and Miller, 1994; Murray, 1997). Moreover, the adverse outcomes are most significant among children who are at greatest risk, including those who are close to domestic and community violence and those who receive less supervision and parental monitoring of such exposure.

Effect of Violence on the Child When the Child Knows the Perpetrator

The impact on children of exposure to violence depends on many factors, including the age of the child, the characteristics of the neighborhood (e.g., degree of community resources), the amount and quality of the support provided by key caregivers and other significant adults, the child's

Table 51–1 • What Do Children Learn From Exposure to Domestic Violence?

- Violence is an appropriate way to resolve conflicts
- Violence is a part of family relationships
- The perpetrator of violence in intimate relationships often goes unpunished
- Violence is a way to control other people

Adapted from The Children of Domestic Violence, a report by the Massachusetts Coalition of Battered Women Service Groups and the Children's Working Group, 1995.

experience of previous abuse, the child's proximity to the violent event, and his or her level of familiarity with the victim or perpetrator. The capacity of children to perceive and "remember" a violent experience affects the presence or absence of symptoms, the pattern of the symptoms, and the circumstances under which they are likely to occur. In addition to producing symptoms, contact with violence affects the way children think about themselves and about the world around them, particularly regarding the extent to which they view relationships as trustworthy and dependable.

Whatever protective influence a lack of understanding of violence may afford the very young child, this appears to fail when severe trauma occurs, especially when the child witnesses the murder of a parent. Posttraumatic stress–like symptoms, including sleeplessness, disorganized behavior, and agitation, are often observed, although caretakers and others in the child's environment may tend to deny these problems (Pynoos, 1993; Osofsky and Fenichel, 1994). Many of these children show a reaction to viewing violence similar to that of having been abused themselves (Fantuzzo et al, 1991; Jaffe, Wolfe, and Wilson, 1990; Kashani et al, 1992).

Young children may be especially vulnerable to domestic violence. Reports based on clinical experience with the Boston City Hospital Child Witness to Violence Project emphasize that domestic violence can be particularly damaging for young children when they see assaults between people to whom they are emotionally attached (Groves et al, 1993; Zuckerman et al, 1995). This is corroborated by other evidence that children's psychological reactions to trauma are likely to be more intense if they know the victim or perpetrator (Pynoos and Eth, 1986). In our own work, we have found that both parents and police perceive observing violence against a parent to have a much greater impact on a child than violence against a stranger. Our data show further that children are likely to show the strongest negative reactions when violence involves a parent or caregiver (Osofsky, 1997).

Developmental Impact on Children of Exposure to Violence

Reactions to exposure to violence vary depending on the child's age and developmental level. Children in the first 3 years of life show increased irritability and sleep disturbances as well as fears of being alone (Osofsky and Fenichel, 1994). Exposure to trauma can interfere with their normal development of trust and later emergence of autonomy through exploration. Regression in developmental achievements such as toileting and language is common (Drell, Siegel, and Gaensbauer, 1993). For preschoolers, cognitive confusion is common, with a decrease in verbalization and more precocious use of trauma-related expressions in play and language. Again, sleep problems, night terrors, and other manifestations of increased anxiety are common (Osofsky et al, 1993). School-aged children also experience increases in anxiety and trouble with sleeping. They may have difficulty paying attention and experience intrusive thoughts. For preschoolers as well as school-aged children, there is often a decrease in mastery motivation, including a lack of pleasure in exploring the physical environment. For adolescents, learning problems are common, with difficulties in concentration, school decline, and failure. Resulting secondary problems with self-esteem often lead to increased risk of aggressive acting-out behaviors, substance abuse, and secondary psychiatric morbidity. It is important to recognize that any evaluation of the effects on children of proximity to violence must consider that their parents or caregivers also are numbed, frightened, and depressed and often are unable to be available emotionally to their children. When they cannot depend on the trust and security that comes from caregivers who are emotionally accessible, children at any age may withdraw and show disorganized behaviors.

SHORT-TERM SYMPTOMS

Overall, most children demonstrate the same patterns of behavioral and physiologic reactivity and symptoms following trauma that have been observed in adults. Many show an increase in anxiety at bedtime, exaggerated startle reactions, persistent hypervigilance, difficulty in regulation (including either increased aggression or social withdrawal), and, especially for young children, new fears (including fear of being alone). Posttrauma psychopathology may include posttraumatic stress disorder symptoms, phobic and overanxious disorders, depression, substance abuse, and dissociative or somatization disorders.

Recent empiric studies, as well as clinical reports, have provided important descriptive data on the symptoms of very young children who have been close to significant forms of violence. These findings demonstrate that infants and toddlers have fewer ways of expressing their feelings than even slightly older children, who are able to use words, play, or drawings to communicate their experience. Many kinds of stress, including contact with violence, can contribute to sleep and eating difficulties, withdrawal, nightmares, and night terrors in children of all ages. There is some indication of sex differences in the responses of school-aged children, with boys more likely to show aggressive responses and girls more likely to withdraw. Although rigorous research in this area is just beginning, it is important to recognize that violence may contribute significantly to the development of secondary symptoms and problematic behaviors. Indeed, clear associations have been found between children's exposure to violence and posttraumatic symptoms and disorders in children ranging from early childhood well into adolescence. A consensus seems to be emerging about the types of symptom clusters associated with posttraumatic stress in children (Drell, Siegel, and Gaensbauer, 1993). These include reexperiencing the traumatic event (e.g., nightmares or play that includes reexperiencing the trauma); avoidance of people or situations that remind the child of the fearful event; numbing of responsiveness (e.g., emotionally subdued, socially withdrawn, constricted in play); and increased or decreased arousal (e.g., hypervigilance, exaggerated startle responses, night terrors, increased aggression or withdrawal).

LONG-TERM SEQUELAE

Less is known about children's later adaptation and the long-term sequelae of exposure to violence. Retrospective studies of prisoners and psychiatric patients indicate that a majority experienced some (or often many) forms of exposure to violence earlier in their lives. Follow-up studies of children who have been maltreated, as well as investigations of those who have been close to a homicide of someone familiar to them, indicate that they have more difficulty with later school adjustment, peer relationships, and interpersonal relationships in general. Longer-term outcomes for children are likely to be related to the child's gender, age at exposure, frequency and type of contact, comprehension of danger, developmental status and functioning before the experience, and available supports after the event. There is general agreement among clinicians that the nature of the supports available to the child following exposure to violence is likely to be crucial for facilitating adaptation. For treatment to be successful, it is crucial that the child be able to experience some sense of safety in his or her environment. Further, the parents' or caregivers' ability to deal with their own trauma and grief is extremely important for their children's progress, so that the children will be able to express anxieties, fears, and concerns with people they trust. Prospective studies of the longer-term effects of violence exposure for children, as well as evaluations of the effects of early intervention services, have not been conducted.

Other Risk Factors

Many other factors contribute to children's involvement with violence. Paramount among these are (1) the ready availability of guns; (2) youth involvement with drugs, both as consumers and in other aspects of the drug economy; (3) peer pressures; (4) fragmented and, at times, inadequate family, school, and community supports; and (5) individual issues related to developmental factors. Guns are more freely available, with a number of studies demonstrating high frequency of children's seeing guns in schools (Christoffell, 1997). Data link this gun availability with students' fears for safety, their feelings that they need to have protection, and their exposure to violence. Greater youth involvement with drugs also appears to link directly or indirectly to interaction with violence. Dukarm and colleagues (1996) analyzed data from a nationally representative sample of over 12,000 high school students to investigate the relationship between substance use, weapon carrying, and physical fighting among male and female adolescents. They used the 1991 Centers for Disease Control and Prevention's Youth Risk Behavior Survey. They found that a significant increase in the number of male and female adolescents carrying weapons and physically fighting was associated with all forms of substance use. The risk of violent behavior increased significantly, and was of equal magnitude, for adolescent females and males who were users of illicit substances.

It is important to recognize not only fragmented supports for many of our youth but also the impact of peer pressures and risk taking, both of which are important contributors to behavior, especially during adolescence. Peer pressures with the wish to be liked and respected contribute to risk taking and exposure to drugs, violence, and violent behaviors. Further, adolescents, based on developmental factors, are likely to minimize vulnerability and engage in high-risk behaviors. In that light, the Youth Risk Behavior Surveillance System (Kann et al, 1995) includes both a national school-based survey conducted by the Centers for Disease Control and Prevention and state and local school-based surveys conducted by state and local education agencies. The results of their 1995 national survey conducted with over 10,000 students in grades 9 through 12 indicated that 72% of all deaths among school-aged youth and young adults result from four causes: motor vehicle crashes, other unintentional injuries, homicide, and suicide. The survey data suggest further that many high school students practice behaviors, including illegal behaviors, that may increase their likelihood of death from these four causes: 22% had rarely or ever used a safety belt; in the 30 days preceding the survey, 39% had ridden with a driver who had been drinking alcohol, 20% had carried a weapon, 52% had drunk alcohol, 35% had smoked cigarettes, and 25% had used marijuana; 9% had attempted suicide during the 12 months preceding the survey. Significant morbidity and social problems among school-aged youth and young adults also result from unintended pregnancies and sexually transmitted diseases, including human immunodeficiency virus infection. In 1995, 53% of high school students surveyed had had sexual intercourse; 46% of sexually active students had not used a condom at last intercourse. A significant percentage of students also participated in behaviors that placed them at risk for later adult illnesses. These survey data are being used to alert health and education officials about improving national, state, and local policies and programs that might reduce the risks associated with leading causes of mortality and morbidity.

The Youth Risk Behavior Survey supplement to the National Health Interview Survey was done to examine the relationship between socioeconomic status and risk behaviors for chronic disease among a nationally representative sample of 6300 adolescents, ages 12 to 17 years (Lowry et al, 1996). Most of the adolescents (63%) reported having two or more of the five risk behaviors, including cigarette smoking, sedentary lifestyle, insufficient consumption of fruits and vegetables, excessive consumption of foods high in fat, and episodic heavy drinking of alcohol. The study found further that among adolescents, these risk behaviors for chronic disease are inversely related to socioeconomic status. They suggested that improved community- and school-based programs to prevent such behaviors among adolescents are needed, especially for lower socioeconomic groups.

These data on risk behaviors among youth in general, and their specific relationship with violent behaviors, are of particular importance for health care providers, especially pediatricians who may be the first to come in contact with these young people. These contacts may provide an especially important opportunity for both prevention and intervention.

The Role of Health Care Providers

Health care providers who work with inner-city children (and, at times, with youth living in more privileged communities), often have to deal with violence as part of their clinical practice experience. Both pediatricians and nurses come in contact with other risk behaviors with some frequency (Jones, 1997; Zuckerman et al, 1995). Health care providers who work with children and adolescents who witness violence need to understand and recognize symptoms of mental and emotional distress from association with violence. Sharing of knowledge and skills is crucial to enhance prevention and intervention strategies. Concurrent with the problems faced by children who have been exposed to violence directly and who are exhibiting risky behaviors, pediatricians and other health care providers increasingly are confronted with the concerns of parents and other caregivers who may have difficulty handling their children and their behaviors as well as coping with their own fears. At times, it might seem easier to address the immediate presenting symptoms in the child and avoid the deep-seated sequelae that relate to violence contact and risk-taking behaviors. If the doctor feels that he or she cannot change the situation for the family, there is more of a tendency to simply treat the child's symptoms and go no further.

It is important for pediatricians to keep developmental and behavioral issues in mind as they are confronted with children and youth who have been exposed to violence and who exhibit risk-taking behaviors. Problems that may arise include regressions in communicative ability, loss of previously established bladder and bowel control, sleep disturbances, feeding problems, somatic complaints including headaches and stomachaches, excessive clinging and fear of separating from the primary caregiver, learning difficulties, and generally more difficult patterns of behaviors. Excessive risk-taking behavior may also occur in response to chronic or even acute proximity to violence. When parents bring these concerns to the attention of the pediatrician, it is important to be aware that exposure to violence may be playing an important etiologic role.

An important decision regarding the treatment of children who have closeness to violence and those engaging in risky behaviors relates to who should do the treating and when a referral to a mental health professional is indicated. The more awareness the pediatrician has about the effects of exposure to violence and possible etiology of the risk-taking behavior, the better equipped he or she will be to deal directly with the problem or to make an appropriate referral. Many children who are associated with violence do not receive the help that they need. For those who consistently exhibit risk-taking behavior, it may be a desperate plea for help. In some cases, parents may want to avoid dealing with the experience and the behaviors themselves and may not realize that the child has been traumatized or that something can be done to help ameliorate the consequences. Further, many parents, teachers, community workers, and health care professionals often are not sure of how to deal with the problem and may prefer to avoid it entirely. Pediatricians are in a unique position to intervene early after a trauma occurs. Experience with children who have been traumatized indicates that, in most circumstances, the earlier intervention takes place, the better the outcome for the child and family.

Any child who has been exposed to a significant level of violence and who is symptomatic should be referred to a mental health specialist, preferably one who has had experience treating such children. Many children who grow up with chronic violence in their homes and neighborhoods exhibit patterns of symptoms or behaviors that generally are difficult for their parents or caregivers to manage. If the pediatrician is trained to deal with such complexities, management may begin in the primary care setting. In most instances, however, significant problems require referral to a mental health specialist. Although supportive empirical data are not yet available, clinicians working in this area believe that early referral for treatment may be an important determinant of both short and longer term outcomes.

Need for Prevention and Early Intervention

Violence in the United States has grown to epidemic proportions. Not only is the homicide rate far higher than in any other highly industrialized country, but it affects increasingly younger perpetrators and victims. News reports of shootings involving preadolescents are no longer rare. Even babies are killed by random bullets. And yet it is still not understood in our nation that the true "solutions" to the sequences of these tragedies rest with early preventive efforts rather than reactive criminal justice responses.

Effective pediatric advocacy can best be focused in three main areas: (1) a family-centered approach to the prevention of violence and treatment of its aftermath; (2) a public health approach toward decreasing risk behaviors; (3) a national campaign to change attitudes toward violence and tolerance of violent behavior; and (4) informed public policy at all levels of government designed to reduce and prevent the roots of violence.

There are no simple solutions to the complex issues surrounding violence. However, we have a responsibility as health care professionals and citizens to learn as much as we can to help the youngest victims of violence in the United States.

REFERENCES

Carlson BE: Children's observations of interparental violence. *In* Roberts AR (ed): Battered Women and Their Families: Intervention Strategies and Treatment Programs. New York: Springer, 1984, pp 147–167.

Centers for Disease Control and Prevention: Homicide among 15–19 year old males: United States 1963–1991. MMWR 43: 725–727, 1994.

Chalk R, King PA (eds): Violence in Families: Assessing Prevention and Treatment Programs. Washington, DC, National Academy Press, 1998.

Christoffel KK: Firearm injuries affecting US children and adolescents. *In* Osofsky JD (ed): Children in a Violent Society. New York, Guilford Press, 1997, pp 42–71.

Drell M, Siegel C, Gaensbauer T: Post-traumatic stress disorders. *In* Zeanah C (ed). Handbook of Infant Mental Health. New York, Guilford Press, 1993, pp 291–304.

Durkarm CP, Byrd RS, Auinger P, Weitzman M: Illicit substance use, gender, and the risk of violent behavior among adolescents. Arch Pediatr Adolesc Med 150:797, 1996.

Fantuzzo J, DePaola L, Lambert L, Martino T: Effects of interparental violence on the psychological adjustment and competencies of young children. J Consult Clin Psychol 59:258, 1991.

Fingerhut LA, Kleinman JC: International and inter-state comparisons of homicide among young males. JAMA 265:3292, 1990.

Garbarino J, Dubrow N, Kostelny K, Pardo C: Children in Danger: Coping with the Consequences of Community Violence. San Francisco, Jossey-Bass, 1992.

Groves B, Zuckerman B, Marans S, Cohen D: Silent victims: children who witness violence. JAMA 269:262, 1993.

Huesmann LR, Miller LS: Long-term effects of repeated exposure to media violence in childhood. *In* Huesmann LR (ed): Aggressive Behavior: Current Perspectives. New York, Plenum, 1994, pp 61–90.

Hurley D, Jaffe PG: Children's observations of violence: II. Clinical implications for children's mental health professionals. Can J Psychiatry 35:471–476, 1990.

Jaffe PG, Wolfe DA, Wilson SK: Children of Battered Women. Newbury Park, CA, Sage, 1990.

Jenkins EJ, Bell CC: Exposure and response to community violence among children and adolescents. *In* Osofsky JD (ed): Children in a Violent Society. New York, Guilford Publishers, 1997, pp 9–31.

Jones FC: Community violence, children, and youth: considerations for programs, policy, and nursing roles. Pediatric Nurs 23:131, 1997.

Kann L, Warren CW, Harris WA, Collins JL, Williams BI, Ross JG, Kolbe LJ: Youth Risk Behavior Surveillance: United States, 1995. Centers for Disease Control and Prevention, September 27, 1966. Morbid Mortal Wkly Rep 45(No.SS-4), 1996.

Kashani J, Daniel AE, Dandoy AC, Holcomb WR: Family violence: impact on children. J Am Acad Child Adolesc Psychiatry 31:181, 1992.

Lowry R, Kann L, Collins J, Kolbe L: The effect of socioeconomic status on chronic disease risk behaviors among US adolescents. JAMA 276:792, 1996.

McKibben L, DeVos E, Newberger E: Victimization of mothers of abused children: a controlled study. Pediatrics 84:531, 1989.

Murray JP: Media violence and youth. *In* Osofsky JD (ed): Children in a Violent Society. New York, Guilford Press, 1997, pp 72–96.

Osofsky JD: Children in a Violent Society. New York, Guilford Press, 1997.

Osofsky JD, Wewers S, Hann DM, Fick AC: Chronic community violence: what is happening to our children. Psychiatry 56:36, 1993.

Osofsky JD, Fenichel ES: Caring for Infants and Toddlers in Violent Environments: Hurt, Healing, and Hope. Zero to Three. Arlington, VA; National Center for Clinical Infant Programs Publications, 1994.

Pynoos RS: Traumatic stress and developmental psychopathology in children and adolescents. *In* Oldham JM, Riba MB, Tasman A (eds): American Psychiatric Press Review of Psychiatry, Vol 12. Washington, DC, American Psychiatric Press, Inc., 1993, pp 238–272.

Pynoos RS, Eth S: Witness to violence: the child interview. J Am Acad Child Adolesc Psychiatry 25:306, 1986.

Straus MA, Gelles RJ, Steinmetz S: Behind Closed Doors. New York, Anchor, 1980.

Zuckerman B, Augustyn M, Groves BM, Parker S: Silent victims revisited: the special case of domestic violence. Pediatrics 96:511, 1995.

52 *Attention and Dysfunctions of Attention*

Melvin D. Levine

 In all likelihood, difficulties with the controls of attention represent the most common developmental-behavioral complaint confronting primary care physicians. This chapter avoids the simplistic labels of "ADD" and "ADHD" in order to examine in detail the very specific constituents of normal and dysfunctional attention among children. This approach emphasizes the heterogeneity of manifestations and associated dysfunctions encountered among children with attentional difficulty. Assessment and management are geared to the specific breakdowns that impede organized and goal-directed attention during the school years. This chapter stresses the need for high specificity in assessing the nature of a child's attentional difficulties.

Clinicians are seeing increased numbers of children and adolescents who are suspected of having attention deficits, or "ADD." Even though a group of these patients seem to meet traditional criteria for a syndrome-like diagnosis, many of them appear to be struggling with various aspects of attention without manifesting a full-blown picture of behavioral and cognitive turmoil. This chapter addresses problems of attention without making use of labels, such as ADD (attention-deficit disorder) or ADHD (attention-deficit hyperactivity disorder). Instead, a model of the normal underlying mechanisms is presented and the many different phenomena associated with the many different forms of attentional dysfunction are explored. In this way, attention is viewed as an area of development (like language and motor function), and persons with problems with attention are seen to have a weakness or delay in this aspect of their functioning (rather than manifesting a true "syndrome").

The limitations of the labels ADD/ADHD are considerable.

- The labels are restrictive, implying that one can have attentional problems only if he or she manifests a list of specific behaviors. In particular, students who have trouble concentrating and who would benefit from management of their attention may not "qualify" because of their lack of behavior problems.
- The manifestations of attentional dysfunction are nonspecific. That is, they may appear as part of a multitude of different conditions and states, including depression, language processing dysfunction, temperamental traits, or a combination of these conditions.
- Children with attentional dysfunction usually have other neurodevelopmental dysfunctions (Chapter 54) in addition to their attentional problems. Once the label is applied, consideration and management of associated dysfunctions may never occur.
- The label is too vague. To offer optimal management of an affected child, there is a critical need to specify which aspects of attention are not functioning.
- There is no real evidence that this is a distinct syndrome, as opposed to being a commonly clustered group of traits that may stem from a multitude of etiologies and mechanisms.
- The labels are intrinsically pessimistic and often negativistic in their connotations, thereby obscuring the collection of remarkable strengths found in these children.

EXAMPLE

Joe is an 8-year-old boy who is beginning the third grade. He is having serious academic difficulties. Joe is delayed in reading and written output. He is close to grade level in arithmetic but is seriously deficient in his spelling. His teachers have noted that Joe is highly distractible. He seldom concentrates and keeps missing important details. Furthermore, he is highly fidgety in class. He frequently annoys others and has trouble staying in his seat. His teachers and parents have to repeat directions several times for Joe to process them. During an evaluation of his learning, Joe was demonstrated to have significant problems with language processing. These dysfunctions were impeding his academic progress. Meanwhile, another clinician had seen Joe and had his parents and teachers fill out a questionnaire, the results of which led to a "diagnosis" of ADHD. The clinician did not consider Joe's language function. Joe's parents were confused, wondering whether their son had an attention deficit plus a language disability or whether the attentional problems were a direct result of his difficulties processing language. Eventually Joe was placed on medication, which helped somewhat, but he continued to have trouble learning as well as intermittent difficulties with behavioral adjustment in school.

Attention as a Control Panel of the Mind

Attention can be conceptualized as a network of highly interactive controls over conscious mental functioning.

499

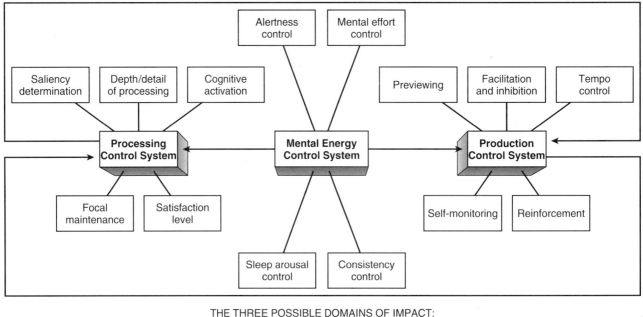

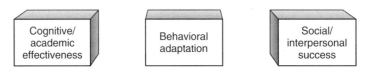

Figure 52–1. Various attention controls. These controls can break down in varying combinations to cause children to have difficulty with various aspects of attention.

Problems with attention, or attention deficits, represent breakdowns in various of these controls. The specific attention controls play a strictly managerial role in the human mind. That is, they do not actually interpret incoming information or implement actions and reactions; rather, the attention controls activate, regulate, and monitor those parts of the brain that are more directly involved in performance. For example, the attention controls do not enable one to understand language but, instead, they regulate the intensity and selectivity of listening, which secondarily impacts comprehension.

The controls of attention can be grouped into three systems: mental energy control, processing control, and production control (Fig. 52–1). The following section explores these three control systems and the individual controls that comprise them. Normal functioning of each control is described, as are the phenomena that are observable when that control chronically breaks down.

Control Systems and Their Breakdown Points

The three control systems are highly interactive. Mental energy controls regulate the initial flow, allocation, and maintenance of an energy supply necessary to foster alertness and facilitate the exertion of effort. Processing controls regulate the uptake of information as well as its further interpretation. Production controls oversee the mind's output. A reasonable flow of mental energy is needed for optimal processing and production. It is also the case that efficiency and selectivity of uptake and output can "conserve fuel."

Each of the three control systems has three relevant domains of impact, namely, cognition and academic effectiveness, behavioral adaptation, and interpersonal (social) effectiveness. Thus, problems with specific attention controls may negatively affect one or more of these domains.

The following discussion looks at the three control systems and their constituent individual controls. In each case, normal function and dysfunction are discussed.

Mental Energy Controls

Recently, there has been considerable interest in the ways in which the mind acquires and uses the energy needed for thinking and for intellectual productivity (Sergeant, 1996). The term *cognitive energetics* is often applied to the study of such processes. There is evidence to suggest that the central nervous system has finite energy resources that must be properly mobilized and allocated to meet task demands (Gopher and Navon, 1980). Sergeant notes, "The resource model of selective attention conceives attention as a general pool of energy that is limited but can be distributed over simultaneous demands."

The mental energy controls regulate the distribution of resources needed for concentration and goal-directed action. The control system can be divided into two components: (1) arousal and alertness control and (2) mental effort control.

AROUSAL AND ALERTNESS CONTROL

The ability to initiate and maintain concentration is essential for success in schoolwork as well as in most other pursuits. This function includes the capacity to fend off the ever-present threat of mental fatigue and the ability to remain focused without experiencing excessive tiredness, which, in turn, could lead to a loss of concentration. The function also involves the capacity to regulate the flow of mental energy such that a heightened state of arousal can be attained under circumstances that demand particularly intense concentration or vigilance.

Arousal and alertness control (Table 52–1) is closely tied to the regulation of sleep and the maintenance of appropriate daily rhythms of sleep and wakefulness. In other words, this control ensures that an individual is sleeping adequately at night and feeling sufficiently awake during the day. Sleep and arousal are regulated within the reticular activating system and the locus ceruleus, two areas within the brainstem. Variations in neurotransmitter metabolism and release during the day and night are associated with patterns of sleep and wakefulness.

Dysfunctions of Arousal and Alertness Control

Children with dysfunctions of arousal and alertness control endure excessive mental fatigue in the classroom. They experience intermittent difficulty with concentration and therefore have problems sustaining their focus on relevant information. The manifestations of their mental fatigue are sometimes misleading or even paradoxical. They may fidget, squirm, and become hyperactive, seemingly an attempt to combat the uncomfortable feeling of fatigue. Rather than acknowledging explicitly that their minds feel tired in school, they are apt to lament that "school is too boring." Many such children can be observed to yawn and stretch in class more often than their peers.

A subgroup of children with attention deficits manifests a sleep-arousal imbalance. They fail to sleep adequately at night and have trouble sustaining their alertness during the school day. Often it is hard for them to fall asleep at night; they may be wide awake at midnight. It might be difficult for them to get out of bed in the morning. Once at school, these children may display varying patterns of insufficient alertness, such as trouble getting started in the morning, difficulty focusing after lunch, or a tendency to keep tuning in and out.

Table 52–1 • Alertness and Arousal Control

Form	Explanation	Applications
Alertness	Maintenance of sufficient energy for concentration	Listening to instructions in a classroom setting
Sleep-arousal balance	Sleeping adequately at night; feeling alert during day	Being sufficiently well rested to focus effectively in school
Arousal regulation	Being able to increase level of arousal when needed	Increasing level of attention when heeding a warning

Table 52–2 • Mental Effort Control

Form	Explanation	Applications
Working capacity	Ability to engage in activities requiring effort	Completing homework; studying for tests
Behavior	Capacity to exert effort needed to comply/adapt	Accepting limits in school
Consistent output	Maintenance of a steady level of performance	Schoolwork revealing a steady level of effort and quality

Children with weaknesses of alertness and arousal control may also have trouble regulating and modulating the level of their alertness. They may not become sufficiently aroused during important events (such as studying for a major examination) or they may become overaroused (too excited and invested) at unimportant moments (e.g., while watching television). Thus, they exhibit a lack of ability to match the intensity of the flow of mental energy to the particular context or circumstance.

MENTAL EFFORT CONTROL

The ability to exert mental effort (Table 52–2) when called for is critical as children develop a cognitive working capacity during their school years. They need to be able to delay gratification, struggle through sometimes frustrating intellectual challenges, and create academic products that demand considerable energy. Their effort needs to be sustained and goal directed. The ability to initiate, allocate, maintain, and terminate (at the right time) a flow of mental effort is tightly linked to academic productivity and success. Often mental effort entails the ability and willingness to do "things you don't feel like doing," presumably to satisfy some greater and often delayed good that will result from the effort or to avoid negative consequences, such a punishment. In scientific terms, mental effort has been conceptualized as the energy "required when the current state of the organism did not meet the state required to perform a task" (Sanders, 1983).

There is a reciprocal relationship between mental effort and motivation. When an individual feels highly motivated to undertake and complete an activity, relatively little mental effort is required. If motivation is low, far greater mental effort is demanded. When a child perceives a task as difficult and unexciting, great mental effort may be needed to complete it. Motivation may dwindle in part because the effort required is so great.

Dysfunctions of Mental Effort Control

For some children, work is too much work. They have a great deal of trouble exerting mental effort, accomplishing assignments, or fulfilling responsibilities that are not particularly entertaining or immediately motivating. They may appear to be lazy or oppositional. They are apt to be negligent in completing assignments. They often require heavy prodding and coercion of various types to accomplish work. Battles over homework completion commonly disrupt their families, especially as these children pass through the middle grades. Feelings of fatigue and boredom seriously compromise their productivity in school and elsewhere.

Some individuals with weak mental energy control have trouble getting started with tasks or activities; they seem to require excessive coercion or a "jump start" to begin doing homework or fulfilling domestic responsibilities. At other times, they may be able to begin an activity but are unable to sustain the effort or finish what they start. Poor control over mental effort may also be associated with behavior problems. An affected child may seem to lack the energy needed to control behavior. His or her fatigue may actually lead to a loss of behavioral control with a resultant outpouring of negative actions.

The Enigma of Performance Inconsistency

Children who experience problems with mental energy control do not endure these problems all of the time; they manifest these deficiencies much of the time and often during moments when alertness or mental effort is needed. Because of the intermittence of their inattention, affected children exhibit considerable performance inconsistency. They can be alert and productive on some days or during some hours, but at other times they display mental fatigue and a lack of effort. This inconsistency is most often highly erratic. Some children "tune in and tune out" for periods of seconds or minutes during much of the school day. Or, they may have hours, days, or weeks during which they function well, only to disappointment the adult world with their seeming inability to perform during other hours, days, or weeks. Such patterns of inconsistency may be reflected in inconsistent test scores over a semester or, alternatively, by inconsistent error patterns within tests. For example, a student may correctly answer two questions, incorrectly answer the next three, then err on the next three. That same student may be accurate on some difficult questions and then show poor performance on easier ones, the random error pattern suggesting variable attention.

Performance inconsistency is frequently misinterpreted by adults. The fact that a child can succeed admirably some of the time often elevates general expectations, so that when the child is out of focus, she or he may seem to be "not really trying." Such children grow up with the constant refrain, "We know she can do it when she sets her mind to it," with the underlying misguided implication that the consistency of performance is totally within the control of the child.

Processing Controls

EXAMPLE

Bonnie is a 13-year-old seventh-grader whose parents and teachers are completely confused by her. On some days, she is well-behaved, conscientious, and focused. On other days, she "just can't get her act together." Her teachers have had trouble dealing with Bonnie's inconsistency. They note that she concentrates effectively and gets her work done with care and attention to detail whenever she makes up her mind to do well. At other times, she

does not care and fails to take responsibility for her actions. They know she can function well when she wants to. Her parents are not so sure of this. They were recently sent an attention questionnaire to complete for their physician. They joked that the results of the questionnaire would be determined by the day on which they choose to fill it out.

Processing controls are a set of regulatory functions that depend heavily on the controls of energy distribution and maintenance already described. The processing controls regulate information uptake and utilization. The information may be used as a basis for learning, as guidance for behavior or compliance, or as input needed for relating reciprocally to others (as occurs during the processing of conversation). The processing control system contains five basic controls: (1) saliency determination, (2) processing depth and detail, (3) cognitive activation, (4) focal maintenance, and (5) satisfaction control.

SALIENCY DETERMINATION

The discrimination between important and unimportant information is essential. Human processing systems simply cannot handle the information overload that floods the consciousness without some control over what gets interpreted, stored, and used from moment to moment. That control is what is meant by saliency determination, sometimes referred to as *selective attention*. The concept of selectivity forms a critical component of most scientific models of attention (Mirsky, 1996).

Table 52–3 summarizes the different forms of sali-

Table 52–3 • Saliency Determination

Form	Explanation	Applications
Distraction filtration	Focusing on a purposeful information source or currently meaningful sensory pathway	Listening to the teacher instead of looking out the window; ignoring irrelevant background noises
Task analysis	Focusing on relevant data to meet current expectation	Following directions so as to complete an assignment
Rank ordering	Determining relative levels of importance; prioritizing	Knowing what to study for a test
Main points identification	Deciding what is most significant in a message	Summarizing, paraphrasing, underlining
Vigilance	Being able to be alert to important, rarely occurring stimuli	Proofreading
Divided attention	Being able to focus on multiple important "targets" simultaneously	Listening and writing at the same time (e.g., while taking notes)
Experience analysis	Knowing what was relevant or important in an occurrence (post hoc)	Learning from experiences

Table 52–4 • Common Forms of Distractibility

Form	Manifestations
Visual	Tendency to focus on nonrelevant sights or trivial visual detail
Auditory	Tendency to focus on background sounds; trouble with sustained listening
Tactile	Tendency to keep touching and handling objects instead of attending
Temporal	Tendency to keep focusing on the future rather than present activities
Somatic	Tendency to focus on body feelings, trivial pains, discomforts, scabs, scars
Social	Tendency to keep focusing on peers, ignoring other stimuli

ency determination in which a child must engage. Saliency determination involves the constant review of available stimuli and the rejection of those stimuli that are not sufficiently relevant or needed to accomplish a goal. At the same time, data that are deemed important are selected or highlighted for further processing and utilization. Mirsky and colleagues (1991) characterized the process, which they termed *focus-execute*, as "the ability to select target information from an array for enhanced processing."

Saliency determination, like other processing controls, must interact with other neurodevelopmental functions. Thus, to make rational determinations of saliency, there is a need for some preliminary interpretation. For instance, to know what is important in a paragraph, one must possess some understanding of its content. It is also the case, however, that the ability to identify a main point greatly enhances comprehension of that paragraph. So it is that saliency determination, like all of the attention controls, works reciprocally with other needed neurodevelopmental functions.

Dysfunctions of Saliency Determination

Children with weaknesses of saliency determination often show signs of overt distractibility. In addition or instead, they may reveal problems that are less obvious, difficulties often related to rank-ordering stimuli, identifying main points, dividing their attention effectively, and analyzing tasks and experiences.

Many children with attention deficits are described as "distractible." That is, they keep focusing on seemingly irrelevant stimuli. Within a population of children with attention deficits, different patterns of distractibility are found. Some common patterns are described in Table 52–4.

The individual forms of distractibility listed in Table 52–4 may be more or less prominent in individual children. The inability to filter out totally irrelevant stimuli may seriously impede learning and day-to-day classroom engagement and participation. On the other hand, distractibility and creativity may sometimes go hand in hand. Some distractible children are capable of making observations and sensing similarities that elude other children. They can be highly observant, noticing things that others might miss.

As noted, children and adolescents with weaknesses of saliency determination may also manifest more subtle

problems, sometimes referred to as difficulties with significance determination. It may be hard for them to identify main ideas in a story or paragraph. When confronting a word problem in arithmetic, they may struggle to determine what information is needed to solve the problem and what is irrelevant. Older students may have great difficulty studying for a test, that is, reading a text and deciding what is most important or relevant and therefore most likely to be asked on the examination. History textbooks are often the downfall of students with saliency determination problems; such children have great trouble deciding what is most important amid the plethora of information. Note-taking and underlining (highlighting) may also represent elusive challenges for these individuals. Problems with vigilance may make it hard for them to proofread, especially if they also have difficulty with self-monitoring.

Students with weak saliency determination may show unorthodox patterns of memory, which may manifest as a tendency to remember trivial details better than critical details, a phenomenon often referred to as *incidental learning*.

DEPTH AND DETAIL OF PROCESSING

If salient information is to be understood and used fully, it must be registered in consciousness with adequate depth. That is, the individual must concentrate hard enough on the incoming stimuli. Such concentration in depth helps a student to hold incoming information in place, enter it in short-term memory, and begin to interpret it.

Depth of processing (Table 52–5) strongly influences the appreciation of internal detail, that is, the fine-grained information contained within an array of data. The more deeply a person is concentrating, the more effectively he or she will assimilate fine detail. As processing depth diminishes, internal detail becomes increasingly vague. An analogy might be the use of a postmark on an envelope; if it has not been stamped hard enough, much of the fine detail of the imprint may not be discernible, and only its rough outline may be visible. It could be determined that the letter had been canceled, but the date or name of originating post office would be unreadable.

Dysfunctions of Processing Depth and Detail

It is common for children with attention deficits to show shallow processing and a lack of focus on detail. Their

Table 52–5 • Depth and Detail of Processing

Form	Explanation	Examples
Concentration depth	Processing with sufficient intensity	Listening carefully to directions
Concentration balance	Seeing the big picture without losing the internal detail	Reading for meaning
Registration in short-term memory	Processing with enough depth to retain information	Remembering material while studying
Attention to detail	Focusing enough to appreciate fine detail	Attending to operational signs in arithmetic

shallow processing creates situations in which information "goes in one ear and out the other." Such children are likely to need repetition of instructions and explanations. They may not fully process the instructions for a homework assignment. Much of their listening and watching is likely to occur at a superficial level of intensity.

Children so affected may reveal a lack of awareness of fine detail, along with a much greater appreciation of the "big picture." Their minds are apt to be more like a wide-angle than a telephoto lens. In solving a series of arithmetic problems, such a student may demonstrate a good understanding of the concepts and processes but have trouble dealing with small details, such as the difference between a plus sign and a minus sign or between the numbers 23 and 32. As a result, they are prone to commit careless errors even in the face of strong understanding.

Because depth and detail of processing is an actual control, it can, so to speak, be turned up too high or down too low. Consequently, there are some children with attention deficits who are said to "overattend." They become bogged down in fine detail and have trouble perceiving the great significance or "big picture." They may function slowly, spending too much time on small details. Some students seem to alternate between being too attentive and too detailed at some times and then becoming highly superficial and "wide angle" at other times. They have trouble regulating the depth and detail of their processing.

Shallow processing also takes a toll on short-term memory function. This phenomenon is often seen in children with attentional dysfunction who, as a result, may have trouble responding to recently delivered directions. Their short-term memory deficits may also make it hard for them to study. They may review material repeatedly and still not register it with sufficient depth in short-term memory. This frustrating predicament becomes evident when the student is quizzed on information that he or she is studying at the moment.

Shallow processing may sometimes lead to apparent noncompliant behavior. A student may violate limits in school because he or she never fully processes the rules, warnings, and admonitions articulated by the teacher. The resulting transgressions may be misinterpreted as intentional violations rather than unintended failure to appreciate the described behavioral implications.

COGNITIVE ACTIVATION

When new information enters the mind, it should activate and connect to prior knowledge and experience. An actively engaged mind takes in new material and recalls relevant preexisting facts and ideas, often using the new input to reconstruct somewhat related prior knowledge. This form of cognition is known as *active learning* or *active processing* (Table 52–6). It involves complex interactions between processing control and memory. An active processor keeps on connecting and associating. Cognitive activation helps a student form connections between bits or areas of knowledge. The control over this activity is an essential part of attention, because it is important for cognitive activation not to be calibrated at a level that is either too high (overactive) or excessively low or passive. When

Table 52–6 • Cognitive Activation Control

Form	Explanation	Examples
Association	Active linking of new inputs to prior knowledge	Associating something in class with a recent television show
Connection	Thinking about relationships between areas of learning	Connecting fractions with decimals
Elaboration	Interpreting actively, relating inputs to personal ideas/values	Forming an opinion about something the teacher communicates
"Free flight" inhibition	Preventing excessive activation	Recognizing that an idea has triggered daydreaming and then refocusing

optimally established, active processing adds to the enjoyment of intellectual content, enabling students to formulate interesting contrasts and comparisons as they learn. However, overly active processing may actually distract a student or distort the intended meaning of incoming information. The inhibition of such "free flights of ideas" is another responsibility subsumed under cognitive activation control.

Dysfunctions of Cognitive Activation

Some students with attention deficits tend to be passive processors. When new knowledge is imparted, not much occurs within the mind of the student. Few if any associations and connections are forged. Such a child may seldom elaborate on knowledge, failing therefore to mingle his or her own perspectives with new inputs. Showing a marked overreliance on rote memory in school, these students often seem to regurgitate knowledge on tests or when called upon in class without fully understanding or integrating it. They have a tendency to be nonelaborative, and they are likely to feel understimulated and unfulfilled in school.

The opposite phenomenon also commonly occurs in students with attention deficits, namely a tendency to overactivate their minds, to experience the "free flight of ideas" in school and elsewhere. When some new data bit enters their minds, it automatically elicits an extended chain of associations, which can be irrelevant to the topic at hand. For example, a teacher may say something about a bird, which reminds the child of a duck, which, in turn, leads to thoughts about Donald Duck, which reminds him of his trip to Disneyworld, which makes him think of the vacation he will be taking next summer to the Grand Canyon where you ride a mule into the canyon, which makes him wonder how big mules are. Over a brief span, thoughts of birds have been transformed into mule speculations.

Children who have trouble inhibiting such "free flights" are often highly imaginative and fanciful. They often make comments in class that seem to have little or nothing to do with current topics or activities. They may gravitate toward the back of the room where they create surrealistic drawings or pursue in other ways their rich fantasy lives.

Some children with dysfunctions of cognitive activation harbor manifestations at both extremes; at times, their minds are passive and, at other times, far too active. It seems hard for them to match the level of mental activity with current circumstances or demands.

FOCAL MAINTENANCE CONTROL

The ability to match the duration of focus to the demands posed by incoming information is yet another parameter of optimal attention. Many investigators have studied the processes involved in sustained attention. There is widespread agreement that the ability to sustain a focus is an important and distinct component of attention (Halperin, 1996). Certain forms of input demand extended concentration if they are to be processed with accuracy, whereas other circumstances call for briefer attention with more frequent changing of focus. Thus the length of concentration (sometimes known as *attention span*) has to be tailored to task demands and the nature of the subject matter. Focal maintenance also entails the ongoing monitoring of attention, so that it continues when it is yielding useful information and terminates when that is no longer the case. Table 52–7 summarizes the forms of focal maintenance control that are needed for effective attention.

Dysfunctions of Focal Maintenance Control

It is common to describe children with attention deficits as having "short attention spans." Many of them do manifest this trait. However, it is also true that such children may perseverate, concentrating too long on certain kinds of stimuli and not long enough on other (perhaps more worthwhile) inputs. They may show evidence of perseveration some of the time. They are likely to have trouble with set maintenance, losing focus too soon when needed information is continuing to arrive and/or concentrating too long when there is no longer a flow of useful data. It may be hard for them to shift attention smoothly from one target to the next.

Table 52–7 • Focal Maintenance Control

Form	Explanation	Examples
Sustained attention	Focusing long enough to process fully	Listening to entire set of instructions from the teacher
Shifts of attention	Changing focus when mission is completed; not perseverating	Shifting from reading story to listening to directions for next activity
Set maintenance	Continuing focuses that are working well and discontinuing those no longer leading to a set goal	Focusing on dictionary long enough to find word or shifting to other source when word cannot be located

Table 52–8 • Satisfaction Control

Form	Explanation	Examples
Gratification delay	Ability to postpone rewards	Studying for test to get pleasure from good grades
Appetite dampening	Reducing intensity of material/experiential wants	Doing homework while wanting to go shopping
Appetite termination	Being able to cease or curtail gratification	Being able to stop playing and start other activity
Motivation	Feeling motivated to focus	Wanting to study
Focus under moderate-to-low excitation conditions	Being able to feel satisfied in the absence of high levels of excitement	Behaving well under peaceful conditions in the current environment

SATISFACTION CONTROL

Children are likely to vary in what it takes to satisfy their attention (Table 52–8). The processing controls operate best under conditions in which they are felt by their user to be fulfilling or gratifying in some way. The controls are likely to operate most effectively in contexts in which the individual derives interest and a reasonable level of excitement from the content at hand. Certainly, not all information input and daily experience can be romantically attractive and fun. It is possible and common for incoming data to be important but not exciting or especially alluring to the processor. Nevertheless, it is worthy of attention. Satisfaction control enables an individual to exercise good processing control even when the inputs are not particularly exciting. Thus, satisfaction control becomes an important ingredient of intrinsic motivation. Furthermore, it allows for delay of gratification, for the dampening of immediate wants and appetites, and for the allocation of mental energy to the processing of relatively low interest information or stimuli. In other words, this control facilitates a sense of satisfaction and fulfillment that can occur under conditions of attention without high excitation.

Dysfunctions of Satisfaction Control

Many children with attention deficits have been described as "insatiable."

They are exceedingly hard to satisfy. They crave intensity and feel unfulfilled and restless unless the conditions surrounding them are conducive to high levels of fun and immediate gratification. Their insatiability can impede the function of their processing controls, because they are unable to attend effectively in a classroom setting unless the subject matter is particularly entertaining.

There are two common forms of insatiability: material and experiential. Children harboring material insatiability want *things* much of the time. When they want something, they crave it. They may have great difficulty postponing gratification, needing to have the object of their yearning immediately. Yet, almost as soon as they get what they want, they start the quest for another material acquisition. They have trouble functioning when they want something; they can wear out their parents until they receive what they have been seeking. They are often accumulators and collectors, because they appear to lust after and hoard material possessions.

Children with experiential insatiability seem to hunger for intensity of experience. They want excitement, and when none is available at the moment, they are likely to create the excitement, often by committing provocative acts, just "to stir things up." This phenomenon is associated with some loss of behavioral control. Their need for excitement also impairs concentration in school. In a sense, they are distracted by their own appetites. They are able to concentrate, but only when the material is sufficiently compelling or romantically attractive to them. Unfortunately, no educational system can sustain such a high level of romantic attractiveness throughout the school day. There is a great deal of material that simply is not exciting but needs to be learned nonetheless. Children with experiential insatiability experience their greatest difficulty with such relatively low motivational content.

EXAMPLE

Ramon is a 7-year-old boy in the second grade. He has seemed to acquire early reading, spelling, and mathematics abilities fairly well, but Ramon has had chronic behavior problems in the classroom and at home. He is described as restless, provocative, and whiny. Ramon wants things all of the time, and as soon as he obtains what he seeks, he immediately becomes fixated on further acquisitions. Ramon loves excitement. When things are quiet, he is capable of creating tense and turbulent moments by saying and doing things that are inappropriate and unsettling. He never knows when to stop. His teacher and school principal view him as a "troublemaker." His mother describes Ramon as a boy with an incredibly active mind that needs constant stimulation to feel satisfied.

As insatiable children reach adolescence, they are likely to engage in risk-taking behaviors, which may help to satisfy their insatiable hunger for excitement. This trait also places them at risk for substance abuse and some antisocial behaviors. Insatiability during childhood and adolescence may ultimately evolve into productive drive and ambition in an adult. Thus, the trait is not necessarily negative, but it carries with it some substantial risk.

Production Controls

This section delineates the control over output, the regulatory effects of the production controls. Processing controls and production controls are highly interdependent, in that effective output often depends on accurate and efficient interpretation of information. Likewise, production is a way of learning. People are constantly processing or interpreting for themselves and others what they are doing. Thus, processing and production enhance each other's roles.

The production controls govern the multiple pathways of output; they regulate the creation of products (such as writing reports for school), the implementation of

behaviors (such as acting appropriately in class), and the formation and nurturance of relationships (such as maintaining a close friendship). Much of what is included under the category of production controls coincides with what is called *executive functions*. However, there is considerable disagreement among investigators and clinicians regarding the components of these varied managerial functions of the mind. Denckla (1996) provides a good review of the issues. Five production controls are described in this section: (1) previewing control, (2) facilitation and inhibition control, (3) tempo control, (4) self-monitoring control, and (5) reinforcement control.

PREVIEWING CONTROL

Previewing control (Table 52–9) is a function that helps predict the outcomes of planned actions. As such, it represents the mind's facility with forethought and foresight. Denckla (1996) refers to this form of control as "attention to the future." It enables us to anticipate an occurrence or event in order to plan a response likely to engender a positive outcome. Thus, through previewing, an individual is able to look ahead, to estimate outcomes, and to be ready for upcoming circumstances and challenges.

Good previewing helps a student academically in many ways. She or he can have an idea of what a report will be like once the topic is selected. A student uses previewing to study for a test, to estimate answers in mathematics, and to decide what books and papers to bring home to accomplish various assignments. In the latter case, the student forms a picture of the evening "study scene" and fills in the materials needed.

Previewing helps with transitions. By picturing what is coming next, a student can be better prepared to move smoothly into a new activity.

Previewing plays a significant role in behavioral adaptation as well. It enables children to consider the "What if I . . . ?" question. "What if I say this, will I get into

Table 52–9 • Previewing Control

Form	Explanation	Examples
Quantitative prediction	Estimating final numbers in calculations	Knowing roughly the answer to a math problem
Social prediction	Foreseeing effects of one's actions on relationships	Predicting whether others will laugh at a joke
Behavioral prediction	Foreseeing the consequences of an action	Realizing that punishment results when one cheats
Anticipation	Having an awareness of what might come next	Recognizing that someone is about to start teasing
Product outcome vision	Having an idea of what a product will be like when finished	Picturing what an art project will look like when it is completed
Transition readiness	Looking ahead to prepare for a new activity/challenge	Knowing what is needed to take to class

trouble?" "What if I fail to hand in this assignment, what will happen to me and how will my parents react when they find out?" These kinds of questions also relate closely to social skills. To relate effectively to others, it is necessary to keep predicting with accuracy the reactions of others to things one is about to say or do in their presence. "What if I tell my friends that I caught a huge fish last weekend? Will they think I'm excellent or will they think I boast too much?"

Dysfunctions of Previewing Control

Children with poor previewing may endure considerable academic trouble. They may have no idea of how a report or project is going to turn out; instead, they proceed with little sense of a destination or outcome. This can lead to disorganized output that strays from the topic and has poorly defined goals. Some of these children have trouble estimating answers in mathematics, such that their responses on assignments and quizzes can be bizarre and nowhere near correct.

Weak previewing also engenders behavioral maladaptation in some children. They commit aggressive or antisocial acts without first predicting the responses of others. In other words, they get into trouble because they did not foresee the consequences of their actions. They may also have trouble with anticipation, so that it may be hard for them to prepare an appropriate behavior in advance of an occurrence. They may not be able to think, for example, "I heard my new science teacher is very strict, so I better not fool around much in his class." Social anticipation may be impaired as well, preventing a child from thinking, "I bet she's going to invite me to her party, but I don't want to go. What should I say when she asks me?" Because of their weak previewing, such children seem to be taken by surprise; they are unready to respond in the most appropriate manner.

Many children with previewing problems have trouble with transitions. Because they fail to foresee next events, they are apt to lack the materials or preparation needed to deal with them. They may arrive in class without a pencil, come home with the wrong books, and be reluctant to move from one activity to another because they have not thought about what the transition might entail. Sometimes their lack of readiness creates in them a high level of anxiety at times of transition.

FACILITATION AND INHIBITION CONTROL

Just as saliency determination control facilitates the sorting out of possibilities for the uptake of information, facilitation and inhibition control (Table 52–10) allows one to review possibilities for output or action, facilitating the best possibility while inhibiting the others. Whereas saliency determination control allows for *selective attention*, facilitation and inhibition control promotes *selective intention*.

Facilitation and inhibition control enables an individual to review options for behavior, for verbal communication, for undertaking a task, or for various forms of problem solving and then to facilitate the possibility that is most likely to succeed while inhibiting (i.e., eliminating or postponing) the other choices. The concept of response inhibition is closely related and involves the capacity to delay or abort first reactions to stimuli, at least long enough to consider other possible responses. For example, in solving a word problem in arithmetic, instead of using the first method to come to mind, it might be wise to wonder, "What are the ways I could solve this problem and what is the very best way?" If a child pushes and shoves a fellow student, the victim may react immediately and aggressively or else make use of facilitation and inhibition control to quickly review the behavioral options of the moment and select the best one for implementation.

The review of options and selection of best choices can be important for problem solving, for coping with stress, and for thinking through various study skills and learning strategies (e.g., "Let's see, what's the best way to remember these French vocabulary words?").

Facilitation and inhibition control also relates to the level and efficiency of motor activity. When operating well, this control inhibits excessive motor activity, thereby conserving physical energy. It also serves to inhibit muscle groups that need not participate in a particular action, while

Table 52–10 • Facilitation and Inhibition Control

Form	Explanation	Examples
Response inhibition	The delaying of a response long enough to review additional options	Not reacting immediately when insulted by a peer
Temptation resistance	Avoidance of seductive but ill-advised activities	Refraining from smoking in early adolescence
Stress management	Reviewing possible solutions when feeling sad or apprehensive; developing frustration tolerance	Thinking of various ways to catch up with overdue work
Strategy development and problem solving	Considering various approaches before undertaking task/project	Figuring out how to study for a particular test in school
Verbal regulation	Thinking about how and whether to communicate a message	Modifying or canceling a statement to avoid hurting someone's feelings
Voice control	Adjusting the loudness of one's voice	Not yelling or shouting needlessly
Behavioral regulation	Canceling or curtailing an inappropriate/ineffective behavior	Reducing one's aggression on the playground
Affective control	Separating an emotional response from the immediate emotional content of the stimulus	Trying not to display automatic, immediate anger at a person who shows anger toward you
Motor regulation	Control over the level and efficiency of motor output	Slowing down when starting to become hyperactive

simultaneously activating those muscle groups that are critical to the performance. Such neuromotor facilitation and inhibition potentiates smooth and efficient motor output.

Dysfunctions of Facilitation and Inhibition Control

Various forms of disinhibition can be especially problematic during childhood. Children may exhibit verbal, behavioral, affective, and/or motor control weaknesses. Thus, they may get into difficulty for saying things they should not have said (and would not have said had they thought about them). Analogously, they may transgress in school and at home because they keep acting without sufficient premeditation. They may also reveal a lack of response inhibition and temptation resistance, tending to act and react in a way that reflects the first possibility that comes to mind rather than engaging in a review of behavioral options.

Some students with weak facilitation and inhibition functions may reveal a low frustration tolerance. They may "fly off the handle" or lose interest when things are not going their way. In some cases, this is a direct result of not actually having alternatives or strategies that can be thought about to deal with setbacks or frustration.

Weak facilitation and inhibition control can also exact an academic toll. A child may solve a mathematics problem or meet some other scholastic challenge by doing the first thing that comes to mind rather than surveying the possible problem-solving routes and selecting the best one. Poor study skills may be a result of a chronic inability to seek best methods before engaging in an academic pursuit.

A lack of sufficient motor inhibition may result in hyperactivity or a tendency to move around too quickly and without purpose. However, not all children with attention deficits display this phenomenon. Some children with attention deficits are indeed hyperactive, whereas others are normally active or even, in some cases, underactive. Of interest is the fact that the population of normally active and underactive children with attention deficits includes a higher proportion of females than is seen in the hyperactive group. Also, older adolescents (of both genders) with attention deficits often do not show signs of hyperactivity.

Weak motor facilitation and inhibition also can result in motor inefficiency. Overflow movements, a tendency for some children to engage in a motor act and have it mirrored in the mouth or opposite limb may be a manifestation of deficient facilitation and inhibition. That is, instead of activating only the specific muscle groups needed to accomplish a task, the central nervous system induces movement in superfluous muscle groups. Sometimes it is possible to observe an affected child playing a sport, riding a bicycle, or running and detect all of the extraneous movement that occurs as a result of weak motor inhibition.

Other possible signs of poor facilitation and inhibition include loud speech, emotional overreaction to stimuli, tactless responses, and generally deficient problem-solving skills.

Barkley (1997) has evolved an encompassing theoretical basis for attentional difficulty. Limiting his discussion to the label "ADHD" (comprising children who have attention deficits plus hyperactivity), he cites a fundamental deficiency in inhibitory functions as a central mechanism. Barkley's formulation is very similar to problems with the production controls.

TEMPO CONTROL

In general, the production controls enable a person to function slowly and deliberatively. They decelerate responses to allow for more deliberative, thought-out actions. Tempo control (Table 52–11) involves several closely related forms of regulation. First, tempo control entails the selection and application of the appropriate rate for completing a task or engaging in an activity. The pace should not be excessively fast or slow; it should be matched to task demands and available time.

Second, tempo control relates to the synchronization of multiple functions. This control is essential, because virtually all activities require the collaborative participation of multiple neurodevelopmental functions. These functions need to operate together at the same or otherwise compatible rates. For example, the flow of ideas that occur while speaking needs to be synchronized with the encoding of those ideas in language (which, in turn, demands the synchronization of word finding with sentence formulation with narrative organization).

Finally, tempo control is associated with an appreciation of time in general. It helps to regulate the allocation of time to tasks at hand, the prediction of time required, and the ability to use time as a medium to facilitate productivity (i.e., time management). Tempo control also instills a sense of "step-wisdom," the conceptualization that many activities need to be undertaken in a series of steps or stages rather than all at once. Such "step-wisdom" greatly enhances productivity and makes sizable tasks more manageable.

Dysfunctions of Tempo Control

Tempo control difficulties are commonly concomitant with attentional dysfunction. These children may do many things much too quickly, thereby committing careless errors and performing at a level inferior to what would be seen with more deliberative pacing. Frequently, they may appear to

Table 52–11 • Tempo Control

Form	Explanation	Examples
Pacing	Performing at a rate appropriate to the task and available time	Using right amount of time on a test
Synchronization of functions	Inducing functions to operate at same rate during a task	Synchronizing motor function, language, ideation, and memory while writing
"Stepwisdom"	Being able to break down and perform tasks in stages	Doing a project in manageable steps over time
Time management	Appreciating and working with time intervals	Meeting deadlines; allocating time for homework

be in a hurry to get things over with. At other times, they may operate too slowly, seldom functioning at a rate that is well matched to current conditions and needs.

Many children with tempo control problems have a diminished appreciation of time and its optimal utilization. They may have trouble staging tasks, difficulty meeting deadlines (procrastinating endlessly), and problems scheduling or allocating time to meet demands. They may be said to be in a "time warp." Frequently, these children are apt to falter when undertaking tasks that require the synchronization of multiple functions, at which times they are likely to feel overwhelmed and discouraged. Most commonly this is manifest when they are expected to write large amounts. They may encounter problems trying to synchronize the multiple subskills and functions needed for efficient and satisfying written output (see Chapter 71).

Hyperactivity and Impulsivity

It is common for children with attention deficits to be described as "hyperactive" and/or "impulsive." These terms correspond to some of the control problems already described. A child may be hyperactive because of several control weaknesses. Hyperactive behavior may sometimes stem from a child's need to "wake himself up," to become more aroused and alert through physical activity. Hyperactivity may also represent a form of motor disinhibition or it can be a manifestation of poor tempo control. Impulsivity is likely to represent an amalgam of poor previewing, weak facilitation and inhibition, and problems with the control of tempo. Thus, an impulsive child is apt to have trouble looking ahead and predicting an outcome before acting. She or he may also manifest difficulty inhibiting first responses along with problems adjusting the tempo sufficiently to reflect before undertaking a cognitive/academic task, responding with a behavior, and/or putting forth a social initiative. Hence, the child is perceived (correctly) as impulsive.

SELF-MONITORING CONTROL

Self-monitoring serves as a quality control mechanism (Table 52–12) because it enables an individual to know how she is doing during an activity and how she just did right after the activity. Self-monitoring allows for self-regulation.

Table 52–12 • Self-Monitoring Control

Form	Explanation	Examples
Social feedback reception	Reading cues that indicate social success or failure	Noticing when anyone else laughs when one acts silly
Academic error detection	Detecting work errors/proofreading	Recognizing a spelling error while or after writing
Behavioral regulation	Noting the effects of one's behaviors	Realizing that one is getting into trouble on the playground
Motor feedback	Sensing the location and activity of one's muscles	Localizing fingers during writing (see Chapter 53)

It affords the child an opportunity to get back on course when straying from the accomplishment of a goal. For example, while writing a report, a child may notice that she is no longer on the topic she set out to pursue. While driving a car, the driver might notice that he or she is slightly out of the driving lane and then make a precise correction. A child who is talking in class may recognize that the teacher is becoming irritated and may then stop the behavior. So it is that self-monitoring constitutes a feedback loop, a servomechanism that fosters quality control during and immediately after various activities and the creation of products.

There are many forms of self-monitoring that are needed for optimal behavior, interpersonal relationships, and school performance. The ability to detect one's own errors plays an indispensable academic role in all subject areas. Behavioral and social self-monitoring are needed to comply with rules of discipline and to relate effectively to others. Human neuromotor systems require constant feedback; while the child plays a sport or writes, the involved muscle groups need to report back to the brain on their current locations, so that they can be "told" where to go next (Chapter 53). These self-monitoring activities need to occur "on line" and post hoc. That is, there is a need to know how a task or activity is proceeding while it is being undertaken and there is a need to evaluate its degree of success or failure once it is completed. Self-monitoring control, when working properly, serves these purposes.

Dysfunctions of Self-Monitoring

Poor or absent self-monitoring can have a range of effects on behavior and academic performance. Affected students are prone to make frequent careless errors when they work. They have difficulty with proofreading, a process they often vociferously avoid. They may diverge markedly from the directions for an assignment without realizing that they are no longer doing what they were instructed to do. Their lack of awareness prevents them from self-righting while performing. Some students are chronically unable to evaluate their own performance; after taking a test in school, such a student may report having done extremely well, while actually having failed the examination. Their inability to know how they are doing over time can make it difficult for such students to allocate effort, to know, for example, that they will need to study harder for the next test because they are getting farther and farther behind in a course.

EXAMPLE

Alma is 18 years old and a senior in high school. She has had a lifelong history of problems with organization. It is hard for her to keep track of time. She is late for everything and seems to have no ability to do things in a logical, stepwise manner. Schedules, deadlines, and work plans make little sense to her. She does everything at the last minute. In addition, Alma has trouble knowing how she is doing. Right after a test in school, she often comments that the examination was "cinchy," only to discover subsequently that she received a failing grade. She seems to have problems evaluating how she is doing with any undertaking. Alma has never shown signs of behavioral problems or hyperactivity. Recently, Alma was in a serious automobile accident during which she "totaled" the family car and was speeding and taking needless risks without actually realizing it. Her parents wonder whether it will ever be safe for Alma to drive.

Behavioral and social difficulties can result from poor self-monitoring. A child may keep repeating an action that was initially amusing without detecting the anguish of those around him. Some of these children seem oblivious to social feedback cues, such as can be read in the facial expressions, vocal inflections, and body movements of those with whom one is interacting.

Poor feedback from muscles can result in writing difficulties (finger agnosia), while diminished body position sense can be one source of gross motor dysfunction in some children with poor self-monitoring due to attention deficits.

REINFORCEMENT CONTROL

The extent to which previous experience is used to guide current output is within the domain of reinforcement control (Table 52–13). Just as previewing represents foresight, reinforcement control makes use of hindsight. It enables individuals to base current responses and actions on previous (negative and positive) experience. This regulatory component enables an individual to learn from punishment and reward, to be sensitive to positive and negative reinforcement. Such sensitivity facilitates the use of previous outcomes of one's actions to influence current or anticipated actions. If a child behaved in a way that got her into trouble yesterday, she had best not repeat that pattern of behavior this afternoon. If a student found an excellent way to solve a particular mathematics problem last week, that method should then be used to solve a similar arithmetic challenge he now faces. That is, the new method that led to success and gratification should be reinforcing enough to be included in the student's future repertoire of strategies. If a particular experience has occurred repeatedly, the child might even derive a rule from such past experience, for example, "Whenever Mom's in a bad mood, hold off on

telling her you lost something on the way to school." Through good reinforcement control, past experiences connect to current decision making. In this way, precedents and learned rules can help to steer behavior and academic output.

Dysfunctions of Reinforcement Control

There are many children with attention deficits who are described as weakly reinforceable. They get into trouble one day and then reenact similar violations shortly thereafter. At times, they seem not to react to punishment. Likewise they may show a diminished response to praise or rewards. Organized reward systems for good behavior or academic productivity may be short-lived in these cases, because the children reveal their underresponsiveness to such positive and negative reinforcement programs. Their actions often seem disconnected from previous experience. They simply are not making sufficient use of the outcomes of past behaviors to determine current behavioral output.

Many children with weak reinforcement control encounter learning difficulties that are based, in part, on their inadequate use of past successes and failures to shape their approaches to learning. They often appear unable to assimilate new techniques or strategic approaches that have facilitated work when they have tried them in the past. As a result, they do too many things the hard way. They do not acquire a rapidly growing repertoire of academic output tactics that should be emergent from direct experience. Such children may also reveal a reduced appreciation of rules that govern behavior. They may have trouble generalizing from one situation to another, a process that is greatly facilitated by developing rules and applying them in relevant contexts or circumstances.

Table 52–13 • Reinforcement Control

Form	Explanation	Examples
Sensitivity to reward and punishment	Tendency of an individual to respond adequately to reward and/or punishment	Not repeating an action for which discipline resulted yesterday
Rule guidance	Ability to use experience to form rules that guide current and future output	Using the fact that certain behaviors inevitably lead to certain positive or negative reactions from others
Academic outcome use	Incorporation of academic methods that have worked	Using a study technique that worked well on last quiz

---

> ***The Attention Controls: Some General Considerations***
>
> Some general points should help refine one's thinking about the attention controls and their breakdowns:
>
> 1. The individual attention controls are highly interdependent. Thus, effective previewing enhances facilitation and inhibition, good self-monitoring makes an individual more reinforceable, and well-regulated mental energy control helps to establish optimal levels of cognitive activation. Consequently, the attention controls compose an overall system rather than a set of isolated regulatory functions. This is analogous to many other systems in the human body. For example, in the cardiovascular system, the heart and the aorta are distinct entities, but their functions are tightly interdependent such that a problem in one can cause damage to the other, and a strength in one can help to compensate for a problem in the other.
> 2. An individual attention control, such as saliency determination, may be weak while others appear to function adequately. In such cases, one should consider sources of difficulty aside from generalized attention deficits. For example, saliency determination may be weak because a child has a language disorder and reduced understanding of certain subject matter; it is impossible to make good determinations of saliency when understanding is very poor.

3. The attention controls may work under certain conditions but not in other contexts. A child may have problems with attention at school but not at home. In part, this too may result from problems processing information and meeting expectations in school. A child's attention controls are apt to reveal higher-than-usual effectiveness: under high-interest conditions (e.g., while working on a hobby), when utilizing strengths (e.g., while a highly skilled athlete plays a sport), and when motivation levels are elevated (e.g., while seeking a short-term reward). A child's attention controls may deteriorate when he or she is placed in a setting that is ill matched to the child's personality, current neurodevelopmental profile, or cultural background. Breakdowns in attention controls can result when a teacher's teaching style is disparate from a child's manner of learning. This is especially common when attention is somewhat weak to begin with.

4. The attention controls collaborate closely with other neurodevelopmental functions in all activities. Sometimes there are distinct breakdowns in the relationships between attention and other functions. For example, attention and memory may not interact properly. At times it can be hard to decide whether a child is not remembering because she is not concentrating or if she is not concentrating because she is having trouble stabilizing information in short-term memory. Similarly, interactions and potential breakdowns at the junctions exist between attention and all of the other neurodevelopmental functions. The production controls relate constantly to higher-order cognitive functions in the generation of rules, the application of strategies, the use of problem-solving skills, and the development of metacognition.

5. Acute or chronic anxiety can interfere significantly with the attention controls. For instance, mental energy may be diverted or exhausted when a child is worried or intensely preoccupied with personal problems or fears. It can be difficult sometimes to differentiate between attention deficits and affective disorders during childhood.

6. When assessing a child's attention controls, it is critical to ask the following questions: Does this child have a breakdown in one, several, or most of the attention controls? (The more controls affected, the more likely it is that the child has primary attention deficits as opposed to attention deficits mainly as a result of a processing problem or anxiety.) Are there indications that this child's attentional problems manifest themselves only in certain contexts or situations? Are there contexts in which the attention controls work especially well? Are there any forms of processing (e.g., language or visual-spatial) that either bring out or minimize the child's problems with attention? To what extent is anxiety impairing the operation of the attention controls? These and other questions form the basis for assessment of a child with signs of attentional difficulty.

The Attention Controls and Their Brain Locations

There is still much to be learned regarding the neuroanatomy of attention. In recent years, however, there has grown a body of knowledge that has helped in the understanding of which parts of the human brain are responsible (or, more often, partially responsible) for each control.

The mental energy controls are largely under the influence of nuclei located in the brainstem. Specifically,

the reticular activating system and the locus ceruleus are centers of activity that contain nerve cells that are rich in the neurotransmitter dopamine. These cells play a significant role in promoting "nonspecific arousal." That is, they activate higher cortical cells with no specific target in mind; they simply wake up consciousness. Interestingly these brainstem cells have rich connections with the prefrontal cortex (Pennington et al, 1996), which governs the production controls.

The processing controls are the most diffuse in their localization. That is, their functions are carried out in various remote brain sites. The controls pertaining to specific modalities (such as visual or verbal processing) are located in association areas adjacent to the parts of the brain responsible for perceiving those specific forms of input. Mirsky (1996) describes components or factors that compose attention and has investigated their neuroanatomic connections. Table 52–14 summarizes some of his findings.

The aforementioned functional localization is not always the case. As Mirsky (1996) notes, "the system organization allows for shared responsibility for attentional function, which implies that the specialization is not absolute and that some structures may substitute for others in the event of injury."

The production controls are more centrally located than the processing controls. For the most part, these controls have their headquarters in the prefrontal cortex. The production controls closely parallel what are sometimes called the executive functions. Many studies have documented problems with these controls in patients who have had damage to this part of the brain. As Tranel, Anderson, and Benton (1995) note, ". . . there is rarely a discussion of disturbances of executive functions that does not make reference to dysfunction of prefrontal brain regions."

Assessment of Attention

There are many different ways to assess the attention controls and uncover attention deficits in children. Each

Table 52–14 • Anatomic Sites of Some Processing Controls

Function (Mirsky's Terms)	Related Attention Controls	Neuroanatomic Sites
Focusing on environmental events	Saliency determination, depth of processing	Superior temporal and inferior parietal cortices, plus structures in the corpus striatum
Sustaining focus	Focal maintenance	Rostral midbrain structures, as well as other thalamic and brainstem areas
Shifting focus	Focal maintenance	Prefrontal cortex, including the anterior cingulate gyrus
Encoding or *stabilizing*	Processing depth and cognitive activation	Hippocampus and amygdala

has its distinct advantages and disadvantages. Considerable caution is called for in interpreting the results of assessments of attention. Many biases can distort the findings.

RETROSPECTIVELY COMPLETED QUESTIONNAIRES

Questionnaires are usually behavioral checklists that are filled out by parents and teachers. In general, they correspond to the symptoms of "ADD" as delineated in the *Diagnostic and Statistical Manual of the American Psychiatric Association.* The Conner's Questionnaire (short and long forms) is the most commonly used. Most of these questionnaires are not sensitive to the cognitive effects of attention deficits and therefore are apt to detect mainly, if not exclusively, those individuals whose weak attention controls are precipitating behavior problems. Additionally, these tools fail to look closely at the status of the individual controls of attention. I have developed a section of the ANSER System questionnaires (Levine, 1996) to meet the need for amore fine-grained analysis. The ANSER System questionnaires contain separate forms that are completed by a child's teachers and parents as well as a form on which children age 9 years and older rate their own attention. The ANSER System also closely examines various neurodevelopmental functions (Chapter 53) as well as many components of academic performance, health, and overall behav-

```
┌─────────────────────────────────────┐
│            RATING KEY               │
│                                     │
│  3 = Never or almost never evident  │
│  2 = Occasionally evident           │
│  1 = Evident often                  │
│  0 = Evident all or almost all the time │
└─────────────────────────────────────┘
```

PART I — MENTAL ENERGY CONTROLS
(Alertness, Arousal, Mental Effort)

	Con	Trait	Effects on Schoolwork				Effects on Behavior				Effects on Peers			
			0	1	2	3	0	1	2	3	0	1	2	3
AC01	AL	Has trouble staying alert												
AC02	AL	Attention hard to attract												
AC03	AL	Loses focus unless very interested												
AC04	CO	Has unpredictable behavior/schoolwork												
AC05	CO	Has excellent days and poor days												
AC06	CO	Keeps "tuning in and tuning out"												
AC07	ME	Has trouble finishing things he/she starts												
AC08	ME	Has difficulty getting started with homework												
AC09	ME	Has a hard time exerting effort/doing work												
AC10	SL	Has trouble falling/staying asleep at night												
AC11	SL	Has trouble getting up in the morning												
AC12	SL	Looks tired												

Abbreviation Key

Con	Attention controls	Forms of mental regulation
AL	Alertness control	Being able to become and remain alert
CO	Consistency control	Performing and behaving in a consistent manner
ME	Mental effort control	Working, putting forth effort
SL	Sleep control	Sleeping well at night, awake enough during the day

Figure 52–2. Part of the ANSER system Parent Questionnaire for elementary school-aged children. The grid is one portion of the section on attention. The items refer to the specific controls of attention. Similar items are used on the ANSER system questionnaires for teachers and for the children themselves. (From Levine MD: The ANSER System. Cambridge, MA, Educators Publishing Service, 1996.)

ATTENTION CHECKPOINT FOUR (Visual Processing)

OBSERVATION	SCORE			DESCRIPTION
Impulsivity	0	1	2	Started task in an unplanned manner or answered too quickly—compromising quality
Frenetic tempo	0	1	2	Paced task too quickly
Poor attention to detail	0	1	2	Missed relevant detail during task
Distractibility	0	1	2	Became distracted during task or seemed not to listen
Mental fatigue	0	1	2	Yawned, stretched, otherwise showed fatigue during task
Deterioration over time	0	1	2	Lost focus as task progressed or had difficulty sustaining attention
Performance inconsistency	0	1	2	Showed erratic error pattern during task
Poor monitoring	0	1	2	Performance impaired by poor monitoring or made careless errors
Gross overactivity	0	1	2	Displayed extraneous large muscle motion during task, e.g., appeared restless, left seat
Fidgetiness	0	1	2	Displayed extraneous small muscle motion during task, e.g., appeared fidgety, squirmy

Figure 52–3. This grid is completed by a clinician performing a neurodevelopmental examination (PEERAMID 2). The examiner makes these judgments at four points during the assessment. In this way it is possible to detect students whose attentional problems are most obvious when they are confronted with certain specific demands (such as the need to process language). (From Pediatric Neurodevelopmental Examinations [PEEX 2 and PEERAMID 2]. Cambridge, MA, Educators Publishing Service, 1995.)

ior. A sample section of the ANSER System is shown in Figure 52–2.

DIRECT MEASURES OF ATTENTION

Direct methods of measuring attention are often computerized and tend to detect weaknesses of vigilance, impulsivity, deterioration of attention over time, and weak focus on detail. Examples include the Gordon Diagnostic Test and the TOVA (Test of Vigilance and Attention). The vigilance tests on PEEX 2 (Pediatric Early Elementary Examination) and PEERAMID 2 (Pediatric Examination of Educational Readiness at Middle Childhood) represent examples of less extensive direct tests of attention (Levine, 1995). Largely for research purposes, there exist a multitude of tests that relate to the specific controls of attention. These include tests of vigilance or continuous performance, assessments of impulsivity versus reflectivity, and a range of tests for cognitive flexibility, strategy use, and other dimensions of production control. A number of these tests have been extensively reviewed by Barkley (1994).

GUIDED OBSERVATIONS OF ATTENTION

Guided observations of attention stress the prospective inspection of attention over time. The Teacher's View (from the SCHOOLS ATTUNED Project) is an instrument used in the classroom to guide teachers' observations of patterns of attention. During the performance of the pediatric neurodevelopmental examinations (PEEX 2 and PEERAMID 2), there are systematic observations of attention during the

performance of specific tasks. The observation grid that is used is shown in Figure 52–3.

Precautions Regarding the Assessment of Attention

1. Some questionnaires may be more calibrated to detect behavior problems and less sensitive to the cognitive/academic manifestations of attentional dysfunction. These questionnaires may tend to identify all children with serious behavior problems as having "ADD." After all, it is hard even to imagine a child with serious misbehavior who is seldom impulsive, who concentrates well, and who does not talk out of turn.

2. Questionnaire scoring systems may not be valid. Many questionnaires are based on the underlying (questionable) assumption that the number of traits manifest determines whether or not a child has an attention deficit. However, a child may have relatively few incapacitating symptoms and not "qualify" as having attention deficits. Cutoff points may be arbitrary and not clinically valid or helpful.

3. The validation of attention questionnaires makes use of imperfect methods. There is no gold standard against which to establish their accuracy.

4. The agreement between observers is often poor. A school questionnaire may suggest the presence of attentional difficulty, whereas the parent questionnaire may paint a different picture of the child. Even individual teachers may reveal disagreement; similar disparities may be found between parents.

5. Direct tests of attention may be too dependent on the current state of the child. Because attention deficits repre-

sent a chronic problem and because performance inconsistency is the rule, an isolated test of attention may not detect the problem. Also, such tests assess only a few of the attention controls; manifestations such as weak reinforceability and poor previewing are not included. Furthermore, some children may be romantically attracted to the testing situation, as a result of which their attentional difficulties are obscured by the high motivational experience of the test itself. In general, children with attention deficits perform much better on a one-to-one encounter than they do in a group; this too can distort the results of direct testing.

6. Direct observations also can be problematic. They may be highly subjective and too dependent upon the tolerance, the astuteness, and the level of experience of the observer. Attention can be affected by the complexity and level of interest derived from the content and expectations a child is confronting. Some children, for example, may exhibit attentional difficulty in settings that are highly verbal and detail laden but not in other environments. During testing or direct observations, the evaluator must always take into consideration the particular characteristics of the setting that may be influencing attentional function.

The most valid and reliable assessments of attention are likely to be those that combine several methods, such as the use of questionnaires (completed by more than one source) plus direct observations.

FOCUS OF ASSESSMENT

Assessment should be focused on evaluating the status of the specific attention controls as they affect academic performance, behavioral adaptation, and social interaction. An accurate description of strengths and weaknesses in the specific controls is likely to be far more helpful than a score or a label. This description of attentional controls can then be integrated with descriptions of the child's strengths and weaknesses. Attention should never be assessed in isolation. It is critically important to evaluate a child's attention along with his or her current competency in other areas of neurodevelopmental function (Chapter 53). A child who has attention deficits plus a language disorder needs very different management from a child who has an attention deficit in the presence of strong language abilities. Most children who have attention deficit also harbor one or more other areas of neurodevelopmental dysfunction. To manage the attention deficit without tending to the associated dysfunctions is likely to result in eventual treatment failure.

The end product of an assessment of attention should be a descriptive profile of the child's attention controls, their strengths and deficiencies. In most cases it is not possible to decide on a cause for the child's attention deficits. Nevertheless, it is important to seek possible causes or closely associated conditions that may be present.

Management of Attention Deficits

The management of weak attention controls must be one part of the management of a child's overall neurodevelop-

mental profile. The following discussion contains suggestions for the management of the attentional issues specifically.

DEMYSTIFICATION

Children with attention deficits can benefit from a substantial emphasis on learning about the attention controls. They need to understand the workings of normal attention as well as the specific breakdowns that are causing them difficulty in life. They should acquire a vocabulary regarding attention. The concepts and terminology they learn should be used as well by their teachers and parents.

Demystification can be achieved by having the child read relevant information about attention. *Keeping a Head in School* (Levine, 1990) (for middle and high school students) and *All Kinds of Minds* (Levine, 1994a) (for elementary school children) may be helpful. The Concentration Cockpit (Fig. 52–4) has been developed to help children conceptualize the attention controls by likening them to the controls in an airplane cockpit. Children rate themselves on each of the controls by marking their pointer with a magic marker in each meter. The adult explaining the controls can document the child's responses in an administration booklet, which can augment assessment as well as demystification. For older adolescents and young adults, a more straightforward explanation is used with graphic representation (Fig. 52–5).

Demystification needs to be reviewed periodically with a clinician, parent, and/or teacher. Children should feel comfortable reporting specific examples of times when their attention controls have worked well, as well as instances when breakdowns have occurred. Having provided demystification, the clinician or teacher is in a much better position to enact bypass strategies and interventions at the breakdown points. Such management techniques are likely to be most effective when the child understands the reasons for their use. Thus, demystification strongly fortifies other forms of intervention.

BYPASS STRATEGIES AND INTERVENTIONS AT THE BREAKDOWN POINTS

Once the attention controls that need to be worked on are identified, it is possible to devise specific strategies, some of which bypass weak attention controls and some of which directly strengthen the attention controls. The following suggestions are a starting point for teachers and clinicians, who can add to the list the techniques that they find most effective in the settings in which they work. The measures discussed herein are apt to be most effective when the child understands what each applied intervention is intended to accomplish. In other words, demystification is an essential accompaniment of each management strategy.

I. Dysfunctions of mental energy control
   A. Inconsistent alertness
      1. A child may benefit from preferential seating in class. Being close to the teacher may help a student sustain alertness.
      2. There should be careful management of any

THE CONCENTRATION COCKPIT
Attention Controls for Behavior, Learning, and Getting Along with People

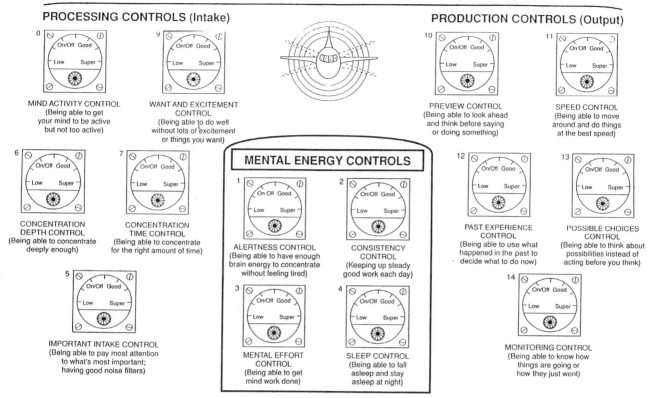

Figure 52–4. The concentration cockpit is used to "demystify" children who have attentional problems. An examiner reviews each of the meters on this diagram, following which the child draws in his or her needle, indicating whether that particular control is perceived as weak or strong by the child. The concentration cockpit is available in a Mylar-coated poster, which children can write on with a felt-tipped pen. (From Levine M: The Concentration Cockpit. Cambridge, MA, Educators Publishing Service, 1995.)

sleep and arousal imbalance, including consistent bedtimes, the use of white background noise for sleep, reassurance of the child to alleviate anxiety over sleep, and, in some cases, medication to facilitate falling asleep (Catapres in small doses at bedtime has been recommended and used for this purpose—see Chapter 82)

3. Teachers and parents should aim for "chunk size reduction," frequent breaks from homework, and in class, shorter assignments.
4. It is good to encourage the use of hands for physical activity (modeling clay, doodling) while concentrating; moving feet or tapping them rhythmically may also help.
5. Stimulant medication may significantly increase alertness (see Chapter 82).
6. Exploitation of strong modalities/affinities in school can strengthen focus.

B. Inconsistent effort
  1. It is good to avoid using inconsistency as a "moral" issue (i.e., "we know you can do better; we've seen you do it when you really want to . . .").
  2. There may be a need for staged approaches to task completion with scheduled work breaks, following which effort may be fortified.

3. There should be conscious attempts to document graphically on a calendar or in a diary "on times" and "off times" for effort.
4. Students should try to describe—verbally and/or in writing—exactly what it feels like to be running out of mental effort.
5. There should be a legitimate search for tactics to make effort increasingly less effortful (i.e., What can you do to make work easier for yourself?).
6. Rotating work sites at home is often helpful; a child should try studying for 10 minutes in the bedroom, 15 minutes on the living room floor, 10 minutes in the kitchen, and so on.
7. A child may benefit from nonaccusatory assistance at work initiation ("jump starting" effort); that is, a parent may need to write the first line of a report or help with the first mathematics problem.
8. Stimulant medication may be helpful in improving mental effort.

II. Dysfunctions of processing control
  A. Poor saliency determination
    1. There should be a stress on development of paraphrasing and summarization skills.
    2. The child can play video games that demand vigilance and attention to relevant detail.

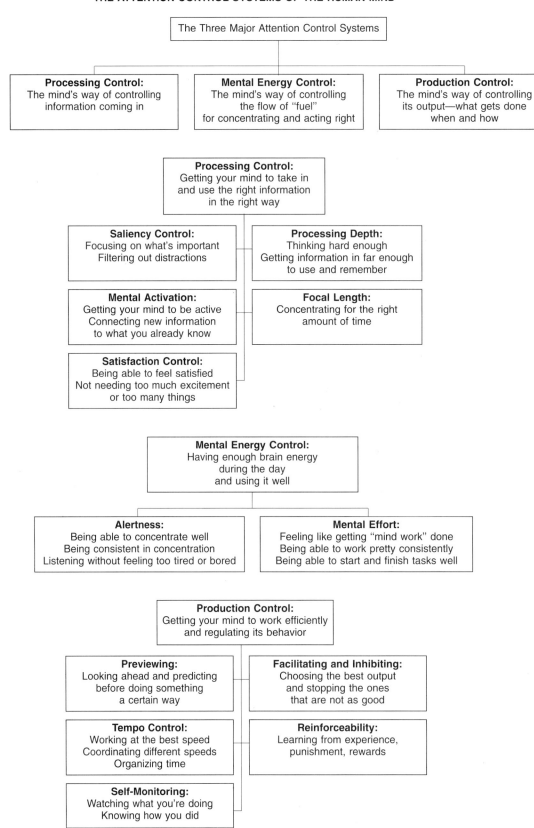

Figure 52–5. Materials used to help "demystify" adolescents with attention deficits. They can be used for patient education with older students. After learning about the various attention controls, adolescents can take greater "ownership" of their problems and devise ways to improve their function.

3. Underlining and circling skills should be encouraged during reading.
4. There can be practice crossing out superfluous information (e.g., word problems containing too much information can be devised).
5. Efforts should be aimed at minimizing specific vulnerable pathways of distraction in work settings at home and at school.
6. Use of consistent background sounds (e.g., music) for study may be helpful in some cases.
7. There should be breaks during which the facilitated distraction pathway is consciously pursued (e.g., chance for a visually distractible child to look out the window during a work break).
8. A child may need subtle/inconspicuous reminders to tune back in during periods of high distraction; a tap on the shoulder may work.

B. Superficial or excessively deep processing
1. The child should learn and apply rehearsal strategies (see Chapter 53)—subvocalization, visual "scratch pad" use, and note taking (even primitive forms thereof).
2. Self-testing techniques should be encouraged as part of studying.
3. Paraphrasing what is heard or read can increase the depth of processing.
4. There may be a need for repetition of instructions and explanations.
5. The child should be encouraged to make good eye contact while listening.
6. When processing is too deep, the student should be encouraged to read or work at a more rapid pace, and when necessary, time limits should be imposed.

C. Passive or extremely active processing
1. Reminder cards can be used—attached to a desk or notebook. ("Am I being passive or is my mind active or maybe *too active*?")
2. There should be disciplined elaboration activities to make the mind a more active processor. ("What are the things you already know that this new stuff reminds you of? How is it pretty much like it? How is it new and different?")
3. The acquisition and longitudinal (long-term) pursuit of expertise may encourage active processing; the child starts by processing actively in an area about which he or she knows a great deal and has strong interest.
4. The child should try to keep score of "canceled mind trips" and/or "wake-up calls" (attempts to get his or her mind back on track).
5. One should actually create opportunities for a child to use the creative/imaginary propensities inherent in "free flight" tendencies; these children desperately need creative outlets.
6. One should encourage high-quality "top-down" processing (i.e., free associating and infusing of one's own ideas, values, and perceptions into what is being read or listened to).

D. Focal maintenance problems
1. The child should be praised whenever he or she sustains attention appropriately.
2. There may need to be an explicit reminder when it is time to change focus.
3. Using computer software for learning may be a way to extend attention in many children.
4. The suggestions for "inconsistent alertness" also pertain to focal maintenance problems.

E. Insatiability
1. High motivational content should be used to bolster learning.
2. There should be an emphasis on the "ethics" of sharing and taking the perspective of others.
3. Parents and teachers should be explicit about delays of gratification (e.g., telling the child that he or she can play football in 40 minutes, but not before then).
4. The child should be helped to identify and acknowledge low-motivational processing tasks (things that make the child feel a little bored when he or she listens to or reads about them).
5. Specific times at home should be designated as "getting satisfied times"; other times should be periods of gratification delay.
6. There should be everyday use of the word "insatiability" with minimal moralization. ("How has your insatiability been going today? Do you think it's a little out of control?")

III. Dysfunctions of production control
A. Poor previewing
1. Parents and/or teachers can institute "what if?" exercises in behavioral, social, and/or cognitive-academic domains (e.g., "What if you call your friend a 'dummy'? What will that do to how he feels about you?").
2. There should be a stress on articulating and describing *final products*. ("What do want this to look like when it's finished? What is it you want to say in this report? What do you want this girl to think about you? How would you like your behavior to be in the lunch room?")
3. The child can practice writing or telling stories that end with a particular sentence (e.g., "George's gerbil will never eat that again!"), or the child can write reports creating the last paragraph first.
4. A student may benefit from practice estimating answers to quantitative questions.

B. Weak facilitation and inhibition
1. The child is likely to benefit from specific training in problem-solving skills (Levine, 1994b) applied across social, behavioral, and academic domains.

2. In confronting new challenges, there should be a systematic review of alternative (cognitive-academic, social, and/or behavioral) strategies and selection of "best bet"—and back-up—strategies.

3. Hypothetic case studies can be used to practice problem solving.

4. Problem-solving techniques can be applied post hoc in reviewing a student's previous misconduct or poor performance on a test or assignment. ("Let's go back and review how you could have done better if you had stopped and thought carefully about the problem.")

5. The child should submit work plans and/or "social survival plans" describing how he or she will go about tackling a serious problem or challenge. The Problem Solving Planner may be used for this (Levine, 1994b).

6. The child might try diagramming possible pathways of facilitation and inhibition (flow charts) for specific academic assignments and behavioral dilemmas.

7. Stimulant medication may help to "decelerate" a child and allow for more reflective thinking and behavior; it may simultaneously help with pacing.

C. Improper pacing
1. Time management (scheduling) procedures should be instituted at home and in school.

2. The student should serve as a time manager in school (e.g., working out schedules for putting on a play, doing a class project, or going on a field trip).

3. At home and in school there can be some stress on time estimation. ("How long should this take me?")

4. Parents and teachers should avoid providing incentives for frenetic pacing, so that there are no advantages to finishing first or "getting it over with."

5. Time landmarks can be used for writing, reading, and doing projects (i.e., where the child should be when).

6. The student should learn to write in stages (see Chapter 71).

7. There should be regular discussions regarding time and time management.

8. Stepwise approaches to tasks should be modeled for the student whenever possible.

D. Deficient self-monitoring and self-righting
1. Teachers and parents should remind students to engage in midtask and terminal self-assessment. ("How am I doing?" or "How do I think I did?")

2. A child should do some self-grading and commenting (on the quality of the work) *before* submitting tests and assignments—with extra credit given for accurate self-appraisal.

3. Proofreading exercises should be used, with credit being given for finding and correcting mistakes (of self and others).

4. There should be a requirement for proofreading of one's own work at least 48 hours after completion (note that it is very hard and probably unwise to proofread something you have just created).

5. Hypothetic case studies can be used to demonstrate the impacts of poor self-monitoring of behavior and interpersonal relating. The crucial role of self-monitoring while driving a car can be used as an example and metaphor to make students more aware of the process.

6. In devising work plans (for a project or a report), students should always include "quality control" measures.

7. Students should examine their work and try to explain *why* they think they made a particular error or where they think they went astray.

E. Low reinforceability
1. There should be a stress on *very consistent* consequences for improper actions.

2. Parents and teachers may need to keep modifying incentives or rewards to sustain a child's motivation.

3. Personal diaries on paper or audiocassette can be used to help a student review events of past days and talk about how those events should affect future actions.

4. A student might maintain lists of "What I've done right today" and "Where I went astray today," with a stress on lessons learned for the future in the development of a cognitive and behavioral repertoire.

5. An affected child might benefit from having an individual (mentor) in school to whom he or she can relate and from whom he or she can receive official recognition for improvement.

OTHER FORMS OF MANAGEMENT

Other modalities of management often warrant consideration in children with attention deficits. The following are some of the more important options.

Counseling

Children with attention deficits who also have significant problems relating to their families may benefit from a course of counseling from a mental health professional. The whole family may need to participate. The counseling can help to elaborate on and extend the demystification process. It can also deal with issues of day-to-day behavioral management and the resolution of family conflicts. In some cases, the siblings of a child with attention deficits need individualized help in understanding and dealing with that brother or sister. The siblings of highly insatiable children are often very resentful and angry; counseling can be especially needed in such instances.

Educational Help

Because it is rare to encounter a child with attention deficits who has no other dysfunctions or subskill weaknesses, educational help is often required. The nature of such support is dependent on the profile of the child with attention deficits.

Social Skills Training

When a child with attention deficits is experiencing substantial interpersonal difficulty, help with social cognition can be beneficial. Such training is often provided in small groups, using standard curriculum materials (see Chapter 54).

Parent Groups

Parents of children with attention deficits may derive support from opportunities to meet with other parents who are facing similar challenges. These groups are often led by an experienced parent and/or professional.

Medication

The psychopharmacology of attention deficits has been the subject of considerable scientific and clinical scrutiny (Green, 1995). Unquestionably, drugs, especially the psychostimulants, have a role to play in the management of children with attention deficits. A clinician prescribing such medications should try to abide by the guidelines set forth in Chapter 82 of this book. Some possible indications for the use of medication are as follows:

- Persistent mental fatigue in school
- Hyperactivity and frenetic pacing
- Extreme and frequent impulsivity (cognitive and/or behavioral)
- Trouble focusing that cannot be accounted for by other dysfunctions or anxiety
- Inexplicable serious inconsistencies in school function

Long-Term Follow-Up and Advocacy

Children with attention deficits are likely to endure rather turbulent school years. The issues and the decision-making dilemmas undergo constant change. There is a need for professionals, such as pediatricians or mental health spe-cialists, to offer ongoing support while representing the rights of these children. Ideally, they should be seen at least three times a year for follow-up and timely advice. Periodic complete physical and neurologic examinations are indicated as part of their close monitoring.

REFERENCES

Barkley RA: Behavioral inhibition, sustained attention, and executive functions: constructing a unifying theory of ADHD. Psychol Bull 121:65, 1997.

Barkley RA: The assessment of attention in children. *In* Lyon GR (ed): Frames of Reference for the Assessment of Learning Disabilities. Baltimore: Paul H. Brookes, 1994.

Denckla MB: A theory and model of executive function. *In* Lyon GR, Krasnegor NA (eds): Attention, Memory and Executive Functions. Baltimore: Paul H. Brookes, 1996.

Gopher D, Navon D: How is performance limited: testing the notion of central capacity. Acta Psychologica 46:161, 1980.

Green WH: Child and Adolescent Psychopharmacology, 2nd ed. Baltimore: Williams & Wilkins, 1995.

Halperin JM: Conceptualizing, describing, and measuring components of attention. *In* Lyon GR, Krasnegor NA (eds): Attention, Memory and Executive Function. Baltimore: Paul H. Brookes, 1996.

Levine MD, Reed M: Developmental Variation and Learning Disorders. Cambridge, MA, Educators Publishing Service, 1998.

Levine MD: The ANSER System. Cambridge, MA, Educators Publishing Service, 1996.

Levine MD: All Kinds of Minds. Cambridge, MA, Educators Publishing Service, 1994a.

Levine MD: Educational Care. Cambridge, MA, Educators Pubishing Service, 1994b.

Levine MD: Pediatric Neurodevelopmental Examinations (PEEX 2 and PEERAMID 2). Cambridge, MA, Educators Publishing Service, 1995.

Levine MD: Keeping a Head in School. Cambridge, MA, Educators Publishing Service, 1990.

Mirsky AF: Disorders of attention: a neuropsychological perspective. *In* Lyon GR, Krasnegor NA (eds): Attention, Memory and Executive Function. Baltimore: Paul H. Brookes, 1996.

Mirsky AF, Anthony AJ, Duncan CC, et al: Analysis of the elements of attention: a neuropsychological approach. Neuropsychol Rev 2:109, 1991.

Pennington BF, Bennetto L, McAleer O, Roberts RJ: Executive functions and working memory. *In* Lyon GR, Krasnegor NA (eds): Attention, Memory and Executive Function. Baltimore: Paul H. Brookes, 1996.

Sanders AF: Towards a model of stress and perfomance. Acta Psychologica 53:61, 1983.

Sergeant J: A theory of attention. An information processing perspective. *In* Lyon GR, Krasnegor NA (eds): Attention, Memory and Executive Function. Baltimore: Paul H. Brookes, 1996.

Tranel D, Anderson SW, Benton AL: Development of the concept of executive function and its relationshop to the frontal lobes. *In* Boller F, Grafman J (eds): Handbook of Neuropsychology, Vol 9. Amsterdam: Elsevier, 1995.

53 Neurodevelopmental Variation and Dysfunction Among School-Aged Children

Melvin D. Levine

 There are more ways to be different than there are to be the same. It is likely that no two children are "wired" identically. This chapter guides the reader through the complex central nervous system circuitry through which such differences are manifest. The pages that follow explore the neurodevelopmental variations that, in some cases, come to represent dysfunctions and disabilities that evolve into significant handicaps. It is through the understanding of neurodevelopmental variations that clinicians can develop a keen appreciation of the wide-ranging and often subtle learning disorders that deprive so many young children of success and productivity during their school years. Like the chapter on attention, this contribution offers a way of understanding school problems without needing to reduce children to rather arbitrary labels.

At any point during the school years, a child's neurodevelopmental profile is a conspicuous marker of health and function. A school-aged child's ledger of assets and dysfunctions is likely to serve as a critical mediating agent between experiential and genetic inputs and performance outcomes (Fig. 53–1). The neurodevelopmental profile consists of a child's balance sheet of abilities within the following interrelated constructs: attention, memory, language, temporal-sequential ordering, spatial ordering, neuromotor skill, higher cognition, and social cognition (Levine and Reed, 1998). Weaknesses in one or more of these areas may be associated with academic underachievement, behavioral difficulties, and problems with social adjustment. It has been estimated that between 5% and 15% of school-aged children harbor low-severity impairments of neurodevelopmental function. The actual prevalence may be even higher when one takes into consideration discrete dysfunctions that lead to a transient self-limited problem within a particular subject area.

Neurodevelopmental variations are associated with a wide range of possible learning styles and impediments (Table 53–1). A variation that represents a developmental weakness (such as a problem with expressive language) is considered a dysfunction. If that dysfunction interferes with the acquisition of a particular skill (such as writing), it becomes a disability. If the skill impaired by the disability is particularly germane to productivity and the acquisition of reasonable gratification in our society, the disability constitutes a handicap. Neurodevelopmental variations also include areas of unusual strength or talent. In describing a child's neurodevelopmental profile, therefore, it is important to take into consideration his or her functional assets (such as creativity, strong spatial ordering, or excellent nonverbal problem-solving abilities).

Most children who experience academic difficulties harbor more than one neurodevelopmental dysfunction. The additive effect of multiple dysfunctions is sufficient to impair the innate developmental resiliency of a child,
thereby generating academic underachievement. It is likely that most children are able to circumvent a single neurodevelopmental dysfunction to attain at least passable academic achievement.

Neurodevelopmental dysfunctions are most likely to result in the delayed or laborious acquisition of academic skills and in a notably reduced level of productivity from day to day in school. When neurodevelopmental dysfunctions are overtly disruptive of learning, these problems are often referred to as *learning disabilities* (Kavanagh and Truss, 1988). Other terms, such as *attention-deficit disorder, dyslexia,* and *minimal cerebral dysfunction,* have also been applied to children with "low-severity" dysfunctions. Such diagnostic labels may be important for obtaining services for a child in school and for receiving reimbursement for services outside of school; however, the diagnostic criteria for such labels are highly controversial and constantly changing. There are many children with serious academic problems who fail to meet the standard criteria for such labels and therefore tend to "fall between the cracks," while their needs go unrecognized and unfulfilled. Not only that, there are serious dangers inherent in applying fixed labels to children. These hazards include self-fulfilling prophecies, an inherent pessimism, a tendency to ignore multifactorial causes and manifestations of a child's problems (i.e, reductionism), and a widespread practice of neglecting children who are struggling but who fail to meet a school's criteria for service eligibility. Consequently this chapter shuns such labels and offers an empiric approach to the neurodevelopmental dysfunctions that cluster to generate discrete disabilities and significant handicaps.

Etiologies

Diverse etiologies underlie the neurodevelopmental dysfunctions of childhood. In some cases, genetic causes have been documented. Strong family patterns of reading and

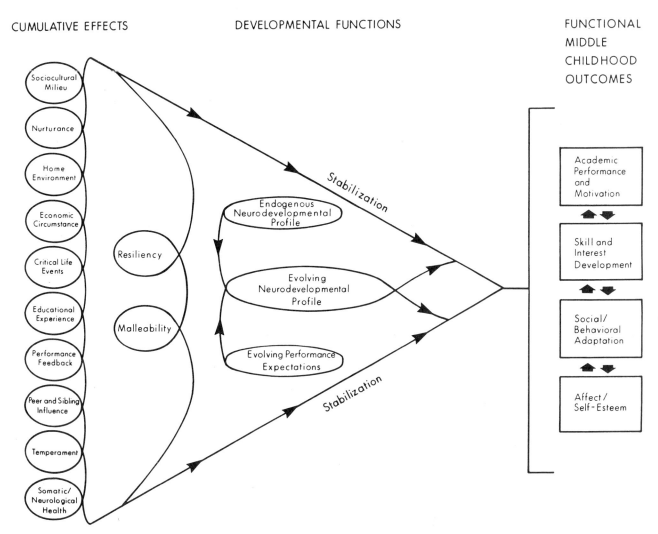

Figure 53–1. This diagram portrays the manner in which multiple cumulative effects interact and transact with a child's inborn profile of neurodevelopmental strengths and weaknesses to generate significant outcomes during middle childhood.

spelling disabilities are demonstrable. Other studies have suggested causal associations between specific dysfunctions and abnormal chromosomal patterns (Chapter 23), low-level lead intoxication (Chapter 30), recurrent otitis media (Chapter 34), meningitis, acquired immunodeficiency syndrome (AIDS) (Chapter 28), intraventricular hemorrhage, serious closed-head trauma (Chapter 27), and low birth weight (Chapter 26). Poor nutrition (Chapter 29) and sociocultural deprivation have also been implicated etiologically or at least as potentiators of neurodevelopmental dysfunction. In most individual cases, an irrefutable etiology cannot be established.

It is important to acknowledge that neurodevelopmental variations are not generated in a vacuum. Their effects are shaped by environmental circumstances, cultural values (Chapter 10), physical health factors, temperament (Chapter 8), critical life events (Chapter 14), and evolving academic expectations. Therefore a low-severity neurodevelopmental dysfunction commonly exerts its most profound influence when it occurs in a context of environmental turmoil or deprivation (Levine et al, 1985). Analogously, the effects of a neurodevelopmental dysfunction may be minimized under optimal environmental conditions.

Clinical Manifestations of Dysfunction

Children with neurodevelopmental dysfunctions vary widely with regard to the clinical symptoms they manifest.

Table 53–1 • Hierarchy of Neurodevelopmental Status

Variation	An unusual pattern of neurodevelopmental function (e.g., a higher divergent mind)
Dysfunction	A distinct weakness within a neurodevelopmental function (e.g., weak retrieval memory)
Disability	A performance deficiency caused (at least in part) by a neurodevelopmental dysfunction (e.g., trouble throwing a ball)
Handicap	A disability occurring in a much-needed or critical performance area (e.g., a significant reading problem)

Their specific patterns of academic performance and behavior represent final common pathways, the convergence of the multiple factors delineated previously. In addition, the manifestations of a particular dysfunction vary depending on a child's strengths or weaknesses in other neurodevelopmental areas. Thus a memory dysfunction will present differently in a child with strong language skills, good attention, and excellent thinking skills than in a child whose memory problems are intensified by weaknesses of attention and delays in receptive language acquisition. Consequently our full understanding of a child with neurodevelopmental dysfunction must include consideration of strengths and weaknesses in the components of all eight key areas of neurodevelopmental function, which are summarized in Table 53–2. In the following section, we look at the basic manifestations of deficits and strengths in each of the key neurodevelopmental areas.

ATTENTION

Dysfunction of attention are, in all likelihood, the most common neurodevelopmental problems affecting children. Weaknesses of attention are especially incapacitating and are likely to have a broad, although often subtle and insidious, impact on day-to-day performance. Neurodevelopmental dysfunctions of attention are so common and pervasive that they are dealt with separately (see Chapter 52).

MEMORY

Memory development during childhood entails the acquisition of a complex array of subskills (Weinert and Perlmutter, 1988). As children proceed through school, there is a progressively increasing and potentially incapacitating strain on memory (Levine and Reed, 1998). Students are expected to be selective, systematic, and strategic in entering skills and facts into memory. They must be equally effective in their use of long-term and short-term memory and in the precise recall of stored rules, data, concepts, and procedures. By secondary school, rapid and accurate recall is an indispensable requisite for acceptable academic performance. Not surprisingly, some students experience tremendous frustration when their memory dysfunctions prevent them from meeting ever-intensifying academic demands (Swanson and Cooney, 1996).

There are students who experience difficulty with the initial registration of information or skill in short-term memory (Table 53–3). They have trouble keeping pace with the information flow in a classroom. In some cases, children with attention deficits are insufficiently selective, alert, and reflective to register the most salient information in memory. They are likely to have generalized deficiencies of the initial registration process. Other students have more

Table 53–2 • Neurodevelopmental Constructs

Attention	Temporal-sequential ordering
Memory	Neuromotor function
Language	Higher order cognition
Spatial ordering	Social cognition

Table 53–3 • Four Levels of Memory and Signs of Dysfunction

Level	Signs of Dysfunction
Short-term memory	Trouble following directions; need for repetition, difficulty studying for tests
Active working memory	Problems with mathematic computation; trouble remembering while reading; problems with writing
Consolidation in long-term memory	Overreliance on rote memory; inconsistent long-term recall; disorganization
Retrieval from long-term memory	Slow recall; problems in writing and mathematics

specific registration weaknesses (Vallar and Papagno, 1995). Some may have trouble only with registering visual-spatial data in memory, whereas others may be ineffective at the registration of sequences of data or of verbal material. There are some children who ultimately can register data in short-term memory, but they cannot do so quickly enough. They are constantly struggling to keep pace with instructions, explanations, and material they need to copy rapidly from a board. Others have trouble capturing data that are presented in "large chunks"—they simply are unable to register sizable portions of new material.

Many children experience problems with active working memory. They have difficulty suspending information in memory temporarily while they are working with it or developing it. Ideally, active working memory enables a student to keep in mind all the different components of a task, such as a mathematics problem, while working to complete it. A student with an active working memory dysfunction, on the other hand, might carry a number and forget what he or she intended to do after having carried the number. Active working memory enables children to remember the beginning of a paragraph until they arrive at the end of it. Thus children with active working memory disorders can have trouble performing computations in mathematics and difficulty remembering or retelling what they have read.

EXAMPLE

Meg seems to be a very bright and articulate girl. She has always been advanced in her ability to decode words for reading. During the early grades, she was near the top of her class in mathematics and she demonstrated excellent writing skills. Meg has always been very well organized and a really effective strategist.

Meg does not present a behavior problem in school. She is extremely conscientious. Her teachers feel that she is rather hard on herself. She shows considerable performance anxiety, especially when she takes tests. Although she does not appear nervous before a test, while taking an examination she obviously "tenses up." The teachers feel that her anxiety actually interferes with test-taking performance. Meg has always done quite well on multiple choice tests. However, math quizzes have been problematic for her. Her group achievement test scores have all been very high, even in math. Likewise, Meg's reading comprehension scores are excellent, although she claims reading is a problem for her. In fact, despite her positive attitude toward school, she clearly hates to read. Her teachers feel that Meg understands what she reads, but that she does not retain or apply very much of it.

Meg's mathematics teacher observes that she is well prepared for tests but that she has difficulty taking them. Meg herself claims that things get "all jumbled up" when she does math tests. She points out that she keeps forgetting important things while she is working on problems. When she does one step in a problem, she loses track of what she had intended to do next.

Meg's parents are totally confused by her. Meg has two older sisters who have excelled academically. Meg's parents are convinced that Meg is brighter than either of the older sisters, yet there seems to be something missing, some elusive barrier that is preventing her from succeeding and feeling sufficiently good about school.

Some children have particular problems consolidating information in long-term memory. They may have little or no trouble registering data initially in memory, but their long-term storage is undependable. Ordinarily consolidation of data in long-term memory takes from hours to days and is accomplished in one or more of four ways: (1) pairing two bits of information together (such as a cluster of letters with the sound it represents), (2) classifying data in categories (such as filing all insects together in memory), (3) linking new information to established rules (so-called rule-based learning), and (4) arranging knowledge or skills in logical chains (such as the months of the year, the steps needed to tie shoelaces or form a letter, or the sequence of events in a story). Some students struggle in vain with specific paired associations, category filing, rule-based learning, or the formation of procedural/causal/chronologic chains.

Although they seem able to register and consolidate information in memory, some children have inordinate difficulty recalling data or skills on demand. Their recall may be painfully slow or inaccurate. Some of them encounter serious problems with simultaneous recall; they cannot recall several facts or procedures at once. This shortcoming can be especially disabling when it comes to writing, a task necessitating the concurrent recall of spelling, capitalization, letter formation, punctuation, facts, ideas, vocabulary, and the directions or topic for the assignment. Consequently many children with simultaneous-recall deficits are disabled in their written output. When they try to write, they experience a disheartening memory overload, often manifesting as illegibility (owing to a crowding out of memory for letter formation), poor use of punctuation and capitalization, deficient spelling, and surprisingly primitive ideation. These children may be accused of a lack of motivation or a failure to strive because legibility or spelling is so poor in a paragraph and so far superior in isolation (such as on a list of spelling words). Some of these children also fare poorly in mathematics, in which the rapid and simultaneous recall of previously learned facts and skills is a daily necessity.

As children proceed through their school years, they do not develop more memory capacity per se. Instead they become increasingly adept at using memory. It has been found that they do so through the deployment of an ever-expanding repertoire of mnemonic strategies (Torgeson, 1985). Most children spontaneously develop facilitative techniques to register new data more deeply in memory, to consolidate new data within multiple preexisting categories of knowledge, to visualize what they hear or to verbalize what they see in preparation for its entry into memory, and to consciously plan the process of memorization. In the last case, students become increasingly deliberative and systematic in studying for tests. By adolescence, learners with good memory strategies are able to decide what is most likely to appear on a test, what they will be able to figure out during the test, what they will need to memorize, how long it will take to memorize the material, what techniques will help to register the information in memory, and how they will test themselves to determine if (and when) they know what they thought they needed to know. Unfortunately, some students with memory dysfunctions have few or no mnemonic (or other learning) strategies (Meltzer, 1996). They are lacking in metamemory, or a sense of how memory works and how they can maximize its operation. Such "non-methodologists" struggle academically. In some cases, the failure to develop strategies is limited to the memory domain; in other instances, students fail to use strategies in a wide range of circumstances, including memory, problem solving, and even in the face of social conflict.

Students with memory strengths can deploy these assets to overcome weaknesses or potential deficits in other domains. For example, a child who has difficulty understanding certain concepts in mathematics may compensate (at least in part) by having an excellent recall of mathematic facts and rules.

LANGUAGE

Linguistically competent children have a distinct advantage in school, since much of what gets taught is encoded in literate language. All of the basic academic skills are conveyed largely through verbal expression. Many important thinking skills are conveyed and applied through language (Nelson, 1996). Therefore it is not surprising that children with language dysfunctions are susceptible to tumultuous academic careers (Wallach and Butler, 1994).

There are many forms or levels of language dysfunction. These are summarized in Table 53–4 (see also Chapter 63). Some children have problems with phonology, so that they experience problems appreciating and manipulating individual language sounds. They may have trouble discriminating between and forming associations with the sounds of their native language. Problems with phonologic awareness have been studied extensively in recent years

Table 53–4 • Common Forms of Language Dysfunction

Poor phonologic awareness: a lack of appreciation of language sounds
Semantic deficiency: trouble acquiring, recalling, and/or using vocabulary
Syntactic problem: difficulty dealing with word order (affecting sentence comprehension and/or formulation)
Weak metalinguistics: a diminished sense of how language works

and have been identified as one of the most common forms of learning disorder in childhood. Affected students have difficulty perceiving some or many of the 44 language sounds (phonemes) in the English language. In some cases, there may be evidence of problems processing the transitions that bind acoustic signals within a language sound (such as the "d" and the "uh" in the phoneme "duh" as in "dull") (Tallal, Sainburg, and Jernigan, 1991). Children with reduced phonologic awareness are vulnerable to problems learning to decode words for reading and to encode words during spelling. They may rely too much on visual and context clues during reading. For many of them it is hard to hold language sounds in active working memory firmly enough to break a word down into its component sounds and reblend them, a skill needed to decode new multisyllabic vocabulary. It is common for children and adolescents with even mild phonologic difficulties to endure frustration and failure when they attempt to master a second language. Some bilingual children who have school problems do so because of phonologic dysfunctions in their underlying primary language.

Difficulty with semantics is another common language breakdown. Students so affected have rigid and restricted notions of word meanings. It is hard for them to acquire new vocabulary, which becomes a very serious liability in high school and college, where there is a virtual explosion of key technical words that are essential for understanding complex subject matter.

Other language-based problems are in understanding and using syntax (word order), a poor appreciation of how language works (weak metalinguistics), and trouble with "higher language." The last includes such functions as the understanding and formulation of abstract language, the detection and resolution of ambiguity, the drawing of inferences (i.e., supplying missing information), the use of symbolic language (e.g., metaphors, analogies), the use of language to form abstract concepts, and the mastery of a second language. The attainment of these higher language levels becomes vital for success during secondary school. Students who proceed through high school lacking higher language sophistication often experience failure and commonly also develop signs of behavioral maladjustment.

A distinction is usually made between receptive language dysfunctions (those affecting comprehension) and expressive language dysfunctions (those thwarting language production or communication). Children with primarily receptive language problems may have serious difficulty following instructions in the classroom, understanding verbal explanations, and interpreting what they read. Those with expressive weaknesses include children with oromotor problems affecting articulation and verbal fluency. In addition, some display weaknesses of word retrieval; despite an adequate vocabulary, their dysphasias make it hard for them to recall exact words on demand. This impairment can make it embarrassing and difficult for an affected student to participate in class discussions or come up with precise answers on a quiz. Still others with expressive dysfunctions have trouble formulating sentences, using grammar effectively, and organizing spoken (and often written) narrative.

Children with expressive language problems are likely to be hesitant when they speak. They may overindulge in circumlocutions. Their spoken narrative is often lacking in cohesive ties; it sounds as if they are reading a list of sentences when they talk. Words such as "then," "as soon as," "before," and "next" are used sparsely (if at all), resulting in a lack of narrative cohesion. Some students with expressive language problems may become passive, taciturn, and chronically nonelaborative in their communications. When asked what he or she did in school today, such a student is likely to respond: "stuff!" Sometimes a child with expressive language dysfunctions speaks fluently with peers and family members, making use of limited vocabulary and simple or repetitive syntactical patterns. These same students may be poor at using more literate language.

EXAMPLE

Laura has never had an easy time in school; however, she did best in kindergarten and first grade. She seemed highly motivated at that time, and she was near the top of her class in several of her readiness skills, including number and letter recognition. On the other hand, her teachers always felt that she acted as if she were confused. They found themselves repeating directions to her, a practice that has had to continue up through the present.

Laura seems to be verbally fluent. She is especially expressive when she is with her friends. She is also fairly articulate in class. At this time, there are concerns about Laura's reading comprehension and decoding skills. She is said to be nearly 2 years delayed in all aspects of reading. Her spelling is likewise problematic. Her errors are usually good visual approximations, but her renditions are unpronounceable in the English language. Laura's performance in English class has been problematic. She has had tremendous difficulty understanding grammatical rules and parts of speech. She gets confused about her assignments. Moreover her poor reading is a major impediment. On the other hand, Laura has always been a proficient mathematics student. She likes math and has done above-average work. However, during the current year (eighth grade), there has been discernible slippage in mathematics as well. This has been especially discouraging to Laura.

Laura has been showing progressive signs of inattention. She seems to be daydreaming in class and is looking increasingly tired. While she does not really doze off, she yawns, stretches, and stares into space with some regularity. Frequently she seems confused and preoccupied. She is starting to lose her motivation. Currently, she appears to be interested only in her friends. In addition, she is having increasing difficulty completing homework assignments. This is especially the case in social studies and in a science course. In both areas, Laura has said there are just too many ideas and facts to figure out.

Language dysfunctions range from blatant to subtle to barely discernible. They are frequently diagnostically elusive. Some students with mild language difficulties function reasonably well in school until they are required to master a second language. Other students with language dysfunctions may succeed until they reach late elementary or middle school, when language becomes increasingly decontextualized. That is, they can do well when language is used to describe familiar contents. When it becomes less predictable, such as when a teacher describes events that occurred long ago and far away, a language-impaired child may experience a steep decline in comprehension.

Students with strong language function may make use of their linguistic facility to overcome other learning problems. For example, it may be possible to verbalize one's way through the mathematics curriculum, thereby overcoming a tendency to be confused by some primarily nonverbal concepts (such as ratio, equation, and circumference).

It is important to be aware of the fact that some children may show a disparity between their receptive and expressive language abilities. In particular, a child may be highly expressive verbally but may not be particularly skilled at interpreting other people's language. Such a youngster may impress everyone during a class discussion or an informal conversation and yet do quite poorly when processing a teacher's verbal explanations or understanding what he or she reads in a text. It is also possible for a student to comprehend verbal information but be relatively poor at expression. These two patterns may be deceptive and confusing to parents and teachers.

SPATIAL ORDERING

Visual-perceptual abilities entail the appreciation of spatial attributes. Most spatial data enter the nervous system through visual pathways, but some are mediated through nonverbal conceptualization or propriokinesthetic pathways. Shape, position, relative size, foreground/background relations, and form constancy (the notion that a shape retains its integrity regardless of its position in space) are among the constituents of visual-spatial ordering. Young children with visual-spatial dysfunctions may encounter problems with letter recognition. Spelling may ultimately emerge as a deficit, since affected children commonly are vague in their recall of the visual configurations of words. In general, however, those who are confused about spatial attributes are unlikely to have long-standing or devastating academic problems, unless their visual-spatial weaknesses are complicated by other neurodevelopmental dysfunctions. At one time, it was thought that visual-spatial dysfunctions were a common cause of reading disabilities. Most recent research has refuted this view.

Children with spatial ordering dysfunctions may be late in discriminating between left and right. They may exhibit fine or gross motor clumsiness, or both, as they struggle to make use of visual-spatial data to program motor responses.

Students with particularly keen spatial ordering may possess artistic talents. They may be able to use visualization to enhance their learning of even highly verbal concepts. This bypass route can be especially redemptive for students with strong visual-spatial ordering in the presence of a language disability.

TEMPORAL-SEQUENTIAL ORDERING

The appreciation and application of time and sequence constitutes an important neurodevelopmental function. Students need to be able to preserve and manage a vast range of practical and abstract sequences. They must tell time, process and produce multistep explanations and procedures, and register lengthy sequences in short-term memory. The curriculum demands the preservation of serial order in spelling, in narrative, and in various mathematic algorithms. An inability to deal with sequences is likely to be associated with problematic writing, with mathematic deficiencies, and with generalized organizational problems.

Children who have difficulties with temporal-sequential ordering may be delayed in learning to tell time. They can also become confused over multistep inputs of various types. Thus it is not unusual for a child with temporal-sequential disorganization to experience trouble in following multistep instructions and processing complex sequential explanations. Sequencing weaknesses often result in trouble learning the multiplication tables and performing multistep procedures in mathematics. Over time such dysfunction can interfere with a student's ability to organize tasks in stages and to allocate time effectively. Thus it is not unusual for children with temporal-sequential dysfunctions to be poor at time management as they proceed through school.

NEUROMOTOR FUNCTION

A child's motor skills can play a significant role in a wide range of academic and nonacademic pursuits (Denckla, 1985). Productivity in school becomes very dependent on efficient writing skills. The motor aspects of writing are known as *graphomotor function,* a set of capacities that differ from fine motor function. In fact, it is not at all unusual for a student to display good fine motor function (such as in art and in repairing things) in the presence of poor graphomotor function. Because writing demands rapid and precise graphomotor coordination, it is not surprising that students with certain forms of dysfunction are prone to substantial academic underachievement. Such students have been described as having "developmental output failure." They seem to have much more trouble with productivity than with actual learning. The graphomotor dysfunctions that affect writing can be divided into eight subtypes, which are described as follows (Table 53–5):

1. Some children have finger agnosia; they have trouble localizing their fingers in space while they write. There appears to be a breakdown of propriokinesthetic (reafferent) feedback resulting in poor appreciation of the precise location of the point of the writing utensil at any particular instant. Because of their impaired tracking, these children need to maintain their eyes very close to the page. Ultimately their writing becomes agonizingly slow and laborious. Often these students develop a fistlike pencil grip that causes them to write with their wrists and their elbows rather than the distal joints of their digits. The wrists and elbows clearly have wider excursions during writing, so that propriokinesthetic feedback will be less subtle. Regrettably the awkward pencil grip itself is a liability, making writing agonizingly slow, uncomfortable, and laborious. In particular, these students are likely to have trouble with lengthy writing, such as is needed to complete book

Table 53–5 • Subtypes of Graphomotor Dysfunction

Parameter	Weak Visualization	Procedural Sequencing Weakness	Verbal:Motor/ Eye:Motor Incoordination	Production Deficit	Finger Agnosia	Pseudomotor Dysfunction	Functional Undermining
Writing speed	Variable	Variable	Variable	Slow	Slow	Rapid	Load dependent
Legibility	Poor	Poor	Adequate	Variable	Adequate	Poor	Load dependent
Grip	Tight or appropriate	Tight or appropriate	Appropriate	Hooked, tight, or distal	Fistlike	Variable	Usually normal
Mechanics	Variable	Variable	Consistent, adequate	Adequate	Decline over time	Careless errors	Load dependent
Organization of ideas	Adequate	Often poor	Adequate	Adequate	Adequate	Often poor	Often poor
Cursive writing	Avoided	Avoided	Preferred	Sometimes avoided	Used	Variable	Used
Spelling	Usually poor	Variable	Variable	Adequate	Often a problem	Adequate	Load dependent
Mathematics	Adequate	Often a problem	Variable	Adequate	Often a problem	Adequate	Often a problem
Reading	Adequate	Adequate	Variable	Adequate	Often a problem	Adequate or advanced	Adequate
Speech	Normal	Normal	Adequate	Possible problems	Normal	Possible early stammering	Adequate

reports in junior high school. Additionally children with finger agnosia tend to have other neurodevelopmental dysfunctions resulting in broad delays in academic performance.

2. Graphomotor production deficits affect many children, who have difficulty implementing the coordinated motor movements for writing. It is inordinately difficult for them to decide which muscles to facilitate (and which to inhibit) to form specific letters. It is hard for them to assign certain muscles to the stabilization of the writing utensil and others to its movement. They are motorically indecisive. During the early grades they often exhibit an unstable pencil grip (occasionally dropping the pencil in the middle of a sentence). Eventually they compensate, often by developing a perpendicular, excessively tight and distal (or hooked) grasp as a means of overstabilizing the utensil, which can result in awkward, laborious movement. Many of these students also display an oral-motor production deficit, resulting in speech articulation defects as well as writing problems.

3. Some students harbor a previsualization dyspraxia. They have difficulty visualizing and therefore planning the configurations of letters and words they are about to form. Because they do not have a clear and consistent visual plan or blueprint, their written output tends to be poorly or inconsistently legible. Often the same problem they experience when visualizing letters impedes the ability to visualize entire words. Consequently they frequently exhibit spelling errors as well as legibility problems. Their spelling errors are likely to be phonetically correct but visually poor approximations (e.g., "brawt" for "brought"). Of interest is the fact that many children with previsualization weaknesses fluctuate in their picturing of letter configurations. As a result, their writing is inconsistent; while forming a letter they often (but not always) forget the gestalt of that letter. Therefore their writing is marked by hesitation, retracing, and erratic letter formation.

4. Some students have procedural memory dyspraxias. They are unable to recall and therefore plan the precise sequences of motor movements required to form letters. These children also show letter formation inconsistencies, a poor writing rhythm, and erratic legibility. Their motor sequential recall may fluctuate from word to word or even letter to letter. They (as well as students with previsualization weaknesses) commonly prefer printing (manuscript) to cursive writing. Often students with procedural memory dyspraxias also endure difficulties in mathematics as a result of their weak recall of the multistep procedures in that content area.

5. Visual-motor dyspraxia occurs in children who have a great deal of difficulty using visual information to program a motor response. In this case, memory is not required. The child must copy from a board or a book with the information remaining in front of him or her. Some youngsters will have great difficulty making use of visual configurational data and the act of writing. They are likely to have trouble copying quickly and accurately in school.

6. Verbal-motor dyspraxia is found in students who appear to have tremendous difficulty listening and writing at the same time. They may experience extreme agony in trying to take notes in high school or in college. Some of these youngsters have underlying language problems. Others have difficulty with immediate verbal memory or active working memory. But in many cases they are students with good language and memory abilities who simply are unable to integrate verbal inputs with motor responses.

7. Pseudomotor dysfunction is encountered in children whose ideational fluency far exceeds the normal ca-

pacity of their fingers to transcribe thoughts on paper. Sometimes these students have excellent verbal abilities, fertile imaginations, and notable verbal fluency. Graphomotor output simply cannot keep pace with the accelerated rate of their thought processes. Sometimes these children exhibit stammering or stuttering during their preschool and early elementary school years. This too is a manifestation of a disparity between rapid ideational fluency and relatively slow motor (i.e., oral-motor) speed. When they are able to decelerate their thought processes, both articulation and writing are likely to improve substantially.

8. Sometimes graphomotor abilities are compromised by functional undermining. In this case, one or more of the nonmotor components of writing are siphoning so much effort that motor precision is compromised. If a student has to struggle inordinately with the simultaneous memory demands of writing (as described previously in this chapter), letter formation may be secondarily compromised. That same student may be able to write a list of words legibly, that is, when he or she does not have to deal with multiple other simultaneous demands.

A student with a writing disability may suffer from one or more of the eight basic graphomotor dysfunctions. It is important to recognize that many such students excel at fine motor activities that do not involve writing. Thus a child with a procedural memory dyspraxia or with finger agnosia may be an excellent artist or mechanic despite difficulties with writing. Alternatively a student may have eye-hand coordination problems but good motor memory and nonvisual finger localization. Such a child may be excellent at writing but clumsy or awkward when it comes to artistic endeavors, building a model, fixing things, or working with a computer.

EXAMPLE

Carlos is an aggressive and controlling youngster. He is very well developed physically, and he uses his muscles rather liberally in school. Other students are frankly frightened of him.

Carlos' schoolwork has been problematic. His teachers have difficulty knowing whether Carlos does poorly because he does not try or whether he has stopped trying because he does poorly. Writing is a particularly humbling experience for Carlos. His handwriting is nearly illegible. He holds the pencil very close to the point and perpendicular to the page. He writes painfully slowly and therefore can never finish tests on time. He becomes quite embarrassed and defensive about this.

Carlos is also a reluctant participant in class discussions. He has a noticeable speech impediment for which he used to receive speech therapy. Although he has a fairly good vocabulary, Carlos does not say much in class.

Carlos is frequently late for class. His mother reports that Carlos seems to be late for everything at home as well. He has always been confused about time. He has trouble following multistep directions and carrying out multistep processes. He keeps getting things in the wrong

order. Moreover, Carlos still does not know the months of the year.

Carlos would like very much to have friends. However, he keeps alienating everyone without realizing it. He seems to be socially "tone deaf." He is unaware of how he is affecting other students. His aggressiveness and bullying tactics have made him many enemies. He was described by one of his guidance counselors in elementary school as "insensitive to the needs of other people." In addition, Carlos seems to have trouble using language effectively in relating to other people. This has made some adults wonder whether Carlos has some kind of language disability. He constantly says inappropriate things to people. He sounds hostile for no apparent reason and without any provocation. He also keeps thinking other people are saying things that are hostile toward him. A great deal of misunderstanding ensues and sometimes ends up in physical or verbal conflict. Of interest is the fact that in other contexts, Carlos seems to have excellent language skills. He is fluent in Spanish and English. His reading comprehension is nearly 2 years above grade level. Carlos loves to read and is constantly taking books out of the library. On a one-to-one basis, when Carlos is not feeling self-conscious about his speech articulation, he exhibits excellent verbal fluency, advanced vocabulary for his age, and a great deal of sophistication in his verbal conceptualization.

Some children harbor underlying gross motor dysfunctions with or without fine motor or graphomotor incoordination. They may exhibit generalized gross motor delays or highly specific deficits (Sugden and Keogh, 1990). Some cannot program accurate motor responses based on the processing of certain kinds of input data. For example, some children have difficulty using visual-spatial information to guide their gross motor actions. Consequently they are inept at catching or throwing a ball. They simply do not make accurate judgments or estimates about trajectories in space. Others are poor at using "inner spatial" data, so they have trouble interpreting proprioceptive and kinesthetic information emanating from their muscles and joints. They are said to be lacking in body position sense, an impairment that compromises activities requiring balance and keen awareness of one's body movements. Still other children show evidence of a gross motor dyspraxia and have trouble implementing complex motor procedures demanding precise mobilization of specific muscle groups. They may be slow at acquiring skills for swimming, gymnastics, and dancing. Closely related to this phenomenon is one in which children cannot master gross motor sequences. They have trouble forming, automatizing, and sustaining complex rhythms.

Children with gross motor problems are at risk. Many of them suffer a significant loss of self-esteem, while their feelings of inadequacy erode self-concept (Shaw, Levine, and Belfer, 1982). They may incur considerable embarrassment in physical education classes. Their gross motor dysfunctions result in specific athletic disabilities, which, in turn, can become handicaps when they perpetuate social rejection or withdrawal.

Children who exhibit motor strengths have access to some valuable modes of gratification in life. Students who have academic disabilities and motor talents can use the latter to preserve their self-esteem while struggling with coursework. Motor competency can also enable a child to feel efficacious artistically as well as in the mechanical-spatial realm.

Higher-Order Cognition

Higher-order cognition is composed of a range of sophisticated thinking skills. Included in this category of neurodevelopmental function are concept acquisition, problem-solving skill, critical thinking, brainstorming (including creativity), metacognition, various forms of reasoning, and rule recognition and application.

Children vary considerably in their capacities to understand the conceptual bases of skills and content areas in school. Concepts are groupings of ideas that somehow fit together. For example, the concept of furniture includes tables, chairs, beds, and bookcases. As students progress through their education, the concepts they encounter become increasingly abstract and complex. New concepts often contain preexisting concepts, and students are continually adding new elements to preexisting conceptual frameworks. Over time they can identify perfect prototypes of a concept as well as imperfect prototypes of that concept, and they become increasingly able to distinguish between an idea that fits a concept and one that is beyond the realm of that concept. Such conceptual ability is critical for truly in-depth learning. Unfortunately some students acquire only a tenuous grasp of concepts. Those who hold such chronically tenuous grasps are most likely ultimately to underachieve. Some of them may exhibit pervasively weak grasps, whereas others may have difficulty with conceptual grasps in circumscribed domains (such as mathematics, social studies, and science). There are students who much prefer to conceptualize verbally, whereas others are more comfortable forming concepts without the interposition of language. Many of the best students try to portray or ponder concepts both verbally and nonverbally. Some students have serious trouble mastering abstract concepts. They tend to be overly concrete. Such a student may struggle to assimilate concepts such as liberalism, internal combustion, or equation.

Problem-solving skills are an important part of mathematics as well as virtually every other content area in school. Students with well-developed problem-solving skills are keen strategists. They are generally excellent at previewing or estimating answers, thinking about multiple alternative techniques to solve a problem, selecting the best technique, and monitoring what they are doing while they are doing it (Bloom and Broder, 1950). Poor problem solvers, on the other hand, tend to be rigid, unsystematic, or impulsive. They often mismatch time allocation to the task at hand, allowing either too much or too little time for problem solving. They fail to consider alternative strategic approaches, instead irreversibly committing themselves to an initial approach whether or not it is working. These students may encounter significant problems in coursework that requires methodical strategy deployment and flexible thinking.

Brainstorming skill is needed to derive a topic for a report, to think about the best way to undertake a project, and to deal with a variety of other open-ended academic and nonacademic challenges. Some children have difficulty generating original ideas. They much prefer to be told exactly what to do. They would rather comply than innovate. They balk at having to choose a topic, speculate, develop an argument, or think freely and independently. They have trouble confronting a blank page and generating the ideas to fill it.

Critical-thinking skills represent another higher cognitive acquisition during childhood. Successful students often demonstrate keen abilities to evaluate statements, products, and people, deploying objective criteria in doing so. They are able to tease out their own personal biases and the viewpoints of others. They are effective in comparing and contrasting their values and views with those of an author. They can think about and talk about the qualities of a person. They become adept at assembling criteria to judge the products they see in a store or on television. But some students are notably weak in their critical thinking. They have difficulty analyzing issues, developing arguments, and evaluating ideas. This can be especially handicapping in subjects (such as social studies) that often demand critical reading and analytical abilities.

Some children and adolescents experience difficulty with specific forms of reasoning. They may have trouble reasoning with analogies or using deductive or inductive logic. Their reasoning gaps may constrain mathematical proficiency most conspicuously.

Metacognition has received considerable attention in recent years. A child's metacognitive ability refers to his or her capacity to think about thinking. Children with strong metacognition are able to observe themselves thinking or studying. In this way they develop an understanding of thought processes, enabling them to enhance their personal learning strategies and become more efficient and productive students. Those who lack metacognition tend to perform many intellectual tasks the hard way. They are unlikely to use facilitative techniques to study for a test, to write a report, or to meet other complex academic challenges.

Rule development and application is another key component of higher-order cognition. Students who are effective in this domain are acutely sensitive to regularity and irregularity. They are able to develop their own rules based on consistent judgments or observations they have made. When two phenomena are seen as invariably associated, they may adhere as a rule in the mind of a student. Rules generally assume the configuration of "if . . . then." Students who are quick to discover rules are likely to have the learning process greatly facilitated for them. A student may come to notice that every time he or she encounters the name of a city in a book it is capitalized. Such a student may discern this regularity before the formal rules of capitalization are explained by a teacher. In addition to being able to discern regularities or rules, students must understand and apply the rules they are taught. For some children rules are appealingly logical. Some even crave rule-based learning. Others experience agonizing frustration in subjects that demand substantial rule application. Somehow grammatical rules, mathematic rules, and foreign language rules fail to clarify phenomena for them.

It should be clear that a student's strengths in any of the six higher cognitive functions can go far to bypass weaknesses in other domains. Someone who is excellent at conceptualizing may not need to process or memorize verbal material as thoroughly as a learner who is weak at conceptualizing. The strong conceptualizer does not need to rely as much on rote memory as does the student who has a poor or tenuous grasp of concepts. Similarly good problem-solving ability, brainstorming effectiveness, meta-cognition, and rule application can be facilitators of learning and academic productivity. They too can enable a student to bypass weaknesses in other neurodevelopmental areas. On the other hand, a student with higher cognitive weaknesses as part of a cluster of neurodevelopmental dysfunction is at a distinct disadvantage academically.

Social Cognition

A student's social abilities are stringently tested throughout the school day. There exists a discrete neurodevelopmental function of social cognition. Some children are extremely adept in their social cognitive abilities, whereas others exhibit debilitating social skill deficits. Social skill variations are discussed in detail in Chapter 54. An account of a child's social abilities is a critical component of any complete description of his or her neurodevelopmental profile.

Academic Impacts

The neurodevelopmental functions that have been enumerated are represented in varying clusters (of strengths and of weaknesses) within individual children. In fact, there are so many different combinations of dysfunctions operating in such diverse environmental and cultural contexts that an endless variety of performance and behavioral patterns is encountered. This heterogeneity constitutes further justification for avoiding the simplistic labeling or categorizing of school-aged children. Clusters of neurodevelopmental dysfunctions commonly result in academic delays, particularly in the basic skills of reading, spelling, writing, and mathematics. Although there exists considerable variation, the following is a general description of some common associations between neurodevelopmental dysfunctions and academic skills.

READING

Reading disabilities may be associated with a range of neurodevelopmental dysfunctions (Johnson, 1988):

1. Most often, subtle or blatant language dysfunctions are found among children with substantial reading delays. Initially many language-impaired students have difficulty with phonologic awareness. They may endure debilitating problems forming associations in memory between language sounds (phonemes) and specific combinations of letters (graphemes). This associative memory gap results in delayed skill acquisition at the level of decoding individual words.

An affected child may have trouble with his or her word analysis skills (the ability to break down words into their sound units) and be slow to acquire a sight vocabulary (i.e., a repertoire of words that can be identified instantly). Decoding ability involves the capacity to translate individual written words into their appropriate language sounds and meanings. When decoding skills are delayed or not well automatized, sentence and passage comprehension is likely to be compromised because so much cognitive effort and attention are being allocated to decoding that few, if any, resources remain for understanding.

2. Occasionally students with spatial ordering dysfunctions have trouble learning to read, but this is now thought to be a relatively rare cause of chronic reading difficulty. Affected students initially have difficulty with whole-to-part spatial relationships (i.e., what goes with what to form a discrete spatial entity), which later gives way to problems recognizing visual patterns, making it hard for a student to develop an automatic sight vocabulary for reading.

3. Children with weaknesses of temporal-sequential ordering may have some difficulty breaking down words into their component sounds (phonemes) and then reblending them while preserving correct sound sequences.

4. Memory dysfunction can cause insidious problems with reading recall, with the aforementioned associative memory for phonemes and graphemes, and with the acquisition of a reading vocabulary. As noted previously in this chapter, some children with active working memory weaknesses may have trouble remembering the beginning of a passage by the time they read the end of it. They may also be poor at decoding multisyllabic words. Some students exhibit weak or slow recall from long-term memory, which can impair reading comprehension in the upper grades because learning from textbooks demands rapid activation of prior knowledge during reading.

5. Some students with higher cognitive deficiencies experience trouble comprehending or applying what they read because they lack a strong grasp of the concepts in the text. Reading ability is greatly enhanced by the capacity to activate just the right preexisting facts and concepts while reading. Students who have a poor grasp of what they have learned in the past may derive relatively little meaning from what they are currently reading. They are often described as passive learners; little of what they read resonates with prior experience or education.

Frequently children with reading disabilities do whatever they can to avoid reading. They undertake virtually no reading for pleasure. Thus it is not unusual for a poor reader to superimpose a lack of reading practice over an underlying reading disability. Consequently the child's delay becomes increasingly pronounced over time, as other students not only can read better but are also benefiting from more reading practice. Such a reading inhibition can also ultimately compromise overall language skills, since reading experience is a continuing source of linguistic knowledge and skill.

SPELLING

Impairments of spelling take various forms, depending in part on the nature and extent of a child's neurodevelopmental dysfunctions:

1. Students with language disorders may have trouble applying a knowledge of phonology to spelling. They may overuse a visual (gestalt) sense of word configuration, so that their spellings are phonetically inaccurate yet visually comparable to actual words (e.g., "taugh" for "tough").
2. Others seem to have trouble with visualization or the recall of word configurations. Some of them have pervasive visualization weaknesses, as described previously in this chapter. Others have effective visually driven motor memory but have difficulty visualizing correct spellings. Their errors tend to be phonetically correct but visually discrepant (e.g., "tuff" for "tough").
3. Children with certain memory disorders can spell words adequately during a spelling bee or on a spelling list, but then they misspell the same words when writing a paragraph. Such functional undermining was described previously in this chapter. As noted, in these cases an overburdened memory is unable to sustain several distinct operations concurrently during the act of writing.
4. Some students commit mixed spelling errors. Usually these children harbor multiple dysfunctions of memory and language. They generally have the worst prognosis with regard to the acquisition of spelling skills.
5. Some children consistently generate "illegal" spellings. They deploy letter combinations that do not exist in English. They are likely to ignore spelling rules. For example, the long vowel rule dictates that when a letter is to be pronounced in its long form, there needs to be an "e" at the end of the word. Thus the word "cute" must have an "e" at the end if the "u" is to be pronounced in the long form. A student with a poor grasp of rules might spell the word "cut" instead of "cute."
6. Erratic spelling is very common in children with attention deficits. Because they are tuning in and out of focus, their spelling is unpredictable. Moreover a lack of consistent self-monitoring ensures they are unlikely to detect and correct spelling mistakes as they commit them.
7. There are students whose spelling problems are a part of a broader difficulty with the mastery of "linear chunks" of data. These children or adolescents omit letters from the middle of words, showing greater accuracy with word beginnings and endings.

WRITING

Writing is commonly the heaviest of burdens for many children with neurodevelopmental dysfunctions. Since the demand for written output grows exponentially during one's school career, children with writing disabilities are likely to experience increasing agony and underachievement. To write effectively, a student must be able to coordinate four levels of fluency: ideational fluency, verbal fluency, mnemonic fluency, and graphomotor fluency. Ideational fluency refers to the speed and richness with which ideas get generated. Verbal fluency relates to the speed and precision with which language is produced to encode those ideas. Mnemonic fluency comprises the speed and accuracy of recall for the various subcomponents of writing (e.g., letter formation, spelling, punctuation). Finally graphomotor fluency entails the rapid muscular coordination and neuromotor efficiency needed to keep pace with the flow of ideas, language, and mnemonic elements. When one or more of these fluencies is errant or too slow, children are likely to experience significant problems with written output. Sometimes a particular function proceeds too quickly, a phenomenon that may also result in impaired writing. As noted, some children with very rapid ideational fluency lack the mnemonic and graphomotor speed and precision needed to keep up with the vast outpouring of thoughts.

Some neurodevelopmental underpinnings of writing disability include the following:

1. In many cases writing is too laborious because of one or more underlying graphomotor dysfunctions. In such instances, a child's graphomotor fluency lags behind ideation and language production. Thoughts are simplified, literally forgotten, or under-elaborated during writing because the mechanical effort of transcription is so taxing.
2. Just as students with simultaneous memory deficiencies experience problems spelling in paragraphs, they are also prone to more global writing problems. Their written output is often inconsistent in its legibility, ideation, and conformity to rules.
3. Children with sequential ordering problems may have difficulty organizing their ideas effectively when they write. Their narratives may be free-associative. They may have trouble making use of a lead paragraph and a concluding statement. It may be hard for them to sequence events or facts in the correct order while summarizing a book. They commonly have trouble adhering to a topic while writing.
4. Written language is probably the most sophisticated of all linguistic demands. Children with language dysfunctions may be poor at expressing their ideas on paper.
5. The attentional demands of writing are formidable; therefore many children with attention deficits experience writing problems. They have trouble, in particular, utilizing the production controls or executive functions during writing. They are easily overwhelmed by the organizational demands imposed by writing.

MATHEMATICS

Delays in mathematical abilities can be especially refractory. In a recent community study, it was discovered that students delayed more than 6 months in mathematics in sixth grade almost never caught up. Mathematics becomes an emotionally painful pursuit for many children. It has been reported that during elementary and junior high school, children regard mathematic ability as the ultimate criterion of whether they have intellectual ability. The subject assumes so much importance that some individuals become phobic about mathematics. Anxiety over mathematics frequently aggravates underlying mathematics disabilities.

The following are some of the common neurodevelopmental dysfunctions that deter learning in mathematics:

1. Some children experience mathematics failure because they fail to grasp certain arithmetic concepts. Good mathematicians are able to employ both verbal and nonverbal conceptual abilities to master firmly such concepts as decimal, proportion, volume, and place value. Ineffective mathematicians may have serious difficulty moving back and forth from abstract to concrete concept formation. As a result, it may be hard for them to apply concepts effectively in solving word problems or when confronted with practical situations. These students may then rely too much on rote memory. They may deceive themselves into believing that if they can state the definition of a concept, they truly understand it. Others may apply concepts in highly stereotypical ways, thereby sacrificing their versatility or applicability in diverse situations. For example, a student may learn to add and multiply fractions without ever fully comprehending what a fraction is or knowing what is happening to the value of a fraction during addition or multiplication.

2. Circumscribed memory weaknesses often compromise mathematic performance. Affected students have trouble automatizing mathematics facts (such as the multiplication tables). It simply takes them too long while solving a problem to recall that $8 \times 4 = 32$. So much effort is devoted to the recall of mathematics facts that attention to problem solving is sacrificed. Some students have difficulty with the precise recall of procedural sequences (such as the serial steps involved in solving a long division problem). They tend to perform computations in the wrong order or with agonizing hesitancy. Others may harbor weaknesses in active working memory, so that when they focus on one step in a mathematics problem, they are likely to forget other components of that same problem.

3. Some students with language dysfunctions underachieve in mathematics because they have problems understanding their teachers' verbal explanations of quantitative concepts and operations. These students also commonly experience frustration in their attempts to solve word problems.

4. Many students with attention deficits falter in mathematics classes because of their trouble focusing on precise detail (such as operational signs). Consequently they frequently commit careless errors. Often these students possess divergent thinking and memory patterns. They balk at the highly precise convergent demands in mathematics.

5. Some children are poor at mathematics because of their underdeveloped problem-solving skills. In many instances they are too impulsive to be systematic. They have trouble making clear determinations of what is being asked in a problem. It is hard for them to estimate answers, to detect helpful clues in the wording of a problem, to activate just the right prior skill or knowledge, to consider multiple strategies for solving the problem, and to self-monitor while they are working. Students with underdeveloped problem-solving skills may be inflexible or unsystematic in their approaches to mathematics tasks.

CONTENT AREAS

Children with neurodevelopmental dysfunctions may experience difficulty in a wide range of academic content areas. The sciences may be problematic, especially as they necessitate the processing of dense verbal material in textbooks and the rapid convergent recall of facts. Social studies courses often entail sophisticated language, systematic memorization, and the mastery of abstract verbal concepts (such as totalitarianism, separation of church and state, and balance of power). Social studies also entails good visualization skills, particularly when geographic relationships need to be learned and recalled. Historical texts often stress sequential memory and causal reasoning.

Foreign language learning can create a painful crisis for a student with even subtle language dysfunctions or memory dysfunctions. Some students have trouble mastering the sound system (phonology) of a second language. Others struggle in vain with the cumulative memory demand; they have difficulty recalling in April what they learned the previous October. Because foreign language learning is cumulative, memory shortcomings may be particularly disabling. Other students simply cannot master the grammar of a foreign language. In many cases, they have not totally assimilated the grammatical system in their native language either. Some children have great difficulty acquiring new vocabulary in their native language; they are especially vulnerable to failure in their attempt to master a second language. Clinicians need to be alert to students with mild or severe language dysfunctions and early foreign language failure. Such students should postpone the learning of a foreign language until late in high school; in some cases, they may need to be granted foreign language waivers to graduate from high school and further their education. Clinicians can be very helpful in writing letters and providing justification for such waivers.

Many students with attention deficits can succeed only in content areas that they find romantically attractive. They exhibit disappointing performance in courses that contain substantial quantities of (not very exciting) detail. They may have trouble distinguishing salient data from trivia in texts because their selective attention is too diffuse to make such fine distinctions.

Students with organizational problems commonly suffer in content area subjects. They often lack effective learning strategies. Some are far too impulsive to make use of systematic techniques to facilitate studying and work output. Others struggle because they are unable to maintain a usable notebook, record assignments properly, arrive at places on time, meet deadlines, locate books and utensils, organize a locker or desk, and remember what materials to take home from or bring to school. They are often unclear about their assigned work. Many seriously disorganized students also have trouble studying for tests. They seem not to know how and what to study or for how long. They frequently lack appropriate self-testing skills.

Nonacademic Impacts

Neurodevelopmental dysfunctions often culminate in problems that extend well beyond the classroom and the school day. Some nonacademic impacts are indigenous to the dysfunctions themselves, whereas other sequelae are secondary to persistent failure, embarrassment, and frustration. Children with attention deficits (Chapter 52) are particularly prone to both academic and nonacademic effects of their dysfunctions. In some cases, their impulsivity and lack of effective self-monitoring techniques lead to behavioral maladaptation. A student with attentional dysfunction may be aggressive or disruptive in the classroom and at home. He or she may be unable to accept behavioral limits, assume responsibilities, and delay gratification. Children with social cognitive weaknesses (Chapter 54) may show evidence of social withdrawal, or, alternatively, they may deploy disruptive or "weird" behaviors in a desperate and misguided attempt to lure friends.

In some instances, children with neurodevelopmental dysfunctions harbor excessive performance anxiety, overt clinical depression, or both. Sadness, self-deprecatory comments, diminished self-esteem, chronic fatigue, loss of interests, and even suicidal ideation may result. Not uncommonly, children with neurodevelopmental dysfunctions lose motivation. They are apt to give up and exhibit "learned helplessness," as they assume they have no personal control over their destinies (Diener and Dweck, 1978). As a result, they feel no need to expend effort. Learned helplessness ultimately can promote depression, a loss of motivation, pessimism, dependency, or withdrawal.

Many studies have documented a relationship between learning disorders (LD) of various types and juvenile delinquency (JD). The so-called JD-LD link can occur on many levels. Highly impulsive children may be more likely to commit crimes. Those who experience excessive academic failure and embarrassment may feel a need to engage in "macho" acts aimed at impressing a peer group, since they are unable to acquire respect through other means.

There is a close association between language dysfunctions and delinquent behavior. In some instances, a child or adolescent may commit antisocial acts simply because he or she cannot control circumstances verbally; more physical means then come forth. It is unlikely that learning disorders actually cause juvenile delinquency. On the other hand, they certainly represent risk factors that may be actuated, especially amid depriving or stressful environmental circumstances.

Assessment

Children with possible manifestations of neurodevelopmental dysfunction require meticulous multidisciplinary evaluations based on differential diagnoses appropriate for chronologic age and grade level. It is unlikely that any single professional can adequately assess the diverse sources and broad effects of academic underachievement. An optimal evaluation team should consist of a pediatrician or nurse, a psychologist or psychiatrist, and a psychoeducational specialist. The last should be either a special educator or an educational psychologist who can undertake a fine-grained analysis of academic skills. Other professionals can become involved as needed in individual cases. These additional clinicians include a speech and language pathologist, an occupational therapist, a neurologist, and a social worker. The exact composition of teams and outside consultants depends largely on local needs and accessible resources in the school and in the community.

Many children undergo evaluations within a school setting. Such assessments are an entitlement in the United States under Public Law 94-142. Multidisciplinary evaluations conducted in schools are usually very helpful and are a requirement if a child is to qualify for special services. However, evaluations in school are susceptible to some biases or conflicts of interest. Available therapeutic resources, rigid regulations, and funding constraints may unduly influence the outcome of a school-based evaluation. Because of such limitations, there has been a growing demand for independent evaluations, for second opinions outside of the school. Often pediatricians are asked to become involved in such independent evaluations.

Commonly children are determined to be eligible for services if they exhibit a significant discrepancy between intelligence quotient (IQ) test results and achievement test scores. Such a discrepancy is interpreted as an indication of "learning disability." Unfortunately, by the use of this paradigm, many dysfunctioning students are likely to "fall between the cracks" and not qualify for services. Certain clusters of neurodevelopmental dysfunctions may fail to create a sufficient disparity between an IQ result and an achievement test score. Clinicians need to be aware of those students who have significant neurodevelopmental dysfunctions and yet are ineligible to receive help in school.

The evaluation of a child with suspected neurodevelopmental dysfunctions should include a complete physical, neurologic, and sensory examination. Standardized questionnaires can be used to obtain historical data from the school, the parents, and even the child. Several pediatric neurodevelopmental examinations exist for those clinicians who wish to make direct observations of neurodevelopmental function. These examinations include the PEET, the PEER, the PEEX 2, and the PEERAMID 2. They allow pediatricians or other clinicians to observe or directly sample key neurodevelopmental functions, such as attention, memory, language, and motor skills. Examinations of this type also permit direct behavioral observations as well as assessments of minor neurologic indicators (sometimes called "soft signs") frequently associated with certain neurodevelopmental dysfunctions. These indicators include associated movements, or synkinesias.

Intelligence testing can be helpful. Although an overall IQ may be misleading, the results of specific subtests often are helpful in providing evidence for one or more specific neurodevelopmental dysfunctions. Psychoeducational testing can yield highly relevant data, especially when such testing includes error analyses that pinpoint discrete breakdowns in reading, spelling, writing, and mathematics (Chapter 71). A psychoeducational specialist, making use of input from multiple sources, can help to formulate specific recommendations for regular and special educational teachers.

A mental health professional is valuable in identifying family-based issues complicating or aggravating neurodevelopmental dysfunctions. That professional also can diagnose any specific psychiatric condition contributing to the clinical picture in a child with academic problems.

Management

Just as assessment demands a multidisciplinary approach, the management of children with neurodevelopmental dysfunctions necessitates multimodal intervention. Most children with neurodevelopmental dysfunctions require at least several of the following 10 forms of intervention:

1. Demystification. Many children with neurodevelopmental dysfunctions have little or no understanding of the nature or sources of their difficulties. Once an appropriate descriptive assessment has been performed, it is especially important to explain a child's dysfunctions and strengths to that child. This explanation should be provided in nontechnical, optimistic, concrete, and nonaccusatory terms. Children can also be given an opportunity to read about the subject of neurodevelopmental dysfunction (Levine, 1990; Levine, 1994). Parents and teachers also need to become knowledgeable (Levine, 1995).

2. Bypass strategies (accommodations). Numerous techniques can enable a child to circumvent neurodevelopmental dysfunctions. Ordinarily such bypass strategies should be encouraged in the regular classroom, while individualized intervention in other settings is aimed at strengthening deficient functions. The general forms of bypass are summarized in Table 53–6. Examples of specific bypass strategies include using a calculator while solving mathematics problems, writing essays with a word processor, presenting oral instead of written reports, assigning fewer mathematics problems, seating a child close to the teacher to minimize distraction, offering visually presented demonstration models of correctly solved mathematics problems, and granting permission for a student to take scholastic aptitude tests (SATs) untimed. These bypass strategies do not "cure" neurodevelopmental dysfunctions, but they minimize their academic and nonacademic impact.

3. Remediation of skills and subskills. Tutorial programs are commonly used to bolster deficient academic skills. Reading specialists, math tutors, and other such professionals can make use of diagnostic data to select techniques that take advantage of a student's neurodevelopmental strengths and content affinities in an effort to improve decoding skills, writing ability, or mathematic computation. Often remediation takes place in a resource room or learning center at school. Remediation need not focus exclusively on specific academic areas. Many stu-

Table 53–6 • General Forms of Bypass Strategy Used in the Management of Children With Neurodevelopmental Dysfunctions

Form	Description or Examples
Rate adjustment	Allowing a child more time on a test or a longer interval to answer a question or presenting instructions/explanations more slowly
Volume adjustment	Reducing the length of a report or number of items on a test
Complexity adjustment; prioritizing	Simplifying directions or explanations, stressing or grading on fewer task components (such as ignoring spelling errors and emphasizing good ideas in a report)
Staging	Performing tasks in specific prescribed steps
Format shift	Presenting information in a child's strong learning mode (e.g., visually demonstrating a mathematic process to a child with a language dysfunction)
Affinity use	Teaching skills with materials that tap a child's interests or areas of expertise

dents need assistance to acquire study skills, cognitive strategies, and organizational habits.

4. Developmental therapies. Considerable controversy exists regarding the efficacy of treatments to enhance weak neurodevelopmental functions. It has not been demonstrated convincingly that it is possible to substantially improve a child's fine motor skills, memory, problem-solving proficiency, or temporal-sequential ordering abilities. Nevertheless some forms of developmental therapy are widely accepted. Speech and language pathologists commonly offer intervention for children with language dysfunctions. Occupational therapists strive to improve the motor skills of certain students with writing problems or gross motor clumsiness. Recently there has been considerable interest in social skills training that usually takes the form of small group sessions in which school-aged children are helped to become more aware of the dynamics of social interaction. Cognitive-behavioral therapy is another recently introduced intervention. In this modality of treatment, children learn about their neurodevelopmental dysfunctions and are given specific exercises aimed at enhancing the weak areas. For example, a child with attention deficits may be taught about his or her impulsivity and then provided with exercises that encourage reflection, planning, and a less frenetic tempo.

5. Curriculum modification. To succeed, many students with neurodevelopmental dysfunction require alterations in the school curriculum. For example, high school students with memory weaknesses may need to have their courses selected so that they do not have to cope with cumulative memory overload in any one semester. The timing of a foreign language course, the selection of a mathematics curriculum, and the choice of science courses are critical issues for many underachieving students.

6. Strengthening of strengths. In all cases students with neurodevelopmental dysfunctions need to have their affinities and potential or actual talents identified and exploited. It is as important to strengthen strengths as it is to remedy deficiencies. Athletic skills, artistic inclinations, leadership abilities, creative talents, or mechanical aptitudes are among the potential assets of certain students who are underachieving academically. Parents and school personnel need to create opportunities for such students to build on these proclivities and to savor respect and praise for their efforts. The strengthening of strengths is an essential process for sustaining self-esteem and motivation.

7. Individual and family counseling. When learning difficulties are complicated by family problems or identifiable psychiatric disorders, psychotherapy may be indicated. Clinical psychologists or child psychiatrists are able to offer long-term or short-term therapies. Such interventions can involve the child alone, an entire family, or a small group of children with similar problems. It is essential that the therapist have a firm understanding of a child's neurodevelopmental dysfunctions. The parents and child can become seriously confused if a psychotherapist attributes the child's learning difficulties exclusively to environmental factors, thereby ignoring the potent influence of underlying dysfunctions of attention, language, or memory. Most families do not require a heavily psychoanalytical or psychodynamic approach but instead can benefit from a counseling program that offers practical advice on behavioral management.

8. Advocacy. Children with developmental dysfunctions require informed advocacy. They must have their rights upheld in the school, in the family, and in the community. A physician can be especially helpful in advocating for a child in school. Some children, for example, are devastated by retention in a grade. The likelihood of benefit is minimal. A physician may need to represent the rights of a child in opposing such grade retention as well as other acts of public humiliation. A physician may also need to advocate strongly so that a child can receive services in school or benefit from modifications in the curriculum. Physicians can also advocate by becoming vocal citizens of their communities. Serving on a school board, for example, a physician can exert a major influence on local policy and on the allocation of resources to school-aged children with special educational needs.

9. Medication. Certain psychopharmacologic agents can be especially helpful in lessening the toll of neurodevelopmental dysfunctions. Most commonly, stimulant medications are used as part of the management of attention deficits. They are never a panacea, since most children with attention deficits have other associated dysfunctions (such as language disorders, memory problems, motor weaknesses, or social skill deficits). Nevertheless the use of medications such as methylphenidate, dextroamphetamine, and pemoline can be an important adjunct to treatment because they seem to help youngsters focus more selectively and control their impulsivity. When depression or excessive anxiety is a significant component of the clinical picture, antidepressants can be prescribed. Pharmacotherapy is discussed in greater detail in Chapter 82. Children receiving medication need regular follow-up visits that include a review of current behavioral checklists, a physical examination, and appropriate modifications of medication dose. Treated children should be given periodic "medication holidays," drug-free intervals so that they can strive to be in control of themselves.

10. Longitudinal case management. All children with neurodevelopmental dysfunctions can benefit from the support and guidance of a service coordinator, a professional who can offer advice in a continuing manner and be available to monitor function over the years. The pediatrician may be an ideal professional to assume this responsibility. New questions inevitably emerge as a child's neurodevelopmental dysfunctions evolve while academic expectations undergo progressive change. Because children with neurodevelopmental dysfunctions represent such a heterogeneous group, no two individuals require the same management plan. Nor is it possible to predict with certainty at age 7 what the needs of a youngster will be when he or she is 14. Consequently, affected children and their families require vigilant follow-up and individualized objective advice and informed advocacy throughout their years in school.

REFERENCES

Bloom BS, Broder L: Problem Solving Processes of College Students. Chicago, University of Chicago Press, 1950.

Denckla M: Motor coordination in dyslexic children: theoretical and clinical implications. *In* Duffy FH, Geschwind N (eds): Dyslexia: A Neuroscientific Approach to Clinical Evaluation. Boston, Little, Brown, 1985, p 187.

Diener CI, Dweck CS: An analysis of learned helplessness: continuous changes in performance, strategy and achievement cognitions following failure. J Person Social Psychol 5:541, 1978.

Johnson DJ: Review of research on specific reading, writing, and mathematics disorders. *In* Kavanagh JF, Truss TJ (eds): Learning Disabilities: Proceedings of the National Conference. Baltimore, York Press, 1988.

Kavanagh JF, Truss TJ (eds): Learning Disabilities: Proceedings of the National Conference. Timonium, MD, York Press, 1988.

Levine MD: Keeping a Head in School: A Student's Book About Learning Abilities and Learning Disorders. Cambridge, MA, Educators Publishing Service, 1990.

Levine, MD: All Kinds of Minds. Cambridge MA: Educators Publishing Co, 1994.

Levine MD: Educational Care. Cambridge MA: Educators Publishing Co, 1995.

Levine MD, Reed M: Developmental Variation and Learning Disorders, 2nd ed. Cambridge, MA, Educators Publishing Service, 1998.

Levine MD, Karnisky W, Palfrey J, et al: Risk factor complexes in early adolescent delinquents. Am J Dis Child 139:50, 1985.

Meltzer L: Strategic learning in children with learning disabilities. Adv Learn Behav Disabil 108:181, 1996.

Nelson K: Language in Cognitive Development. Cambridge, England: Cambridge University Press, 1996.

Shaw L, Levine MD, Belfer M: Developmental double jeopardy: a study of clumsiness and self-esteem in learning disabled children. J Devel Behav Pediatr 4:191, 1982.

Swanson HL, Cooney JB: Learning disabilities and memory. *In* Reid DK, Hresko WP, Swanson HL (eds): Cognitive Approaches to Learning Disabilities, 3rd ed. Austin, Tx, Pro-Ed, 1996.

Sugden DA, Keogh JF: Problems in Motor Skill Development. Columbia, SC, University of South Carolina Press, 1990.

Tallal P, Sainburg RL, Jernigan T: The neuropathology of developmental dysphasia: behavioral, psychological, physiological evidence for a pervasive temporal processing disorder. Read Writ Interdisc J 3:363, 1991.

Torgeson JK: Memory processes in reading disabled children. J Learn Disabil 18:350, 1985.

Vallar G, Papagno C: Neuropychological impairments of short-term memory. *In* Baddeley AD, Wilson BA, Watts FN (eds): Handbook of Memory Disorders. New York, John Wiley, 1995.

Wallach GP, Butler KG (eds): Language Learning Disabilities in School-Age Children and Adolescents. New York, MacMillan, 1994.

Weinert FE, Perlmutter M: Memory Development: Universal Changes and Individual Differences. Hillsdale, NJ, Lawrence Erlbaum Associates, 1988.

54 Social Ability and Inability

Melvin D. Levine

Day in and day out, school-aged children contend with intense and unrelenting social pressures. At the same time, they crave meaningful relationships with individual peers. Some children are highly successful in the social realm, as they obtain lofty levels of personal gratification from their interactions. Regrettably, a subgroup of school children receives failing grades in social cognition and performance. They fail to understand the dynamics of successful relating. Many such children achieve a suboptimal reputation and are forced to endure bullying, verbal abuse, and the pain of rejection. In this chapter, the elements of social cognition are described, along with some of the common breakdowns that thwart successful relationships and reputations for some children. Social failure is common, yet it is a surprisingly neglected subject within the field of pediatric health care.

The social lives of school-aged children may lead to abundant gratification or to incapacitating frustration and anxiety. A school-aged child encounters a relentless succession of social tests each day, facing highly judgmental scrutiny by peers and adults alike. A child's social abilities allow him or her to gain a respectable reputation among peers while facilitating the formation and maintenance of friendships. Considerable research conducted in recent years has enabled us to understand the critical functions that are needed for social success in childhood. At the same time, we have learned a great deal about the social cognitive dysfunctions that impair some children. This chapter explores various components of social cognition and the common breakdowns in these functions that cause many children and adolescents to experience social failure and suffering.

Student Subgroups

Within any school culture, the students can be divided into groups that characterize their levels of social success. Many studies have focused on these subgroups and the behaviors that often characterize their members (Asher and Coie, 1990). The groups are as follows:

- Popular students: These are children who are well liked and respected by their peers. They are apt to influence public opinion and occupy leadership roles. They receive many invitations and telephone calls.
- Amiable students: These are children who are inoffensive and likable but not actively sought after for friendship.
- Controversial students: These are children who are popular with some students and unpopular or even actively rejected by others.
- Neglected students: These are children whom no one or hardly anyone knows. Either they are inconspicuous and withdrawn by nature or they consciously seek to maintain a low profile.

- Rejected students: These are children who are excluded by their peers. They may endure verbal and physical abuse from others. Rejected students can be further divided into those who show many aggressive behaviors and those who are rejected but are nonaggressive in their behaviors.

Over the years, social psychologists and other investigators have been interested in how students gain social acceptance, how they become amiable or popular and elude rejection. In various studies, a series of social cognitive functions have been identified. Weaknesses in these specific social abilities appear to underlie the interpersonal failure of some individuals (Levine, 1995). The social cognitive functions and dysfunctions can be subdivided into verbal and nonverbal traits. They are summarized in Table 54–1.

Nonverbal Social Cognition

Many social abilities do not entail overt verbal communication. These nonverbal functions comprise a range of social interpretations and actions that can help children gain peer acceptance and true satisfaction from their interactions. On the other hand, when these abilities are deficient or seemingly absent, the social life of a child becomes a persistent source of anguish. The important nonverbal social cognitive abilities include the following:

- Greeting skill: This entails the ability to sense the prevailing tone emanating from a group of children and produce a behavior that fits in with it effectively. A child with weak greeting skill may act silly when peers are trying to be serious.
- Reinforcing and reciprocal behaviors: These are ways of acting to make another person feel good about herself. A child with a diminished sense of the need for reciprocity and reinforcement may show excessive egocentricity, taking things from others, refusing to share, and doing little to make another child feel good.

Table 54–1 • A Checklist of Social Cognitive Functions

Student's Name _____ Grade _____ Date _____

Observer's Name _____ Position _____

A. Nonverbal Functions

Specific Function	Description of Function	Adequacy of Current Practice		
		−	±	+
Greeting skill	"Reading" a social scene and acting in a way that fits into it	Weak	Adequate	Strong
		−	±	+
Reinforcing behaviors	Making someone else feel good about himself/herself	Weak	Adequate	Strong
		−	±	+
Reciprocal behaviors	Showing altruism (e.g., sharing, praising), especially with close friends	Weak	Adequate	Strong
		−	±	+
Collaborative behaviors	Being effective at cooperating in play and/or work activities	Weak	Adequate	Strong
		−	±	+
Nonverbal cueing	Using appropriate eye contact and body movements in relating to others	Weak	Adequate	Strong
		−	±	+
Timing and staging	Pacing relationships; not expecting too much too soon	Weak	Adequate	Strong
		−	±	+
Social feedback sensitivity	Knowing how one is faring during or immediately following an interaction	Weak	Adequate	Strong
		−	±	+
Behavioral interpretation	Being able to discern reasons for or intent of a peer's actions	Weak	Adequate	Strong
		−	±	+
Awareness of impacts	Having awareness of one's reputation and "usual" effects on peers	Weak	Adequate	Strong
		−	±	+
Conflict resolution	Resolving social conflicts without resorting to aggression	Weak	Adequate	Strong
		−	±	+
Social control level	Relating to peers without demanding too much or too little control	Weak	Adequate	Strong
		−	±	+
Recuperative strategies	Coping with, recovering from social setbacks	Weak	Adequate	Strong
		−	±	+
Self-marketing skill	"Packaging" one's image to be socially acceptable to peers	Weak	Adequate	Strong

B. Verbal Functions

Specific Function	Description of Function	Adequacy of Current Practice		
		−	±	+
Feelings conveyance	Expressing feelings accurately, preventing misinterpretation	Weak	Adequate	Strong
		−	±	+
Feelings interpretation	"Reading" language cues to infer the feelings of others	Weak	Adequate	Strong
		−	±	+
Lingo fluency	Using the language of one's peer group (fluently and credibly)	Weak	Adequate	Strong
		−	±	+
Topic selection and maintenance	Knowing what to talk about when, with whom, and for how long	Weak	Adequate	Strong
		−	±	+
Humor utilization and calibration	Employing the right kind or level of humor in a current social context	Weak	Adequate	Strong
		−	±	+
Code switching	Modifying language expression to "fit" the expectations of a current audience	Weak	Adequate	Strong
		−	±	+
Perspective taking	Knowing what others know and what they need to know from you	Weak	Adequate	Strong
		−	±	+
Requesting skills	Asking for something in a nonoffensive manner	Weak	Adequate	Strong
		−	±	+
Communication repair	Revising misinterpreted language or fixing miscommunication	Weak	Adequate	Strong
		−	±	+
Affective matching	Creating language that complements the prevailing mood(s) of others	Weak	Adequate	Strong

This grid comprises a checklist that can be used as a clinical inventory of verbal and nonverbal social abilities. The list is not meant to be scored but rather to yield a qualitative view of those functions that may require further social skills training.

- Nonverbal cueing: Socially competent students have ways of making eye contact and regulating body movements to present a friendly, attractive, and compatible image to peers. Some children have problems putting forth such positive signals. In some cases they show evidence of dyssemia, a condition in which an individual has no control over the social implications of body movements. Such an individual may seem "weird" or out of step to others without understanding why.
- Timing and staging: Socially proficient people understand how to pace their relationships. Some children with social cognitive deficits take liberties too early in friendships or they seem to "wear out" their peers with the frenetic intensity of their interactions.
- Social feedback sensitivity: In the social domain, feedback is critical. An individual must know how a relationship is going. There are children who have difficulty processing social feedback. They may be unable to recognize that they are displeasing their peers or saying things that are offensive to others. For example, they may have serious problems "reading" the facial expressions of others as a part of their insensitivity to social feedback cues.
- Awareness of impacts: Closely related to social feedback sensitivity is an individual's ability to gauge her or his overall reputation or standing within a group. Some children with social cognitive weaknesses show insufficient awareness of their social status within a classroom, neighborhood, or other milieu.
- Conflict resolution: Socially adept people are apt to be skilled at dealing with interpersonal conflicts. Many children who have social difficulty appear unable to resolve conflicts without resorting to aggression. In the face of social stress, they may be highly volatile, aggressive, or self-destructive. They simply lack a repertoire of amicable solutions to social conflicts.
- Social control level: Socially successful people are usually able to exercise an optimal level of control over their relationships with others; they are neither too dominant or bossy, nor totally submissive or passive. Some individuals with social cognitive problems have trouble maintaining this balance. Some are too passive in their social behaviors, while others can relate only by taking complete command of any interaction.
- Recuperative strategies: Everyone encounters social setbacks, embarrassing incidents, or disappointing social outcomes. A socially resilient person can recover readily and not brood excessively. Some children seem to lack the social recuperative ability to "bounce back" from a setback. Social defeats may leave needless scars and cause a child to withdraw or become extremely anxious for a prolonged period.
- Self-marketing skill: Socially skilled people develop an image that is reasonably appealing to the outside world. They may do so consciously, semiconsciously, or unconsciously. They know how to dress, tend to personal hygiene, develop personal interests, and comfort themselves in a manner that is attractive to others. Many children with social cognitive weak-

nesses have serious self-marketing problems. They are likely to project an image that is distasteful to others, often without realizing that they are doing so.

EXAMPLE

Brenda is a 14-year-old eighth-grader. Her parents and teachers are very concerned because they perceive her as becoming increasingly withdrawn and faltering in her self-esteem.

Brenda is a very good artist and an average student. She spends a great deal of time by herself and forms very few relationships with other teenagers. At home she seldom receives or makes telephone calls. Nor does she get invited to social activities.

Brenda is extremely awkward in her relationships with peers. It is hard for her to initiate contact with other students. She seems overly intrusive when she encounters students interacting with each other. She tends to barge in and take little notice of ongoing social scenarios. Sometimes she rushes (and quickly wears out) relationships.

It has been hard for Brenda to "market herself." Her clothing, her hairstyle, and her mannerisms fail to fit in with those of her classmates. As a result, she is considered an oddball. Some girls just don't want to be seen with her. She has been explicitly excluded.

There is no evidence that Brenda has much insight into her social difficulties. She has told her parents she would like to have friends but that no one wants to be near her. She blames the school, stating that there are many "snobs."

Recently Brenda has been gaining a great deal of weight. She is now moderately obese, which is making life harder for her.

Verbal Social Cognition

Language ability plays a key role in the generation of social success during childhood. The capacity to deploy language effectively within social contexts is known as "verbal pragmatics." A child's verbal pragmatic abilities enable him or her to understand and say the right things at the right times while interacting with others (Ninio and Snow, 1996). Verbal pragmatic dysfunctions are commonly present in children with social difficulties (McTear and Conti-Ramsden, 1992). Sometimes such weaknesses are part of a broader picture of language dysfunction, but at times problems with the social aspects of language occur in an individual who displays good language function for academic activities. The following are some major verbal pragmatic functions and signs of dysfunction:

- Conveyance and interpretation of feelings: Language communication often conveys an individual's feelings or moods. A child with good verbal pragmatic skills is able to exercise control over expressed feelings, so that an intended sentiment is properly expressed. Some people with verbal pragmatic difficulties sound angry, hostile, or abrasive when they do not mean to project such feelings. They are often misinterpreted because the tone of their voices, their choices of words, or their inflections give forth unintended (often negative) feelings that may seriously alienate others. Many such children also have difficulty inferring other people's feelings from their language expression. They therefore are apt to believe falsely that someone is angry or disapproving.

- Lingo fluency: It is common for children as a group to share certain fashionable linguistic patterns. Various words, sentence constructions, and even inflections often contribute to the contemporary lingo that is applied, in particular, when children are relating to each other. Some young people with verbal pragmatic dysfunctions have great difficulty using the lingo convincingly and credibly. When they try to do so, they sound awkward and unnatural. Some do not even attempt it.

- Topic selection and maintenance: The ability to know what to talk about when and for how long is an essential component of verbal pragmatics. Some children have a propensity to select inappropriate subjects for conversation, given the particular people, settings, or contexts within which they are conversing. They may also have difficulty knowing how much or how long to talk, as they sometimes perseverate and seem unable to conclude their coverage of a topic.

- Humor utilization and calibration: The effective use of humor is another important verbal pragmatic function. Some children with impaired verbal pragmatic abilities frequently use humor inappropriately, as they seem unable to match their form of humor with a current audience. Thus, they may tell jokes or make comments that are in poor taste or just plain out of step with the sophistication and tastes of others. Sometimes these same children are poor at interpreting the humor of others; they may have trouble understanding jokes or witty comments. Such humor comprehension failure can compromise peer interactions.

- Code switching: In a sense, everyone is constrained to speak in several different language codes. A child does not use the same expressions, vocabulary, and intonation to talk to his grandmother that he might use with friends or with a teacher or when speaking to a policeman. With good verbal pragmatics it is possible to switch from one language code to another in response to changing audiences or circumstances. Unfortunately, some children find it hard to manipulate multiple language codes. For example, when with their peers, they may sound excessively adult or pseudosophisticated in their speech.

- Perspective taking: Verbal pragmatics includes an ability to know what it is that a listener knows and what she or he needs to find out from the speaker. In this way, a child does not use terms or refer to people that are unknown to others, at least not without some explanation. Likewise, a verbal pragmatist is carefully not to provide too much information that the listener obviously already possesses. Some children with verbal pragmatic dysfunctions reveal an apparent inability or reluctance to evaluate the needs of a listener during conversation.

- Requesting skills: It is important to be able to ask for something in a manner that makes it likely the request will be satisfied and that the recipient of the request will not be annoyed or offended. There are children who have persistent trouble knowing how to ask for something. When they try to do so, they may be abrasive or evasive. Their requests are therefore more likely to be denied.

- Communication repair: Everybody commits the occasional faux pas or regrets having said something or feels that an idea "did not come out right." A person with good verbal pragmatic skills recognizes the communication gap and is able to revise a previously articulated statement so that it can work better socially. A child with deficiencies of verbal pragmatics may fail to notice the communication error or may not know how to correct it.

- Affective matching: Language can be used to match feelings with others in a social situation. If others are joking, then a person can use language humor to fit in. If two people are commiserating over a sad event, then a third person entering the scene can match their feelings with language of similar tone and content. When a child has trouble with verbal pragmatics, it may be hard for him to sense the prevailing tone and match it accurately. Thus, when his friends are acting angry or sad, he may try to tell a joke. When they are engaged in slapstick humor, he may utter some profound and serious thoughts. In other words, the affect of his language is too often poorly matched to the moods of those to whom he is trying to relate.

EXAMPLE

Scott is an 8-year-old boy with a vivid imagination and a highly fertile fantasy life. He excels academically, having had no trouble acquiring basic skills in the early grades. He also is a wellspring of knowledge, especially when it comes to nature and the environment. Scott has a special interest in turtles (which he collects). When he expounds on these and other amphibians, he sounds like an adult, a "little professor."

Developmentally, Scott has done well with the exception of his gross motor coordination, which is notably delayed. Perhaps as a result, he has always shied away from athletic pursuits.

During the current year, Scott has become the victim of some verbal abuse by his classmates. They have derided him during physical education classes. His peers talk of Scott (openly) as being really weird.

In class discussions, Scott is extremely vocal, but he easily gets off track and likes to discuss issues or topics that would seem more appropriate for adults. Sometimes Scott acts silly and tells jokes, without noticing that he is the only person laughing at his witticisms. At other times, he tries to sound "macho" or tough, but he totally lacks credibility when he does so.

Scott's parents report that he is quite irritable when he gets home. He is very aggressive toward his younger sister and has begun to be oppositional toward his parents.

Scott has no real friends in the neighborhood. He relates best to younger children and adults. His parents' friends seem to adore him. Scott's mother and father sometimes feel that Scott is too "gifted" to relate meaningfully to children of his own age. They state that he "marches to his own drummer."

Assessing Social Cognitive Function

In reviewing the history of a child with learning or behavioral adjustment problems, possible difficulties with social cognition may become evident. Behavioral questionnaires, such as the ANSER System (Levine, 1996) may elicit signs of social failure. When this is the case, a more specific inventory of social traits can be completed by a child's teacher. Such an inventory can enable a clinician to target for management specific gaps in a child's social repertoire (see Table 54–1).

Social cognitive dysfunctions frequently are part of a cluster of neurodevelopmental dysfunctions (Chapter 53). For example, it is common for children with weak attention controls to have difficulty slowing down and engaging in behaviors that are sufficiently reflective to allow for good social judgment and output. Although they may possess social skills, they seem unable to apply them as needed. Some children with language dysfunctions endure deficiencies of verbal pragmatic function that result in significant interpersonal failure. Likewise, other dysfunctions, such as gross motor incoordination or memory weakness, may be associated with social problems. Therefore, any evaluation of a child with apparent social cognitive weaknesses needs to take into account the role of the child's overall neurodevelopmental profile.

The following questions should be addressed in the assessment of a child with social cognitive weaknesses:

1. What traits of social cognitive dysfunction can be documented in this child (see Table 54–1)?
2. Does she or he show areas of social strength?
3. How aware and insightful is the child with regard to the social stress being endured?
4. What additional neurodevelopmental or behavioral difficulties are present?
5. What assets does this child possess that ultimately might be used to make him or her more appealing to peers?

In some instances it may be discovered that a child with social cognitive weaknesses shows evidence of frank autism (Chapter 60). In milder cases, there may be a temptation to label an individual as having *Asperger syndrome*. This appellation is rather arbitrary as well as pessimistic and is unlikely to be of any direct benefit to the child or family.

Managing Social Cognitive Failure

A number of therapeutic options exist for children with social cognitive problems. They can often benefit from a sensitive and sympathetic program that includes the following components:

- Demystification: When a child is found to have social cognitive problems, it is important that he or she learn very specifically about those areas of weakness that need to be worked on. Affected children need to learn about their areas of social weakness. They need to acquire the vocabulary that describes their dysfunction with specificity. It is nearly impossible to work on a weakness for which you have no word.
- Social skills training: A number of organized curricula exist to teach affected children the social abilities they seem to lack. Most often the training takes place in small groups with a trained adult at the helm. In many cases the children pursue activities and discussion, some of which may be videotaped for future scrutiny and discussion by participants. In this way the children attain a higher level of conscious awareness of key aspects of forming and maintaining meaningful relationships. Children can also read about social cognition. I have written two children's books that contain chapters on social skills and social difficulties (Levine, 1990, 1994).
- Individual counseling: Some children with social cognitive failure need one-to-one counseling. A relatively short course of therapy may be beneficial, especially if the professional involved can offer the student specific advice related to the actual people with whom a child is relating inadequately.
- School-based intervention: At times there may need to be some strong advocacy within a school for a child who is experiencing overt rejection and verbal or physical abuse (bullying). A teacher or school principal may need to address an entire class or group of children to alert them to the cruelty of their actions against a child who may be friendless. Ideally, all schools should offer courses on social cognition to all children, so that they might have a better understanding of intricacies of social life.
- Parent support: Parents need to play a substantial role in supporting a child who is being rejected by peers. On a regular basis, a mother or father can spend time reviewing a child's social experiences with her or him. A trusting relationship can evolve around social issues, so that the child feels comfortable confiding about specific incidents that have been social setbacks. Parents should be good listeners to these stories and should avoid preaching, excessively reassuring, and offering glib advice. These children need to know that their parents are sympathetic and on their side.
- Marketing assistance: Affected children can benefit from measures that enable them to become more appealing to others of their age. In particular, it can be helpful if their parents and teachers can discover activities or endeavors that will encourage meaningful and congenial interactions. It is especially important to help the rejected child use his or her strengths to develop products or abilities that will be impressive to others. A major role in a school play, success in a sport, or some form of conspicuous

creative output can make a great difference. A child may also need advice on physical appearance, on what musical instrument to play, and on other ways of becoming "cool" (if this is desired).

REFERENCES

Asher SR, Coie JD (eds): Peer Rejection in Childhood. Cambridge, England, Cambridge University Press, 1990.

Levine MD: Keeping a Head in School. Cambridge, MA, Educators Publishing Company, 1990.

Levine MD: All Kinds of Minds. Cambridge, MA, Educators Publishing Company, 1994.

Levine MD. Educational Care. Cambridge, MA, Educators Publishing Service, 1995.

Levine MD: The ANSER System. Cambridge, MA, Educators Publishing Service, 1996.

McTear MF, Conti-Ramsden G: Pragmatic Disability in Children. San Diego, Singular Publishing Group, 1992.

Ninio A, Snow CE: Pragmatic Development. Boulder, CO, Westview Press, 1996.

55 Maladaptation to School

Mark Ruggiero

 School is a theater in which many developmental and behavioral issues are on stage. From the earliest grades, children must adapt to this setting in which they are required to act autonomously—without the visible accompaniment and support of their parents. This chapter reviews some of the clinical patterns that clinicians face when children fail to adapt to educational constraints and opportunities. This chapter also offers clinicians some practical interventions that can foster adaptation or "re-adaptation" in school.

Humans are products of the complex interplay between genetic potential and various environmental influences. In addition to the effects of family and culture on a child's development, the educational experience is one of the most important stages on which the players' "nature" and "nurture" exert influence. The school experience not only offers children the knowledge they need to gain success but also reinforces and heightens their developing sense of self-worth. Students' judgments about themselves are molded by constant feedback from peers and teachers, giving them clear input regarding their personal assets and shortcomings in the social, emotional, and academic domains (Jackson, 1983). Maladaptation to school, a type of "failure to thrive" in the school setting, can therefore occur as a result of a broad range of negative influences. In many children, this maladaptation leads to school disinterest, disengagement, and subsequent attendance problems. Because it is clearly found that excessive absences and school failure are associated with an increased risk of later psychiatric disorders and increased dropout rate, the individual and societal implications of this heterogeneic problem are striking (Berg et al, 1993).

Classification and Diagnostic Criteria

There is a long history of disagreement among professionals regarding the terms used to describe different manifestations of school maladaptation. Most of the confusion in this subject area involves the terminology used to describe problematic absenteeism. Broadwin (1932) first described "a special kind of truancy," in which a child's absence is consistent and the parents know where the child is at all times. Because the root of this "special truancy" problem appeared to be grounded in unreasonable fears, clinicians and researchers began using the term *school phobia*, indicating its neurotic nature and as a distinction to the "truancy" associated with conduct problems in older children. Later, after it was recognized that some of these "phobic" children in reality had separation anxiety problems, the term *school refusal* was preferred so that both fear and anxiety-based problems would be accounted for. The more general terms *school avoidance* and *school absenteeism*

have also been used interchangeably with school refusal and school phobia, but unlike the latter two terms, they also include the problem of truancy.

Three manifestations of maladaptation to school are discussed in this chapter: (1) school disengagement, (2) school avoidance, and (3) dropout. In this chapter, the term *school avoidance* is used to describe an extreme reluctance to attend school for a sustained period of time. Both *school refusal* (which is used synonymously with *school phobia*) and *truancy* are considered as two subtypes of school avoidance, each resulting in subsequent absenteeism. School disengagement often leads to school avoidance of either type, and both school avoidance and school disengagement often lead to dropout.

The fact that none of the aforementioned terms appears as a separate diagnosis in either the *International Classification of Diseases (ICD-10)* or the *Diagnostic and Statistical Manual of Mental Disorders*, 4th edition, (*DSM-IV*) adds to the ongoing confusion and disagreement regarding terminology and diagnostic criteria. In the *ICD-10*, problematic school absenteeism is classified as one of the following: separation anxiety disorder of childhood, phobic anxiety of childhood, or social anxiety of childhood. The *DSM-IV* also uses the classification of separation anxiety disorder for the younger child who specifically fears separation from parents, but if the child does not meet those specific *DSM-IV* criteria, a diagnosis of another anxiety disorder or a specific phobia is suggested. There are no specific diagnoses for school disengagement or dropout.

Prevalence

The prevalence of school maladaptation is difficult to assess because of its varied sources and manifestations. Truancy prevalence is difficult to measure because of the child's attempt at secrecy, but it is found in surveys to be alarmingly common. About 75% of adults admit to manifesting this behavior during childhood, and in some studies truancy was admitted to by as many as 50% of teenaged boys. School refusal (school phobia) occurs in less than 1% of the population. Most cases occur in children between the ages of 7 and 12 years, usually boys. Between 5% and 7% of all children referred to behavioral clinics were found to have school refusal. There is no way to estimate the prevalence of school disengagement that does not also show significant absences, but the prevalence of two frequent sources of disengagement (learning disabilities and attention deficits) are estimated to occur in 5% to 10% of the school-aged population.

In any case, it is clear that virtually all teachers, school counselors, school psychologists, and pediatric health care providers encounter children with maladaptation to school on a relatively regular basis. Despite the frequency of this problem and the gravity of its consequences, however, identification of primary presenting characteristics and appropriate evaluation and treatment practices are often unclear to those professionals who initially address this population. In addition to the disagreement regarding terminology and diagnoses, information is not as readily available in this arena as compared with other more specific emotional and behavioral problems identified in school children. Although it is often one or more of these more specific underlying emotional and behavioral difficulties that are among the sources of the maladaptation, it has been found that a significant percentage of children with maladaptation do not have associated psychiatric disorders (Kearney and Beasley, 1994).

Sources

A variety of sources can lead to maladaptation to school (Table 55–1).

PSYCHIATRIC AND EMOTIONAL DISTURBANCES

Many children with school refusal or avoidance have personal problems and conflicts that they are unable to resolve, creating mood disturbances or one of several anxiety disturbances. As many as 40% of school-aged children with severe attendance problems have psychiatric disorders (Berg et al, 1993). Many children who are described as having school phobia in reality have either generalized anxiety or separation anxiety difficulties. Disruptive behaviors are associated with conduct disorder and oppositional defiant disorder. A behavioral history looking at causes and timing of anxiety as well as signs and symptoms of depression helps identify these difficulties. Because these problems can be genetically as well as psychodynamically based, a careful family and social history is also important in the diagnoses of these sources.

TEMPERAMENT

Many children have temperaments that make the school experience difficult and frustrating (Chapter 8). For example, a child may have much difficulty managing routines and schedules, making the daily logistics of school seem impossible. Some students may be sensitive to criticism and live in constant fear of embarrassment during the school day, which may be self-defeating by engendering a conservative, or non–risk-taking, attitude. Others may react unusually negatively to difficulties in the social and academic domains, draining their motivation and leading to a feeling of learned helplessness. An affected child feels that his or her success in school is determined solely by external forces, which can often lead to reactive depression and anxiety disturbances. Identification of these difficulties and appropriate counseling can help the child and parents understand the role that temperament can play in contributing to school maladaptation.

SOCIAL IMBALANCES

Some children have social relatedness problems, which often result in rejection by their peers (Chapter 54). Perceived conflict and lack of personal support in friendships is associated with multiple forms of school maladaptation, including loneliness and avoidance (Ladd, Kochenderfer, and Coleman, 1996). Conversely, some children

Table 55–1 • Sources of School Maladaptation

Psychiatric/emotional disturbances	Neurodevelopmental dysfunctions
Affective disorders/disturbances	Learning difficulties
Depression	Attention deficits
Bipolar disorder	Gross and fine motor deficits
Anxiety disorders/disturbances	Sociocultural influences
Phobias (specific school phobia, social)	Inability to identify with education
Obsessive-compulsive disorder	Permission granted by family (to stay out of school)
Panic disorder	Normal peer behavior is not attending school
Separation anxiety disorder/disturbance	Family/environmental stressors
Conduct disorder	Parental marital problems
Oppositional defiant disorder	Sexual/physical abuse
Sleep disorders	Neglect
Temperamental difficulties	Realistic fear of harm from violence in school setting
Difficulty with routines	Other family dysfunction (spousal abuse, substance abuse)
Sensitivity to criticism	Chronic disease and those physically challenged
Fear of humiliation	Diabetes, cystic fibrosis, cerebral palsy, vision or hearing impaired, spina bifida
Conservative non–risk-taking	Drug-induced
Low motivational states	Prescribed medications (e.g., haloperidol, propranolol)
Social imbalances	Recreational drugs (e.g., marijuana, alcohol)
Social cognitive deficits	School effects
Social infatuation	Specific school factors affecting attendance are not yet clearly identified.

experience excess social gratification and may occasionally become less interested in their academic performance. During the family interview, specific questions about a student's friendships and activities help identify children with social imbalances.

NEURODEVELOPMENTAL DYSFUNCTIONS

Many children with learning, attention, or motor deficits have feelings of being overwhelmed (Chapter 53). These underlying problems can make the school experience humiliating, both in the classroom and in the gymnasium. Early identification is extremely important to prevent such problems from leading to poor self-esteem and decreased motivation. Poor academic performance, attentional or behavioral difficulties, and complaints of coordination or writing problems may be identified through a careful history or questionnaire. Neurodevelopmental, educational, speech/language, and cognitive testing are other tools used to identify specific neurodevelopmental strengths and weakness.

SOCIOCULTURAL INFLUENCES

Many children do not have academic role models at home or in the community. They may therefore have difficulty identifying with education as it relates to providing opportunities for a more productive and stable future. In addition, cultural and/or community norms may indicate that "hanging out" around the neighborhood instead of going to school is the accepted behavior. Children who "skip" school are not thought to be truant; rather they are looked upon as "normal." Families vary significantly in their ideas regarding appropriate circumstances that are required to allow a child to stay home from school. Many parents, for example, give permission to their children to stay home from school to help with cleaning, shopping, or babysitting younger siblings. Asking a family about these "rules" as well as their values regarding education and careers helps identify these influences.

FAMILY/ENVIRONMENTAL STRESSORS

Children who are heavily preoccupied with family stressors may have serious difficulty concentrating in school. A child may feel guilty for going to school in the morning, or anxious and fearful of going home at the end of the day. Careful attention should be made to always consider and rule out the possibility of the child's suffering from neglect or abuse. It is also important to ask the child whether he or she feels physically threatened at school. In some cases referral to family therapy, to marital counseling, or to the child protective services may be warranted.

CHRONIC DISEASE AND PHYSICAL CHALLENGES

Children whose condition makes them look different or who use adaptive equipment may have difficulty feeling comfortable in school. Some children who have very serious chronic illnesses, including rheumatic and orthopedic conditions as well as cystic fibrosis and leukemia, may have excessive amounts of time out of school to attend to legitimate medical treatment. Many of these children, however, have been found to have absence rates that far exceed what can be accounted for by their illness. However, many surveys have shown that the majority of children with chronic illness and physical handicaps have only a few additional days of absence than what is the average for all students. Because many children who avoid school tend to complain of being ill, it is recommended that sources other than just chronic illness be considered in all children showing excessive absences resulting from complaints of illness (Berg, 1992).

SCHOOL EFFECTS

Irrespective of the characteristics of children, there are significant differences between schools in the prevalence of attendance difficulties and dropout rate. It is not clear, however, which aspects of school life account for these differences (Berg, 1992).

Maladaptation may be manifested by social and academic disengagement and specific school phobia and may lead to subsequent school avoidance, refusal, and absenteeism. Without early identification and appropriate interventions, the resulting cycle of further absenteeism, which increases the probability of school failure, increases the risk of dropout. Figure 55–1 is a schematic of the sources of school maladaptation that lead to different manifestations and the complex and cyclic nature of this problem. Children are usually seen with the general manifestations, but the multitude of possible sources and the frequency of multiple overlapping causes can make evaluation and identification difficult. It is not surprising, therefore, that school maladaptation can be a challenging issue for professionals (see Fig. 55–1).

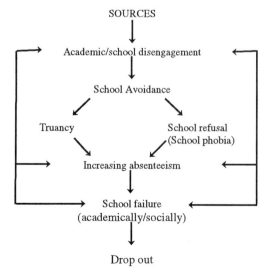

Figure 55–1. Schematic of the sources of school maladaptation leading to different manifestations and the complex and cyclical nature of this problem.

Manifestations of Maladaptation

When considering various forms of maladaptation to school, regardless of the choice of terms used (school phobia, school refusal, truancy), the research and discussion in this area is generally limited to the exploration of excessive absenteeism. It is clear, though, that the manifestations of maladaptation to school also include difficulties such as school disengagement (which does not necessarily result in absenteeism) and school dropout (the extreme of absenteeism, which is usually considered a separate discussion).

School/Academic Disengagement

EXAMPLE

Twelve-year-old Joey was in seventh grade and was brought for evaluation of increasing difficulties with sleep, poor academic performance, and possible attentional deficits. He had been missing school more and more over the past few months. He wrote:

> *"I DON'T LIKE SCHOOL BECAUSE THE TEACHEARS, THEY DON'T TAKE ENOUGE TIME TO EXPLANE WHAT OR HOW TO DO THE WORK."*

Joey had been identified as having learning disabilities in the past, but he was not receiving any services at the time of the evaluation. He was receiving "D" and "F" grades in most of his subjects including math, science, social studies, and written language, but he reported that he enjoyed and was doing fairly well in shop and physical education. He was having significant difficulty falling asleep at night, often not drifting off until 1 AM or 2 AM. He reported falling asleep and daydreaming in class often during the day, and he estimated that he slept an average of 3 to 4 hours during the day. Joey had a fairly good appetite, but had been feeling "down" since his recent move immediately before the school year started and since hearing that one of his old friends had committed suicide. Joey was living with his mother who had dropped out of school but eventually received her GED. His 15-year-old brother was not living at home and was involved with drugs. Joey admitted to smoking cigarettes but denied alcohol or drug use. He was also awaiting a court date for shoplifting.

Academic disengagement can take the form of disruption or withdrawal. When a child is disruptive, it is important to make the distinction between oppositional and defiant behaviors, impulsivity associated with attention deficits, and premeditated aggressiveness. Although each of these behaviors can be disruptive to the individual or interfere with the learning of other students, the approach of management can be very different. Joey was exhibiting withdrawing behaviors as evidenced by his sleeping and daydreaming in class. Students like Joey derive so few benefits from their school experience that they find ways of maintaining a low profile with the conscious or unconscious goal of remaining disconnected from the educational experience. As was the case with Joey, disengagement often leads to increasing absenteeism and increased risk of dropout (Levine, 1987).

CLINICAL EVALUATION

In assessing children with academic/school disengagement, as with each manifestation of maladaptation, a clinician should consider each of the aforementioned sources. In the vignette about Joey, the following sources should be considered:

1. Underlying neurodevelopmental dysfunctions causing learning problems
2. Sociocultural or familial stresses
3. Temperamental difficulties
4. Affective disorder
5. Sleep disorder
6. Recreational drug use
7. School factors

Behavioral inventories were completed by Joey's mother and teachers, and a multidisciplinary team took part in his evaluation. Cognitive testing found that Joey was in the normal range of intellectual functioning. Educational testing identified significant deficits in mathematics calculation and written language. There was evidence of mild attentional deficits. His behavioral inventories and subsequent interview found Joey to be moderately depressed, which could account for his sleep and attentional concerns, and was consistent with his recent environmental and emotional stressors. In addition, Joey grew up in a family in which finishing school had a diminished importance, making his identification with the importance of education difficult. Commonly children unfairly blame teachers for their difficulties, as did Joey in his note. In this case, however, Joey's claim was valid in that he was not receiving the resource help he needed in the classroom for his underlying learning difficulties.

MANAGEMENT

Treatment of academic disengagement in children is treated based on underlying sources, as is the case with each manifestation of school maladaptation. The goal of management is prevention of further disengagement, which can lead to school avoidance and dropout. The following are some general treatment guidelines:

1. Behavioral intervention. For disruptive students, behavioral contracts between teachers, parents, and the student can be effective. Positive reinforcement and consistency are essential for success. Children who are too disruptive to the other students often must be placed in a special classroom with more structure. If impulsivity is determined to be the cause of the disruptive behavior, a trial of stimulant medication may be appropriate.
2. Developing strengths. Self-esteem can suffer greatly in children who are disengaged from school, especially those with learning problems. These children should be encouraged to develop specialties in an area of strength or interest, so that they can feel good about themselves.

3. Neurodevelopmental intervention. Special education focused on skill development and bypass strategies is important once the breakdowns in learning are identified. Language, occupational, and physical therapy may also be indicated.
4. Counseling. Intervention in the form of counseling should be focused on a student's gaining insight into the relationship between behavior and possible underlying emotional difficulties.
5. Social skills training. Many students are withdrawn because of social skills difficulties. Children with attentional difficulties also often benefit from help in this area. Some schools have social skills groups, but often this particular area of intervention is only available privately.

In Joey's case, his depression was treated initially while behavioral interventions were implemented for his sleep and attention difficulties. Counseling was started and antidepressant medication was recommended. Also, his learning difficulties were addressed in the classroom with the appropriate resource help.

School Avoidance

EXAMPLE

Jenny was a very mature and bright 13-year-old. She was an only child of working professional parents. Since moving to a new city and starting a new school she began to have more and more frequent illnesses and subsequent absences. After a negative medical work-up for abdominal pain and a possible "immune deficiency," she was referred to a psychologist.

Jenny was thought to be somewhat of a perfectionist and introverted. Although she was doing well academically, her teachers had noted that she seemed to be somewhat anxious in class. She was having some trouble making friends. During psychological testing, Jenny showed some significant performance anxiety. She said that she felt she had to "get A's" so that her parents would be proud of her. She also was told by her violin teacher that she "could do much better if she could just relax." Jenny's parents were mystified about the whole situation. Her mother left for work before her father, who was described as a "softy" when it came to his little girl. Jenny also confided that, unlike her old school, her new school insisted all students "dress out" for physical education class. This made her very uncomfortable and embarrassed.

School avoidant behavior includes school refusal (school phobia) and truancy and essentially describes a child's resistance or refusal to attend school. This resistance may manifest in different ways, ranging from a child's exhibiting somatic symptoms such as stomachache, to blatant refusal, to secretive attempts at skipping school as in truancy. School avoidance occurs in both sexes and in children of all ages, although it is more common in children 10 years of age or older. There is some evidence that lower socioeconomic status increases the likelihood of truancy, but this has not been found to be the case with school refusal (Berg, Nichols, and Pritchard, 1969). Truant children were 73% more likely to show conduct problems, and school refusal children were 62% more likely to have anxiety difficulties (Berg et al, 1993).

There have been many attempts at identifying subtypes of school refusal. Early investigators identified type I, the acute incident child, and type II, the chronic school refusal (school phobia) child (Table 55–2). Even though many children do not fit either type precisely, these criteria can be used to help determine interventions and prognosis. Type I has an excellent prognosis, often responding well to a behavioral approach or clearing spontaneously, and type II often requires long-term intensive treatment.

Most researchers agree that there are three peak ages of presentation of school avoidant behavior:

1. Age 5 or 6 years (shortly after school entry)—more often related to separation anxiety
2. Age 11 to 13 years—complex presentations related to school refusal (phobia), anxiety, and affective difficulties
3. Age 14 years and older—more associated with truancy and more likely to be the precursor of more serious mental illness.

In studies looking at children referred to school avoidant behavior clinics, about half were diagnosed with anxiety disorders, and half of these also had a major depressive disorder. Because only a small minority had oppositional behavior or other conduct problems, again, one must question the choice of the term *school refusal* to describe this heterogeneous group of children (Bernstein, 1991). Furthermore, investigators have found that, indeed, severe school avoidance (including both refusal and truancy) can occur in the absence of associated psychiatric disorders. A study of 100 children being seen for school attendance problems found that only half of the school refusers met ICD-9 criteria for psychiatric disorders (Bools et al, 1990). This finding supports the contention that the aforementioned sources of maladaptation that are not

Table 55–2 • Subtypes of School Refusal

Type I	Type II
Acute onset	Incipient onset
Lower grades	No clear precipitating experience
Depressed affect	Upper grades
Parents well adjusted	Poor school performance
Help sought by parents	History of school refusal
Good school performance	Parent with emotional/personality problems
Feelings of isolation	Parental/marital problems
Presence of trauma or loss	History of prolonged family crisis
	Personality disturbance in child
	Parents difficult to work with
	Referral from outside the family

Adapted from Kennedy WA: School phobia: rapid treatment of fifty cases. J Abnorm Psychol 70:285–289, 1965, and Paccion-Dyszlewski MR, Contesa Kilus MA: School phobia: identification of subtypes as a prerequisite to intervention. Adolescence 22:378–384, 1987. Copyright 1965 by the American Psychological Association. Adapted with permission.

Table 55–3 • Motivational Subgroups of School Avoiders and Possible Sources of Maladaptation

Type	Descriptions	Sources
1. Proactive attraction to alternatives to school	Desire to stay with family, watch television, or "hang out" with peers (truants or dropouts)	Sociocultural influences, conduct disorder, oppositional defiant disorder
2. Reactive avoidance of experiences at school	Feeling of incompetence and humiliation, fear for personal safety, fear of not being liked or accepted	Neurodevelopmental dysfunctions, environmental stressors, school effects, chronic disease
3. Reactive avoidance of control by others at school	Power struggle between student, teacher, and parents	Temperamental difficulties and family stressors
4. Reactive avoidance in response to overwhelming anxiety or fear	Feelings of incompetence, fears and anxiety not matching reality, persistent somatic symptoms such as stomachaches	Neurodevelopmental dysfunctions and social imbalances, emotional disturbances (anxiety and affective disorders)
5. Needs related to family members and events	Keeping child home to baby-sit, for company, or filling other parental needs	Family stressors, sociocultural influences

Adapted from Taylor L, Adelman HS: School avoidance behavior: motivational bases and implications for intervention. Child Psychiatry Hum Dev 20:219–233, 1990.

considered psychiatric disorders (such as neurodevelopmental dysfunctions) lead to school disengagement and often precede school avoidance and frequent absenteeism. Taylor and Adelman (1990) identified motivational subgroups of school avoiders. Table 55–3 lists characteristics of these motivations and their possible sources.

CLINICAL EVALUATION

The assessment of a child who is showing school avoidance should begin by making a distinction between school refusal (phobia) and truancy. Although some children show both behaviors, most follow one general pattern. The clinician must still look for the underlying sources of maladaptation, but this distinction helps the clinician focus on certain issues.

Clinical Evaluation Checklist

1. Were there previous absence problems and when did they occur?
2. When did the present school attendance problem start?
3. On school mornings, is the child openly reluctant to go to school?
4. Does the child cry or appear otherwise emotionally upset?
5. Does the child complain of headaches, stomachaches, other physical problems?
6. Does the child often refuse breakfast and deny being hungry?
7. Where is the child when not in school?
8. How did the parents become aware of the problem?
9. Does the child miss school on the same day each week?
10. How often is the child accompanied to school by parents or caretakers?
11. Who takes the child to school?
12. Who has been contacted for help?
13. Are parents worried about the problem?
14. Who takes responsibility for getting the child to school?
15. Does the child complain of being bullied?
16. Is someone at home mornings with the child?
17. Does the child tell lies or steal?
18. Are there other behavioral problems?
19. Has the child had trouble with police?
20. Are there many children in the neighborhood who are truant or who have dropped out of school?
21. If so, does the child "hang out" with these children when not in school?
22. Does the child appear to be sad or anxious?
23. Does the child have difficulty relating to peers or adults?
24. Does the child have learning, attentional, or physical problems?
25. Are there significant family stressors (marital problems, abuse, neglect)?
26. Is the child afraid of being physically harmed in school?
27. Does the child have a chronic illness?
28. Does the child have difficulty with a specific teacher?
29. Does the child have feelings of inadequacy in a particular domain?

The checklist can be completed by the child's parents with other standardized child behavior checklists and questionnaires filled out by both parents and teachers to aid in identifying areas of concern and possible sources of the school avoidance behavior. A complete social history is important, and educational, language, and neurodevelopmental testing may be helpful in identifying learning disabilities and attention deficits.

Jenny's case illustrates how a series of events coupled with a particular personality and family system can compound and produce school refusal. Jenny's case shows that the precipitating experience was the family move and subsequent change to a new school. Jenny's "type A" personality and social difficulties made these changes difficult. Her performance anxiety could also signal an underlying anxiety disorder, which was exacerbated by the embarrassment of dressing out for physical education class. The family dynamics of her parents' being "high achievers" as well as her father's role of being the parent responsible for getting her to school were thought to have significantly contributed to the outcome of school avoidance and refusal.

MANAGEMENT

There has been ongoing controversy with regard to management of school avoidance behavior. Numerous studies examining responses to various treatment approaches have been flawed methodologically and often lack detailed long-term follow-up. Both psychodynamic and behavioral approaches have shown some success, but questions still remain:

- Should the child be treated before returning to school, or should treatment be started while an initial attempt at return is made?
- Who should be involved in treatment?
- Should the attempt at return be incremental or immediate and enforced?

The psychodynamic literature has usually emphasized community-based outpatient treatment, but hospitalization has been recommended in some difficult cases. Although the outcome of inpatient treatment has generally not been good, outpatient treatment coordinating family-based treatment with school personnel involvement has been successful. In the family systems model, the real problem of most school avoidance is seen to be in the relationships between family members rather than in the child, the parents, or a specific relationship between just two family members. For example, Skynner (1974) used an enforced return to school treatment model as a focus for exposing and confronting inappropriate communications between family members and found success in 87% of cases.

Behavioral treatment programs include the following methods of behavioral intervention and techniques: (1) *systematic desensitization* using humor, role reversal, and imagery (classic conditioning), (2) *flooding* (an immediate return to school using an escort if necessary), (3) *contingency management* at home and school (to deal with somatic complaints and the reinforcement of appropriate behaviors), and (4) *positive reinforcement* for school attendance (operant conditioning).

Comparative studies looking at psychodynamic versus behavioral approaches generally find the behavioral interventions more clinically effective and cost effective (Blagg and Yule, 1984). Most clinicians agree, however, that depending on the specific problems confronting a child and family, often the implementation of a combination of behavioral and psychodynamic approaches, while ensuring a cooperative effort between school personnel and clinicians, best facilitates reentry of a child with school refusal. It is also widely accepted that a child should be guided sensitively, but also firmly and quickly, back to school. The child should be given positive reinforcement for each step of going back. Depending on the particular child and situation, an immediate (flooding) or a stepwise approach can be adopted. In making management decisions, it is important to approach each case by addressing the complex overlapping issues involving the child, family, school, community, and possible medical factors. In addition to psychodynamic and behavioral approaches to treatment, the following are some specific interventions that should be addressed by the clinician:

1. When a child is being bullied and is fearful of being harmed, the clinician should empathize and assure confidentiality regarding his or her concerns. The child can be counseled to face the problem or can be helped to circumvent the situation. All efforts should be made so that a child feels as safe as possible in the school setting.

2. Somatic symptoms must be taken seriously. Psychosomatically rooted complaints such as abdominal pain, although often not the primary reason for school avoidance, may, in fact, be symptoms of real illness. For example, a child's heightened anxiety may lead to refusing meals and subsequent gastritis. These manifestations should be managed as part of the treatment plan of school avoidance.

3. Socially charged school arenas such as the bus stop, the bus, physical education class, and the lunchroom may need to be sidestepped until a child feels more confident.

4. Psychoactive medications may be helpful in alleviating anxiety in some difficult cases. Antidepressant treatment (e.g., imipramine up to 5 mg/kg) is usually considered if school absenteeism exceeds 2 weeks, and it can be very effective when treating school refusal and absenteeism with mood and anxiety disturbances as their underlying sources. Parents should also be referred for treatment when appropriate, and benzodiazepines have also been found to be effective for the "anticipatory anxiety" that can occur when first going back to school. Buspirone and fluoxetine might also be considered.

5. Some children are afraid to return to school because they fear criticisms or other negative comments by

Table 55–4 • Risk Factors for School Dropout

Lower socioeconomic status
    Significantly affects dropout rates for whites and Hispanics, but not blacks
Family process factors
    Poor parental academic support, supervision, and lower educational expectations
Grade retention
    The single most powerful predictor in many studies
Changing schools
    Relates to the finding that frequent moving was related to a host of education problems
Discipline problems
    Predictive when problems existed in both elementary and high school
Poor academic performance
    Children with significant learning problems that are either not identified or not understood
High absenteeism (truancy and school refusal)
    Greatly increases the odds of dropping out in all groups
Employment
    Students who are attracted to full-time employment are at higher risk
Pregnancy
    Pregnant teenagers have a high likelihood of dropout.
Substance abuse
    Chronic substance abuse is a strong risk factor for dropout.
Family history of dropout
    Students with family members who have left school early have a tendency to do the same.
Gang membership
    Students who are actively involved in gangs have a high risk of leaving school.
Psychiatric disorders
    Students with disorders such as depression or anxiety are at greater risk.

their peers. It can be helpful for a child to be coached or to rehearse confident responses to possible comments.

6. Arranging for a sensitive peer to accompany the child around school during the settling-in period can also be helpful in making the transition easier. Sometimes a child may be picked up by an individual from school each day until the child becomes more confidant.

7. The use of an electronic beeper to make a child feel that his or her parents are easily accessible can also make the transition back to school easier.

8. Children with social cognitive deficits should be referred for social skills individual or group therapy.

9. Children with neurodevelopmental dysfunctions benefit from various learning interventions and bypass strategies as well as behavioral and medication interventions. A clumsy child who has fear of humiliation during physical education may receive adaptive physical education with other children in the class. These classes offer alternative activities and sports that may not require children to perform skills that are too difficult for them, such as those that do not require hand-eye coordination.

10. For children with chronic illnesses, school attendance should be planned so that their time in school is affected as little as possible by their illness or disability. Special concessions should be made to ensure that their medical care or medication regimen does not unnecessarily call attention to them or disrupt their experience.

School Dropout

Western culture has for centuries greatly valued formal education. In fact, a legal framework exists to help ensure that children are educated. In some areas of the United States, parents can be issued a fine if their child has frequent absences. In spite of our goal as a society to educate all our children, the problem of school dropout continues to be one of the major policy issues facing American educators today. The U.S. Census Bureau estimated that 11% of all youth aged 16 to 24 years in 1992 had dropped out of school. And while the proportion of students completing high school continues to improve overall, there remains widespread variation among social groups and schools. For example, for some urban schools, the dropout rate is as high as 40%. A school dropout has devastating individual and social consequences. Individuals who drop out of school are more likely than graduates to be unemployed long-term, have health problems, engage in criminal behavior, and become dependent on welfare and other government programs. In one city, it was estimated that a year's cohort of dropouts from that city would eventually cost $3.2 billion in lost earnings and $400 million in social services (Caterall, 1987). The number of children who are found to be at higher risk for dropout, approximately 30% of the nation's students, is continuing to increase at an alarming rate. In the absence of effective intervention, future demographic changes in our society such as an increase in the proportion of racial and ethnic minorities, low-income families, and single-parent households could significantly increase the number of dropouts over the coming years. Table 55–4 outlines risk factors for school dropout. Research has shown that dropping out of school, like school disengagement and school refusal, is caused by a wide range of factors and sources associated with students, families, the schools, and their communities.

MANAGEMENT

Management for school dropout really denotes *prevention*. Because dropping out is increasingly being viewed as a

---

Table 55–5 • Propositions for Successful Schools for Students at Risk

School autonomy and flexibility
Schools are encouraged to autonomously pursue the development of relevant programs for students. They need to have the power to be more flexible in their curricula. Programs should give students a choice in what is offered, show diversity in content, and allow flexibility in delivery. Successful programs for at-risk students create a good fit between school and career. Vocational programs, for example, demonstrate clearly to students a direct personal benefit from staying in school. A clinician can play an active role in policy by serving on the school board or advocating for students at risk.

School involvement
Successful schools take a proactive approach to maintain a supportive environment for at-risk students as well as identifying needs. The willingness and ability to adapt all school practices to individual differences will create conditions that foster self-esteem and are conducive to personal growth. This includes making an effort to find specific areas of interest and academic content for which a child has an affinity (such as sports, dance, music, theater, or shop).

Student and parent involvement
Successful schools enlist the assistance of parents in working on solutions or problems that affect the lives of their children. They also encourage teachers and students to work together in the academic and social aspects of school activities.

Career counseling
Students at risk should be offered career counseling and vocational assessments. Counseling should be reality based and emphasize the relevance of an education and how staying in school can affect future contentment and socioeconomic status.

Early intervention
Enriched preschool education programs such as Head Start may reduce dropout rates for those children who are at-risk socioeconomically or medically.

Grade promotion
Students should generally not be retained, because such a practice has been shown repeatedly to be concomitant to dropout. Retention in kindergarten or first grade may be justifiable in certain circumstances, but repetition of a grade in middle and upper grades has significant impact on a student's mental health and subsequent academic achievement.

Dropout prevention programs
An increasing number of school systems are providing advocates within the school and community to students at risk. Such support entails guiding the student in all aspects of the school experience, from helping with daily attendance to making sure their needs are met. The advocates encourage participation and protect them from embarrassment and humiliation.

long-term process of disengagement from school that often begins in elementary school, early identification of school disengagement is thought to be paramount in prevention. Although research has helped identify more clearly the risk factors and characteristics of students who drop out, the focus has been mainly on their social, family, and personal characteristics. These findings do not often carry any implications for shaping school policy and practice (Wehlage and Rutter, 1986). Some researchers think that the focus should be less on the pathology associated with dropout and more on a positive paradigm that looks at what keeps students in school. Table 55–5 outlines propositions for successful schools for students at risk (Renihan and Renihan, 1995).

One important proposition would be to increase school's autonomy and flexibility so that students with strengths in areas other than traditional academics can be offered curricula with more emphasis on vocational and technical training. This would give many students with learning disabilities and other high-risk factors for dropout an opportunity for success in an area of interest at an earlier point in their educational lives. This success and subsequent improvement in self-esteem would significantly change their experience in school for the better and therefore would likely decrease maladaptation and dropout. The importance of this increase in flexibility of curricula becomes even more evident as our changing industry and economy are making technical skills more of a necessity for competition in our increasingly high-tech society.

REFERENCES

Berg I: Absence from school and mental health. Br J Psychiatry 161:154–166, 1992.

Berg I, Butler A, Franklin J, et al: DSM-III-R disorders, social factors and management of school attendance problems in the normal population. J Child Psychiatry 34:1187–1203, 1993.

Berg I, Nichols K, Pritchard C: School phobia—Its classification and relationship to dependency. J Child Psychol Psychiatry 10:123–141, 1969.

Bernstein GA: Comorbidity and severity of anxiety and depressive disorders in a clinic sample. J Am Acad Child Adolesc Psychiatry 30:43–50, 1991.

Blagg NR, Yule W: In Ollendick TH, King NJ, Yule W (eds): International Handbook of Phobic and Anxiety Disorders in Children and Adolescents. New York, Plenum Press, 1994.

Bools C, Foster J, Brown I, Berg I: The identification of psychiatric disorders in children who fail to attend school: a cluster analysis of a non-clinical population. Psychol Med 20:171–181, 1990.

Broadwin IT: A contribution to the study of truancy. Orthopsychiatry 2:253–259, 1932.

Catterall JS: On the social costs of dropping out of school. The High School Journal 71(1):19–30, 1987.

Jackson P: The daily grind. In Giroux H, Purpel D (eds): The Hidden Curriculum and Moral Education. Berkeley, CA, McCutchan Publishing, 1983.

Kearney CA, Beasley J: The clinical treatment of school refusal behavior: a survey of referral and practice characteristics. Psychology in the Schools 31:128–132, 1994.

Kennedy WA: School phobia: rapid treatment of fifty cases. J Abnorm Psychol 70:285–289, 1965.

Ladd GW, Kochenderfer BJ, Coleman C: Friendship quality as a predictor of young children's early school adjustment. Child Dev 67:1103–1118, 1996.

Levine MD: Developmental Variation and Learning Disorders. Cambridge, MA, Educators Publishing Service, 1987.

Levine MD: Maladaptation to school. In Levine M, Carey W, Crocker A (eds): Developmental-Behavioral Pediatrics. Philadelphia, WB Saunders, 1991.

Paccione-Dyszlewski MR, Contesa-Kilus MA: School phobia: identification of subtypes as a prerequisite to intervention. Adolescence 22:378–384, 1987.

Renihan FI, Renihan PJ: Responsive high schools: structuring success for the at-risk student. The High School Journal. Oct/Nov:1–13, 1995.

Skynner ACR: School phobia—Babel of tongues. Br J Med Psychol 47:1–16, 1974.

Taylor L, Adelman HS: School avoidance behavior: motivational bases and implications for intervention. Child Psychiatry Hum Dev 20:219–233, 1990.

Wehlage G, Rutter R: Dropping out: how much do schools contribute to the problem? Teachers' College Record 87:374–392, 1986.

56 *Mental Retardation**

Allen C. Crocker • Richard P. Nelson

 Categorical presentations about mental retardation (including this one) may be useful for study and planning, but one then quickly moves on to a personalized consideration of the circumstances and needs for each individual child.

If the job is well done within the context of native talents, and if the pursuit of happiness and the best quality of life is honored, the measured features of performance are not important.

In establishing arrangements for the necessary support systems for their children with special needs, parents suddenly become expert "caregivers" and even "case managers."

The assignment of prevention, basically, is to provide protection and sustenance to the developing central nervous system. In the larger arena, this means support to pregnant women and little children.

Definition of Mental Retardation

The term *mental retardation* is an incomplete and unsatisfactory descriptor. It has a role in psychological (and other clinical) nosology but has too often been employed in a fashion that is prejudicial and personally limiting. A central element is obviously an exceptionality in cognitive function, although this need not be inscrutable. One must acknowledge but challenge the lore of retardation and to look freshly at the settings of this individual manifestation, knowledge about its natural history, approaches to supportive intervention, and its cultural importance. Categorical presentations about mental retardation (including this one) may be useful for study and planning, but one then quickly moves on to a personalized consideration of the circumstances and needs for each individual child.

In current times, much thought has been given to establishing a more functionally oriented and dynamic definition of mental retardation. To this end, an ad hoc committee of the American Association on Mental Retardation (AAMR; the leading professional organization in this field) has proposed the following description:

> Mental retardation refers to substantial limitations in present functioning. It is characterized by significantly subaverage intellectual functioning, existing concurrently with related limitations in two or more of the following applicable adaptive skill areas: communication, self-care, home living, social skills, community use, self-direction, health and safety, functional academics, leisure, and work. Mental retardation manifests before age 18 (AAMR, 1992).

Of critical importance are the following four assumptions; they are viewed as essential to the application of the definition:

1. Valid assessment considers cultural and linguistic diversity as well as differences in communication and behavioral factors.
2. The existence of limitations in adaptive skills occurs within the context of community environments typical of the individual's age-peers and is indexed to the person's individualized needs for supports.
3. Specific adaptive limitations often coexist with strengths in other adaptive skills or other personal capabilities.
4. With appropriate supports over a sustained period, the life functioning of the person with mental retardation will generally improve (AAMR, 1992).

The characteristics and measurement of intelligence are considered in Chapters 70 and 72, with both the utility and the limitations presented there relating to the concept of the *intelligence quotient* (IQ). While these constraints are admitted, the basic degree of cognitive disability is commonly discussed in terms of IQ ranges. An accepted convention is to view intelligence in a distribution, with the retardation level commencing at 2 standard deviations below the median and with subsequent categories charted at 3, 4, and beyond. In applying results from the Wechsler Intelligence Scale for Children, these groups would be as follows:

- Mild retardation: IQ 70–50
- Moderate retardation: IQ 49–35
- Severe retardation: IQ 34–20
- Profound retardation: IQ below 20

It has long been usual practice to refer to IQ measurements of 70 or lower as compatible with mental retardation. The new AAMR recommendations are to acknowledge the imprecision of IQ determination and use "approximately 70 to 75 or below" as the psychometric boundary. If taken literally, this would move many persons from the borderline normal range into retardation, but the point is well taken that preoccupation with small number differ-

*Preparation of this material was supported in part by the US Department of Health and Human Services, Maternal and Child Health Bureau (Project MCJ-259150), and Administration on Developmental Disabilities (Project 90DD0357).

ences does not do justice to the basic principles of this field. Between 1% and 2% of the population, at any age, tests in the "significantly subaverage" level, with the majority (85–90%) falling in the area of "mild" disability.

In earlier times, there was a commanding hierarchy of social and educational policy implications deriving from the mental retardation classification. *Mild retardation* was traditionally referred to as "educable mental retardation" in schools, and such a child was considered to be eligible for partial integration and limited achievement. *Moderate retardation* was viewed as "trainable mental retardation" a condition then usually handled in segregated classes and thought to be inconsistent with mastery of useful reading or independence. *Severe* and *profound* retardation had become associated with a defeatist prospect, below the level of justification for energetic educational investment. These perceptions have become archaic. The use of segregated classes is greatly reduced altogether, and expectations for achievement are now much more open and supportive (see Chapter 79).

The "adaptive skills" concerns in the definition of mental retardation acknowledge that "retardation" has cultural and personal aspects as well. Some of these components are easier to measure than others. Relevant instruments exist for the general assessment of adaptive behavior, such as the Vineland Social Maturity Scale and the AAMR Adaptive Behavior Scale. In typical situations, adaptive and social skills parallel rather closely the intellectual capacity of the young person. In exceptional situations (with unusually creative or unusually desultory support, or in some idiosyncratic settings) there may be notable deviation. The assumptions given with the new AAMR definition absolutely require that one reflect on the setting of learning and living for the person being discussed, that evaluation be carried out in an equitable fashion, and that real needs for services and supports be evaluated.

In the young child, *adaptation* implies achievement of useful coordinated psychomotor skills, then communication capacity, and finally gains in "activities of daily living" (self-help and independence in eating, dressing, and toileting). These obviously are related to basic neurologic issues as well. Later one looks to broad social skills, accommodation to the educational environment, achievement of prevocational and vocational competence, and then ability to manage outside living requirements. In the latter sequence, experiential and mental health factors are important.

Persons who are retarded, those who are related to persons with retardation, and those who are involved in professional or voluntary efforts for persons with retardation come to realize that there is a "world" of "mental retardation." For all these people, the categories and definitions are inadequate. There is a subculture associated with "significantly subaverage intellectual functioning" among humans. It has its own special warmth and special desperation. The awakening of human rights efforts in the past 3 decades has brought a particular grace to the field of mental retardation. One can hope that the new atmosphere of individual consideration, active support, and freedom from prejudicial generalizations will prevail in our culture.

Origins of Mental Retardation

When mental retardation is identified in a child, there is a sense of urgency to determine the causative factor or factors. This derives primarily from a need to guide and counsel the family accurately but also pertains to the eventual ability to plan appropriate interventions and training. In the broader view, the settings for retardation must be understood as a basis for public health and preventive activities (Crocker, 1989).

It is often stated that the etiology of mental retardation is usually unknown. Such an assertion is only part of the story. It is true that in the majority of children with very mild disabilities, one can make only somewhat vague conclusions about background issues of inferred relevance, the so-called cultural-familial factors. Discrete elements of importance become more apparent as the degree of disability increases. The varying populations are on a continuum, however, and a thoughtful search for contributing conditions is justified in all instances. In young children, in those in whom direct contact is possible with the parents, in those for whom full historical information is available, and in those in whom modern biomedical pursuit can be undertaken, the yield of accurate surmise about causation is high. Retrospective studies of older persons, such as those in state residential facilities, are of restricted value. In any instance, one may be limited to declarations about the probable setting, and uncertainty may remain regarding the precise pathogenesis. Such information is still helpful to the family, as is also their ability to dismiss some of their own fears about other possible causes in which they may be accusing themselves of having an operational role.

Impressions about the mechanisms of mental retardation are influenced by the circumstances in which children are seen. Professionals who work in the child study sections of school systems see large numbers of children with mild, more dynamic disabilities of apparent cultural and environmental origin. Workers in community health clinics or mental health clinics are impressed by the frequency of troubled support systems for families and of polygenic inheritance. Pediatricians and hospital clinicians, on the other hand, see a disproportionate number of children with organic difficulties and complications of illness. Finally child development centers and mental retardation institutes tend to draw the complex child, with mixed biological and social liability, who has bewildered the educational and health care systems. It is in the latter setting that some of the most analytical studies are undertaken, and the lessons from this work are emphasized here. Table 56–1, for example, reflects the diagnostic experience of a university-affiliated program for mental retardation, as it carefully evaluated children referred for developmental review from community, school, and residential programs.

Any schema that outlines the backgrounds for the occurrence of mental retardation inevitably becomes a checklist for disordered human development in general. As such, it chronicles all the steps in the developmental sequence at which pernicious influences can intrude. The clinical outcome may well be predominantly mental retardation, but it may just as well be cerebral palsy, epilepsy, blindness, deafness, physical disability, or even emotional

Table 56–1 • Settings in Which
Mental Retardation Occurs*

	Percentage of Total Group

HEREDITARY DISORDERS
(preconceptional basis; variable expression, multiple somatic effects, sometimes a progressive course)
    Inborn errors of metabolism (e.g., Tay-Sachs disease, Hurler syndrome, phenylketonuria)
    Other single gene abnormalities (e.g., neurofibromatosis, tuberous sclerosis, diverse syndromes)
    Chromosomal aberrations, including translocation, fragile X syndrome
    Polygenic familial syndromes
	5

EARLY ALTERATIONS OF EMBRYONIC DEVELOPMENT
(sporadic events affecting embryogenesis; phenotypic changes, usually a stable developmental disability)
    Chromosomal changes, including trisomy (e.g., Down syndrome)
    Prenatal influence syndrome (e.g., intrauterine infections, drugs, unknown forces)
	32

OTHER PREGNANCY PROBLEMS AND PERINATAL MORBIDITY
(impingement on progress of fetus during the second half of pregnancy or in the newborn period; neurologic abnormalities frequent, disability stable or occasionally with increasing problems)
    Fetal malnutrition—placental insufficiency
    Perinatal difficulties (e.g., prematurity, hypoxia, trauma)
	11

ACQUIRED CHILDHOOD DISEASES
(acute modification of developmental status; variable potential for functional recovery)
    Infection (e.g., encephalitis, meningitis, encephalopathy of human immunodeficiency virus infection)
    Cranial trauma
    Other (e.g., asphyxia, near drowning, intoxications)
	4

ENVIRONMENTAL PROBLEMS AND BEHAVIORAL SYNDROMES
(dynamic influences, operational throughout development; commonly combined with other disabilities)
    Psychosocial deprivation
    Parenteral neurosis, psychosis
    Emotional and behavioral disorders
    Autism, childhood psychosis
	18

UNKNOWN CAUSES (no definite hereditary, gestational, perinatal, acquired, or environmental issues; or else multiple elements present)	30

*Experience of the Developmental Evaluation Center, Children's Hospital, Boston (3000 children with retardation).
Adapted from Crocker AC: The causes of mental retardation. Pediatr Ann 18:623, 1989.

disturbance or learning disability (with any combinations thereof). Reference is made to numerous other chapters in this book (Chapters 22 through 26 and 57 through 62) for further discussion about related situations and syndromes.

HEREDITARY DISORDERS

Hereditary disorders as a background for significant mental retardation are much less frequent than popular belief

would indicate. Single gene aberrations with biochemical markers, the so-called inborn errors of metabolism (such as Tay-Sachs disease, Hurler syndrome, phenylketonuria, and galactosemia), can produce a devastating cerebral handicap but are of very low incidence. The phakomatoses, including neurofibromatosis and tuberous sclerosis, are more frequent but have a wide variation in developmental effect. Occasional families are found who demonstrate unique patterns of cortical disorder with recessive or dominant inheritance, and certain notable pedigrees show apparent polygenic or variable expression genetic liability. (See Chapter 22 for a full review of hereditary concerns.)

CHROMOSOMAL ABERRATIONS

Chromosomal aberrations are probably underestimated as a source of serious developmental disability (see Chapter 23). Down syndrome has long been identified as one of the major discrete biomedical origins of retardation. Technologic advances in recent years have provided evidence that other chromosomal rearrangements lie behind the problems of many troubled young people. The incidence of the fragile X syndrome appears to equal that of Down syndrome in males; the Prader-Willi syndrome is commonly generated by chromosomal change; and other moderate chromosomal variations are now being identified when carefully sought in syndromes associated with retardation.

CONGENITAL ANOMALY SYNDROMES

"Birth defects," as they were formerly called, or prenatal influence syndromes—the outcomes of embryodysgenesis—constitute a notably important background for developmental disability, as discussed in Chapter 25. In some instances, these involve a cluster of dysmorphic features of familiar nosology, one of the named syndromes. More commonly, however, one encounters the small child with various mild phenotypic variations who also has developmental delay, with the assumption implicit that the central nervous system has shared in the malformation complex. Topographic indicators include changes in the position or configuration of the eyes or ears, midface deficiencies, an unusual palatal shape, a small mandible, changes in the digits, palmar creases, dermatoglyphics, hernias, genital variation, or unusual feet. The child may have a normal birth weight or be small for dates; body growth is commonly slowed; and head size is often small (but sometimes proportionate to small bodily growth). Computed tomographic scanning studies or magnetic resonance imaging of the central nervous system usually reveals normal findings unless there is an odd cranial configuration, and the brain changes can be assumed to be in cortical organization or at other subtle levels. It is a rare experience when one is able to provide the family with a presumed mechanism for these first (or second) trimester influences.

FETAL MALNUTRITION

Fetal malnutrition refers to diminished support for fetal growth as pregnancy proceeds, especially regarding factors in placental integrity or vascular configuration. Reduced size of the infant or the early onset of labor may result, sometimes with untoward developmental consequences directly or as listed in the following section.

PERINATAL STRESS

Perinatal stresses, considered in detail in Chapter 26, affect particularly the vulnerable infant. Perinatal stress refers to premature birth or obstetric complications in the full-term infant. There is a potentially compromising complex of troubling events—anoxia, trauma, central nervous system hemorrhage, acidosis, hypoglycemia, and sometimes infection—that can operate negatively on the extrauterine adjustment of the immature infant brain. These important issues can produce immediately recognizable complications for development or place the child in an uncertain "at risk" status.

ACQUIRED CONDITIONS

Specific conditions acquired in childhood cause mental retardation in relatively few instances. Most significant are complications of central nervous system infections (encephalitis, meningitis) and cranial trauma (household and motor vehicle accidents); see Chapter 27. The role of toxins is often less discrete but unquestionably important (see Chapter 30).

DEPRIVATION

Deprivation in children constitutes a vast area of varying characteristics, which include psychosocial disadvantage and disordered parenting. Specific issues of inadequate stimulation, deficient interpersonal nurturance, physical abuse, and malnutrition may be operative. Family chaos, cultural maladjustment, poverty, and inept support systems are common. (See Chapters 16 and 29 for specific analyses of these potential developmental deterrents.) Such situations may also complicate the course in children who already have specific disabilities.

PSYCHIATRIC DISORDERS

Various psychiatric disorders in child, parents, or both can also lead to a modified developmental course and ultimate mental retardation. Maternal schizophrenia can be such a setting, as can also a serious intrinsic psychic atypicality in the child. Childhood autism has puzzling origins, some hereditary elements, and a moderately dynamic prospect for outcome. Its best place in the classification schema is unclear. (See Chapters 60 and 64 for further discussion.)

A detailed search for the factors just described may yield negative or inconclusive results in an appreciable number of children with significant mental retardation, and one is required to list the apparent causation as unknown. In the experience reported in Table 56–1, this represented almost one third of the total. In some of these children, multiple factors may be present, but none of ascendant importance, and no final conclusions can be drawn. In others, historical review and current study provide no viable hypothesis regarding the route of developmental disability. Here, as mentioned, one can nonetheless discount

certain parental fears. Otherwise such children stand as testimony to the incomplete knowledge that presently exists about the vulnerabilities and liabilities of the small maturing human.

Meaning of Retardation for the Child and Family

PSYCHOLOGY OF EXCEPTIONALITY

Children and adults with mental retardation share an attribute with all other minority groups: They are different. The difference may be real or perceived, but the effect is substantial. Difference begins with the altered expectations of parents when they learn about retardation. The newborn infant with Down syndrome may lack none of the capabilities of other newborns, yet that infant is perceived as different. Deeply entrenched cultural attitudes may serve to assign a disappointing and negative connotation to this difference and reinforce the parents' sense of alarm. Counselors assisting parents during the period of diagnostic crisis, whether this be in early infancy or in later years, must reckon with the personal significance of difference.

When one examines the characteristics of difference for an individual with mental retardation, one notes several components, all of which are to some extent dynamic. First is the matter of *achievement* and *performance*, in the measured or standard sense. This is linked to the functional limitation present, of cortical origin. As mentioned previously, however, the final effects of constraints in intelligence are modulated by concurrent attainments in adaptation. If expectations remain low, elements of self-fulfilling prophecy will intrude on performance.

The second dissimilarity is that of *requirements for services* provided to the person and family to allow maximal realization of potential. This is real and not always easy but fits justifiably within the spectrum of contributions expected among people and their agencies. All of us draw on inside and outside services in this social world; for persons with significant exceptionality the urgency is greater.

A third difference can be that of *participation* in life events and sequences, or involvement in the usual experiences of growth and daily living. For the child with retardation, this has a considerable cultural prescription. Descriptors such as normalization, communitization, least restrictive environment, and inclusive society speak to the current resolve to provide an enhanced setting for participation in usual form. Further, in the external sense, the victories of the past several decades in the human rights area provide assurance that joining in school, community, and residential settings will be guaranteed. The right to establish contracts (such as marriage and ownership), with guidance as appropriate, also assists in the reversal of historic limitations.

The fourth or final difference could be that of *connectedness*. Here there can be no fundamental or primary defense, although societal weakness or clouded vision has often deprived us all of full fellowship.

It is conceded, of course, that difference is present in the best of times. Thinking about the difference in the context of its components (mentioned previously) may diminish the first impressions of oppressiveness and give some guidance about best plans for helpful actions. When one shares time and experiences with families who have children with mental retardation, one is taught some precious lessons about the ultimate meaning of the residual differences. It becomes clear that the importance of less-than-superior skills is a matter of personal interpretation and is not absolute. If the job is well done within the context of native talents, and if the pursuit of referenced happiness and best quality of life is honored, the measured features of performance seem less prominent. Diversity among humans is a richness. When appropriate support systems are in place and a cordial environment exists, parents come to assign uncommon value to their exceptional family member. The differences are often accommodated with grace. In fact, professionals frequently damp the natural strengths of families to love and succeed.

INFANTS AND YOUNG CHILDREN AT RISK FOR MENTAL RETARDATION

For the past 25 years, a great deal of attention has been focused on infancy and toddlerhood, acknowledging this period as dynamic for the establishment of developmental patterns. Serious concerns are raised by the presence of congenital anomalies and chromosomal aberrations; bewilderment exists about possible sequelae from stressful perinatal experience; and there is discomfiture about dysfunctional circumstances of infant nurturance and stimulation. The impression persists that devoted investment in infant support and training can draw on a measure of plasticity still present in the young nervous system and avoid or reduce the occurrence of developmental disability.

Early speculation in this area devised a concept of particular infants being specifically "at risk" for developmental disorder. Three categories of circumstances have been widely employed in research and planning. The first refers to infants at *established risk*, by virtue of the presence of biomedical conditions known to affect personal progress. The second, that of *biological risk*, speaks to children who have had a history of events with a significant potential for brain impairment or whose early functioning gives concern about development. And the third, or *environmental risk*, notes young children being reared with incomplete supports or compromised settings.

It is difficult to produce certain figures for the prevalence of these situations. The smallest number would be those with established risk. Down syndrome, with its 1 in 1000 birth incidence, accounts for 0.1% of newborns. Other congenital anomaly syndromes are individually less frequent but in the aggregate represent an additional 0.2% to 0.3%. Serious inborn errors of metabolism and prenatal syndromes producing hypotonia or cerebral palsy-like pictures may add another 0.1% to 0.2%. In sum, those with established risk are well below 1% of infants.

Infants born prematurely are the major component for those regarded to be at biological risk. From the large number with nominal low birth weight (6–7%), only a fraction are developmentally threatened (possibly 15%), particularly those most seriously preterm (see Chapter 26). Hence, 1% or so of all infants qualify for inclusion in biological risk. Another 0.5% may have developmental delay of diverse origins and be at biological risk as well.

Reckoning is notably difficult in the area of environmental risk. Teenaged motherhood (13%), single parenthood (20%), childrearing in poverty, illicit drug use, and developmental disability in the parents, singly or in combinations, can easily add to 10% or more of young children with serious concern in current times. The meaning, or irreversibility, of those risks is unknown, but experience suggests that at the moment mental retardation is disproportionately represented among the outcomes.

Public and private programs of "early intervention" (training, health promotion, family support) have been widespread in the United States for more than 20 years. In these activities, infants typically receive home visits by educators or therapists in the early months and training in small groups in centers as the next several years proceed. At the present time various states have enrolled from 2% to 6% of all infants in early intervention programs. This usually accounts for one half or more of those at established or biological risk, but irregular or smaller numbers from the environmental risk category. New commitments from Public Law 105-17 embody involvement of a larger percentage of infants and toddlers, especially from the latter category. This is a courageous and commendable resolve. Results from early intervention efforts have been difficult to ascertain but are encouraging (Guralnick, 1997). See Chapter 80 for more discussion of early education.

The current concern with services for infants in educationally oriented programs has served other purposes as well. For families, this interest has provided endorsement of their own hopes for the children's best progress. Direct family assistance in practical matters, personal counseling, and parenting instruction has relieved isolation and troubled circumstances. Physicians have been involved in "child find" screening and infant tracking activity, which have given particular attention to medical interventions as well (Nelson, 1989). Preventive health care has been reinforced and monitored, including consideration of hearing, vision, seizures, orthopedic issues, nutrition, growth, intervention for physical anomalies, and behavioral issues.

EFFECTS OF MENTAL RETARDATION AND ITS CAUSES ON THE CHILD

Obviously the central figures in this life-story are the young persons themselves. While we analyze the consequences of exceptionality, they are living it. It seems reasonable to state that the results are better than we as "others" might have predicted. Some of the poignant aspects of being different have been mentioned; they are not all necessarily unfavorable. The key issues are understanding, support, and respect. The social revolution of the 1960s and 1970s infused our culture with a critically valuable and long overdue level of compassion for rights and opportunities. For children with mental retardation, the new world has been more nurturant; the quality of life has gained greatly.

Much of the action in the child's life plays out in the school. What was formerly a curtailed number of years has now come to extend from infancy to early adulthood. School districts have gradually moved their pupils with special needs from segregated to mainstreamed to integrated class designs, with increasing capacity for a common learning environment and social experience. The most creative conception, the truly inclusive class, has a challenging assignment and a growing adherence (see Chapter 79). These later models have a potential for familiarity and friendships among students with and without special needs (and out of school as well), with each learning from the other. The degree of attainment of the hoped-for outcomes varies, as could be expected. Certainly the old isolation has been permanently relieved.

In current times, about 10% to 20% of school children have special "education plans," formulated jointly by the school district and the families. Most of these are for students with learning disabilities or speech or language impairments; about 18% are for children with mental retardation. These plans contain concrete information on educational techniques and goals, with a capacity for assessment and modification as required. In a 1990 study of five large school districts, Palfrey and colleagues (1990) found that most students with mental retardation were being provided concurrent habilitative therapies—18% received occupational or physical therapy, 34% had counseling services, and 57% participated in speech and language therapy. Such studies have demonstrated that for children with particular developmental needs, the schools continue to be the major providers of therapeutic services.

As personal progress in education has moved forward, the process of inclusion can be felt in the community also. Children with mental retardation and other developmental disabilities are increasingly a part of neighborhood life, and as they reach young adulthood they often look to the prerogatives of more independent living. Many have become spokespersons, locally or with a larger audience (books, television, national groups). Special cause for celebration is the strength seen now from the 20 years of growth of the self-advocacy movement. The various People First organizations, and others such as Self Advocates Becoming Empowered, are assisting all of us toward better understanding (Dybwad and Bersani, 1996).

NEEDS OF FAMILIES AND THEIR RESPONSES

In establishing arrangements for the necessary support systems for their children with special needs, parents suddenly become expert "caregivers" and even "case managers." It is an enormous tribute to their love and resiliency that this adaptation is achieved so strongly (Taylor, Epstein, and Crocker, 1990). Among the many assignments they characteristically carry out are those that relate to

- Physical maintenance of the child (diets, adaptive equipment, home modifications, access to specialized health care).
- Emotional and psychological support (assistance in emerging self-concept, personality definition, developing autonomy, and interactive skills).
- Ensuring access to appropriate education (advocacy, conferencing, monitoring).
- Social and recreational opportunities (finding possibilities for groups, camps, sports).
- Ensuring the transition to adulthood (living, vocational, and personal components).

Coordination of medical care may also be a major responsibility. The professions have traditionally underestimated the magnitude of parental contributions to the success of a child's course (Crocker, 1992, 1997).

When one interviews families about the pressures felt and the supports desired, the most prominent strategic requirements are the following:

- Parent education of rights and entitlements
- Financial counseling
- Information on community resources
- Recreational opportunities
- Parent support groups
- Parent training for child's health needs
- Transportation
- Respite care
- Legal services

These reflect the diverse areas of activity and outreach enjoined by a family with a child who has a developmental disability. The search for special knowledge is splendidly discussed in two books by and for parents: Featherstone, *A Difference in the Family: Life with a Disabled Child* (1980), and Callanan, *Since Owen* (1990).

Particular regard is due for brothers and sisters, as they grow up and help in households with members who have retardation (Powell and Gallagher, 1992). These young persons will ultimately have the longest-term relations with the special child, and their understanding and support have traditionally not received appropriate attention. Brothers and sisters must often deal with alterations in the normalcy of family rhythm, competition for parental resources and attention, possible misconceptions about the origins or outcome of the syndrome of the involved child, a requirement to act as a surrogate parent, an obligation to meet enhanced parental expectations, and bewilderment about their parents' conflicts (Crocker, 1983). They may also receive mixed messages about double standards on compliance and behavior and on the competency of the affected child. The brothers and sisters gain significantly by being provided meaningful information in suitable form, being involved in decision making, and having counseling or group activity with like peers when appropriate. The majority of studies actually show a favorable long-range adaptive outcome for these siblings, which is a tribute to their strength and to the complex, often positive, effects of living with difference.

During the past 25 years there has been a slowly growing number of families who have adopted children with mental retardation or other developmental disabilities. Although to some degree this outreach has been promoted by the reduced availability of normal infants and children, another more specific motivation is generally at work. The children with special needs are discretely chosen in an earnest expression of caring, and many times more than one is eventually taken (Lightburn and Pine, 1996). The families are predominantly from moderate-income to low-income groups. As Lewis (1989) states, "very often they have had experience with mental retardation in the past. These experiences have left them hopeful, not bitter, comfortable with differences, and eager to be more personally involved." Physician assistance is needed, both in preadoption reformation transfer and in postplacement supportive services, but pediatricians have been slow to realize the extent of this movement. In many metropolitan areas there are actually waiting lists for infants and young children with Down syndrome, for example, a fact that should be acknowledged during genetic counseling. The adoption of children with mental retardation validates their dignity and provides credibility to their value in the family's community.

TRANSITIONS

In the first full definition of developmental disabilities, included in 1978 in Public Law 95-602, it is indicated that the need for special services is "lifelong." Our school and agency programs tend to build discrete units of activity oriented to particular age periods—infancy, preschool, school years, young adult, adult, and elderly—with limited provision about coordination of the carry-over periods. The two periods of transition for young persons with mental retardation that prove to be the most pressing are (1) movement from early intervention services to public preschool at 3 years of age, and (2) graduation of youth from education services (and entitlements) at 21 years or so into the potential for further vocational training and employment as an adult.

For youth and young adults in the latter circumstance, there are many chances for discontinuity. Further, this is an interval of notable personal challenge for intrinsic reasons. Adolescents with mild and moderate retardation are confronted with difficulty in relating to their impetuous normal peers. Their thinking may be immature, concrete, passive-dependent, or compulsive, which results in increased isolation and diminished self-image (Szymanski, 1983). The emergence of sexual feelings is bewildering because these are seldom realistically acknowledged by parents or service providers. Silence, overprotection, and covert alarm are often extended to pubertal persons with retardation by our society; the converse would be meaningful exchange and education, plus the guided opportunity for positive experience.

In the search for suitable autonomy, youth with retardation have need of numerous assisted preparations. As conceptualized by Turnbull and Turnbull (1985), these involve *consent and choice* (training for skills in problem solving and choice making), *personal life planning* (exploring one's identity, aspirations, and potential), *social support networks* (peer groups, peer counselors, neighbors, relatives, and service providers), and *self-advocacy* (learning to carry out self-assistance and promotion). It can be claimed that we are often guilty of holding young people hostage to dependency, and in this sense society has a developmental disability.

Since the 1970s, important changes have occurred in the fields of rehabilitation and vocational counseling, including stronger identification with young persons who have mental retardation. There have also been improvements in the commitment to prevocational and vocational training in the public schools. It is now generally conceded that with the development of assisted employment and supported employment, virtually all persons with mental retardation can be established in gainful jobs (Kiernan, 1992). At the moment, however, this has been achieved

only for a minority. Yet further facilitation is needed in the early and continuing school vocational experiences, with thoughtful personal choices and broadly based counseling assured. State mental retardation agencies must also begin promptly with their incorporation of young adults in community support services, to avoid possible waiting list involvement. Of importance, a greater variety of options for community living has made transitional planning more comprehensive than during times past.

CONSUMER ACTIVISM AND ORGANIZATIONS

Finally, vigorous accolades must be paid to the army of parents, relatives, friends, and sympathizers who have done so much to change the milieu in which children with mental retardation now live. Singly or in small groups they have worked as program volunteers, advocates, peer supporters, and authors. They have served endlessly on advisory groups, human rights committees, and developmental disabilities councils. In many communities parents have performed the necessary work to begin group homes, including arrangement for property acquisition, long-term financing, and staffing. Their public voice has served to hearten other, less articulate, families; to educate government officials and agency personnel; and to prod the conscience of professionals. They have planned programs, written legislation, and launched class action suits. Such private persons have raised money for research, joined in projects, and been responsible for the creation of prevention endeavors. Needless to say, their activities have gone far beyond any prospects of particular assistance to their own family members. The list could be vast, but special acknowledgment must be made at least to The Arc (national, state, local), United Cerebral Palsy Association, Epilepsy Foundation, National Down Syndrome Congress, Parent to Parent, Federation for Children with Special Needs, TASH, Association for the Care of Children's Health, Alliance of Genetic Support Groups, National Tay-Sachs and Allied Diseases Association, and the National MPS Society.

Severe and Profound Retardation

In the total spectrum of mental retardation there exists a minority within the minority whose disability is of unusually serious nature: children (and adults) who have severe or profound retardation. This group—at most 5% of all persons with cognitive disabilities—raises special issues because of the magnitude of their quantitative and qualitative atypicality. It can be fairly said that their need for us to teach them is extraordinary, and that their ability to teach us is equally remarkable. The general public, and many professionals as well, are bewildered by individuals with IQs below 35 (or, particularly, below 20) and lack frames of reference for interaction with them. Some of their notable features are the following:

1. Lack of self-care and even survival skills. These are persons with a truly pervasive disability who often are not able to dress, feed, or toilet themselves, even

in adult life, and who have a compelling dependency on others throughout their lives.

2. Communication blockade. Inadequate language is invariable, and often there is no successful verbal communication whatsoever. This can lead to social difficulties, complicated by the incomplete ability of others to interpret the person's feelings.

3. Deviant behavior. With blunted exchange and reward on other levels, there is often a resort to bizarre repetitive or stereotypic behavior, sometimes self-stimulating. This can include rocking, twirling, and posturing, with alarm induced when actions become self-injurious.

4. Serious organic pathology. Although severe or profound retardation is found in all segments of the causation schema (see Table 56–1), it is more frequent in those with hereditary or malformation problems. Usually there are combined disabilities (including seizures and sensory problems) and many times serious health issues as well. Motor function difficulties or complications often reduce the person's potential for ambulation.

5. Greater commitment for intervention. Incidental learning (such as that from ambient experiences and social exchange) is reduced, so that efforts for progress require more discrete programming.

6. Teacher confusion regarding potential. Standard test instruments are less relevant at this far end of the spectrum, and personal progress and its documentation are slow and irregular. Disagreements have often erupted in determination of public policy regarding the educational investment.

Persons with these serious degrees of developmental disability raise special personal challenges. It is axiomatic in human development (and in education) that continued learning and progress are a fundamental response to adequate stimulation for all except those who are in coma, but in these situations the gains can be painfully slow and the feedback not of the conventional sort. Individual interactions have their own language and their own special rewards. Most clinical psychologists restrict the use of the term *profound mental retardation* to individuals in whom the adaptive components are extremely restricted, rather than utilizing the IQ definition primarily. Dybwad (personal communication, 1981) has pointed out that profound mental retardation is probably not in itself a useful term; *profound disability* is more reasonable because in these persons complexity of problems is the rule. Since the 1970s, the promulgation of "no reject" programs for education, family support, and general activities has allowed many quiet miracles of personal triumph to occur. This refers to fulfillment for the individuals with severe special needs as well as for those who relate to them or work with them.

The ultimate role of the large public residential institutions—the "state schools," "training schools," or, in the modern idiom, "developmental centers"—is dubious. These troubled facilities were initially established, beginning at the turn of the century, with the alleged purpose of providing specialized treatment (Nelson and Crocker, 1978). It soon became apparent, however, that programs

were severely compromised by the many hundreds (even thousands) of needy humans domiciled there, with the attendant management complications. When enrollment reached almost a quarter million persons in the early 1960s, a reaction developed to further admission, and the philosophical position of "deinstitutionalization" began. As the population in the state residential facilities declined (now nationwide about 65,000), those remaining were increasingly the complex older individuals with severe or profound retardation. Most people believe that even these clients are best served in smaller, more normalized environments within the community. There is currently a firm resistance to admitting children to state schools; the same basic reasons apply to adults as well.

Prevention of Mental Retardation

On first consideration, the achievement of prevention regarding mental retardation would seem to consist of identifying a causation of relevance, devising an interventionist strategy, and then applying the strategy in the appropriate setting. In practice this only occasionally works. Problems come in the wide variety of etiologies, some of them multifactorial, frequent conundrums about affecting the process, and competition for resources or priority for application. Actually, we have done quite well in a number of low-volume–high-intensity disorders with retardation (e.g., molecular, viral), but in the subtler, high-volume dilemmas we are not doing so well.

The assignment, basically, is to provide protection and sustenance to the developing central nervous system. In the larger arena, this means support to pregnant women and little children (Crocker, 1992; Wallace and Nelson, 1994). It is generally felt that the basic maternal and child health services construct must be maintained, and that the particular activities of greatest ultimate value are (1) family life education in public school (in parenting skills), (2) early, high-quality, and affordable prenatal care, (3) regional newborn intensive care units, (4) generously supplied early intervention programs, (5) a "medical home" for each small child, with continuity of care, and (6) effective services for children and families where there is disability. With moderately diligent utilization of these principles, many of the most important risk indicators are not changing appreciably (teenage fertility, racial disparity in infant morality, preterm birth, child abuse) (Crocker, 1994). In recent times much energy has been given to the prevention of secondary conditions (complications or contingencies of primary disabilities), and this can be expected to have valuable conserving effects.

Here is the current scorecard on prevention work:

NEARLY TOTAL ELIMINATION

- Congenital rubella, by early immunization and antibody screening.
- Retardation in phenylketonuria, galactosemia, and congenital hypothyroidism, by newborn screening followed by dietary management or replacement therapy.

- Kernicterus, by reduction of sensitization through the use of globulin therapy.

MAJOR REDUCTION

- Tay-Sachs disease, by carrier screening and prenatal diagnosis in persons with increased risk.
- Morbidity from prematurity, through newborn intensive care nurseries.
- Measles encephalitis and *Haemophilus influenzae* meningitis, by early vaccination.

SIGNIFICANT CURRENT EFFORTS UNDER WAY

- Neural tube defects, by folic acid supplementation and by maternal serum alpha-fetoprotein screening and prenatal diagnosis.
- Down syndrome, through counseling of older pregnant women and prenatal diagnosis guided by marker screening.
- Lead intoxication, by environmental improvement, screening of lead levels, and chelation when necessary.
- Fetal alcohol effects and syndrome, by public education.
- Morbidity from head injury, via the use of child restraints in automobiles.
- Child neglect and abuse, through family life education in public schools that assists young people in preparation for parenthood.

SPECIAL ASSISTANCE AND RELIEF

- Prompt identification and early intervention for infants with disability or at risk.
- Support to families with children who have disabilities, to provide guidance and resources.
- Genetic counseling when special risk is involved.
- Improved management for difficult pregnancies.

Regrettably there are many children whose disability cannot be prevented by usual means. These include the majority with congenital anomalies from unknown prenatal influences, most nonfamilial chromosomal disorders (including the children with Down syndrome born of younger mothers—80% or more of the total), most serious childhood neuroses and psychoses, which interfere with development, and the very substantial number of children in whom the basis of retardation cannot be identified at all, even on careful study.

The outlook is good for continuing improvement in the prevention of mental retardation syndromes. Child care professionals can assist in this movement by the promotion of immunization, newborn screening, guidance during pregnancy, and the use of child safety measures. Gains will also be made through the wider employment of early developmental screening, comprehensive assessment of children with known disabilities, and thoughtful genetic counseling. Public support should be marshaled for programs for the infant and young child. Basic and applied research regarding the nature of cortical impairment must not lapse (Crocker, 1990).

REFERENCES

AAMR: Mental Retardation: Definition, Classification, and Systems of Supports. Washington, DC, American Association on Mental Retardation, 1992.

Callanan CR: Since Owen: A Parent-to-Parent Guide for Care of the Disabled Child. Baltimore, Johns Hopkins University Press, 1990.

Crocker AC: The impact of disabling conditions. *In* Wallace HM, Biehl RF, MacQueen JC, Blackman JA (eds): Mosby's Resource Guide to Children with Disabilities and Chronic Illness. St. Louis, Mosby–Year Book, 1997, pp 22–29.

Crocker AC: Prevention of disability. *In* Wallace HM, Nelson RP, Sweeney PJ (eds): Maternal and Child Health Practices, 4th ed. Oakland, CA, Third Party Publishing Co, 1994, pp 705–710.

Crocker AC: Data collection for the evaluation of mental retardation prevention activities: The Fateful Forty-Three. Ment Retard 30:303, 1992.

Crocker AC: Societal commitment toward prevention of developmental disabilities. *In* Pueschel SM, Mulick JA (eds): Prevention of Developmental Disabilities. Baltimore, Paul H. Brookes Publishing Co, 1990, pp 337–343.

Crocker AC: The causes of mental retardation. Pediatr Ann 18:623, 1989.

Crocker AC: Sisters and brothers. *In* Mulick JA, Pueschel SM (eds): Parent-Professional Partnerships in Developmental Disabilities. Cambridge, MA, Ware Press, 1983, pp 139–148.

Dybwad G, Bersani H (eds): New Voices: Self-Advocacy by People with Disabilities. Cambridge, MA, Brookline Books, 1996.

Featherstone H: A Difference in the Family: Life with a Disabled Child. New York, Basic Books, 1980.

Guralnick MJ: The Effectiveness of Early Intervention. Baltimore, Paul H. Brookes Publishing Co, 1997.

Kiernan WE: Vocational rehabilitation. *In* Levine MD, Carey WB, Crocker AC (eds): Developmental-Behavioral Pediatrics, 2nd ed. Philadelphia, WB Saunders Co, 1992, pp 734–736.

Lewis RG: Adoption and mental retardation. Pediatr Ann 18:637, 1989.

Lightburn A, Pine BA: Supporting and enhancing the adoption of children with developmental disabilities. Children and Youth Services Review 18:139, 1996.

Nelson RP: Community services for children with mental retardation. Pediatr Ann 18:615, 1989.

Nelson RP, Crocker AC: The medical care of mentally retarded persons in public residential facilities. N Engl J Med 299:1039, 1978.

Palfrey JS, Singer JD, Ralphael ES, Walker DK: Providing therapeutic services to children in special educational placements; an analysis of the related services provisions of P.L. 94-142 in five urban school districts. Pediatrics 85:518, 1990.

Powell TH, Gallagher PA: Brothers and Sisters: A Special Part of Exceptional Families, 2nd ed. Baltimore, Paul H. Brookes Publishing Co, 1992.

Szymanski LS: Emotional problems in a child with serious developmental handicap. *In* Levine MD, Carey WB, Crocker AC, Gross RT (eds): Developmental-Behavioral Pediatrics, 1st ed. Philadelphia, WB Saunders Co, 1983, pp 839–846.

Taylor AB, Epstein SG, Crocker AC: Health care for children with special needs. *In* Schlesinger M, Eisenberg L (eds): Children in a Changing Health Care System: Prospects and Proposals. Baltimore, Johns Hopkins University Press, 1990, pp 27–48.

Turnbull AP, Turnbull HP: Developing independence. J Adolesc Health Care 6:108, 1985.

Wallace HM, Nelson RP: Emerging priorities in maternal and child health services. *In* Wallace HM, Nelson RP, Sweeney PJ (eds): Maternal and Child Health Practices, 4th ed. Oakland, CA, Third Party Publishing Co, 1994, pp 120–130.

57 Hearing Impairment

Desmond P. Kelly

Profound hearing loss is relatively rare, but milder degrees of hearing impairment, particularly secondary to otitis media with effusion, are commonplace.

Fifty percent of childhood hearing impairment is due to genetic factors, more than 20% is due to prenatal, perinatal, or postnatal environmental influences, and 30% is of unknown cause.

Early diagnosis and intervention are central to achieving optimal outcome in the language and social areas.

In reading comprehension, the mean grade equivalent for 18-year-old deaf students in special education settings is at the fourth-grade level, and mathematics is at the seventh-grade level.

The goal is universal detection of infants with hearing loss as early as possible, with screening for all infants admitted to neonatal intensive care units and screening of all other infants within the first 3 months of life.

Hearing impairment poses a grave threat to language, social, and emotional development and academic achievement. Early diagnosis of this sometimes hidden aberration is vital, and appropriate early intervention will significantly improve developmental outcome. Individual variations among children with hearing impairment bear close attention, and the adaptability and successes of many of these children highlight the potential for neuronal plasticity as well as individual resilience.

Although profound hearing loss is relatively rare, milder degrees of hearing impairment, particularly secondary to otitis media with effusion, are commonplace. Estimates of the prevalence of hearing impairment are beset by inconsistencies in classification and reporting. While 1 to 2 per 1000 children in developed countries have bilateral sensorineural hearing loss of a moderate degree or greater (above a threshold of 50 dB), 5 to 10 times as many experience lesser degrees of diminution (Brookhouser, 1996). In underdeveloped countries, sensorineural hearing loss is almost twice as common, with greater risk of suppurative complications of otitis. Although preventive techniques such as rubella immunization and improved antibiotic and surgical interventions have lowered the incidence of some forms of hearing impairment, the increasing number of children surviving extreme prematurity or complex medical conditions suggests that the overall prevalence is unlikely to decline significantly.

Terminology

Although the term *hearing impairment* covers the range from mild to profound hearing loss, the designation *deaf* (used as an adjective, and not appropriately as a noun) is generally reserved for those children whose hearing loss is in the severe to profound range, and who can at best hear only a few prosodic and phonetic elements of speech. Children who are *hard of hearing*, with hearing loss below the severe range, can at least partially understand spoken language. Sounds consist of complex combinations of pure tones that vary in frequency (or pitch) and intensity (or loudness). Hearing is commonly measured by pure tone audiometers and graphically reported by means of pure tone audiograms. Typical conversational speech occurs in the range of 30 to 50 dB. Figure 57–1 illustrates the loudness and pitch of common sounds with the functional impact of varying degrees of hearing loss. Classification systems are usually based on the average hearing threshold in decibels for pure tones presented at 500, 1000, and 2000 Hz. The range for normal hearing is 0 to 15 dB. Although the threshold for classification as hearing impaired has generally been defined as 25 dB, most experts agree that any hearing loss above 15 dB in an infant or young child could impede speech perception and language development. Further degrees of hearing loss can be functionally categorized as follows (Roeser, 1988):

1. Mild hearing loss (26 to 40 dB): difficulty with soft-spoken speech.
2. Moderate (41 to 55 dB): able to understand speech between 3 and 5 feet from source; some articulation deficits.
3. Moderate to severe (56 to 70 dB): hear only loud sounds and experience difficulty understanding speech in groups; limited vocabulary with articulation disorders.
4. Severe (71 to 90 dB): may understand loud speech at 1 foot; may distinguish vowels, but have trouble, even with hearing aids, distinguishing consonants; voice quality and articulation defective.
5. Profound (greater than 90 dB): auditory channel can-

Audiometric Characteristics of Speech Sounds and Functional Impact of Hearing Loss

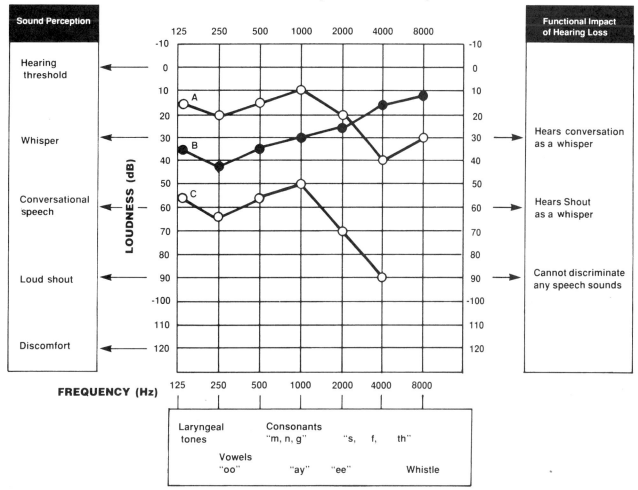

Figure 57–1. Audiometric characteristics of speech sounds and functional impact of hearing loss. Audiograms A and C reflect mild and moderate-to-severe hearing loss, respectively. Note the greater deficits in the higher-frequency ranges that particularly affect appreciation of consonants. Audiogram B, mild conductive loss, is notable for greater involvement at lower frequencies. (Adapted from information in Ballantyne J, Martin JAM: Deafness, 4th ed. New York, Churchill Livingstone, 1984.)

not serve as primary mode of communication; reliant on visual perception for communication.

Although hearing loss is traditionally subtyped as either conductive or sensorineural, a combination of these components, mixed hearing loss, is not infrequent. Conductive hearing loss reflects an interruption in the mechanical conducting components, which include the pinna, external ear canal, eardrum, ossicles, and the middle ear cavity. Children with conduction defects generally experience loss across the frequency ranges and can discriminate speech if it is loud enough. In turn they may be soft-spoken, as they hear their own voice more loudly. The degree of conductive loss is usually limited, with some bone conduction occurring if sounds are louder than 50 dB. Sensorineural hearing loss results from dysfunction of the inner ear (cochlear apparatus) or nerve pathways. The higher frequency ranges are usually affected most. Comparison of air and bone conduction levels is used to differentiate the type of loss. In the treatment of children with sensorineural hearing

loss, the clinician should monitor for any associated conductive hearing loss that might be amenable to medical or surgical intervention.

Etiology

Despite advances in knowledge and diagnostic techniques, etiology remains undetermined in up to one third of children with significant hearing loss. Most studies estimate that 50% of childhood hearing impairment is due to genetic factors and that 20% to 25% of cases are due to perinatal, prenatal, or postnatal environmental influences. The recent advances in molecular genetics have greatly increased knowledge of inherited causes of hearing loss. Autosomal recessive inheritance accounts for 80% of genetic hearing loss. Half of these patients have no additional organ system involvement (nonsyndromic) and probably constitute many of the cases of hearing loss of unknown cause. Genetic

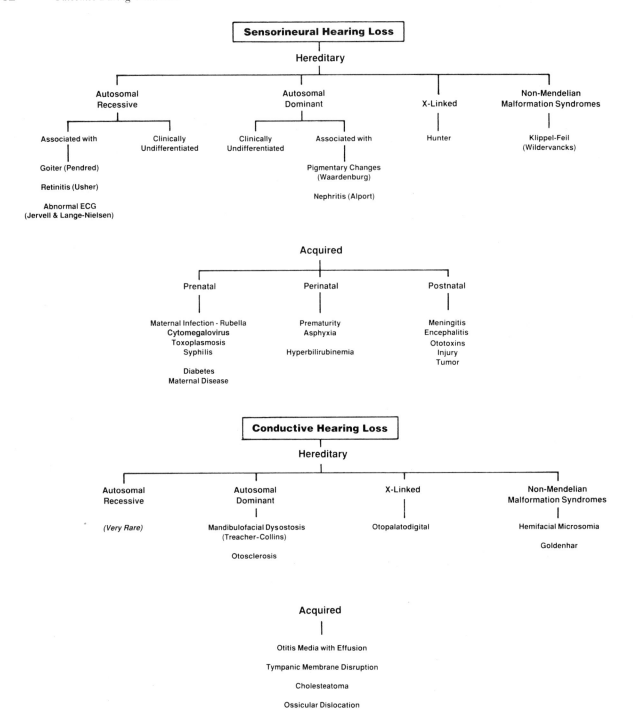

Figure 57–2. Overview of more common causes of hearing impairment, etiologic classification. (Based on information in Fraser GR: The Causes of Profound Deafness in Childhood. London, Bailliere-Tindall, 1976.)

linkage studies have already enabled identification of more than 20 genes responsible for nonsyndromic hereditary hearing loss, and estimates of the total number of such genes range up to 200. Progress in gene localization and identification holds great potential for increased understanding of the pathophysiology of hearing loss, for identification of at-risk individuals, and for devising strategies for intervention and treatment (Brookhouser, 1996). Figure 57–2 provides some idea of the spectrum of established causes, including a wide range of hereditary syndromes and

potentially preventable congenital and postnatal acquired conditions (Konigsmark and Gorlin, 1976). The heterogeneity of the population with hearing impairment is thus clearly underscored.

Developmental-Behavioral Impacts

The hidden nature of hearing impairment can influence both diagnosis and later life experiences. The health professional has to be alert to sometimes subtle signs of hearing loss in children with no external physical manifestations, to make an appropriate early diagnosis. In turn, persons with hearing impairment are not automatically afforded special consideration by individuals with whom they have contact in day-to-day life and who might not be aware of the extent of their disability. It has in fact been noted that one of the useful purposes of hearing aids is to function as an external marker of hearing deficits.

There are so many variables influencing the impact of hearing loss on development that generalizations regarding outcomes for children with deafness are largely unrealistic. Each child deserves individual consideration. Factors that have been clearly implicated can be categorized as follows (Meadow, 1980):

1. Degree of hearing loss. The child with a mild hearing loss corrected by amplification at an early age will be at very little risk developmentally, in contrast to the profoundly deaf youngster who has to learn visual and manual forms of communication.
2. Etiology. Children with inherited deafness whose parents are deaf by and large fare better academically and behaviorally than those with acquired deafness. It has been assumed that this reflects the benefits of early diagnosis and appropriate communication and family support. It should be recognized, however, that children with acquired deafness, such as that secondary to a congenital infection, are at higher risk for additional neurologic dysfunction. Maternal rubella has been a prototypical example of the acquired etiology with potential for multisystem involvement, including visual problems, heart disorders, mental retardation, and emotional and behavioral problems.
3. Age at onset of deafness. Lack of exposure to language during the critical early developmental years places those who are prelingually deaf (generally defined as less than 2 years of age) at significant disadvantage compared with those who have been able to assimilate a language structure prior to losing their hearing.
4. Family climate. Children born into families with other members who are deaf generally benefit earlier from adaptations and efforts to facilitate communication and other aspects of development. In families without prior experience of deafness, early efforts by parents and other members to learn sign language and foster communication will provide similar benefits. In contrast, many educators of children who are deaf will bear testimony to the frustration of observing children making significant gains in the educational setting only to regress following time spent away from school in an understimulating home environment where they are unable to engage in any substantive communication. Such children, coping with the multiple disability of sensory and psychosocial deprivation, are at grave risk for poor outcome.
5. Timing and appropriateness of educational interventions. Early diagnosis and intervention are central to achieving optimal outcome in the language and social areas. Controversy persists regarding which educa-

tional settings facilitate optimal development, and again individual factors need to be considered.

COMMON DEVELOPMENTAL PROFILES

Language

In children who are profoundly deaf the primary impact is not merely that they are unable to hear sounds, but that their ability to develop spoken language is impeded. As Sacks notes, children who are prelingually deaf are deprived of auditory memories, images, and associations. Not only are they unable to communicate their thoughts and needs or readily acquire information verbally, but inner language development, including the ability to translate experience into verbally mediated thoughts and memories, is also impeded. The role of standard language in thought processes and "intelligence" remains unestablished. Studies of children with deafness show that they place greater reliance than hearing children on visual-spatial short-term memory than on temporal-sequential coding (Marschark, 1993).

It is known that infants can recognize their mothers' voice from birth, and much of early parent-child interaction involves soothing talk and vocal interactions. It is indeed a marvel to realize that by 4 years of age the average child will have a complete grasp and knowledge of his or her native language that has been assimilated without the aid of any formal teaching. This illustrates the disadvantage that a child with profound deafness would be at without appropriate efforts to foster communication (such as very early exposure to sign language in the home and later in the educational setting).

Cognitive Development

Determination of the intellectual abilities of children who are deaf can prove elusive. The majority of the test instruments in common use are based on the ability to read a standard language, and comparison of verbal intelligence scores is thus not practical. On the nonverbal, or performance, sections of tests, children who are deaf generally fall within the normal range of intelligence but score consistently below hearing age-mates (Marschark, 1993). Again one is faced with the fact that expression of many abstract concepts is dependent on a system of symbolic language that the child with deafness might not have had the opportunity to develop. Although expert opinions have varied over the years, it is now agreed that deafness per se does not impart limitations to intelligence. However, children who are deaf show qualitative differences in the interrelations among their abilities. In particular, they are likely to be less competent in their language abilities and cognitive flexibility. Measured levels of academic achievement are generally lower for deaf school-aged children. Early schooling for children with deafness concentrates heavily on development of communication skills, leaving less time for instruction in other areas. Leaders in deaf education have also voiced concern that goals and expectations for students with deafness are unnecessarily low. In reading comprehension, the mean grade equivalent for 18-year-old students with deafness in special educational settings is at the fourth-grade level, with math at the seventh-grade level. There is also the risk that some children with deafness will have difficulty with balance, equilibrium, and other motor skills reflecting associated vestibular dysfunction (Rapin, 1993). In contrast, research has suggested the development of compensatory skills in those deprived of hearing. Some studies indicate more efficient visual processing abilities. By use of brain electrical activity mapping techniques, investigators have demonstrated differences in cortical organization between deaf and hearing children, with the former generally showing compensatory changes in the right hemisphere and visual processing areas (Wolff and Thatcher, 1990). History is replete with accounts of "deaf and dumb" individuals who were considered to be severely retarded and lacking in all social skills before it was discovered that they were deaf. Although such drastic examples are uncommon these days, there is still a wide variation in outcomes for children with deafness based on timing and effectiveness of interventions.

Social and Emotional Development

Although generalizations are to be strongly avoided, studies have suggested that persons with deafness are less "socially mature" (a culturally derived term). This global description would seem to reflect the fact that opportunities for usual social interaction are limited and parents generally tend to be more protective of children who are deaf. Language and communication is, of course, a central component of all social exchanges. Other descriptors include egocentricity, rigidity, and suggestibility. In extensive studies of children with deafness secondary to rubella, Chess and Fernandez (1980) noted deficits in internal controls, or impulsivity with aggressive behavior. These findings were more common in those with associated physical disabilities. It has been postulated that deficits in verbal mediation of self-control contribute to increased levels of impulsivity and that aggressive behavior might reflect frustrated attempts to express emotions verbally (Cohen, 1980). Even in nonconfrontational interactions, children who are deaf are likely to initiate more physical contact, such as touching others to gain their attention.

Associated Challenges

Not unexpectedly, the percentage of hearing-impaired school-aged children with educationally significant associated disabilities is considerably higher than that for the general population. The Annual Survey of Hearing-Impaired Children and Youth continues to report such difficulties in up to 30% of deaf children, with many of these problems being related to the same factor that caused the deafness (1994). The unfortunate term *multiply handicapped hearing-impaired children* has evolved to describe this group. Such additional conditions include visual problems, epilepsy, cerebral palsy, mental retardation, and specific learning disabilities (Mencher and Gerber, 1983). It is thus important to evaluate each child fully and to be aware of conditions that might have an impact on development and performance. For example, a child with deafness and associated visual-perceptual deficits might have great difficulty processing sign language and speech reading. Such a child might be incorrectly classified as cognitively impaired. Although there has been a paucity of research regarding attention deficits in children who are deaf, it is clear that a youngster who is reliant on visual input for learning and communication would be at double jeopardy for learning problems if he or she had attentional weaknesses. Studies at a residential school for children who are deaf utilizing parent and teacher questionnaire ratings have suggested that although the overall prevalence of attention deficits in children who are deaf is not higher than for the general population, those children with acquired deafness, such as secondary to bacterial meningitis, are at significantly increased risk (Kelly et al, 1993).

Evaluation

SCREENING AND DIAGNOSIS

The health professional must maintain an index of suspicion regarding hearing loss in infants and young children. Careful consideration of risk factors coupled with astute observation and attention to parental concerns is the key to successful early diagnosis. Unfortunately the average age of diagnosis of significant hearing loss remains unacceptably high at 2 1/2 years. There have therefore been renewed efforts to promote early diagnosis. The use of a "high risk register" was previously promoted to identify those children at most significant risk for hearing loss who should have evaluation of hearing and close follow-up. The factors recommended by the Joint Committee on Infant Hearing in 1990 were revised and expanded in a 1994 position statement. These "indicators" are intended for utilization in development of a screening program and are as follows:

1. Neonates (birth through 28 days)
   a. family history of hereditary childhood sensorineural hearing loss
   b. In utero infection associated with hearing loss
   c. Presence of craniofacial anomalies
   d. Birth weight less than 1500 g
   e. Neonatal jaundice at a serum level requiring exchange transfusion
   f. Ototoxic medications
   g. Bacterial meningitis
   h. Evidence of severely depressed physiologic status at birth (e.g., Apgar score 0 to 4 at 1 minute or 0 to 6 at 5 minutes)
   i. Mechanical ventilation lasting 5 days or longer
   j. Physical findings of a syndrome known to be associated with hearing loss
2. Infants (age 29 days through 2 years) with certain health conditions that require rescreening of hearing
   a. Parent or caregiver concern regarding hearing, speech, language, or developmental delay
   b. Bacterial meningitis and other infections associated with hearing loss
   c. Head trauma associated with loss of consciousness or skull fracture
   d. Stigmata of a syndrome associated with sensorineural or conductive hearing loss
   e. Ototoxic medications

f. Recurrent or persistent otitis media with effusion for at least 3 months
3. Infants (age 29 days through 3 years) who require periodic monitoring of hearing
   a. Family history of hereditary childhood hearing loss
   b. In utero infections such as cytomegalovirus, rubella, syphilis, herpes, or toxoplasmosis
   c. Neurofibromatosis type II
   d. Recurrent or persistent otitis media with effusion
   e. Anatomic deformities and other disorders that affect eustachian tube function
   f. Neurodegenerative disorder (progressive conductive and sensorineural hearing loss can occur in disorders such as Hurler and Hunter syndromes)

As only 50% of infants or young children with profound hearing loss will manifest one of these risk factors, there have been renewed efforts to promote universal screening of newborns for hearing loss. A National Institutes of Health consensus panel made this recommendation in a 1993 statement (National Institutes of Health, 1993). In 1994 the concept was endorsed by a Position Statement of the Joint Committee on Infant Hearing. The goal is universal detection of infants with hearing loss as early as possible, with screening for all infants admitted to Neonatal Intensive Care Units and screening of all other infants within the first 3 months of life. The Joint Committee also addressed the importance of identifying those children whose hearing loss might not develop until after 3 months of life. This group is incorporated in Section 3 of the risk indicators. It is recommended that all infants be tested by means of otoacoustic emissions testing with follow-up auditory brainstem response testing of those who fail initial testing. These recommendations have given rise to debate related to expense and reliability of techniques and the challenge of retesting those who might have had false positive results on screening. Nevertheless such universal screening is being widely implemented. In those settings in which there is not universal screening, programs should be developed to ensure hearing testing of all children with any of the risk indicators. In all situations, the health professional must initiate further testing if there is any degree of parental concern, or any suspicion of hearing loss.

Delayed acquisition of language skills may be the first sign of hearing impairment. It is strongly recommended that the physician use some objective measure of language development as a means of screening and charting rates of development. Such instruments include the Early Language Milestone (ELM) Scale or the Clinical Linguistic and Auditory Milestone Scale (CLAMS). The revised Denver Developmental Screening Test (Denver II) has an expanded language section that can also facilitate screening for early delays. Informal assessments of hearing in the office setting such as reactions to a bell or jingling keys can be misleading given the high intensity and limited frequency range of many of these noises. Office screening of hearing using portable screening devices with cooperative preschoolers is a valuable adjunct to the well-child evaluation, but if there is any question about hearing abilities, evaluation by an experienced audiologist is essential.

If hearing loss has been confirmed, the medical evaluation should be directed toward establishing a cause as well as ruling out any associated health problems that could further impede communication or have long-term health implications. Evidence of a potentially correctable condition such as middle ear dysfunction warrants consultation with an experienced otolaryngologist to elucidate potential benefits of surgical intervention. Determination of etiology has important implications with regard to genetic counseling and prognostication regarding potential outcomes or associated physical problems. Routine evaluation should include close attention to vision status, given the vital importance of this sensory modality to persons who are hearing impaired. Early diagnosis of a condition such as Usher syndrome, with progressive loss of vision in addition to deafness, would have important treatment implications. It is widely recommended that children with hearing impairment have an assessment of vision annually, both to monitor visual acuity and to check for retinal changes. Other aspects of the medical examination warranting close attention include possible craniofacial anomalies, presence of goiter (Pendred syndrome), pigmentary changes (Waardenburg syndrome), and assessment of renal function (Alport syndrome). A history of syncopal episodes or other unexplained changes in level of consciousness should raise suspicion of cardiac arrhythmias secondary to prolongation of the QT interval seen in Jervell and Lange-Nielsen syndrome. Detailed neurologic examination is also necessary, particularly in those with acquired deafness who might be at risk for other neurologic or vestibular dysfunction. Further special investigations are dependent on individual circumstances. A computer tomographic scan of the temporal bone region could help to identify structural anomalies of the inner ear that would have management implications.

The child with otitis media and persistent effusion raises special concerns because a conductive loss of 20 to 30 dB, and even up to 50 dB, can be associated with middle ear effusions. Many questions remain regarding the impact of fluctuating degrees of conductive hearing loss on subsequent language and learning abilities. There is support in the literature that otitis media with effusion is one of multiple risk factors that influence the development of language (Roberts and Wallace, 1997). There also appears to be a correlation between early and persistent otitis media with effusion and subsequent attention deficits (Ultmann and Kelly, 1991). Children with persistent middle ear effusions, especially during the critical early years of language development, should be referred for audiologic evaluation.

EVALUATION OF HEARING

There are persisting misperceptions that hearing cannot be accurately tested in very young children. However, with appropriate equipment and professional expertise, reliable assessments can be carried out at any age. Even antenatal diagnosis of hearing loss in high-risk pregnancies is becoming an accepted procedure. Movement of the fetus in response to sound and auditory evoked potentials is used to assess hearing in the third trimester (Isaacson, 1988).

In infants under 6 months of age, objective measurements of hearing abilities by means of auditory brainstem evoked potentials is preferred. This method enables differentiation between conductive and sensorineural loss, as well as diagnosis of unilateral hearing loss. For children older than 6 months, full evaluation of hearing involves three potential measurements, including behavioral audiometry, impedance testing, and use of auditory brainstem response testing (Ruben, 1987).

Audiometry measures the response of the child to sound presented either through headphones or through speakers. In children less than 2 years of age, behavioral conditioning by use of visual reinforcers can be used to train the children to localize by turning their heads to the direction of the sound. Depending on the skill and persistence of the audiologist, very reliable estimates of hearing can be obtained in young children. From 2 years of age, children can be engaged in play audiometry, in which they are conditioned to provide a specific response to sounds. In older children, speech recognition threshold is tested by having them repeat words or carry out performance tasks such as pointing to body parts or pictures.

Tympanometry assesses middle ear status by determination of whether a normally mobile tympanic membrane is absorbing acoustic energy, or whether this energy is being reflected back by an immobile membrane. Measures include the flow of acoustic energy into the middle ear system (static admittance), an estimate of middle ear pressure (the location of the peak pressure when admittance is highest), ear canal volume, and the presence and threshold of the acoustic reflex. Physical conditions such as middle ear fluid, negative pressure, and ossicular discontinuity can be measured. Although the acoustic reflex does correlate with hearing capacity, it should not be used as an indicator of normal hearing.

Auditory brainstem response testing has been used increasingly as an objective measure of hearing abilities. This procedure makes use of surface recording electrodes and microcomputer averaging and enhancement of signals to extract the responses of the brainstem to sound. Potentials evoked by up to 2000 separate auditory stimuli are stored and averaged to produce one wave form, which is then analyzed for its overall morphology. This wave form contains seven peaks, of which three are analyzed closely for latency and amplitude characteristics. One of the most significant benefits of this test is that it does not rely on the cooperation of the patient. However there are pitfalls, including subjectivity involved in interpretation of the wave forms and the fact that other conditions affecting the brainstem might result in abnormal wave forms, while behavioral audiometry reveals normal hearing. Conversely, because responses are being measured below the level of the auditory cortex, this test does not necessarily indicate that the subject is correctly interpreting sounds.

Evoked otoacoustic emissions testing is a physiologic test that is being used more frequently, especially in screening for hearing loss. Evoked otoacoustic emissions are a form of acoustic energy produced by active movements of the outer hair cells of the cochlea in response to sound. Testing involves measurement of emissions from the inner ear following presentation of a click from a probe placed in the ear canal. The technique does not require advanced training and is sensitive to hearing loss above 30 dB. There have been concerns regarding its specificity and risk for false positive results. Refinements in the procedure and technologic advances are increasing its accuracy.

DEVELOPMENTAL ASSESSMENT

Formal assessment of cognitive, language, and social abilities should be carried out by professionals who have experience in testing children with hearing impairment. Tests of cognition include the Hiskey-Nebraska Test of Learning Aptitude (specifically developed for children with hearing impairment), the performance scales of the Weschsler Intelligence Scales (WISC III), the Leiter International Performance Scale, and the Kaufman Assessment Battery for Children. Visual-motor tasks including the Bender-Gestalt and Developmental Test of Visual Motor Integration are also used frequently. Projective techniques can be helpful (if not entirely reliable) in assessing emotional status, in addition to use of instruments such as the Meadow/Kendall Social-Emotional Assessment Inventory for Deaf Children (Meadow et al, 1980).

EXAMPLE

Mary was born at term without apparent medical complications. She had very frequent episodes of otitis media during the first year of life. Her parents are medical professionals. At 15 months of age she was not using any single words and her parents had concerns about her response to environmental sounds. Behavioral audiometry indicated hearing loss, and auditory brainstem response testing at the time of myringotomy and insertion of ventilation tubes indicated severe hearing loss in one ear and profound loss in the other. Mary was fitted with hearing aids and an FM system and was enrolled in an intensive program of speech and language therapy, including the use of sign language. Her parents decided at an early stage to promote oral communication as much as possible. After initial gains in language skills (using a limited one-word vocabulary consistently) there was regression in communication abilities. Repeated testing indicated progression of the hearing loss to a profound degree bilaterally. Mary's parents had her evaluated at a number of centers and she was deemed eligible for cochlear implantation. At surgery there was evidence of new bone formation in the cochlea, suggesting an infectious etiology for the deafness, probably bacterial meningitis (although there had been no recognized symptoms of such an illness). Immediately following the implant, Mary demonstrated improved perception of environmental sounds. Language skills progressed slowly initially. Evaluation at another center indicated a need for remapping of the processor. Mary has since made steady gains. She receives individual and group speech and language therapy and separate weekly sessions of auditory-verbal training in a nearby city. She has attended regular preschool classes and is currently functioning well in a prekindergarten educational program at a private school. Two years after receiving the implant, her expressive language has advanced to two- to four-word combinations. Receptively she is able to identify two-key verbal elements such as "red book" without any visual cues. Her cognitive abilities have been measured to be in the average range and she increasingly enjoys academic activities. There are mild behavioral challenges with limit-testing and occasional noncompliance. She enjoys social interaction.

Mary's history highlights many key issues, including the challenge of early diagnosis, the risks of progressive hearing loss, multiple modalities of treatment, and the large commitment of energy and resources by parents seeking an optimal outcome for their child.

Management

Optimal outcome for the child with hearing impairment will be facilitated by attention to all areas of functioning, as illustrated in Figure 57–3.

MEDICAL ROLE

Preventive efforts are crucial, including rubella immunization and other measures to decrease the risk of prenatal infections and minimize the other risk factors previously listed. Immunization against *Haemophilus influenzae* type B infection has significantly decreased the incidence of this form of bacterial meningitis and the deafness associated with it. The physician should also counsel regarding risks of exposure to loud noises such as firecrackers and loud music. Routine health screening and prompt treatment interventions should be coupled with focused anticipatory guidance. The primary care physician is in a unique position to interpret findings of other specialists during the diagnostic process and to function as care coordinator. Other medical management might include surgical interventions by an otolaryngologist or continued ophthalmo-

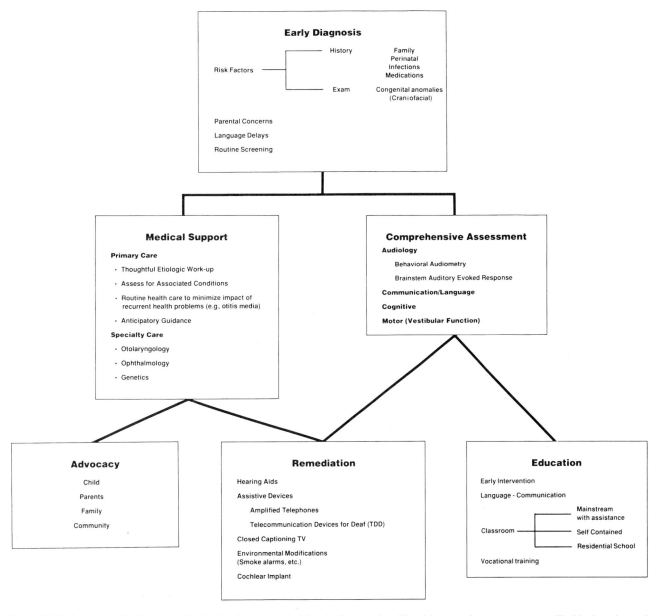

Figure 57–3. Steps to optimal outcome for the hearing-impaired child. An integrated multimodal approach to management will aid adaptation and achievement of full potential.

logic follow-up. The physician should ensure that there are no delays in having the child who is deaf fitted with hearing aids, and he or she can consult with an audiologist in this regard.

Cochlear implants can provide useful hearing to selected children with profound hearing loss. This treatment modality has received much attention and evoked considerable debate in recent years and is being performed with increasing frequency. The device consists of an internal component that is surgically implanted and an external component that is worn by the child. Sounds are received through an external microphone and then processed and encoded into radio frequency signals that are transmitted across the skin to a magnetic receiver situated near the mastoid. In turn an electrical signal is sent to a multichannel electrode that is implanted in the cochlea through the round window. The electrode directly stimulates the spiral ganglion cells of the cochlear nerve, with higher frequency sounds stimulating the basal turn and lower frequencies activating the apical turn. Candidates for cochlear implantation should be carefully selected from among children older than 24 months who have bilateral profound sensorineural hearing loss and have shown little or no benefit from hearing or vibrotactile aids. Associated cognitive or behavioral problems must be considered, and there must be family commitment to the intensive training and habilitation program that is an essential component of the process. Follow-up studies have indicated promising results related to better appreciation of environmental sounds and significant long-term gains in speech perception and intelligibility and in expressive language abilities (Langman et al, 1996).

In addition to specialized interventions, children with hearing impairment require the same routine health supervision and management of acute illnesses that any other children do. Special consideration is required to ensure that the child who is deaf is not excluded from conversations with parents during these encounters. Use of interpreters should be considered, especially for prolonged discussions, such as preparation for surgery (Lotke, 1995). The pediatrician or family physician should also provide anticipatory guidance regarding behavioral and developmental challenges. Inadequate communication between parents and child can heighten the stresses associated with mastering skills such as toilet training. The physician might also be called on to advise regarding treatment of more significant neurobehavioral problems, such as attention deficits. Although controlled studies are lacking, it appears that medications such as stimulants have a similar spectrum of activity and efficacy in children with hearing impairment.

EDUCATION

Three factors have been described that have central implications for optimal development of children who are deaf and should be incorporated into management plans (Marschark, 1993). *Early language experiences*, particularly linguistic interaction with parents from an early age, are critical. These interactions result in gain of facts, cognitive strategies, and social skills, as well as knowledge of self and a sense of being part of the world. The second factor is *diversity of experience* that shapes basic perceptual, learning, and memory processes. Active exploration

of the environment and experience with people promotes problem-solving skills and flexibility. *Social interaction* is the third essential element. In addition to the cognitive functions of social interactions, these relationships help to develop bases for exploration and provide emotional support. In turn, self-esteem, motivation, and moral development are promoted. Early intervention should thus focus on development of communication skills for both the child and the parents. Opinions have differed among the deaf community and educators regarding most appropriate instructional methods. The first efforts at deaf education by French monks in the late 1700s expanded on the native forms of sign language already being used by persons with deafness. The concept of "Oralism" subsequently came to fore in the United States. This approach uses lip reading and vocal expression rather than manual signs and was advocated as offering the best opportunity for integration of children who are deaf into society. However, acquisition of understandable speech proves an almost insurmountable task for children with profound prelingual deafness without treatment such as a cochlear implant. In contrast, proponents of manual communication point out that children who are deaf may develop a broader appreciation for "language" much earlier through the use of signs and can more easily communicate with other persons with deafness with whom they might share a common identity (Ziring, 1983) or with hearing persons who have signing skills. "Total communication," which combines speech reading, manual communication, and oral expression, has emerged as a compromise and is the predominant approach used in deaf education at this time. There is also considerable disagreement regarding sign language, however. There is no universal sign language, with each country having its own adaptations and forms of sign. In the United States, American Sign Language (ASL) is a unique form of communication and a complete language system of its own that is used by many members of the deaf community as an alternative to "Signed English" or other manual communication such as fingerspelling. In this regard, it is important to note that a growing number of persons with hearing impairment identify themselves as members of a deaf community with a distinct set of cultural values and ways of behaving. For them, ASL is a mark of distinction and a source of pride (Moores, 1987).

The passage of Public Law 94-142, the Education for All Handicapped Children Act, since reauthorized as the Individuals with Disabilities Education Act (IDEA), has had a significant impact on deaf education. Free public education for all students who are deaf has broadened the available services and opportunities. Part H of this legislation mandates services from infancy, or the time of diagnosis. Families are entitled to assistance from a multidisciplinary team of professionals who can determine eligibility for services and work with the family to develop an individualized family service plan (IFSP). Ideally this team should consist of a physician with expertise in otologic disorders, an audiologist, a speech-language pathologist, and an educator. Primary care physicians should consult and collaborate with this team in the development of treatment and education plans. As children approach school age, parents will encounter differences of opinion among professionals regarding whether special school programs or mainstreaming in regular school programs provides the better educational environment. Residential schools for children who are deaf have been the traditional means of providing education for those who have profound hearing impairment and usually number teachers who are deaf among their faculty. With interpreters and other increased services for students who are deaf provided by public schools, as well as the mandate for education in the least restrictive environment, has come an increasing emphasis on mainstreaming of students who are deaf. The majority of children with hearing impairment receive their education in regular school settings. However, this does carry the risk of social isolation inherent in being one of a small number of, or the only, student who is deaf in a school or classroom. The final decision regarding which educational setting is most appropriate for the individual child is influenced by many factors including the resources and qualifications of professional staff in the different potential settings, the philosophy of educational approaches, goals of parents and educators, and the capability of the family to invest fully in the supportive components. Regardless of the setting, it is crucial that young children with hearing impairments receive appropriate intensive training in language development.

Increasing numbers of students who are deaf are pursuing higher education. There is a wide variety of post-secondary education programs for students who are deaf, and over 1000 colleges and universities in the United States report supportive programs, including note-taking and interpreter services and availability of telecommunication devices. Gallaudet University in Washington, DC, and the National Technical Institute for the Deaf in Rochester, New York, serve over one half of the students who are deaf now in college.

HABILITATION

There are many resources available for maximizing hearing potential. Hearing aids consist of a microphone for converting acoustic energy into electric energy, an amplifier powered by a battery, and a receiver or earphone for converting the amplified electrical energy back into acoustic energy and channeling this into the child's ear canal. If there is absence of the ear canal, a bone conduction oscillator is used. There are four different types of hearing aids, including body-worn (with a flexible cord leading from the microphone and amplifier to the button-sized receiver, used mostly by younger children), behind-the-ear (with all components contained in a small curved case), in-the-ear (with all components contained within a plastic shell fitted into the outer ear), and eyeglass aids (with the components built into the frame). The amount of sound amplification (gain) and the frequency response of the aid can be varied depending on the characteristics of the individual's hearing loss. In general, higher frequencies are amplified more. Free-field FM systems can be used in the classroom setting as an effective means of amplification. These operate like a miniature radio transmitter with a unit worn by the teacher transmitting the speech to a receiver worn by the student that amplifies and transfers it to small earphones or the student's own hearing aid.

Other assistive listening devices and systems include telephone hand set amplifiers or hearing aid compatible telephones. Telecommunication devices for persons who are deaf (TDDs) use a keyboard and a screen or paper printout to convey messages via tone telephone. Closed caption television supervised by the National Captioning Institute (established by Congress in 1979) has significantly increased access to news and entertainment. Alerting and warning assistive devices include those that convert the ring of a telephone into a low-pitched warble, strobe light, or flashing household lamp. Similar devices are available for doorbells, wake-up alarms (including vibrotactile devices), smoke detectors, and adverse weather warning systems.

New technologic developments continually broaden the horizons of those with many forms of impairment, and this is no less true for persons with hearing impairment. As computers assume more central roles in day-to-day life, the only limit is the creativity and ingenuity of program developers. A prototype that might not be too far from reality is that of reading glasses with a receiver that translates spoken input into printed representations of words, displayed on a screen across the bottom of the lenses.

SUPPORT AND ADVOCACY

Comprehensive management of the services needed by a child with hearing impairment mandates a commitment to advocacy and support. In addition to medical management, the health professional can fill an important role as educator, not only of the family but also of the community, regarding the special needs of these children. Families of children with hearing impairment need support, guidance, and training during many difficult periods of adjustment. More than 90% of children who are deaf are born to hearing parents, and the resultant changes in the family milieu are far-reaching. The diagnostic process is often delayed and traumatic for parents who might have previously received false reassurances for their concerns. With a number of different specialists, including audiologist, otolaryngologist, and pediatrician or family practitioner, involved, it is not unusual for parents to receive the diagnosis in a fragmentary way with continuing hope that yet another specialist will be able to offer a cure. There is much new information to be learned regarding all aspects of hearing impairment. Enrollment in an early intervention program carries additional burdens with many prescriptions and suggestions that might seem overwhelming or conflicting to parents. As children progress through school, questions arise regarding the most appropriate educational approaches and services, and the controversies within the deaf education community in this regard only add to the uncertainty faced by parents. The advent of adolescence raises more questions regarding how much independence to allow a child who is deaf and highlights the conflicts and concerns faced by all parents at this developmental stage. If the parents are fluent in their child's primary language, the issues may be comparable to those in a hearing family. In all these areas, empathy and advice from the primary physician who has ongoing contact with the family can be of substantive assistance.

Ziring (1983) noted the special difficulties faced by children with deafness in hospital wards or emergency rooms, where communication problems add stress and where preparation of the nursing staff or provision of an interpreter is of such importance. Similarly, consultation with educators and other professionals regarding medical issues affecting children who are deaf is another important support component.

Ultimately the unique characteristics and strengths of each child must be fostered as he or she grows into adulthood and plans for an independent life and career. Role models such as deaf lawyers arguing cases before the Supreme Court, artists receiving national awards, and successful professionals or artisans in all walks of life underline the growing opportunities available. The challenges are real, but the outlook is promising.

REFERENCES

Annual Survey of Hearing-Impaired Children and Youth, 1992–1993: Characteristics of deaf and hard of hearing students in four special education program types. Am Ann Deaf 139(2):242, 1994.

Brookhouser PE: Sensorineural hearing loss in children. Ped Clin North Am 43(6):1195, 1996.

Chess S, Fernandez P: Impulsivity in rubella deaf children: a longitudinal study. Am Ann Deaf 125:505, 1980.

Cohen BK: Emotionally disturbed hearing impaired children: a review of the literature. Am Ann Deaf 125:1040, 1980.

Isaacson G: Antenatal diagnosis of congenital deafness. Ann Otol Rhin Laryngol 97:124, 1988.

Joint Committee on Infant Hearing 1994 Position Statement. Pediatrics 95(1):152, 1994.

Kelly DP, Kelly BJ, Jones ML, Moulton NJ, et al: Attention deficits in children and adolescents with hearing loss: a survey. Am J Dis Child 147:737, 1993.

Konigsmark BW, Gorlin RJ: Genetic and Metabolic Deafness. Philadelphia, WB Saunders, 1976.

Langman AW, Quiglet SM, Souliere CR: Cochlear implants in children. Ped Clin North Am 43(6):1217, 1996.

Lotke M: The sounds of silence: the hearing impaired child. Contemp Peds 12(10):104, 1995.

Marschark M: Psychological Development of Deaf Children. New York, Oxford University Press, 1993.

Meadow KP: Deafness and Child Development. Berkeley, CA, University of California Press, 1980.

Meadow KP, Karchner MA, Petersen LM, Rindner L: Meadow/Kendall Social Emotional Assessment Inventory for Deaf Students. Washington, DC, Gallaudet College Press, College Programs, 1980.

Mencher GT, Gerber SE: The Multiply Handicapped Hearing Impaired Child. New York, Grune & Stratton, 1983.

Moores DF: Educating the Deaf, 3rd ed. Boston, Houghton Mifflin, 1987.

National Institutes of Health: Early Identification of Hearing Loss in Infants and Young Children: Consensus Development Conference of Early Identification of Hearing Loss in Infants and Young Children, Bethesda, MD, National Institutes of Health, 1993.

Rapin I: Hearing Disorders. Pediatr Rev 14(2):43, 1993.

Roberts JE, Wallace, IF: Language and otitis media. In Roberts JE, Wallace IF, Henderson FH (eds): Otitis Media in Young Children. Baltimore, Paul H. Brookes Publishing Co, 1997, p 133.

Roeser RJ: Audiometric and immittance measures: principles and interpretation. In Roeser RJ, Downs MP (eds): Auditory Disorders in School Children, 2nd ed. New York, Thieme, 1988.

Ruben RJ: Diagnosis of deafness in infancy. Pediatr Rev 9(5):163, 1987.

Ultmann MH, Kelly DP: Attention deficits in children with hearing or visual impairments. In Accardo P, Whitman B (eds): Early Diagnosis and Intervention in Attention Deficit Hyperactivity Disorder. New York, Marcel Dekker, 1991, pp 171–187.

Wolff AB, Thatcher RW: Cortical reorganization in deaf children. J Clin Exp Neuropsych 12:2, 1990.

Ziring PR: The child with hearing impairment. In Levine MD, Carey WB, Crocke AC, Gross RT (eds): Developmental-Behavioral Pediatrics, 1st ed. Philadelphia, WB Saunders, 1983, p 770.

SUGGESTED READING

Sacks O: Seeing Voices: A Journey into the World of the Deaf. Berkeley, CA, University of California Press, 1989.

58 *Visual Impairment and Blindness**

Philip W. Davidson • Christine M. Burns

 About 1 in 1600 children has significant visual impairment.

Retinopathy of prematurity (ROP) and congenital cataracts are the leading causes of childhood blindness.

In general, significant delays are found in infants with blindness in the development of locomotion, prehension skills, and attachment behavior. The infant eventually develops all these functions during the 2nd and 3rd years of life.

The literature relating to the development of receptive and expressive language in infants and young children with blindness indicates a parity with sighted children.

The teaching of braille reading is often idiosyncratic from school to school and teacher to teacher, and not all readers ever obtain maximum efficiency.

Evaluation of the child with visual impairment is best done by an interdisciplinary team.

In North America it is estimated that the prevalence of blindness and serious visual impairment in the pediatric population is between 30 and 64 children per 100,000 population. Another 100 children per 100,000 have less serious visual impairment. Hence it is quite likely that every pediatrician or family medicine specialist in a primary care setting will have at least several children with serious impairment in his or her practice. The child with blindness, like any other youngster with a lifelong disability, presents special social, educational, and psychological needs, which if identified and met can reduce the degree of handicap associated with the disability.

Definitions, Incidence, and Prevalence

No common worldwide definition of blindness exists. Member countries of the World Health Organization (WHO) have agreed to the following definition (always with reference to the better of two eyes):

1. Visual impairment: Snellen acuity no better than 6/18 m (corrected) or visual field no better than 20 degrees.
2. Social blindness: Snellen acuity no better than 6/60 m (corrected) or a visual field no better than 20 degrees.
3. Virtual blindness: Snellen acuity no better than 1/60 m or a visual field of less than 10 degrees.
4. Total blindness: no light perception.

The United States Public Health Service defines blindness as the best corrected acuity in both eyes of 6/60 m or visual fields of less than 20 degrees bilaterally. Using this definition, Goldstein (1980) compiled incidence and prevalence rates for the United States from a number of primary demographic resources. About 1 in 1600 children was significantly visually impaired (about 50,000), and only about 10% of all expected cases of blindness in the total population occurred in children and adolescents.

Robinson, Jan, and Kinnis (1987) reported the prevalence in British Columbia of congenital blindness from all causes to be about 3 per 10,000 live births. This represents a significant decline since the 1940s, as a result in part of a reduction in lens disorders caused by maternal rubella infections and in part of a lowered number of cases of retrolental fibroplasia.

Table 58–1 shows estimates of the prevalence of congenital blindness as reported by Robinson, Jan, and Kinnis (1987). The most common types of lesions include those of the retina, optic nerve, lens, and eyeball in general. Retinopathy of prematurity (ROP) and congenital cataracts are the leading causes of childhood blindness, although the incidence of both diseases has declined over the past 25 years (Robinson, Jan, and Kinnis, 1987). ROP still occurs (Phelps, 1994) and the improved survival rates for very low birth weight infants has caused an increase in cases of ROP relative to other causes (Phelps, 1989). The leading causes are accidents, brain trauma, and neoplasms affecting the visual system (Robinson and Jan, 1993).

About 20,000 school-aged children require braille (or other tactual system) as a reading medium and must be taught as children who are nonseeing. Most of these children are now receiving and will in the future receive their education in the public educational system as mainstreamed students in local school districts, since most states use schools for the blind for only a very small number of children with blindness and multiple disabilities.

*Preparation of this material was supported in part by Grant MCJ 369341 from the Maternal and Child Health Bureau, HRSA, DHHS.

Table 58–1 • Prevalence of Congenital Ocular
Blindness by Site and Type of Lesion*

Site	Type	Percent of Cases
Retina	Retrolental fibroplasia	22.0
	Macular degeneration	1.7
	Retinitis pigmentosa	0.5
	Other	5.9
Optic nerve	Optic nerve atrophy	12.2
	Other	7.5
Lens	Cataract	18.8
	Other	0.1
Eyeball in general	Albinism	6.2
	Hydrophthalmos	3.0
	Myopia	2.6
	Other	4.3
Uveal tract	Absence of iris	2.1
	Chorioretinitis	1.4
	Other	1.2
Cornea, sclera	—	0.9
Vitreous	—	0.5
Other	Nystagmus	7.8
	Other	1.2

*A survey of all children born in British Columbia, Canada, between 1945 and 1984.
Adapted from Robinson GC, Jan JE, Kinnis E: Congenital ocular blindness in
children, 1945 to 1984. Am J Dis Child 141:1321–1342. Copyright 1987, American Medical Association.

Developmental Issues Relating to Visual Impairment

The deprivation of vision has important implications for development. It is known from studies of normal child development that visual experience facilitates (and probably underlies) many important concepts of space and form that are in turn important to the development of perception and perhaps even intelligence itself. When a child is forced to interact with the world without vision, he or she is doing so without the sensory system most adapted for spatial and shape information gathering. Total blindness may have very different consequences in terms of child development compared with partial vision loss. Children who have even limited visual function may still experience the development of spatial reasoning based on visual referents and may function much more like sighted peers than do children with total blindness. How well these functions can be subsumed by other perceptual modalities such as touch and audition seems to depend on the nature of the task, the adaptability of the child, and the way in which the residual modalities are enriched by experience.

Little evidence has emerged to demonstrate sensory compensation, such as changes in fingertip sensitivity, in persons blinded so severely as to necessitate use of the hands as the primary modality for perceiving shape. However, much research suggests that perceptual learning can occur with increased usage of a perceptual modality. This learning tends to increase the user's attention to attributes of a stimulus that differentiate one shape from another and improve the information pick-up process in that modality. Most researchers now agree that this learning explanation accounts for observations of compensation.

It has been learned that interactions between infant and caregiver during the immediate postpartum period and thereafter form the basis for attachment, a very important cornerstone of social development. A significant element of this interaction is visually mediated via face-to-face contacts. The consequences of a lack of visual mediation in the case of the blind infant are unclear, but data indicate substantial delays, which if not corrected may have as yet unknown effects on social and emotional development.

Children who are blinded after 1 to 2 years of age are generally referred to as being adventitiously blind. A considerable period of the early development of these children is accomplished with vision available. A sizable number of studies have compared the developmental course in such children with that of children who are born blind. In general, adventitiously blind children perform most tasks of spatial and form perception more accurately than congenitally blind children and often do not differ in performance from blindfolded sighted children (Hatwell, 1978; Worchel, 1951). The finding is not universal, and the outcome of specific experiments depends on certain task and subject variables, such as the amount of specific visual experience with the stimuli being used and the particular attribute of shape or space being perceived. Particularly important in explaining the effects of early visual experience are the data indicating negative instances. Greater early tactile experience sometimes outweighs early visual experience and sometimes makes no difference. Ultimately the explanation probably relates to the efficiency of the principal perceptual system being used by the subjects (Davidson, 1976). Hence there is a need to compare the capacities of perceptual systems.

Haptic and Auditory Perception

The term *haptic* refers to the process of actively exploring an object or perceptual space with the hands. The haptic perceptual system combines input from tactile sensations and kinesthesis. Active movement enables the individual to identify distinctive characteristics of the stimulus, such as relationships between parts of a form, that are not perceptible without movement. The hands gather information from disparate points in a haptic array successively. The perceptual process is much slower by hand than by eye. Also successive prehension of different parts of a shape by the hand places an extra burden on short-term haptic memory to integrate the parts in a whole percept.

It appears that seeing persons develop visual perceptual proficiency at a faster rate than nonseeing persons develop haptic proficiency, a finding of considerable importance in understanding developmental delays in children with visual impairment. There is also a hint that the haptic system may develop differently when vision is available compared with when it is not. The hand is used more for orienting stimuli for the eye when both are present but is used for active primary information gathering when vision is absent. Perceptual development probably proceeds in a similar sequence and follows the same rules of information processing for the eye and the hand; hence enrichment strategies for visual learners (such as educationally disadvantaged or developmentally delayed seeing children) and for haptic learners may be qualitatively similar.

Haptic perception is adapted only for proximal stimulus prehension. In the absence of vision, the auditory system is the only remaining means a person with visual impairment has of gathering information about distal space. However the ideal stimulus for specifying spatial information is light, not sound. Few distinctive aspects of space, such as distance, depth, symmetry, and motion, are detectable ordinarily by auditory cues alone. The person with visual impairment must learn to use the auditory cues available to facilitate the localization and tracking of spatial attributes and, when none are available, to supply his or her own.

One of the best examples of an adequate substitution of auditory for visual cues in determining spatial properties is the phenomenon of echo location. In avoiding collisions with obstacles during locomotion, persons with visual impairment who are skilled in mobility use the reflections of self-produced sounds to judge distances of objects in their paths. The skill is similar to echo location behavior in bats and is learned through attention to differential loudness of the reflected sounds. It can be acquired surprisingly quickly by naive blindfolded sighted subjects.

Unfortunately not all spatial features can be detected by audition or touch, and this situation may be responsible for some developmental delays in early infancy and childhood for blind youngsters.

Development of the Child With Blindness

INFANCY

A number of comparisons have been made of various developmental milestones in blind and sighted infants. In general significant delays have been found in infants with blindness in the development of certain gross motor behavior patterns related to the development of locomotion, in prehension skills, and in the development of attachment behavior. The infant with blindness eventually develops all these functions during the 2nd and 3rd years of life. However, many links probably exist between such early behavior and the normal development of important cognitive, perceptual, and personality functions, suggesting that the infant with blindness ordinarily may be considered at risk for later developmental delays without adequate parental education and specific intervention in infancy.

Gross Motor Development

Table 58–2 shows a comparison of gross motor milestones in infants who are blind and those who are sighted as reported by Fraiberg (1977). There is a uniform delay of gross motor functions in this series of 10 infants with blindness. The greatest delays occur in mobility-related and locomotion-related behavior, including precrawling, sitting, pulling to standing, and walking. Ninety percent of Fraiberg's babies with blindness were substantially delayed in the onset of walking and independent walking, which did not appear until a median age of almost 20 months (1977).

Prehension of objects by the hands is also delayed in the infant with blindness. This response appears in its completed form by about 6 months of age in infants without blindness; major milestones in its achievement include bringing the hands to the midline, hand-in-hand play, grasping and transfer from hand to hand, gross swiping, and finally reaching accurately to a target with coordinated prehension. The essential ingredient in the normal emergence of this sequence is coordination of eye and hand, an impossible task for the blind child. As a result, such a child generally does not show a completed prehension response until about 9 months of age, and some 1-year-old babies with blindness still do not show the response. Of considerable importance is the potential effect of these prehension delays on the development of haptic exploratory skills. The blind infant paradoxically may show poorer haptic skill than sighted infants.

Fraiberg (1977) attributes these gross motor and

Table 58–2 • Gross Motor Items and Age Achieved by Children Who Are Blind (Child Development Project) and Those Who Are Sighted (Bayley)

Item	Age Range*		Median Age		Difference in Median Age
	Sighted	*Blind*	*Sighted*	*Blind*	
Elevates self by arms, prone†	0.7–5.0	4.5–9.5	2.1	8.75	6.65
Sits alone momentarily	4.0–8.0	5.0–8.5	5.3	6.75	1.45
Rolls from back to stomach†	4.0–10.0	4.5–9.5	6.4	7.25	0.85
Sits alone steadily	5.0–9.0	6.5–9.5	6.6	8.00	1.40
Raises self to sitting position†	6.0–11.0	9.5–15.5	8.3	11.00	2.70
Stands up by furniture (pulls up to stand)†	6.0–12.0	9.5–15.0	8.6	13.00	4.40
Stepping movements (walks hands held)†‡	6.0–12.0	8.0–11.5	8.8	10.75	1.95
Stands alone†	9.0–16.0	9.0–15.5	11.0	13.00	2.00
Walks alone, three steps†	9.0–17.0	11.5–19.0	11.7	15.25	3.55
[Walks alone, across room]†	[11.3–14.3]	12.0–20.5	[12.11]	19.25	7.15

*All ages given in months. Ages rounded to nearest 1/2 month. Three cases corrected for 3 months' prematurity. Age range includes 5–95% of Bayley sample, 25–90% of Denver sample, and 10–90% of Child Development Project sample.
†One child had not achieved by 2 years.
‡Not observed for one child prior to walking alone.
[ ]: Item from Denver Developmental Screening Test.
Adapted from Insights from the Blind: Comparative Studies of Blind and Sighted Inputs by S. Fraiberg. Copyright © 1977 by S. Fraiberg. Reprinted by permission of Basic Books, Inc., a division of HarperCollins Publishers.

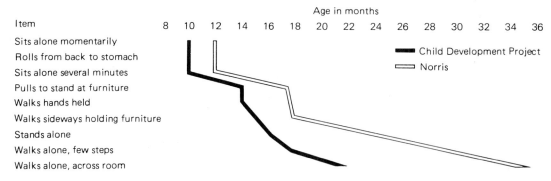

Figure 58–1. Comparison of two groups of infants who are blind. One group (n = 10) received developmental intervention (dark line). The other group (n = 66) received no such intervention (light line). (From Fraiberg S: Insights from the Blind: Comparative Studies of Blind and Sighted Infants. Copyright © by S. Fraiberg. Reprinted by permission of Basic Books, Inc., a division of HarperCollins Publishers.)

guidance response delays to the forced substitution of auditory for visual cues to identify distal shapes and spatial properties. Distal objects not prehensible by nonmobile blind infants probably are not recognized as features of a permanent world until much later in development.

Developmental interventions in infancy that are designed to enhance the development of aurally based object permanence have been successful. Figure 58–1 shows data from one such intervention program designed and implemented by Fraiberg in her well-known Michigan Child Development Project. The 10 babies with blindness in Fraiberg's apparently successful program are compared with another series of 66 infants with blindness who did not receive interventions, reported by Norris, Spaulding, and Brodie (1957). The essence of the intervention program was the introduction of paired auditory-tactual cues to sustain the infant's interest in and contact with the distal world and encouragement of physical activity. The data show a substantial acceleration of gross motor functions in Fraiberg's series, but all milestones are still delayed in relation to sighted babies. Unfortunately, because no follow-up data for Fraiberg's babies are available, one cannot say anything about durability of the intervention effects.

Development of Attachment

With infants who are sighted, the infant and caregiver develop a pattern of reciprocal reactions that lead to the emergence of attachment. The milestones include smiling at the familiar face (6 months), stranger avoidance (7 to 15 months), and distress at separation from the caregiver (6 to 9 months). The infant with blindness, however, shows a different pattern. Smiling (developed as a response to a familiar voice) occurs only inconsistently, even in 12-month-old infants with blindness. Exploration of the caregiver's face and smiling in response to familiar tactile-kinesthetic handling occur, however, at the same time as does smiling at a caregiver's face in the sighted child. Anxiety toward strangers appears at 1 year of age in the child with blindness, but a reaction to separation is not apparent until 11 to 20 months of age (a 6-month delay compared with the typical sighted infant). These delays are

no doubt related to the inability of the blind infant and caregiver to "communicate" by visual face to face contact. The typical infant with blindness may make his or her needs for attachment and comforting known through a sign system of hand gestures, which include "tactile seeking." These gestures, if unknown by the caregiver, may be misconstrued as a sign of disinterest (Erwin, 1994).

Language Development

The literature relating to the development of receptive and expressive language in infants and young children with blindness indicates a parity with sighted children. There are some exceptions, however. Infants blinded as a result of retrolental fibroplasia may show a more limited vocabulary development than other blind children. The important variable here may be an increased anticipation by the caregiver of the congenitally blind child's needs, thus decreasing the demand for language production.

Intervention

As pointed out previously, most of the delays in early sensorimotor development in the infant with visual impairment occur as a result of a deprivation of visual information. Substitution systems can be effectively taught to the infant and the expected defects can be reduced. Fraiberg (1971) has developed a comprehensive intervention protocol. Although limited evidence is available to document its effectiveness, the data relating to outcome are encouraging, and the protocol is in wide use in programs for infants with visual impairments in the United States. Fraiberg (1977) has also published a popular text readable by parents and other caregivers that highlights areas of concern and suggests some remediation techniques. Of considerable importance to the primary care provider is the counseling of parents regarding special differences between infants with visual impairments and sighted infants, such as the use of a tactile sign system discussed previously. Without this basic information, delays in social, cognitive, and perceptual development may be exacerbated.

Olson (1987) and Davidson and Harrison (1997) recently provided comprehensive reviews of the literature pertaining to the effectiveness of early intervention for children with visual impairments. In general, this literature is descriptive, involves very small samples, and rarely provides empiric data addressing efficacy. Nevertheless, both home-based and center-based intervention models have been described to stimulate specific developmental domains that are at high risk for delays owing to visual impairments, such as mobility, sensory-motor development, language, and social communication.

CHILDHOOD

The period between 1 and 6 years of age in the development of the child with visual impairment has rarely been studied. A considerable amount of literature is available on social, cognitive, and perceptual development in the school-aged child with visual impairment, however.

Cognitive and Perception Development

In general, patterns of cognitive and perceptual development in otherwise unaffected children who are blind and nonblind run a parallel course for auditory-based functions. Children with visual impairment appear to have somewhat better auditory attention, but tasks involving abstract reasoning with either tactual or auditory verbal material are equivalently performed. If any discrepancies do exist, they usually can be explained by the sometimes limited experience of children with visual impairment with stimulus materials being used.

Tests of abilities, including intelligence quotient (IQ) tests as well as functional batteries, have been used to estimate the pattern of global intellectual development in children with blindness. Several conclusions are of importance. First, as is seen in a subsequent section, few IQ tests are available with normative data relating to individuals with blindness or that are "culture fair." Hence comparing blind and sighted persons on the basis of IQ is very difficult and probably inappropriate. Second, certain etiologies for blindness lead to either increased or decreased overall cognitive potential. For example, a sizable number of studies have shown that children blinded as a result of retinoblastoma may have a significantly higher level of ability than children blinded by other conditions. In several studies, the mean Hayes-Binet IQ for patients who were bilaterally enucleated because of retinoblastoma was about 120, or 21 points above that of a control group of patients without retinoblastoma as well as that of a control group with unilateral retinoblastoma. The advantage probably reflects a combination of genetic and environmental factors as yet only partially understood. A second example is the incidence of lowered IQ scores in children blinded by ROP. In several series of such children, as many as 35% showed neurologic abnormalities, and more than 40% had IQ scores below the average range. Some controlled series have also indicated that the probable reason for lowered IQ is not the ROP per se but possibly the neurologic sequelae of prematurity. Phelps (1994) reported that these infants typically have the most difficult course while hospitalized in neonatal intensive care units.

The most significant deficits in cognition and percep-tion in children with blindness occur in tasks that are aided by vision or visual experience. The best-studied example of this phenomenon is the development of conservation. Conservation refers to a cognitive concept or rule of perceptual transformation: A physical property (such as the amount of solid or the volume) remains invariant even though its perceptible shape or appearance is transformed. A block of clay loses no mass if it is rolled into a wiener shape, even though its physical dimensions have been altered and it looks different. The seeing child makes this judgment correctly at about 8 to 9 years of age, coincident with the onset of the Piagetian cognitive stage of concrete operational thought. The child with blindness, in repeated studies, has been shown to lag behind in the onset of this response by 2 to 3 years.

Other concepts in the child with blindness are delayed, such as seriation and certain classification abilities that are significantly dependent on visual experience. The delays are much less significant, or nonexistent, in youngsters who are adventitiously blind, reinforcing the experiential hypothesis.

Functions of Haptic Exploratory Search

Sighted preschoolers tend to be very passive when asked to use their hands to explore a shape, pressing down or squeezing it and paying little attention to critical details that distinguish the shape from others. Between about 5 and 8 years of age, sighted children increase their active exploration, using styles that globally search the shape in a comparative fashion. By the age of 12 years, haptic search ability is quite well developed.

Some studies suggest that it may take the child with visual impairment longer than the sighted child to develop coordinated haptic exploration. By age 10 or 12, however, the child with visual impairment shows haptic search ability that appears to be more active and more efficient than sighted children's efforts at isolating features and discriminating different shapes. The proficient blind haptic explorer also tends to remember what was felt more accurately than the sighted child.

Some Educational Issues

To be an effective advocate, the primary care provider of a child with visual impairment must be familiar with several special needs in the child's education.

Reading. Many children who are legally blind can read normal newspaper print with some additional magnification, but others require large print texts and newsprint. Some but not all reading materials are available in large print. As mentioned, about 20,000 school-aged children in the United States have visual impairments severe enough to require alternatives to print to read. The most widely used system, of course, is braille. Despite its universality, braille suffers from some serious systematic deficiencies. First, the reading rate for even the best braille readers is about one third as fast as that in the visual reading of print. Second, not all materials are available in braille and transcription. The American Printing House uses computerized transcription, but there is a delay in obtaining this service. Third, the space required for storage of braille books is considerable (one 250-page print book may require 12 or more volumes of braille pages), preventing most individuals from maintaining large libraries at home. Finally there is a very poor understanding of the basic perceptual and linguistic mechanisms underlying the acquisition of braille reading skill. As a result, the teaching of braille reading is often idiosyncratic from school to school and teacher to teacher, and not all readers ever obtain maximum efficiency.

Alternatives to braille have been developed. The talking book program has existed for some time and is available in most libraries. The Stanford Research Institute has developed a device called OPTACON (Optical to Tactile Converter), which receives optical input from a standard printed text and converts it to a tactual dot figuration, which can be distinguished by the finger. The device is portable but expensive (about $1000). Also because it senses only one character at a time, it leads to very slow reading rates (about 35 words per minute). It does not do well with print that is not clear and sharp; hence one can read a newspaper only with difficulty.

Grunwald has developed a reading machine that reproduces braille from material coded on tape and passes the resulting signals across the reader's fingertips passively. This device is inflexible insofar as it does not allow the finger to search a text; the finger can "read" in only one direction, one cell at a time, as the materials come off the tape.

Print-to-speech converters, such as the Kurzweil device, are in many public libraries. This device accepts a print format and "reads aloud" to the user.

Despite new developments, it is very likely that braille will continue as the principal medium for nonvisual reading for some time to come.

Orientation and Mobility. Although guide dogs are in wide use among adults with visual impairment, most school-aged youngsters with visual impairment use the long cane as an aid.

Orientation and mobility instruction can be started in most public school settings very early in the child's educational career and is provided in most states through cooperative arrangements between schools and agencies for blind persons.

Alternatives to the conventional mobility aide are being developed. The most promising such device is a computer that converts visual images, sensed by a microcomponent video camera mounted in a pair of glasses, to actual impressions on the back. Also, a system has been developed in which the input from the camera is transmitted directly to the central nervous system by means of optic nerve electrode implants.

Sensory aids have been developed to assist young children with visual impairments to acquire mobility skills. The Canterbury Child's Aid (Strelow and Boys, 1979) and the Sonic Guide (Ferrell, 1980) are based on sonar wave emissions that are converted to audible stimuli with pitch scaled to distance from obstacles that can be discriminated even by young children. The date reported on efficacy of these devices are limited and inconclusive (Davidson and Harrison, 1997).

Residential Versus Public School. Prior to 1974, the majority of children with significant visual impairment were educated in state-operated or private residential schools. Along with the general movement toward mainstreaming children with disabilities in public educational facilities, which occurred after 1974, virtually all children with visual impairment have been returned to their local districts for schooling. The residential school populations are made up of children who have visual impairment along with multiple disabilities. In a number of states, the residential units have been refurbished and reclassified as intermediate care facilities for persons with mental retardation.

The public educational sector has been successful in providing the specialty programs once offered at the state schools. Braille and orientation and mobility instruction are usually provided by itinerant teachers; few districts have self-contained classes for children with visual impairment. Nearly all such children are provided for through the local district's Committee on Special Education (CSE) or by a Commission for the Blind, and parents often need help in seeing that their child receives the proper support for an appropriate education.

Blindness and Associated Disabilities

In recent years most researchers assume that the early delays in visual function are a reflection of more global developmental delays secondary to developmental neurologic disorders (Hoyt and Good, 1993; Kivlin et al, 1990; Tresidder, Fielder, and Nicholson, 1990). About 50% of children with visual impairment have associated disabilities (Robinson, Jan, and Kinnis, 1987). About 20% to 25% of all blind children in the Robinson series are thought to have some degree of mental retardation. Black and Sonksen (1992) reported that children with congenital retinal dystrophies such as Leber congenital amaurosis have coincident mental retardation in about 60% of cases. In general the person with mental retardation and blindness is probably far more disabled than someone with either one or the other disorder and is at high risk for severe educational and vocational impairment unless specialized services are provided.

At least three significant series of patients with ROP have been reported in which about 15% showed autistic behavior, including withdrawal, noncommunication, stereotypy, and self-injurious activity. The origin of this correlation is unknown, but some interplay between central nervous system damage, parent-child relationships, and sensory deprivation is suspected. Early diagnosis and intensive treatment are keys to anything other than a guarded prognosis for these children. In many children with visual impairment, there is a relatively high prevalence of repetitive head and body, limb, and hand movements, actions sometimes referred to collectively as "blindisms." Such socially inappropriate behavior also occurs in children with other disabilities, but usually only in those who are the most severely mentally retarded; therefore its occurrence in the child with visual impairment is of some concern. The patterns of stereotypy occur in infants and continue through childhood and adolescence unless treated. Their origin is unclear, but most of the literature points to a compensatory response to increased sensory stimulation.

There is no indication that blindisms are necessary to the overall functioning of the child with visual impairment; these behavior patterns respond favorably to straightforward operant behavior therapy and should be treated.

Developmental Evaluation of the Child Who Is Visually Impaired

Assessment of the child's developmental status is of great importance in proper educational and habilitative planning. Evaluation of the child with visual impairment is best done by an interdisciplinary team.

Few causes of visual impairment result in total loss of vision; therefore most patients have some useful vision. Assessment of functional vision in the infant, however, is difficult. Obviously, early and careful assessment can lead to maximization of early partial sight. In addition to ophthalmologic studies, a number of visually guided behavior patterns are useful in estimating infant visual status. For example, visually guided reaching and its precursors, such as swiping, cannot occur on time without vision. Infants with partial vision develop these responses normally; hence their presence implies functional vision. Often infants with field defects are identifiable by visually guided responses that occur only in functioning fields or only when targets are at specific distances. Finally the presence of a gaze disorder in infancy should not be confused with functional blindness.

As has been noted, infants with visual impairment are at risk for significant developmental delays; therefore, some attempt should be made within the first 3 to 6 months of life to obtain a baseline measurement of the infant's gross motor development. The Denver Developmental Screening Test or other similar developmental checklists can be useful for in-office screening. Referral to Early Intervention Programs (created in 1987 as a part of PL 99-457, The Individuals with Disabilities Education Act) will access physical therapy, occupational therapy, special education, speech therapy, and audiologic consultations to provide more information to the parents in regard to intervention. Parents should be counseled about their child's possible developmental delays and what they can do about it. Finally an assessment of cognitive and emotional functioning should be obtained within the 1st year of life from a pediatric psychologist or other developmental specialist. Not every such specialist has training or experience with visually impaired infants and young children.

Follow-up with most children with visual impairment should be periodic, from preschool years through the early grades, because developmental problems may persist. Most school districts provide specialized teams of allied health and educational professionals who can accomplish the evaluations and help in the planning process for the child. However, few persons on such teams have extensive experience with children who have visual impairment, and one might seek additional expertise with the help of the local Association for the Blind. This agency can also usually provide assessments of orientation and mobility, braille reading readiness, and other haptic skills, all of significance to the thorough evaluation of children with visual impairment.

Community Resources for Persons Who Are Visually Impaired

As should be evident from the discussion to this point, the child with visual impairment and his or her family need a variety of nonmedical services, including educational, social and recreational, vocational, orientation and mobility, and financial services. As is true for almost every developmental disability, the provision of services in these areas has evolved from separate and often noncommunicating sectors complicated by multiple age-specific entitlement programs. Included in the mix are agencies of federal, state, or local government and private not-for-profit providers. Some agencies offer comprehensive services in a particular area of specialization, such as state education departments, which operate state schools for the blind and programs for children who are hearing and visually impaired. Other agencies provide only specialized service (the Commission for the Blind in some states offers only advocacy assistance). There is overlap at times, and obtaining services can be a confusing and time-consuming activity for the family of a child with visual impairment. The primary care provider can facilitate the process by assisting the family in obtaining accurate information about services and helping them to contact relevant agency counselors.

Education of children with visual impairment between birth and 21 years in all states is a public responsibility. Children under 3 years of age with visual impairment are served by Early Intervention Programs. Those 3 to 5 years of age are served by local schools and by different state agencies. Any educational needs of a school-aged child should be referred to the chairman of the local school district's Committee on Special Education (or its equivalent). Social, recreational, and sometimes special educational and vocational needs of children with visual impairment are usually met by either state or local governmental or private agencies, such as the Lighthouse or other local Associations for the Blind.

Vocational needs, although they are the responsibility of the Office of Vocational Rehabilitation, may also be met in part by the Association for the Blind and Visual Impaired. Financial aid via the federal Disabled Children's Program, Physically Handicapped Children's Program, Medicaid, and Supplemental Security Income are administered by the state Departments of Social Services and Health.

Advocacy groups and agencies may be operated by states or may involve parent support organizations. They may offer services specifically for persons with visual impairment or to all the individuals with disabilities. Advocates can often help a client obtain services and can take on responsibilities that otherwise would fall to the primary care provider. They can be particularly helpful when the child has multiple needs or when multiple disabilities exist, requiring transactions with numerous agencies. They may also provide parent training and other family support services. Advocacy agencies are accessible through the Association for the Blind.

Associated Issues

Prevention of developmental delay secondary to blindness is still an evolving field. The most effective tool is early habilitation. An increasing number of communities have home-based early intervention programs specialized for infants and preschoolers with visual impairment as a part of the Early Intervention Program. Without such programs, infants and their families may not obtain educational-habilitative services until the child can begin a day program at age 2 or 3 years, and valuable time is lost.

Another important secondary and tertiary preventive mechanism is parent education. The infant and young child with visual impairment have special needs, which, if not met, can lead to developmental disability. The primary care provider must take time to counsel parents about such needs and act as a continuing resource for developmental consultation if necessary. Such advocacy may be needed through the early elementary school years for children with visual impairment and requires more continuous patient contact than would be dictated by well-child care schedules.

REFERENCES

Black M, Sonksen P: Congenital retinal dystrophies: a study of early cognitive and visual development. Arch Dis Childh 67:262, 1992.

Davidson PW: Some functions of active handling: studies with blinded humans. New Outlook for the Blind, May, 1976, pp 196–202.

Davidson P, Harrison G: The effectiveness of early intervention for children with visual impairment. *In* Guralnick M (ed): The Effectiveness of Early Intervention. Baltimore, Paul H. Brookes Publishing Co, 1997, pp 483–495.

Erwin E: Social competence in young children with visual impairments. Infants Young Children 6(3):26, 1994.

Ferrell KA: Can infants use the Sonic Guide? Two years' experience of Project View! J Visual Impairment and Blindness 74:209, 1980.

Fraiberg S: Insights from the Blind: Comparative Studies of Blind and Sighted Infants. New York, Basic Books, 1977.

Fraiberg S: Intervention in infancy: a program for blind infants. J Am Acad Child Psychiat 10:381, 1971.

Goldstein H: The reported demography and causes of blindness throughout the world. Adv Ophthalmol 40:1, 1980.

Hatwell Y: Form perception and related issues in blind humans. *In* Held R, Leibowitz H, Teuber HL (eds): Handbook of Sensory Physiology, Vol 8. Perception. New York, Springer-Verlag, 1978.

Hoyt C, Good W: Visual factors in developmental delay and neurological disorders in infants. *In* Simmons K (ed): Early Visual Development, Normal and Abnormal. New York, Oxford University Press, 1993, pp 505–512.

Kivlin J, Bodnar A, Ralston C, Hunt S: The visually inattentive pre-term infant. J Pediatr Ophthalmol Strabismus 27:190, 1990.

Norris M, Spaulding P, Brodie F: Blindness in Children. Chicago, University of Chicago Press, 1957.

Olson M: Early intervention for children with visual impairments. *In* Guralnick M, Bennett F (eds): The Effectiveness of Early Intervention for at Risk and Handicapped Children. New York, Academic Press, 1987, pp 297–324.

Phelps D: Retinopathy of prematurity: a neonatologists perspective. *In* Isenberg SJ (ed): The Eye of Infancy, 2nd ed. St. Louis, Mosby–Year Book, 1994, pp 437–447.

Phelps D: Retinopathy of prematurity: a neonatologist's perspective. *In* Isenberg SJ (ed): Acquired Ocular Disorders of the Newborn. Chicago, Year Book, 1989, pp 417-427.

Robinson G, Jan J: Acquired ocular visual impairment in children: 1960–1989. Am J Dis Child 147:325, 1993.

Robinson G, Jan J, Kinnis C: Congenital ocular blindness in children, 1945 to 1984. Am J Dis Child 141:1321, 1987.

Strelow ER, Boys JT: The Canterbury Child's Aid: a binaural spatial sensor for research with blind children. J Visual Impairment and Blindness 73:179, 1979.

Tresidder J, Fielder A, Nicholson, J: Delayed visual maturation: ophthalmic and neurodevelopmental aspects. Dev Med Child Neurol 32:872, 1990.

Worchel P: Space perception and orientation in the blind. Psychol Monogr, 1951.

59 *Cerebral Palsy*

Stephen A. Back

Although perinatal complications were previously judged to be the single most important factor in the subsequent development of cerebral palsy (CP) in the full-term infant, a variety of epidemiologic studies now indicate that a minority of cases of CP are strongly related to full-term intrapartum asphyxia.

The primary concerns in management of the motor complications of CP are to optimize limb mobility and postural stability and prevent the development of joint deformity, joint dislocations, and scoliosis.

Although spastic quadriplegia is the most uncommon form of CP, it is the most severe and debilitating.

There is clearly a tremendous range of potential developmental outcomes within any given subtype of CP.

General Implications for Development

Cerebral palsy (CP) refers to a group of nonprogressive disorders that arise because of injury to the developing brain. Brain injury may occur prenatally, perinatally, or during the first years of life and invariably affects motor function. Given the large number of potential causes of injury to the developing brain, the spectrum of CP is broad. From a practical standpoint it encompasses those conditions in which the predominant needs of the individual relate to motor disabilities. Each form of CP also carries a risk for a variety of other developmental deficits. These include difficulties with vision, speech, language, behavior, epilepsy, learning, feeding, and gastrointestinal function. Despite significant motor impairment, many children with CP are of normal intelligence.

Paradoxically, advances in newborn medicine and concomitant reductions in infant mortality have not resulted in a decline in the overall incidence of CP, which has remained stable in developed countries between the 1950s and the present. Although perinatal complications were previously regarded as the single most important factor in the subsequent development of CP in the full-term infant, a variety of epidemiologic studies now indicate that a minority of cases of CP are strongly related to full-term intrapartum asphyxia (Roland and Hill, 1997). These studies have directed attention to various maternal and prenatal factors (Table 59–1) that may contribute to the development of fetal brain injury that manifests as a neonatal encephalopathy (Dammann and Leviton, 1997). Despite these continuing controversies regarding etiology, several groups of newborns should be monitored for a variety of developmental disabilities related to CP. The first are infants with a birth weight of less than 1500 g for whom the timing of injury is primarily postnatal. Of the 85% of these infants who survive the neonatal period in the United States, 5% to 15% develop CP. Comparable numbers of survivors of term intrapartum asphyxia are affected. Infants who undergo cardiac bypass surgery in the first weeks of life for congenital heart disease are at significant risk for selective injury to the basal ganglia (du Plessis, 1997), as are infants who develop kernicterus secondary to hyperbilirubinemia.

Although CP is defined as nonprogressive in nature, the distinction from a progressive neurodegenerative condition is not always clear. Progressive gliosis, cavitation, and atrophy may occur for months after brain injury and result in an initial picture of evolving motor disability. In some forms of CP, largely normal or stable periods of motor development may precede the onset of unexpected new disabilities. The timing of the new disability may coincide

Table 59–1 • Risk Factors Associated with Cerebral Palsy

Maternal Factors
Multiple gestation pregnancy
Preterm labor/threatened abortion
Premature placental separation
History of fetal loss
Prenatal Factors
Intrauterine growth retardation
Congenital malformations
Twin gestation
Perinatal Factors
Prolonged, precipitous, or traumatic delivery
Apgar score <3 at 15 minutes
Venous cord blood pH <6.9
Premature or postmature birth
Abnormal fetal presentation
Postnatal Factors
Hypoxic-ischemic encephalopathy with multiorgan failure
Periventricular leukomalacia
Intracranial or intraventricular hemorrhage
Hyperbilirubinemia

with that period in brain development when a particular neural system normally matures. Such is the case, for example, in hemiplegic CP, in which the onset of upper extremity spasticity occurs after a period of normal motor development in the first months of life and coincides with the appearance of the hand grasp. In some children with dyskinetic CP, a worsening of the movement disorder may occur for unknown reasons after a stable course of many years. Progressive deterioration in a child with CP may also herald a new pathologic process related to the prior injury. The onset of posthemorrhagic hydrocephalus, for example, may rarely be delayed up to a year after intraventricular hemorrhage. Clinical deterioration can also follow a bout of status epilepticus that caused further brain injury.

Diagnostic Considerations

Several considerations arise when a diagnosis of CP is suspected. The first is to establish that the child's presentation is consistent with a static brain disorder. Importantly, a diagnosis of CP must be made as a diagnosis of exclusion. In support of the diagnosis may be a variety of risk factors associated with CP elicited from the mother's or infant's history (see Table 59–1). In most situations, an overt history of perinatal factors will be lacking. In about half of all the children, no etiology will be identified. Very rarely will a familial genetic condition be identified as the cause of CP (e.g., a familial spastic paraparesis syndrome), but this should be suspected if multiple family members are affected. Central nervous system malformations may produce a clinical picture resembling CP. Congenital spinal cord malformations (e.g., diastematomyelia) should be considered when spastic diplegia presents without upper extremity involvement in a patient who lacks other risk factors. When clinically indicated, care must also be taken to consider a variety of metabolic or degenerative conditions that can mimic CP (Table 59–2), and in atypical cases, one should not hesitate to revisit these considerations as the child's development progresses, to ensure that the diagnosis of a progressive disorder has not been missed (Volpe, 1995).

When a diagnosis of CP is made, the family's response is often one of shock and disbelief. It may be helpful to begin by discussing the features of the child's motor delay that are consistent with CP. The initial visit can be tailored to the family's perceived need for education about what CP is and is not. Families will want to know what they can anticipate for their child's future and what can be done immediately to improve their child's condition (Miller and Bachrach, 1995).

For those occasions in which the type of CP may be uncertain, discussion of those aspects of the child's motor development that are consistent with CP may bring the diagnosis more into focus than will an attempt to give a firm label. As discussed earlier, changes in muscle tone and function may continue to manifest during the first several years of life and may require revision of the diagnosis of the type of CP as well as raise new therapeutic considerations. This approach may prevent needless doubts or confusion from arising for the family, should the diagnosis of the type of CP later require revision.

Table 5–2 • Differential Diagnosis of Cerebral Palsy

CP Type	Differential Diagnosis
Infantile hypotonia with delayed motor development	Chromosomal disorders
	Hypothyroidism
	Neuronal migration disorders
	Congenital brain malformations
	Congenital myopathies
Spastic types	Leukodystrophies
	Multicystic encephalomalacia
	Congenital brain malformations
	Congenital spinal cord tumors
	Familial spastic paraparesis
	Familial microcephaly syndromes
	Intrauterine infections
	Hydrocephalus
Dyskinetic types	Kernicterus
	Hyperthyroidism
	Dopa-responsive dystonia
	Lesch-Nyhan syndrome
	Glutaric acidemia type 1
Ataxic	Urea cycle disorders
	Aminoacidopathies
	Mitochondrial myopathies
	Peroxisomal disorders
	Ataxia-telangiectasia
	Angelman syndrome

General Approach to Management

IMPAIRMENT IN MOTOR DEVELOPMENT

Once a diagnosis of CP has been made, a careful assessment is required of the child's level of motor function within the context of his or her global development. Consideration must also be given to the general health of the child and the degree to which recurrent or debilitating conditions associated with CP (e.g., respiratory compromise, failure to thrive, or epilepsy) may be affecting developmental progress (Table 59–3). The extent of motor delay, as well as abnormal patterns of motor development, must be identified to organize an optimal therapeutic plan. It is also important to assess whether motor impairment may impede the child's ability to perform during cognitive testing. When a selection or matching task is presented, for example, some children with severe dystonic CP may show

Table 59–3 • Cerebral Palsy–Associated Complications

Gross motor	Speech and language
Joint deformity	Dysarthria
Joint instability	Dysphasia/aphasia
Scoliosis	Visual impairment
Limb asymmetries	Strabismus
Fine motor	Field defects
Cortical fisting	Visual-perceptual deficits
Absent pincer grasp	Cortical blindness
Epilepsy	Sensorineural hearing deficits
Cognitive/behavioral	Systemic complications
Learning disabilities	Failure to thrive
Mental retardation	Gastroesophageal reflux
Attention-deficit hyperactivity disorders	Constipation
Adjustment disorders	Aspiration pneumonia

a delay of a minute or more before the initiation of a reaching response. These same children may also be unable to verbally communicate their response because of the inability to coordinate the muscles required for speaking.

The primary concerns in management of the motor complications of CP are to optimize limb mobility and postural stability and prevent the development of joint deformity, joint dislocations, and scoliosis (Dormans, 1993; Barry, 1996; DeLuca, 1996). Serial orthopedic evaluations are essential as early in the course as significant changes in tone are identified. Ideally, the initial assessment involves an orthopedic surgeon and a physiatrist in conjunction with physical and occupational therapists. A variety of approaches are available to prevent or forestall the development of joint deformites that otherwise will require surgical correction. These approaches seek to restore the balance between opposing muscle groups by either diminishing the overly active agonist muscles or strengthening the antagonist muscles. Interventions include physical therapy, bracing, serial casting, oral medications, intrathecal baclofen, neuromuscular blockade, and selective dorsal rhizotomy.

During infancy the initial orthopedic approach is conservative. Emphasis is placed on training caregivers to integrate a daily stretching program into the child's routine (e.g., at diapering). Proper positioning is also essential to achieve joint alignment and postural stability as well as to optimize the child's interactions with the environment. Growth velocity is monitored for the onset of growth spurts that can cause joint instability owing to an imbalance in the forces exerted on the joint by agonist and antagonist muscle groups. Periods of accelerated limb growth during infancy may, in particular, be associated with progressive hip adductor spasticity. Hip instability carries a significant risk for femoral head subluxations and should be evaluated with regular hip films. If positioning and stretching prove insufficient to control the progression of spasticity, the surgeon may intervene with orthoses, splints, or serial casting. Skeletal alignment, improved mobility, and better postural control may also be promoted with adaptive equipment, including standers, prone boards, and side-liers.

Medical therapies may be introduced prior to or concurrent with orthopedic interventions (Pranzatelli, 1996). The selection of agents for CP-related spasticity or movement disorders is dictated by the predominant clinical problem. In general, the drugs currently available for CP-related complications are not the mainstay of therapy but are used as an adjunct to orthopedic interventions. Oral medications are of partial benefit, and dosing is limited by unacceptable side effects including sedation, increased oral secretions, and nausea. The most commonly used agents for spasticity are baclofen, the benzodiazepines, and dantrolene. The treatment of CP-related dyskinesias includes baclofen, benzodiazepines, and trihexphenidyl and must be tailored to the particular movement disorder. Recent promising trials of intrathecal baclofen in patients with CP have demonstrated improved control of spasticity and dystonia at lower doses that avoid more of the systemic side effects of oral baclofen (Albright, 1996).

Neuromuscular blockade weakens agonist muscles and is another important means to transiently improve function, diminish pain, and slow the progression of joint deformity (Koman, Mooney, and Smith, 1996). The longer-acting neuromuscular blocking agents in current practice are ethyl alcohol, aqueous phenol, and botulinum A toxin. These agents transiently weaken selected muscles for several months, thereby providing the opportunity to intensify physical therapy in an attempt to delay or assess the potential benefits of surgical interventions. Unlike alcohol or phenol, botulinum A toxin has the advantage that direct injection does not require deep conscious sedation or general anesthesia. Given that the generally accepted maximal dosage is 6 U/kg, the number of target muscles that can be safely injected is limited. Moreover, the injections are given at least 1 month apart to reduce the risk of production of antibodies to the toxin. Most patients require injection at 3- to 6-month intervals. When multiple or large muscle groups require treatment, phenol motor point blocks of selected nerves may be preferable to circumvent the dose-limitations of botulinum A toxin.

Surgical interventions in the form of various combinations of tendon releases or transfers may be inevitable if significant contractures develop despite conservative measures (DeLuca, 1996). Operations are generally not planned before the patient is 4 or 5 years old, when growth begins to slow, to avoid the need for an early revision. Planning of operations may be greatly assisted by a gait laboratory evaluation. For carefully selected patients in whom spasticity does not provide a gain of function, dorsal rhizotomy may be beneficial to achieve functional ambulation; in these same patients dorsal rhizotomy may be harmful in other settings, where a loss of spasticity might actually reduce function by unmasking underlying weakness or by causing hip instability (Abbot, 1996).

Regular attention should be focused on three major areas of common disability: functional use of the hands, the acquisition of optimal seating, and ambulation. The success of therapeutic interventions for a dysfunctional hand may be better if the origin of the fisting stems from spasticity rather than from dystonia. Wrist or hand splints are useful to prevent contractures. Focal injection of botulinum A toxin into the wrist or hand flexors may assist in determining the degree of functional use of the extensor muscles after the antagonists have been transiently weakened. Such a trial can also permit intensified physical therapy to strengthen the hand and to assess the potential benefits of surgical interventions.

Independent sitting is commonly delayed in CP and may not be achieved. Malpositioning secondary to poor head and trunk support can produce fatigue and irritability, contribute to poor feeding, exacerbate gastroesophageal reflux, seriously hamper reaching and exploration of the environment, and increase the risk of the child's developing hip dislocation or scoliosis. Poor seating can also promote the development of maladaptive patterns of movement, such as preferred head turning, through repetition of primitive automatisms (i.e., an asymmetric tonic neck response). Remedies include a well-outfitted wheelchair that provides good head and trunk support. For those with weakness of the head and trunk, a soft spinal orthosis can improve the positioning of the trunk so that the child may dedicate more energy to achieving head control. Often multiple strategies need to be formulated to discourage maladaptive patterns of movement from becoming persistent learned behaviors.

Whether a child will achieve functional or independent ambulation is a common concern for the family of a child with CP. For a child using a wheelchair, functional ambulation is defined as the ability to execute independent transfers over short distances. Independent ambulation is defined as long-distance walking done with or without crutches or other assistive devices. Both increased extensor tone of the lower extremities and low truncal tone influence the success of ambulation. In addition, the persistence of primitive automatisms or the failure to develop protective postural responses negatively correlates with eventual walking. The likelihood of walking has been correlated with the persistence or absence of certain developmental motor patterns (Bleck, 1987) (Table 59–4). In general all but the most severely affected children with spastic diplegia or hemiplegia will be functional ambulators. The outcome is more variable with other forms of CP. At some point consideration must be given to the actual benefit to the child of independent ambulation if exhaustive effort must be expended to the detriment of other activities. For some children, mobility with a wheelchair is preferable so that their energy may be directed toward the activities they enjoy.

PSYCHOSOCIAL DEVELOPMENT

Cerebral palsy poses a lifelong series of adjustments for the individual and the family. As the child's development progresses, the challenge to the clinician is to identify newly emerging disabilities and coordinate the necessary services to meet the child's needs (Blum et al, 1991).

During infancy, appropriate strategies must be developed to enable a child with significant motor impairment to maximize his or her cognitive potential. Because an infant with CP may appear "weak" or "helpless" to caregivers, they may, perhaps unconsciously, reduce their efforts to provide appropriate infant stimulation. All infants should have the benefit of an early intervention program, which provides ongoing evaluation of developmental needs within the context of physical, occupational, and cognitive stimulation programs. An in-home assessment by an infant

developmental specialist can ensure that such needs as interactive play and visual and tactile exploration of the child's surroundings are encouraged. Toward this end, it is important for the child to have seating that optimizes head and trunk support so that positioning that forces the child into maladaptive reflex postures is avoided. A child with dystonic CP, for example, whose attempts at grasping are accompanied by adventitious head movements that trigger an asymmetric tonic neck reflex, will be unable to functionally reach or visually direct the hand toward the desired target.

During the 2nd year of life, communication can become a source of great frustration for a child with CP. Language delay may be multifactorial stemming from discoordination of the muscles of speech and phonation as well as from deficits in vision or hearing. Early evaluation by a speech therapist and, where indicated, by an ophthalmologist or audiologist is required before the communication potential of the child can be determined. If it becomes clear that spoken language will be impossible, alternative forms of communication should be investigated. Children with dyskinetic CP, for example, may effectively communicate using sign language. The recent advent of computer-driven language boards offers a wealth of new opportunities for effective alternative forms of communication that allow the child to enjoy greater social interactions and provide enhanced prospects for eventual job opportunities.

Entry into school is often a crisis point for both the child with CP and the family. For some families the realization comes that their child will face new difficulties in school. At this time a variety of learning disabilities may begin to be identified. As a result of the underlying brain injury, behavior problems are also more likely to manifest in the genetically predisposed child. Children with CP have a higher incidence of most kinds of behavior problems, including attention and hyperactivity disorders. In addition, entry into school confronts the child on a daily basis with his or her physical or intellectual differences from peers. Thus the child may experience mounting frustration and a sense of isolation due to his or her inability to keep up with play, athletic activities, and homework assignments. Some peers may be frightened by or shun the child because of deformities, shorter stature, abnormal movements or speech, or the need for orthotic devices. The beginning of school thus forces the recognition that the physical differences are permanent and may further promote a reluctance to attempt assimilation with peers. Some children develop a denial of their CP and no longer cooperate with physical therapy.

Anger and depression are common responses for the child that can wreak havoc on the family life. The family may become completely absorbed in dealing with the child's behavior, which may then engender hostility between the child and siblings. It is thus of vital importance that the child's emerging crisis be identified early so that supportive counseling or psychiatric intervention can be arranged.

For the adolescent with severe disability, for whom increasing difficulties associated with transfers, dressing, and transportation may occur, it can be unrealistic for the family to attempt to care for the child entirely without the assistance of in-home nursing or a community care facility.

Table 59–4 • Seven Predictors of Walking by 7 Years in a Child with Cerebral Palsy*

Abnormal If Present After 6 Months	Abnormal If Absent	Presence Always Abnormal
Asymmetric tonic neck reflex	Foot placement reaction	Extensor thrust
Symmetric tonic neck reflex	Parachute reaction	
Moro reflex		
Neck-righting reflex		

*The tests permit a 95% prediction of walking by 7 years of age. Each abnormal response is scored one point. The prognosis for independent ambulation with or without crutches is good with a score of zero. Prognosis is guarded with a score of one point, and a score of two or more points indicates a poor prognosis.
Adapted from Bleck E: Orthopedic Management in Cerebral Palsy. Philadelphia, JB Lippincott, 1987.

For many less disabled adolescents with CP, there is a growing awareness of the potential limitations of their condition on future independence, gainful employment, and meaningful interpersonal relationships. Concerns with body image, weight gain, and sexuality affect self-esteem and compound the issues of adolescence that center around independence. Social activities such as school dances and weekend outings may be restricted because of impaired or awkward ambulation. Isolation increases as the peer group becomes more athletically advanced. The adolescent may become more passive, withdrawn, and dependent in reaction to a perceived helpless situation. Families should work closely with their child's school to identify activities that encourage integration into a peer group and involvement with extracurricular and social programs. Families should be provided with access to vocational and career guidance and, when needed, individual or group therapy.

Clinical Forms of Cerebral Palsy

A variety of classification schemes are currently in use based on the patterns of motor findings that may be recognized in CP. Several types of motor disability in CP are more commonly encountered (i.e., spastic diplegia, hemiplegia, spastic quadriplegia, and dyskinetic CP). These arise mainly from either corticospinal tract injury, with resultant spasticity, or extrapyramidal motor system injury, with resultant dyskinesia (e.g., dystonia or athetosis). Injury to cerebellar pathways gives rise to an uncommon form of ataxic CP that will not be dealt with here. Not uncommonly, a "pure" form of CP cannot be identified. In these cases, a mixed form of CP combines elements of spasticity and dyskinesia. It is thus of practical value to determine whether each of a child's motor disabilities is largely spastic or dyskinetic, because the management of motor disabilities differs for treatment of spasticity or dyskinesias.

SPASTIC DIPLEGIA

Spastic diplegia refers to a pattern of weakness that disproportionately involves the lower extremities relative to the upper extremities or the face. Spastic diplegia is overwhelmingly a disorder affecting children of premature birth. Paradoxically, the incidence of spastic diplegic CP has not decreased with the advent of improved survival of premature infants. This reflects the fact that the sick premature infant is prone to development of a pressure passive cerebral circulation. The resultant fluctuations in cerebral perfusion may cause two distinct forms of subcortical white matter injury: germinal matrix hemorrhages (i.e., periventricular hemorrhagic infarction) and infarction of the periventricular white matter (i.e., periventricular leukomalacia) (Volpe, 1997). Since these infants may be subject to recurrent episodes of cerebral hypoperfusion, white matter injury may become cumulative over time; hence the ultimate impact on motor development is variable.

Close developmental follow-up is mandatory for any infant with a history of premature birth. Diplegia may develop despite the lack of detectable lesions by ultrasonographic or computed tomographic scan in the newborn period. Alternatively, echogenic lesions detected by ultraso-

nography may disappear without development of diplegia. The first signs of nascent spastic diplegia in the neonate may include hypotonia or poor feeding. Not uncommonly, however, the onset of hypotonia is delayed until 2 to 3 months of age. Thereafter, the onset of hypertonia is often heralded by episodes of generalized increase in tone triggered by changes in the infant's posture. Other signs include increasing difficulty with diapering owing to progressive hip adductor spasticity and a pseudoprecocious ability to roll from supine to prone. The latter reflects increased truncal hypertonia or even frank opisthotonus such that the infant assumes excessive postural extension of the trunk and lower extremities. This hypertonic stage is followed by the development of frank spasticity. In a seated position, the posture is dominated by flexion of the knees and hips. A standing posture or vertical suspension triggers extension of the lower extremities with crossing of the legs (i.e., "scissoring"), inward rotation of the legs, and equinus posturing of the feet with plantar extension. These signs reflect the development of spasticity in the hip adductors, hamstrings, and heel cords.

Management of spasticity is directed toward the goal of achieving functional ambulation (Fig. 59–1). Independent ambulation is achieved in all but the most severe

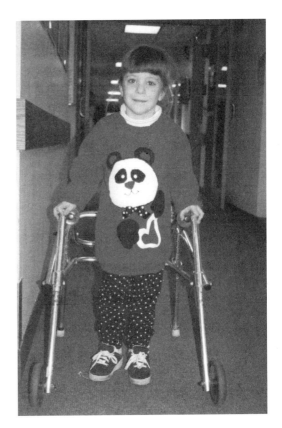

Figure 59–1. This 5-year-old girl has age-appropriate development with the exception of motor delay due to spastic diplegia acquired following complications related to premature birth at 27 weeks' gestation. As a neonate she had a ventricular peritoneal shunt placed for posthemorrhagic hydrocephalus, and her cranial MRI was consistent with bilateral periventricular leukomalacia. Although she ambulates independently with the aid of ankle-foot orthoses, her gait is labored and she uses a walker for long distances. She has reached the age at which she is under consideration for orthopedic surgery to improve her gait.

situations and is characterized by a flexed posture at the hips and knees while walking up on the toes with absence of consistent heel strike. The approach in infancy is initially conservative. A program of daily physical therapy is essential to prevent the development of joint deformity. Caregivers should be taught by their physical therapist a stretching program that can be incorporated several times a day into the infant's daily routine, such as when diapering or after the bath. Close developmental and orthopedic follow-up is important to monitor the success of the program. The high risk for occult femoral head subluxation should be addressed with regular hip radiographs. If spasticity progresses despite physical therapy, the antispasticity agents valium, baclofen, or dantrolene may be tried. Most children will be fitted with ankle-foot orthoses or night casts to oppose plantar flexion of the foot. Focal injections of botulinum A toxin into the gastrocnemius muscle will weaken these muscles for 3 to 6 months, thereby potentiating the success of physical therapy to strengthen the antagonist muscles. Surgical heel cord lengthening and hip adductor or hamstring releases are generally delayed until school age to avoid the need for early revision.

EXAMPLE

John is a handsome, articulate 10-year-old boy from an academic family who was born at term following a pregnancy notable for frequent episodes of threatened preterm labor during the third trimester. Despite repeated reassurances by his pediatrician that he would catch up, his mother remained concerned about floppiness in the first months of life. This progressed by 1 year of age to increasing stiffness in the lower extremities that made diapering difficult. John was slow to sit and was referred to a neurologist when he was not crawling or walking at 16 months. A diagnosis of spastic diplegia was made, and a cranial magnetic resonance image showed discrete foci of periventricular leukomalacia bilaterally with slightly enlarged ventricles. John began to commando crawl by 2 years of age and at 4 years was able to walk with long leg braces. Language was also delayed. At 2½ years, he had only three words and training in sign language was begun. A year later he was speaking in full sentences.

When we saw him at 8 years of age, he had not been seen by his orthopedist in over a year owing to relocation of his family. His mother felt that his walking, with the aid of ankle-foot orthoses, had worsened. Examination revealed weakness of the hip abductors, marked tightness of the hip flexors, hamstrings, and heel cords, and a crouched gait with poor endurance. Questioning revealed that although John was doing above average in school, he seemed troubled by his physical differences from his peers and had become more oppositional and less motivated in class. His mother started him on piano lessons in the hope that his self-esteem would improve. These he greatly enjoyed, but to the detriment of his CP condition. His mother admitted that in striving to increase her son's upper extremity accomplishments, she had largely neglected his daily physical therapy routine.

Intensive physical therapy was resumed to strengthen the hip girdle and stretch the hamstrings and heel cords. Improved ankle dorsiflexion was achieved with a trial of botulinum toxin to the gastrocnemius muscles followed by serial casting. Although John was able to walk 40 feet without assistance, his gait remained crouched. At 10 years of age, he underwent an iliopsoas tenotomy, tendon transfers, and hamstring and heel cord lengthening. Currently he walks with minimal assistance and enjoys swimming, piano playing, and horseback riding.

There are several patterns of deficits that may present in association with spastic motor deficits of the lower extremities. The upper extremities and face are often involved to variable degrees. Functional use of the hands is the rule, although rapid or alternating hand movements are commonly impaired. Speech and swallowing are often minimally affected and a horizontal smile may be the only sign of facial weakness. Epilepsy is uncommon with this form of CP and is generally easy to control when it occurs. Visual-spatial deficits may initially go undetected unless strabismus develops. These arise from injury to the periventricular white matter of the occipital hemispheres. Injury to the optic pathways may be detected early as visual field defects by confrontation testing or visual perimetry. Otherwise injury may not be recognized until school age, when visual-spatial deficits that affect hand-eye coordination, reading, and object-pattern recognition are detected.

The cognitive deficits associated with spastic diplegia often manifest during the school-age years. Although it has been widely held that the majority of children with diplegia develop normal or near-normal intelligence, it is now clear from numerous reports that careful psychometric testing reveals a variety of mild to moderate learning disabilities. These principally include deficits in mathematics and visual-spatial processing that affect reading and pattern recognition. The pathophysiologic basis for these learning disabilities is unclear given the lack of apparent cerebral cortical injury. It has been suggested that injury to subplate neurons may account for these deficits, since they are situated at the junction between the gray and white matter of the hemispheres (i.e, at sites of predilection for periventricular leukomalacia) and play a critical role in neuronal migration and the organization of neuronal circuitry (Volpe, 1996). Loss of these neurons might have wide-reaching impact on early brain development. This represents a critical area for future research to account for disabilities that affect up to half of the children with a history of premature birth.

A variety of psychosocial adaptations confront the child with diplegia. Some children achieve a wide variety of gross motor activities that they learn to do at their own pace. A significant challenge is coping with the pressure of family or peers, either real or perceived, that the child cannot keep up with play activities. The child may also feel pressured to develop "adaptive" skills not involving the legs to compensate for the shortcomings imposed by the diplegia. There may be considerable parental encouragement for the development of upper extremity skills such as playing a musical instrument or writing. Emphasis on these new endeavors may come at the expense of continuing physical therapy, however, with a resultant worsening in spasticity. Hence the clinician must work supportively to encourage the child and family to accept responsibility to integrate continued physical therapy into the daily routine without its becoming a troubling reminder to the child that he or she is different at a time when acceptance by the peer group becomes increasingly important.

DYSKINETIC (DYSTONIC OR ATHETOID) CEREBRAL PALSY

Dyskinetic CP arises when there is significant involvement of the extrapyramidal motor system. Injury to the basal ganglia and thalamus as a result of hypoxia-ischemia most commonly occurs in the full-term infant. The deep gray matter appears to be particularly vulnerable to energy failure as a result of sustained hypoxia-ischemia, because of high concentrations of excitatory amino acid receptors that are transiently expressed at term. The resulting injury to regions modulating control of movement of the face, neck, trunk, and limbs is variable, and disorders of tone, posture, and movement may all be superimposed. Dyskinetic CP is probably the most underrecognized or misdiagnosed form of CP, in part because spasticity may be readily confused with dystonia early in the course. However, it is important to make this distinction early, because the impact on motor development is quite different, as may be the approach to the treatment of spasticity or dystonia.

Diagnosis of dyskinetic CP can be aided by identification of one or more of the etiologic risk factors. With the advent of more sensitive modalities to image the brain, it has become increasingly apparent that persistent injury to the basal ganglia and thalamus predominates in many survivors of full-term perinatal asphyxia. Kernicterus was previously an important cause of dyskinetic CP in the full-term infant that manifested as the relentless slow writhing movements of choreoathetosis. The incidence of kernicterus in the full-term neonate has decreased dramatically due to heightened vigilance in the early detection and treatment of indirect hyperbilirubinemia. The onset of dyskinetic CP in an infant with a history of prematurity should continue to raise suspicion for kernicterus. The hypoxic premature infant is at increased risk to develop kernicterus, even at levels of indirect bilirubin that would not normally be toxic to the full-term infant. Finally, a severely debilitating and sometimes fatal form of dyskinesia may develop in some survivors of cardiac bypass surgery.

Early in infancy there may be no specific signs to point to a diagnosis of dyskinetic CP. Infants are usually alert and interactive and seizures are uncommon, consistent with the relative sparing of the cerebral cortex. Variable degrees of hypotonia and postural instability may be an early sign. The onset of abnormalities in muscle tone and adventitious movements begins insidiously around the latter half of the 1st year and may continue to progress throughout the 2nd year. The rapid increase in dyskinesia early in infancy should raise suspicion for an alternative diagnosis such as a neurodegenerative disorder or an inborn error of metabolism (see Table 59–2). An important manifestation of dsykinetic CP is fluctuations in tone that increase with dynamic motor activity. Hence the hands may be held open at rest but become fisted when motor activity is initiated. This is an important distinction from spasticity, in which fisting is persistent and is not affected by the level of motor activity. Similarly, later in childhood, extensor posturing of the foot (i.e., a dystonic foot) may be more prominent with walking and may be mistaken for spasticity. In general, dyskinetic rigidity or hypertonia is more prominent when awake and will diminish or disappear when the child is asleep. Another diagnostic clue is the presence of motor restlessness or akisthisia that manifests as intermittent or persistent movement of the head, neck, limbs, hands, or feet. Often caretakers may be aware of, but not mention, fine restless movements of the hands or feet and attribute them simply to the child's being very active. Other characteristic extrapyramidal signs include tongue thrusting, chewing movements, orofacial grimacing, and dystonic posturing of any part of the body (Fig. 59–2).

One of the more debilitating features of dyskinetic CP is marked hypotonia of the neck and trunk. The resultant limitations imposed on the child's exploration of the environment are considerable. Neck hypotonia is accompanied by maladaptive posturing of the head and neck. Good midline head support is therefore essential to prevent asymmetric dystonic posturing of the head that can trigger a

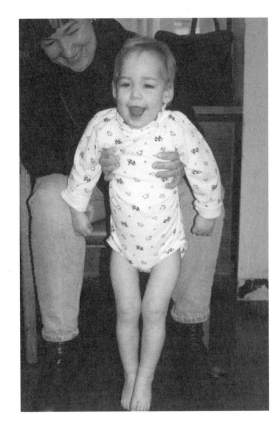

Figure 59–2. This 2-year-old girl is visually impaired, has a well-controlled seizure disorder, and has global developmental delay. She shows signs of mixed CP acquired following an intrauterine course complicated by twin-twin transfusion and threatened fetal hydrops. Her cranial MRI at 12 months old was consistent with bilateral periventricular leukomalacia and showed cortical white matter loss. The plantar hyperextension is a characteristic feature of the spastic motor weakness seen in this form of CP. The fisted hands and dystonic posturing of the face manifest when she is animated and are a sign of extrapyramidal motor system injury. She participates in an infant stimulation program where she receives physical, occupational, and speech therapy and also attends a school for children who are blind.

tonic neck reflex that misdirects visual gaze and impairs hand-eye coordination. Truncal hypotonia further restricts the child's interactions with the environment, and when it is severe, functional ambulation is often not possible because the combination of severe truncal hypotonia and dyskinesia prevents a stable standing position. For these children, a custom-designed wheelchair that provides good trunk and head control can allow the child multidirectional control of the chair through head movements. Medical management of the movement disorder in most children is difficult. Anticholinergic agents are the mainstay of treatment, but the response is often limited, and unsatisfactory side effects, particularly sedation, limit their usefulness. Other agents that are variably effective are benzodiazepines and baclofen.

Special attention should be directed in infancy to language and communication. Children with dyskinetic CP are often markedly impaired in their ability to articulate language, because of involvement of the musculature of the speech apparatus. Associated hearing loss may be contributory. Drooling can also be a major problem. Attempts at spoken language trigger facial grimacing and slow dystonic sounds, which, in combination with odd patterns of movement, give the child an unfortunately subnormal appearance. Careful testing, however, will often demonstrate that receptive language skills and intelligence approach normal in the majority of children. The frustration that these children experience because of their inability to communicate is considerable. If it becomes apparent that spoken language will be severely limited, efforts toward this end should be abandoned in favor of alternative means of communication. For some, sign language becomes an effective form of communication. For the most severely affected child, computer-driven language boards are a viable form of effective communication that can be tailored to individual needs. Visual disturbances that may impair symbolic recognition or reading should not be overlooked. Strabismus is the most common problem. The child with kernicterus may have a supranuclear gaze palsy presenting as impaired voluntary horizontal or vertical eye movements.

Throughout the school-age years and adolescence, family and teachers must continue to reassess the impact on these children of the disparity between the motor and cognitive potentials. The motor disability can be quite isolating and seriously erode the child's self-esteem. Special attention should be given to ensuring that the child meets his or her fullest cognitive potential. Social integration is important, including for those children with potential for advanced vocational or college education.

EXAMPLE

Michael is a 5-year-old boy with mixed CP whose birth at 41 weeks' gestation was complicated by fetal bradycardia, a tight nuchal cord, no spontaneous respirations at delivery, and seizures within the 1st hour of life. His motor development has been globally delayed from the first months of life. He cannot sit without support or pull to stand due to marked axial hypotonia. The use of his limbs is further limited by marked dystonic posturing that misdirects his limbs when he attempts to use them. He has a raking hand grasp and bilaterally adducted thumbs that prevent the effective use of a cup or utensils. He tries hard to communicate vocally by imitating facial expressions and mouth movements. However, marked oral-motor discoordination prevents him from articulating sounds and has also made eating a slow, laborious process. He is a bright and interactive child who delights in the company of others and clearly understands much spoken language. He correctly recognizes multiple shapes, numbers, letters, colors, and body parts.

Michael is a lovable child with an engaging smile and unflagging determination, who has stolen the hearts of the people in the small New England town where he lives. Both his parents and the town have worked hard through fundraisers and persistence with government agencies to obtain much of the costly equipment he needs to further his development. His daily life greatly improved after he received a custom-designed motorized wheelchair that he has learned to operate with movements of his head. He has also learned to direct a lamp on his head to point to objects that he wants. With the aid of a home computer, he is learning to communicate using language boards that speak for him. Currently, Michael tolerates, as well as any 5-year-old can, various interventions to relieve the spasticity in his limbs. He has undergone serial casting to maintain range of motion in his ankles. Physical therapy has become easier with injections of botulinum A toxin into the gastrocnemius muscles and into his adducted thumbs and injections of phenol into the hamstrings and hip adductors. He is attending a preschool 5 days a week where he enjoys the company of his classmates and receives physical, occupational, and speech therapy.

HEMIPLEGIC CEREBRAL PALSY

In hemiplegic CP, injury localizes predominantly to one cerebral hemisphere and results in unilateral spastic motor weakness. The distribution of injury is variable and may be cortical or subcortical depending on etiology. Hemiplegic CP arises from heterogeneous etiologies and encompasses both congenital and acquired conditions. It is thus not possible to generalize about outcome. Among the congenital group, the majority are full-term infants in whom cortical injury results from apparent prenatal factors, although identifiable etiologies, such as brain malformations, are in the minority. Among full-term infants, intrauterine vascular embolic catastrophes are commonly suspected on the basis of imaging findings that may demonstrate cystic encephalomalacia in the territory of the middle cerebral artery to be already present at the time of birth. Perinatal injury is uncommon and arises most commonly from intracerebral hemorrhage. Among preterm infants, unilateral periventricular leukomalacia, often in combination with a hemorrhagic venous infarction, is the typical pathologic entity. Acquired hemiplegic CP can arise from any of a wide variety of causes of stroke in childhood.

With hemiplegic CP, abnormal motor development is rarely suspected in the newborn, for whom a period of deceptive normality is usually present. Even in the presence of documented lesions, abnormalities are uncommonly detected until 4 to 5 months of age, at which time the infant's attempts at grasping always occur on the same side. The presence of an early hand preference, abnormal before about 18 months, is accompanied by an evolving picture of weakness on the affected side. Typical early features include distal upper extremity spasticity manifested as fisting and a delayed or absent pincer grasp. Later, the affected upper limb is held in abduction with flexion at the wrist and hyperextension of the fingers. In general, spasticity with contractures is the primary concern, whereas weakness is often relatively mild. Ultimately, decreased growth of the arm and hand (with smaller nail beds) is often seen on the affected side. Functional impairment of the hand ranges from mild to severe. When mild, a pincer grasp is possible, as are individual hand movements, whereas in more severe situations the hand may be nonfunctional.

Involvement of the lower extremity may not be appreciated until walking begins. In those of full-term birth, the lower limb is usually much less affected than the upper. By contrast, in those of preterm birth, the lower limb may be more involved, perhaps as a result of greater involvement of the periventricular lower extremity fibers due to hydrocephalus or leukomalacia. Overall, in up to half of children walking begins within the normative time, and, except for the most severely affected children, ambulation is always achieved. Facial weakness, when it occurs, is generally mild.

The likelihood of normal intelligence is quite variable and is correlated with the severity of the hemiplegia and the presence of epilepsy. Those with severe hemiplegia tend to have worse social and employment prospects, and mental retardation is likely to occur together with epilepsy in this group. Intellect may be further compromised by the potential sequelae that arise from severe epilepsy. In most cases, intractable epilepsy does not develop and seizures are readily controlled. Deficits in speech and language may occur with injury to either hemisphere and are also more prominent when the hemiplegia is severe.

QUADRIPLEGIC CEREBRAL PALSY

This pattern of motor impairment involves the head and neck as well as all four limbs. Although it is the most uncommon form of CP, it is the most severe and debilitating. The degree of cognitive impairment is variable and is influenced by the underlying pattern of brain injury. Spastic quadriplegia predominantly occurs in the full-term infant as a result of parasagittal cortical injury arising from complications of hypoxia-ischemia. A similar clinical presentation may arise, in addition, from a variety of prenatal or postnatal insults (see Table 59–1). Less commonly, the premature infant will present with significant involvement of the upper and lower extremities rather than the more common diplegic picture. These infants may have a relative preservation of cognition that reflects the primarily subcortical pattern of injury. In some cases of prematurity, an asymmetric pattern of weakness may be observed with, for example, greater involvement of the upper than lower extremities. In such atypical occasions in which a diagnosis of CP is called into question, a prolonged neonatal course with repeated bouts of hypoxia-ischemia may account for the unusual clinical presentation.

The clinical features in spastic quadriplegic CP in the full-term infant typically include some degree of mental retardation ranging from mild to severe that may be exacerbated by recurrent seizures. Motor impairment frequently is compounded by dystonic features secondary to injury to the basal ganglia or thalamus. Epilepsy can be of multiple types that include generalized tonic-clonic seizures, myoclonic seizures, infantile spasms, the Lennox-Gasteaux syndrome, and status epilepticus. The orthopedic complications of spastic quadriplegia include joint instability (e.g., femoral head subluxation and hip dislocation), joint contractures, and scoliosis. Pseudobulbar weakness of the facial and pharyngeal musculature is universal and may be accompanied by dysphagia, gastroesophageal reflux, recurrent aspiration pneumonia, and failure to thrive. A further complication of generalized spasticity is a paucity of lower extremity movement with resultant constipation or fecal impaction. In the most severe instances, these problems may be further compounded by cranial nerve palsies and bulbar paralysis. The failure to acquire complex speech or language is common and may be compounded by a variety of sensory impairments, including cortical blindness or sensorineural hearing loss.

The outlook for survival beyond the neonatal period is variable and is greatly influenced by the degree of systemic complications. Given the wide range of potential outcomes the clinician may need to anticipate and advocate for services including regular orthopedic attention to joint deformities, a custom-outfitted wheelchair, devices to assist with transfers, a communication enhancement program, or neurologic management of epilepsy and behavioral difficulties. For the less severely affected child, appropriate training should be arranged as early as possible to assist the child to reach the highest degree of functional independence and social adaptation. This includes education to attend to personal hygiene, physical transfers, and optimal communication skills. Early schooling will have the added benefit of improved self-esteem through regular social interactions with other children.

For the most severely affected children, total care is required throughout life. The considerable demands on the family to maintain round-the-clock supportive care at home are usually untenable without relief provided by skilled nursing care or outside assistance. These children optimally are followed by a multidisciplinary team that coordinates the services required to address their complications.

PROGNOSIS

Predicting long-term outcome remains a difficult problem for those caring for children with CP. There is clearly a tremendous range of potential developmental outcomes within any given subtype of CP. Although parents will likely ask for prognosis early on, it is appropriate to feel uncomfortable delivering even general prognostic statements such as "favorable," "guarded," "poor," or "devastating." It may be several years before the child's ultimate outlook becomes clear. During the clinical course, the team must take into account a variety of factors in assessing developmental prognosis. The clinical history and examination findings remain the most reliable factors in formulating a general sense for clinical outcome (Olsen et al, 1997).

Clearly, with significantly abnormal results of a neurologic examination accompanied by systemic complications, neonatal seizures (see Table 59–3), or abnormal cranial imaging findings, one can predict from the outset that a child is likely to have important problems. However, the scope of those problems is impossible to predict. It is thus often quite humbling for even the seasoned clinician to retrospectively compare the child's developmental gains with what parents will recount as the prognostic statements made in the first days of life. Moreover, the early findings for many children are not so straightforward. As a result there is an increasing reliance on neuroimaging to predict outcome. Not uncommonly, however, there is a disparity between serial cranial magnetic resonance imaging findings and the child's clinical course. In fact, one recent study found that long-term follow-up with cranial magnetic resonance imaging was no better than the clinical examination to predict learning problems at school age in a group of children with a history of premature birth and risk factors for periventricular leukomalacia (Olsen et al, 1997).

There are additional "intangible" factors that, from clinical experience, would appear to influence outcome. We have all encountered families in which the optimism or pessimism of parents and other caregivers shapes the attitude and will of the child to deal with his or her physical impairments. In our current climate of shrinking resources for children with disabilities, the parents play the central role in fighting for services and equipment that are essential to both minimize CP-related complications and optimize the child's developmental progress. Hence clinicians must follow more closely those children for whom parental denial of illness is likely to have a negative impact on development. Rejection of illness may be expressed, for example, as a parental perception that the child does not require daily physical therapy, thereby placing the child at risk for joint deformities and a decreased likelihood of ambulation.

The most elusive factor in the developmental "equation" is, of course, the child. That each child has a unique developmental potential in the presence of brain injury is supported by clinical experience as well as the wellspring of recent research in neurobiology. Injury to the developing nervous system occurs against the backdrop of a remarkably "plastic" nervous system, with varying individual potential to respond to injury through mechanisms of repair and reorganization. The timing of injury is just one factor of critical importance in determining the impact of a given pattern of injury on future motor and cognitive development. Clearly the complexity of these factors ultimately makes predictions of prognosis unreliable except in the most severe cases of brain injury and underscores the importance of close developmental follow-up to reassess with each visit the adequacy of the therapeutic plan to meet the evolving needs of the child.

REFERENCES

Abbot R: Sensory rhizotomy for the treatment of childhood spasticity. J Child Neurol 11(Suppl 1):S36, 1996.

Albright A: Baclofen in cerebral palsy. J Child Neurol 11:77, 1996.

Barry MJ: Physical therapy interventions for patients with movement disorders due to cerebral palsy. J Child Neurol 11(Suppl 1):S51, 1996.

Bleck E: Orthopedic Management in Cerebral Palsy. Philadelphia, JB Lippincott, 1987.

Blum RW, Resnick M, Nelson R, St Germaine A: Family and peer issues among adolescents with spina bifida and cerebral palsy. Pediatrics 88:280, 1991.

Dammann O, Leviton A: The role of perinatal brain damage in developmental disabilities: an epidemiologic perspective. MRDD Res Rev 3:13, 1997.

DeLuca PA: The musculoskeletal management of children with cerebral palsy. Ped Clin North Am 43(5):1135, 1996.

Dormans J: Orthopedic management of children with cerebral palsy. Ped Clin North Am 40:645, 1993.

du Plessis A: Cardiac surgery in the young infant: an in vivo model for the study of hypoxic-ischemic brain injury. MRDD Res Rev 3:49, 1997.

Koman L, Mooney J, Smith B: Neuromuscular blockade in the management of cerebral palsy. J Child Neurol 11(Suppl 1): S23, 1996.

Miller F, Bachrach S: Cerebral Palsy: A Complete Guide for Caregivers. Baltimore, Johns Hopkins University Press, 1995.

Olsen P, Vainionpaa E, Pyhtinen J, Jarvelin M-R: Magnetic resonance imaging of periventricular leukomalacia and its clinical correlation in children. Ann Neurol 41:754, 1997.

Pranzatelli M: Oral pharmacotherapy for the movement disorders of cerebral palsy. J Child Neurol 11(Suppl 1): S13, 1996.

Roland E, Hill A: How important is perinatal asphyxia in the causation of brain injury? MRDD Res Rev 3:22, 1997.

Volpe JJ: Brain injury in the premature infant: neuropathology, clinical aspects and pathogenesis. MRDD Res Rev 3:3, 1997.

Volpe JJ: Subplate neurons: Missing link in brain injury of the premature infant? Pediatrics 97:112, 1996.

Volpe JJ: Neurology of the Newborn. Philadelphia, WB Saunders, 1995.

60 Autism and Related Disorders

Stuart W. Teplin

There is increasing evidence for the role of genetic factors in the etiology of autism, although no single mode of inheritance or gene abnormality accounts for the diverse spectrum of autistic disorders.

Contrary to "dogma" about children with autism, very few of them are so socially isolated that they fail to interact with a loved family member.

The use of various forms of consistent positive and negative reinforcements has long been a mainstay of intervention for children with autism.

In contrast to more dismal outcome reports prior to 20 years ago, reviews from the past 10 years have documented greater percentages of individuals with autism going on to "good" outcomes.

Autism describes a spectrum of clinical conditions of neurobiological origin that are characterized by (1) qualitative dysfunctions of social interaction, (2) qualitative impairments in communication abilities, and (3) unusual or restricted ranges of play and interests. The totality of these impairments, though quite variable from person to person, is usually a lifelong condition that results in some degree of social isolation and varying amounts of unusual behavior. The current American definition of autism (Table 60–1) rests on three main clinical pillars; however, it is now viewed as one subcategory under the broader diagnostic umbrella known as *pervasive developmental disorders* (PDD) (Table 60–2).

The current definitions are the latest in a series that has evolved over the last half-century. As with many other developmental disabilities, we are still early in the process of understanding the underlying core dysfunctions and their neuroanatomic and neurochemical bases.

Historical Overview

In 1943, Leo Kanner first described 11 children with what he called "infantile autism," a constellation of behavioral symptoms that distinguished this from other psychiatric conditions of childhood. Although our current understanding of autism has undergone changes, those original descriptions still capture key clinical elements. These in-

Table 60–1 • Diagnostic Criteria for Autistic Disorder

A. A total of six (or more) items from (1), (2), and (3), with at least two from (1), and one each from (2) and (3):
  1. Qualitative impairment in social interaction, as manifested by at least two of the following:
    a. Marked impairment in the use of multiple nonverbal behaviors such as eye-to-eye gaze, facial expression, body postures, and gestures to regulate social interaction
    b. Failure to develop peer relationships appropriate to developmental level
    c. A lack of spontaneous seeking to share enjoyment, interests, or achievements with other people (e.g., by a lack of showing, bringing, or pointing out objects of interest)
    d. Lack of social or emotional reciprocity
  2. Qualitative impairments in communication as manifested by at least one of the following:
    a. Delay in, or total lack of, the development of spoken language (not accompanied by an attempt to compensate through alternative modes of communication such as gesture or mime)
    b. In individuals with adequate speech, marked impairment in the ability to initiate or sustain a conversation with others
    c. Stereotyped and repetitive use of language or idiosyncratic language
    d. Lack of varied, spontaneous make-believe play or social imitative play appropriate to developmental level
  3. Restricted repetitive and stereotyped patterns of behavior, interests, and activities, as manifested by at least one of the following:
    a. Encompassing preoccupation with one or more stereotyped and restricted patterns of interest that is abnormal either in intensity or focus
    b. Apparently inflexible adherence to specific, nonfunctional routines or rituals
    c. Stereotyped and repetitive motor mannerisms (e.g., hand or finger flapping or twisting, or complex whole-body movements)
    d. Persistent preoccupation with parts of objects
B. Delays or abnormal functioning in at least one of the following areas, with onset prior to age 3 years: (1) social interaction, (2) language as used in social communication, or (3) symbolic or imaginative play.
C. The disturbance is not better accounted for by Rett's Disorder or Childhood Disintegrative Disorder.

From American Psychiatric Association: Diagnostic and Statistical Manual of Mental Disorders, 4th ed. Washington, DC, American Psychiatric Association, 1994.

cluded onset during infancy; delayed acquisition of language that, when present, was often unusual, echolalic, and noncommunicative; significant difficulties in establishing reciprocal relationships with others; a tendency to engage in repetitive, stereotyped, nonimaginative play; and an apparent "need for sameness." These children had no dysmorphic features and tended to have excellent rote memory.

During subsequent decades, various authors emphasized different aspects of Kanner's original description. These observations helped to clarify distinctions between autism and superficially similar conditions, including mental retardation, schizophrenia, and language disorders. Initial theories espousing environmental or psychosocial causation were eventually abandoned in light of overwhelming evidence of the neurologic basis of the condition. Since 1980, the task of revising the American definition of autism has been assumed by the American Psychiatric Association, as documented in their periodically updated *Diagnostic and Statistical Manual of Mental Disorders*, most recently in its fourth edition, *DSM-IV* (American Psychiatric Association, 1994). Classification remains a controversial area, and varying terminology in the clinical and research fields reflects current professional confusion regarding the core concepts of autism.

Epidemiology

PREVALENCE

In contrast to earlier prevalence estimates of 4 to 5 per 10,000, recent epidemiologic studies, utilizing more inclusive definitions of autism, suggest a prevalence rate of 10 to 20 per 10,000 (Gillberg, Steffenburg, and Schaumann, 1991). There is no predilection for any particular social strata. The prevalence appears to have increased during the past decade, perhaps due to (1) greater awareness about autism and its symptoms, (2) more-inclusive recent definitions, and (3) possibly a true increase in incidence. Overall, the ratio of males to females is about 3:1 to 4:1. Among those individuals with the most severe levels of associated mental retardation, however, the sex ratio is closer to equal; as a group, females with autism tend to have a higher rate of mental retardation and associated neurologic disorders (Ritvo, Freeman, and Pingree, 1989).

GENETIC FACTORS

There is increasing evidence for the role of genetic factors in the etiology of autism, although no single mode of

Table 60–2 • Subcategories of Pervasive Developmental Disorder

Autistic disorder
Rett disorder
Childhood disintegrative disorder
Asperger disorder
Pervasive developmental disorder not otherwise specified (including atypical autism)

From American Psychiatric Association: Diagnostic and Statistical Manual of Mental Disorders, 4th ed. Washington, DC, American Psychiatric Association, 1994.

inheritance or gene abnormality accounts for the diverse spectrum of autistic disorders. Apart from the autism sometimes associated with specific syndromes of known genetic origin (e.g., fragile X syndrome, tuberous sclerosis), the empiric recurrence risk for autism in a family with one autistic child ranges from 2% to 8.6% (Smalley and Collins, 1996). A subgroup of autistic spectrum disorders is closely linked to positive family histories for major affective disorders, particularly bipolar disease.

OTHER BIOLOGICAL FACTORS

Whether adverse obstetric and perinatal factors such as maternal age and parity, obstetric instrumentation, birth weight, gestational age, and previous fetal loss are associated with later development of autistic disorders remains a matter of speculation (Nelson, 1991). The fact that the concordance rate for autism between monozygotic twins is not 100% suggests that at least some, as yet unknown, intrauterine environmental factors play an etiologic role.

Diagnostic Criteria

Generating a rational taxonomy to describe the highly heterogeneous group of individuals who have autistic and "autistic-like" features has continued to be a vital and controversial effort. Following extensive field-testing, recently revised criteria were published in 1994 as the *DSM-IV* (American Psychiatric Association, 1994) and were purposely written to coincide with the latest *International Classification of Disease*, 10th edition (the *ICD-10*) (World Health Organization, 1992). The *DSM-IV* modifications of the concept of PDD include elevation of PDD to an umbrella category that encompasses autism and other nonautistic conditions (see Table 60–2), restricting the criteria for diagnosing autism, and increasing the age by which symptoms must occur to 3 years.

Table 60–3 summarizes examples of behaviors within each of the three primary domains that make up the current definition.

LANGUAGE DEFICITS

Although language dysfunction is one of the core deficits in autism, the wide variability in severity and quality of these deficits reflects the marked heterogeneity of children within the autistic spectrum. For those who are the most severely involved (roughly half of children with autism), verbal language never develops (Coleman, 1989). At the other end of the spectrum, the child may be able to speak very coherently and meaningfully, with only the most subtle deviations of social or prosodic nuances reflecting the underlying autistic disorder (see Table 60–3). In children with autism, receptive language is as delayed or even more delayed than expressive language. This pattern differs from the more typical reverse pattern seen in children with mental retardation who do not have autism, who can understand language at a higher level than they are able to express it. This finding is partly a function of the way that language is typically assessed, particularly in young children. The relatively high scores in expressive language

Table 60–3 • Main Characteristics and Examples of Autistic Behaviors

Impaired Social Interaction	Verbal and Nonverbal Communication Dysfunction	Restricted, Repetitive Interests & Behaviors
Poor eye contact Little or no interest in establishing friendships Difficulty with reciprocal social interaction Limitations in emotional empathy	Diminished or absent verbal expression or gestures and poor comprehension of other's speech and body language Impaired "pragmatics" of initiating/sustaining conversation Stereotyped, "robotic," or idiosyncratic speech Echolalia and rote imitation of words or dialogue Unusual prosody of speech (sing-song, monotone)	Perseveration or preoccupation with certain topics; restricted interests (e.g., weather, schedules) Preference for routines; need for sameness Over-focus on parts of toys, rather than usual function of toy Difficulty with transitions Stereotypic behaviors (e.g., hand flapping)

can be a diagnostically misleading consequence of the child's excellent rote memory and echolalic expression of previously heard speech. Parents of verbal children with autism are often initially surprised to be informed that their child has language difficulties. In fact, they are often quick to point out the child's excellent memory and speech but may be unaware of the less apparent deficits in the child's understanding of what he or she is hearing and use of language in socially appropriate ways (the pragmatics of language). Some more capable individuals with autism do communicate and have relatively normal understanding and use of the phonologic aspects, syntax (grammar), and some aspects of the semantics (meaning) of language. However, their language deficits are marked by difficulty gauging their listener's perspective, realizing meaningful implications of what is said, using language toward social goals, and understanding and conveying shades of meaning through speech prosody (stress, pitch, and intonation in voice quality). One example of this is the difficulty that children with autism who are verbal have in appreciating and appropriately using humor, which often relies on an understanding of social contexts and verbal ambiguities.

SOCIAL DEFICITS

Dysfunctions in a variety of social and interactional skills are a hallmark of autism. When questioned carefully, parents may recall that their child showed signs as early as infancy. The young child may be described as "preferring to play alone," making little or no eye contact with other people, appearing to be deaf when his or her name is called, or lacking in empathy for another person's emotional perspective, such as another's pain.

Other social deficits in children with autism are a lack of joint attention, an apparent disinterest in imitating others, and an evident failure to acquire the normally automatic skill of "reading" nonverbal emotional cues, particularly others' hand gestures and facial expressions. Joint attention is a normal, spontaneously occurring behavior in which an infant or toddler (as young as 6 to 8 months) tries to share interest, amusement, or apprehension about an object by purposefully looking back and forth between the object of interest and the eyes of a nearby caretaker or playmate. Such behavior seems to imply a fundamental realization that the other person's perspective or attention

is important and desirable. Lack or marked infrequency of joint attention is a characteristic of young children with autism. Consider, for example, an adult and child engaged in a bubble-blowing activity. If an adult is blowing bubbles with a child who is nondisabled or mentally retarded and nonautistic, the child will spontaneously look back and forth between the bubbles and the eyes of the adult in glee or anticipation of the next bubble barrage. A child with autism might also enjoy this activity but would be much more likely to focus visually on the bubbles, perhaps fleetingly looking at the adult's mouth as the "cause" of the bubbles, but with little or no reference to sharing the fun with the partner.

Contrary to "dogma" about children with autism, however, very few of them are so socially isolated "in their own world" that they fail to interact with a loved family member. Over many months and years, some parents unconsciously adapt to their child's unusual style of showing or accepting affection, not realizing how different this can be from that expressed by peers who are not autistic. There is increasing evidence, however, that even more children who are severely autistic can show definite signs of attachment, secure relationships, and comfort with familiar people. Such behaviors might include crying upon separation from the mother or proximity-seeking toward the parent upon reunion. What is important to determine is the extent to which that activity was initiated and structured by the adult. For the child who is autistic, purposeful social interaction, other than for specific "needs" (e.g., bringing an adult's hand to a container that the child wants to have opened), is usually muted or fleeting. And without the emerging sense of the other's perspective, these children fail to form the typical basis for generalization of normal social relationships with others (Sigman and Capps, 1997).

RESTRICTED INTERESTS AND BEHAVIORAL PROFILE

All children within the autistic spectrum show one or more behaviors or interests that are unusual and often repetitive. These often take the form of stereotypic movement rituals, unusual perceptual routines, or perseverative preoccupations with certain ideas or objects.

The motor stereotypies appear to be self-stimulating and are often manifest at times of increased arousal, such as intense interest, excitement, or anxiety over something occurring in the immediate environment. For some children, particularly those with more cognitive disability, these may also take the form of self-injurious behaviors. Head banging, face or body slapping, self-pinching, and self-biting are examples. Other stereotypic behaviors center around peculiar sensory or perceptual arousal. Some children may tend to visually inspect objects out of the corner of their eye (using peripheral rather than central vision), such as holding a toy up to the side of their face to examine it. Other unusual visual phenomena include preoccupation with edges of objects, spinning objects (e.g., fans, wheels of toy cars), shiny surfaces (e.g., windows, mirrors, chrome fenders), or particular shapes. One young child insisted on holding the same type of object in each hand, such as a triangular block. He got very upset if he could find only one of the pair. Other unusual sensory behaviors include auditory responses, such as appearing to be deaf at times, while tuning in to more distant or irrelevant sounds at other times. Sniffing objects, refusing to eat foods with certain tastes or textures, screaming whenever shirt tags are touching the back, and compulsive touching of certain textures are other commonly noted sensory rituals.

For children who are older or cognitively more able, the preoccupations are often less motoric and more symbolic. These include fascination with numbers, letters, license plates, train schedules, weather patterns, or subtypes of any classification (e.g., dinosaurs, cars, dogs). Hyperlexia, a type of learning style characterized by apparently advanced reading skills, is sometimes seen in children with autism, even during the preschool years. Although this skill initially amazes and delights parents, the reading is usually very concrete, with minimal understanding of the purpose of reading or the ability to comprehend the written words at the same level. One young child's father expressed amazement that he and his 5-year-old son could play chess together. Upon further questioning by the clinician, however, his father acknowledged that their chess "games" were re-enactments of specific chess moves on specific pages of a certain chess book that his son had rotely memorized. The child had little awareness of the way that chess pieces are moved and in fact did not understand that the "game" involves "winning" or "losing." He would become very upset if someone tried to play a "regular" game of chess with him or with his father.

Further behavioral difficulties often arise from the typical resistance to change and apparent need for sameness that characterizes most individuals with autism. Transitions between activities may present problems for the toddler and preschooler. "Needing" to always eat the bread *before* the salad and "insisting" on driving the same route to school are examples. This lack of flexibility is one of the most troubling features of autism in adolescents and adults. At times it may be difficult to differentiate these rigidities from more classic obsessions or compulsions. In individuals without autism, however, the latter symptoms are felt as intrusive and distressing.

One important "window" through which clinicians can observe the core autistic features of a child is how the child spontaneously plays, both with objects and with other people. Instead of inventing a story of a truck delivering supplies to another location (complete with engine and brake sound effects), the child with autism is more likely to repeatedly move the truck back and forth on the floor in silence, perhaps looking at it out of the corner of his eye, or becoming fascinated with spinning the truck's wheel. For an older and higher-functioning child with autism, pretend play may, on the surface, appear to be quite complex and imaginative. However, further inquiry of the caretaker may reveal that this same scenario and dialogue is played out over and over again in a rote fashion, often accompanied by echolalic imitation of dialogue from a favorite video or TV show.

Associated Findings

A number of associated clinical features of autism are quite variable in their frequency and intensity. They are not essential criteria for the diagnosis, yet their presence often lends further credence to assigning such a label.

"SAVANT" SKILLS

Splinter skills in a person with autism are sometimes mistaken for evidence of high intelligence but represent only excellent rote skills or highly specialized nonverbal talent within a very restricted range of interests. They are particularly striking when compared to the individual's otherwise limited abilities to apply these skills to meeting real-life challenges. For example, the character Raymond, an autistic savant in the 1988 film *Rain Man*, displayed an uncanny ability to perform complex calculations in his head (predicting accurately what day of the week any date in the past or future would fall on), yet he could not figure out how to pay for a meal in a restaurant. Some parents (and professionals) mistakenly assume that individuals with autism have such "hidden intelligence." Other "savant" abilities include hyperlexia and unusual talent in music or art.

SEIZURES

The discovery of the higher incidence of seizures in populations of persons with autism was one of the first clues that autism is, in fact, a biological disorder rather than a primarily emotional or "psychological" one. Approximately one third of children within the autistic spectrum develop a seizure disorder (Tuchman, Rapin, and Shinmar, 1991a, 1991b). Seizures are more likely to emerge during infancy or adolescence.

MENTAL RETARDATION

Approximately 75% of individuals with autism are also mentally retarded. In young children, it is sometimes difficult to differentiate which aspects of behavior are truly autistic and which are a function of the child's mental retardation. The level of mental retardation often determines, to a large extent, the ultimate severity of the individual's ability to adapt and function relatively independently as an adult.

SENSORY AND PERCEPTUAL PROBLEMS

Hearing. As noted earlier, for many parents of children with autism, one of the first concerns they raise with the child's primary care physician is a suspicion that the child might be deaf. Sometimes the same child seems hypersensitive to certain types or frequencies of sounds (e.g., distant fire engines or thunderstorms) yet strangely unresponsive to nearby or loud noises that would ordinarily startle other children.

Vision. Reduced eye contact with people and unusual side-glancing at objects of interest have already been mentioned. In addition, some children with autism show extreme interest in the visual qualities of objects, such as certain colors or sizes of objects. They might become remarkably adept at matching visually similar objects or demonstrate uncanny memory for the location or direction of places.

Touch. Strong preference or aversions for certain textures may be noted and may change over time. Light touch may be experienced as strongly painful, whereas deep pressure has been described by verbal individuals with autism as providing a calming feeling. Many parents comment that their child who has autism seems to be indifferent to pain.

Smell and Taste. Parents often worry about the insistence of their child who has autism on eating only certain foods. At times, such perseverations seem to grow, with increasingly limited repertoires of tolerated foods. An unusual preoccupation with sniffing or licking nonfood objects (e.g., licking mirrors, sniffing other people, pica) may occur.

SELF-INJURIOUS BEHAVIOR

Self-injurious behavior can be one of the most difficult symptoms for parents to endure. Some view this as an extension of self-stimulatory behaviors such as hand flapping, spinning, or finger flicking. Most commonly, the behavior includes the child's biting his wrists or hands, banging his head, picking at his skin, or hitting his face with his open hand or fist. The trigger for such behavior may be predictable, such as frustration or anxiety, or it may remain unknown and seemingly random.

OTHER

To a variable extent in any individual or sample of children or adolescents who have autism, other comorbid behavior problems may be present. These include anxious behavior, labile affect, attention deficits, and aggressive behavior.

Associated Medical Conditions

An ever-enlarging list of medical conditions in which a subgroup has autistic features highlights the importance of the medical work-up as part of the diagnostic evaluation of any individual with autism. Although only 5% to 20% of children with a particular condition (e.g., fragile X syndrome, phenylketonuria, or tuberous sclerosis) may have autistic elements, together these account for a small but significant subgroup among all children with autism. Table 60–4 lists examples of these medical conditions. In some regards, it can be considered that these disorders produce a phenocopy of autism.

Clinical history and findings consistent with the autistic spectrum should prompt the clinician to consider the possibility that the autistic features are symptoms of one of these potentially diagnosable conditions.

Searching for the "Core" of Autism

Investigators from a diverse array of scientific disciplines are vigorously pursuing the fundamental question as to what the underlying core deficit is in autism. From a histoanatomic standpoint, interesting leads have emerged regarding abnormal cell size and distribution in the circuits of the limbic system and cerebellum. Positron emission tomography studies have shown evidence of disruptions in the connections between cortical and subcortical structures. Hypotheses regarding abnormal synapse pruning and growth are currently under investigation. Neuropharmacology, molecular genetics, and neurochemistry are all fields in which active research is ongoing. Neurophysiologic studies have suggested abnormal hemispheric lateralization during linguistic tasks.

Other interesting hypotheses in the neuropsychological domain are also being explored. Prominent among these are abnormalities in "theory of mind" (being able to think about thinking); underdevelopment of "eye-direction detectors," which disrupts attention and understanding of others' intentions; and primary deficits in the ability to plan ("executive dysfunction"). Another theory points to abnormal

Table 60–4 • Medical Conditions Sometimes Associated With the Presence of Autistic Features

Chromosomal and single gene abnormalities
Fragile X syndrome (q27)
Other X chromosome abnormalities
Down syndrome
Prader-Willi syndrome
Williams syndrome
Duchenne muscular dystrophy
Neurocutaneous disorders
Tuberous sclerosis
Neurofibromatosis
Hypomelanosis of Ito
Inborn errors of metabolism
Phenylketonuria
Lesch-Nyhan syndrome
Infections
Congenital rubella
Congenital cytomegalovirus
Postnatal herpes simplex
Perinatal disorders
Hypoxic encephalopathy
Prematurity
Other disorders
de Lange syndrome
Leber amaurosis
Rett syndrome
Moebius syndrome
Tourette syndrome

coordination between affective and cognitive processing (Sigman and Capps, 1997). Eventually there may be convergence of all these fields as our understanding of autism unfolds.

Differential Diagnosis

OTHER PERVASIVE DEVELOPMENTAL DISORDERS AND THE AUTISTIC SPECTRUM

In contrast to the *DSM* system of classification, some experts advocate an alternative system that puts less emphasis on divisions between what they view as somewhat artificially rigid categories, particularly in the distinctions between the more capable levels of autism, Asperger syndrome, and not-otherwise-specified PDD (PDD-NOS). Instead they propose to view the conditions seen as parts of an autistic spectrum, with ill-defined boundaries between varying levels of involvement. Figure 60–1 is one researcher's interpretation of the ways that various PDDs and language disorders may have overlapping boundaries.

This remains a controversial area (Frith, 1991) that continuing research should help to clarify. Wing (1997) has proposed a classification system relying more on the notion of a "spectrum" than the *DSM* system does. She also suggests a different type of classification based on social interaction styles. The three subgroups are (1) the Aloof group, (2) the Passive group, and (3) the Active-but-Odd group (Wing, 1997). Definitions in future editions of the *DSM* will no doubt evolve as debate on this important issue comes to some resolutions. In the meantime, clinicians must try to use the present *DSM* system, although phrases such as "marked impairment," "social interac-tion," and "abnormal in intensity" remain ambiguously subject to variations in interpretation.

ASPERGER SYNDROME

In 1944, the year after Kanner's classic description of children with "infantile autism," Hans Asperger, an Austrian pediatrician, published a paper depicting a group of children with some features overlapping those described by Kanner, yet differing in a number of important ways. It was not until the early 1980s, however, that Asperger's ideas were brought to wider public attention and further described by Wing (1981).

Like children with classic autism and other PDDs, those with Asperger syndrome also have qualitative deficits in verbal and nonverbal communication, social interaction, and imaginative and play activities. Children with Asperger syndrome, however, tend to have much better facility with the mechanics of verbal expression, are without mental retardation, and have a greater interest in interpersonal social activity, although they are driven to pursue this activity almost solely around their current obsessive, often bizzare, preoccupation. Their verbal skills lack the deviancy noted in classically autistic children (e.g., they usually do not have trouble with pronoun reversals or echolalia), although their language pragmatics (initiating and maintaing conversations, recognizing and helping to "repair" communicative breakdowns) are deficient, often interfering with the establishment of successful social interactions. Children with Asperger syndrome engage much more frequently in imaginative or pretend play than children with classic autism and generally show less perseveration with physical aspects of objects such as spinning wheels or strings. However, as noted, their obsessive fascination with certain themes dominates their play, resulting in perseverative repetitions of the same litany of facts or memorized script of a favorite TV program or movie. Unlike other children in the autistic spectrum, these children rarely have a clear-cut history of altered social interactions as young children. Parents do not typically report early problems with eye contact, affection, or joint attention. As they enter preschool and school, however, their social interactions become strained by their apparent aloofness and difficulty in fitting in with others. They seem to want this contact, but they lack the social skills to achieve it easily.

Despite the apparent clarity of the most recent revisions of diagnostic terminology *(DSM-IV)*, controversy remains around the theoretical and practical issues of whether Asperger syndrome is a distinct entity or simply the highest end of the autistic spectrum, just beyond "high-functioning" autism and perhaps shading into "normal but shy/eccentric."

> Kanner's cases are so well known that they will always remain prototypes for new similar cases. Children who do not talk or who parrot speech and use strange idiosyncratic phrases, who line up toys in long rows, who are oblivious to other people, who remember meaningless facts—these will rightly conjure up Leo Kanner's memory. Children and adults who are socially inept but often socially interested, who are articulate yet strangely ineloquent, who are gauche and impractical, who are specialists in unusual fields—these will always evoke Hans Asperger's name (Frith, 1991).

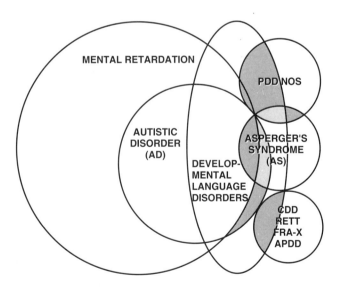

Figure 60–1. A theoretical representation of various autistic spectrum disorders and related developmental disorders. APDD = atypical pervasive developmental disorders; CDD = childhood disintegrative disorder; FRA-X = fragile X syndrome; PDD NOS = pervasive developmental disorders, not otherwise specified. (From Siegel B: The World of the Autistic Child: Understanding and Treating Autistic Spectrum Disorders. New York, Oxford University Press, 1996, p 11. Copyright © 1996 by Oxford University Press, Inc. Used by permission of Oxford University Press, Inc.)

RETT SYNDROME

Rett syndrome is a neurologic disorder of girls, characterized by early normal development and head growth, followed, between 6 and 48 months, by regression in language and social function, loss of previously acquired hand function (associated often with stereotypies involving the hands, such as perseverative hand wringing), and deceleration of head circumference growth leading to microcephaly. Progressive spasticity and severe to profound mental retardation are typical long-term sequelae.

CHILDHOOD DISINTEGRATIVE DISORDER (CDD)

Unlike most children with the form of autism characterized by early normal development, children with childhood disintegrative disorder are usually speaking in full phrases and often in sentences prior to the loss of language, which heralds their neurologic deterioration. This normal phase may last from 2 to 10 years, but usually the disintegration in function occurs by 5 years of age.

NOT-OTHERWISE-SPECIFIED PERVASIVE DEVELOPMENTAL DISORDER

The clinician is often faced with a child or adolescent whose behavioral idiosyncrasies, language quirks, and odd ways of relating to others emerged during the early years and are reminiscent of those seen in autism, yet are qualitatively or quantitatively insufficient to meet the *DSM-IV* criteria for autistic disorder or any of the other specific PDD subcategories listed in Tables 60–1 and 60–2. Such children may be described as having PDD-NOS. Unlike the other subcategories, this is more a diagnosis of exclusion of the better-defined conditions. From a clinical standpoint, this terminology is ambiguous and its borders are "fuzzy," intentionally allowing a broad spectrum of behaviors. Perhaps as the task of subtyping these behaviors progresses, more specific syndromes will be carved out, just as Asperger and Rett syndromes were when *DSM-III* gave way to *DSM-IV*. The science of this nomenclature is too preliminary to clarify with certainty the border between behavior that is simply an "odd" or "eccentric" variation of normal, as distinct from a very mild or "borderline" form of autism.

Further problems of nomenclature arise as professionals from related disciplines also attempt to develop their own classifications of disorders. Thus, for example, the same child who might be legitimately described by a physician as having "PDD-NOS" could also understandably be found to have a "semantic-pragmatic" language disorder by a speech and language pathologist or perhaps Asperger syndrome by a psychiatrist. Another clinical situation for which the PDD-NOS designation might be appropriate is the child whose behaviors are typical of one of the PDD conditions except for a failure to meet the age-of-onset criterion, that is, the symptoms did not become apparent until after the first 3 years of life (but are not severe enough to qualify as childhood disintegrative disorder).

Sometimes the PDD-NOS diagnosis provides a convenient but temporary way of asserting that a child's social and behavioral atypicalities are of concern and need to be monitored, pending collection of further evidence to support a more specific type of PDD classification (Towbin, 1997).

Some conditions currently outside the PDD spectrum, characterized by disturbances in reciprocal social interactions, also border on the PDD-NOS designation and are often difficult to diagnose with certainty. These include developmental language disorder, semantic-pragmatic disorder, reactive attachment disorder, schizotypal disorder, and avoidant disorder.

Mental Retardation

Since the majority of children who are autistic are also mentally retarded, there is certainly a great deal of overlap between these two clinical entities. Some clinical conditions commonly associated with mental retardation, such as Down syndrome, may occasionally also be associated with autism. For children and adolescents without autism who are severely or profoundly mentally retarded, some autistic-like behaviors, such as stereotypic hand movements, body rocking, or occasional self-injurious behaviors, may be present. However, the differentiation from autism is the fact that these individuals' social responsiveness and communication efforts are generally appropriate for their developmental level.

Obsessive-Compulsive Disorder

Obvious similarities exist between the obsessive thoughts and compulsive, repetitive actions characteristic of obsessive-compulsive disorder and the preoccupations and stereotypic behaviors prominent in the autistic spectrum disorder. Particularly for individuals at the capable end of autistic functioning and those with Asperger syndrome, the overlap can make the distinctions quite difficult. To the extent that it can be determined, individuals with obsessive-compulsive disorder find their symptoms to be distressing and wish they did not "have" to carry them out; that is, they are "ego-dystonic." This contrasts with most individuals within the autistic spectrum, who, even when their cognitive abilities are high enough to allow them awareness of their differences, do not appear to want to change their own odd preoccupations or repetitive mannerisms. Unfortunately, for individuals who are nonverbal or mentally retarded, making these distinctions is difficult.

Sensory Impairments

Children with hearing impairment may show somewhat similar "unresponsiveness" to that of autism, and one study found that in one third of the children who were diagnosed as autistic, parents had expressed concern about their child's hearing. In general, however, children who are not autistic but have hearing impairments have excellent eye contact and facial expressions, indicative of their intent to communicate (i.e., using their available sensory abilities to "connect" with the environment). Of course it is also possible for a child to have multiple disabilities, including the combination of hearing impairment and autism, each exacerbating the effects of the other.

In children with known visual impairments, particularly those that are more severe, self-stimulatory behaviors are sometimes noted, such as body rocking, eye pressing, and flicking fingers in front of bright lights. These may appear to be typical autistic-like behaviors but should not be considered such unless other evidence about the child's cognitive, social, and language functions also point in that direction. Once again, it is possible for a child to be both visually impaired and autistic. Sometimes what a parent attributes to the child's visual problem is actually more a function of autism. Some eye conditions may be more frequently associated with autism. These include cortical visual impairment, retinopathy of prematurity, Leber amaurosis, and rubella encepalopathy.

Language Disorders

Certain children with severe developmental language disorders can appear to be very similar to children within the autistic spectrum, particularly if their long-standing language deficits have secondarily interrupted their social relationships. The major distinction for clinicians to make, however, is whether the individual has the *desire and intent* to communicate (including use of body language, gesture, and facial expression), whether he or she can establish and maintain social relationships, and whether he or she demonstrates other evidences of imaginative play (e.g., elaborate representational play). Children with so-called semantic-pragmatic language disorder can look like those with Asperger syndrome in that they both have competent expressive language structure and vocabulary but cannot use language effectively in the service of social relationships (Rapin and Allen, 1983). The main difference, however, is that in the former condition, social impairment is not a paramount issue. Unfortunately for primary care clinicians and specialists as well, making such distinctions in the real world of children and their variable ways of relating to others can be very difficult.

Landau-Kleffner Syndrome

Landau-Kleffner syndrome is a condition characterized by acquired aphasia with epilepsy (multifocal spike and wave pattern on electroencephalogram). While the regression in language can superficially mimic the onset of autism, the distinctions are usually evident in the relatively spared interest in communication and use of nonverbal means to communicate. Also, the history usually shows completely normal development well beyond the child's third birthday. Occasionally, however, other autistic-like behaviors are seen, making the differentiation of syndromes more difficult.

Attention Disorders

Children with autistic disorders often have apparent difficulties with sustained attention, overactivity, impulsivity, and distractibility. Physicians may be so struck by the more obvious attentional problems that they might miss the more subtle problems of autism in some children. Furthermore, certain children with attention-deficit hyperactivity disorder have comorbid difficulties with social skills and verbal expression. Except for some children at the most capable end of the autistic spectrum, however, the clinical pictures are different enough that differentiation of these two symptom complexes can be made.

Tourette Syndrome

Characterized by chronic persistence of both motor and vocal tics and frequently accompanied by obsessive-compulsive behaviors, Tourette syndrome can sometimes overlap autistic conditions (i.e., these can occur in the same child). Confusion between motor tics and stereotypic movements is sometimes a problem for clinicians, but with experience, the distinctions can usually be made.

Schizophrenia

Although schizoprenia is historically confused with autism, these two conditions are recognized to be very distinct. Schizophrenia has different epidemiologic characteristics, usually has its onset in adolescence, is not typically associated with mental retardation, and has a lower male to female ratio. People with autism have no greater risk for developing schizophrenia than those individuals without autism. Adults who are autistic are sometimes mistakenly assumed to be schizophrenic, particularly when no developmental history is available to help make the distinction.

Developmental Pathways Through Childhood and Adolescence

MODES OF PRESENTATION

After diagnosis, some parents might be able to recall certain behaviors or developmental quirks that puzzled or concerned them when their affected child was an infant. However, many children who are ultimately diagnosed as autistic do not present to a physician because of such problems until sometime between 15 and 36 months of age. At times, the story is one of an infant who was always very "good," undemanding of attention, and overly content to play by himself or herself. Other infants may start out with a temperament that is extremely difficult, exhausting parents with frequent episodes of inconsolable crying and unpredictable moods. There may or may not be a history of early social "aloofness" or difficulty getting the infant to establish eye contact during interactions.

The parents often have wondered whether their young child is hearing impaired because of limited responsiveness or attention to their calling his or her name or to other surrounding events. Early motor milestones have remained unremarkably normal, although unusual motor behaviors sometimes are retrospectively recalled, such as hand flapping when excited, spinning around, or head banging. Often there is an early proclivity toward visual-motor tasks such as solving puzzles or figuring out how to operate electronic devices, or an unusual interest in the orderly lining up of toys in very particular ways. Over time, an array of strong sensory preferences or intolerances may emerge, ranging from insistence on or rejection of certain food textures, colors, sounds, or smells. And finally, as expectations for useful language increase during the second year of life, the parents often experience a growing awareness of the toddler's delay or deterioration in this developmental domain. Around the same time, the most alarming symptom, social withdrawal, becomes painfully apparent.

CHANGES THROUGH THE LIFE SPAN

Infanthood and Preschool Years

The majority of young children with autism have a history of delayed or unusual development from early infancy. However, in approximately one third of children with autism, the presenting clinical picture is a toddler with previously normal development who is now showing developmental regression in language, social relatedness, and behavior. This regression becomes apparent between 1 and 3 1/2 years of age (Kurita, 1985) and occurs equally among boys and girls. There is no apparent correlation between the type of onset (early vs. late) and severity of the autism. For children who are eventually diagnosed with Asperger syndrome, however, in which initial language milestones are normal, early symptoms may not be apparent to teachers or parents until closer to 4 to 6 years of age.

Characteristic Features

During infancy, parents may notice that their baby resists cuddling or avoids eye contact with them, although these behaviors are not universal. The infant tends to be content with passive play and lacks the typical driving curiosity or initiative to explore. The baby's body posture may be unusual, such as failing to spread the arms in anticipation of being picked up by a parent. Studies utilizing retrospective use of families' home videotapes of their infants (Osterling and Dawson, 1994) have documented that as early as 1 year of age, social behaviors (e.g., looking at others and orienting to name) and the infant's initiating of joint attention with adults were already different from those of infants who do not have autism.

Delays and deviations in language development usually become apparent during the child's 2nd or 3rd year and are commonly the point of concern that leads parents to seek professional help. Unlike children with other causes of language dysfunctions (e.g., hearing impairment, mental retardation, and specific language disabilities), autistic children not only have abnormal verbal language (e.g., echolalia) but also are likely to lack even the *intent* to communicate. Sometimes parents are proud of their child's exceptional memory, as exemplified by his or her ability to mimic perfectly the dialogue of a repeatedly viewed videotape or parental speech patterns and phrases. The latter might be characterized by pronoun reversals. As noted before, young children may also show unusual sensory perceptions.

School-Age Years

The family must now collaborate with the school system to arrive at the most suitable educational setting, with agreement that modifications may be necessary as class-room learning and behavioral issues become better clarified with time. In light of the vast heterogeneity of language, social, and learning abilities among autistic children, there is no one "prescribed" educational setting. As discussed later, various combinations of specialized and integrated settings and programs will need to be molded to the individual needs of each child.

The degree of accompanying mental retardation determines to a large extent the goals and methods of formal education in elementary schools. If an autistic child is moderately mentally retarded, he or she may acquire rudimentary skills to read "survival" words by rote recognition and concrete concepts of quantity using manipulatives. Acquisition of verbal language, even if characterized largely by rote phrases, may signal capabilities to learn rudimentary reading, writing and mathematics skills. Such children may be placed in classes with other children with language impairment or mild mental retardation. More capable children with autism, Asperger syndrome, or PDD may attend resource classes designed for children with learning disabilities. The potential for "full-inclusion" for such children is a matter of active consideration in current times. The unique characteristics of children in this spectrum generally defy many of the usual principles of classroom learning. Unusual processing of sensory information (overreactions to sounds or smells), resistance to transitions, and limited efficacy of traditional incentives for learning (e.g., working for positive social reinforcements) may counteract any advantages of traditional inclusion in regular academic classrooms. For more severely involved children, there may be continued stereotypic motor movements such as rocking, spinning, or hand flapping, but often as the child matures, these tend to diminish in frequency and intensity. Other nonmotor, repetitive obsessions or compulsions may replace these motor behaviors, however. For many children with autism who are more capable or for those with Asperger syndrome, these elementary school years are characterized by an increase in the frequency and intensity of obsessive preoccupations or ritualistic compulsions to touch, hold, or collect unusual objects.

Parental patience and tolerance for their child's differentness, particularly in public places, may be challenged. Having to respond to perseverative questions and comments about the same topic becomes stressful; yet the child appears unaware that he asked the very same question (for which he already knows the answer) 5 minutes earlier. It is also common for one topic or preoccupation to wax and wane in its intensity. Often, however, as one interest fades, another replaces it. These often have an element of anxiety attached to them as well. For example, one family chose to put their annual Christmas tree in the front yard one year, instead of the usual spot in the living room. This provoked marked anxiety in their 7-year-old son with autism, who for months afterward commented to family members and strangers alike that the tree should be in the house. As this obsession finally diminished, it seemed to shift to a related one regarding gifts.

Adolescence

Depending on the overall cognitive level of the individual adolescent with autism or related disorders, many of the normal tasks of adolescence can be distorted or delayed well beyond the time of biological maturation.

In the social domain, the teenager with autism who has attained some verbal skills is likely to be confused by the more abstract humor, sarcasm, and irony typical of the higher language skills seen in teenagers without disabilities. Adolescents with autism may have a vague sense of wanting to be "with the group," but they increasingly realize that this is very difficult and fraught with risks of misunderstanding and rejection. They are likely to have difficulty processing nonverbal cues of everyday social interactions, particularly when there are rapid shifts between visual and auditory cues (Fullerton, 1996).

Social interactions may be further obstructed by the adolescent's difficulty in putting himself or herself "in the shoes" of another person, and by the other person's views of the individual's unusual sensory and perceptual reactions. The organizational and attentional problems often accompanying autism may further interfere with smooth interactions. Often the adolescent and young adult with autism appear unintentionally aloof to others, the product of not being able to coordinate words, feelings, and facial expressions. Some verbal adolescents with autism are at risk for developing depression as they struggle with normal desires to be part of the group while sensing that they lack the requisite skills that everyone else seems to have so naturally (Szatamri, 1991).

One behavior that tends to improve during childhood is hyperactivity. In fact several observers have noted that adolescents with autism are often underactive. Data are mixed as to whether aggressive and self-abusive behaviors increase during childhood, but in view of the higher stakes involved with adolescents and young adults, the impacts of such behavior are greater. The rate of ritualistic and compulsive behaviors that had increased during childhood tends to decrease again during adolescence.

Diagnostic Issues and Assessment

CLINICAL ASSESSMENTS

Even though parents may raise concerns by the time their child is 18 months old, physicians often fail to make the appropriate referrals or diagnosis until 1 to 2 years later, sacrificing valuable time that could have been used for early intervention (Siegel et al, 1988). No single screening test has both high sensitivity and specificity; however, brief instruments such as the Checklist for Autism in Toddlers (CHAT) (Baron-Cohen, Allen, and Gillberg, 1992), designed to screen for autism in 18-month-olds, can be a useful start. On the CHAT, a parent's answer of "no" to more than two of five questions is suggestive of autism. The questions address pretend play, pointing to an object of interest, social relation to peers, interest in social games like "peek-a-boo," and joint attention with a parent (bringing an object over to show it to a parent).

Other screening tools for identifying possible autism are currently undergoing standardization and appear to be promising (Siegel, 1998; Stone, 1998).

For children who are 3 to 7 years of age and had no apparent prior developmental problems, a recent history of social isolation, pedantic, echolalic speech patterns, or preoccupation with certain topics might suggest Asperger syndrome or PDD-NOS.

Differentiating a disorder within the autistic spectrum from the previously mentioned related conditions can be extremely difficult and often requires a lengthy period of observation and review of prior developmental history. This is often best accomplished by an interdisciplinary team, preferably one with experience in the assessment of young children and expertise regarding the autistic spectrum. The team can supplement their observations with other standardized instruments such as the Childhood Autism Rating Scale (CARS) (Schopler et al, 1980), the Autism Diagnostic Interview (ADI) (LeCouteur et al, 1989), and the Autistic Battery for Children (ABC) (Krug, Arick, and Almond, 1980), in addition to behavioral observations. A team evaluation can also include general developmental or cognitive tests, as well as assessments of motor and language abilities.

For those young children whose development seems to begin normally, the emergence of symptoms suggestive of autism may be subtle at first, encouraging parents, physicians, or both to take a "wait and see" approach. Physicians often feel uncertainty in view of the child's young age and the variability of normal language milestones and temperamental styles. However, as noted earlier, waiting too long can be detrimental. If the child's delays and distortions in behavior and language development show persistence, autistic disorders and other conditions in the differential diagnosis must be considered, including a specific language disability, mental retardation, and hearing loss. The possibility that the new symptoms might reflect the earliest expression of a neurodegenerative disease requires consideration as well.

PHYSICAL EXAMINATION

For most children who have a disorder within the autistic spectrum, results of the physical and neurologic examinations will be entirely normal. However, checking specifically for signs and symptoms of medical conditions known to be associated with autism is important. For example, small or large head circumference, neurocutaneous signs of tuberous sclerosis, and facial features typical of fragile X syndrome can provide valuable clues.

LABORATORY AND IMAGING AIDS

The question of whether to obtain various laboratory or brain imaging studies remains controversial. While some experts advocate obtaining an electroencephalogram and brain magnetic resonance image for most children newly suspected of having autism, others advise tailoring the tests to specific questions raised by the history and physical examination. In the absence of any history suggestive of seizures, it is doubtful that an electroencephalogram will yield useful information, although a low threshold for checking an electroencephalogram is wise in view of the risk of seizure disorder in this population. Similarly, no "routine" laboratory tests seem necessary, but close attention to possible genetic or metabolic indicators should guide the clinician's actions. In particular, testing for fragile

X syndrome should be readily considered in view of the critical implications for family planning that such a diagnosis would yield. When in doubt, or when the family is particularly concerned about these issues, referral to a geneticist for further evaluation can be very helpful.

Management Issues

Although no definitive "treatments" are yet availabe, remarkable progress in the area of intervention has occurred, particularly during the 1980s and 1990s. Primary modalities include (1) educational programs, including early intervention, school-based programs, and prevocational services; (2) behavioral techniques; (3) speech and language therapy programs; (4) family support services; and (5) adjunctive psychopharmacologic management of specific symptoms. The physician caring for the child with autism should also become familiar with the growing interest among families and some professionals in various "alternative" or nontraditional treatment programs.

EDUCATIONAL PROGRAMS

In most communities, the primary intervention approach for children with autistic disorders is through educational programs. In the United States, legislation (Public Laws 94–142 and 99–457 and their legislative successors) guarantees a free and appropriate education for all children with disabilities beginning at the age of 3 years. Many states also provide services for infants and toddlers. Accumulating evidence supports the efficacy of these intensive early intervention programs in reducing inappropriate and stereotypic behaviors, enchancing more socialized play, promoting independence in self-help skills, and advancing more successful verbal and nonverbal communication skills. This is often accomplished within the context of an "integrated" daycare or preschool program along with typically developing children. With the current educational emphasis on "inclusion" of children with disabilities, this approach has been increasingly popularized for school-aged children with autism. Controversy remains, however. The potential benefits attributable to modeling the behavior of children without disabilities and the availability of "normalized" social milieux must be weighed against the advantages of a more individualized approach in a special education setting, which allows a teacher to provide the needed intensity, repetitions, and behavioral reinforcements so critical to learning in many autistic children.

Educational approaches need to accommodate any associated limitations, such as the presence of mental retardation or a lack of functional language skills. Similarly, for more verbal children, balancing their needs for academic advancement with help in pragmatic language skills and socialization efforts requires committed teamwork among school personnel, family, and involved professionals. The educational goals for any child with autism will need to be tailored to his or her unique profile as spelled out by the Individualized Educational Program. This individualized developmental approach, along with a commitment to the importance of family members as primary interventionists, is the hallmark of the widely disseminated approach of the TEACCH (Treatment and Education of Autistic and related Communication handicapped CHildren) program from the University of North Carolina at Chapel Hill (Schopler, Reichler, and Lansing, 1980).

Key principles of classroom intervention include a high level of consistency and structure, a curriculum that is developmentally appropriate, emphasis on social interaction and multimodal learning (visual and tactile cues accompanying verbal information), peer modeling with typically developing children, and strong family involvement in daily teaching. Physicians and parents can advocate for year-round schooling to avoid considerable loss of skills learned during the standard 9-month school year. The quantity and quality of educational programs varies tremendously according to location, socioeconomic factors, theoretical beliefs about the underlying dysfunctions in autism, and philosophies regarding special education among various school systems.

BEHAVIOR THERAPY

Using various forms of consistent positive and negative reinforcements has long been a mainstay of intervention for children with autism. Initially applied as a way of decreasing negative behaviors such as self-injurious or self-stimulating mannerisms (sometimes including aversive techniques that are no longer considered acceptable), these methods have become useful in promoting positive behaviors, including eye contact, use of verbal communication, and initiating social interaction.

Several university-based centers (e.g., TEACCH and the Princeton Child Development Center) throughout the United States have special assessment and intervention programs for children with autism. An increasingly renowned model is the Young Autism Project at UCLA, headed by Ivar Lovaas, a research psychologist. This is a system of intensive (35–40 hours per week), home-based teaching of young children with autism through "applied behavioral analysis." In this method, many tasks are broken down into small increments of behavior, each of which is intensively reinforced before the therapist moves on to the next step in the chain. Tasks range from simple or concrete actions (e.g., imitation of facial movements or following one-step instructions) to more complex and abstract skills (e.g., initiation of asking "wh-" questions or describing how to make a peanut butter and jelly sandwich). Eventually, the trainer's verbal and physical prompts are systematically faded.

Initial research on the outcomes of this approach has yielded impressive results in a small cohort, with significant short- and long-term gains (over a comparable control group) in cognitive, social, and language development (Lovaas, 1987; McEachin, Smith, and Lovaas, 1993). Some critics have questioned the validity of the outcome measures and whether the study sample is representative of most other populations. Many researchers, however, now feel that intervention that is early (in the first 2 to 3 years), intense, and individualized to the child's responses can yield significant improvements in many children with autism. Unavailability of adequately trained therapists, cost, and insufficient intensity are potential obstacles to success, however.

Table 60–5 • Selected Drugs Used in the Treatment of Behaviors in Autistic Spectrum Disorders

Indications	Medications	Classification	Affected Neurochemical System or Central Nervous System Action	Target Symptoms	Potential Side Effects (Selected)	Comments
Stereotypic, self-injurious, and/or aggressive behavior	Buspirone (BuSpar)	Anxiolytic (atypical)	Serotonin-1A receptor (partial agonist)	Aggression, Anxiety, Adjunct, Treatment for obsession/compulsion	Drowsiness, disinhibition	May allow for reduction in dose of neuroleptic
	Carbamazepine (Tegretol)	Anticonvulsant	Reduces polysynaptic responses; blocks post-tetanic potentiation	Aggression, Self-injurious behavior	Dizziness, drowsiness, nausea, bone marrow suppression	Incidence of blood dyscrasias are very rare, but periodic follow-up of complete blood count is recommended
	Clomipramine (Anafranil)	Antiobsessional	Tricyclic; probable serotonin-reuptake inhibitor	Stereotypic behaviors, Self-injurious behavior	Gastrointestinal disturbances, anorexia, sedation, dizziness, sleep disturbances, dry mouth	Some improvement in core symptoms of autism (including deviant speech) reported in small studies
	Clonidine (Catapres)	Antihypertensive	Centrally acting alpha agonist	Aggression, Impulsivity, Tics, Hyperactivity	Sedation (frequent), hypotension (rare)	Some children develop tolerance for beneficial effects
	Fluvoxamine (Luvox)	Antiobsessional	Selective serotonin-reuptake inhibitor (but chemically unrelated to other selective serotonin-reuptake inhibitors)	Stereotypic or compulsive behaviors, Obsessional thinking, Depression, Anxiety, Aggression	Headache, nausea, insomnia, somnolence, nervousness, dizziness, sweating	Can improve social relatedness in autistic adults; side effects are mild and rare in adults; no controlled trials of use in children with autism
	Guanfacine (Tenex)	Antihypertensive	Centrally acting alpha-2 agonist	Aggression, Impulsivity, Tics	Sedation	Less sedation than with clonidine
	Haloperidol (Haldol)	Neuroleptic	Dopamine antagonist	Agitation, Hyperactivity, Aggression, Stereotypic behaviors, Mood lability, Short attention span, Social withdrawal	Extrapyramidal reactions, weight gain, sedation, increasing risk of tardive dyskinesia with long-term treatment	Older children respond better than younger children (preschoolers)
	Naltrexone (ReVia)	Opioid agonist	Opioid agonist	Stereotypic behaviors, Self-injurious behavior, Aggressive/disruptive behavior, Social withdrawal	Sedation (mild)	Treatment efficacy has been correlated in one study with blood beta endorphin levels; bitter taste

Indication	Drug	Class	Mechanism of action	Target symptoms	Side effects	Comments
	Propranolol (Inderal)	Beta-blocker	Beta-blocker	Aggressive behavior Impulsive behavior Self-injurious behavior	Hypotension	May allow for reduction in dose of neuroleptic; seems to alleviate "chronic hyperarousal" (McDougle, 1997)
	Risperidone (Risperdal)	Neuroleptic (atypical)	Serotonin 5HT2-receptor blockade Dopamine D-2-receptor blockade Alpha-1 and alpha-2 adrenergic Antihistaminic activity	Self-injurious behavior Aggressive behavior	Sedation, headache, dry mouth, constipation, blurred vision, urinary retention Theoretical risk of tardive dyskinesia	Risk of tardive dyskinesia appears to be lower than for other neuroleptics
Hyperactivity, short attention span, and/or impulsivity	Dextroamphetamine (Dexedrine, Dextrostat, Adderall*)	Stimulant	Norepinephrine-reuptake inhibition Dopamine-reuptake inhibition	Short attention span Hyperactivity Distractibility Impulsivity	Appetite suppression, sleep disturbances, headache, dysphoria, rebound	Higher risk of exacerbating hyperactivity, mood lability, and irritability in autistic (vs. nonautistic) children; need to monitor growth velocity
	Methylphenidate (Ritalin)	Stimulant	Norepinephrine-reuptake inhibition Dopamine-reuptake inhibition	Short attention span Hyperactivity Distractibility Impulsivity	Appetite suppression, sleep disturbances, headache, dysphoria, rebound; possible deceleration of growth velocity	Higher risk of exacerbating hyperactivity, mood lability, and irritability in autistic (vs. nonautistic) children; need to monitor growth velocity
Depression, anxiety, and/or obsessiveness (see also above-noted drugs for stereotypic behaviors)	Fluoxetine (Prozac)	Antidepressant	Selective serotonin-reuptake inhibitor	Depression Anxiety Ritualistic behavior Impulsivity Short attention span	Agitation, hyperactivity, decreased appetite, insomnia, drowsiness, nausea, diarrhea, excessive sweating, sexual dysfunction	
	Paroxetine (Paxil)	Antidepressant	Selective serotonin-reuptake inhibitor	Depression Anxiety Obsessive/compulsive symptoms	Nausea, dry mouth, somnolence, dizziness, sexual dysfunction	
	Sertraline (Zoloft)	Antidepressant	Selective serotonin-reuptake inhibitor	Depression Anxiety Obsessive/compulsive symptoms	Anxiety, gastrointestinal disturbances, sedation, dizziness, insomnia, sexual dysfunction	Preliminary studies in autistic adults show improvement in social interaction, aggression, and repetitive behavior

*Adderall is a combination of two salts of dextroamphetamine and two salts of amphetamine. See McDougle, 1997 for additional details.

SPEECH AND LANGUAGE THERAPIES

Enabling children with autism to communicate more effectively is another primary focus of intervention. Success in this area may diminish self-injurious and other atypical behaviors to the extent that these may have been the only forms of communication available to the child. Even for those children who may never acquire speech, therapies can help provide nonverbal forms of communication. On the other hand, children who have speech, even when it is nonecholalic, will need help with functionally using that language in the real-world venue of social interaction (language pragmatics), a task that often remains challenging throughout the child's life.

FAMILY SUPPORT

Another critical goal of intervention is to help the child's family. To optimally encourage their child, the family needs support in understanding the nature of the autistic spectrum, their own child's unique behavioral and developmental strengths and limitations, and concrete techniques for promoting learning and adaptive skills. Stresses encountered by families are particularly likely to occur around the time of diagnosis, at times of major transitions (e.g., moving from preschool to elementary school or at school graduations), when sexuality and other adolescent-onset milestones occur, and whenever there are additional medical complications (e.g., the onset of seizures). Support should also include discussions about possible family counseling, respite services, contact with formal or informal parent support groups (e.g., the Autism Society of America) and sibling support services, and provision of written materials (both hard-copy books and articles and online resources through the Internet). Some of these resources are included at the end of this chapter. Goals of intervention are facilitation of coping, improving advocacy skills, emotional support, parent education, and helping brothers and sisters deal with their sibling's behavior and their perceived loss of parental attention.

PSYCHOPHARMACOLOGIC MANAGEMENT

Medication is not a primary treatment for autism but can be useful as an adjunct to other therapies in targeting specific symptoms, particularly aggressive, self-injurious, stereotypic, anxious, or hyperactive behaviors. Table 60–5 lists many of the psychopharmacologic agents currently being used, as well as their indications and potential side effects.

Although older neuroleptics such as haloperidol have been found to be effective in ameliorating many of these behaviors in children with autism, there is a cumulative dose-related risk of significant and permanent neurologic deficits, particularly tardive dyskinesia, rendering such medications suitable only for short courses and for the most severely incapacitating behaviors. Some medications, such as the psychostimulants, may be useful in treating significant hyperactivity, distractibility, and impulsivity in children with autism, but parents should be informed that there are risks of exacerbation of stereotypic or self-injurious behaviors. Cautious monitoring is warranted.

Primary care physicians are encouraged to use only those medications with which they are familiar. Consultation with a child psychiatrist or developmental pediatrician regarding further psychopharmacologic management is recommended.

"ALTERNATIVE" AND UNORTHODOX TREATMENTS

Learning quickly that there is no consensus within the mainstream medical and educational establishment regarding the fundamental causes or treatments for autism, yet hopeful that there are more effective ways to help their children progress or even be "cured," parents are often tempted to pursue "alternative" treatments. These encompass a wide variety of theoretical bases and modalities. As is happening with all other aspects of health care in the United States, parents are becoming more secure and outspoken as advocates and consumers for their family members with autism. While still committed to excellent medical care, they may also be open to these less orthodox treatments, despite professionals' skepticism or outright condemnation. Parents often learn about such treatments from other parents, through parent groups, popular books, parent conferences, local and national newsletters, and even television "news magazines" and movies. The Internet also provides a rapidly growing and changing marketplace for these ideas, opinions, and programs, complete with anecdotal reports of success and opportunities to make instant credit card purchases. Family members are often reluctant to mention to their doctors that they are considering such treatments, apprehensive that the physician may automatically condemn the treatment or chastise them for considering such "unscientific" programs. What can the physician do to help families navigate through the myriad treatment programs they will encounter?

The list in Table 60–6 includes some treatment programs being promoted at the time of the writing of this chapter (late 1997). The reader should note that new treatments come and go quite frequently. These programs are mentioned to help readers understand the types of treatment options that many parents encounter; listing them here should not be interpreted as implying endorsement. The purported rationale for some of the treatments listed in Table 60–6 are briefly described here.

Table 60–6 • "Alternative" or Unorthodox Treatments for Autism

Auditory training	Sensory integration therapy
Facilitated communication	Patterning (Doman-Delacatto)
Dietary modifications	Holding therapy
Vitamins and minerals	Craniosacral therapy
Casein (milk)/gluten elimination	Optical therapies
Synthetic coloring elimination	Tinted lenses
Enzymes	Special prisms
Elimination of sulfur-containing	Melatonin
foods	Dimethylglycine (DMG)
Anti-yeast therapy	Intravenous immune globulin
Defeat Autism Now! (DAN!)	Steroids (autism vs. Landau-
Protocol	Kleffner syndrome)

Auditory Integration Training

Auditory integration training is a form of sensory-integration therapy that is based on the rationale that distortions of hearing can contribute to inappropriate or antisocial behavior. By systematically listening to appropriately frequency-filtered music, the individual's brain auditory centers are said to "normalize" the hearing and thereby the resuting behaviors.

Facilitated Communication

Facilitated communication, popularized in the early 1990s, is a method of assisting individuals with disabilities to communicate via a portable keyboard or communication device. A "trained facilitator" steadies the individual's hand or arm as he or she types a message with an outstretched index finger. Sensationalized television testimonials and "docudramas" of this technique played to the fervent hope of many parents that there is a "normal" child in some fashion locked within. Multiple controlled studies have shown the claims of the proponents of facilitated communication to be false.

Dietary Changes

There have been many claims for the alleged "cure" of autism through one or more dietary modifications. These have included megadoses of vitamins (e.g., vitamin C, vitamin B_6 with magnesium) or the exclusion of certain food colorings. Based on unsubstantiated theories of a "leaky gut" in autism, some writers advocate systematic desensitization or administraton of formulated enzymes. Others link this with a disturbance of the endogenous opioid system leading to problems with socialization, pain insensitivity, repetitive behaviors, and so forth. They recommend elimination of casein (milk products) and gluten. Scientific support remains sketchy and poorly controlled.

Anti-Yeast Therapy

Advocates of a combination of a low-yeast diet and the administration of systemic anti-yeast medications claim that individuals with autism have candidal overgrowth, which is perhaps related to an underlying immune deficit or the excessive use of antibiotics.

Defeat Autism Now! (DAN!) Protocol

This is a collection of various "biological" techniques for assessing the basis for autism and purportedly could lead to specific treatment regimens. The approach involves extensive laboratory work-ups obtainable through certain recommended reference laboratories.

Summary

Pediatricians and other health care providers need to be alert to current trends in therapeutic approaches, even when they are not necessarily described in scientific publications. Ideally, through the parent-physician alliance, an open communication about these alternative theories and therapies

can take place. Parents can be encouraged to exercise caution, to remember that placebo effects can be every bit as real as treatment effects, and to be as objective as possible in evaluating purported results. Hopefully, parents' pursuit of such treatments will not preclude treatment programs that do have proven efficacy and will not initiate repeated cycles of trying unusual therapies. Several descriptions of the overall issue of "alternative therapies" for autism have been provided in literature for parents (Siegel, 1996).

DEMYSTIFICATION

In view of the shifting definitions of autism and the recent expansion of the concept to include an autistic "spectrum," it is understandable that professionals, including physicians, struggle with the key concepts. The struggle is even greater for most parents upon receiving the diagnosis regarding their son or daughter. Taking time to first listen to parents' own understanding of what autism is can form the foundation for a meaningful interpretive discussion. The clinician needs to set aside sufficient time to explain the changing and often-confusing terminology (e.g., PDD, autism, autistic spectrum) and expose the common myths (e.g., that most autistic people are brilliant but "trapped" in their "prison," or that no change is possible). Other roles for the physician include ensuring that the child receives appropriate primary care (e.g., including dental visits, immunizations, and treatment of routine medical problems), providing advocacy in helping the family secure needed school and community services, and providing referral to appropriate specialists when indicated.

Prognosis

Given the heterogeneous population of individuals identified as being within the autistic spectrum, it should not be surprising that there is a wide range of possible functional outcomes as these children age into adults. However, in contrast to more dismal outcome reports prior to 20 years ago (Lotter, 1978), reviews from the past 10 years have documented greater percentages of individuals with autism going on to "good" outcomes (4–32% vs. 5–17%) and fewer with "poor" to "very poor" outcomes (20–48% vs. 61–73%) (Stone and Ousley, 1996). More emphasis on and enthusiasm about the benefits of early intervention as well as greater legal and community supports for group homes and supported job opportunities for people with autism have contributed to this somewhat brighter picture of the future. The potential outcomes are even more positive for those individuals with autism whose intelligence quotient scores were greater than 60 to 65 as young children and who acquired functional language by their early school years. In recent studies of a small sample of these individuals as young adults, roughly 33% were employed, 9% to 31% were living independently, and 11% to 50% were attending college (Stone and Ousley, 1996).

There is reason to hope that in the future, current trends in greater understanding of underlying neuropsychological bases of autism, improved educational programs, and more available community resources can further boost the prognosis for individuals with autism and related disorders.

REFERENCES

American Psychiatric Association: Diagnostic and Statistical Manual of Mental Disorders, 4th ed. Washington, DC, American Psychiatric Association, 1994.

Baron-Cohen S, Allen J, Gillberg C: Can autism be detected at 18 months? The needle, the haystack, and the CHAT. Br J Psychiat 161:839, 1992.

Coleman M: Young children with autism or autistic-like behavior. Infants Young Children 1:22, 1989.

Frith U: Asperger and his syndrome. *In* Frith U (ed): Autism and Asperger syndrome. Cambridge, UK, Cambridge University Press, 1991, pp 11–12.

Fullerton A: Who are higher functioning young adults with autism? *In* Fullerton A, Stratton J, Coyne P, and Gray C (eds): Higher Functioning Young Adults and Adolescents With Autism: A Teacher's Guide. Austin, TX, Pro-Ed, 1996, p 15.

Gillberg C, Steffenburg S, Schaumann H: Is autism more common now than ten years ago? Br J Psychiatr 158:403, 1991.

Krug DA, Arick JR, Almond PG: Behavior checklist for identifying severely handicapped individuals with high levels of autistic behavior. J Child Psychol Psychiatr 21:221, 1980.

Kurita H: Infantile autism with speech loss before the age of thirty months. J Am Acad Child Psychiatry 24:191, 1985.

LeCouteur A, Rutter M, Lord C, et al: Autism diagnostic interview: a standardized investigator-based instrument. J Aut Dev Disord 19:363, 1989.

Lotter V: Follow-up studies. *In* Rutter M, and Schopler E (eds): Autism: A Reappraisal of Concepts and Treatment. New York, Plenum Press, 1978, pp 475–495.

Lovaas OI: Behavioral treatment and normal educational and intellectual functioning in young autistic children. Consul Clin Psychol. 55:3, 1987.

McDougle CJ: Psychopharmacology. *In* Cohen DJ, Volkmar FR (eds): Handbook of Autism and Pervasive Developmental Disorders. New York, John Wiley & Sons, 1997, pp 707–729.

McEachin JJ, Smith T, Lovaas OI: Long-term outcome for children with autism who received early intensive behavioral treatment. Am J Ment Retard 4:359, 1993.

Nelson KB: Prenatal and perinatal factors in the etiology of autism. Pediatrics 87:761, 1991.

Osterling J, Dawson G: Early recognition of children with autism: a study of first birthday home videotapes. J Autism Dev Disorders 24:247, 1994.

Rapin I, Allen D: Developmental language disorders: nosologic considerations. *In* Kirk U (ed): Neuropsychology of Language, Reading, and Spelling. London, Academic Press, 1983, pp 155–183.

Ritvo ER, Freeman BJ, Pingree C: The UCLA–University of Utah epidemiological survey of autism: prevalence. Am J Psychiatry 146:194, 1989.

Schopler E, Reichler RJ, De Vellis RF, et al: Toward objective classification of childhood autism: childhood autism rating scale (CARS). J Aut Dev Disord 10:91, 1980.

Schopler E, Reichler RJ, Lansing M: Individualized Assessment and Treatment for Autistic and Developmentally Disabled Children: Vol 2. Teaching Strategies for Parents and Professionals. Baltimore, University Park Press, 1980.

Siegel B: Early screening and diagnosis in autism spectrum disorders: The Pervasive Developmental Disorders Screening Test (PDDST). Unpublished, 1998.

Siegel B: Non-mainstream treatments for autism. *In* Siegel B (ed): The World of the Autistic Child: Understanding and Treating Autistic Spectrum Disorders. New York, Oxford University Press, 1996, pp 321–332.

Siegel B, Pliner C, Eschler J, et al: How children with autism are diagnosed: difficulties in identification of children with multiple developmental delays. J Dev Behav Pediatrics 9:199, 1988.

Sigman M, Capps L: Children With Autism: A Developmental Perspective. Cambridge, MA, Harvard University Press, 1997, pp 54–58; 149–163.

Smalley SL, Collins F: Brief report: genetic, prenatal, and immunologic factors. J Autism Dev Disorders 26:195, 1996.

Stone W: Descriptive information about the Screening Tool for Autism in Two-year olds (STAT). Unpublished, 1998.

Stone WL, Ousley OY: Pervasive developmental disorders: autism. *In* Wolraich ML (ed): Disorders of Development and Learning: A Practical Guide to Assessment and Management, 2nd ed. St. Louis, Mosby, 1996, pp 379–405.

Szatmari P: Asperger's syndrome: diagnosis, treatment, and outcome. Psychiatric Clin North Am 14:81, 1991.

Towbin KE: Pervasive developmental disorder not otherwise specified. *In* Cohen DJ, Volkmar FR (eds): Handbook of Autism and Pervasive Developmental Disorders. New York, John Wiley & Sons, 1997, pp 123–147.

Tuchman R, Rapin I, Shinnar S: Autistic and dysphasic children: II. Epilepsy. Pediatrics 6:1219, 1991a.

Tuchman R, Rapin I, Shinnar S: Autistic and dysphasic children: I. Clinical characteristics. Pediatrics 88:1211, 1991b.

Wing L: Syndromes of autism and atypical development. *In* Cohen DJ, Volkmar FR (eds): Handbook of Autism and Pervasive Developmental Disorders. New York, John Wiley & Sons, 1997, pp 148–172.

Wing L: Asperger's syndrome: a clinical account. Psychol Med 11:115, 1981.

World Health Organization (WHO): The ICD Classification of Mental and Behavioral Disorders: Clinical Descriptions and Diagnostic Guidelines, Geneva, WHO, 1992.

RECOMMENDED READING

Books

Frith U (ed): Autism and Asperger's Syndrome. Cambridge, UK, Cambridge University Press, 1991.

Maurice C (ed): Behavioral Intervention for Young Children with Autism: A Manual for Parents and Professionals. Austin, TX, Pro-Ed, 1996.

McDonnell JT: News from the Border: A Mother's Memoir of her Autistic Son. New York, Ticknor and Fields, 1993.

Miller S: Family Pictures. 1990.

Powers MD: Children with Autism: A Parents' Guide. Bethesda, MD, Woodbine House, 1989.

Schopler E (ed): Parent Survival Manual: A Guide to Crisis Resolution in Autism and Related Developmental Disorders. New York, Plenum Press, 1995.

Siegel B: The World of the Autistic Child: Understanding and treating Autistic Spectrum Disorders. New York, Oxford University Press, 1996.

Sigman M, Capps L: Children with Autism: A Developmental Perspective. Cambridge, MA, Harvard University Press, 1997.

Williams D: Nobody Nowhere: The Extraordinary Autobiography of an Autistic. New York, Avon, 1992.

Newsletters and Journals

The Advocate: Newsletter of the Autism Society of America; free to members (see below for ASA address and phone number)

Autism Research Review International: publication of the Autism Research Institute, directed by Dr. Bernard Rimland, a psychologist and parent of an adult son who has autism. 4182 Adams Avenue, San Diego, CA 92116.

Journal of Autism and Developmental Disabilities: Pelnum Publishing, 233 Spring St. New York, NY 10013, (212) 620–8468.

The MAAP: Newsletter focusing on "More Able Autistic People." Susan J Moreno, P.O. Box 524, Crown Point, IN 46307.

The Morning News: a newsletter by Carol Gray, an educator who publishes creative curricular materials for students with autism, 2140 Bauer Road, Jenison, MI 49428, (616) 457–8955, or FAX (616) 457–4070.

Parents' Newsletter on Special Education Law: published by an attorney who is the father of a child with autism. Focuses on advocacy and legal issues. P.O. Box 4571, Chapel Hill, NC 27515–4571.

RECOMMENDED WEBSITES

Moreno S, O'Neal C: Tips for teaching high functioning people with autism. http://www.udel.edu/bkirby/asperger/moreno tips for teaching.html

TEACCH home page. http://www.unc.edu/depts/teacch/

TEACCH: Nonverbal thinking, communication, imitation, play (practical interventions for helping young autistic children). http://www.unc.edu/depts/teacch/Develop.html

Temple Grandin: An inside view of autism. ftp//ftp.syr.edu/information/autism/an inside view of autism.txt

Williams K: Understanding the student with Asperger syndrome: Guidelines for teachers. http://www.udel.edu/bkirby/asperger/karen williams guidelines.html

ORGANIZATIONS

Autism Society of America (ASA), 7910 Woodmont Avenue, Suite 650, Bethesda, MD 20814; 1–800–3–AUTISM (1–800–328–8476).

Founded in 1965, this organization is the primary national support agency for individuals with autism and their families. Many states have state and local chapters as well.

Autism Society of Canada, 129 Yorkville Ave, Suite 202, Toronto, Ontario M5R 1C4 Canada; (416) 922–0302.

Autism Society of North Carolina (ASNC), 3300 Woman's Club Drive, Raleigh, NC 27612–4811; (919) 571–8555 or FAX (919) 571–7800.

A state chapter of the Autism Society of America. Publishes a comprehensive catalog of books pertaining to autism and related developmental disabilities.

TEACCH (*T*reatment and *E*ducation of *A*utistic and related *C*ommunication handicapped *Ch*ildren), CB# 7180, University of North Carolina at Chapel Hill, Chapel Hill, NC 27599–7180; (919) 966–2174 or FAX (919) 966–4127.

This division of the Department of Psychiatry of the School of Medicine at UNC-CH is a comprehensive, community-based program that includes direct services for children, adolescents, and adults with autism or related communication disabilities and their families; consultation to other programs and classrooms throughout the state of North Carolina; research; and professional training. They offer a limited number of evaluation slots to out-of-state children.

61 *The Child With Multiple Disabilities*

Richard P. Nelson • Allen C. Crocker

Functional impairment and the extent of required interventions are more central to a child's living circumstances than a specific medical diagnosis.

The child must have access to all of the venues that characterize development opportunity: the circle of family and eventually the "schoolyard" of other childhood experience.

Psychiatric treatment facilities have traditionally been skittish about accepting clients with retardation, and classes for children with mental retardation have been bewildered when atypical behavior is prominent.

An emerging major population of children with multiple disabilities are those individuals who have daily special health care procedure requirements, including the need for life function support by machines or other equipment.

The child with a serious health condition or multiple disabilities faces diverse challenges in functional living. The rigors of daily activity, whether time with playmates and friends or the more formal expectations of school, require focus, energy, and resolve. The child must also have access to all of the venues that characterize developmental opportunity: the circle of family and eventually the "schoolyard" of other childhood experience.

Whereas most children who have chronic illness or physical limitation can accommodate the need for medication or clinical treatment, other children must cope with extraordinary functional compromise. For these children, the routine of daily life is anything but routine. Their day may revolve around periodic medical therapies (such as chest percussion for the chronic lung disease of cystic fibrosis), mobility aids (a wheelchair for motor deficits), or the obligatory assistance of a ventilator (as, for example, following a cervical spine injury). These children often have extensive health care needs, and their families may require other support services to preserve their functionality (Taylor, Epstein, and Crocker, 1990; Newacheck and Stoddard, 1994; Crocker, 1997).

The Issue of Definition

Who are these children with lasting and diverse issues? How do we identify them? Are they receiving necessary care and services? These straightforward-sounding questions unfortunately do not stimulate ready answers. Over recent years it has become increasingly important to seek a definition, not only as a measure of whether children are receiving services to which they are entitled under a public program or a health care financing plan, but also to evaluate the effects of care and services (Epstein et al, 1989).

Early attempts to categorize the children based on medical diagnosis alone have been recognized to have limited utility. The condition "cerebral palsy" illustrates this limitation. Even specific diagnostic descriptions of the type of cerebral palsy do not adequately define severity. Similarly, one child with asthma is asymptomatic on minimal medication, while another child with the same diagnosis may require intermittent steroids to control life-threatening bronchospasm.

Functional impairment and the extent of required interventions are more central to a child's living circumstances than a specific medical diagnosis. Such observations have led to formal attempts to define this population of children to better characterize their needs. In 1995, the Maternal and Child Health Bureau of the federal Department of Health and Human Services published the following definition:

> Children with special health care needs are those who have or are at increased risk for chronic physical, developmental, behavioral, or emotional conditions and who require health and related services of a type or amount beyond that required by children generally.

This definition is broadly quoted among public program advocates working in state maternal and child health programs supported by the federal Title V legislation. Yet others have sought to construct a more objective definition that has utility in identifying, serving, and monitoring the status of this population. Stein and colleagues (1993) structured a framework for ongoing health conditions that encompasses functional limitations, a requirement for compensation for the limitation, and a description of the need for services (Table 61–1).

Functional Effects of Multiple Disabilities

There is a specific or actual additive constraint to human development caused by the presence of more than one

Table 61–1 • Definition of Chronic or Special Health Care Conditions

1. Have a biologic, psychologic, or cognitive basis, and
2. Have lasted or are virtually certain to last for at least 1 year, and
3. Produce one or more of the following sequelae:
   a. Limitation of function, activities, or social role in comparison with healthy age peers
   b. Dependency on one of the following: medications, special diet, medical technology, assistive devices, personal assistance
   c. Need for medical care or related services

Adapted from Stein REK, Bauman JJ, Westbrook LE, Coupey SM, Ireys HT: Framework for identifying children who have chronic conditions: The case for a new definition. J Pediatrics 122:342, 1993.

disability. When a deaf child cannot utilize manual language because of visual impairment or a motor dysfunction, the child is further restricted. The complication of a serious mobility limitation intrudes upon the potential of a child with mental retardation for access to learning experiences. Far more significant than these concrete elements, however, have been the societal, political, and even professional reactions to children with a multiplicity of disability. Three prototypic situations illustrate the traditional dilemmas of compounded disability.

DEAFNESS WITH OTHER PROBLEMS

In earlier times, children with early-onset "pure" deafness were educated for the most part in segregated and highly structured "schools for the deaf." The minority who had other difficulties in addition generally melded with the population who had serious mental retardation, by default. The huge rubella epidemic of 1963–64 created a sudden and dramatic increase in the numbers of children with sensorineural deafness, many of whom had visual disabilities, central processing problems, behavioral atypicality, and sometimes mental retardation. The flexibility of the deaf school criteria was critically challenged, and many small new educational facilities were created to develop experimental curricula that could reach out and meet the needs of deaf children with multiple disabilities. In Massachusetts, the names of those freshly formed (Little People's School, Learning Center for Deaf Children, and Willie Ross School—named after an involved child, for example) reflected a more expeditious approach to child needs than had the traditional institutions (e.g., Boston School for the Deaf). Beyond this a federal program reflected specific Congressional support for the education of children with deaf-blindness. When an inventory was established of these young people with double sensory disabilities, it was found that many were already grouped with persons who were severely or profoundly mentally retarded in state residential facilities, without cognitive impairment ever having been demonstrated.

SERIOUS PHYSICAL DISABILITY (INCLUDING CEREBRAL PALSY) AND MENTAL RETARDATION

The difficulty in making an accurate determination of intellectual function in a child with very substantial physical disability often led to educational nihilism if some evidence of mental retardation was detected. In earlier decades, many young people with borderline or mild retardation who had striking cerebral palsy were allowed to languish in state residential facilities, to have their true learning potential uncovered only when the movement of "deinstitutionalization" got under way. Further, until the advent of PL 94-142, it was usual to exclude from early educational efforts children who had major bodily disabilities that could lead to fragility of health or a fatal outcome, such as those with the Cornelia de Lange syndrome or Hurler syndrome. This deprived the child and family of coordinated supports and reinforcement of personal progress within the years available. Finally, until the revision of federal guidelines, it was difficult to obtain vocational rehabilitation services for a young adult with physical limitations if a significant degree of retardation was also present.

MENTAL RETARDATION ACCOMPANIED BY BEHAVIORAL DISTURBANCE

The classic instance of programmatic confoundment, and often rejection, has been that seen in the presence of the "dual diagnosis" of mental retardation and mental illness. Psychiatric treatment facilities have traditionally been skittish about accepting clients with retardation, and classes for children with mental retardation have been bewildered when atypical behavior is prominent. The usual cause in current times for referral of children with retardation to residential schooling is the inability of community programs to deal with serious behavioral disturbance. The urgent need for coordinated effort between mental health and retardation resources is demonstrated as well by serious childhood psychosis (and autism), in which retardation is often a sequela.

The ultimate additive disadvantage for a child with disability, of course, is social and personal. For a child from a minority group, the vulnerability is yet greater. If the family is in chaos, support systems are ineffective, and the child experiences devaluation and social isolation, a critically compromising group of complications can ensue. A loss of individual compensation and personality integration will place serious limits on the child's adaptive outcome.

Special Health Care Requirements

The support system for a population of children with disability must provide assistance in a predictable group of continuing health needs. Mental retardation programs, for example, make an important contribution in the treatment of emotional disturbances, motor function and orthopedic problems, and seizures. The most widespread of these is emotional difficulty, of significance in half or more of the persons, and varying from mild behavioral disturbance to depression, acting out, self-abuse, or even overwhelming thought disorder. These issues are discussed further in Chapter 62.

Other complications commonly encountered in children with disability, influenced in part by their special lifestyle, include nutritional difficulties (both feeding problems and obesity), chronic ear infections, pulmonary infection or fibrosis, dental or periodontal disease, injury, and pica. Some special syndromes have obvious liabilities regarding cardiac disease, hydrocephalus, urinary tract infections, growth failure, or reduced fertility. Strabismus, undescended testes, and scoliosis are frequent anomalies. (See reviews in Rubin and Crocker, 1989; Crocker, 1992; Capute and Accardo, 1996; and Batshaw, 1997.)

An emerging major population of children with multiple disabilities are those individuals who have daily special health care procedure requirements, including the need for life function support by machines or other equipment (Nelson, 1989). This latter group of children is generally referred to as technology-assisted or -dependent. The federal Office of Technology Assessment has developed a useful classification of these children, summarized in Table 61–2. Nationally, as many as 100,000 children may be included in these groupings (Palfrey et al, 1994; Porter et al, 1997). The requirements of care at home and in school may be considerable, but the healthy adaptation of these children to extraordinary circumstances is an increasing phenomenon, as represented by the ventilator-assisted child depicted in Figure 61–1.

Children with these needs may or may not have coincident developmental disabilities that shape their functional attributes. Systemic failure (as in primary respiratory insufficiency) almost always compromises some aspect of physical function, even when there is no direct involvement of the brain or musculoskeletal tissues. Such children often lack stamina, may be chronically undernourished due to diminished appetite, and may develop depression or other emotional difficulties. A direct neurologic or physical impairment will affect developmental progress, can limit basic skills (eating, fine motor abilities, communication, and mobility), and can increase the requirements for personal and professional care.

An illustration of the needs of children with multiple disabilities can be constructed by considering the spectrum of services appropriate for a child at different ages. Table 61–3 presents a listing of services and professionals that a child with a neuromotor disorder (such as cerebral palsy)

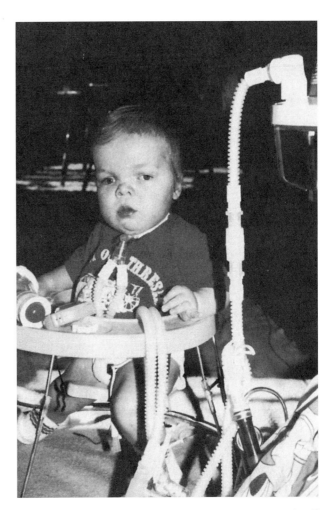

Figure 61–1. Darrin, a 2-year-old boy with chronic respiratory insufficiency due to pulmonary hypoplasia.

and concurrent related developmental disabilities might receive at three different ages (in early and middle childhood and adolescence). Not only are the needs diverse, but they often become more complex over time. Some newly

Table 61–2 • Classification of Technology-Dependent Children

Group	Definition
I	Children dependent on mechanical ventilators at least part of each day
II	Children requiring prolonged intravenous administration of nutritional substances or drugs
III	Children with daily dependence on other device-based respiratory or nutritional support, including tracheostomy tube care, suctioning, oxygen support, or tube feeding
IV	Children who require daily or nearly daily nursing care with prolonged dependence on other medical devices that compensate for vital body functions: Infants requiring cardiorespiratory monitors Children requiring renal dialysis Children requiring other devices such as urinary catheters or colostomy bags as well as substantial nursing care in connection with their disabilities

Table 61–3 • Services and Professionals Utilized by the Child With Multiple Disabilities*

Early Childhood	Middle Childhood	Adolescence
Primary physician	Primary physician	Primary physician
Orthopedist	Orthopedist	Orthopedist
Neurologist	Neurologist	Psychiatrist
Physical therapist	Physical therapist	Physical therapist
Occupational therapist	Occupational therapist	Adaptive physical educator
Speech-language therapist	Speech-language therapist	Adaptive communication specialist
Early intervention teacher	Learning disabilities resources	Prevocational program
Nutrition-feeding team		Community social activities

*Example: child with a neuromotor disorder.

available interventions have multiple potential applications and should be explored more extensively. An example would be therapeutic horseback riding, now shown to be valuable in many syndromes with associated chronic physical or emotional disability.

Children With Multiple Conditions

A vast number of diseases and syndromes cause multiple disabilities. The conditions discussed in this section are representative. They include conditions amenable to habilitation and a productive life (such as the myelodysplasias and intrauterine drug exposures) in addition to other fixed disorders necessitating lifelong comprehensive services (e.g., Prader-Willi syndrome). Progressive conditions (e.g., mucopolysaccharidoses) create a different set of dynamics in health care (Fig. 61–2).

INTRAUTERINE ALCOHOL EXPOSURE

While not completely novel to this time, an emerging threat to the health and well-being of innumerable children has occurred as a direct consequence of the use of alcohol during pregnancy. Not uncommonly, other drugs and medications are involved as well. The teratogenic impact of these materials has undoubtedly affected newborn infants since antiquity, but only recently have physicians noted patterns of malformation and developmental outcomes in relationship to specific substances. Although the long-term and basic neuropathologic effects of opioids, such as cocaine, are still quite puzzling, there is important evidence that ethanol alters basic neural development during fetal life, with resulting severe disability.

Characteristics

A constellation of sometimes subtle craniofacial and other anomalies has been observed in infants born to women with flagrant alcohol abuse during pregnancy. The abnormalities include microcephaly; dysmorphic facial features (flattened midface, narrow palpebral fissures, hypoplastic maxillae, and thin upper lip); prenatal and postnatal growth deficiency; skeletal, cardiac, and urogenital abnormalities; and mental retardation. There is no single pathognomic feature, and therefore, in the collective, an affected infant or child is described as having fetal alcohol syndrome.

The cause of the syndrome is multifactorial. Some fetuses appear to be severely affected by only modest alcohol use, while other infants of mothers with chronic alcoholism seem to have suffered no identifiable effect of the alcohol abuse. In involved infants, a pattern of midline brain anomalies has been identified using magnetic resonance imaging (Swayze et al, 1997). The anomalies include partial to complete callosal agenesis and cavum septi pellucidi. These anomalies are associated with facial abnormalities, a finding consistent with known patterns of embryonic development (see Chapter 25).

As might be expected in a condition of varying severity, children with this syndrome have widely disparate outcomes. Children with the most mild involvement, to the point where the diagnosis itself is in dispute, may have no discernable compromise of organ systems and a pattern of development that cannot be assigned wholly to the syndrome. Other children, especially those with microcephaly, will have notable compromise, requiring special services and supports throughout life.

Establishing the diagnosis of this syndrome should be approached with caution by the physician, especially when the features are mild or the clinical history of mater-

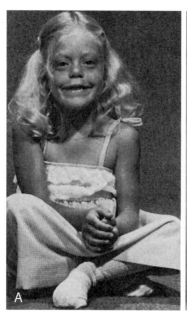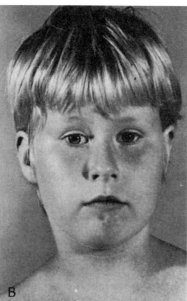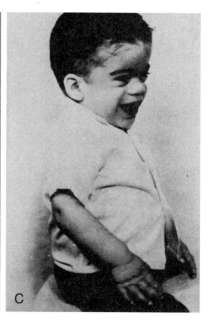

Figure 61–2. Children who have multiple disabilities. *A*, Lisa, 6 years old, with myelodysplasia (lower extremity paralysis, bladder incompetence, shunt for hydrocephalus). She attends first grade, with a resource room. *B*, Susan, 7 years old, with Prader-Willi syndrome (mild retardation, excessive appetite), doing well on a diet for weight control. *C*, Roland, 3½ years old, with Hurler syndrome (skeletal changes, developmental delay, hepatosplenomegaly). He died from congestive heart failure a few months after this photo was taken.

nal alcohol use is inconclusive. For the mildly affected infant or child, once internal organ abnormalities are excluded, assignment of the diagnosis probably has no medical therapeutic value and may convey a self-fulfilling prophecy to parents and teachers who then interpret every childhood difficulty as an unsolvable limitation. From the perspective of the mother (and other family members) the diagnosis attributes responsibility and guilt. Again, in situations in which the maternal history suggests minimal alcohol use, this labeling may be not only unfair but also destructive to maternal nurturance.

Treatment

Medical, educational, and social interventions should respond to the specific needs of the child. Early childhood developmental services are almost always warranted. If maternal alcohol abuse is well-documented, considerable effort is warranted to protect the fetuses in any additional pregnancies, as affected multiple offspring have been documented in numerous families.

MYELODYSPLASIA

Disturbances in the orderly development of the neural tube create the largest group of major malformations known in humans. The spectrum of anomalies ranges from defects of the cephalad neural tube incompatible with extrauterine life (such as anencephaly), to occult spina bifida, usually a serendipitous finding on pelvic radiographic examination. Collectively these conditions, variously referred to a meningocele, myelomeningocele, or spina bifida, or by other specific terms, are called the myelodysplasias.

Neural tube defects occur at a rate of 1 to 2 per 1000 births. Anencephaly or other multiple malformation syndromes, which result in early neonatal death, account for almost 70% of the instances of neural tube variants. The survival rate in infants with encephalocele or myelomeningocele is about 80%.

Characteristics

A majority of children with myelomeningocele survive long-term and have physical disability necessitating assistance with ambulation. The neurologic deficit and associated medical problems are the primary determinants of functional outcome. Neurologic difficulties involve both motor and sensory problems corresponding to the denervated segmental levels. Motor function is characterized by a flaccid muscular paralysis. A combination of spastic and flaccid paralysis is present in 10% to 40% of the children. Abnormal limb positions result from muscle imbalance. Children with disorders at the lumbar and sacral spinal levels may require surgical and orthotic management to permit functional ambulation. Children with lesions at spinal levels above the lumbar region usually are not effective ambulators and require a wheelchair or other adaptive means of locomotion.

Children with spina bifida have a greater incidence of congenital malformations of other neuroectodermal and mesodermal tissues. Seventy percent of children with myelomeningocele are likely to have hydrocephalus; 50% to 80% of these require shunting. Revisions of the shunts are frequently required, especially before the age of 4 years. Hydrocephalus and its treatment complications are the major cause of death in infancy and the preschool years.

The principal sources of morbidity and mortality among children with myelomeningocele beyond 3 years of age are pyelonephritis and renal failure. Urologic evaluation and management should be begun early in the neonatal period. The management of the neurogenic bowel and bladder remains a lifelong process. Depending on the level of the lesion and the associated denervation of bowel and bladder, specific techniques and surgical procedures have been devised to optimize continence and prevent renal deterioration.

The capability for making a prenatal diagnosis of these anomalies now hinges on the observation that an open neural tube defect leaks large quantities of alpha-fetoprotein in the amniotic fluid and across the placenta; elevated amounts are measurable in the maternal serum late in the first trimester. The widespread use of fetal ultrasonography has also facilitated prenatal diagnosis.

Recently a reduction in prevalence of neural tube defects has been demonstrated when pregnant women have diets adequate in folic acid. This observation has prompted scientists to recommend that a ubiquitous foodstuff, such as commercially baked bread, be supplemented with folic acid in a population-based effort to prevent neural tube defects.

Treatment

Aggressive neonatal management of liveborn infants with myelomeningocele is desirable. Care includes repair of the myelomeningocele and shunting of hydrocephalus if the condition is severe or progressive in the first weeks or months.

The goal of comprehensive habilitation of the child with myelodysplasia is to provide an environment facilitating the achievement of maximal levels of motor, intellectual, and social functioning. The immediate and long-term functional goals are established through an understanding of the neurologic dysfunction, the associated medical problems, the level of cognitive function, and psychosocial adjustment (Akins, Davidson, and Hopkins, 1980). The major efforts are to prevent or reduce deformities, to train the child in adaptive functioning and self-care skills, to achieve some means of independent locomotion, to control the elimination of urine and feces, to foster the best possible personal adjustment, and to provide proper education and vocational training.

Experience has shown that guidance of the child with myelodysplasia is best done through a team approach. The team works with the child, family, and primary care physician to develop a management strategy. The clinic team typically includes specialists in pediatrics, physical medicine and rehabilitation, neurosurgery, orthopedics, urology, genetics, nursing, physical and occupational therapy, psychology, and social services.

DUCHENNE TYPE OF MUSCULAR DYSTROPHY

The Duchenne type of muscular dystrophy is a progressive disorder that results in loss of ambulation, eventual total physical incapacitation, and death in late adolescence or early adulthood. In contrast to most of the other conditions discussed in this section, this disorder disrupts the apparently normal development of the young child by superimposing a chronic loss of function.

The disease is evidenced initially by the onset of weakness, generally most obvious in the proximal muscles of the legs. The characteristic "waddling gait" is a manifestation of weakness in the hip girdle area and is a consequence of alternating weight transfer from hip to hip. In the Duchenne type of dystrophy, the myopathy appears to be a primary disease of striated muscle. Variations of the disease or other dystrophies may be secondary to other biochemical or neurophysiologic changes and have different clinical manifestations.

Characteristics

The progressive loss of function in children with Duchenne dystrophy generates an increasing disability. At diagnosis, the child's gait and ability to climb stairs may appear to be normal to the casual observer. Eventually, because of muscle weakness, the child will use a railing or other assistance in negotiating a stairway. The rate of climb slows as weakness progresses. Walking continues to be accomplished unassisted, as are other gross motor maneuvers such as rising from a chair, but ultimately the child loses the ability to lift his or her legs and climb steps. As the disease continues, the child is not able to rise from the sitting position but is able to walk. Thereafter walking depends on stabilization in the lower legs through the use of braces and assistance in balance using a walker. Then the child will be able to stand in bracing support but will be unable to walk even with assistance. Finally the child is confined to a wheelchair and useful motor activity is restricted to the upper extremities.

Progressive physical incapacity can easily lead to withdrawal from social interaction, the fostering of dependence on parents and other family members, and the onset of troubled interpersonal relationships that may reflect the child's preoccupation with the disease process. The basic developmental performance of a specific child relates most directly to the family circumstances and the child's effectiveness in coping with his or her condition. With progressive disability, the likelihood of a severe respiratory compromise or the onset of characteristic cardiomyopathy determines the child's longevity. When the child intellectually grasps the course of his or her disease, there may be chronic depression. Family counseling and a unified strategy in working with the child become essential to maintaining an equilibrium of emotions at home and in preventing unfavorable reactions from brothers and sisters as well as between parents.

Diagnosis and Treatment

The toddler or young preschool child who clinically is suspected of having dystrophy should be the subject of intensive scrutiny to specify the type of dystrophy, which establishes the prognosis. Careful physical examination that centers on the neuromuscular status of the child is indicated. Absence of reflexes or pathologic neurologic signs are not characteristic of the Duchenne type of dystrophy in the early stages of this disease. Gowers' maneuver may be used to demonstrate the pattern of proximal weakness. In this maneuver the child must use his hands and arms to push off the floor from a sitting position to rise to standing, to compensate for the loss of proximal muscle strength in the thighs. The hypertrophic appearance of calf muscles is the classic presenting physical sign. The creatine phosphokinase level should be measured in the serum. Intermediate levels of this enzyme may indicate another type of dystrophy or another myopathy. The disease should be confirmed by muscle biopsy, which in the Duchenne type of dystrophy shows a variety of degenerative changes.

Once the diagnosis is established, the general therapeutic course should be discussed at length with the family. Eventually the child himself will ask direct questions deserving a response. In the early years, the overall goal of treatment is to maintain ambulation and the child's normal daily activities. This includes school attendance and participation in community activities. With progressive weakness, the habilitative measures necessary for the maintenance of ambulation may be undertaken. At this point, the child clearly will recognize the presence of disability and must become an active participant in treatment. Physical therapy to prevent the onset of lower extremity contractures and the maintenance of an active life pattern are overall goals.

The specter of terminal disease makes it difficult to consider the future in the usual sense. Since the child will function well intellectually until the final stages of the disease, it is important to maintain an active personal and family life. The outlook may be defined in achievable increments of weeks or months, giving the child expectations for specific events and activities. Many families consider it important to emphasize the needs of brothers and sisters. If there is more than one affected child in the family, professional counseling and support may be critical for maintenance of family function. Denial of reality is at all times inappropriate; progression should be confronted in a supportive yet determined manner.

PRADER-WILLI SYNDROME

Children who present with a history of infantile hypotonia, obesity, short stature, hypogonadism, and mental retardation share a disorder described as Prader-Willi syndrome.

Characteristics

Owing to the irregular expression of the syndrome, it is still common for some individuals not to be diagnosed until adolescence or early adulthood. With the current emphasis on careful developmental evaluation of young children, this may be less so in future years. The infant who is hypotonic because of a muscular disorder and who shows evidence of delay in other areas of development may well fall into a course consistent with the syndrome. It has been recognized that many of these children show peculiar food-related behavior patterns that can be documented prior to the onset of obesity, including the sneaking of food, gorging at meals, consumption of food products not normally considered appetizing to children, and a general preoccupation with food, food storage, and eating.

Diagnosis and Treatment

Concomitant delays in general development are typical in children with mild to moderate mental retardation. These require that the clinician be aware of the overall pattern of development and issues surrounding eating and weight gain in order to be suspicious of the diagnosis. There are no pathognomonic diagnostic features, although studies usually show specific deletions on chromosome 15 in individuals with Prader-Willi syndrome (see Chapters 23 and 25).

The treatment for individual children centers on their specific cognitive and nutritional needs. The approach to special learning needs resulting from the mental retardation is similar to that in other children with the same degree of disability. Strenuous approaches are advocated to control weight gain. Such measures may include the temporary placement of a child in a controlled environment, generally a specialized residential program, to monitor food intake and institute appropriate dietary change reinforced by behavior modification techniques. A protein-sparing, modified fast has been reported to yield at least temporary success in some individuals who normally have not experienced satiety in their typical eating environment. The complications of extreme obesity, including poor skin hygiene, clinical diabetes mellitus, and stress to the cardiovascular system, are all positively affected by weight control and weight loss when such approaches have been attempted. Radical changes in the home environment, including the locking of refrigerators or the elimination of food from the house, generally place great stress on other family members and result in hostility toward the affected child.

Maintaining motivation and a successful control of weight for the young person with the Prader-Willi syndrome may make possible much more comprehensive integration into community life, including supported employment and semi-independent residential living. Without weight control, severe obesity can readily shorten life expectancy and create major problems in ambulation and other areas. A comprehensive approach to behavior management and activities of daily living is beneficial (Greenswag, 1990).

HURLER SYNDROME

Hurler syndrome is produced by a rare inborn error of metabolism involving mucopolysaccharides. These are large carbohydrate-based polymers with important structural functions in connective tissue, cartilage, cornea, heart, and cerebral cortex. The eponym derives from a Swiss pediatrician, Gertrud Hurler, who described a brother and sister with this disease in 1919. Involved children have a characteristic bodily appearance, which denotes serious accompanying disabilities. Death typically occurs in middle childhood. As with many inborn errors, there is autosomal recessive hereditary transmission. The parents (heterozygotes) are not clinically affected, but in the child with the double (homozygous) abnormality there is an absence of "iduronidase" activity. It is the critical deficiency of this enzyme that leads to all the subsequent complications.

Characteristics

Appearance in the newborn period is nearly normal, but in the months that follow there is a gradual change. The head is relatively large, with a prominent forehead, a broad nose, and a rather flat facial contour. Enlargement of the liver and spleen gives an appearance of fullness to the abdomen. There may be inguinal or umbilical hernias. A limitation in all the joints causes flexion contractures, preventing normal extension of the elbows, fingers, hips, and knees. There is an unusual configuration of certain vertebral bodies, with a "kyphos" in the midback. The corneas are cloudy, although this does not seriously compromise vision. Linear growth is enhanced at first, with most children being well above the 90th percentile at their 1st birthday. Because of the cartilage disturbance at the epiphyses, there follows a gradual growth arrest (by about 3 years). There is hirsutism of the limbs and trunk, chronic nasal discharge is usual, hearing impairment is frequent, and seizures may occur. Cardiac abnormalities are produced by changes in the structure of the valves, subintimal deposits in the coronaries and aorta, and mucopolysaccharide accumulations within the myocardial cells. Repeated respiratory infections are common.

The early developmental progress is nearly normal, but the children come to follow the usual decelerating "metabolic" developmental course. Although independent walking may be achieved by the age of 1 to 1½ years, motor skills generally remain limited. Some words will be learned at a later age, but language development is severely constrained. Toileting independence is rarely acquired. After about 3 years, further learning is sporadic, and one begins to see the loss of previously learned skills. The ability to walk is gradually lost, facility with language recedes as well, and the child shows increasing lack of interest in the environment. Death occurs from chronic pulmonary disease, refractory congestive heart failure, or the complications of decerebration.

Diagnosis

Hurler syndrome is usually diagnosed in the second half of the 1st year of life, at which time the pediatrician and others become concerned by the remarkable appearance of the child (as well as the enlargement of the liver and spleen). By this time, radiologic study of the skeleton reveals many changes (particularly in the metacarpals, spine, and hips). A screening test is available for the detection of increased mucopolysaccharide excretion in the urine (Berry spot test), but precise identification of the syndrome requires documentation of an iduronidase deficiency in the white blood cells or cultured skin fibroblasts. Iduronidase analysis can be performed by an experienced laboratory on cultured amniotic cells as well, providing the capacity for prenatal diagnosis in subsequent pregnancies.

Treatment

Respiratory infections and middle ear infections require diligent treatment. Hernia repair may be required, but incarceration virtually never occurs and anesthesia represents a significant risk. The nasal discharge and obstructive sleep apnea are partially relieved by adenoidectomy, an approach not always justified. Heart failure responds at first to the use of digitalis. Subarachnoid cysts may produce increased intracranial pressure and hydrocephalus, sometimes requiring shunting operations. The ultimate hope for therapy would be the prompt and effective provision of enzyme replacement. Many dozens of children with Hurler syndrome have now had such a therapy sought through bone marrow transplantation. This procedure is ardous, but provocatively useful results are often achieved.

The young child with the Hurler syndrome benefits substantially from a developmental training program. The child has excellent social interactions and gives back a bouyant fellowship. There will be gains in language, motor, and self-help skills and the acquisition of limited preacademic competence. These are precious accomplishments and a store against the coming times when learning is diminished. Medical problems (infections, cardiac disease) may be intrusive, and coordination is needed between the clinical and educational resources. Because of the progressive cerebral disease, there should be a realistic tailoring of goals. The limitation in joint motion cannot be effectively modified by physical therapy. It is appropriate to keep the child's world from shrinking as skills diminish, but eventually the activities possible become very limited.

REFERENCES

Akins C, Davidson R, Hopkins T: The child with myelodysplasia. *In* Scheiner AP, Abroms IF (eds): The Practical Management of the Developmentally Disabled Child. St Louis, Mosby, 1980.

Batshaw ML (ed): Children With Disabilities, 4th ed. Baltimore, Paul H. Brookes Publishing Co, 1997.

Capute AJ, Accardo PJ (eds): Developmental Disabilities in Infancy and Childhood. 2nd ed. Baltimore, Paul H. Brookes Publishing Co, 1996.

Crocker AC: The impact of disabling conditions. *In* Mosby's Resource Guide to Children with Disabilities and Chronic Illness. St Louis, Mosby–Year Book, 1997, pp 22–29.

Crocker AC: Expansion of the health-care delivery systems. *In* Rowitz L (ed). Mental Retardation in the Year 2000. New York, Springer-Verlag Publishers, 1992, pp 163–183.

Epstein SG, Taylor AB, Halberg AS, et al: Enhancing Quality: Standards and Indicators of Quality Care for children With Special Health Care Needs. Boston: New England SERVE, 1989.

Greenswag LR: A community outreach program for individuals with Prader-Willi syndrome. J Ped Health Care 4:32, 1990.

Nelson RP: Community services for children with mental retardation. Ped Ann 18:615, 1989.

Newacheck PW, Stoddard JJ: Prevalence and impact of multiple childhood illnesses. J Pediatrics 124:40, 1994.

Palfrey JS, Haynie M, Porter S, et al: Prevalence of medical technology assistance among children in Massachusetts in 1987 and 1990. Public Health Rep 109:226, 1994.

Porter S, Haynie M, Bierle T, et al (eds): Children and Youth Assisted by Medical Technology in Educational Settings: Guidelines for Care, 2nd ed. Baltimore, Paul H. Brookes Publishing Co, 1997.

Rubin IL, Crocker AC (eds): Developmental Disabilities: Delivery of Medical Care for Children and Adults. Philadelphia, Lea & Febiger, 1989.

Stein REK, Bauman LJ, Westbrook LE, et al: Framework for identifying children who have chronic conditions: The case for a new definition. J Pediatrics 122:342, 1993.

Swayze VW, Johnson VP, Hanson JW, et al: Magnetic resonance imaging of brain anomalies in fetal alcohol syndrome. Pediatrics 99:232, 1997.

Taylor AB, Epstein SG, Crocker AC: Health care for children with special needs. *In* Schlesinger M, Eisenberg L (eds): Children in a Changing Health Care System: Prospects and Proposals. Baltimore, Johns Hopkins University Press, 1990, pp 27–48.

62 Emotional Problems in Children With Serious Developmental Disabilities

Ludwik S. Szymanski

 In studies of populations of children and adolescents with mental retardation, the prevalence of psychopathy diagnosed by standard criteria has been as high as 64%.

The diagnostic process is similar to the evaluation of children who are not retarded brought in by parents who are the principal informants.

It is now well accepted that all forms of mood disorder can be seen in persons with Down syndrome, although the diagnosis is often missed.

Referral for child psychiatric consultation is indicated if the child's distrubance is pervasive or functionally limiting.

Behaviors, Emotions, and Mental Disorders in Children With Mental Retardation

Behavioral problems are one of the most frequent, if not the most frequent, impediment to the progress and adaptation of children who have mental retardation. Whereas disruptive behaviors are the usual reason for referring the child for mental health consultation, less obvious symptoms such as lack of motivation, depression, or anxiety may impair adaptation as well. Terms such as *behavioral disorders, emotional disorders,* and *mental disorders* have been used in these instances, although they have not been defined, except for the latter, which refers to behavioral or psychological patterns of an individual associated with present distress or disability (*DSM-IV,* 1994). Thus, any behavioral problem serious enough to require treatment might be included here. The term *behavioral disorder* is often used for problems thought to be a reaction to an environmental situation and not given a formal psychiatric diagnosis. However, this is an artificial distinction and not particularly helpful (Szymanski, 1994).

It is now generally agreed that the prevalence of mental disorders in persons with mental retardation is higher than in comparable groups of persons without retardation. In the classic Isle of Wight study of Rutter and coworkers in 1976, of the total population of children 9 to 11 years of age, psychopathology was several times more frequent in children with mental retardation. In studies of selected and representative populations of children and adolescents with mental retardation, the prevalence of psychopathology diagnosed by standard criteria has been as high as 64% (Bregman, 1991). All types of mental disorders have been described; and there is no evidence of occurrence of disorders unique to this population. Among 99 children and adolescents (under 18 years of age) with mental retardation referred to the Developmental Evalua-

tion Center at the Children's Hospital in Boston, the most frequent diagnosis was one of a pervasive developmental disorder (PDD) (in 32%).

DIAGNOSTIC ASSESSMENT OF CHALLENGING BEHAVIORS

Persons with mental retardation are usually multiply disabled, with dysfunctions in several areas contributing to the behavioral manifestations. Thus, the assessment should be comprehensive and not limited to the formal "label" and coding. The recent diagnostic manual of the American Association on Mental Retardation (AAMR, 1992) specifies assessment of mental retardation in four dimensions: intellectual and adaptive, psychological and emotional; physical, health, and etiology; and environmental. Szymanski and Crocker (1989) described the concept of "expanded" diagnosis, which includes description of the clinical presentation justifying the diagnosis, the patient's strengths and liabilities, and comprehensive recommendations. Such diagnostic statements may resolve doubts and anxiety about otherwise incomprehensible behaviors as well as lead to an appropriate treatment or prevent an inappropriate one. A "generic" diagnosis, such as of "aggression," will not lead to a proper treatment, since aggressive behavior might be associated with depression, psychosis, personality disorder, and so on, each requiring different treatment (Szymanski et al, 1997). For instance, an aggressive youngster who is in a behavioral program because of "attention-getting" may actually be psychotic and in need of relevant treatment, whereas another one, with superficially similar symptoms and treated with an antipsychotic drug, might not have a psychotic illness but may be reacting to institutional boredom and deprivation.

PRINCIPLES OF PSYCHIATRIC DIAGNOSTIC ASSESSMENT OF PERSONS WITH MENTAL RETARDATION

In most cases, the diagnosis can be made using the standard diagnostic schema of the *DSM-IV* (*DSM-IV,* 1994). Certain modifications might be necessary, depending on the patient's level of development, and communication skills in particular (just as with young children without mental retardation). The assessment is done in the context of the total clinical picture (including developmental levels in various domains, associated disabilities, and psychosocial factors). Thus considerable clinical expertise with this population and interdisciplinary collaboration of several specialists may be necessary. The diagnostic process is similar to evaluation of children who are not retarded, who are brought in by parents who are the principal informants. The history has to be comprehensive, starting with the reasons for referral at this time (especially if the problem has existed for some time). Multiple informants (such as parents, teachers, and therapists) might provide better description of the problem, such as in what situations it does and does not occur.

The clinical interview with the patient is essential, starting with the observation of a child's interaction with parents and peers in the waiting room, where one may obtain more data than attempting to interrogate a frightened child in the examining room. In any case, sufficient time should be taken. Impressionistic, instant diagnoses should be avoided. The level and quality of a child's communication patterns should be recognized, perhaps by watching how the parents and the child communicate. With verbal children, an interview conducted in a supportive, friendly manner, with some directiveness and structure, in concrete language understandable to the child, may yield significant information. The best opening gambit is to focus on the child's strengths and successes rather than on failures. Nonverbal techniques, such as observation of the child's play, are also helpful. The findings should be compared with descriptions of the child's behavior at home and at school. Rating scales, such as Conners Rating Scales (parents' and teachers' versions), Reiss Screen, and the Aberrant Behavior Checklist, may supplement the clinical observations (Reiss, 1994).

OUTLINE OF ASSESSMENT OF CHALLENGING BEHAVIORS

The following is a general guide to obtaining the history and clinical observations that are needed for the diagnostic assessment and treatment planning.

1. Presenting complaints
   a. Description of the problems: since when did they exist, environmental and other events prior to or around time of onset, detailed and concrete description of behavioral manifestations, in what situations they occur and do not occur
   b. Caregivers' expectations of this referral (including overt and "hidden" agenda)
   c. Past management: concrete description, consistency of implementation, results
   d. Psychotropic medications: dosages, length of use, response and adverse effects
   e. Other medications: dosages, length of use and relationship to presenting symptoms, possible psychotropic side effects
2. Past History

   a. Etiology of the disability (if unknown, adequacy of past assessments)
   b. Developmental and health history
   c. Educational/habilitative history; services received, progress
   d. Environmental-psychosocial history (family composition, living situation, support system and services)
   e. Possibility of exposure to abuse (sexual and other)
3. Personal characteristics
   a. What is the child like: strengths, skills (verbal and nonverbal communication, self-care, social, work, others), attention span, predominant mood and mood stability over time and in various situations vs. cyclicity
   b. Awareness of own disability, motivation for independence vs. dependency
   c. Interpersonal relating: eye contact, expression of affection, trust, personal attachments, separation anxiety, peer relationship and friendships
   d. Affective expression: includes verbal and nonverbal expression of emotions, self-control, impulsivity
   e. Sexually related behaviors and interests: developmental appropriateness, appropriateness of expression
4. Family/caregiver's assessment
   a. Understanding of, and feelings about, child's disability
   b. Child management patterns: limits, consistency, expectations, empathy, promoting independence
   c. Family history of developmental and mental disorders
   d. Effects of child's disability on family's functioning
   e. Brothers and sisters: adjustment and attitudes to the disabled child
5. Psychiatric "review of systems"
   a. Mood: appropriateness to developmental level, cyclicity, predominance of dysfunctional moods (depression, anxiety, agitation)
   b. Delusions, hallucinations
   c. Fears/phobias, obsessions and compulsions, stereotypic, self-stimulatory, self-injurious behaviors, motor tics
   d. History of regression: loss of skill and/or memory
   e. Substance use and abuse
   f. Symptoms suggesting reaction to abuse, such as vigilance, flashbacks, frightening dreams, reenacting traumatic event, avoidance of certain stimuli, places, and persons
   g. Are there clusters of symptoms suggesting a diagnosis of a specific mental disorder according to the *DSM-IV* criteria?

DIAGNOSIS OF SPECIFIC MENTAL DISORDERS

In the following section, some of the main categories of mental disorders are briefly reviewed. The focus is on adaptation of the *DSM-IV* diagnostic criteria to persons with developmental disabilities.

Pervasive Developmental Disorders

Autistic disorder was first described in 1943 by Kanner. Later, he and his followers believed that it was associated with normal or above-normal intelligence and that it was caused by inappropriate parenting patterns. Both beliefs were disproved by later research. It is currently accepted that 75% to 80% of children with autism have also comorbid mental retardation. Thus these diagnoses are not mutually exclusive. The current tendency is to view autism as a behavioral syndrome, probably consisting of subsets with different etiology. The diagnosis of autism was made "formal" only in 1980, when the *DSM-III* introduced a category of *pervasive developmental disorders,* which included infantile autism. Currently, in the *DSM-IV* the PDD category includes autistic disorder, Rett's disorder, childhood disintegrative disorder, Asperger disorder, and PDD not-otherwise-specified (PDD-NOS). The diagnosis of autistic disorder requires qualitative impairment in social interaction (such as in eye contact, peer relationships, sharing emotions); qualitative impairment in interpersonal communication; and restricted, repetitive, and stereotyped patterns of behavior (such as preoccupation with restricted patterns of interest, nonfunctional routines, motor mannerisms). The onset of at least some of the symptoms must be prior to 3 years of age. Children with significant mental retardation alone might also engage in stereotypic behaviors, but they do not show symptoms of the first or second group of these criteria, although their patterns of relating and communication are immature for chronologic age. Children with Asperger syndrome by definition have no significant delay in language and cognitive development. The PDD-NOS subcategory does not really have diagnostic criteria. It should be used when criteria for autistic disorder are not fully met, such as because of time of onset or atypical or less severe symptomatology; however, there should be a pervasive impairment in the development of reciprocal social interaction (not just shyness). Thus the diagnosis of PDD-NOS should not be used for children who relate appropriately to their developmental level but who have poor language skills or self-stimulatory behavior. Furthermore there is no diagnosis simply of PDD, as this terms applies to a category and not to a single disorder.

The further details on PDD are contained in Chapter 60.

Mental Disorders Due to a General Medical Condition

This term replaced in the *DSM-IV* the previous one of "organic" mental disorders and syndromes. The latter had been often inappropriately used in children with mental retardation instead of a more specific diagnosis. The premise was that their behavioral problems must also be the result of the brain pathology that caused mental retardation. The "organic" diagnoses were used liberally, even though in children without mental retardation the same behavioral presentation would be given different diagnosis. The *DSM-IV* requires clinical, historical, or laboratory evidence, or a combination of these, that the mental disorder is the direct physiologic consequence of a medical condition (which is listed separately on Axis III). Such a medical condition

might include brain traumas, infections, tumors and vascular disorders, and medication intoxication.

Another problem is with differentiation between mental retardation and dementia. By definition, the diagnosis of mental retardation can be made only if the onset is prior to the age of 18 years, whereas dementia can be diagnosed at any age. The diagnosis of dementia requires that there will be deterioration of memory as well as personality, abstract thinking, judgment, or other cognitive functions. Assessing this in young children may be difficult. According to the *DSM-IV*, diagnosis of dementia might not be appropriate before the age of 4 to 6 years, and it does not have to be made if the condition is sufficiently characterized by the diagnosis of mental retardation alone.

EXAMPLE

A 19-year-old woman with Down syndrome was referred because of noisy grunts, self-stimulation, swearing, and stubbornness, all of which interfered with her schooling. On examination, abrupt movements of shoulders and arms as if she were shrugging, often accompanied by grunts, were noticed. Diagnosis of Tourette disorder was made. On 1.5 mg thioridazine, the movements and grunts disappeared. Behavioral measures helped her to develop better behavioral adjustment.

Behavioral disorders that result from intake of, or withdrawal from, a medication should be mentioned here. This is particularly relevant for persons with significant mental retardation who often have associated medical disorders and are on multiple medications. A full list of such drugs and their effects would be beyond the scope of this chapter. Hyperactivity resulting from phenobarbital, depression from beta-blockers, atropine psychosis from antiparkinsonian agents, and irritability with sleep and eating disorders following an abrupt discontinuation of antipsychotics may serve as examples.

Psychotic Disorders

Schizophrenia and other psychotic disorders may be difficult to diagnose accurately in persons who have significant retardation, since, in the absence of language skills, recognizing hallucinations, delusions, and thought disorder in general may not be possible. In such patients, the less specific diagnoses of undifferentiated schizophrenia or psychotic disorder "not otherwise specified" might have to be made based on behavioral changes as compared with premorbid behavior. In particular, the appearance of symptoms of social or affective withdrawal, bizarre behaviors not seen before, and deterioration in the level of functioning may raise the suspicion of such diagnosis. On the other hand, psychosis should not be diagnosed in a person with significant mental retardation merely on the basis of self-stimulatory or aggressive behavior.

EXAMPLE

A young man, age 17 years, with moderate retardation due to the fragile X syndrome was referred because of aggression. He had done very well at school until a week prior to referral, when he reportedly attacked his gym teacher. The history clarified that he felt very embarrassed because she demanded that he jump rope, which was difficult for him. When she prompted him physically, he pushed her away. This was interpreted as aggression, and male teachers were called, who restrained him on the floor. After that he started to believe that the teachers put him down in order to rape him, and that music broadcast at the school had coded messages to that effect. Diagnosis of a brief psychotic disorder was made. He was treated with thioridazine and supportive therapy, and within 2 months recovered completely.

A severe disorder of young children, thought to be an early stage of one form of schizophrenia, has been described (Cantor, 1988). These children are usually markedly hypotonic and have early sleep disorder, unusual fears, social withdrawal, and at a later age symptoms of thought disorder. They often are seen first in developmental disabilities clinics because of the motor and cognitive abnormalities.

Mood Disorders

Although earlier literature questioned whether persons with retardation could at all suffer from depression, it is now well accepted that all forms of mood disorder can be seen in this population, including persons with Down syndrome, who are usually considered happy and social (Sovner and Hurley, 1983; Szymanski and Biederman, 1984). This diagnosis is often missed, however, for several reasons. Depressed persons with mental retardation are often ignored, since they may be quiet and do not disturb their caregivers. As with psychoses, verbal productions cannot be used to assess the affective state in persons with limited or no language. However, most of the diagnostic criteria for mood disorders in the *DSM-IV* can be satisfied on the basis of observations made by persons other than the patient (such as caregivers). These include observations of vegetative signs (sleeping and eating disorders), irritability, psychomotor retardation, agitation or aggressive behaviors, withdrawal, anhedonia, and general appearance of sadness. Persons with mental retardation who have even limited language skills can provide quite good information about their feelings, although they are apt to use concrete and simple descriptions (such as stating that they feel sick or not good, rather than depressed).

EXAMPLE

A 17-year-old woman who is nonverbal and has severe mental retardation was admitted because of progressive refusal to eat, weight loss, and crying of several months' duration. Results of medical evaluation were negative. Psychotic depression was diagnosed and on imipramine she did well and gained weight. Several weeks later she became agitated and aggressive and did not sleep. She gradually improved when the medication was tapered and stopped, but 3 weeks later the original, preadmission symptoms returned. Atypical bipolar disorder was diagnosed, supported by family history. Lithium was started and the patient improved, returned to her premorbid state, and remained well.

Stereotypic Movement Disorder and Self-Injurious Behaviors

This disorder is characterized by motor behaviors, such as persistent rocking, that are repetitive, driven, and result in significant functional impairment. A specifier "with self-injurious behavior" (SIB) is used if the behavior (such as self-hitting, head banging) results in an injury requiring medical care. Serious damage may result from these behaviors, such as retinal detachment and blindness. Often the individual may switch from one type of behavior to another. Stereotypic behaviors occur in up to one third of persons with mental retardation, and severe SIB in 2% (Reiss, 1990). SIB is more common when the retardation is severe and in certain mental retardation syndromes, such as Lesch-Nyhan and Cornelia de Lange. The causes of these behaviors are still a matter of controversy and psychological mechanism or disorder in endogenous opioid and serotonin systems have been postulated (Harris, 1995). The true cause is probably multidetermined, with neurobiological and environmental factors playing a role. The latter (e.g., the secondary gain of attracting the caregivers' attention) may maintain such behavior. In some nonverbal individuals, the SIB may be related to pain from a medical condition.

Treatment Interventions

TREATMENT PLANNING

Clinicians should resist the temptations and pressure to immediately "prescribe something to take the edge off" challenging behaviors before the total clinical picture and factors involved are understood. The first step is, of course, assessment of immediate safety of the patient and others and, if necessary, implementing measures to ensure that safety, which may include close supervision, medication, and hospitalization. The following are the general principles in treatment planning:

1. Comprehensive, diagnostic assessment as delineated previously.
2. Incorporating the mental health intervention into the comprehensive treatment and habilitation program that should address patient's needs in all areas.
3. Addressing the environmental and management issues that might be causing and maintaining the presenting symptoms.
4. Starting with treatment modalities with best risk-to-benefit ratio.
5. Establishing clear goals and priorities of the treatment and means of monitoring its effectiveness and side effects.
6. Ensuring that the caregivers and the patient, if capable, participate in the development of the treatment program, understand it, and effectively collaborate in its implementation.
7. Continuing the treatment only if it is proven effective and the side effects are acceptable.
8. Ensuring that human rights and legal aspects are respected.

SPECIFIC TREATMENT MEASURES

Psychotherapies

Psychotherapy with persons with mental retardation may be very effective if it is goal-oriented, uses communication measures appropriate for the patient, and has structured approaches. The patient should have some degree of language (including speech, sign language, computer typing) that permits effective communication with the therapist (Szymanski, 1980; Sigman, 1985). Group therapy may be very effective, as it provides peer support and social opportunities.

Psychotropic Drugs

The periodic use of these drugs is described in detail in Chapter 82. There is no evidence that they have a unique action in persons with retardation. In using these drugs, one must follow the same principles of sound medical practice as with patients who do not have mental retardation. Unfortunately the psychotropic drugs have often been misused, particularly in institutions, under pressure from the administration and the nonmedical staff to render the clients docile and "compliant." These drugs should be prescribed (as any other drug) by a physician who is thoroughly familiar with them. They should be a part of a comprehensive treatment program, not a substitute for it. One should remember that various treatment modalities such as psychotherapy, milieu therapy, and behavior modification have a synergistic effect with the medications. As much as possible, these drugs should be used for their designated action in specific disorders. For example, thioridazine should be used as an antipsychotic and not as a nonspecific "major tranquilizer." When used in this way and in proper dosage, these drugs are often very effective and permit the patients to participate meaningfully in a variety of treatment and educational activities. For instance, there is no specific drug for aggression. Aggressive behavior may be caused by psychosis, depression, a painful condition, anger, or reaction to environmental conditions, each of which requires quite different interventions. High doses of an antipsychotic drug might suppress any aggressive behavior, but at the cost of side effects and suppressing the person's general functioning.

The most common reasons for failure of psychopharmacologic treatment include improper indications due to lack of accurate diagnostic psychiatric assessment; using the drugs as the sole treatment while ignoring other problems, such as environmental factors; continuation of treatment not proven efective; and lack of caregivers' cooperation. Persons with mental retardation are often given multiple drugs for various purposes. Whenever possible, consideration should be given to the use of a fewest number of drugs. For example, a patient treated with phenytoin for seizures who develops a bipolar disorder might be switched to carbamazepine, which has both anticonvulsant and mood stabilizing effects, rather that being given lithium in addition to phenytoin.

Another caveat in the use of drugs in this population concerns side effects. Nonverbal persons may have considerable difficulty in reporting side effects. They should be monitored carefully, according to predetermined criteria and baseline data. Some side effects may mimic original symptoms; for example, akathisia may look like an increase in preexisting agitation, especially if the persons cannot describe how they feel. The involuntary movements of tardive dyskinesia may be difficult to differentiate from preexisting stereotypies. Videotaping the patient's behavior prior to starting the drug may help in this differentiation.

Prevention of Emotional Maladjustment

THE PEDIATRICIAN'S ROLE

Pediatricians have the best opportunity to provide the family of a child with mental retardation with support and guidance, which is most important in preventing a child's emotional and behavioral problems. Most parents understand that pediatricians cannot cure most cases of mental retardation, but they want from them explanations of the child's problems, support, guidance, and education as to what they can do for the child. The not uncommon statement of the physician, "There is nothing you can do," is particularly destructive because it conveys an attitude of helplessness and hopelessness.

What the family needs, first of all, is to learn from the pediatrician to regard the child as an individual who has human worth as does any other child. The physician who inquires about and points out the child's personal characteristics and strengths (rather than focusing on the impairments only), who talks to the child and responds with understanding to parental questions, conveys the message of individualization. Providing the parents with up-to-date information about the child's condition, referring them for a second opinion to a specialized clinic and for support to a parents' group, advising on services, and giving "permission" to set limits and proper expectations for the child are all important. The pediatrician can teach the family to provide the child with appropriate stimulation, to set the necessary limits, to promote the child's independence, and to focus on the child's strengths rather than disabilities. All of this will help the child to develop a positive self-image.

The pediatrician should also be able to provide early identification of behavioral problems that are related to environmental situations or to normal developmental crises. It is important to help the parents learn to pay most attention to the child when he or she behaves appropriately, rather than to discuss only what they should do when the child misbehaves.

UTILIZATION OF PSYCHIATRIC CONSULTATION

If there is a suspicion of a more pervasive, functionally limiting, behavioral or emotional disturbance, referral for child psychiatric consultation is indicated. One should avoid the common tendency to refer only patients who are disturbing to others, while neglecting those who are otherwise disturbed. Choice of a consultant is important, since most child psychiatrists have little experience and training in developmental disabilities. Psychiatrists associated with the University Affiliated Programs (for developmental disabilities) are usually familiar with this population. The success of a consultation depends to a considerable degree on good communication between the pediatrician and the child psychiatrist. A clear statement of the reasons for consultation is necessary, as are a developmental and medical history and careful assessment for possible medical conditions that might be related to the behavioral symptoms. The child should not be referred for "medication review," but for a comprehensive assessment. Conversely, prompt and preferably detailed feedback by the consultant is important. The psychiatrists are expected to synthesize the available information about the child into a comprehensive assessment rather than limit themselves to prescribing medication or making psychological interpretations only.

REFERENCES

American Association on Mental Retardation (AAMR): Mental Retardation: Definition, Classification, and Systems of Supports. Washington, DC, AAMR, 1992.

Bergman J: Current developments in the understanding of mental retardation: Part II: psychopathology. J Am Acad Child Adolesc Psychiatry 30:861, 1991.

Cantor S: Childhood Schizophrenia. New York, Guilford Press, 1988.

Diagnostic and Statistical Manual of Mental Disorders, 4th ed (DSM-IV): Washington, DC, American Psychiatric Association, 1994.

Harris J: Developmental Neuropsychiatry. New York, Oxford University Press, 1995.

Reiss S: Prevalence of dual diagnosis in community-based day programs in the Chicago metropolitan area. Am J Ment Retard 94:578, 1990.

Reiss S: Handbook of Challenging Behavior: Mental Health Aspects of Mental Retardation. Worthington, OH, IDS Publishing Co, 1994.

Rutter M, Tizard J, Yule W, et al: Isle of Wight Studies, 1964–1974. Psychol Med 6:313–332, 1976.

Sigman M: Individual and group psychotherapy with mentally retarded adolescents. *In* Sigman M (ed): Children with Emotional Disorders and Developmental Disabilities. Orlando, Grune & Stratton, 1985.

Sovner R, Hurley AD: Do the mentally retarded suffer from affective illness? Arch Gen Psychiatry 40:61, 1983.

Szymanski LS: Mental retardation and mental health: concepts, aetiology and incidence. *In* Bouras N (ed): Mental Health in Mental Retardation: Recent Advances and Practices. Cambridge: Cambridge University Press, 1994.

Szymanski LS: Individual psychotherapy with retarded person. *In* Szymanski LS, Tanguay PE (eds): Emotional Disorders of Mentally Retarded Persons. Baltimore, University Park Press, 1980.

Szymanski LS, Biederman J: Depression and anorexia nervosa of persons with Down's syndrome. Am J Ment Defic 89:246, 1984.

Szymanski LS, Crocker AC: Mental Retardation. *In* Kaplan HI, Sadock BJ (eds): Comprehensive Textbook of Psychiatry, 5th ed. Baltimore, Williams & Wilkins, 1989.

Szymanski LS, King B, Goldberg B, et al: Diagnosis of mental disorders in people with mental retardation. *In* Reiss S, Aman MG (eds): Psychotropic Medications and Developmental Disabilities: The International Consensus Handbook. Columbus, OH, Ohio State University, 1998.

63 Disorders of Speech and Language

Desmond P. Kelly • Janine I. Sally

The development of effective communication skills represents one of the more formidable hurdles in child development. In this chapter, a broad array of disorders of speech and language are explored in a systematic fashion. Clinicians need to be skilled at the early detection of such breakdowns in human communication. This chapter offers a convenient classification system that can enable providers of health care to be responsive when parents and schools express concern over a child's acquisition of language and effective speech.

Language is fundamental to learning, social interaction, and development of personal identity. Disorders of communication are the most common developmental problems in preschool-aged children, and 7% to 10% of children are considered to be functioning below the norm in some aspect of speech or language ability. Three percent to 6% of children are affected by a specific expressive or receptive language disorder and are at increased risk for later difficulties in reading and writing (Bashir, Stark, and Graham, 1992). Health professionals working with children should be acutely attuned to variations in language development and early signs of communication difficulties. Early diagnosis and initiation of therapeutic and educational interventions offer the best chance of optimal outcome for children with disorders of speech and language.

Definitions

The child who is not developing communication skills along typical trajectories presents a complex challenge to the clinical skills of the practitioner. Equally challenging is the terminology used in this field of study.

Language is a system of symbolic representation that is used to communicate meanings, feelings, ideas, and intentions. *Speech* is the expression of language in the verbal mode and can be more specifically defined as the production of an acoustic signal. Patterns of sound are grouped to form acoustic symbols that convey meaning according to the rules of the listener's language. *Phonemes* are the units of sound in speech. *Phonology* refers to the order in which the speech sounds form the language symbols or words. A *morpheme* is the smallest unit in a language that conveys meaning. *Semantics* refers to words and their meaning. These meanings will vary depending on the *morphology* of the word (e.g., prefixes, suffixes, inflection). *Syntax* is the order in which words are grouped to form sentences and convey messages. Syntax is bound by the grammatical rules of specific languages. *Discourse* is the organization of larger volumes of language into paragraphs, passages, stories, directions, or explanations. *Pragmatics* is the social use of language and is related to the meaning of messages in various contexts. This is the

communicative use of language and is a fundamental component. *Metalinguistics* is an understanding of how language works. *Expressive language,* or language production, entails the ability to form words from sounds (phonology) and combine words with correct meaning (semantics) into sentences (syntax) that are appropriate to the social situation (pragmatics). *Receptive language,* or language processing, likewise entails the ability to process sounds and recognize the meaning of words being spoken (semantics and vocabulary) and how these are combined in sentences and discourse (comprehension) and to interpret the ideas and feelings of others through language (pragmatics).

Speech has a number of specific components and qualities. *Articulation* is the process by which the speech signal is formed by the movements of the oral structures. *Voice* refers to vocalization, or the production of the sound created by vocal fold vibration. *Phonation* is the physical and physiologic process of vocal fold vibration. *Resonance* is the amplification and filtering of sound waves produced by vocal fold vibration. Resonators include the oral and nasal cavities. *Fluency* is a reflection of the appropriate rhythm and flow of the speech signal. Dysfluencies can present as inappropriate pauses in speech with a halting pattern, or as rapid repetitions of units of speech such as occurs in stuttering. *Prosody* refers to the intonation, inflection, and cadence of speech.

Development

Language development combines verbal and nonverbal components in a dynamic and interactive process that begins with the earliest developmental experiences and follows a predictable course. The rate of acquisition of language skills can vary quite broadly, however, and it is affected by a number of biological and environmental factors. It appears that there are sex differences in the patterns of development and the functional organization of the brain for language. Recent research utilizing functional magnetic resonance imaging has demonstrated more diffuse activation of neural systems in females compared with males during phonologic processing tasks. In males, brain activation appears lateralized to the left inferior frontal gyrus regions, in contrast to females, in whom both the left and right regions are active (Shaywitz et al, 1995). This bilateral representation of language in girls might explain why they are less likely than boys to manifest language problems in early childhood.

PRELINGUISTIC PERIOD (BIRTH TO 12 MONTHS)

During the prelinguistic, or preverbal, stage, the social use of language (pragmatics) emerges. Communicative intents are initially nonverbal (such as making eye contact and smiling), but the expectations are that children will eventually be able to code their intents and apply specific discourse rules through the language code. For example, the game of "peek-a-boo" between a caretaker and a child is a joint activity that provides a framework for turn-taking behavior in conversations. The preverbal stage is also characterized by the beginnings of phonologic development, and a systematic evolution of productive vocalizations appears over the first year. Repetitive vocalizations at 3 to 4 months evolve into babbling of chains of consonant-vowel combinations at 8 months. By the age of 12 months, the child is using single words specifically as well as nonverbal gestures and responds to simple requests such as waving good-bye or pointing to pictures.

EARLY LINGUISTIC PERIOD (1 TO 3 YEARS)

During the early linguistic period, children use words to code what they know through concepts. The child's interactions are initiated by words that are initially child-centered such as "all gone," "more," or "no," and she responds to the communicative partner with these words, following rules of discourse. The nonverbal formats continue and are used in conjunction with words as phonology, semantics, and pragmatics also develop interactively. Between 12 and 18 months of age, the child uses single words, with a vocabulary growing to 20 words. During the two-word stage from 18 to 24 months of age, syntax begins to emerge as children combine and order words into patterns. Usually the word patterns relate knowledge about something such as a specific topic. Vocabulary grows from a few dozen to several hundred words, with two to three exchanges per topic and increasing imitative abilities. The child shows much more flexibility in his ability to communicate interaction more precisely. The three- to four-word stage, from 24 to 36 months of age, marks a great deal of expansion of vocabulary and extended application of previously learned words. The final linguistic component, morphology, also emerges, such as expressing intent and numbers (e.g., two cookies). The child becomes more adept at using words in the appropriate order and using specific patterns to communicate feelings, desires, and interests, while using nonverbal formats more supportively. The 3-year-old child is able to say her name, age, and sex, recognize common objects and pictures, and follow two- to three-step commands.

PRESCHOOL YEARS (3 TO 5 YEARS)

During the preschool years, more complex language forms emerge such as prepositional phrases ("on the table"),

conditionals ("if . . . then"), and connectors ("because," "therefore," "but"). During this time the child becomes more efficient in accurately coding intent and meaning and in adjusting pragmatically to different social situations. Preschool children are able to tell stories and follow three-component commands and to anticipate future events ("tomorrow we're going to . . ."). They can respond to questions such as "who," "where," and "what" but may still have difficulty with "how" and "why" (although frequently asking "why?"). By 4 years of age, speech should be almost fully intelligible to a stranger (Haynes, Pindzola, and Emerick, 1992). Warning signs of delayed acquisition of early language skills are listed in Table 63–1.

EARLY SCHOOL YEARS (5 TO 12 YEARS)

Upon school entry, new demands are placed on all language systems. The child will be required to pragmatically adapt to the new context of the classroom and other school setting which are very different from the home environment. In large groups, turn taking will be expected, and the ability to adapt the discourse rules and flexibility in conveying ideas will also be required to ensure academic and social success. The expansion of skills takes place through semantics. New words related to specific academic content must also be learned and used. Directions and new information will have to be comprehended to master the specific academic areas. By 7 to 8 years of age the child is using language symbolically, with the ability to use language to think about language (metalinguistics). By the time a child reaches the age of 12, he has many of the cognitive and linguistic skills of an adult.

Differential Diagnosis

The differential diagnosis of speech and language disorders encompasses a wide spectrum of conditions that can result in dysfunction of the neural systems and the peripheral structures responsible for the perception, processing, and production of speech and language. There is considerable overlap of these influences, which hinders precise categorization or subtyping. Systems of classification of speech and language disorders vary depending on the professional background of the authors. Medical classification systems focus on causes of language disorder, whereas linguistic classifications focus more on observed patterns of disorder. Figure 63–1 is an attempt to depict the domains of dysfunction that can interact to impede speech and language abilities.

EXAMPLE

John is an 18-month-old boy whose parents are concerned that he does not say any words clearly. He was the full-term product of an uncomplicated pregnancy, and his early development appeared to progress normally. At 11 months of age he was hospitalized with fever and emesis. He experienced two prolonged seizures at that time and has been on anticonvulsant medication since then, with no further seizures. He has been noted to have decreased strength and coordination of the right arm and

Table 63–1 • Warning Signs of Speech or Language Disorders

Age Range	Signs
First 12 months	Does not smile at familiar faces or voices by 2 months
	Does not smile at other people by 3 months
	Does not try to imitate any sounds by 4 months
	Does not babble by 8 months
	Shows no ability or interest in games such as "peek-a-boo" by 8 months
	Uses no single words by 12 months
	Does not use any gestures such as waving "bye-bye" or shaking head by 12 months
	Does not point to any objects or pictures by 12 months
12–24 months	Does not use at least 15 words by 18 months
	Prefers gestures instead of vocalizing wants or needs by 18 months
	Struggles when attempting to imitate sounds or has a limited or a restricted use of consonants and vowels by 18 months
	Sequences of sounds in familiar words are unclear, not understood by 2 years
	Does not use two-word utterances by 2 years
	Does not imitate words or actions by 2 years
	Does not follow simple instructions by 2 years
24–36 months	Does not combine words into short phrases or sentences by 3 years
	Does not initiate interactions with others by 3 years
	Is not able to use the sounds /p, h, m, n, t, d, k, g/ correctly before 3 years
	Frequent expression of frustration in communicative situations
	Restricted or repetitive play with toys
	Limited vocabulary, possibly use of nonspecific vocabulary (e.g., "this," "that one")
	Does not interact or play with others
	Unable to understand and answer simple questions
4 years	Unable to be understood by people outside of family
	Cannot retell simple stories or recall recent events clearly
	Sentences seemed unorganized, with a lot of errors
	Sentences contain many sound errors, either substitutions or omissions

leg. He has received physical therapy and occupational therapy, and motor skills are progressing. He has had some difficulty chewing and swallowing solids, and there is increased drooling. There are no behavioral concerns. He is described as affectionate, seeking out social interaction and expressing his needs by gesture and vocalization. Two or three words are distinguishable (e.g., "juice" and "bye"). His parents question whether there is a need for further language testing or therapy.

John's history raises questions about a number of possible conditions that could be contributing to his language delay.

HEARING LOSS

Significant hearing loss, either sensorineural or conductive, which is congenital or sustained prior to development of language, is invariably associated with some degree of language impairment. Some studies of children with language delay have identified hearing loss as a contributing factor in up to 50% of cases. The severity of language impairment is influenced by multiple factors, including the degree of hearing loss, age at diagnosis, and timing and appropriateness of interventions to amplify hearing and to establish systems of communication. This subject is addressed in greater detail in the chapter on hearing impairment (Chapter 57).

The conductive hearing loss that accompanies recurrent and persistent episodes of otitis media with middle ear effusion (OME) can also potentially impede early speech and language development. Although conductive losses generally do not exceed 20 to 30 decibels (dB), with a maximum loss of 50 dB, speech discrimination can be affected significantly. Studies of the long-term effects of OME on language development have yielded conflicting results. Language difficulties associated with OME most often appear to manifest as expressive delays in early childhood and phonologic problems in the early school years (Roberts and Wallace, 1997).

There has also been study of the mechanisms of auditory perception and discrimination. Central auditory processing problems have been hypothesized as reflecting potential difficulties in discriminating, analyzing, and storing auditory stimuli, especially in the presence of competing sounds.

INTELLECTUAL IMPAIRMENT

The most common cause of delayed acquisition of language skills is a generalized impairment of cognitive abilities, or mental retardation. Language delays are frequently the first manifestation of such a problem. Language skills will generally follow normal patterns of progression, but at a slower rate, and problems will become most apparent as the complexity of language demands increases.

Some chromosomal and genetic disorders are associated with particularly increased risk of language dysfunction. Children with Down syndrome often have a disproportionate degree of language disability, which can compound developmental and behavioral challenges. In fragile X syndrome, children show unique patterns of language dysfunction involving prosody as well as content.

AUTISTIC DISORDER

Communication disorder is a core feature of autism, along with impairment in ability to relate socially to others and

DYNAMICS AND DOMAINS OF DYSFUNCTION IN SPEECH-LANGUAGE DISORDERS

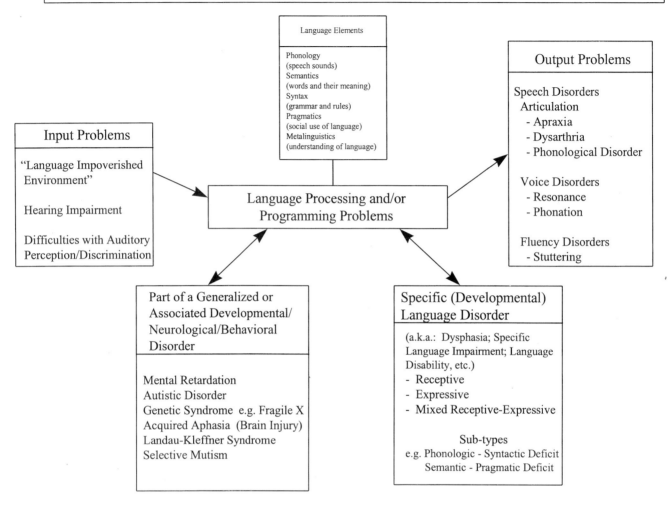

Figure 63–1. Multiple factors can contribute to delayed or disordered development of speech and language. Although some of these conditions can occur in isolation, there is usually a combination of interrelated areas of dysfunction.

rigid, perseverative responses to the environment. Language impairment can range from a total lack of comprehension and a nonverbal state to atypical patterns in which speech is overly formal or pedantic, with stilted prosody. Pragmatic skills are invariably affected. There may be echolalia with perseveration as well as impaired nonverbal communication with little reciprocal eye contact and limited use of facial expressions and social gestures.

NEUROLOGIC DISORDERS

Interruption of the neuromotor pathways responsible for production of speech is commonly seen in children with cerebral palsy. Articulation difficulties are frequent and receptive abilities can be stronger than expressive language skills. The neurologic basis for specific language disorders has defied attempts at discrete identification. Localized left hemisphere brain lesions in children usually do not result in the specific dysphasic symptoms seen in adults. Congenital strokes have complex, and usually subtle, effects on language development. Children with left hemisphere lesions

generally have more difficulty with language and academic skills such as reading and writing than do children with right hemisphere lesions, although problems can occur in both groups. These findings reflect the plasticity of the immature brain as well as the contribution of the right hemisphere to acquisition of language skills (Nass, 1997). *Acquired childhood aphasia* is the term used to describe language deficits that follow a brain lesion (such as trauma or tumor) sustained after a child has developed language skills to the degree of speaking in sentences. Symptoms and syndromes of aphasia can be classified as sensory aphasia (an auditory comprehension disorder in children with fluent speech), anomic aphasia (difficulty formulating an appropriate name for a target), conduction aphasia (difficulty retrieving words), or motor aphasia (nonfluent, laborious language). Prognosis for language skills and academic progress appears less favorable than previously supposed (Van Hout, 1997). A rare neurologic cause of language disorder that has received increased attention recently is the syndrome of acquired aphasia with convulsive disorder, or Landau-Kleffner syndrome. This syndrome affects previously normal children who undergo a regression of receptive or expressive language abilities, or both, which can range in severity to the extreme of auditory agnosia (inability to identify environmental sounds). All affected children have abnormalities on electroencephalography (bilateral spike and slow waves), and at least two thirds have seizures of varying types. Some children can recover language skills but most reports indicate that one half of the patients have severe residual language deficits (Feekery, Parry-Fielder, and Hopkins, 1993). Some children with hydrocephalus have been described as manifesting the "cocktail-party syndrome," using long and complicated sentences with sophisticated vocabulary but limited content.

BEHAVIORAL DISORDERS

There is a significant association between language disability and behavioral problems. The behavioral difficulties are frequently secondary to communication problems, manifesting either as an apparent inability to follow directions or as externalizing behaviors reflecting frustration at the inability to communicate feelings and wishes. Rates of anxiety disorders, conduct disturbance, and attention-deficit disorders are higher in children with language disorders. In turn, delayed or disordered language development can follow significant emotional trauma or psychosocial adversity (Rutter and Lord, 1987). *Selective mutism* is a rare condition with onset usually before the age of 5 years, in which there is a persistent failure to speak in certain social situations such as at school. These children generally have normal language skills but may occasionally have a related communication disorder. The symptoms usually resolve within a few months. True mutism is very rare and usually results from large frontal or midbrain lesions or diffuse axonal shearing, resulting in a total lack of spontaneous language.

ENVIRONMENTAL DEPRIVATION

The rate at which children acquire vocabulary and language correlates with the number of words their parents use in interactions with them and how their attempts at verbal communication are repeated and expanded by adults (Huttenlocher et al, 1991). Language skills are not well acquired from sources such as television or radio. Children raised in an environment in which exposure to language is impoverished will lag in language development. Such children are the ones who will show most dramatic response to early therapeutic intervention and stimulation of language abilities. The role of a bilingual family environment as a possible cause of language delays has been debated. In general this does not appear to be a significant contributory factor.

EXAMPLE

John revisited: Hearing evaluation was normal. A brain scan showed bilateral temporal lobe atrophy with atrophic changes of the left motor cortex. Subsequent special investigations confirmed a diagnosis of glutaric aciduria. Speech and language evaluation indicated oral-motor dysfunction with weakness and apraxia. Expressive and receptive language abilities were delayed. There was good

intentional communication. John made progress in individual and group speech and language therapy as well as occupational and physical therapy to increase trunk control and stability. His parents have provided much language stimulation in the home environment, and he interacts very appropriately with family members and peers. At 4 years of age his receptive language abilities are in the low-average range. Speech remains slurred, with distortions, substitutions, and omissions. There is early evidence of other learning problems.

Speech Disorders

The verbal expression of language can be impeded by dysfunction at various points along the complex and coordinated pathways responsible for formation of the acoustic signal.

DISORDERS OF ARTICULATION

The term *articulation disorder* is applied to children who misarticulate sounds, by substitution of one sound for another ("wabbit" for "rabbit"), omission of a sound ("kool" for "school"), distortion or nonstandard production of a sound, or addition of a sound ("puhlese" for "please"). A useful guide to assessing development of articulation is the so-called Rule of Fourths. The average 2-year-old child should be intelligible to strangers half the time (2/4), a 3-year-old, three quarters of the time, and a 4-year-old, all the time.

Articulation requires the integration of a number of key functions. The basic structures for articulation include the vocal tract, the articulators, and intact neural pathways mediating precise motor function. Cognitive and linguistic skills are required to process pragmatics, semantics, and syntactics and apply the rules of phonology. Finally, there is a sensorimotor-acoustic component that allows for motor programming and motor learning of the sequences of physical movement in a variety of phonetic contexts (Creaghead, Newman, and Secord, 1989).

The articulatory errors can be organic or functional. The organically based articulation disorders fall into the areas of apraxia and dysarthria.

Apraxia refers to a motor disorder of speech involving the central programming for the production of phonemes and the sequencing of the voluntary muscle movements for the production of words. The voluntary control of the lips, tongue, and palate during speech is impaired, but automatic movements such as licking, eating, and drinking are intact. Imitation of syllables, single words, and short phrases may be normal, but spontaneous speech is often unintelligible. On clinical evaluation, children with apraxia of speech will have great difficulty repeating the sequence "pa, ta, ka" rapidly. Prosody is often affected, with the child having difficulty maintaining a rhythmic speech pattern. Children with apraxia of speech often manifest associated dyspraxias such as fine motor problems or "soft neurologic signs." The neurologic dysfunction often persists, and progress in therapy is usually slow. There is also an increased risk for a concurrent language problem. Receptive skills are usually a relative strength, but as the apraxia resolves, other language problems can emerge, sometimes not manifesting until the third or fourth grade, where the child might have difficulty with higher-order processing of language such as categorizing, organizing, and abstracting (Esckelson, 1990).

Dysarthria results from difficulty in the actual production of speech sounds, rather than the programming. Dysarthria includes disorders of phonation, articulation, resonation, and prosody that occur singly or in combination as a result of weakness, altered tone, and incoordination of the muscles used in speech production. It is seen most often in adults as a result of a neurologic impairment caused by a stroke, head trauma, or a progressive disease. In childhood, dysarthia is most often associated with cerebral palsy. Often articulation is hampered by involuntary movements or limitations in range, strength, and direction of the movements. Many nonspeech skills are incorporated into appropriate articulation, such as head control and a coordinated pattern of respiration and phonation. These abilities are also impaired in many children with dysarthria (Creaghead, Newman, and Secord, 1989).

Phonologic disorder refers to functional problems that involve multiple phoneme errors. Table 63–2 lists the upper age limits for consonant production.

There are a number of key phonologic processes that can be dysfunctional in children with phonologic disorder. The child might delete final consonants or use voiced consonants to begin words instead of voiceless consonants ("gup" instead of "cup"). Other dysfunctional processes include palatal fronting ("su" for "shoe") or velar fronting ("tup" for "cup") as well as stridency deletion ("tichen" for "chicken") or cluster simplification ("bush" for "brush"). "Liquid simplification" refers to the relatively common error of producing "liquid" sounds /l and r/ as "glides" /w and j/ (Khan and Lewis, 1986). A number of other specific phonologic disorders can be identified during evaluation by a speech and language specialist.

DISORDERS OF VOICE

Voice disorders can also be functional or organic and are characterized by deviations of pitch, loudness, quality, and resonance. These problems can exist by themselves but are frequently combined with other speech or language problems to form a complex communication disorder.

The most common voice quality problem is *hoarseness*. Persistent or progressive hoarseness, especially if associated with airway symptoms such as stridor or audible breathing, indicates the need for further otolaryngologic evaluation. Fiberscopic examination might reveal edema related to allergies or specific lesions such as laryngeal papillomas, congenital glottic webs, or vocal nodules.

Nodules are believed to result from harsh mechanical contact between the edges of the vocal folds and are seen more frequently in children who are loud or incessant talkers. Vocal fold paralysis usually presents with a weak, breathy cry or soft or absent voice or cry. The laryngeal paralysis can be congenital or acquired and unilateral or bilateral. Genetic syndromes such as cri du chat syndrome are associated with voice disorders and laryngeal paralysis (Gray, Smith, and Schneider, 1996).

Resonance is a process whereby sound is generated in the larynx and modified as it passes through the upper respiratory tract. The most obvious resonance effect is the formation of vowels. Most disorders of resonance are characterized by either too much or too little nasal resonance. The only sounds of the English language in which air is sent purposefully through the nose are /m, n, ing/. *Hypernasal* speech occurs when an abnormal amount of air flows through the nasal cavity during the formation of other sounds. The velopharynx usually forms a muscular valve separating the oral and nasal cavities during speech (as well as during swallowing, blowing, and sucking). Velopharyngeal inadequacy results in hypernasality and may be caused by cleft palate, submucous cleft palate, congenital palatal incompetence, and neurologic dysfunction affecting the precision and timing of velopharyngeal closure. This problem can be precipitated by adenoidectomy in children with previously undetected palatal incompetence or a submucous cleft. *Hyponasal* (or denasal) speech occurs when there is less than the expected amount of nasal resonance. This is the quality of a voice when someone has a severe upper respiratory infection or rhinitis. Usually when the denasality is chronic, it is caused by enlargement of the adenoids. There are clearly therapeutic implications to the diagnosis of disorders of resonance (such as whether an adenoidectomy is indicated). The nasometer, a microcomputer-based instrument, can measure sound energy emitting from the oral and nasal cavities and aid differentiation and diagnosis (Gray, Smith, and Schneider, 1996).

DISORDERS OF FLUENCY

Dysfluencies include pauses, hesitation, interjections, prolongations, and repetitions that interrupt or disrupt the flow of speech. Dysfluent speech often begins in early childhood between the ages of 2½ and 4 years. During this time, a certain amount of repeating, stopping, or pausing is to be expected. When the frequency of these behaviors becomes excessive or when the types of behaviors seem different from the other children, the child maybe showing early signs of *stuttering*. If these danger signs are detected early enough, stuttering in young children can be prevented. If help is not available, often the signs increase in severity, interfering with social interaction and academic achievement. Stuttering affects approximately 1% of the population, with 85% of cases beginning in the preschool years. Boys often outnumber girls by a ratio of 4:1. The following are danger signs that should be recognized.

1. *Repetitions* can be normal in children as speech and language develop; however, repetitions that are too frequent, more than 50 per 1000 words, indicate a need for intervention.

Table 63–2 • Milestones for Consonant Production

By age 3: /p, m, h, n, w/
By age 4: /b, k, g, d, f, y/
By age 6: /t, ng, r, l/
By age 7: /ch, sh, j, v, voiceless th/
By age 8: /s, z, v, voiced th/

2. *Prolongation* occurs with pulling out a sound with prolonged attention and forcing on the initial sound of a word, e.g., "fffffffish."
3. *Struggle* and intention include facial contortions, jaw jerks, wide-open mouth, protrusion of the tongue, rolling of the eyes, and a combination of struggle behaviors. Often children who are at this level are highly aware of their difficulty.
4. *Avoidances* are a set of complex behaviors that can be used by children to cope with and hide some of the stuttering behavior. Usually they are learned behaviors whose efficiency is temporary.

The reaction of the listeners has a significant impact on the progression of symptoms in many children who stutter. Often the longer the stuttering problem exists the more likely the child is to develop associated emotional problems (Pindzola, 1997).

Language Disorders

Terminology and definitions used to describe language disorders have varied, and there is still no universal agreement among experts. Some of the terms used have included developmental language delay, developmental aphasia, dysphasia, and specific language impairment. The medical term currently most commonly used is *developmental language disorder*. The diagnosis of developmental language disorder is made in the absence of the known associated factors discussed earlier. In particular, children with language disorders manifest a specific discrepancy between cognitive functioning (such as score on a nonverbal or performance measure of intelligence) and measured language skills (Hall, 1997). The causes of developmental language disorders are generally unknown. Use of sophisticated imaging techniques such as functional magnetic resonance imaging, single photon emission spectroscopy, and positron emission tomography has provided more information regarding the neurologic underpinnings of language. The left perisylvian regions have been implicated in the processing of phonemes and auditory information, and areas of the planum temporale and angular gyrus have been found to have altered function in children and adults with language impairment or closely related disorders such as dyslexia (Semrud-Clikeman, 1997). Similar functional variations in family members of individuals with language problems suggest a genetic component to some of these disorders. Other studies have also demonstrated an increased prevalence of language problems and related learning disorders among family members of children with language disorders.

EXAMPLE

Andrew is a 4 1/2-year-old boy who is experiencing difficulties following directions at home and in preschool and is manifesting hyperactivity and aggression. Medical history was unremarkable and hearing is normal bilaterally. A speech and language evaluation had indicated delays in expressive and receptive abilities as well as apraxia of speech. Fine and gross motor skills were also delayed. He displayed a lot of jargoning in his attempts to communicate.

Andrew was enrolled in speech and language therapy. His auditory processing and receptive language skills improved and there was a significant improvement in his speech intelligibility with a decrease in jargoning. Andrew continued in individual and group speech and language therapy and was enrolled in a preschool early intervention program. At follow-up 1 year later, his overall language abilities were in the average range, although there were still difficulties with processing and memory. Andrew was experiencing difficulty with reading.

In describing children with language deficits, the terms *language delay, language disorder,* and *language difference* are often used. A language delay describes a language learning sequence that is normal but with a slower rate of acquisition. For example, a child of 5 years of age would be functioning linguistically like a child 4 years of age. A language difference describes a child who comprehends and uses the language code of the group, but dialectical differences are present. Lastly, a language disorder denotes a sequence of language development that differs from normal, with language learning strategies frequently being different.

Language disorders can be classified as either receptive or expressive or a combination of both. The disorder usually affects all of the linguistic components, including pragmatics, semantics, and syntax. Often, one of the components may be age-appropriate, while others may be significantly delayed or nonexistent. Language disorders can also occur along a continuum of severity from mild to severe depending on the extent to which communication is affected. An extreme end of the continuum may be represented by autism, and at the mild end would be an articulation problem with mild sound substitutions. The language disorders that occur in one linguistic component often will affect the development of another component. For example, a child with a restricted syntactic rule system will not have a large variety of phrases or sentences available to code meaning and intent as may be necessary. A disorder in the pragmatic area encompasses the rules for discourse and intent, and when a child fails to understand these areas there is a disruption in the foundations for interaction. A child with a severe pragmatic disorder often is behaviorally inappropriate and does not understand the rules for interaction across the domains. A semantic disorder often is reflected in limited vocabulary by which the child is restricted or is unable to understand the symbols represented in the vocabulary. Lastly, a morphologic disorder is present when a child does not have the phrases or sentence complexity to adequately communicate intended meaning. Often the sentences may be fragmented and lack appropriate morphologic markers to be understood by a listener.

Table 63–3 lists many of the common types of language difficulties found in school-aged and adolescent children. All of the difficulties span all areas of language to include semantics, pragmatics, morphology, reading, writing, cognitive abilities, and general language processing. There may also be specific difficulties with understanding and using appropriate syntactic rules.

Table 63–3 • Language Disorders in School-Aged Children

Linguistic Area	Disorder
Semantics	Word finding/retrieval deficits
	Use of a large number of words in the attempt to explain a concept because the name cannot be recalled
	Overuse of limited vocabulary
	Difficulty recalling names of items in categories (e.g., animals, foods)
	Difficulty retrieving verbal opposites
	Limited vocabulary
	Use of words lacking specificity (e.g., "thing," "stuff")
	Inappropriate use of words (selection of wrong word)
	Difficulty defining words
	Less comprehension of complex words
	Failure to grasp double word meaning (e.g., "can," "file")
Syntax/morphology	Use of grammatically incorrect sentence structures
	Simple, as opposed to complex, sentences
	Less comprehension of complex grammatical structures
	Prolonged pauses while constructing sentences
	Semantically empty place holders (e.g., filled pauses, "uh," "er," "um")
	Use of many stereotyped phrases that do not require much language skill
	Use of "starters" (e.g., "you know . . .")
Pragmatics	Use of redundant expressions and information the listener has already heard
	Use of nonspecific vocabulary such that the listener cannot tell from prior conversation or physical context what is referred to
	Less skill in giving explanations clearly to a listener (lack of detail)
	Less skill in explaining something in a proper sequence
	Less conversational control in terms of introducing, maintaining, and changing topics (may get off the track in conversation and introduce new topics awkwardly)
	Rare use of clarification questions (e.g., "I don't understand")
	Difficulty shifting conversational styles in different social situations (e.g., peer vs. teacher; child vs. adult)
	Difficulty grasping the main idea of a story or lecture (preoccupation with irrelevant details)
	Trouble making inferences from material not explicitly stated (e.g., "Sally went outside. She had to put up her umbrella." Inference: It was raining)

Adapted from Haynes W, Moran M, Pindzola R: Communication Disorders in the Classroom. Dubuque, IA, Kendall-Hunt, 1990; and Haynes WQ, Pindzola RH, Emerick L: Diagnosis and Evaluation in Speech Pathology, 4th ed. Englewood Cliffs, NJ, Prentice-Hall, 1992.

Classification systems have been proposed that delineate subgroups of deficit or dysfunction, and there is ongoing research regarding subtyping. Some of the categories of mixed receptive-expressive disorder that have been proposed include *verbal auditory agnosia,* severe impairment of the abilities to decode phonology through the auditory channel, which results in the child's understanding little or nothing of what is heard; and *phonologic-syntactic deficit,* in which children have difficulty producing language, with dysfluency and use of simplified sentences. Comprehension is variable and speech onset is delayed. Disorders of central processing and formulation include *semantic-pragmatic deficit,* in which children are fluent (often hyperverbal) with a large and sophisticated vocabulary but have limited comprehension, perseverate, and lack pragmatic skills such as appreciating the rules of turn taking in conversation. These patterns are more typical in children with hydrocephalus or high-functioning autism. *Lexical-syntactic deficit* involves difficulty finding words in discourse or putting ideas into words (Allen, Rapin, and Wiznitzer, 1988).

Evaluation of the Child With Disordered Speech or Language

The key to successful outcome in children with disorders of speech and language is early identification of problems, accurate diagnosis, and implementation of appropriate management interventions. All professionals working with infants and young children should be vigilant for signs of speech or language dysfunction.

The primary care physician who has regular interactions with young children bears unique responsibility in this regard. Compared with surveillance of development in other domains such as motor skills, monitoring of acquisition of language skills is particularly challenging. Typical toddlers rarely display their expressive language abilities in a medical office setting, and the clinician is largely dependent on historical information from parents and caregivers for assessment. A variety of factors, as noted earlier, can influence language development. Warning signs of early language disorders are listed in Table 63–1. Primary markers for disordered language development include the child who is not babbling by 10 months, using single words at 18 months, or using phrases at 24 months of age. Atypical patterns of language that are also red flags include echolalia or unintelligible speech by 4 years.

The standard components of medical assessment will assist greatly in untangling the complex differential diagnosis and ruling out potentially associated medical and environmental factors. Assessment of language and play patterns should occur prior to physical and neurologic examination. Atypical patterns of behavior or social interactions might suggest autistic disorder. Aspects of family history or physical appearance might prompt further testing for a genetic syndrome. The general physical examination should include evaluation of oral-motor status. A bifid uvula might indicate a submucous cleft of the palate. Problems with drooling or swallowing could reflect structural defects or a bulbar palsy. Any problem with language development is an indication for formal evaluation of hearing. Informal assessment of hearing in the office setting (with a background noise level of up to 50 dBs) is notoriously inaccurate. A loss of skills necessitates further special investigations such as electroencephalography or metabolic testing.

SCREENING OF LANGUAGE DEVELOPMENT

Although retrospective recall of early milestones is difficult, it is important to delineate the progression of language development as carefully as possible. Parent inventories such as the MacArthur Communicative Development Inventory can help parents report their child's abilities with regard to established and emerging skills (Fenson et al, 1993). It is helpful to elicit specific examples from parents of a child's current capabilities for self-expression (such as describing experiences or asking questions) and to comprehend (following simple or complicated instructions, answering questions). Developmental screening tests such as the Denver II (Frankenberg, 1992), the Early Language Milestone (ELM) scale (Coplan 1987), and the Clinical Linguistic and Auditory Milestone Scale (CLAMS) (Capute and Accardo, 1978) provide a structural approach to such language assessment. The older child can be asked questions of increasing complexity, depending on age, and should be asked to repeat phrases. Again, screening instruments such as the Sentence Repetition Screening Test can provide a structured means of assessing and monitoring progress (Sturner, Funk, and Green, 1996). Children will often be anxious, reticent, or uncooperative in the office setting, precluding formal language assessment. Video or audio recordings of language samples from the home setting can help. Observations of pretend play can add significantly to information about the child's concepts of his or her world and cognitive development. Questions should be open-ended and focused. Interaction with the child in context of play can also help in exploring language skills (e.g., "where is the car?"; "feed the baby"; "put the cup behind the chair"). Suspicion of a significant delay in language development necessitates referral for formal speech and language evaluation by a specialist.

FORMAL SPEECH AND LANGUAGE EVALUATION

The assessment of communication disorders can be broadly categorized into four areas: language, articulation, fluency, and voice. The purpose of the assessment is to determine specifically whether a problem or a specific risk status exists and to help in prioritizing specific intervention goals. A combination of caregiver interview, language sampling, and formal assessment tools provides the most comprehensive information. The assessment should be an ongoing process with involvement of caregivers in an informal role with the evaluator. As is the case with screening in the primary care setting, evaluation by a speech and language pathologist incorporates a variety of strategies and involves an interview technique with significant others as well as observation of communication, play, and language during spontaneous interactions in natural environments. The communication skills are related to other developmental domains of cognition (sensorimotor, symbolic, and constructive play) and motor and social interaction.

The best representative sample of a child's language function, whether it be spoken or signed, is the most important component of a language evaluation. The structured formalized tests that focus on language form and context usually give only partial data as to the child's communication ability. The spontaneous conversational sample allows the child the freedom of expression in a more realistic and relaxed context. It also displays how he or she understands a language code and the use of the linguistic components as well as nonverbal communication abilities. The language sample is then analyzed across the parameters of pragmatics, semantics, and syntax. The traditional assessment tools incorporate normative data, which can be used to quantify a child's developmental level. They are usually easy to administer and are fairly reliable across different examiners. Further, the standardized measures of language can also be useful when establishing eligibility for services, comparing children to a normative group, and documenting change over time. Table 63–4 lists evaluation tools according to specific language areas.

Management

General approaches should focus on interventions to maximize opportunities for language development. Parents should be directed in techniques of providing a language-rich environment, using language in a reciprocal and eliciting manner with their child.

MEDICAL ROLE

Medical management should be directed at correcting any underlying or associated medical problems. The primary care physician can play an important role in referring to and coordinating specialized services. Psychological testing could help to delineate specific cognitive abilities. Abnormal medical findings might necessitate further evaluation by a neurologist or assessment of voice or resonance problems by an otolaryngologist. Evaluation by a multidisciplinary team at a medical center could help to clarify the diagnosis and plans for management. Children with language disabilities are more likely to pose behavioral challenges, and anticipatory guidance in regard to behavior management techniques could prevent secondary problems. There is also a need for vigilance regarding learning problems, especially in reading and writing, which are more prevalent in children who have had delays in early language development (see Chapter 53). School entry thus brings new challenges for families and opportunities for guidance and advocacy by the primary care physician.

Table 63–4 • Standardized Tests of Language Skills

Skill	Test (Age)
Pragmatics	Test of Pragmatic Skills, Revised (3–8 yrs)
Semantics	Peabody Picture Vocabulary Test, Revised (2–21 yrs)
	Expressive One-Word Picture Vocabulary Test, Revised (2–11 yrs)
	Receptive One-Word Picture Vocabulary Test (2–11 yrs)
	Test of Word Finding (6–13 yrs)
	Boehm Test of Basic Concepts, Preschool (3–5 yrs)
	Test of Adolescent Word Finding (12–21 yrs)
Syntax and morphology	Multi-Level Informal Language Inventory (4–12 yrs)
Auditory processing	Test of Auditory Comprehension of Language, Revised (3–21 yrs)
Comprehensive language test	Preschool Language Scale, III (0–6 yrs)
	Reynell Developmental Language Scale (1–7 yrs)
	Sequenced Inventory of Communication Development, Revised (4–48 mo)
	Preschool Language Assessment Instrument (3–6 yrs)
	Clinical Evaluation of Language Fundamentals, Preschool (3–6 yrs)
	Clinical Evaluation of Language Fundamentals, Revised (6–21 yrs)
	Clinical Evaluation of Language Fundamentals, III (6–21 yrs)
	Test of Adolescent Language, II (12–18 yrs)
	Test of Language Development Primary, II (4–8 yrs)
Metalinguistic and problem solving	Test of Problem Solving, Elementary (6–11 yrs)
	Test of Language Competence (9–19 yrs)
Nonverbal skills/preverbal skills	Communication and Symbolic Behavior Scales (8–24 mos)
	The Non-Speech Test for Receptive-Expressive, Revised (0–48 mos)
	Uzgiris and Hunt Scales of Infant Psychological Development (0–3 yrs)
	Communication Placement Assessment for Severe to Profound (0–21 yrs)
	Evaluating Acquired Skills in Communication (0–21 yrs)

SPEECH AND LANGUAGE THERAPY

Therapy by a speech and language pathologist usually incorporates objectives established from a formal language evaluation and should reflect appropriate expectations, being "child centered, child initiated, and child directed." Without this particular focus, a child may in fact be taught nonfunctional vocabulary, interactions, or sentence structures. All of the linguistic components of pragmatics, semantics, and syntax are interrelated and function in that way. Pragmatic language targets should always have priority over semantic and syntactic targets. If deviant interactional behaviors are present, they need to be changed before vocabulary and grammar are targeted. A language program must be established to provide additional stimulation to facilitate language learning. This needs to include the combined effort of parents, teachers, and therapists in the creation of a positive language facilitation environment. This does not mean individual drill, but activities initiated to focus on interaction so that the children can experience a realistic and functional communicative environment. Guidelines should incorporate the following principles:

1. Maintenance of developmental sequence. Normal children learn language in a universal sequence, and this order should also be maintained with children with language disorders. For example, a child's basic pragmatic abilities must be present before he then can develop semantics, and subsequently develop syntax and morphology.
2. Correction of errors. Errors within a child's language rules system that might limit effectiveness of communication should be corrected by means of modeled forms in a natural context.

3. Introduction of meaning form and structures. The forms and structures that carry specific meaning should have a high priority.
4. Development of structural flexibility. Flexibility allows a child to communicate more effectively in different situations. For example, a child wishing to communicate that he is hungry can be taught in different ways such as "want to eat," "hungry," or "want food."
5. Refinement of established abilities before introduction of new targets. The new abilities should be developed and based on an established performance.

Use of prior knowledge and ability can allow the child to build on foundations that are already present in his or her communication system. Children always learn through past experiences and acquire new information based on these past experiences. Modeling should always be combined with an expansion of the child's vocalization or utterance. The modeling can serve to correct form and structures; the content is expanded and the topic can be maintained to allow the child the appropriate interaction. Vocabulary that is targeted should be functional and useful for the child. The functional vocabulary should be words that the child can code and that have the most relevance for him or her (e.g., "more," "help," "open"). Finally, reinforcement is another important consideration for targeting and facilitating language learning. Feedback is given through fulfillment, manipulation of others, and accomplishment of specific tasks. Combining language learning on an individual basis with other therapy such as occupational and physical therapy can also enhance the overall language learning process.

Parents and caregivers play a large role in the child's

language development. The following are natural reinforcements techniques that can be used to facilitate and reinforce language; join in a child's play and follow his lead; comment on the child's activities; expand or extend the child's utterances for more information; and reflect on the child's utterances and model correct production. Finally, since language facilitation occurs in a natural environment, stimulating children's language in a group format provides a good avenue for language learning. Additional language facilitation techniques include playing with the appropriate toys, using a computer, and reading to the child. The stories in books or on the computer provide rhythm and rhyming forms and are often easily stored in memory for later practice and processing of linguistic information. The group format provides reinforcement for acquiring new language through the use of questions by the child or other children in the group. It also provides the ability for the child to become more independent in language usage by learning to monitor and correct himself or others through the group interaction. All of these delivery models provide an avenue to facilitate and structure the child's linguistic environment within the context of a variety of communication interactions.

Summary

Speech and language disorders are complex, diagnostically challenging, and far-reaching in their potential to impede development. Crucial developmental domains are at risk, including social abilities, emotional and behavioral adjustment, and academic achievement. Early signs of dysfunction are subtle, and in the majority of cases there are no physical clues or markers. Early identification is essential and accurate diagnosis requires skill and patience. The differential diagnosis is broad and requires consideration of interrelated contributory factors. Clinical manifestations vary over time, and certain developmental sequelae may emerge only after school entry. There is no standard battery of medical investigations. Hearing must be tested in all children with language problems. Interventions must be family centered and usually incorporate a number of disciplines. Response to treatment interventions is variable, and prognostication is difficult. Health professionals have a critical role to play in diagnosis and management and in providing support and advocacy for the child and family through evolving developmental stages and challenges.

REFERENCES

Allen DA, Rapin I, Wiznitzer M: Communication disorders of preschool children: the physician's responsibility. J Dev Behav Peds 4(3):164, 1988.

Bashir AS, Stark RE, Graham JM: Communication disorders. *In* Levine MD, Carey WB, Crocker AC (eds): Developmental-Behavioral Pediatrics, 2nd ed. Philadelphia, WB Saunders, 1992, p. 557.

Capute AJ, Accardo PJ: Clinical linguistic and auditory milestones during the first two years of life: a language inventory for the practitioner. Clin Pediatr 17:847, 1978.

Coplan J: The Early Language Milestone Scale (revised). Austin, TX, Pro-Ed, 1987.

Creaghead A, Newman W, Secord A: Assessment and Remediation of Articulatory and Phonological Disorders, 2nd ed. Columbus, OH, Merrill Publishing Company, 1989, p. 274.

Esckelson D: Developmental Apraxia: A Clinical Handbook. Las Cruces, New Mexico, Language Pathways, 1990.

Feekery CJ, Parry-Fielder B, Hopkins IJ: Landau-Kleffner syndrome: six patients including discordant monozygotic twins. Pediatr Neurol 9:49, 1993.

Fenson L, Dale PS, Roznick JS, et al: MacArthur Communicative Development Inventories, User's Guide and Technical Manual. San Diego, Singular Publishing Group, 1993.

Frankenberg WK, Dodds J, Archer P, et al: Denver II: a major revision and restandardization of the Denver Developmental screening test. Pediatrics 89:91, 1992.

Gray SD, Smith ME, Schneider H: Voice disorders in children. Ped Clin North Am 43(b):1357, 1996.

Hall NE: Developmental language disorders. Semin Pediatr Neurol 4(2):77, 1997.

Haynes W, Moran M, Pindzola R: Communication Disorders in the Classroom. Dubuque, IA, Kendall-Hunt, 1990.

Haynes WO, Pindzola RH, Emerick L: Diagnosis and Evaluation in Speech Pathology, 4th ed. Englewood Cliffs, NJ, Prentice-Hall, 1992.

Huttenlocher J, Haight W, Bryk A, et al: Early vocabulary growth: relation to language input and gender. Dev Psychol 27:236, 1991.

Khan LM, Lewis N: Khan-Lewis Phonological Analysis. Circle Pines, MN, American Guidances Services, 1986, p 4.

Nass R. Language development in children with congenital strokes. Semin Pediatr Neurol 4(2):109, 1997.

Pindzola R: Stuttering Intervention Program. Tulsa, Oklahoma, Modern Educational Corporation, 1987.

Roberts JE, Wallace IF: Language and otitis media. *In* Roberts JE, Wallace IF, Henderson FH (eds): Otitis Media in Young Children. Baltimore, MD, Paul H. Brooks Publishing Co, 1997, p 133.

Rutter M, Lord C: Language disorders associated with psychiatric disturbances. *In* Yule W, Rutter M (eds): Language Development and Disorders. Oxford, UK, MacKeith Press, 1987, p 206.

Shaywitz BA, Shaywitz SE, Pugh KR, et al: Sex differences in the functional organization of the brain for language. Nature 373:607, 1995.

Semrud-Clikeman M: Evidence from imaging on the relationship between brain structure and developmental language disorders. Semin Pediatr Neurol 4(2):117, 1997.

Sturner RA, Funk SG, Green JA: Preschool speech and language screening: further validation of the sentence repetition screening test. J Dev Behav Peds 17(6):405, 1996.

Van Hout A: Acquired aphasia in children. Semin Pediatr Neurol 4(2):102, 1997.

64 *Major Psychiatric Disorders in Childhood and Adolescence*

David Brent • Harris Rabinovich • Boris Birmaher •
John Campo

 For the most part, the major psychiatric disorders that occur in childhood and adolescence require highly specialized care. Most primary care providers and even most developmental-behavioral pediatricians need to be aware of the manifestations and early signs of these severe conditions. In most instances, their management may need to be turned over to individuals who are knowledgeable and comfortable at this extreme end of the morbidity spectrum. This chapter offers an overview of major psychiatric disorders. It is written by psychiatrists, using the conceptual model that is most widely accepted within that specialty. An understanding of the model and of the clinical morbidity described herein can facilitate communication and collaboration between child psychiatrists and pediatric health care providers.

Psychiatric disorders in children and adolescents are defined as disturbances of thought, emotions, or behavior that result in impaired functioning with family, with peers, or at school. General issues of the epidemiology and classification of child and adolescent psychiatric disorders are discussed in this chapter, as is the role of the pediatrician in the detection of such disorders. Sections about specific mood, anxiety, somatoform, and psychotic disorders follow, in which each disorder is discussed with regard to its definition, descriptive epidemiology, risk factors, clinical picture, course, identification, and management. For more detail, refer to two of several excellent textbooks of child psychiatry (Lewis, 1996; Rutter, Taylor, and Hersov, 1994).

Child Psychiatric Nosology and Epidemiology

CURRENT CHILD PSYCHIATRIC NOSOLOGY

Modern child psychiatric approaches to nosology began with Rutter and colleagues' (1970) Isle of Wight epidemiologic study. This study first demonstrated that children and their parents could reliably report on symptoms of emotional and behavioral disorders when interviewers used a semistructured diagnostic interview. From this work evolved a multiaxial approach to child psychiatric nosology, currently embodied in the *Diagnostic and Statistical Manual*, 4th edition, revised (*DSM-IV*) (American Psychological Association, 1994). The *DSM-IV* has symptom criteria for each disorder in order to standardize diagnostic classification. *DSM-IV* diagnoses are multiaxial, with five axes in total: I, psychiatric disorder; II, developmental difficulties; III, medical disorder; IV, significant stressors; and V, level of function. Alternative classification systems exist (e.g., *International Classification of Diseases [ICD-*

10]), but all conform to the idea of standardized criteria for specific diagnoses.

EPIDEMIOLOGY

Population studies have estimated that the prevalence of child and adolescent psychiatric disorder is about 15% to 20% in the population (Anderson et al, 1987; Costello et al, 1988a, 1988b; Offord et al, 1987; Rutter, Tizard, and Whitmore, 1970). Early investigations by Rutter and colleagues (1970) demonstrated that child psychiatric disorders can be divided into two broad types: "emotional" and "behavioral." Emotional disorders, often referred to as *internalizing disorders*, have symptoms of worry, fear, sadness, and somatic complaints as a prominent part of their clinical pictures, and they tend to be overrepresented in female patients, particularly after puberty. The emotional disorders to be discussed in this chapter include mood, obsessive-compulsive, anxiety, posttraumatic stress, and psychosomatic disorders. Behavioral (or *externalizing*) disorders refer to difficulties with attention and behavior, such as conduct disorder, oppositional defiant disorder, and attention deficit-hyperactivity disorder (ADHD), and are more common in boys. Aggressive behavior and attention deficits are discussed in more detail in Chapters 49 and 52, respectively. Both of these broad classifications can be assessed with high reliability, correlate with distinct demographic and psychosocial risk factors, and tend to be relatively stable over time. Persons with mixed emotional and behavioral disorders tend to have a course more similar to those with pure behavioral disorders (Rutter, Tizard, and Whitmore, 1970).

NEW HIDDEN MORBIDITY

Even though the American Academy of Pediatrics has taken a strong stand in emphasizing the importance of the detection of this "new morbidity" of pediatric psychiatric disorder in the training and practice of modern pediatricians, Costello and colleagues (1988a) have observed that as yet, this new morbidity remains largely undetected. In a study of psychiatric disorder in a Health Maintenance Organization (HMO) pediatric practice, pediatricians identified only 13% of 7- to 11-year-old children with psychiatric disorder, as diagnosed by research interviews. In another study, primary care providers correctly identified 54% of those screening positive on the Pediatric Symptom Checklist (Kelleher et al, 1997). Patients who were better known to the pediatrician and who had come in for well-child visits as compared to being seen at an acute care visit were more likely to be identified (Kelleher et al, 1997).

DEVELOPMENTAL PERSPECTIVE

The evaluation of symptoms and functional impairment in children and adolescents must occur in the context of a developmental framework. For example, although the anxiety that keeps the 8-month-old infant clinging to its mother when confronted by an adult stranger is very common in the general population of infants and is considered normal, the same is not true of an 8-year-old who is too frightened to greet an unknown adult and clings to his mother. Temper tantrums in a 2-year-old are a common sight, whereas if the same tantrum were to occur in that child 6 years later, it could be representative of a pathologic condition. However, the concept of the developmental mediation of the symptomatic expression of psychopathology has been overrated and has contributed to the perpetuation of nosologic confusion in child psychiatry. Only in preschoolers do developmental factors strongly alter the expression of psychopathology, and these effects decrease quickly with increasing age. However, whereas the manifestation of these disorders does not change greatly over childhood and adolescence, the risk for many major psychiatric disorders increases after puberty.

SCREENING INSTRUMENTS

The most widely used and carefully researched instrument for screening of psychiatric disorder is the Child Behavior Checklist (CBCL) (Achenbach, 1991). This 113-item parent report has been found to be internally consistent, to be reliable, and to discriminate well between clinic-referred and nonreferred children. Age and gender norms exist for children aged 6 to 16 years. A parallel teacher report for 6- to 16-year-olds and a youth self-report for ages 11 to 18 years have also been developed. The instrument provides measures of social competency and broad-band internalizing (emotional) and externalizing (behavioral) disorders. One psychiatric survey of an HMO pediatric practice found that a pathologic score on the CBCL identified 79% of those diagnosed as disordered on interview, but with a positive predictive value of only 39% (Costello et al, 1988b). Other valid and reliable screening instruments include the 35-item Pediatric Symptom Checklist (PSC). The PSC has been shown to have strong internal consistency, test-retest reliability, and convergent validity (Jellinek and Murphy, 1990).

DIAGNOSTIC INTERVIEWS

For a review, see Hodges (1994). There are two fully structured instruments with well-demonstrated reliability: the Diagnostic Interview for Children and Adolescents (DICA) and the Diagnostic Interview for School Age Children, Revised (DISC-R). Both instruments are suitable for lay interviewers and give separate diagnoses for parent and children interviews. The latter is one of the most commonly used instruments in epidemiologic studies. There are several semistructured psychiatric interviews; the most widely used is the Schedule for Assessment of Depression and Schizophrenia in School Age Children (K-SADS). This interview has a current and lifetime version and involves the administration of this schedule by a clinically trained interviewer to both parent and child. A current *DSM-IV* version of the instrument, the K-SADS-PL (Kaufman et al, 1997), integrates the present and lifetime versions and demonstrates good interrater reliability as well as discriminant and convergent validity. In contrast to the DISC and DICA, the interviewer attempts to resolve discrepancies between the two informants and generate "best-estimate" diagnoses.

Mood Disorders*

CLASSIFICATION

Mood disorders are classified on the basis of severity, course, and presence or absence of mania. The diagnosis of major depressive disorder (MDD) requires at least 2 weeks of depressed mood during most of the time and four additional depressive symptoms. A more chronic, intermittent disorder such as dysthymic disorder may have periods of depression interspersed with normal mood. Adjustment disorder is a still milder disturbance of mood that follows a serious life stressor. A history of manic symptomatology in a person with dysthymia or major depression confers a diagnosis of bipolar affective or cyclothymic disorder, respectively.

DESCRIPTIVE EPIDEMIOLOGY

Mood disorders are relatively rare in prepubertal children, with estimates of point prevalence of MDD ranging from 1.8% to 2.5%, "minor" forms of depression, including dysthymia of 2.5%, and bipolar illness of 0.2% to 0.4% (Fleming and Offord, 1990). The point prevalence of mood disorder is estimated to be about three to four times more common in adolescence, with estimates for the frequency of current or recent-onset MDD ranging from 2.9% to 4.7%, and dysthymia, 1.6% to 8.0%. Depression is equally common among prepubertal boys and girls, whereas among adolescents, depression is more common in girls. The prevalence of bipolar disorder (including cyclothymic and milder bipolar disorder) among adolescents is estimated at around 1% and is equally common in boys and girls.

---

*Sections on Mood Disorders and of Suicide and Suicidal Behavior are adapted from Brent DA: School age and adolescence: Mood disorders and suicide. *In* Green M, Haggerty RJ, Weitzman ML (eds): Ambulatory Pediatrics, 5th ed. Philadelphia, WB Saunders, 1999. Adapted with permission.

However, in one community study, a larger proportion (5.7%) were found to have some criteria of bipolar disorder, such as expansive or irritable mood and evidence of impaired functioning.

RISK FACTORS

For a review, see Brent and colleagues (1995). The most potent risk factor for development of a depressive disorder in childhood is having at least one parent, particularly the mother, with a history of depression. The increased risk of depression is greater and age of onset of depression is younger when there are higher familial rates of depression, earlier age of onset of depression in parents, and a family history of either bipolarity or recurrent unipolar disorder (Brent et al, 1995). Family problems, including discord, divorce, parental death, and dissatisfaction with family role, predict adolescent depression, as does the presence of anxiety symptoms in childhood. Bipolar illness, which occasionally occurs with a negative family history, may be inherited in a major single locus, dominant pattern, whereas unipolar depression appears to have a much more multifactorial etiology. Among the psychosocial factors associated with depression are stressful life events, family discord, and physical or sexual abuse. The incidence of depression is increased in patients with certain chronic illnesses, such as epilepsy, inflammatory bowel disease, and juvenile-onset diabetes. Medications that may predispose the child to depression include antihypertensive agents, phenobarbital, and steroids, the latter of which may also predispose the child to mania. Although the etiology of depression is unknown, it is likely that biological factors play an important role, in light of familial aggregation and neuroendocrine and biological markers that have been described in early-onset depression.

BIOLOGICAL CORRELATES

For a review, see Brent and colleagues (1995). There is consistent evidence for blunted growth hormone (GH) response to provocative challenge in prepubertal depressed patients after administration of clonidine, growth hormone–releasing hormone, or insulin-induced hypoglycemia, which is consistent with an alteration in noradrenergic neurotransmission. Abnormal response of prolactin and cortisol in response to L-5 hydroxytryptophan in prepubertal depressives indicates an associated abnormality in serotonergic neurotransmission. These same findings have been identified in nondepressed children at very high risk for depression owing to heavy familial loading for mood disorders, suggesting that an alteration in serotonergic neurotransmission may *antedate* the onset of depression.

The "classic" sleep electroencephalographic (EEG) correlates of depression—namely decreased rapid eye movement (REM) latency, increased REM density, and increased sleep latency—are not found among prepubertal depressive children, unless they have been inpatients, suicidal, or severely depressed. In general, these findings of decreased REM latency, increased REM density, and increased sleep latency first emerge in later adolescence. Decreased REM latency in depressed adolescents may also predict future recurrences of depression.

CLINICAL PICTURE

The presentation of depressive disorders in children and adolescents is similar to that described in adults (Ryan et al, 1987). Because "depressed mood" can refer to sadness, irritability, or boredom, inquiry about depression should include the different labels youngsters may use, such as sad, depressed, low, down, down in the dumps, empty, blue, very unhappy, or having a "bad feeling inside" that he or she cannot get rid of. Patients with either dysthymia or major depression frequently have other comorbid psychiatric disorders: anxiety disorders, attention deficit disorder, conduct disorder, and substance abuse (Angold and Costello, 1993; Ryan et al, 1987).

Clinical surveys of prepubertally depressed patients frequently report associated psychotic features, specifically, mood-congruent delusions (of guilt, sin, poverty, somatic illness, persecution, or unrealistic expectations), self-deprecatory auditory hallucinations, and paranoid ideation (Ryan et al, 1987). Psychosis is not only thematically linked with depression but also associated temporally. Psychotic features in depression are often a harbinger of future episodes of mania, and additional features of bipolar depression include hypersomnia, hyperphagia, and psychomotor retardation.

Mania may be characterized either by expansive mood, silliness, euphoria, and grandiosity or by anger and irritability. Symptoms of mania and hypomania (a milder form of mania without the degree of functional impairment) may occur separately from depressive episodes, or they may occur with them. The simultaneous occurrence of manic and depressive symptoms is known as a "mixed state." Early-onset bipolar disorder often presents with a mixed state, accompanied by marked irritability and mood lability, comorbid disruptive disorders, substance abuse, and lack of clinical response to lithium. Such patients are at particular risk for suicide and suicidal behavior. Delusions, associated with either grandiosity or paranoia, often accompany severe mania, particularly if prolonged sleep deprivation has occurred (Carlson, 1973).

DIFFERENTIAL DIAGNOSIS

Within depressive disorders, the main differential diagnosis is among depression, dysthymia, and adjustment disorder with depressed mood. Dysthymia is a more chronic and intermittent form of mood disorders than major depression, although the two disorders can coexist (major depression developing "on top of" dysthymia, so-called double-depression).

Adjustment disorder with depressed mood (reactive depression; acute depressive reaction) generally has less severe mood disturbance, fewer symptoms, and a self-limited course, generally 3 months or less (Kovacs et al, 1984). The depressive symptoms are precipitated by psychosocial stressors such as parental separation or divorce, death of a loved one, break-up of an adolescent love affair, disruptive geographic move, or failure in school. The phenomenon has not been well studied, probably because only a small proportion of these children ever reaches psychiatric attention. For that reason, the incidence of adjustment disorder is hard to estimate, but it is likely that it affects a substantial proportion of children in view of the frequency of the aforementioned psychosocial stressors. Although the disorder is self-limited, the provision of support and an opportunity to ventilate by the parent and pediatrician may be of benefit. More intensive mental health intervention is in order when there is significant disturbance of social relations or school performance or a poor parent-child relationship.

However, the presence of the stressor before the onset of depression does *not* invalidate making a diagnosis of MDD. The grief of bereavement may be indistinguishable from depressive symptomatology. If bereavement is associated with severe functional impairment, suicidal ideation, psychotic features, worthlessness, and prolonged course (greater than 4 weeks), the diagnosis of depression may be made. Previous psychiatric disorder and a family history of depression predispose the child to depression following bereavement.

Various other psychiatric disorders may also have associated mood disturbances. Patients with learning disabilities or attention deficit disorder may suffer from poor self-esteem and demoralization, but such patients should not be diagnosed as being depressed unless they meet criteria for this condition. Children with separation anxiety disorder (SAD) are often quite dysphoric when separated from their parents, but, in the absence of comorbid depression, the dysphoria is relieved by reunion with the parent. Patients with anorexia nervosa, particularly if malnourished, may show a markedly depressed affect. However, a diagnosis of depression should not be made until nutritional status is normalized. Patients with drug and alcohol abuse often show disturbance of mood. At times, the mood disorder may antedate, and even predispose the child to, substance abuse, but the mood disorder may also occur secondary to substance abuse and subside within a month of detoxification. The differential diagnosis between depression and chronic medical illness can be difficult, given that the incidence of depression may be higher in certain illnesses and that chronic illness may have effects on sleep, appetite, and energy similar to those seen in depressed patients. Symptoms of guilt, feelings of worthlessness and hopelessness, and suicidal thoughts are unlikely to be attributable to the chronic illness itself and, if present, strongly suggest the presence of a depressive disorder.

Mania can be indistinguishable from stimulant abuse (e.g., cocaine, amphetamine). Irritability can be a symptom of either mania or depression, so that the differential diagnosis between the two rests on whether the preponderance of associated symptoms are those of mania or of depression. As discussed, it is also possible for mania and depression to occur together in a so-called mixed state. Irritability, anger, and poor judgment may also be prominent features of conduct disorder, but the absence of changes in energy, sleep, sexuality, and thought patterns generally excludes mania. Similarly, the features of attention deficits (Chapter 52) may suggest mania, but manic patients are more likely to have had mood swings and neurovegetative symptoms (i.e., changes in sleep and appetite) and are more likely to show elated mood, hypersexuality, and inappropriate joking and punning. In the case of a patient who fails to respond to stimulants, the diagnosis of bipolar disorder should be considered, particularly when associated with some of the aforementioned clinical features or a positive family history of mania.

CLINICAL COURSE

Naturalistic studies indicate that depressive disorders in children and adolescents run a chronic and recurrent course. According to one longitudinal study, untreated MDD lasts an average of 7.2 months and dysthymic disorder an average of 45.9 months (Brent et al, 1995). Those patients with both MDD and other comorbid diagnoses (e.g., anxiety disorder, substance abuse) may show a more prolonged course, as can those depressed youth with family discord and disorganization and with depressed parents (Brent et al, 1995). On the average, 40% of depressed children experience a recurrence within 2 years. Earlier age of onset, co-occurrence of an underlying dysthymic disorder, and adverse psychosocial factors (e.g., family discord and criticism) increase the risk of depressive recurrences.

Certain features of depressive disorder predict future mania: psychotic features, comorbidity with attention deficits, heavy family loading for bipolar disorder, hypersomnia, hyperphagia, and anergia. Earlier age of onset of mania, presence of nonaffective comorbidity, and presence of a mixed state or rapid cycling seem to predict a more prolonged course of mania that may be more refractory to lithium (Strober et al, 1988).

Even after recovery from depression, prepubertal children show significant social impairment (Puig-Antich et al, 1985). Adolescents who have "recovered" from a depressive episode still show evidence of multiple types of impairment, including substance and tobacco use (Rohde, Lewinsohn, and Seeley, 1994). The adult sequelae of adolescent depressive symptomatology include drug and alcohol use, development of antisocial behavior, impairment in work, and interference with interpersonal relationships. Moreover, depression confers a substantially increased risk for suicide in both male and female adolescents, particularly if accompanied by comorbid substance abuse (Brent, 1995; Shaffer et al, 1996).

IDENTIFICATION OF DEPRESSED PATIENTS IN PEDIATRIC SETTINGS

Any disturbance in mood that is associated with functional impairment should be considered a psychiatric disorder until proven otherwise. Parents and children alike frequently have a tendency to mislabel bona fide depressive disorders as "the ups and downs" of childhood or adolescence, yet epidemiologic studies have conclusively demonstrated that serious depression in childhood and adolescence is *not* normative. Mood disorders should be a strong consideration for any child with unexplained somatic complaints, decline in school performance, apathy and loss of interest, social withdrawal, increased irritability or tearfulness, sleep and appetite changes, or suicidal ideation or behavior. Moreover, depressive illnesses are frequently accompanied by tobacco, alcohol, and drug abuse, promiscuous sexual behavior, and excessive risk-taking behavior. Depressive disorders may follow bereavement, particularly if the patient has a personal or family history of depression, and may follow other severe stressors, such as physical or sexual assault. The pediatrician should be aware of a family history of depression or bipolar disorder, because this increases the risk of depressive disorder substantially.

MANAGEMENT

Children and adolescents with mood disorders are best managed by a clinician with expertise in this area. Generally, psychiatric intervention has three components: (1) family psychoeducation, (2) psychotherapy, and (3) pharmacotherapy. Most patients with mood disorders can be managed as outpatients. Inpatient referral should be reserved for those who are psychotic, acutely suicidal, acutely manic or in a mixed state, or abusing substances or for whom less restrictive levels of care have been unsuccessful.

Family Psychoeducation

Family psychoeducation approaches depression as a chronic illness, with its aim to instruct family members about the nature and course of the illness (Brent et al, 1993). Such an approach is likely to improve compliance with treatment and reduce the risk of relapse. Psychoeducation is also aimed at reducing the tensions of living with a person with a mood disorder by altering familial expectations. This alteration involves parents' accepting the illness and making appropriate expectations of the patient and themselves. Finally, psychoeducation should enable the child and family to identify early signs of recurrence of the disorder and to seek treatment before the recurrent mood disorder becomes severe.

Psychotherapy

Psychotherapy should be directed at ameliorating the interpersonal and social deficits associated with depressive symptoms. Cognitive behavioral therapy, which aims at correcting the cognitive distortions associated with the depressive state, has been shown to be efficacious for depressed adolescents. Individual brief cognitive behavior treatment, around 3 months in duration, has been shown to be more efficacious than either family or supportive treatment for the relief of adolescent depression (Brent et al, in press). Group cognitive-behavioral treatment has also been shown to be helpful both in the treatment of depression and in the prevention of depression in youth with subsyndromal depression (Clarke et al, 1995; Lewinsohn et al, 1990). The response rates for psychotherapy and pharmacotherapy appear to be similar, although they have not been compared directly. Therefore, for mild-to-moderate, nonpsychotic, nonbipolar, depressive patients, we generally begin with psychotherapy and add pharmacotherapy if no response is seen in 4 to 6 weeks.

Pharmacotherapy

For a review, see Rosenberg, Holttum, and Gershon (1994) and Green (1995). Fluoxetine, a selective serotonin-reuptake inhibitor (SSRI), has been shown to be more effective than placebo for child and adolescent depression (Emslie et al, 1997). SSRIs have a more favorable side effect profile than tricyclic antidepressants (TCAs), their most notable advantage being their lack of fatality in overdose. However, SSRIs may cause agitation, sleep problems, and gastrointestinal complaints.

TCAs are no longer first-line agents for early-onset depression insofar as no study has shown a difference between TCAs and placebo, and because of their danger of fatality in overdose. However, TCAs may be useful for the treatment of ADHD with comorbid anxiety or depression. Their use requires careful monitoring for cardiovascular side effects, with a baseline electrocardiogram, pulse and sitting or standing blood pressure, and regular follow-up rhythm strips and vital signs.

Treatment of bipolar disorder consists of use of mood stabilizers for prophylaxis, as well as the acute treatment of manic or depressive episodes. Traditionally, lithium has been the mainstay of mood stabilization, but this agent may be less effective than valproate or carbamazepine for patients in mixed states and who have rapid cycling, both of which may be more common in juvenile populations.

With regard to the use of lithium, blood levels for lithium should be monitored to check compliance and to avoid toxicity. Renal effects of lithium are rare, aside from polyuria, but kidney function should be monitored by urinalysis, blood creatinine, and blood urea nitrogen assays. Hypothyroidism can complicate lithium treatment, so thyroid function tests should be performed at 4- to 6-month intervals in patients who receive maintenance lithium. Other frequent side effects of lithium include tremor, nausea, diarrhea, weight gain, acne, and psoriasis. For manic patients who do not respond to lithium alone, it may be necessary to add or substitute valproate or carbamazepine. Lithium is contraindicated in the first trimester of pregnancy, as its use is associated with congenital malformations, namely Ebstein's anomaly. Patients with bipolar disorder who experience depressive symptoms should be continued on lithium and an antidepressant should be added. In patients with a "bipolar-type" depression (anergia, hypersomnia, hyperphagia, psychotic symptoms), particularly in those with a positive family history of mania, it may be optimal to begin with a mood-stabilizing agent and then adding an antidepressant to avoid precipitating mania.

Valproate has become more frequently used as a first-line agent in juvenile bipolar disorder. The most significant side effect is that of hepatotoxicity, and the drug is contraindicated in persons with liver disease. The risk of liver damage is greatest in children younger than age 2 years and in the first 6 months of use. Thrombocytopenia and other hematologic abnormalities have been reported, necessitating monitoring of complete blood counts and liver function tests. Other side effects include sedation, weight gain, hair loss, and nausea and vomiting, with nausea and vomiting generally being transient. In girls with significant weight gain, polycystic ovary syndrome has been reported. Because of the increased risk of congenital malformations, the use of valproate is contraindicated during pregnancy. In adults, valproate was found to be superior to lithium in the treatment of mania complicated by depression. Plasma valproate levels of 50 to 110 μg/ml are considered in the therapeutic range.

Carbamazepine has also been used for the treatment of bipolar illness refractory to lithium, particularly for patients with rapid cycling or mixed states. Therapeutic level is from 4 to 12 μg/ml. The most common side effects of carbamazepine are dizziness, drowsiness, nausea, and vomiting. The most dreaded side effect is hematologic, namely, aplastic anemia and agranulocytosis, necessitating frequent monitoring of complete blood count at regular intervals.

The role of neuroleptics in the management of early-onset mania is somewhat controversial given their long-term complications of tardive dyskinesia. However, they can be of great benefit in the initial stabilization of profoundly manic, agitated, and psychotic patients. Neuroleptics may also be useful in outpatients to circumvent increased manic symptoms when it is not feasible to increase the dosage of lithium. The newer neuroleptics, such as Risperdal and olanzapine, have a more favorable side effect profile (e.g., less sedation, rare extrapyramidal side effects), but experience is limited with these agents in children and adolescents. Alternatively, the temporary use of potent benzodiazepines (e.g., clonazepam) has been advocated.

Psychoeducation is critical in the management of bipolar disorder in order to improve compliance with medication in what may well be a lifelong condition. It is also important to help the bipolar youth and family establish regular routines and good sleep hygiene, because sleep deprivation can precipitate a manic episode.

Suicidal and Suicidal Behavior*

EPIDEMIOLOGY

Suicide is the third-leading cause of death among youth aged 15 to 24 years. The rate of suicide among 15- to 24-year-olds has increased nearly fivefold from 2.7 per 100,000 in 1950 to 13.2 per 100,000 in 1990. This increase may, in part, be related to increased availability and use of alcohol and firearms among minors (Brent, Perper, and Allman, 1987). Suicidal behavior has also become increasingly common, to the point where 1.7% of high school students have made a suicide attempt within the previous 12 months, and 7% to 8% have made a suicide attempt at sometime in their lifetime (Centers for Disease Control, 1991; Lewinsohn, Rohde, and Seeley, 1996). However, only one in four adolescents who attempt suicide ever comes to medical attention (Centers for Disease Control, 1991).

Age

Within the child and adolescent range, the suicide rate and the rate of attempted suicide increases with age (Brent, 1997; Lewinsohn, Rohde, and Seeley, 1996). Prepubertal

children may be protected against suicide by their cognitive immaturity, which prevents them from planning and executing a lethal suicidal attempt, despite suicidal impulses. After puberty, the incidence of mood, psychotic, and substance abuse disorders increases substantially, thereby increasing the risk of suicide. When suicidal behavior is observed in preschool children, it is often associated with physical or sexual abuse.

Sex

The suicide rate is five times higher among boys than girls, whereas the suicide attempt rate is two to three times higher among girls. This may be related to the male tendency to use more violent means of suicide (Centers for Disease Control, 1991; Lewinsohn, Rohde, and Seeley, 1996).

Race and Socioeconomic Status

The suicide rate is higher among whites than African Americans, although there has been a dramatic increase in the suicide rate among African American adolescent males in recent years (Shaffer, Gould, and Hicks, 1994). Young native Americans have a very high suicide rate, especially within tribes that have experienced erosion of traditional culture and that have high rates of delinquency, alcoholism, and family disorganization. Suicidal behavior (but not suicide) may be more common among Hispanic youth compared to whites and African Americans (Centers for Disease Control, 1991).

CLINICAL PICTURE

Precipitants

The precipitants for suicidal behavior and suicide among children and adolescents most frequently involve problems such as interpersonal conflict, interpersonal loss, or disciplinary crises (Brent, 1995; Gould and Shaffer, 1986).

Method

In the United States, firearms are the most common method of suicide, followed by hanging, jumping, carbon monoxide poisoning, and self-poisoning. Suicide by firearms is associated with availability in the home and with an intoxicated state in the victim (Brent et al, 1987, 1995). By contrast, self-poisoning is the most common method of suicide attempt.

Motivation and Intent

Adolescent suicide victims frequently show evidence of high intent (i.e., a strong wish to die), as manifested by timing the suicide so as not to be discovered, planning ahead, leaving a note, choosing an irreversible method, and stating intent before the actual suicide. Seriously suicidal adolescents frequently confide their suicidal plans only to another friend. In contrast, most adolescent suicide attempts are impulsive, with little resultant threat to the patient's life. Only one third of attempters truly wish to die, and the motivation for most attempts appears to be a

---

*Sections on Mood Disorders and of Suicide and Suicidal Behavior are adapted from Brent DA: School age and adolescence: Mood disorders and suicide. *In* Green M, Haggerty RJ, Weitzman ML (eds): Ambulatory Pediatrics, 5th ed. Philadelphia, WB Saunders, 1999. Adapted with permission.

desire to influence others, gain attention, communicate love or anger, or escape a difficult or painful situation (Kienhorst et al, 1995).

RISK FACTORS

Psychiatric Disorder and Psychological Traits

Based on psychological autopsy studies, most adolescent suicide victims suffer from at least one major debilitating psychiatric disorder, predominantly affective disorder, substance abuse, or conduct disorder, often in combination (Shaffer et al, 1996). At least half have made suicidal threats or attempted suicide in the past. Depression, conduct, substance abuse disorders, and past suicidality also characterize adolescents who attempt suicide (Lewinsohn, Rohde, and Seeley, 1996). Among depressed patients, those with a chronic course (duration of at least 2 years) and with comorbid substance use were most likely to be suicidal (Ryan et al, 1987). Suicidal patients have also been shown, when compared to comparable nonsuicidal patients, to be more hopeless and to show poorer problem-solving and social skills (Lewinsohn, Rohde, and Seeley, 1996).

Family History

The relatives of both adolescent suicide completers and attempters have a high prevalence of affective disorder, alcohol and drug abuse, antisocial behavior, suicide, and suicidal behavior. The familial transmission of suicidal behavior may be separate from that of psychopathology and more related to the transmission of impulsive violence (Brent et al, 1996a).

Family Environment

Both suicide victims and suicide attempters have experienced a high prevalence of divorce, parental absence, and abuse (Brent, 1995; Lewinsohn, Rohde, and Seeley, 1996). Sexual abuse is quite prevalent among suicide attempters, with a population attributable risk of nearly 20% for all suicide attempts in one epidemiologic study (Fergusson, Horwood, Lynskey, 1996). The family environments of suicidal adolescents have been characterized as less supportive, more conflicted, and more hostile than those of comparable, nonsuicidal teens (Lewinsohn, Rohde, and Seeley, 1996).

Exposure to Suicide

Exposure to suicide, either through the suicide of a schoolmate or by viewing fictional or nonfictional television programs about suicide, may also increase the risk for suicide (Gould and Shaffer, 1986; Lewinsohn, Rohde, and Seeley, 1996). Although the close friends and siblings of suicide victims do not appear to be at increased risk of suicide attempts upon 3-year follow-up, depression and posttraumatic stress disorder (PTSD) are frequent complications of exposure (Brent et al, 1996b).

Pediatric Settings

Children with epilepsy have a higher-than-expected suicide attempt rate, in part because of the iatrogenic effects of phenobarbital (Brent, 1986; Brent et al, 1987). In inner-city walk-in clinics, children with a history of suicide attempts were more likely to be seen for recent physical or sexual assault, concerns about pregnancy, or a sexually transmitted disease (Robins, 1989). Adolescents who use the emergency department as their main source of primary care, who are intoxicated or have a history of substance use, who have a history of mental health treatment, and who have poor school performance are more likely to have attempted suicide (Slap et al, 1989).

Risk of Repetition of Suicidal Behavior

In follow-up studies of hospitalized adolescent suicide attempters, the reattempt rate was between 6% and 15% per year, with evidence that this risk was highest close to discharge (Brent, 1997). One community study showed the highest risk of repeated attempt occurring within 3 months of the initial attempt, with about one fourth reattempting during this time period (Lewinsohn, Rohde, and Seeley, 1996). Factors associated with reattempts were high suicidal intent, exposure to suicidal behavior in a friend, serious psychopathology (either depression or substance abuse), hostility and aggression, hopelessness, noncompliance with treatment, social isolation, poor school performance, family discord, abuse and neglect, and parental psychiatric illness (Lewinsohn, Rohde, and Seeley, 1996).

Risk Factors for Completed Suicide Among Suicide Attempters

Among boys, the risk for completed suicide ranges from 0.7% among those seen at an emergency department for an overdose to 10% among psychiatrically hospitalized suicide attempters. Among girls, the risk ranges from 0.1% of attempters seen in an emergency department to 2.9% on follow-up of psychiatrically hospitalized suicide attempters. The risk factors for completed suicide inferred from longitudinal and from case-control studies are male sex, no apparent precipitant, high suicidal intent, "active" method, major depression comorbid with substance abuse or disruptive disorder, and bipolar or psychotic disorder (Brent, 1995, 1997).

Firearms

Case-control studies have demonstrated that the availability of guns is markedly increased in the homes of persons who successfully complete suicide compared to the homes of those who attempt suicide and to community controls. A loaded gun is even associated with suicide even when the victim did not have evidence of serious psychopathology (Brent, 1995, 1997).

Suicidal Ideation

Suicidal ideation, or thoughts about suicide, are even more common than suicidal behavior. Suicidal ideation can be thought of as a continuum from nonspecific ideation (e.g., "Life is not worth living", "I wish I was dead"), specific ideation (e.g., suicidal ideation with intent to die or with a suicidal plan), and finally, actual suicidal behavior. According to one epidemiologic study of adolescents, 19.4% of those studied had a lifetime history of suicidal ideation and 2.7% had current ideation, with a nearly threefold excess among girls (Lewinsohn, Rohde, and Seeley, 1996). Ideation is also common among prepubertal school children. Specific suicidal ideation (e.g., ideation with a concrete suicidal plan), like suicidal behavior, is associated most closely with depression, hopelessness, substance abuse, conduct disorder, and physical or sexual abuse. Because it is rare for those who attempt suicide not to have a previous ideation, and because those with specific suicidal ideation closely resemble those who actually attempt suicide, patients with specific suicidal ideation should be considered to be at high risk to act upon their suicidal thoughts.

Identifying Youth at Risk for Suicide and Suicidal Behavior

There are three categories of personal problems that should induce the physician to probe further for suicidal risk (Table 64–1): (1) psychiatric, (2) social adjustment, and (3) family/environmental. Any child who is suspected of being at risk should be questioned as to suicidal ideation (Table 64–2), moving from nonspecific questions to more specific ones, if the answers to the nonspecific inquiries are positive. There is *no* evidence that asking a child or adolescent about suicidal thoughts in a clinical situation will initiate, encourage, or exacerbate suicidal behavior.

After identification of suicidality, it is important to listen to the patient in a nonjudgmental way. Promises of confidentiality should be avoided, because it may be necessary to break such confidences in order to protect the child and provide proper treatment. The patient's parents should always be given some feedback about the assessment. Upon discovering that a patient is suicidal, it is critical to

Table 62–2 • Interviewing for Suicidal Ideation

1. Have you ever thought that life was not worth living?
2. Have you ever wished you were dead?
3. Have you ever tried to hurt youself?
4. Do you intend to hurt yourself?
5. Do you have a plan to hurt yourself?
6. Have you ever attempted suicide?

From Brent DA: Suicide and suicidal behavior in children and adolescents. Pediatr Rev 4:380, 1993. Reproduced by permission of Pediatrics in Review.

obtain a no-suicide agreement, in which the patient promises to refrain from hurting himself or herself, and to notify the physician or a care-taking adult if he or she does feel suicidal again. In formulation of the no-suicide agreement, the pediatrician should review with the patient those precipitants for the suicidality and rehearse alternative methods for coping with these stressors. It is also important to make sure that firearms are removed from the home. A mental health consultation should be obtained, and then the pediatrician, mental health specialist, and family can conjointly make a decision about the next appropriate step. If mental health treatment is recommended, the pediatrician can play a critical role in monitoring compliance and satisfaction with treatment, because many suicidal patients and their families are noncompliant with treatment. Referral to a psychiatrist, as compared to other mental health professionals, is specifically indicated if the patient is psychotic, has a serious mood or anxiety disorder, requires detoxification from drugs or alcohol, has a medical condition complicating psychiatric presentation, or requires psychopharmacologic intervention.

Referral for Inpatient Psychiatric Treatment

Suicidal children and adolescents who are judged to be at serious risk for committing or attempting suicide are most appropriate for inpatient hospitalization. The specific indications for psychiatric hospitalization are listed in Table 64–3.

Table 64–1 • Circumstances Increasing Suicidal Risk

Psychiatric Difficulties
  Depression
  Bipolar disorder
  Substance abuse
  Conduct problems
  Psychosis
  Past suicidal threats or attempts
Poor Social Adjustment
  School failure or dropout
  Legal problems
  Social isolation
  Interpersonal conflict
Family or Environment
  Interpersonal loss
  Family problems
    Abuse or neglect
    Family history of psychiatric disorder or suicide
  Exposure to suicide (in those already psychiatrically vulnerable)

From Brent DA: Suicide and suicidal behavior in children and adolescents. Pediatr Rev 4:380, 1993. Reproduced by permission of Pediatrics in Review.

Table 64–3 • Indication for Psychiatric Inpatient Hospitalization

Characteristics of Suicidality
  Inability to maintain a no-suicide contract
  Active suicidal ideation (with plan and intent)
  High intent or lethality suicide attempt
Psychiatric Disorder
  Psychosis
  Severe depression
  Substance abuse
  Bipolar illness
  Serious aggression
  Previous attempts
  Previous noncompliance or failure with outpatient treatment
Family Problems
  Abuse
  Severe parental psychiatric illness
  Family unable or unwilling to monitor or protect patient

From Brent DA: Suicide and suicidal behavior in children and adolescents. Pediatr Rev 4:380, 1993. Reproduced by permission of Pediatrics in Review.

Therapeutic Interventions

Treatment of suicidal youth should proceed on three levels: (1) treatment of the underlying psychiatric illness, (2) remediation of social and problem-solving deficits, and (3) family psychoeducation and conflict resolution. (For a review, see Brent, 1997.)

Obsessive-Compulsive Disorder

CLINICAL PICTURE

Obsessive-compulsive disorder (OCD) is a disorder characterized by (1) obsessions, that is, recurrent and persistent thoughts, impulses, or images that are experienced as distressing and senseless, and/or (2) compulsions, that is, repetitive, purposeful, and intentional behaviors performed in a ritualistic and stereotyped manner in response to an obsession. Like obsessions, compulsions are also experienced as irrational. These obsessions and compulsions can be extremely impairing. One common picture is that of intrusive thoughts of uncleanness, accompanied by compulsive handwashing or bathing, with such rituals occurring in up to 85% of those with OCD (Flament, Whitaker, and Rapoport, 1988). Obsessions often involve fears of sexual behavior, aggression, dirt or contamination, noncompletion of tasks, or physical illness. Sexual concerns, particularly guilt about masturbation, or heterosexual or homosexual impulses can be accompanied by complex atonement rituals or handwashing after being touched. Fear of contamination can be accompanied by rituals of compulsive food checking, eating in a rigidly prescribed manner, or complex toileting routines. Another class of rituals are those of task completion, including compulsive checking of lights or gas jets, checking and rechecking school assignments, or ritualistic dressing and undressing. Such rituals can take over a child's entire existence and preclude normal functioning. Moreover, compulsive handwashing can result in skin breakdown. Some researchers think that trichotillomania in some instances is a form of OCD, in which the ritual is the compulsive removal of hair, although the response to pharmacologic treatment has been much less positive than has been found in OCD proper.

DESCRIPTIVE EPIDEMIOLOGY

The point prevalence of OCD among children and adolescents has been estimated at around 0.5% and 1.8%, respectively, and rates of OCD symptoms to be up to 3% (Flament, Whitaker, and Rapoport, 1988; Whitaker et al, 1990). Boys are more common than girls in clinical samples of prepubertal age, whereas the sex ratio approaches unity in adolescent community surveys (Flament, Whitaker, and Rapoport, 1988; Whitaker et al, 1990).

PSYCHOSOCIAL RISK FACTORS

Although the bizarre and explicit nature of OCD patients' symptomatology has elicited many psychological theories about the etiology of this disorder, OCD may be one of the most intrinsic and biological of the child psychiatric disorders. Psychosocial dysfunction in the patient and family is much more likely to be a consequence, rather than a forerunner, of OCD. However, stress may exacerbate symptoms. There is no historical evidence that children with OCD have more rituals, superstitions, or other "subsyndromal" precursors of OCD than control children. Moreover, compulsive personality traits, characterized by a tendency to perfectionism and insistence on sameness, are quite phenomenologically distinct from OCD.

NEUROBIOLOGICAL CORRELATES

There is evidence that OCD may aggregate within families and that there is a biological basis to this disorder involving the basal ganglia (March and Leonard, 1996). Several disorders with basal ganglia involvement are associated with a greater incidence of OCD-like syndromes, including Tourette syndrome (TS), Sydenham chorea, carbon monoxide poisoning, and von Economo encephalitis. Moreover, neuroimaging studies in adults have shown an increased metabolic rate in the left caudate and orbital gyrus of OCD patients compared to normal control subjects. Neuroimaging studies have shown that medication-naive youths with OCD had significantly smaller basal ganglia volume than controls, and that basal ganglia volume was inversely correlated with the severity of OCD symptoms. The caudate is rich in serotonergic fibers, and neurochemical studies suggest that serotonergic functioning is abnormal in patients with OCD, a hypothesis supported by the efficacy of antidepressants with serotonergic agonist properties in the treatment of OCD. There is evidence that some cases of OCD and/or tic disorders could have an autoimmune etiology, in that there are case reports of the onset or exacerbation of OCD/TS associated with beta-hemolytic streptococcal or viral infections responding to plasmapheresis, intravenous immunoglobulin, or immunosuppression (Allen, Leonard, and Swedo, 1995). For example, Sydenham chorea has prominent obsessive and compulsive features that may be explained by antibodies that cross-react against both streptococci and basal ganglia (Kiessling, Marcotte, and Culpepper, 1994). This spectrum of pediatric, infection-triggered, autoimmune neuropsychiatric disorders (PITANDs) and their proper treatment is still under investigation and delineation, and such treatments are currently considered experimental.

COMORBIDITY

In an epidemiologic study of adolescents, 15 of 20 patients with OCD had at least one additional lifetime major psychiatric disorder: eating disorder (25%), depression or dysthymia (30%), overanxious disorder (20%), phobia (12%), and panic attacks (20%) (Flament, Whitaker, and Rapoport, 1988). Whereas most cases of OCD occur in the absence of TS, OCD symptoms are an integral part of the disorder, and in girls with TS or who are first-degree relatives of patients with TS, the OCD symptoms may predominate. Therefore, it is important in movement disorders to examine for evidence of OCD, and conversely in OCD to check for the presence of tics and other movement disorders.

CLINICAL COURSE

There is evidence that untreated OCD will continue unremitting in most cases. However, with behavioral treatment and proper pharmacotherapy, symptoms and social adjustment have been found to improve in most cases.

DIFFERENTIAL DIAGNOSIS

The differential diagnosis of OCD can be challenging, especially in light of the high rates of comorbidity among these patients. The most common differential diagnostic issues are between personality, anxiety, mood, and psychotic disorders and OCD. Compulsive personality traits differ from OCD insofar as personality traits are experienced as acceptable to the patient, whereas the insistence on neatness in a patient with OCD is experienced as intrusive and is usually accompanied by rituals that are very time-consuming and impairing. Patients with OCD often experience worry and fear, both in response to intrusive thoughts and when they are prevented from completing a "required" ritual. On the other hand, the experience of anxiety in patients with overanxious disorder occurs with regard to performance, in patients with separation anxiety in response to separation from a parent, and in patients with phobic disorder in response to a particular trigger (e.g., heights, animals). Patients with OCD may refuse to go to school, not out of fear of separation or of school, but because their rituals prevent them from leaving the house or because they cannot perform their rituals at school. Patients with OCD may experience sadness and demoralization with respect to functional impairment or the nature and unacceptability of intrusive thoughts, and a secondary depression may develop. However, intrusive suicidal thoughts, guilt, and accompanying rituals can be part of OCD, and only when symptoms such as suicidality and guilt become more pervasive can these be considered a symptom of depression. Finally, the bizarre nature of the intrusive, obsessive thoughts may present a differential diagnostic issue with schizophrenia or other psychotic disorders. However, the obsessive thoughts in the OCD patient are usually experienced as unwanted and bizarre, whereas delusions in a schizophrenic patient are more likely to be accepted by that patient as having a basis in reality. However, in younger children and those with chronic OCD, obsessive ideation may not be experienced as irrational.

In addition, the differential diagnosis should consider tic disorders and infectious conditions that may affect the basal ganglia, such as Sydenham chorea and other PITANDs.

IDENTIFICATION AND REFERRAL

The secretive nature of OCD makes identification in a primary care setting difficult. A latency of about 7 years between onset and referral for treatment has been reported. The dermatologic stigma of repetitive bathing or handwashing should raise the index of suspicion for the pediatrician of OCD. A profound deterioration in function, such as inability to complete schoolwork, inability to leave the house, or social withdrawal, should also lead the pediatrician to suspect this disorder. Given the specialized nature of this condition and its treatment, and given the high rate of psychiatric comorbidity, these patients are best managed by a child psychiatrist with experience and expertise with OCD.

TREATMENT

There are three key elements to the treatment of OCD: psychoeducation, pharmacotherapy, and behavioral therapy. Patients and families, by the time they come for treatment, are frustrated, debilitated, and angry. The OCD rituals can take over family life, and parents can see their child as "manipulative" rather than suffering from an illness. The family needs help in supporting the OCD patient and in returning to a normal routine.

The mainstay of pharmacotherapy for OCD are antidepressants with serotonergic properties (March and Leonard, 1996). Clomipramine, a TCA with strong serotonergic reuptake-blocking activity, has been shown to be superior to placebo and imipramine in the treatment of OCD. Similar cautions for use hold for clomipramine as for other TCAs (see Pharmacotherapy). Two SSRIs, fluoxetine and fluvoxamine, have also been shown to be effective in the treatment of this disorder. Because of their more favorable side effect profile, SSRIs are becoming first-line agents for the treatment of OCD.

Behavioral treatments also serve as useful interventions, especially because not all patients respond to, can tolerate, or comply with psychopharmacologic regimens. The types of behavioral therapies most useful for OCD patients include graded exposure with response prevention, in particular in vivo exposure. Behavioral treatment aims to reduce the rate of dysfunctional rituals, whereas the exposure techniques aim to reduce the worries and fears that are associated with the intrusive, obsessive thoughts that maintain these rituals.

Finally, because of the description of PITANDs, all patients with new-onset OCD should have a throat culture and an antistreptolysin-O titer done. Active infection should be treated; some experts advocate penicillin prophylaxis in patients with evidence of more chronic autoimmune phenomena. However, because of the relatively recent identification of these conditions, no clear treatment guidelines are yet in place.

Anxiety Disorders

Considered in this section are the following: SAD, generalized anxiety disorder (GAD), social phobia, panic disorder, simple phobia, and PTSD. What all these disorders have in common is an anxious mood accompanied by fearful and worried cognitions and somatic symptoms of anxiety, such as sweating, sighing respirations, rapid heart rate, and fluttering in the pit of the stomach. However, they can be differentiated on the basis of their pervasiveness or emergence with respect to specific situations. *Separation anxiety* is characterized by anxiety about separation from attachment figures, either actual or anticipated. *GAD* is characterized by pervasive worry about performance, self-efficacy, and future events. *Social phobia* involves excessive shyness with strangers, including peers, although a patient with social phobia may enjoy close relationships with family members. *Panic disorders* involve an acute and intense physiologic activation characterized by palpitations and profound discomfort. *Phobias* are fears of very specific situations, such as high places, animals, or public speaking, accompanied by physiologic distress and avoidance of the precipitant. *PTSD* involves the re-experiencing of anxiety and helplessness following exposure to a life-threatening stress. Each of these disorders is discussed in turn with respect to clinical picture, descriptive epidemiology, differential diagnosis, clinical course, identification, and management.

Although these disorders are discussed separately, they often co-occur, and thus the risk factors and neurobiology of anxiety are discussed here. A tendency to experience anxiety has been noted to manifest very early in life. Kagan, Reznick, and Snidman (1987) termed this tendency *behavioral inhibition*, or an excessive withdrawal and physiologic reaction to strange and unfamiliar situations, and they noted that in about one third of behaviorally inhibited infants, this pattern persists into childhood. These children are characterized by higher baseline heart rate and increased frontal EEG activation, which predicts persistent anxious symptoms. The children of anxious parents are much more likely to be behavioral inhibited, and multiple anxiety disorders are much more likely to develop in behavioral inhibited children (Hirshfeld et al, 1992; Rosenbaum et al, 1993). Very few studies of the neurobiology of anxiety in childhood have been performed, but neuroendocrine challenge studies in adults suggest abnormalities in serotonergic and beta-adrenergic receptors, similar to the findings in depression (Brent et al, 1995). Imaging studies suggest involvement of the amygdala, with a tendency for evidence of greater baseline and stress-related activation. Twin studies in adults suggest that anxiety and depression may be different manifestations of the same genetic diathesis, and longitudinal data suggest that anxiety is often a precursor of depression. Parenting style may also influence the likelihood of development of an anxiety disorder in a temperamentally vulnerable child (Kagan, Reznick, and Snidman, 1987).

SEPARATION ANXIETY

Clinical Picture

It is particularly important to view separation anxiety within a developmental context. Separation anxiety first develops as the infant acquires object permanence, around 6 to 8 months of age. After age 3 years, with the ability to understand that separations from attachment figures are temporary, this developmentally appropriate anxiety diminishes. Therefore, caution should be exercised in making this diagnosis before the age of 5 years, and it should never be made in children younger than 30 months. The symptoms of SAD, according to *DSM-IV*, are listed in Table 64–4; at least three symptoms for a duration of 2 weeks are required to fulfill the criteria for SAD. Functional impairment, such as refusal to attend school or camp or to sleep over at friend's house, is the cardinal manifestation of this disorder. Occasionally, a child with SAD is able to attend school, but he or she is so preoccupied about terrible things befalling his or her parent that the child is unable to concentrate. The anticipation of the separation is the most common precipitant; therefore, it is typical for the disorder to manifest itself on Sunday night or Monday morning, before going to school, or after longer separations—for example, summer vacation or after an illness.

Table 64–4 • Diagnostic Criteria for 309.21 Separation Anxiety Disorder

A. Developmentally inappropriate and excessive anxiety concerning separation from home or from those to whom the individual is attached, as evidenced by three (or more) of the following:
(1) recurrent excessive distress when separation from home or major attachment figures occurs or is anticipated
(2) persistent and excessive worry about losing, or about possible harm befalling, major attachment figures
(3) persistent and excessive worry that an untoward event will lead to separation from a major attachment figure (e.g., getting lost or being kidnapped)
(4) persistent reluctance or refusal to go to school or elsewhere because of fear of separation
(5) persistently and excessively fearful or reluctant to be alone or without major attachment figures at home or without significant adults in other settings
(6) persistent reluctance or refusal to go to sleep without being near a major attachment figure or to sleep away from home
(7) repeated nightmares involving the theme of separation
(8) repeated complaints of physical symptoms (such as headaches, stomachaches, nausea, or vomiting) when separation from major attachment figures occurs or is anticipated
B. The duration of disturbance is at least 4 weeks.
C. The onset is before age 18 years.
D. The disturbance causes clinically significant distress or impairment in social, academic (occupational), or other important areas of functioning.
E. The disturbance does not occur exclusively during the course of a Pervasive Developmental Disorder, Schizophrenia, or other Psychotic Disorder and, in adolescents and adults, is not better accounted for by Panic Disorder With Agoraphobia.

Specify if:
Early Onset: if onset occurs before age 6 years

Reprinted with permission from the Diagnostic and Statistical Manual of Mental Disorders, 4th edition. Washington, DC, American Psychiatric Association, 1994, p 113. Coyright 1994 American Psychiatric Association.

Comorbidity with other anxiety disorders and depression is common.

Descriptive Epidemiology

The 1-year prevalence of separation anxiety in prepubertal children has been reported at 3.5% to 4.1% (Costello et al, 1988b), with the ratio of girls to boys being about 3:1.

Specific Risk Factors

Precipitants for SAD may include a forced separation, such as the death, illness, or divorce of a parent. Such precipitants may be more likely to provoke a separation anxiety response in constitutionally vulnerable children.

Differential Diagnosis

SAD can be differentiated from GAD insofar as the latter consists of more global concerns, mostly around issues of performance, appearance, and competency, whereas those with SAD are concerned primarily with separation. Agoraphobia is relatively rare in younger children but relates to a fear of leaving home or being in open or exposed places, rather than a fear of being away from an attachment figure.

Patients with OCD may experience anxiety associated with leaving home, but it usually relates to a specific obsession or ritual. These patients may refuse to leave home because they need to "finish" a ritual. Anxiety about parents' safety may be a feature of OCD, but these thoughts are experienced as irrational, not relieved by the presence of the parent, and often have a component of fear of the patient's own aggressive impulses toward that parent.

In younger children, refusal to attend school is most commonly due to SAD. However, occasionally, the child may have been traumatized at school or may fear a situation at school, such as being bullied. In these cases, the child may suffer from a phobia of attending school, rather than a fear of separation, particularly if separation from parents in other contexts is not problematic. If a child has serious learning disabilities or peer problems, he or she may refuse to attend school because of the attendant humiliation. Children with conduct disorder may refuse to attend school, but they rarely stay at home and are often truant (and may feign school attendance) with a group of other like-minded peers. Especially when school refusal has its onset in early adolescence, the cause may be related to other psychiatric disorders, namely depression, obsessive-compulsive disorder, or psychosis. Children with depression may refuse to attend school as part of an overall picture of social withdrawal, anhedonia, irritability, or declining school performance, whereas those with incipient psychosis may become overwhelmed, paranoid, and delusional about peers and teachers at school.

Clinical Course

Most longitudinal studies have focused on school refusal rather than separation anxiety. However, the prognosis is good for acute-onset school refusal in young children who return to school relatively early in their course, whereas adolescents with other comorbid conditions who have more difficulty achieving an initial return to school have a more guarded prognosis. As a group, those with separation anxiety as children are at higher risk for the development of anxiety disorders in adulthood.

Identification and Pediatric Management

The hallmarks of separation anxiety are easy to recognize, yet the parent and child may be seen by the pediatrician for somatic complaints upon return to school, especially after a weekend or vacation. By recognizing the pattern of onset of somatic complaints and by inquiring about school attendance and fears of separation, the pediatrician is in an excellent position to identify and manage this problem, particularly in acute cases in younger children with early onset (Schmitt, 1973). Children with recurrent or refractory disorder, with comorbid conditions, or with adolescent onset need more intensive and specialized psychiatric treatment.

The watchwords of pediatric management of this disorder are the following: DO NOT COLLUDE. An anxious parent with an anxious child may pressure the pediatrician to write doctor's excuses for school, treat nonexistent ailments, and obtain homebound instruction. A firm stance about the absence of medical illness, the need for the child to progressively return to school, and the need for the parents to enforce school attendance consistently is what is required. If separation difficulties are primarily with one parent, then the other one may need to enforce school attendance. A contact at the school, preferably the teacher or principal, is essential in order to help the child manage his or her distress, yet stay at school. For example, children with somatic complaints may be allowed a visit to a sympathetic (but firm) school nurse, who can reinforce that the symptoms are real, but caused by worries; then the child should return to the classroom. Sometimes family therapy is required to diminish parental anxiety about separation and to build parental resolve that will not crumble when confronted with a school-refusing child.

Behavioral Management

A number of behavioral management approaches have been used to manage SAD, although their efficacy is supported by case reports and anecdotal reviews rather than by clinical trials. These approaches include desensitization through graduated exposure, and cognitive-behavioral approaches to decrease anticipatory anxiety. The core aspect of all psychosocial treatments of anxiety is gradual exposure, so that the individual can confront the feared situation. Randomized clinical trials have shown cognitive-behavior therapy to be superior to a wait list control for children with a variety of anxiety conditions including SAD (Kendall, 1994). For prepubertal children, family management techniques that help the parents cope with an anxious child augment the impact of cognitive-behavioral therapy (Barrett, Dadds, and Rapee, 1996).

Pharmacotherapy

Imipramine, a TCA, has been used clinically in the treatment of SAD, often to augment the impact of behavioral therapy in cases in which behavioral management alone has not been successful, or when anticipatory anxiety or panic attacks are particularly pronounced. Imipramine has been reported to be of benefit in combination with behavioral treatment for school-refusing youngsters in one double-blind placebo-controlled trial (Gittelman-Klein and Klein, 1971), but this result has not been replicated in three other studies, and at this point, we do *not* recommend it as a first-line intervention. In an open-label study, fluoxetine has shown promise in the treatment of childhood anxiety disorders in anxious patients refractory to behavioral therapy and/or TCAs, but further confirmation must await randomized clinical trials (Birmaher et al, 1994).

GENERALIZED ANXIETY DISORDER

In contrast to SAD, which is highly situation specific, GAD is more pervasive and free-floating, with concerns focusing on performance, self-image, and competency. These concerns include worry over past events or worries about the future, such as upcoming tests, social events, or public performance. Somatic manifestations of anxiety are common, such as a lump in the throat, headaches, dizziness, and gastrointestinal symptoms. The *DSM-IV* criteria for overanxious disorder include 6 months of an anxious mood, accompanied by at least four of the following symptoms:

1. Worry about future events
2. Concern about competence

3. Concern about past behavior
4. Somatic complaints
5. Self-consciousness
6. Continual need for reassurance
7. Constant feelings of tension and/or inability to relax

To qualify for the *DSM-IV* diagnosis of GAD, these symptoms should cause social impairment. According to one study of a clinically referred population, patients with GAD were more likely than patients with SAD to have other comorbid anxiety disorders, such as simple phobia or panic disorder.

Descriptive Epidemiology

The prevalence of GAD among prepubertal children and adolescents has been estimated at 2.9% to 4.1% (Anderson et al, 1987: Costello et al, 1988b; Whitaker et al, 1990). The male to female ratio has been reported as 1.7:1 among prepubertal children in one study (Anderson et al, 1987), but approaches 1:3 among adolescents. Family history of anxiety disorder is associated with GAD in children.

Clinical Course

Little is known about the natural history of GAD in childhood, except that it seems to predict future bouts with anxiety disorders in adulthood.

Differential Diagnosis

The most common differential diagnostic issue in GAD is its differentiation from other internalizing disorders. GAD tends to be pervasive and most closely tied to performance and self-concept. In contrast, separation anxiety occurs in response to anticipated or real separation from attachment figures, and simple phobias represent fears and avoidance of specific objects or situations. Both patients with social phobias and patients with GAD may be concerned about speaking in public, but those with GAD also worry about performance in other spheres, both past and future. Patients with dysthymic disorder often view their performance as inadequate, but in contrast to patients with GAD, their mood is primarily depressed, and symptoms are related to hopelessness and anhedonia rather than to failure to achieve or live up to certain (very high) standards. Patients with ADHD may appear to be agitated, but patients with GAD alone do not have difficulties with inattention or impulsivity. Medical illnesses that are associated with an anxious or hypervigilant state (e.g., hyperthyroidism) should be ruled out.

Identification and Management

Parents often do not complain about children who are too conscientious, although if GAD interferes with sleep, peer relationships, or ultimately, schoolwork, either parents or teachers may suggest a referral. Family therapy has been recommended to reduce unrealistic parental expectations and help parents not to inadvertently reinforce their child's anxiety. Individual cognitive-behavioral therapy has also been advocated to modify the patient's expectations and

dysfunctional responses to performance demands. As discussed, cognitive-behavior treatment with family management has been shown to be efficacious in clinical trials; SSRIs may also be of benefit in treatment-refractory youth.

SOCIAL PHOBIA

Clinical Picture

Social phobia is an anxiety disorder related to excessive embarrassment and shyness in novel social situations. As such, patients shy away from contact with peers or adults with whom they have not had a great deal of previous experience. However, these children do have warm and close relationships with family members and other familiar peers and adults. To make the diagnosis of social phobia, the social behavior must persist for 6 months and be severe enough to interfere with social adaptation, yet be specific to avoidance of novel and public social situations. One extreme manifestation of social phobia in younger children is selective mutism, in which children speak only with a small circle of family and friends.

Epidemiology and Natural History

According to one epidemiologic study, the prevalence is between 0.6% and 1.6% (Costello et al, 1988b). Little else is known about this disorder, except in an anecdotal fashion. Persons with social phobia are often characterized as temperamentally shy and may go on to have an avoidant style as adults. In addition to temperamental differences, catastrophic illness or a move (particularly from another country) may play a role in the development of this disorder. Like the other anxiety disorders, behavioral inhibition as an infant appears to be a precursor.

Differential Diagnosis

The main differential diagnoses are between other conditions that interfere with social relationships. In depression, there may be social withdrawal, but this is often antedated by satisfactory social relationships. Schizoid disorder of childhood is characterized by a lack of interest in social relationships with strangers, whereas socially phobic children both desire and fear contact with same-age peers who are not well known to them. Schizotypal children have evidence of thought disorder such as loosening of associations and magical thinking. Children with autism and pervasive developmental disorders have disordered social relationships but usually show other stigmata of these disorders, such as impaired language development and difficulty in forming and sustaining social bonds.

Identification and Management

Parental or school concerns are the usual cues to the presence of social phobia. Except for the treatment of selective mutism, no controlled treatment trials of this disorder have been reported, but current management includes gradual exposure, social skills and assertiveness training, relaxation training, and cognitive behavior psychotherapy aiming at reducing fears of rejection. Selective mutism has been shown to respond to fluoxetine in a randomized clinical trial (Black and Uhde, 1994).

PANIC DISORDER

Clinical Picture

Panic disorder consists of recurrent, unexpected panic attacks followed by at least 1 month of persistent concern about having another panic attack, worry about the possible implications or consequences of the panic attacks, or a significant behavioral change related to the attacks. A panic attack consists of a state of markedly heightened physiologic activation, in which the patient experiences palpitations, difficulty breathing, a sensation of choking, of "going crazy," and a fear that he or she is going to die (Table 64–5). The panic attack can adversely condition a person to a particular situation (e.g., being in open spaces, bridges, tunnels), so secondary agoraphobia can develop.

Descriptive Epidemiology

The prevalence of panic disorder is unknown but is probably underrecognized. These conditions have been described as highly familial.

Management

Little empiric work has been done on the management of juvenile panic disorder, but adults respond to TCAs, SSRIs, and cognitive-behavioral treatment.

SIMPLE PHOBIAS

Clinical Picture

Phobic disorders are related to avoidance precipitated by certain triggers, such as animals, situations, or places.

Table 64–5 • Diagnostic Criteria for Panic Disorder Without Agoraphobia

---

A. Both (1) and (2)
  (1) Recurrent unexpected panic attacks
  (2) At least one of the attacks has been followed by 1 month (or more) of one (or more) of the following:
    (a) Persistent concern about having additional attacks
    (b) Worry about the implications of the attack or its consequences (e.g., losing control, having a heart attack, "going crazy")
    (c) A significant change in behavior related to the attacks
B. Absence of agoraphobia
C. The panic attacks are not due to the direct physiologic effects of a substance (e.g., a drug of abuse, a medication) or a general medical condition (e.g., hyperthyroidism).
D. The panic attacks are not better accounted for by another mental disorder, such as social phobia (e.g., occurring on exposure to feared social situations), specific phobia (e.g., on exposure to a specific phobic situation), obsessive-compulsive disorder (e.g., exposure to dirt in someone with an obsession about contamination), posttraumatic stress disorder (e.g., in response to stimuli associated with a severe stressor), or separation anxiety disorder (e.g., in response to being away from home or close relatives).

Descriptive Epidemiology

Fears are common among children. Among children aged 7 and 11 years, the prevalence of simple phobias is approximately 2.4% and 0.9% respectively (Anderson et al, 1987). Simple phobia has a marked female preponderance. It is thought that parental history of anxiety disorder (particularly phobias), anxious temperament, and traumatic occurrences (e.g., a dog bite, leading to dog phobia) all play a role in the genesis of phobic disorders.

Identification

Many phobic disorders never come to medical attention, because those suffering from the disorder can simply alter their life to avoid contact with the precipitant for their phobic reactions. However, children with simple phobia that leads to school avoidance often become referred for treatment as "school refusers."

Differential Diagnosis

The differentiation between a fear and phobia is in the degree of anxiety in response to exposure, the extent of the avoidant behavior, and the concomitant functional impairment. School phobia may result in the avoidance of school, but the fear is not related to separation, as in the case of SAD. Social phobia is characterized by pervasive shyness with strangers, concern about rejection, and avoidance of specific public or group activities.

Treatment

Behavioral interventions have a well-documented efficacy in the treatment of phobias. Such interventions include desensitization through graduated imagined or real exposure.

POSTTRAUMATIC STRESS DISORDER

Clinical Picture

PTSD was first described in the context of "traumatic neurosis" of World War I soldiers exposed to life-threatening situations. Since that time, it has been recognized that PTSD can occur in response to a variety of traumatic stressors both in wartime and in the civilian population. The *DSM-IV* defines PTSD as follows:

1. The person has experienced an event that would be experienced as markedly distressing by almost anyone. Examples would include exposure to violence, witnessing a homicide, combat, severe injury, serious accident, sexual or physical assault, or natural disaster.
2. The traumatic event is persistently re-experienced in the form of
  a. Intrusive images
  b. Traumatic dreams
  c. Distress at reminders
3. There is a state of psychological numbing accompanied by avoidance of stimuli that might remind the victim of the trauma:

a. Avoidance of thoughts, feelings, locations
b. Reduced interest in usual activities
c. Feelings of being alone, detached, estranged, reduced emotional range
4. Increased state of arousal:
a. Sleep disturbance
b. Irritability/anger
c. Difficulty concentrating
d. Hypervigilance
e. Exaggerated startle

Epidemiology and Risk Factors

The prevalence of PTSD among children and adolescents is unknown, although one school survey found nearly 5% of youth with significant PTSD symptoms. There is concern that as the number of traumatic events (e.g., abuse, witnessed violence) to which children are exposed increases, so will the incidence of PTSD among children.

In one study of children who had witnessed a sniper attack, the severity of the posttraumatic reaction was proportional to the proximity to the victim, the closeness of the friendship to the victim, the perception of life threat, and, to a lesser extent, to previous accumulated traumas (Pynoos et al, 1987). Studies of PTSD in adults have also found an effect for the proximity and degree of exposure, as well as for preexisting psychiatric morbidity. A tendency to autonomic overreactivity, as indicated by an exaggerated startle, may predispose the person to the development of PTSD. The development of PTSD in children seems to be ultimately related to a feeling of helplessness at the time of the trauma and guilt about not being able to help the victim or themselves (Pynoos et al, 1987). In one study of adolescents who lost a friend to suicide, knowing the suicide plans of the friend and feeling that one could have done something to prevent the death were among the strongest predictors of PTSD 3 years after exposure to suicide (Brent et al, 1996b). Family history of anxiety disorder and previous disruptions of important relationships were also contributory. Biological studies have shown alterations in the noradrenergic function and the adrenocortical axis as a function of exposure to sexual abuse, suggesting long-term and profound impact of abuse.

Clinical Course

The study of the course of PTSD is complicated by its frequent coexistence with anxiety and depression. There is evidence that in some children, symptoms endure as long as 4 years later, as in the cases of children kidnapped and buried underground in a school bus (Terr, 1983).

Differential Diagnosis

Whereas the symptomatic picture overlaps to some extent with depressive or anxiety disorders, the trauma-related nature of PTSD makes it unique and unmistakable. The intrusive thoughts and images are a central feature of this disorder as compared to any other internalizing disorder.

Identification

It is important for the pediatrician who works in an emergency department or intensive care setting to be aware that PTSD could develop in any traumatized child. Studies of adults with PTSD indicate that the optimum period for intervention is during the acute period following the trauma.

Treatment

The most significant aspect of the treatment of the child with PTSD is an opportunity to review and process the traumatic event. Consequently, the child is encouraged to identify traumatic reminders, so as to begin to anticipate and manage his or her exposure to them. Reenacting the experience through drama, art, or talking may help the child to experience more control over an otherwise uncontrollable event. The discussion and management of intrusive imagery is also critical. Parents should be apprised of the aforementioned issues so that they can continue to be supportive and create a secure environment for the traumatized child. If parents also experienced the traumatic event, they will need their own assistance as well.

In patients with prominent sleep, concentration, or arousal difficulties, SSRIs have been reported to be of benefit, although not subjected as yet to clinical evaluation.

Somatoform Disorders

For a review, see Campo and Garber, 1998.

CLINICAL PICTURE

Children with somatic complaints that cannot be attributed to a specific physical illness are common in pediatric practice. Even though clinicians must keep in mind the possibility of undiagnosed physical disease—and somatic complaints may certainly be part of the clinical picture in depression and anxiety—there are those patients whose main symptomatic focus is on physical symptoms that are not attributable to physical disease. By far the most common category is that of somatoform disorder, which is defined by medically unexplained physical symptoms in an individual who does not intentionally produce the symptoms and who does not appear to experience any sense of voluntary control over the symptoms. This contrasts with malingering and factitious disorder, in which an individual may deliberately feign, simulate, or produce illness. In malingering, the motivation is external gain such as drug seeking, compensation, or avoidance of a particular responsibility, whereas in factitious disorder, the motivation is internal, generally a psychological desire to be cared for within the medical setting (American Psychiatric Association, 1994).

The specific somatoform disorders include conversion disorder, pain disorder, somatization disorder, undifferentiated somatoform disorder, hypochondriasis, and body dysmorphic disorder (American Psychiatric Association, 1994) and are conceptually distinct from factitious disorders and malingering.

CONVERSION DISORDER

Conversion disorder (Table 64–6) is characterized by symptoms of a loss or alteration of voluntary motor or

Table 64–6 • Diagnostic Criteria for Conversion Disorder

A. One or more symptoms or deficits affecting voluntary motor or sensory function that suggest a neurologic or other general medical condition
B. Psychological factors are judged to be associated with the symptom or deficit because the initiation or exacerbation of the symptom or deficit is preceded by conflicts or other stressors
C. The symptom or deficit is not intentionally produced or feigned (as in factitious disorder or malingering)
D. The symptom or deficit cannot, after appropriate investigation, be fully explained by a general medical condition, or by the direct effects of a substance, or as a culturally sanctioned behavior or experience
E. The symptom or deficit causes clinically significant distress or impairment in social, occupational, or other important areas of functioning or warrants medical evaluation
F. The symptom or deficit is not limited to pain or sexual dysfunction, does not occur exclusively during the course of somatization disorder, and is not better accounted for by another mental disorder

Adapted with permission from the Diagnostic and Statistical Manual of Mental Disorders, 4th edition. Washington, DC, American Psychiatric Association Press, 1994. Copyright 1994 American Psychiatric Association.

Table 64–7 • Diagnostic Criteria for Hypochondriasis

A. Preoccupation with fears of having, or the idea that one has a serious disease based on the person's misinterpretation of bodily symptoms
B. The preoccupation persists despite appropriate medical evaluation and reassurance
C. The belief in criterion A is not of delusional intensity (as delusional disorder, somatic type) and is not restricted to a circumscribed concern about appearance (as in body dysmorphic disorder)
D. The preoccupation causes clinically significant distress or impairment in social, occupational, or other important areas of functioning
E. The duration of the disturbance is at least 6 months
F. The preoccupation is not better accounted for by generalized anxiety disorder, obsessive-compulsive disorder, panic disorder, a major depressive episode, separation anxiety, or another somatoform disorder

Adapted with permission from the Diagnostic and Statistical Manual of Mental Disorders, 4th edition. Washington, DC, American Psychiatric Association, 1994. Copyright 1994 American Psychiatric Association.

sensory function, thereby suggesting a neurologic or other physical disorder, with examples including pseudoseizures, limb paralysis, or "hysterical" blindness. The symptoms are thought to be related to a psychological stressor and/or conflict. The classic expectation of la belle indifference, or indifference to the symptom, is an unreliable clue to the diagnosis and is often not observed.

PAIN DISORDER

In pain disorder, the patient complains of pain but psychological factors are judged to play a significant role in the pain, which is judged not to be intentionally produced or feigned. Recurrent abdominal pain and headache are common examples (Chapter 36). Pain disorder may be diagnosed in the absence of associated physical disease (pain disorder associated with psychological factors) or when physical disease, if present, and psychological factors appear to play a significant role in the individual's pain (pain disorder associated with both psychological factors and a general medical condition).

HYPOCHONDRIASIS

Hypochondriasis (Table 64–7) consists of a preoccupation with the fear of having a major illness, such as malignancy or cardiovascular disease, based on a misinterpretation of one or more physical symptoms. The fear persists despite medical reassurance and causes significant functional impairment. Hypochondriacal concerns may become the focus of the patient's life. Past personal or family experience with illness may play a role.

SOMATIZATION DISORDER

Somatization disorder (Table 64–8) is characterized by multiple, recurrent somatic complaints over several years' duration, resulting in significant functional impairment.

DSM-IV requires involvement of at least four symptom categories (pain, gastrointestinal, sexual, neurologic) to qualify. The full-blown picture is rarely seen until adulthood.

Table 64–8 • Diagnostic Criteria for Somatization Disorder

A. A history of many physical complaints beginning before age 30 years that occur over a period of several years and result in treatment being sought or significant impairment in social, occupational, or other important areas of functioning
B. Each of the following criteria must have been met, with individual symptoms occurring at any time during the course of the disturbance
   (1) *Four pain symptoms:* a history of pain related to at least four extremities, chest, rectum, during menstruation, during sexual intercourse, or during urination
   (2) *Two gastrointestinal symptoms:* a history of at least two gastrointestinal symptoms other than pain (e.g., nausea, bloating, vomiting other than during pregnancy, diarrhea, or intolerance of several different foods)
   (3) *One sexual symptom:* a history of at least one sexual or reproductive symptom other than pain (e.g., sexual indifference, erectile or ejaculatory dysfunction, irregular menses, excessive menstrual bleeding, vomiting throughout pregnancy)
   (4) *One pseudoneurologic symptom:* a history of at least one symptom or deficit suggesting a neurologic condition not limited to pain (conversion symptoms such as impaired coordination or balance, paralysis or localized weakness, difficulty swallowing or lump in throat, aphonia, urinary retention, hallucinations, loss of touch or pain sensation, double vision, blindness, deafness, seizures; dissociative symptoms such as amnesia; or loss of consciousness other than fainting)
C. Either (1) or (2):
   (1) After appropriate investigation, each of the symptoms in criterion B cannot be fully explained by a known general medical condition or the direct effects of a substance (e.g., a drug of abuse, a medication).
   (2) When there is a related general medical condition, the physical complaints or resulting social or occupational impairment are in excess of what would be expected from the history, physical examination, or laboratory findings.
D. The symptoms are not intentionally produced or feigned (as in factitious disorder or malingering).

Adapted with permission from the Diagnostic and Statistical Manual of Mental Disorders, 4th edition. Washington, DC, American Psychiatric Association, 1994. Copyright 1994 American Psychiatric Association.

UNDIFFERENTIATED SOMATOFORM DISORDER

Undifferentiated somatoform disorder applies to children and adolescents with one or more medically unexplained physical complaints present for at least 6 months (e.g., fatigue, gastrointestinal symptoms, urinary complaints) (Table 64–9).

BODY DYSMORPHIC DISORDER

The essential feature of body dysmorphic disorder is a preoccupation with a defect or perceived defect in appearance. This preoccupation may consume much time in self-examination and result in avoidance of ordinary social activities, hence functional impairment. There are many similarities in presentation to that of OCD, and in adults, treatment with SSRIs and clomipramine has been helpful.

FACTITIOUS DISORDER

Factitious disorder is the diagnosis given when a patient purposefully simulates, feigns, or deliberately causes a medical illness, such as by putting blood into a urine specimen, heating a thermometer to simulate a fever, lying about historic information, or ingesting poisonous materials to induce illness. The goal apparently is to maintain the patient role. Chronic factitious disorder is also known as Munchausen syndrome. Munchausen syndrome by proxy has also been reported, for example, when a parent causes illness in a child.

MALINGERING

In malingering, the patient may also feign, simulate, or induce illness, but for external gain, rather than to maintain the patient role per se. For example, an opiate addict might feign renal colic, even putting blood in his urine, to obtain narcotics.

EPIDEMIOLOGY AND RISK FACTORS

Psychosomatic disorders have not been systematically investigated. However, as many as 10% of pediatric visits may be related to psychosomatic illness (Starfield et al, 1984) and as many as 4.5% of boys and 10.7% of girls may experience a somatic complaint syndrome according to the Ontario Child Health Study (Offord et al, 1987). Symptoms of recurrent pain and common somatic symptoms occur equally in boys and girls until puberty, after which unexplained physical symptoms are more common in girls. Conversion disorder is more common in girls and may be more common among those who are less sophisticated and of lower socioeconomic status. Although it has been reported that somatoform disorders in general may be more common in patients characterized as alexithymic (i.e., having difficulty identifying feelings and putting them into words), this has not been well studied. The families of these patients may be somatically preoccupied, and often those with conversion disorders or psychogenic pain have a model of symptoms in another family member. Children with somatoform disorders are often perceived as especially "sickly" or "vulnerable" by family members, and parents are often viewed as somewhat "overprotective." There often is substantial secondary gain in maintaining the symptoms, in the form of release from normal expectations and increased attention. Stressful life events may trigger the onset of a somatoform disorder, and patients with somatoform disorders have been reported to have high rates of abuse, both physical and sexual (particularly those with somatization and conversion disorders). Family discord is also common, as is comorbid anxiety and depression in both patients and family members. Family studies indicate that somatization disorder is linked to a family history of sociopathy and alcoholism, and that the disorder itself may be linked to impulsive dramatic personality disorders. Persons with factitious disorders have been reported to have had a frequent history of abuse, neglect, and early loss.

DIFFERENTIAL DIAGNOSIS

The most important differential diagnostic consideration in somatoform disorders is physical illness. Moreover, medical and psychiatric illness can co-occur, such as in the case of simultaneous pseudoseizures and actual seizures. In fact, having a medical illness may predispose the patient to the development of somatoform disorders. It is important to recognize that some physical symptoms are simply not easily explained, and in the absence of serious impairment, watchful waiting and reassurance are two of the most important tools available to the pediatrician.

Several psychiatric disorders have somatic concerns or complaints as part of their presentation, including SAD, GAD, OCD, and mood disorder. Anxiety and depressive disorder are often *comorbid* with somatoform disorders. In patients with separation anxiety, physical symptoms often develop in response to real or threatened separation, but otherwise, patients remain relatively free of symptoms.

Table 64–9 • Diagnostic Criteria for Undifferentiated Somatoform Disorder

A. One or more physical complaints (e.g., fatigue, loss of appetite, gastrointestinal or urinary complaints)
B. Either (1) or (2):
   (1) After appropriate investigation, the symptoms cannot be fully explained by a known general medical condition or the direct effects of a substance (e.g., a drug of abuse, a medication).
   (2) When there is a related general medical condition, the physical complaints or resulting social or occupational impairment is in excess of what would be expected from the history, physical examination, or laboratory findings.
C. The symptoms cause clinically significant distress or impairment in social, occupational, or other important areas of functioning.
D. The duration of the disturbance is at least 6 months.
E. The disturbance is not better accounted for by another mental disorder (e.g., another somatoform disorder, sexual dysfunction, mood disorder, anxiety disorder, sleep disorder, or psychotic disorder).
F. The symptom is not intentionally produced or feigned (as in factitious disorder or malingering).

Persons with overanxious disorders often experience somatic symptoms, but these tend to be the physiologic concomitants of anxiety, such as palpitations and "butterflies in the stomach," and are temporally related to anxiogenic experiences. Patients with OCD may be preoccupied about their bodily organs, but the ruminative nature of the thoughts, the recognition of them as irrational, and associated rituals help to differentiate the somatic preoccupations of OCD from somatoform disorders, particularly body dysmorphic disorder and hypochondriasis, although both of these disorders have been considered part of an obsessive-compulsive "spectrum" of disorders. Depressed patients may have somatic concerns, but, as in the case of separation anxiety, the somatic symptoms should follow the same temporal pattern as the overall disorder. Patients with depression or, more rarely, schizophrenia may have somatic delusions about having an incurable illness. Hypochondriasis on the other hand is usually characterized by a preoccupation and concern about illness, but not in the form of a fixed belief. Instead, hypochondriacal patients can be reassured, albeit temporarily. Body dysmorphic disorder needs to be differentiated from anorexia nervosa, wherein the patient is concerned about weight rather than a specific body part, and from OCD, when the checking rituals are not related to a specific body part. Panic disorder is frequently associated with somatization, especially concerns about palpitations and chest pain. Factitious disorder needs to be differentiated from malingering, in which the patient simulates a disease for explicit reasons, such as to obtain narcotics or to avoid jail.

COURSE

Little is known about the course of these disorders in childhood and adolescents. Acute conversion disorder often resolves spontaneously, without serious physical sequelae. On the other hand, a more chronic or subchronic course may predict a lifelong pattern of somatoform or other internalizing psychiatric disorder. Somatization disorder, hypochondriasis, and factitious disorder, by virtue of their severity and chronicity, have more ominous prognoses and are less amenable to brief treatment. Based on anecdotal and retrospective evidence, presentation of somatoform conditions in childhood may predict confirmed difficulties into adulthood.

IDENTIFICATION AND PEDIATRIC MANAGEMENT

Many patients with somatoform disorders can be managed in a pediatric setting. It is important not to challenge the reality and validity of the symptoms, yet at the same time to emphasize that the symptoms do not appear to be explained by a clear-cut physical disease. However, it is critical to communicate that the distress experienced by the patient is real and not viewed as "manipulative." It is useful to identify the secondary gain and try to help the patient obtain that gain (e.g., more attention) in a more direct manner. If a "model" is identified, the model (often a parent) is encouraged not to complain about his or her symptoms in front of the patient.

The patient is to be reinforced by the family for "healthy" behavior and expressions. If the family requires reassurance, it may be helpful for the physician to schedule short telephone appointments with the parents and/or patient in order to do so. It is useful to predict that symptoms may wax and wane, and that the pediatrician, patient, and family will work together to manage the situation. Current life stressors need to be addressed as well. For example, if a patient has just moved and is feeling isolated, coming up with a plan to meet peers is likely to be of help. Children with milder forms of hypochondriasis can be managed similarly. Because parental concerns may have an important role in the perpetuation of somatoform disorders, it is critical to address them as well as the concerns of the child.

Treatment must be centralized with one interested, concerned, nonjudgmental physician to avoid involving multiple specialists; exposing the patient to potentially dangerous, expensive, and unnecessary tests; and giving mixed messages to the family. In Munchausen by proxy, one of the hallmarks is multiple physician and health system involvement. A simple consultation letter from a psychiatrist to a primary care physician outlining an approach to adult somatizing patients was shown to be helpful in improving patient satisfaction, improving physical functioning, and reducing medical costs (Smith, Rost, and Kashner, 1995).

PSYCHIATRIC REFERRAL

Psychiatric referral is indicated for chronic or recurrent somatoform disorders accompanied by significant psychosocial impairment. Comorbid depression or anxiety requires treatment, through behavioral or psychopharmacologic intervention or both. Furthermore, the following principles for treatment apply:

1. Identification and reward of health-promoting behavior and increased patient control and responsibility
2. Reduction of secondary gain
3. Education of patient in how to obtain gains in a more appropriate manner
4. Psychoeducation for parent and family about the relationship between thoughts, feelings, and somatic symptoms
5. Education of the patient in how to identify distressing feelings and how to cope with them
6. Identification of significant stressors and subsequent ways of coping with the stress. (If the stressor is abuse, protection of the child is central.)
7. Diminished exposure to models of behavior within the family

Adults with painful somatic symptoms have been reported to respond, in open trials, to antidepressant medications; anecdotal experience with children and adolescents has been similar. A combination of cognitive-behavioral therapy and relaxation therapy has been used successfully for recurrent abdominal pain. No systematic treatment of somatization disorder or factitious disorder has been reported, but clinical anecdotes indicate that long-term, supportive treatment may be of benefit.

Conduct Disorder

Conduct disorder is a term used to describe children and adolescents who engage in chronic (i.e., at least 6 months) violations of social norms and the rights of others. This condition is described in Chapter 49.

Schizophrenia and Childhood Psychoses

For review, see Jacobsen and Rapoport (in press). Schizophrenia and related disorders, although much more common in adulthood, can have their onset as early as 5 years of age. Schizophrenia (Table 64–10) is defined as a chronic deterioration (at least 6 months) from previous level of functioning, with psychotic features, no evidence of toxic or organic etiology, and the absence of prominent affective (either depressive or manic) symptomatology. Psychotic symptoms may include delusions (e.g., thought broadcasting, thought insertion, being controlled by someone, ideas of reference, or persecutory delusions) or hallucinations (frequently auditory hallucinations such as voices commenting on a person's behavior or two voices having a conversation). Affect is often blunted or inappropriate, and speech is digressive, vague, circumstantial, or incoherent. Although not definitive, evidence points to a continuity between children at risk for schizophrenia, early-onset schizophrenia, and adult-onset schizophrenia.

DESCRIPTIVE EPIDEMIOLOGY

The prevalence of childhood onset schizophrenia is not known, but it is thought to be relatively rare, less than 5 in 10,000. The prevalence appears to be greater among boys, at least in clinically referred cases.

RISK FACTORS AND NEUROBIOLOGY

The risk for development of schizophrenia in the children of a schizophrenic parent is about 10%, or about 10-fold the prevalence in the population. The risk is increased even more if the parent had an especially early age of onset, there was evidence of perinatal distress at birth, and the perinatal stress is accompanied by an enlarged third ventricle and an increased ventricle to brain ratio. There is some evidence that schizotypal traits (e.g., a tendency to prefer one's own company or engaging in fantasy or magical thinking and idiosyncratic speech) represent a precursor of schizophrenia and are found to be much more common in the families of patients with schizophrenia.

Onset of puberty seems to precipitate early onset schizophrenia in girls. Precursors of early-onset schizophrenia include movement disorders, poor sensory-motor integration, and impaired coordination. Neuropsychiatric difficulties, including fine motor problems and visual tracking difficulties, are commonly noted. Imaging studies have shown decreased cerebral volume, increased size of the lateral ventricles, and relative sparing of white matter. Longitudinal studies indicate a concerning trend—an increase in ventricular volume over time.

DIFFERENTIAL DIAGNOSIS

Schizophrenia must be differentiated from other forms of psychosis. Acute psychotic presentation can be associated with various causes of organic brain syndrome, including infection, autoimmune phenomena (e.g., lupus, multiple sclerosis), structural lesions, medications (e.g., steroids), illicit drugs (e.g., PCP), or metabolic disorders (e.g., Wilson disease or porphyria). In many of these disorders, psychosis is accompanied by symptoms of delirium or dementia. Bipolar disorder can be accompanied by psychosis, in either the depressive or manic phase. In the depressive phase, psychoses generally are related to mood, such as in the case of nihilistic or somatic delusions, or self-deprecatory auditory hallucinations. Psychosis during mania is exacerbated by sleep deprivation and tends to be grandiose or paranoid in nature. The course and associated

Table 64–10 • Diagnostic Criteria for Schizophrenia

A. *Characteristic symptoms:* Two (or more) of the following, each present for a significant portion of time during a 1-month period (or less if successfully treated):
   (1) Delusions
   (2) Hallucinations
   (3) Disorganized speech (e.g., frequent derailment or incoherence)
   (4) Grossly disorganized or catatonic behavior
   (5) Negative symptoms (i.e., affective flattening, alogia, or avolition)
   Notes: Only one criterion A symptom is required if delusions are bizarre or hallucinations consist of a voice keeping up a running commentary on the person's behavior or thoughts, or of two or more voices conversing with each other.
B. *Social/occupational dysfunction:* For a significant portion of the time since the onset of the disturbance, one or more major areas of functioning such as work, interpersonal relations, or self-care are markedly below the level achieved prior to the onset (or when the onset is in childhood or adolescence, failure to achieve expected level of interpersonal, academic, or occupational achievement).
C. *Duration:* Continuous signs of the disturbance persist for at least 6 months. This 6-month period must include at least 1 month of symptoms (or less if successfully treated) that meet criterion A (i.e., active-phase symptoms) and may include periods of prodromal or residual symptoms. During these prodromal or residual periods, the signs of the disturbance may be manifested by only negative symptoms or two or more symptoms listed in criterion A present in an attenuated form (e.g., odd beliefs, unusual perceptual experiences).
D. *Schizoaffective and mood disorder exclusion:* Schizoaffective disorder and mood disorder with psychotic features have been ruled out because either (1) no major depressive, manic, or mixed episodes have occurred concurrently with the active-phase symptoms or (2) if mood episodes have occurred during active-phase symptoms, their total duration has been brief relative to the duration of the active and residual periods.
E. *Substance/general medical condition exclusion:* The disturbance is not due to the direct physiologic effects of a substance (e.g., a drug of abuse, a medication) or a general medical condition.
F. *Relationship to a pervasive developmental disorder:* If there is a history of autistic disorder or another pervasive developmental disorder, the additional diagnosis of schizophrenia is made only if prominent delusions or hallucinations are also present for at least a month (or less if successfully treated).

symptomatology, even more than the nature of the psychotic symptoms, determine whether the disorder is schizophrenia or a psychosis related to an affective disorder. In schizophrenia, dysphoria occurs secondary to psychotic disintegration, whereas in depression, the psychotic symptoms have onset coincident with the affective symptoms. In schizoaffective illness, the affective component remits, but the thought disorder persists. Schizophrenia can be differentiated from autism and pervasive development disorders insofar as the pervasive developmental disorders have an earlier age of onset and are frequently associated with seizures, mental retardation, and an almost complete lack of appropriate language or social interactions, and autistic patients do not experience hallucinations or delusions. Schizophrenia may also need to be distinguished from schizotypal personality disorder. The latter may be thought of as a forme-fruste of schizophrenia. Patients with schizotypal personality disorder may be circumstantial without being incoherent, and they may have odd beliefs or magical thinking without truly experiencing psychosis.

COURSE

Little is known of the course of pediatric schizophrenia, except the prognosis is relatively poor and chronic. A disturbing trend in early-onset schizophrenia is the continued loss in intelligence quotient over time (Jacobsen and Rapoport, in press). Patients with prominent negative symptoms (e.g., flat affect, withdrawn) have a particularly poor response to treatment and a refractory prognosis. Suicide is a real risk, especially among young adult men with a previously high level of functioning who have had a chronic and relapsing course. In such patients, comorbid depression and hopelessness have been observed to be associated with suicide.

IDENTIFICATION AND PEDIATRIC MANAGEMENT

Psychosis and bizarre behavior are not difficult to identify. Adolescent patients who refuse to go to school and seem guarded about their reasons for refusing school attendance may have paranoid ideation. Schizophrenia is best managed by a child psychiatrist; however, the families of such patients require pediatric support, and the potential medical complications of neuroleptic treatment should be monitored closely.

TREATMENT

Because of the rarity of this condition among youth, little is known about the optimal treatment of such patients in childhood and adolescence. Recent studies from Rapoport's group have demonstrated the superiority of the clozapine over resperidol for the treatment of chronic early-onset schizophrenia. Clozapine was superior for relief of both negative and positive symptoms but has the serious side effect of blood dyscrasia, necessitating careful monitoring for development of this condition. However, clozapine has no extrapyramidal side effects and presumably has a much lower risk of tardive dyskinesia. Especially if one is using one of the older neuroleptics, the lowest possible neuroleptic dosage should be used because of attendant akathisia, extrapyramidal symptoms, tardive dyskinesia, cognitive slowing, and dysphoria. Hopefully, the newer generation of neuroleptics (e.g., olanzapine, respendol) will prove to be effective without the serious side effects of their predecessors. Family psychoeducation and support to reduce undue criticism to the patient with schizophrenia may also be of benefit. Patients who experience depressive symptoms may benefit from the addition of an antidepressant.

REFERENCES

Achenbach TM: Manual for the Child Behavior Checklist/4-18 and 1991 Profile. Burlington, VT, University of Vermont, Department of Psychiatry, 1991.

Allen AJ, Leonard HL, Swedo SE: Case study: a new infection-triggered, autoimmune subtype of pediatric OCD and Tourette's syndrome. J Am Acad Child Adolesc Psychiatry 34:307–311, 1995.

American Psychiatric Association: Diagnostic and Statistical Manual of Mental Disorders, 4th ed. Washington, DC, American Psychiatric Association, 1994.

Anderson JC, Williams S, McGee R, et al: DSM-III disorders in preadolescent children. Arch Gen Psychiatry 44:69–76, 1987.

Angold A, Costello EJ: Depressive comorbidity in children and adolescents: empirical, theoretical, and methodological issues. Am J Psychiatry 150:1779, 1993.

Barrett PM, Dadds MR, Rapee RM: Family treatment of childhood anxiety: a controlled trial. J Consult Clin Psychol 64:333–342, 1996.

Birmaher B, Waterman GS, Ryan N, et al: Fluoxetine for childhood anxiety disorders. J Am Acad Child Adolesc Psychiatry 33:993–999, 1994.

Black B, Uhde TW: Treatment of elective mutism with fluoxetine: a double-blind placebo-controlled study. J Am Acad Child Adolesc Psychiatry 33:1000–1006, 1994.

Brent DA: School age and adolescence: Mood disorders and suicide. In Green M, Haggerty RJ, Weitzman ML (eds): Ambulatory Pediatrics, 5th ed. Philadelphia, WB Saunders, 1999.

Brent DA: Practitioner review: the aftercare of adolescents with deliberate self-harm. J Child Psychol Psychiatr 38:277–286, 1997.

Brent DA: Risk factors for adolescent suicide and suicidal behavior: mental and substance abuse disorders, family environmental factors, and life stress. Suicide Life Threat Behav 25:52–63, 1995.

Brent DA: Overrepresentation of epileptics in a consecutive series of suicide attempts seen at a children's hospital. J Am Acad Child Psychiatr 25:242–246, 1986.

Brent DA, Bridge J, Johnson BA, et al: Suicidal behavior runs in families: a controlled family study of adolescent suicide victims. Arch Gen Psychiatry 53:1145–1152, 1996a.

Brent DA, Crumrine PK, Varma RR, Allen M, et al: Phenobarbital treatment and major depressive disorder in children with epilepsy. Pediatrics 80:909–917, 1987.

Brent DA, Kolko D, Birmaher B, et al: Predictors of treatment efficacy in a clinical trial of three psychosocial treatments for adolescent depression. J Am Acad Child Adolesc Psychiatry, in press.

Brent DA, Moritz G, Bridge J, et al: Long-term impact of exposure to suicide: a three-year controlled follow-up. J Am Acad Child Adolesc Psychiatry 35:646–653, 1996b.

Brent DA, Perper JA, Allman C: Alcohol, firearms, and suicide among youth: temporal trends in Allegheny County, Pennsylvania, 1960–1983. JAMA 257:3369–3372, 1987.

Brent DA, Poling K, McKain B, Baugher MA: A Psychoeducational program for families of affectively ill children and adolescents. J Am Acad Child Adolesc Psychiatry 32:770–774, 1993.

Brent DA, Ryan N, Dahl R, Birmaher B: Early-onset mood disorder. In Bloom FE, Kupfer DJ (eds): Psychopharmacology: The fourth generation of progress. New York, Raven Press, 1995, pp 1631–1642.

Campo JV, Garber J: Somatization. In Ammerman RT, Campo JV (eds): Handbook of Pediatric Psychology and Psychiatry. Boston, Allyn & Bacon, 1998.

Carlson BA, Goodwin FK: The stages of mania. Arch Gen Psychiatry 28:221–228, 1973.

Centers for Disease Control: Attempted suicide among high school students: United States, 1990. MMWR 40:633–635, 1991.

Clarke GN, Hawkins W, Murphy M, et al: Targeted prevention of unipolar depressive disorder in an at-risk sample of high school adolescents: a randomized trial of a group cognitive intervention. J Am Acad Child Adolesc Psychiatr 34:312–321, 1995.

Costello EJ, Edelbrock C, Costello AJ, et al: Psychopathology in pediatric primary care: the new hidden morbidity. Pediatrics 82:415–424, 1988a.

Costello EJ, Costello AJ, Edelbrock C, et al: Psychiatric disorders in pediatric primary care: prevalence and risk factors. Arch Gen Psychiatry 45:1107–1116, 1988b.

Emslie GJ, Rush AJ, Weinberg WA, et al: A double-blind, randomized placebo-controlled trial of fluoxetine in depressed children and adolescents. Arch Gen Psychiatry, 4:1031–1037, 1997.

Fergusson DM, Horwood LJ, Lynskey MT: Childhood sexual abuse and psychiatric disorder in young adulthood: II. Psychiatric outcomes of childhood sexual abuse. J Am Acad Child Adolesc Psychiatry 34:1365–1374, 1996.

Flament ME, Whitaker A, Rapoport JL: Obsessive compulsive disorder in adolescence: an epidemiological study. J Am Acad Child Adolesc Psychiatry 27:764–771, 1988.

Fleming JE, Offord DR: Epidemiology of childhood depressive disorders: a critical review. J Am Acad Child Adolesc Psychiatry 29:571–580, 1990.

Gittelman-Klein R, Klein DF: Controlled imipramine treatment of school phobia. Arch Gen Psychiatry 25:204–207, 1971.

Gould MS, Shaffer D: The impact of suicide in television movies: evidence of imitation. N Engl J Med 315:690–694, 1986.

Green WH: Child and Adolescent Clinical Psychopharmacology, 2nd ed. Baltimore, Williams & Wilkins, 1995.

Hirshfeld DR, Rosenbaum JF, Biederman J, et al: Stable behavioral inhibition and its association with anxiety disorders. J Am Acad Child Adolesc Psychiatry 31:103–111, 1992.

Hodges K: Debate and argument: reply to David Shaffer: structured interviews for assessing children. J Child Psychol Psychiatr 35:785–787, 1994.

Jacobsen LK, Rapoport JL: Research update: childhood onset schizophrenia: implications of clinical and neurobiological research. J Child Psychol Psychiatr, in press.

Jellinek MS, Murphy JM: The recognition of psychosocial disorders in pediatric office practice: the current status of the pediatric symptom checklist. J Dev Behav Pediatr 11:273–278, 1990.

Kagan J, Reznick JS, Snidman N: The physiology and psychology of behavioral inhibition in children. Child Dev 58:1459–1473, 1987.

Kaufman J, Birmaher B, Brent D, et al: The Schedule for Affective Disorders and Schizophrenia for School-aged Children: Present and Lifetime Version (K-SADS-PL): initial reliability and validity data. J Am Acad Child Adolesc Psychiatry 36:980–988, 1997.

Kelleher KJ, Childs GE, Wasserman RC, et al: Insurance status and recognition of psychosocial problems: a report from PROS and ASPN. Arch Pediatr Adolesc Med 151:1109–1115, 1997.

Kendall PC: Treating anxiety disorders in children: results of a randomized clinical trial. J Consult Clin Psychol 62:100–110, 1994.

Kienhorst I, deWilde EJ, Diekstra FW, et al: Adolescents' image of their suicide attempt. J Am Acad Child Adolesc Psychiatry 34:623–628, 1995.

Kiessling LS, Marcotte AC, Culpepper L: Antineuronal antibodies: tics and obsessive-compulsive symptoms. Dev Behav Pediatr 15:421–425, 1994.

Kovacs M, Feinberg TL, Crouse-Novak MA, et al: Depressive disorders in childhood. I. A longitudinal prospective study of characteristics and recovery. Arch Gen Psychiatry 41:219–239, 1984a.

Lewinsohn PM, Clarke GM, Hops H, Andrews J: Cognitive-behavioral treatment for depressed adolescents. Behav Ther 21:385–401, 1990.

Lewinsohn PM, Rohde P, Seeley JR: Adolescent suicidal ideation and attempts: prevalence, risk, factors, and clinical implications. Clin Psychol Sci Pract 3:25–46, 1996.

Lewis M (ed): Child and Adolescent Psychiatry: A Comprehensive Textbook. Baltimore, Williams & Wilkins, 1996.

March JS, Leonard HL: Obsessive-compulsive disorder in children and adolescents: a review of the past 10 years. J Am Acad Child Adolesc Psychiatry 34:1265–1273, 1996.

Offord DR, Boyle MH, Szatmari P, et al: Ontario Child Health Study: II. Six month prevalence of disorder and rates of service utilization. Arch Gen Psychiatry 44:832–836, 1987.

Puig-Antich J, Lukens E, Davies M, et al: Psychosocial functioning in prepubertal major depressive disorders: II. Interpersonal relationship after sustained recovery from affective episode. Arch Gen Psychiatry 42:511–517, 1985.

Pynoos RS, Frederick C, Nader K, et al: Life threat and post-traumatic stress in school-age children. Arch Gen Psychiatry 44:1057–1063, 1987.

Robins LN: Alcohol, drug abuse and mental health administration. Report of the Secretary's Task Force on Youth Suicide: Strategies for the Prevention of Youth Suicide, Vol 4. (DHHS Publ. No. [ADM] 89-1624). Washington, DC, US Government Printing Office, 1989, pp 94–114.

Rohde P, Lewinsohn PM, Seeley JR: Are adolescents changed by an episode of major depression. J Am Acad Child Adolesc Psychiatry 33:1289–1298, 1994.

Rosenbaum JF, Biederman J, Bolduc-Murphy EA: Behavioral inhibition in childhood: a risk factor for anxiety disorders. Harvard Rev Psychiatry 1:2–16, 1993.

Rosenberg DR, Holttum J, Gershon S: Textbook of Pharmacotherapy for Child and Adolescent Psychiatric Disorders. New York, Brunner/Mazel Publishers, 1994.

Rutter M, Taylor E, Hersov L: Child and Adolescent Psychiatry: Modern Approaches, 3rd ed. Oxford, Blackwell Scientific, 1994.

Rutter M, Tizard J, Whitmore K: Education, Health and Behavior. New York, Wiley, 1970.

Ryan ND, Puig-Antich J, Ambrosini P, et al: The clinical picture of major depression in children and adolescents. Arch Gen Psychiatry 44:854–861, 1987.

Schmitt BD: School phobia—the great imitator: a pediatrician's viewpoint. Pediatrics 48:433–441, 1973.

Shaffer D, Gould MS, Fisher P, et al: Psychiatric diagnosis in child and adolescent suicide. Arch Gen Psychiatry 53:339–348, 1996.

Shaffer D, Gould M, Hicks RD: Worsening suicide rate in black teenagers. Am J Psychiatry 151:1810–1812, 1994.

Slap G, Vorters D, Chaudhuri S, et al: Risk factors for attempted suicide during adolescence. Pediatrics 84:762–772, 1989.

Smith GR, Rost K, Kashner TM: A trial of the effect of a standardized psychiatric consultation on health outcomes and costs in somatizing patients. Arch Gen Psychiatry 52:238–243, 1995.

Starfield B, Katz H, Gabriel A, et al: Morbidity in childhood—a longitudinal view. N Engl J Med 310:824–829, 1984.

Strober M, Morrell W, Burroughs J, et al: A family study of bipolar I disorder in adolescence. Early onset of symptoms linked to increased familial loading and lithium resistance. J Affect Disord 15:255–268, 1988.

Terr LC: Chowchilla revisited: the effects of psychic trauma four years after a school-bus kidnapping. Am J Psychiatry 40:1543–1550, 1983.

Whitaker A, Johnson J, Shaffer D, et al: Uncommon troubles in young people: prevalence estimates of selected psychiatric disorders in a nonreferred adolescent population. Arch Gen Psychiatry 47:487–496, 1990.

65 *The Gifted Child*

Neil L. Schechter • Sally M. Reis • Eve R. Colson

 Giftedness is hardly a developmental-behavioral disorder. Yet, children who are cognitively talented present a series of perplexing challenges to clinicians. The management of excellence is a sensitive and painstaking process. As the authors of this chapter point out, giftedness can have undesirable complications. In particular, the reactions and practices of the parents of gifted children may have unintended untoward consequences. This chapter offers clinicians an approach to their gifted patients and a way of responding constructively to the concerns of their teachers and their parents.

Although developmental and intellectual sophistication is not a disease or illness, this aspect of the spectrum of child development is, surprisingly, a significant area of concern for many parents and is fraught with misconceptions. In this era when parents rely increasingly on health care providers for developmental advice, it is important to have information on the evolving conceptual framework and programming strategies for the approximately 10% of children who are considered gifted. The pediatric literature, however, offers few insights. The psychological and educational literature, although more abundant, remains inconclusive.

This chapter provides information to assist the health care provider in dealing with many of the critical issues facing developmentally advanced or academically superior children. Specifically, this chapter reviews the evolution of the concept of giftedness, outlines current perspectives, and provides an overview of the status of education for gifted and talented youth. In addition, public policy controversies are discussed, as are promising educational alternatives and practical approaches for those who provide care for these children and their families.

Definitions of Giftedness

Many ways of defining giftedness have emerged in the past 2 decades. Educators most often rely on definitions from federal reports. The Marland Report (1972), commissioned by the US Congress, included the first federal definition of giftedness:

> Gifted and talented children are those, identified by professionally qualified persons, who by virtue of outstanding abilities are capable of high performance. These are children who require differentiated educational programs and/or services beyond those normally provided by the regular school program in order to realize their contribution to self and society.
>
> Children capable of high performance include those with demonstrated high achievement and/or potential ability in any of the following areas, singly or in combination: general intellectual ability, specific academic aptitude, creative or productive thinking, leadership ability, visual and performing arts, and/or psychomotor ability.

The departments of education in approximately half of the states have adopted this definition. In the most recent federal report on the status of gifted and talented programs, a new definition is proposed based on insights provided by emerging research in neuroscience and cognitive psychology. The new definition differs from the original Marland Report by specifically emphasizing that talents can emerge over time in a wide variety of areas and within all cultural and economic groups (O'Connell-Ross, 1994).

Aspects of both federal definitions are based at least in part on Howard Gardner's (1983) increasingly popular concept that all normal individuals are capable of seven forms of intellectual intelligences: linguistic, musical, logic-mathematical, spatial, body-kinesthetic, interpersonal, and intrapersonal. These multiple intelligences manifest themselves early in life as abilities to process information in certain ways. Each of these intelligences is valuable in society, and not all can be measured through traditional intelligence testing.

In addition to the federal definitions, a number of more operational definitions have been developed by psychologists and educators and have been adopted in some US school systems. The most popular was conceived by Joseph Renzulli (1978), who integrated various criteria into a single definition. He writes that giftedness

> . . . consists of an interaction among three basic clusters of human traits, these clusters being above average general ability, high levels of task commitment, and high levels of creativity. Gifted and talented children are those possessing or capable of developing this composite set of traits and applying them to any potentially valuable area of human performance. Children who manifest or are capable of developing an interaction among these three clusters require a wide variety of educational opportunities and services that are not ordinarily provided through regular instructional programming.

A number of factors appear to play a role in helping children achieve these levels of accomplishment. Bloom (1985) examined the process by which young people hone their talents. Groups studied include concert pianists, sculptors, research mathematicians, research neurologists, Olympic swimmers, and tennis champions who attained high levels of accomplishment before age 35 years. The researchers found that the home environment, parental encouragement, and the direct involvement of families and teachers all are critical environmental components that contribute to maximizing potential.

The definitions as well as clinical research suggest that beliefs about gifted children have changed dramatically from an emphasis solely on academic ability and intellectual potential to the development of gifted behaviors that may eventually yield social productivity. It appears as though giftedness, similar to learning disabilities, is the product of individual human variation and the interaction of an individual's strengths and weaknesses with the environment.

Development in Gifted Children

As suggested previously, most current theoreticians believe that gifted children are a heterogeneous group who display infinite variation in their development. Much previous research, however, focused on the development of a limited subgroup of gifted children—those who achieve in the superior range on intelligence quotient (IQ) measures. Almost all of this research suffers by comparison with current social science by ignoring socioeconomic status and in its primarily retrospective analysis of early development. These studies often reflect the development of upper class children who tend to do well on IQ measures (30% to 40% in the gifted range, as opposed to a predicted 10% to 20%).

PHYSICAL DEVELOPMENT

Terman's (1925) work, which used intelligence test scores to identify the top 1% of the population, suggested that, as a group, the gifted children he studied tended to be more mature physiologically when compared with his control subjects. On 37 anthropometric measures, Terman's gifted group proved to be superior to children of comparable age in measures of height, weight, lung capacity, and muscular strength. They also walked an average of 1 month earlier than his control population.

In a large retrospective study of children with superior intelligence at age 7 years, Fisch and colleagues (1976) found that favorable parental, social, and educational backgrounds were maximally correlated with superior intelligence, whereas perinatal factors, such as Apgar scores, neurologic or physical abnormalities, infections, anoxia, or trauma, were identical for high-IQ, average-IQ, and low-IQ groups. They found that larger head size at 1 year of age was an early finding associated with superior intelligence, as was greater height and weight at age 4 years.

All of these studies suffer from the significant flaws already described. More recent investigators have demonstrated that if socioeconomic factors are held constant, the differences that have been identified in these studies tend to disappear.

COGNITIVE DEVELOPMENT

Investigations of the cognitive development of gifted children have taken two pathways: the search for qualitative and for quantitative differences in the thinking of these children.

Attempts to find qualitative differences in the thinking of gifted children, that is, different approaches to problem solving, have yielded some success in recent years, particularly with respect to metacognitive issues. Examination of the rate of acquisition of skills, however, has been far more fruitful. It is the rate of knowledge acquisition that is primarily measured when attempting to determine giftedness in a young population.

Both early language development and early reading ability have been assessed as possible markers of later superior cognitive abilities. Terman (1925) and Freeman (1979) found that gifted children spoke approximately 3 1/2 months earlier than children in control populations, and they identified a clear relationship between language complexity and later high IQ. Early reading was also more frequent in Terman's group; nearly half of his group of gifted children had learned to read before entering first grade, and 20% had done so before age 5 years. Jackson and Roller (1993), in a current review of reading and gifted children, indicate that precocious readers almost always remain at least at an average level in their reading ability. By fifth or sixth grade, however, reading performance is much more likely to be within the range of their classmates' performance than it was in kindergarten.

In terms of general cognitive development, Robinson (1981) reported that gifted preschoolers in his study achieved Piagetian conservation and the understanding of gender many months before children of average ability. Gender identification is an aspect of social cognition that has been shown to be related to general intellectual development.

PERSONALITY DEVELOPMENT

In the area of personality development, a discrepancy exists between children with higher IQ scores (IQ greater than 180, or development two times the chronologic age) and children with IQ scores between 130 and 150. The higher-IQ students do not fare as well as those with more moderate abilities. Most recent research on this population finds that many display underachievement and alienation, and some contemplate suicide. Children with extremely high IQs may also find difficulty in finding playmates who were congenial in both size and mental ability (Robinson, 1981; Silverman, 1993).

The research on the personality of gifted children with lower IQ scores is much more positive. They appear to rate significantly higher than peers on measures of earnestness, trustworthiness, honesty, and emotional stability as well as the capacity for objective self-appraisal. Their moral judgment appears to be more mature in regard to distinctions between the intention and outcome of an action and right and wrong behavior.

Other investigators attempted to assess the popularity of gifted children. Prior research and more recent studies have found that the academically most able were generally well liked and were often among the most popular children in the class. A clear positive correlation between group acceptance and academic performance was found.

The classic stereotype regarding the personality of gifted children is that they are social isolates. With the exception of students with IQ scores over 180, who have been found to have an increased number of social and psychological problems, this does not appear to be so in the majority of bright children. As one might expect, they run the gamut of personality styles, from outgoing to retiring, from self-confident and assertive to feeling inferior.

When the literature on gifted children is viewed as a whole, Robinson and colleagues' summary (1979) is most apt:

> While some studies have reported that the average levels of personal and social adjustment, physical health, and the like are slightly higher for gifted children . . . the mean difference favoring the gifted group is appropriately matched for variables such as social class. Much more striking than the mean difference is the variability within the gifted group. In fact, intellectually advanced children are about as heterogeneous as any other population on measures other than those directly related to the instruments used to identify them. There is . . . no such thing as a "typical gifted child."

State of Gifted Education

OVERVIEW

A recent Gifted and Talented Education Report (Council of State Directors, 1994) indicates that 47 states, plus Puerto Rico and Guam, have recognized education of the gifted and talented through specific legislation, and the same number of states have assigned state department of education staff to leadership positions in this area. The report also shows that since 1963, when Pennsylvania was the first to require services for the gifted and talented, 24 other states and Guam have implemented a mandate for services.

This growth has not been constant. Researchers and scholars have pointed to various high and low points of national interest and commitment to educating the gifted and talented (Gallagher, 1979; Tannenbaum, 1983). Gallagher described the struggle between support and apathy for special programs for this population as having roots in historical tradition—the battle against an aristocratic elite and the concomitant belief in egalitarianism. Tannenbaum portrays two peak periods of interest in the gifted as the 5 years following the launch of Sputnik in 1957 and the second half of the 1970s. Tannenbaum described a valley of neglect between the peaks in which the public focused its attention on the disadvantaged and the handicapped. "The cyclical nature of interest in the gifted is probably unique in American education. No other special group of children has been alternately embraced and repelled with so much vigor by educators and laypersons alike" (Tannenbaum, 1983). Purcell (1993) found that programs are also being affected differentially by the economy and the existence of a state mandate to provide services to high-ability students.

Even in the best-funded and most active states, gifted programs are seldom comprehensive. In general, many cities and towns reported some type of gifted program, yet only a handful of school districts offer continuous services in grades 1 through 12. Furthermore, most US gifted programs focus only on the academically able and provide little or no service or attention to artistically talented students or those with potential or demonstrated talent in leadership, specific academic areas, or creative and productive thinking.

IDENTIFICATION OF GIFTED AND TALENTED STUDENTS

Identification of gifted students is usually based on the definition selected by the school district. Many school districts have implemented procedures that continue to identify high-achieving or high-IQ students with little or no attention to the developmental nature of giftedness or the potential to display abilities that are not specified in the federal definition (Reis, 1989).

Districts across the United States generally select one of several different identification approaches. A three-step process including referral, screening, and final selection is most often used. Screening generally consists of the collection and review of various types of data, including individual or group intelligence test, creativity assessments, standardized achievement test, and grades. In addition, some schools also include nominations, rating scales from parents and teachers, product evaluations, and classroom observations. Based on the results of this review, students are selected or denied admission into a gifted program. In most states using this system, 3% to 5% of the population is usually eligible to participate in gifted programs.

A popular alternative to this model is the Schoolwide Enrichment Model (SEM) (Renzulli and Reis, 1985), which has been adopted by hundreds of school districts across the United States. Based on the three-ring conception of gift developed by Renzulli (Fig. 65–1), the SEM establishes a "talent pool" of above-average students without formally identifying that group as gifted. Various types of services are provided to the talent pool, usually 10% to 15% of the population, and an attempt is made to cultivate gifted behaviors or products in that group. Those who benefit from enriched programming thus identify themselves and can participate in additional aspects of special programming. This identification system has been widely recognized as an alternative to the more traditional ones. It urges people to think in terms of gifted behaviors that children may demonstrate at one time and not another and allows for the development of gifted behaviors in a wider pool of students. It suggests that giftedness is not an all-or-none phenomenon and that many more children display gifted behavior than can be identified by intelligence measures.

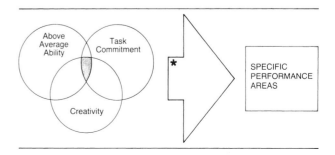

Figure 65–1. The three-ring concept of giftedness.

PROGRAMMING MODELS FOR GIFTED STUDENTS

Many different options exist for the implementation of gifted programs. Some educators advocate an acceleration approach and others advocate an enrichment program; most educators, however, favor a combination approach with elements of both options. More than a dozen educational programming models have been developed for use with this population (Renzulli, 1986). Most program models usually involve a combination of acceleration and enrichment and are usually designed to meet the needs of gifted students either within a resource room in combination with a regular classroom setting or in a separate classroom for gifted students. The decision to separate gifted students is a controversial one, and most programs are provided to gifted students in heterogeneously grouped classrooms.

Some specific programs are of particular note because of their innovative approaches to meeting the needs of gifted children. The Future Problem Solving Program, for example, is a national year-long program in which teams of four students use a six-step problem-solving process to solve complex scientific and social problems of the future such as the overcrowding of prisons or the greenhouse effect. The program challenges students to apply information they have learned to some of the most complex issues facing society. They are asked to think, to make decisions, and, in some instances, to carry out their solutions. Another national program, called Talent Search, actively recruits and provides testing and program opportunities for mathematically precocious 12- to 14-year-old students. They are eligible for multiple options including summer programs, grade skipping, and taking college courses. Another such program, Odyssey of the Mind, encourages teams of students to engage in creative problem-solving activities such as designing structures or vehicles, or creating solutions to complex problems.

A number of challenging curriculum options in science and language arts have been developed under the auspices of the federal Javits Education Act. This federal legislation, enacted in 1990 and funded in 1995, has resulted in the creation of a National Research Center for the Gifted and Talented, which involves five universities, state departments of education, and a consortium of more than 300 school districts from across the country. This center provides current information on research, school-based modifications, and programs for gifted and talented youth. In addition, under the auspices of this legislation, numerous national programs have been developed or implemented for high-ability students in many districts, regional service centers, and states.

Major alternative strategies involving the regrouping or radical reorganization of school structures have been slow in coming. Perhaps this is due to the difficulty of making major educational changes, scheduling, arranging financing, and other issues that have caused schools to substantively change so little in the past half century.

UNIQUE PROBLEMS FACING GIFTED CHILDREN IN SCHOOL

A number of problems in the educational system have made it difficult for children with special gifts and talent to excel in the classroom. Perhaps the most important identified problem is the decreased rigor and level of expectation in school. This is exemplified by the "dumbing down" of textbooks in the past 20 years. Kirst (1982) reported that a sample of US publishers agreed that their textbooks had dropped two grade levels in difficulty over 10 to 15 years. When California educators tried to find textbooks that would challenge the top one third of their students, no publisher had an appropriate book. More recent analyses on the dumbing down of content have yielded similar results (Chall and Conrad, 1991; Reis et al, 1992).

In addition, teachers are sometimes not trained adequately to teach gifted children, and often, necessary classroom modifications are not implemented. The Classroom Practices Observational Study (Westberg et al, 1993) examined the instructional and curricular practices used with gifted and talented students in regular elementary classrooms throughout the United States. The results suggested that there was little differentiation in the instructional and curricular practices, including group arrangements and verbal interactions for gifted students in the regular classroom. The result was that gifted children were often reviewing information that they had already mastered. Recent research has suggested that as a result, some students may be understimulated and begin to act out; behavioral and emotional problems have been found to exist in increasing numbers of gifted students (Reid and McGuire, 1995).

There are two other educational trends that may impact negatively on gifted students. First, the current movement to eliminate "tracking" of students into special classes has resulted in widespread belief that absolutely all forms of grouping have a negative impact on children. Although few educators support the use of tracking, recent research indicates that some forms of ability or instructional grouping are necessary if advanced content is to be provided to high-ability students.

The second movement that may be detrimental to the needs of gifted students is cooperative learning in which groups of students work together on assigned classwork or homework. Some types of cooperative learning may have a negative impact on high-ability students when used for long periods of instruction. For example, in one form of cooperative learning, one bright child, two average children, and one below-average student are placed into a group. Within the group an assumption is made that the bright student will help the others and that all will benefit. However, some gifted students are not interested in teaching others, and some cannot explain how they acquired advanced concepts. Also, this situation may not allow the gifted students to work at their own pace with appropriate challenges.

Finally, gifted and talented students may face the pervasive influence of anti-intellectualism that affects society. Peer pressure may be exerted on gifted students. Labels such as "smarty-pants," commonly used to describe bright students in the 1950s and 1960s, have been replaced by more negative labels such as "nerd," "dweeb," or "dork." The brightest students often learn to avoid answering in class, to stop raising their hands, and to minimize their abilities to avoid ridicule.

A number of ramifications exist for gifted children who face these difficulties in the classroom. First, they are clearly underchallenged, and therefore their development may be delayed or even halted. If instructional materials are not above the student's level of knowledge or understanding, learning is less efficient and intellectual growth may be slowed. Second, too many of the brightest students never learn to work and thus acquire poor work habits. As a consequence, top students in the United States are not achieving at the same level as those in other countries. In mathematics, for example, the top 1% of students in the United States scored very poorly when compared with a similar group of students from 13 other countries.

Special Populations of Gifted Children

CULTURALLY DIFFERENT AND ECONOMICALLY DISADVANTAGED CHILDREN

Minority students are disproportionately underrepresented in gifted and talented programs in the United States. In recent research, Frasier, Garcia, and Passow (1995) clearly indicate that identification and selection procedures are both ineffective and inappropriate for the identification of minority students. Tests traditionally used for identification of gifted students are often biased and inappropriate for use with minority students. Fraiser and Passow (1995) suggest that groups that have been historically underrepresented in gifted programs could be better served through the development of new constructs around the concept of giftedness as well as attention to cultural and contextual variability among students.

Even so, gifted programming for economically disadvantaged and culturally different students has been demonstrated to benefit not only these students but also the general environment in the school. Academic role models are created, and the image of the school as a place where excellence can occur and be nurtured has enormous ramifications for the faculty and students alike.

GIFTED STUDENTS WITH PHYSICAL AND LEARNING DISABILITIES

Many students who are physically disabled are also gifted and talented. Yet because of the high visibility of their physical problem and, possibly, because of the "disability" label and the resulting special program, the needs related to the disability are usually given precedence over academic or artistic potential. Also, the poor self-concept that occasionally accompanies disability may prevent some students from fulfilling their academic or artistic promise. To identify giftedness in students with various types of disabilities, an effort must be made by educators and parents to look for potential, rather than focus on demonstrated ability (Baum, Owen, and Dixon, 1991; Maker, 1977).

Students who have been identified as having a learning disability or as having attention-deficit disorder may also possess high ability and high potential to display giftedness. It is often difficult for teachers to identify these students because their disability may obscure the expression of talent. Inattentive behavior may even be mistaken for lack of interest, and a learning disability may be misinterpreted as lack of motivation. To complicate matters, gifted children may be inattentive because they are underchallenged by their classroom work. In order to sort through these complexities, a multidisciplinary evaluation may be preferable, followed by the development of a multimodal treatment plan that addresses the individual child's needs.

Current research (Reis, Neu, and McGuire, 1993) suggests that some very bright students with disabilities have a difficult time in school. Students and parents often wonder what is wrong with a youngster who appears so bright in some ways but does so poorly on so many types of work in school. Identification of gifted students with learning disabilities is often difficult and should include a wide variety of information, including in-depth assessment of both strengths and weaknesses. Individually administered intelligence and achievement tests pointing to a large discrepancy between verbal and performance scores or between potential and performance scores can be helpful in identifying gifted students with learning disabilities. Programs for gifted students with learning disabilities should focus on the student's strength area and not on the deficit area (Baum and Owen, 1988). These programs enhance self-esteem in this group of youngsters and can be extremely helpful in their academic development.

UNDERACHIEVING GIFTED STUDENTS

Educational psychologists usually define underachievement as academic performance that is lower than might be expected based on a reliable measure of learning potential such as intelligence, achievement, or creativity scores. The underachievement of children of extremely high potential may be one of the most frustrating problems confronting parents. When a parent observes advanced interests and skills in the home that are not accompanied by similar school achievement, frustrations are bound to result.

Gifted underachievers may manifest many patterns of behavioral response to school: noncommunicative and withdrawn behavior, passive compliance to "get by," and aggressive disruptive behaviors (Whitmore, 1980). Underachievement may stem from a variety of causes. Assuming that a learning disability has been ruled out, underachievement might stem from academic deficiencies that resulted from previous developmental delays, poor self-image, motivational problems, or limited environmental reinforcers for academic success.

The identification of giftedness in students who have physical or learning disabilities, who have attention-deficit disorder, or who are underachievers is challenging and requires both additional time and attention to alternative identification procedures, and a commitment to maximizing the potential of these students.

Pediatric Approach to the Developmentally Advanced Child

EXAMPLE

John is a 6-year-old kindergartner who is seen by his pediatrician with his parents for well-child care. John has been seen in this office since birth, and his parents have always been amazed by how quickly he learns. He began speaking at 1 year of age and his language skills developed very quickly. He taught himself to read at age 3 and was quick to grasp math concepts. His preschool teachers all remarked about his advanced abilities.

In the past, John's parents seemed very proud of his accomplishments and never expressed any concerns. This visit is somewhat different. Now John's parents feel overwhelmed by the volume and complexity of his questions. They feel guilty because they have gotten to the point where they do not even want to answer one more question. They also worry about John's need to do everything perfectly and constantly show off his talents. His older sister, who just turned 9, does not like to spend any time with John. He always knows the answers to her homework problems and often makes her feel inadequate. She is also tired of the family making such a fuss over his abilities.

This case is illustrative of some of the problems that families encounter when raising a child with unusual gifts and talents. This section reviews some of the issues that pediatricians face in helping gifted children and their families.

GENERAL CONSIDERATIONS

Although giftedness clearly cannot be construed as a medical problem, pediatricians, in their newly expanded role concerned with quality-of-life issues, may have a part to play in this arena. Families often use the pediatrician as their major child health and development professional, especially before the child reaches school age. Accordingly, the pediatrician may be called on to help the family in sorting out questions concerning giftedness.

The pediatric role in this area appears to have the following components:

1. Pediatricians should be aware of clues that might suggest developmental precocity during their health supervision visits with the child and should help the family recognize those clues as well (Table 65–1).
2. The pediatrician should help families find the appropriate balance between the emphasis on early nurturance and stimulation supported by the recent infant development research and unduly pressuring, overly scheduling, or continuously "teaching" their child.
3. The pediatrician should help the child and family in procuring the most appropriate diagnostic evaluation and educational program, including appropriate referrals when necessary.
4. If the child is eventually identified as being gifted, the pediatrician should support the family and the child in coping with the psychosocial problems that may be part of being different or living with one who is different. The pediatrician should emphasize the fact that the same heterogeneity of development that exists in the general population exists in the gifted population. Stereotypes of academically superior children are inaccurate and misleading.
5. The pediatrician should be aware that there are many

Table 65–1 • Characteristics of Gifted Children

Asynchrony across developmental domains
Advanced language and reasoning skills
Conversation and interests like older children's
Insatiable curiosity; perceptive questions
Rapid and intuitive understanding of concepts
Impressive long-term memory
Ability to hold problems in mind that are not yet figured out
Ability to make connections between one concept and another
Interest in patterns and relationships
Advanced sense of humor (for age)
Courage in trying new pathways of thinking
Pleasure in solving and posing new problems
Capacity for independent, self-directed activities
Talent in a specific area: drawing, music, games, math, reading
Sensitivity and perfectionism
Intensity of feeling and emotion

Adapted from Robinson NM, Olszewski-Kubilius PM: Gifted and talented children: issues for pediatricians. Pediatr Rev 17:427, 1996. Reproduced by permission of Pediatrics in Review.

possible explanations for "boredom" in school, with developmental sophistication being only one of them. Tolerating inappropriate behavior or creating a sense of entitlement is ill-advised, regardless of the explanation.

GENERAL APPROACH

If parents suggest to the pediatrician that they believe their child is gifted and are uncertain how to proceed, the pediatrician should discuss their reasons for believing their child is gifted. What is the child doing that has led them to this conclusion? This necessitates some understanding of the margins of normal development. If the child's development appears to fall within that framework and the pediatrician believes that the child is not exceptional, this opinion should be shared with the family. In this era of increasingly early lessons and academic expectations of children, this is not always an easy task. If the parents still desire a more complete evaluation, or if the physician believes that there is some justification in their claim, the next step is the initiation of the evaluation process. If the child is of school age, responsibility for evaluation of potentially gifted children is defined by individual state law but, when mandated, is usually the responsibility of the local public school. If children are younger than school age, this responsibility is less clear but usually is in the hands of the parents.

Evaluation of younger children most likely consists of the administration of standardized tests that attempt to predict academic potential. These tests may be formal developmental examinations that focus on the child's overall development, or they may be very narrow tests that focus on specific abilities. For example, Fagan and colleagues (1986) have suggested that an infant's performance on a battery of specific visual memory tasks is predictive of subsequent intellectual development. Some have even suggested that this instrument can identify intellectually sophisticated children early on. Such instruments require more research before they can be offered as predictors of giftedness.

In older children, in addition to intellectual testing, achievement tests may be administered and an evaluation of creativity may be performed. If the child has written poems or stories, has done creative work in other fields, or has produced any creative products, these might be considered part of the process to determine giftedness. It should be re-emphasized that certain children with high potential may not produce such work because of their developmental constraints in other areas. As previously stated, there continues to be an enormous controversy over what constitutes giftedness, and in certain communities this may lead to confusion and contradictory statements among professionals and parents involved with the child.

Once the testing has been completed and the child has been categorized as being gifted, the pediatrician should have the child and family visit the office to discuss the implications of this identification. The demystification of the concept is vital. Parents and children have enormous misconceptions about what it means to be gifted. Removal of the stigma attached to the label of "gifted" should be attempted, and the child should be told that he or she is like other children except in having special abilities in certain areas that may enable a different rate of achievement than peers. The child should also be reassured that individual differences are positive and that it is all right to question and perceive the world in a way that is slightly different from one's peers. The child's and family's myths of the development of gifted children should be explored and discussed. The presumed burdens of giftedness should be discussed, and counseling at this point should cover three specific areas: home, school, and the community.

Especially at an early age, a distinction should be made between bright children and those whose abilities are truly unique and extraordinary. Because of the inherent vagueness of testing for giftedness and because of the attractiveness that the concept holds for many parents and the glory that accompanies their child's label, pressure is often put on schools to label many bright children as gifted. Although these children might benefit from the types of services offered in gifted programs, average and poor students might benefit as well from individualization of their curriculum and from the opportunity to explore specific areas in depth. The pediatrician should be aware of these complexities in dealing with families who believe their child may be gifted or talented. The following sections are geared toward those children who are gifted and talented, although the basic principles certainly apply to all children.

Home

Parents often ask the pediatrician for advice when dealing with gifted children at home because few other professionals are in a position to discuss home life intimately with the family. First and foremost, it is important to support the parents in their childrearing practices. Either prior to or as a result of the labeling of their child, parents often develop difficulties in relating to their child. They are fearful that their child is brighter than they are and that they are not adequate to provide the needed stimulation to allow their child's "gift" to blossom. They appear to lose balance as parents and treat their child differently, a ten-dency analogous to that in the vulnerable child syndrome described by Green and Solnit (1964) in children with life-threatening illness. The pediatrician should reassure them that, for their child to have been identified as having special abilities, they must have certainly done something right to the present, and it is important that they be encouraged about their parenting skills.

With regard to stimulation, parents should be instructed not to push their children. A trend has emerged toward the earlier presentation of academic material to children and the simultaneous increase in the scheduling of their free time, allowing limited flexibility and time for play. This situation has been labeled by Elkind as "the hurried child syndrome" (1981), which could be exacerbated by exposing very young children to a variety of experiences in order to cultivate their talents while their brain is considered to be most flexible. Parents may feel extra pressure to begin music lessons as well as introduce math concepts and foreign languages during infancy and the toddler years.

Children labeled as gifted are particularly vulnerable to this type of problem. Stimulation for these children should be centered on their interests, and the child should direct the type of material and the depth of exposure. Material should be flexible and allow for the generation of creative products. Museums, books, and other educational material should be provided in the child's expressed area of interest, and not all areas of endeavor should be foisted on the child. Numerous enrichment experiences within various communities exist and may be pursued either after school or in the summer. Because many children who have great intellectual ability are extremely persistent, they let parents know what they want, if parents are able to listen. Parents should be aware that they may be continually barraged by complex questions and should develop strategies for dealing with them. For example, parents of precocious preschool-aged children often report that they are overwhelmed with questions. Children as young as 3 or 4 years old question parents about issues such as death, war, world hunger, and other issues not usually addressed by children of this age.

It is important as well that there not be undue emphasis on performance in these children, but care should also be taken to challenge children so that they learn how to work. Lask (1988) has reported the histories of a number of children who were talented and gifted on whom undue pressure was brought to bear and in whom a variety of somatic complaints developed in response to the increased pressure for performance.

Parents should be told to treat their child as they do other siblings. It is important that they not focus on the label "gifted" in the presence of the child or in their dealings with siblings. They should be comfortable realizing that there might in fact be areas in which the child's ability surpasses their own and that the child might often ask questions they cannot answer. The parents need to develop the self-confidence to say "I don't know, but let's find out together," instead of the more defensive "because I said so."

The family life of gifted children often becomes complicated. As previously mentioned, parents sometimes forget natural instincts and treat their gifted child differently. Instead of setting appropriate limits, in an effort to be fair, parents may become immersed in interminable discussions because of their respect for the child's intelligence (Robinson, 1996). This may cause struggles between parents. Some data suggest that having a gifted child may have a negative impact on marital relationships.

Siblings of the gifted child often feel inferior because of the special attention focused on a gifted brother or sister. This may be magnified if they are close in age. If the gifted child is surpassing a chronologically older sibling in academic work, it might be particularly painful to the older child, and parents should attempt to find ways to continue to assert that the older brother or sister has the special privileges and responsibilities of age, such as staying up later or doing different chores. It is important to allow and cultivate each sibling's uniqueness and specialness. Special time with parents and the fostering of musical talents or athletic skills of siblings may help them feel more adequate and more involved in family life. As previously mentioned, children with increased intellectual abilities often play with children who are on their developmental level and therefore older. If the sibling of a gifted child is slightly older, his or her friends might well become friends of the gifted child, and this might create further tension, which should be clearly addressed within the family. Other studies of siblings of gifted children suggest that parents tend to see siblings as less competent than in fact they really are. There are increased adjustment problems reported in siblings of gifted children, and they tend to have a higher level of anxiety and a lower self-esteem than the gifted child. The role of parents in this situation is to maintain the self-image and self-esteem of the nongifted sibling while simultaneously presenting opportunities for the gifted child that are unique. It is important that this be done in a way that does not increase the arrogance of the gifted child and does not cause the siblings to feel neglected or incompetent.

Aspects of the child's personality can also cause family tension. Gifted children may tend to be perfectionistic and might want to do things over and over before they are satisfied with their end product. They may continuously ask for additional materials, help, or trips to the library, even though parents and siblings believe the child has done an excellent job already. Some level of perfectionism may be healthy if a child learns to do his or her personal best. Dysfunctional perfectionism, however, can result in a child's never finishing anything or in a child who displays frustration, anger, and animosity.

Parents might wish to read one or more of the periodicals and reference texts that have been developed for parents and teachers of the gifted child (e.g., *Parenting for High Potential*) to allow them further insight into dealing with their child. The National Research Center on the Gifted and Talented also has numerous publications available that parents might find helpful.

SCHOOL

The role of the pediatrician is more limited as a gifted child enters school. Parents receive more advice from teachers and parents of other gifted children at this time, but certain issues do merit discussion.

Continued controversy exists over the appropriateness of acceleration versus enrichment as a cornerstone of the education of gifted children. The pendulum has swung toward enrichment primarily, but for extremely precocious children, acceleration can be very appropriate (Rogers and Kimpston, 1992). Acceleration does not simply imply skipping a grade. In fact, because of the decline in the challenge level of regular curricular materials, skipping only one grade may not meet the needs of advanced students. Instead, acceleration of content for specific subject areas may be appropriate, as may be cluster acceleration, which is the assignment of students to a different grade-level classroom for only one or two subjects. The decision must be individualized for each child depending on the child's chronologic age, personality, and degree of advancement and on school factors.

Educators of gifted children, as all professionals, vary in their enthusiasm, creativity, humor, and intelligence. The emphasis in gifted education should not be on busywork or on a greater quantity of work, but instead on advanced content and projects that expand the child's perspective in a given area. A creative teacher can act as a catalyst and a resource person for the child, helping the child to generate and prove hypotheses. If specific gifted programming does not exist, an experienced classroom teacher may be able to function in this capacity. It is hard for parents to judge the competence of their child's teacher or program.

Certain situations, however, should make the parents concerned about the child's program. For example, excessive homework or additional busywork in school is inappropriate and not to be expected or tolerated. Such work only further develops the intellectual aspect of the child's development at the expense of appropriate play in socially interactive time. If the child appears to be bored with schoolwork, is displaying school avoidance behaviors, such as complaining of stomachaches or abdominal pains on school mornings, or is developing a sense of elitism or peer animosity, the quality and philosophy of the program should be questioned. If boredom in the regular classroom persists, strategies for differentiating or compacting the curriculum should be considered (Reis, Burns, and Renzulli, 1992). In addition, the development of increased distractibility or inattention or signs of depression likewise warrant further investigation of the adequacy of the child's program. Close parent-teacher liaison is vital in working with gifted children, and this should be fostered if it is not already developed.

COMMUNITY

Parents should be urged to join or begin a local chapter of the National Association for Gifted Children or other organizations lobbying for gifted children. Through such an organization, parents can receive suggestions and support from others who are experiencing the excitement and frustration of life with a gifted child. Parent organizations can apply pressure to the school board to create and develop more and better programs for gifted children. Parent groups can generate new ideas for extracurricular activities and help provide the resources, both material and human, to bring them to fruition.

The physician might want to be involved with these parent groups to provide guidance and to learn more about these children and the problems they encounter.

Conclusion

Increasingly, issues surrounding aspects of development, particularly in the preschool years, have fallen under the purview of the physician caring for children. Although the medical role with developmentally sophisticated children is less clear than that with developmentally delayed children, some understanding of the gifted child is important.

As has been suggested in this chapter, major theoretical shifts have occurred in the conceptualization of gifted children. Only recently in this era of individual differences has giftedness been looked at as the interaction of intelligence, creativity, and persistence revealed through a continuum of behavior patterns in a very heterogeneous group of children. A person can be gifted in only one area and only some of the time by these criteria.

New methods of identifying and programming for gifted children have been developed. The most progressive emphasize a type of "self-identification" as manifested by productivity in an enriched environment. In many systems, however, intelligence or achievement tests remain the major criterion for entry into gifted programming. There is limited uniformity in gifted programming, but most models emphasize some combination of enrichment and acceleration.

The field of gifted education has grown dramatically in the 1990s, and there is increasing legislative pressure to mandate gifted education. Federal legislation has been enacted to provide new research and model programs throughout the United States.

The physician's role in this area is to support the families of the children in the inevitable questions that they have and to serve as a resource for the family. The physician should attempt to protect gifted children and all children from inappropriate and overly focused intellectual stimulation and allow the child to grow in all domains. To the extent possible, the young child's academic growth should be child-centered and interest-based. As an independent, knowledgeable, and sensitive individual outside the educational system with a long-standing relationship with the family, the physician is in an ideal position to influence positively the academic development of the child, the stability of the family, and the conceptualization of gifted children within the community.

REFERENCES

Baum SM, Owen SV, Dixon J: To be gifted and learning disabled. Mansfield Center, CT, Creative Learning Press, 1991.

Baum SM, Owen SV: High ability learning disabled students: how are they different? Gifted Child Q 33:321, 1988.

Bloom BS (ed): Developing Talent in Young People. New York, Ballantine Books, 1985.

Chall JS, Conrad SC: Should Textbooks Challenge Students? The Case for Easier or Harder Textbooks. New York, Teacher's College Press, 1991.

Council of State Directors of Programs for the Gifted: The 1994 State of the States Gifted and Talented Education Report. Topeka, KS, 1994.

Elkind D: The Hurried Child: Growing Up Too Fast, Too Soon. Reading, MA, Addison-Wesley, 1981.

Fagan JF, Singer LT, Montie JE, et al: Selective screening device for the early detection of delayed cognitive development in infants at risk for later mental retardation. Pediatrics 78:1021, 1986.

Fisch RO, Bileck MK, Horrobin JM, et al: Children with superior intelligence at seven years of age: a prospective study of the influence of prenatal, medical, and socioeconomic factors. Am J Dis Child 130:481, 1976.

Frasier MM, Garcia JH, Passow AH: A review of assessment issues in gifted education and their implications for identifying gifted minority students (RM 95204). Storrs, CT, University of Connecticut, The National Research Center on the Gifted and Talented, 1995.

Fraiser M, Passow AH: Toward a new paradigm for identifying talent potential. Research Monograph 94111. Storrs, CT, National Research Center on the Gifted and Talented, 1994.

Freeman J: Gifted Children. Baltimore, University Park Press, 1979.

Gallagher JJ: Issues in education for the gifted. *In* Passow AH (ed): The Gifted and Talented: Their Education and Development. Chicago, University of Chicago Press, 1979.

Gardner H: Frames of Mind. New York, Basic Books, 1983.

Green M, Solnit A: Reactions to the threatened loss of a child: a vulnerable child syndrome. Pediatrics 34:58, 1964.

Jackson NE, Roller CM: Reading with young children (RBDM 9302). Storrs, CT, The National Research Center on the Gifted and Talented, 1993.

Kirst MW: How to improve schools without spending more money. Phi Delta Kappan 64:6, 1982.

Lask B: The highly talented child. Arch Dis Child 63:118, 1988.

Maker CJ: Providing Programs for the Handicapped Gifted. Reston, VA, Council for Exceptional Children, 1977.

Marland SP Jr: Education of the Gifted and Talented, Vol 1. Report to the Congress of the United States by the US Commissioner of Education. Washington, DC, US Government Printing Office, 1972.

O'Connell-Ross P: National Excellence, A Case for Developing America's Talent. US Department of Education. Office of Educational Research and Improvement. Washington, DC, US Government Printing Office, 1993.

Purcell JH. The effects of the elimination of gifted and talented programs on participating students and their parents. Gifted Child Q 37(4):177–187, 1993.

Reid BD, McGuire MD: Square Pegs in Round Holes—These kids Don't Fit: High Ability Students with Behavioral Problems (RBDM 9512). Storrs, CT, The National Research Center on the Gifted and Talented, 1995.

Reis SM: Reflections on policy affecting the education of gifted and talented students. The American Psychologist 44(2):299, 1989.

Reis SM, Burns DE, Renzulli JD: Curriculum compacting. Mansfield Center, CT, Creative Learning Press, 1992.

Reis SM, Neu TW, McGuire JM. Talents in two places: case studies of high ability students with learning disabilities who have achieved. Research Monograph 95114. Storrs, CT, University of Connecticut, The National Research Center on the Gifted and Talented, 1995.

Renzulli JS: What makes giftedness: re-examining a definition. Phi Delta Kappan 60:180, 1978.

Renzulli JS, Reis SM: The Schoolwide Enrichment Model. Mansfield Center, CT, Creative Learning Press, 1985.

Renzulli JS (ed): Systems and Models for Developing Programs for the Gifted and Talented. Mansfield Center, CT, Creative Learning Press, 1986.

Robinson HB: The uncommonly bright child. *In* Lewis MB, Rosenblum LA (eds): The Uncommon Child. New York, Plenum Press, 1981.

Robinson HB, Roedell WC, Jackson NE: Early identification and intervention. *In* Passow AH (ed): The Gifted and Talented: Their Education and Development. Seventy-Eighth Yearbook of the National Society for the Study of Education. Chicago, University of Chicago Press, 1979.

Robinson NM, Olszewski-Kubilius PM: Gifted and Talented Children: Issues for Pediatricians. Pediatr Rev 174:427, 1996.

Rogers KB, Kimpston RD: Acceleration: What We Do vs. What We Know. Educational Leadership, pp 58–61, 1992.

Silverman LK (ed): Counseling the Gifted and Talented. Denver, Love Publishing Company, 1993.

Tannenbaum AJ: Gifted Children: Psychological and Educational Perspectives. New York, MacMillan, 1983.

Terman LM: Genetic Studies of Genius: Mental and Physical Traits of a

Thousand Gifted Children, Vol 1. Palo Alto, CA, Stanford University Press, 1925.

Terman LM, Oden MH: Genetic Studies of Genius: The Gifted Group at Mid-life, Vol 5. Palo Alto, CA, Stanford University Press, 1959.

Westberg KL, Archambault FX Jr, Dobyns SM, et al: An Observational Study of Instructional and Curricular Practices Used with Gifted and Talented Students in Regular Classrooms, Research Monograph 93104. Storrs, CT, University of Connecticut, The National Research Center on the Gifted and Talented, 1993.

Whitmore JR: Giftedness, Conflict, and Underachievement. Boston, Allyn & Bacon, 1980.

ADDRESSES

The Gifted Child Today. P. O. Box 6448, Mobile, AL 36660-0448, a publication for parents and teachers.

The National Association for Gifted Children. P. O. Box 66365, Washington, DC 20035, publishes a magazine for parents called *Parenting for High Potential.*

The National Research Center on the Gifted and Talented, 362 Fairfield Road, University of Connecticut, Storrs, CT 06269, publishes research reports and briefs.

PART VI

Assessing and Describing Variation

66 *The Interview*

William Lord Coleman

 A meaningful discussion between a parent and a clinician, or a parent and a child, or a parent and a child and a clinician is a mainstay of developmental behavioral pediatrics. Clinicians who are adept at interviewing are likely to become the most astute diagnosticians and the most effective advice givers. This chapter analyzes the interviewing process. It describes the goals and objectives of such encounters while exploring the different forms of interviewing and the procedures that have the greatest yield during such critical doctor-patient transactions. This chapter helps clinicians to become more consciously aware of the dynamics of interviewing, of the implications of what is said for what is to be done.

The interview is a highlight of the doctor-patient interaction. This is especially the case in developmental-behavioral pediatrics.

Traditionally an interview consists of a doctor's asking a patient about the problem or obtaining a "history of present illness." In this chapter, the term *interview* refers to an overview of doctor-patient communication in which appropriate strategies and techniques engender a satisfying, efficient, and productive interaction. There are three forms of interviews: diagnostic, therapeutic-interpretive, and follow-up. This chapter discusses approaches that are common to all interviews as well as techniques that are unique to each form of interview.

Definition of the Interview

The interview is a conscious, goal-oriented conversation between patient and physician; it is a thoughtful, planned procedure. It is a dynamic, diagnostic, and psychotherapeutic process aimed at obtaining and giving various kinds of information. The interview is art and science, integrating the pediatrician's experience, judgment, skill, knowledge, and individual style. Effective interviewing requires in-depth understanding and knowledge of child behavior and development, medical illnesses, family dynamics, cultural variations, socioeconomic influences, and communication skills; it also requires personal self-awareness and the ability to gain the patient's trust, alleviate anxiety, and instill confidence.

Transference and Countertransference

The interview is an intense personal encounter that often generates feelings in the doctor and the patient or family known as transference and countertransference. These terms refer to the unconscious influences that affect the conscious dynamics of the interview and the doctor-patient alliance. Because every interview evokes some elements of transference and countertransference, physicians are more skillful interviewers if they are aware of and sensitive to these dynamics and feelings.

Transference refers to the influence that past emotional experiences (many of them forgotten) exert on one's contemporary attitudes—including the patient's reaction and feelings toward the physician, who so often is perceived as a parent figure. A specific trait of the physician, age or gender for example, may trigger a transference reaction in the patient. If the patient has unmet needs or perceives the physician as omniscient and omnipotent or like a parent, he or she may try to gain approval and may even change the facts, because the need to please is greater than the need to get appropriate treatment. Stress, which causes patients to regress or feel vulnerable, promotes and intensifies transference. Transference may be "positive," for example, when the patient admires or idealizes the physician and is very motivated to please, or transference may be "negative," for example, when a patient is overtly or subtly angry or hostile, which is more likely if a patient feels disappointed or if hope and expectations are not met immediately. The patient may oppose, question, or not comply with treatment.

Countertransference refers to the physician's past experiences as a child and adult, which, in their sum, exert a strong and particular influence on the way the physician regards various patients. Countertransference is the reaction or remembrance that a patient evokes in the physician, or it may stem from the physician's perspective, bias, or self-image. For example, if the physician sees himself or herself as omnipotent or as a parent figure, he or she may treat the patient like a helpless child. Countertransference may be conscious or unconscious, and if the physician is aware of these feelings, he or she may feel very uncomfortable. Like transference, these feelings may be "positive" (feeling loving, protective) or "negative" (feeling threatened, annoyed), and either of these feelings can interfere with optimal treatment.

Interactive, Spontaneous Process of the Interviews

The traditional medical interview consists of an initial visit composed of two interviews: the diagnostic interview followed by the therapeutic-interpretive interview. The follow-up interview occurs at a subsequent shorter visit. Developmental-behavioral problems, however, often do not fall into a predictable sequence of interviews. Diagnosis and therapy seldom are final processes. Instead, within the biopsychosocial perspective that is central to this aspect of pediatrics, these processes are continuous and evolving. These interview processes are not always or necessarily sequential, linear, forward-moving, predictable, or finite. They may be simultaneous, circular, unpredictable, repetitive, and seemingly infinite. They may follow both pathways. For example, a therapeutic intervention also may serve as yet another diagnostic probe, yielding ever-more knowledge and understanding, redefining expectations and goals, reordering priorities, and continuously driving the interactive process of the interviews.

Communication Skills for All Doctor-Patient Interactions

Effective communication—listening, speaking, observing, and exchanging information and feelings—entails many specific skills. The physician notes what patients say (content) and how they say it (process), for example, opening statements, final statements, pauses, body movements, facial expression, eye contact, family interactions, spontaneous, unsolicited comments, and tone of voice. Patients share their feelings and thoughts if given time and support. The physician's communication skills and interview technique should not be apparent. They should be natural and not obvious. The interview should not be an interrogation, but rather a semistructured conversation, flexible yet organized, using the following 10 selected skills (Table 66–1):

1. *Active listening* is listening and actively responding with visible, audible, discernible reactions to the patient's verbal and nonverbal expressions of thoughts and feelings. The listener conveys interest and support through body language: leaning forward, legs easily crossed or slightly open, good eye contact, appropriate facial expression, and little extraneous movement of hands and feet. Passive listening is reacting minimally and only to words and thoughts.
2. *Reflection* is repeating key words and phrases (using the patient's own words) in order to emphasize their importance or to seek clarification or elaboration.
3. *Elaboration* is describing or amplifying in order to give a richer, more detailed description of a thought

Table 66–1 • Selected Communication Skills

1. Active listening, facilitation. Letting the patient know that he or she is really being listened to by verbal and nonverbal feedback.
2. Reflection, repetition. Repeating or paraphrasing key thoughts and feelings.
3. Elaboration. Encouraging patient to amplify, to describe in more detail.
4. Clarification. Asking for explanations so that both patient and pediatrician understand the information.
5. Empathy. Understanding with emotion. The ability to genuinely feel, without filtering or judging, another's feelings. Acknowledging and responding to another's thoughts and feelings.
6. Confrontation. Resolving an apparent contradiction or a withholding of information.
7. Interpretation. Explaining the phenomenon, making an inference, gaining insight.
8. Silence. Providing periods of silence to encourage the patient to reflect, to organize his or her thoughts and feelings, to speak, to elaborate.
9. Tracking. Adapting one's language and style to that of the patient in a natural, comfortable, subtle manner.
10. Summarization. Recapitulating or distilling the essential information to enhance the patient's attention and memory and to provide an opportunity to ask questions.

or feeling. The physician might encourage the patient to elaborate by saying, "Tell me more." Silence often encourages elaboration.

4. *Clarification* is giving a clearer, more exact meaning or understanding. Both physician and patient need to be clear. The physician should avoid medical or technical jargon, information overload, or a too-rapid rate of speech. The physician should encourage the patient to request clarifications and could ascertain the patient's understanding by asking, "Could you sum up what I said to be sure I explained it clearly?" The physician needs the patient to be clear. For example, layman's terms often have personal meanings (lazy, slow learner, good, sad, never, the rules) so the physician might ask, "What do you mean by 'not acting right'?" Labels (e.g., learning disability or attention-deficit disorder [ADD]) also have different meanings to different people and need to be clarified.
5. *Empathy* is the ability to understand with emotion. It is the ability to feel, to acknowledge, and to respond to the patient's feelings and ideas. It implies a genuine interest and respect for the patient, for example, perceiving or asking how he or she felt about a particular issue or situation. Empathy is the ability to detect the real message behind the indirect message, the emotions that drive the thoughts or behaviors, the real reason for coming to the pediatrician. Questions or statements that demonstrate this ability include "That must have been difficult for you. How did you do it? How did you feel? That must have made you feel [a particular feeling]. You seem to be working hard (not feeling appreciated, feeling criticized)."
6. *Confrontation* is asking a direct question or statement to gain a more truthful answer or to interpret or resolve an apparent contradiction. If the patient's answer appears dishonest or not open, the physician should ask it again (rephrasing it if necessary) and

state its importance, or repeat or rephrase it later when the patient (or physician) is more comfortable. For an apparent contradiction, the physician might state, "When we spoke on the phone, you were very worried, but now you appear very happy. I feel confused. I need to know how you really feel and what you want."

7. *Interpretation* is explaining or demystifying the phenomena so the patient will understand the issues and his or her own actions and feelings in order to gain more meaning and insight. Interpretation is encouraging the patient to share his or her perception or belief in order to better understand orientation or frame of reference. Interpretation also helps the patient make inferences and draw conclusions.

8. *Silence* allows the patient to reflect, to organize thoughts and feelings, to elaborate, to regain composure, and to do most of the talking. Silence is not wasted time. Some patients are uncomfortable with or not used to periods of silence, so the pediatrician initially might use brief periods (5 to 10 seconds) and extend them as appropriate (15 to 30 seconds).

9. *Tracking* is the physician's subtly adapting language, body language, style, and the pace of the interview to that of the family. Its purpose is to put the family at ease and enhance the quality and productivity of the interview. It is done in a natural, nonobvious, respectful manner that is appropriate and comfortable for the physician and the family.

10. *Summarizing* is paraphrasing, condensing, or recapitulating. It serves to correct possible misinterpretations or misunderstandings, to prioritize issues, to give the interview coherence, and to help the patient organize thoughts and feelings. Summarizing enhances the patient's memory and recall of salient information, and it provides an opportunity to ask questions and offer comments. Summarizing may be used intermittently during the interview and should always be used at the conclusion.

Goals of the Interviews

While all three interviews share common goals and skills, each also has its own unique purposes and aspects. The physician can better realize these goals by first appreciating several general interviewing guidelines (Table 66–2) (Korsch, Gozzi, and Vida, 1971).

DIAGNOSTIC INTERVIEW

The goals of the diagnostic interview are the following:

1. To facilitate the formation of a therapeutic, supportive doctor-patient interaction, a complex and intensely personal process that shapes the doctor-patient relationship and is as important to the outcome as prescribed medications or protocols
2. To obtain a complete and accurate history, the nature of the presenting problem, and the patient's and parents' thoughts, feelings, perceptions, and parental knowledge and expectations

---

Table 66–2 • General Interviewing Guidelines

1. Elicit and heed the concerns of the parent and child:
   A. "What caused you to bring your child in today?"
   B. "What worries you the most?"
   C. "Why does that worry you?"
2. Acknowledge the parent's expectations for the visit, perceptions of the problem, and expectations of health and illness.
3. Remember that parents want and need an explanation of the diagnosis, cause, and treatment.
4. Develop the doctor-patient relationship.
5. Minimize the use of medical, psychopathologic, or technical terms.
6. Remember that most patients prefer a friendly, warm, professional attitude, not a formal, businesslike or overly casual approach.
7. Be sensitive to and acknowledge the parents' feelings: happiness, relief, anger, sadness, worry, guilt, tension, and disbelief.

---

3. To make observations of the child and family, their behavior, affect, dress, general appearance, state of health, and interactional patterns, because the normal development of children and families is largely a dynamic, interactive process
4. To identify individual and family strengths and coping abilities
5. To provide sufficient flexibility so that individual needs can be expressed or identified and the chief complaint kept in perspective
6. To maintain the patient's perception of the pediatrician as open and approachable, not as one who is judging the child and parents, nor hiding ignorance or confusion, nor trying to establish power. This last point is especially applicable, because behavioral-developmental-psychosocial issues are often painful and difficult for children and parents to acknowledge or discuss within the family or with an outsider. In one third of these visits, the presenting complaint is not the real problem, and the real reason (the hidden agenda) for seeing the pediatrician is not revealed until the patient and family feel comfortable with the pediatrician (Bass and Cohen, 1982).

THERAPEUTIC-INTERPRETIVE INTERVIEW

The therapeutic-interpretive interview portion of the visit consists mainly of the physician's sharing results (interpretive part), making recommendations (therapeutic part), and suggesting interventions, and, to a lesser extent, the patient's asking questions. Nevertheless, it is termed an interview. The goals of this interview are the following:

1. To provide a variety of indicated treatments
2. To mobilize and nurture the identified strengths and coping abilities
3. To explain or interpret the issues
4. To help the child avoid humiliation
5. To lessen the family's feelings of sadness, disappointment, guilt, inadequacy, or anger
6. To instill hope, confidence, and motivation

FOLLOW-UP INTERVIEW

The follow-up interview occurs on a subsequent visit. The goals of this interview are the following:

1. To obtain an interval history and update the overall developmental and behavioral status of the child
2. To measure and acknowledge improvement (hopefully) in specific targeted behaviors and developmental abilities, emotional status, and family function
3. To assess compliance (child, parent, teacher) with the recommendations
4. To determine the appropriateness and accuracy of the physician's interventions and modify interventions and expectations as indicated
5. To reassess or reconsider the original problems if necessary and assess new ones as they arise
6. To provide anticipatory guidance for predictable developmental changes and environmental challenges
7. To compliment the child and family on their hard work and success

Phases of the Interview

Interviewing is a time-consuming, complex process, and the physician can make it more orderly, efficient, productive, and rewarding for both patient and physician by organizing the interview into its phases and conceptualizing the interview as a connected series of different interviewing skills (diagnostic, therapeutic-interpretive, and follow-up) that are specific for the particular phases of the interview process (Coleman, 1995) (Table 66–3).

Table 66–3 • The Phases of the Interviews

I. The preinterview phase
   A. The diagnostic interview
     1. Telephone call from a parent
     2. Referral from another professional
     3. The family executive: identifying and forming an alliance
     4. Background data
     5. The room and seating arrangement
     6. Tentative hypotheses
   B. The follow-up interview
     1. Chart review
     2. Planning
II. The interview phase
   A. The diagnostic interview
     1. Introduction
     2. Obtaining a description of the problem
     3. Gathering other information
     4. Providing support
   B. The therapeutic-interpretive interview
     1. Providing reassurance
     2. Making recommendations
     3. Providing resources
     4. Making referrals
     5. Providing readings
     6. Summarizing
   C. The follow-up interview
     1. Starting with open-ended questions
     2. Assessing progress and goals
     3. Assessing lack of progress if indicated
     4. Addressing new problems if indicated
     5. Providing anticipatory guidance
     6. Complimenting and following up
III. The postinterview phase
   A. Physician's tasks after all interviews and visits
     1. Revising hypotheses
     2. Dictating a chart note and letter

PREINTERVIEW PHASE

Diagnostic Interview

The preinterview phase of the (initial) diagnostic interview has six components and a variety of strategies: (1) receiving the telephone call, (2) obtaining referral from another professional, (3) identifying the family executive, (4) gathering background data, (5) providing a room and seating arrangement, and (6) forming tentative hypotheses.

Telephone Call From a Parent

The telephone call is really the first interview and should be limited to *only a brief description* of the problem and acknowledgment of the parent's worry or concern. If the child has had previous evaluations, the physician should request copies of the reports or get parental consent to obtain them and to call those professionals, agencies, or schools. The telephone call helps the physician determine the urgency and complexity of the problem, the length of the interview, the time of the visit, and who should attend this particular meeting. The physician must identify the contact person who is responsible for keeping the appointment. The physician should keep the call brief and avoid dispensing advice and stating prognoses.

Referral

The physician should obtain the referring person's impressions of the problem, the child, and the family. If a prior evaluation and treatment plan have been done, the physician should ascertain the family's reaction, acceptance, and compliance and request copies of the report. The physician should determine whether the referral is for consultation only, for collaborative care, or for total care. Follow-up and future communication should be arranged.

Identifying the Family Executive

The family executive is the parent with the power for making childrearing decisions and whose support is critical to the family's acceptance of the physician's evaluation and recommendations. This person is usually the concerned parent who contacted the physician. If the physician suspects the caller is not the executive, the physician must include the executive in the interview. If the executive appears hesitant, uncertain, or opposed to the meeting, the physician should call, answer any questions, and encourage his or her attendance, which allows the physician to form an alliance in the presence of the family and to observe family interactions. The executive may be a "significant other," a grandparent, or another relative and may not even live with the child.

Background Data

Gathering background data saves time and need be neither exhaustive nor completed before the interview. Valuable information can be obtained from the child's medical record, the referring person, previous child/family evaluations, and school reports. Comprehensive parent and teacher questionnaires, such as the ANSER system, are time-efficient, useful supplements to the history (Levine, 1996) (see Gathering Other Information). Parent questionnaires provide current information about perinatal and medical history, family history, behavior, attention, development, temperament, affect, and peer interactions. Observing the fit between the child's and the parents' temperaments is very useful diagnostically and therapeutically (see Chapter 67). Teacher questionnaires provide information about the child's academic skills, study and organizational skills, attention, behavior, emotional status, and peer interactions. Questionnaires may be mailed before the visit or given at the first interview and then either mailed back or brought to the second visit.

Selecting the Room and Seating Arrangement

The pediatrician should select a room that allows everyone to sit comfortably not closer than 3 feet and not farther than 6 to 7 feet from the physician. The room should be quiet and private, free of glaring light or blinding sunlight, and not overly dark or somber, and there should be a place to hang coats. The pediatrician's office or the waiting room after hours might suffice. For several reasons, a separate room or play area should be reserved for the children: the physician may wish to interview the parents alone; parents should be given the opportunity to express worries and confidential information privately; and children should be excused if the parents are angry, critical, or recriminating.

The seats should be comfortable, loosely arranged in a circle, and of a height that allows everyone to be approximately at eye level. The physician should not sit behind a desk, stand, or require other members to stand. If the interview takes place at a table, a round table is ideal, because a round table does not have a head and thus everyone is an equal, respected, and responsible participant.

Materials such as toys and books should be age-appropriate. A box of facial tissues should be handy because interviewing about behavioral and developmental issues often evokes strong emotions.

Establishing Tentative Hypotheses

The physician should form some very general, tentative hypotheses, sort of a broad differential diagnosis, being careful not to draw premature conclusions or make judgments. The physician should construct a general plan and a few specific interview strategies and should set a preliminary goal for the interview. The pediatrician should remain flexible and open-minded in light of increasing knowledge and understanding of the child and family and in view of shifting priorities.

Follow-up Interview

The preinterview phase of the follow-up interview has two components and corresponding techniques: (1) chart review and (2) planning.

Chart Review

The chart should be reviewed to refresh the physician's memory and to note any new information (letters, tele-phone memos, records of previous evaluations, and copies of new evaluations or consultations carried out in the interval).

Planning

The follow-up interview may have a specific purpose—for example, to review diagnostic data with parents, evaluate the child's response to interventions, meet other family members, or address a new issue that may have emerged during the interval or that the family is now willing to discuss. The physician needs to schedule a time that is convenient to the family (especially for parents who cannot leave work early), to schedule enough time (especially for a visit that involves more planning effort and more family members), and to have an adequate and comfortable room for the interview.

INTERVIEW PHASE

Diagnostic Interview

The interview phase of the diagnostic interview has four components and many techniques: (1) introduction, (2) obtaining a description of the problem, (3) gathering of other information, and (4) providing support.

The Introduction

The introduction is important, because impressions formed within the initial moments of the doctor-patient interaction are critical to forming the therapeutic alliance, building rapport, and shaping the relationship. Throughout the entire interview, but starting with the introduction, the family is scrutinizing the physician for signs of support, friendliness, interest, impatience, judgment, or disbelief; they are measuring the physician's every response. A positive introduction actually serves as the first therapeutic intervention.

By being punctual, not keeping the patient waiting, the physician conveys a sense of respect and professionalism. If the physician is late, the parents appreciate being told, especially by the physician himself. They can then make necessary telephone calls, get a snack for the child, or make another appointment if necessary. The parent's time is as valuable as the physician's.

The greeting should be friendly and welcoming. It begins with introductions, handshakes, and smiles. Children should be addressed by name, not "your son," "he," or "she," and parents should be addressed by formal names or titles.

The physician should walk side by side with the family when escorting them to the office, making pleasant conversation (appreciating their taking time and making the effort or their punctuality; being understanding of why they were late; making other appropriate small talk). The physician should review the chart, a confidential document, beforehand and leave it in the office, not rifle through it while walking several steps ahead of the family, hurriedly and silently. This unwelcoming opening conveys a negative impression of physician to the family: disorganized, lack of preparation, "treats us like just another patient," "doesn't care," "doesn't like us."

If observers are present, such as medical students, residents, or visiting practitioners, the physician should introduce them, explain their presence, and seek the family's permission for them to observe (in the room or from a viewing room with a one-way mirror). The family always has the right to decline, and this should be made clear to observers before meeting the family.

Once in the room, the members are invited to sit where they wish. Their seating arrangement itself may reveal something about family relationships. A few minutes of social conversation allows the pediatrician to establish personal contact with each member; overcomes the patient's normal initial tendency to feel nervous, hesitant, and sometimes defensive; and lets everyone (including the physician) settle in and feel comfortable. This is especially important for the first interview. The physician might ask the child what he or she likes to do in and out of school, ask the parents about their occupations, or let them lead the conversation.

Sometimes, children and parents are not sure what a developmental-behavioral pediatrician is all about. It can be helpful for such physicians to explain what kind of doctor they are and what they do. The physician might reassure the child that he or she will not be "giving shots," but if blood tests or procedures might be indicated, if the child appears anxious or asks about them, the physician should promise to address that at the end of the visit. The pediatrician might distract the child or lessen the child's anxiety by engaging the child early in the interview process or offering some activities (books, toys, crayons and drawing paper).

The issue of time, how long the visit will last, should be addressed in the introduction. Making the family aware of the time limitations takes pressure off the physician and the family and allows the family to set their expectations for the visit and "settle in" for the interview. The physician should clearly state that another appointment will be scheduled to provide an appropriate evaluation. Time management is critical because behavioral-developmental interviews generally do not move as fast, smoothly, or predictably as medical visits. In some cases, the issues are painful and difficult for children, adolescents, or parents to acknowledge or discuss within the family or with a physician. In other cases, the family wants to talk and the physician needs to listen. In a general practice, appointments made to address psychosocial-developmental problems are frequently randomly scheduled, often sandwiched between well-child visits and acute illness visits, and are allotted 5 to 10 minutes of the standard medical visit. This is not sufficient time; a first visit usually requires a minimum of 30 to 45 minutes and follow-up visits 20 to 30 minutes.

The physician might schedule these appointments at the end of the day when he or she is not on call, or reserve a half or full day for seeing these patients.

If, early in the interview, the physician realizes that building a therapeutic alliance needs to be the goal of this particular visit, he or she would necessarily slow the pace, and focus on the diagnostic and supportive components in order to develop rapport and trust. The physician should inform the family that this interview is "to understand the issues and hear your concerns," not to prescribe a treatment plan, and that other visits will be scheduled.

In another situation, if the problems are complex or background information is lacking, the pediatrician should tell the family that it is not possible to make an accurate assessment in one visit. Family members respect the need for several visits to carry out a thorough, organized evaluation and to develop an individualized, effective treatment plan, which improves patient outcome and enhances family (and physician) satisfaction.

A clock on the wall, desk, or shelf that is readily visible to the patient helps to prevent the interview from running overtime. A second clock, placed behind the patient, makes time management even easier, because it spares the physician from breaking eye contact to glance at the other clock or sneaking furtive peeks at a wristwatch, which can be distracting or make the physician appear discourteous, uninterested, or hurried. Clocks make it easier for the physician to mention the time limits at the start ("We have till 2:30 for this visit"), to give every member a voice ("We have 10 minutes left and I'd like to hear from Becky"), and to let everyone monitor the time. The physician can use it to pace the interview so it feels organized and ends smoothly and gradually: "As you can see, it's almost time to end. In our last 5 minutes, I'd like to share my thoughts, address your concerns and questions, and plan our next visit."

The mother usually makes most of the childrearing decisions, and she is nominally the "family executive" in this domain of family life. But if the "executive" is not yet known or not present, he or she must be identified by this point. (See Identifying the Family Executive.)

Obtaining a Description of the Problem

The shift to this part of the diagnostic interview, "the history of present illness," must be made clear to the family. The physician might pause and make a transition statement: "Now I'd like us to discuss what brought you here." This part of the interview is devoted to the physician's helping the family in three parts: (1) state the chief complaint or presenting problem, (2) describe the problem in detail, and (3) prioritize the problems (if there are several) and negotiate and agree on a problem (if there is disagreement).

Stating the Chief Complaint or Presenting Problem. The diagnostic interview begins with the physician's eliciting the chief complaint by the use of *open-ended or indirect questions*, for example, "What brings you here today?" "What can I do for you?" or, "How can I help you?" These types of questions clarify the problem and purpose of the visit. Indirect questions or statements may be perceived by the patient as less threatening; they tend to "normalize" problems and may be more effective with children or parents who appear tense, guarded, or slow to warm up (Jellinek, 1990). For example, "Many kids have problems with paying attention. I suppose this paying attention thing might be difficult for you, too. Tell me something about it." Or, "Raising a child is a real challenge for every parent. I see parents every day who want to do the right thing. How would you describe your situation?" The answers to these questions reveal much about the family members' expectations of the physician and the visit, family function, and parental knowledge and perceptions, and they allow the physician to keep the chief complaint in perspective. Close-ended questions (those that can be answered yes or no or with one word) should be avoided at this point, for example, "Do you have a problem with paying attention?" or "How is school going?"

The physician can also begin the diagnostic interview by *restating a known complaint*. The physician either restates or asks the patient to restate a previously expressed complaint. For example, at the end of a previous visit, the parent might mention a problem (the "doorknob" statement), for example, "Oh, by the way, I just want to ask about my son's sleep problems." Or the patient may have telephoned with a specific concern. At the next visit, the physician simply restates the complaint or problem using the parent's own words, "We are here to discuss Barry's sleep problems."

The diagnostic interview should stay on target, stick close to the chief complaint, and avoid wide-ranging exploration, tangential talking, and nonrelated personal topics, especially at the first visit. This focused approach allows the family to organize its thinking, prioritize the problems, settle in, and feel comfortable.

During the diagnostic interview the physician or the parents might prefer to discuss the problem first without the child present. Alone with the parents, the physician can determine what they have told the child, determine their expectations of the child, and explore their feelings about the problem, for example, "What worries you the most?" Or, "Does your child remind you of someone in the family (one who has experienced something similar) or of yourself?" This would also be the time to briefly explore relevant parenting issues, for example, disagreements and conflicts about parenting approaches.

If the parent's own words are too generalizing, critical, or humiliating, for example, "Johnny is always driving me crazy," the physician should "reframe" the complaint and the perception, for example, "So we are here to help the two of you get along better?" Or, "Always? . . . Surely there must be some times you get along." (See Providing Readings and Demystification.)

The physician must be sure that everyone (including himself or herself) understands and is clear about the problem. Words and phrases can mean different things, even to members of the same family. For Johnny's mother, her term "driving me crazy" might mean excessive frustration, but for Johnny it might imply that she is going to be hospitalized, heavily medicated, and never be the same again. The phrase "always failing in school" for the parent might mean getting low passing grades for the past semester. The child might think he has always been a failure and will always fail and disappoint. The physician must seek clarification and elaboration and have each member state his or her version until there is a clear, succinct expression understood by all. See Communication Skills for All Doctor-Patient Interactions.

Describing the Problem in Detail. The physician helps the family describe the problem by using an organized yet flexible method of obtaining a detailed, chronologic history of the symptoms and circumstances. The process begins with open-ended or indirect questions and

then continues with more directed inquires in order to elicit a rich description or history. For example, the physician can elicit a detailed description of a recurrent abdominal pain problem by asking very specific questions as captured by the mnemonic RESSALTQQ (Table 66–4) (Coleman, 1992).

Helping the Family Prioritize and Agree on Problems. Sometimes the family describes many problems and jumps from one to another, and the physician must help them prioritize by considering what is most important at this time and what the family's capabilities are; for example, "Which of these problems is most important to you now?"

If members have different problems or different beliefs and interpretations about a problem, the physician must help them agree on a problem. Each member should state his or her version of the problem, for example, "What do you think is the problem—or reason for this meeting?" If parent and child state two different problems and still cannot agree, the physician can use several strategies to help them negotiate: (1) the physician points out the similarities or "connectedness" of both problems, merges them into one, and gives it a new name; (2) the physician suggests a timetable for addressing both problems, for example, first a few visits for the mother's concern and then a few for the daughter's concern; or (3) the physician suggests they focus on another, different problem but one they all feel is important. Oftentimes, after one problem is resolved and the child is doing better, the other problem seems not so important after all, and the family is content to enjoy its newfound success and happiness.

The pediatrician and family must be willing to change the problem-focus if another problem emerges after the original presenting problem. For example, attention problems (ADD) may be the presenting complaint, but undetected learning disabilities may emerge as the real problem; a complaint of teenage "acting out" may be "the ticket of admission" to the physician's office, but underlying marital conflict may emerge as the real problem or the reason for coming.

Table 66–4 • RESSALTQQ: A Mnemonic for Investigating Recurrent Pain Complaints

R (relief)	Alleviating factors or interventions that the patient has practiced
E (exacerbation)	Factors that tend to worsen the pain
S (situation)	The situation in which the pain tends to occur, including precipitating events and agents and predictability
S (significance)	The context of the pain, the meaning that the pain might convey such as helplessness, fear, need for attention, anxiety, and expectation of relief
A (associated symptoms)	Nausea, vomiting, syncope, pallor, diaphoresis, etc.
L (location)	The point at which the pain starts, radiation of pain, deep or superficial, changing or consistently in one location
T (timing)	Onset, frequency, chronicity, temporal patterns, or cycles
Q (quantity)	The severity of the pain—does it incapacitate the patient or is the patient still functional
Q (quality)	Sharp, burning, dull, achy, throbbing

Sometimes children suddenly are seen for complaints that have been present for weeks, months, or even years. The physician should try to uncover reasons for the delay in seeking professional help (Table 66–5) (Green, 1986).

Observations of parent-child interactions provide valuable diagnostic information. Is the parent loving, respectful, unavailable, intimidating, or domineering? Are the interactions minimal and provocative or appropriate and supportive? Is the child secure enough to express himself or herself and to explore? For behavioral problems especially, the physician should note mutual requests for attention and the responses to those requests.

The physician should ask the parent what he or she thinks is causing the problem. The answer may reveal the level of insight or concern, or a bias or perception that affects the history. The physician should note how the problem affects the rest of the family, for example, the family's response or the secondary gains for the child.

Gathering Other Information

The gathering of other information supplements the problem description by providing a comprehensive assessment and gives a contextual perspective of the child and the problem. The pediatrician would evaluate (1) the child, for example, temperament, medical health, developmental function, and cognitive ability; (2) the family, for example, parenting style, beliefs, and expectations; and (3) the social-environmental situation, for example, community resources, access to health care, presence and support of extended family, and quality of schools. These biopsychosocial data enhance the understanding of the child, aid in the diagnosis, and guide the treatment by yielding a perspective that views the child, the family, and the community as part of a "seamless continuum" (Green, 1994). For example, chronic recurrent pain complaints invariably have a multifactorial etiology (Coleman and Levine, 1986).

Psychosocial factors frequently are associated with developmental and behavioral problems, and the interview should include a screening for situations with psychosocial etiologies. Essentially, five issues should be screened: (1) friends and play, (2) schoolwork, (3) family structure and

Table 66–5 • Reasons Why Children Suddenly Present With Complaints that Have Been Present for Weeks, Months, or Years

1. A family crisis such as divorce, serious illness, death, or economic calamity has occurred recently
2. Feelings of anxiety or depression in a parent or child have amplified the symptoms and magnified the worry
3. School authorities have demanded a medical appraisal because of the child's frequent absences
4. A question of a serious biomedical illness has been raised repeatedly by relatives or friends, or the parents have heard or read a news story and want to be reassured
5. In the absence of a social support network, the parent or child with a need to feel cared for comes to the physician for nurturance
6. The family has reached the limit of its tolerance for the child's problem

From Green M: Sifting the clues to psychogenic illness. Contemp Pediatr 3:9, 1986. Reproduced by permission.

Table 66–6 • Situations When the Symptoms Tend to Have a Psychosocial Etiology

1. When the history and the description of the symptoms do not characterize a biomedical disease with which the physician is familiar.
2. When the reason why the child was brought in remains unclear even after several minutes.
3. When the complaint is associated with frequent absences from school, and neither the parent nor the child spontaneously mentions such absences.
4. When a particular symptom has been present without change for some time.
5. When the complaint itself carries a high probability of a psychogenic etiology.

From Green M: Sifting the clues to psychogenic illness. Contemp Pediatr 3:9, 1986. Reproduced with permission.

function, (4) mood, (5) and communication patterns (Table 66–6).

Because the family is the most enduring and central influence on a child, the physician must determine the impact of the family and home environment on the child's development and future potential (Casey and Bradley, 1982; Cohen and Parmlee, 1983). This important component should include a detailed assessment of the family, for example, the developmental phase in the family life cycle, the family structure and function, and the family medical and social histories. Much of this information can be quickly and systematically obtained by using the Child and Family Evaluation (CAFE). Table 66–7 depicts an abbreviated version of the CAFE.*

Gathering other information often is a cumulative process, requiring several visits and other sources (questionnaires, school records, past evaluations). Much information may be obtained from comprehensive questionnaires such as the ANSER system (Levine, 1996).

Providing Support

Providing support is the interpersonal component of the interview and is critical to building a good relationship with the child or adolescent and the family. Support is a variably significant part of the interview, depending on the circumstances. Support is not glib reassurance and is not measured by time spent with the interview. The physician is supportive when he or she demonstrates empathy, a genuine interest in the child and family, and a respectful, nonjudgmental attitude.

The physician should be sure the child understands the purpose of the visit and inquire about the family's expectations, feelings, and perceptions. Acknowledging the child's feelings builds support by helping the child verbalize feelings represented by the child's behavior or a drawing, for example, "I guess this must be kind of embarrassing." Validating the feelings is also helpful, for example, "Most boys and girls who come here also feel

---

*A complete copy of the CAFE may be obtained free of charge by writing William L. Coleman, M.D., at the Center for Development and Learning, CB 7255, University of North Carolina School of Medicine, Chapel Hill, NC 27514.

embarrassed on the first visit." Reassurance is useful, for example, "By the end of the first visit, these boys and girls feel good because the family is happier, and they are glad they came. Some can't wait to come back."

The physician can elicit or enhance good feelings by smiling, playing with the child, and complimenting the family, parent, or child. Rearranging the seating (or moving himself or herself) in order to bring family members closer to each other or to separate members temporarily improves communication and builds support.

Children and parents feel supported when their intense desire for a diagnosis is addressed. Even when the physician has not yet completed the evaluation or is uncertain of the diagnosis, he or she explains the process, openly states any present uncertainty, and assures the family that he or she will persevere. The physician might say "I know this makes you very worried; however, at this point I can't answer your questions. I need to know more, and I plan to gather additional information (do a screening test, consult with a specialist, make a referral)."

The pace of the interview must be matched to the family's verbal ability and tolerance.

The physician should be aware of an affective-cognitive mismatch in any member, that is, the speaker's affect is inappropriate for or does not fit the content of the talk. This might suggest anxiety, depression, reacting too seriously to a minor problem, an inability to appreciate the serious nature or implications of the problem, or an inability to appreciate and express appropriate emotions about positive attributes, good outcomes, and achievements.

The physician should note recurrent themes, differing priorities of family members, and disagreements between parents' stories. The physician should not criticize anyone or any institution, should not take sides, and should not let members speak for one another or for someone who is not present. If the physician detects inconsistencies, he or she should not point them out right away or accuse anyone of wrongdoing; instead, questions should be asked again in a different way. See Communication Skills for All Doctor-Patient Interactions.

Therapeutic-Interpretive Interview

The therapeutic-interpretive interview has six components, which are the five R's plus summarizing: (1) reassurance, (2) recommendations, (3) resources, (4) referrals, (5) readings, and (6) summarizing.

Providing Reassurance

Providing emotional support is acknowledging and validating a range of feelings experienced by patients and parents.

Table 66–7 • Child and Family Evaluation—CAFE©

EXPLANATION: The family is the most central and enduring influence on a child's well-being. A biopsychosocial perspective allows the family and the physician to appreciate and feel comfortable with a comprehensive approach to child care. This form, representing contextual pediatric care, should be introduced and partially completed on the first encounter. It should be completed by the physician with some input from the family. This may require several visits. This family profile should be updated periodically or as events dictate.

I. THE FAMILY LIFE CYCLE
DIRECTIONS: Explain that all families go through a sequence of predictable developmental stages and expectations/issues/challenges; it is very helpful for the family and the pediatrician to discuss these stages and issues and events and how they affect the child and family. These issues may be contributing to the presenting problem. Families may be in several stages simultaneously. Check (√) the relevant issues.

STAGE	EXPECTATIONS, ISSUES, AND CHALLENGES
1 The new couple	___ Relationship commitment
	___ Marriage/living together
	___ Formation of extended family
2 The birth of children	___ Being both parents and spouses
	___ Sharing tasks
	___ Using extended family supports, e.g. grandparents
3 Families with school-age children	___ More demands on children (school, peers)
	___ More demands on adults (parents, spouses, careers/jobs)
4 Families with adolescents	___ Renegotiation of parent-adolescent relationship (roles and expectations)
	___ Parents support aging relatives (grandparents, others)
5 Mid-life years (parents) Young adulthood (children)	
a. Parents	___ Empty nest; reassess and refocus on marriage, self, and career
	___ Increased support of aging and dying parents (grandparents)
	___ Coming to terms with own aging and physiologic decline
	___ Accommodating new in-laws and grandchildren
b. Young adults	___ Focus on own identity; intimate relationships; marriage
	___ Career development
6 Later life of parents; loss, grieving and death	___ Generational roles change
	___ Adult children care for aging parents
	___ Loss of spouse, siblings, friends; life review; preparation for own death

II. FAMILY GENOGRAM (CAFE©)
DIRECTIONS: With the family's help, first obtain a family history. Then map out the nature of the family relationships (spouses, parents, siblings) and circle those who live in the house. Note any intergenerational processes.

Table continued on following page

Table 66–7 • Child and Family Evaluation—CAFE© *Continued*

FAMILY HISTORY   FAMILY RELATIONSHIPS/BOUNDARIES

M - Medical Problem   L/A - Learning/Attention Problems

E - Emotional Problem   B - Behavioral Problems

ETOH - Alcohol   X - Deceased
(Ask - "How much do you drink?")

D - Drugs

normal
diffuse
affiliation
enmeshed; over involved
estranged
distant
rigid
> coalition

conflict
abuse
separation; divorce
living together; not married
identified patient

Grandparents

Parents

Children

CAFE©

III. COMMUNITY/ENVIRONMENTAL INFLUENCES ON CHILD AND FAMILY HEALTH AND WELL BEING (CAFE©)

    DIRECTIONS: Have the family report on its perception of these influences by using " – " if a risk factor/problem and " + " if a protective factor/strength or NI if not influential.

Extended Family ＿＿	Housing ＿＿	Income ＿＿
Friends ＿＿	Schools ＿＿	Employment/Career ＿＿
Neighborhood ＿＿	Transportation ＿＿	Social Services ＿＿
Cultural System ＿＿	Recreational Resources ＿＿	Health Care ＿＿
Religion ＿＿		(Physical and Mental)

IV. SUMMARY

    DIRECTIONS: Summarize the child-family-community situation

Strengths and Protective Factors   Problems and Risk Factors

1.   1.
2.   2.
3.   3.
4.   4.

Comments ＿＿

V. FAMILY GOALS AND PLANS

The support is offered whenever needed, because, in the case of disappointing outcomes, the family will not be able to "hear" the physician or accept the diagnosis until their feelings are acknowledged and they feel supported. (See Goals of the Interviews.)

Many factors generate the emotions, for example, the nature of the interviewing process, the types and levels of severity of the diagnoses, and the beliefs and expectations of the child and parents. The feelings might be positive (relief, joy, pride, appreciation) or negative (guilt, incompetence, shame, anger, sadness, disappointment).

If a family does not demonstrate an emotional response, several factors might be considered: they might not like or trust the physician; they might not understand or agree with the diagnosis; they may be in shock and unable to respond; they may feel they do not have "permission" to show their emotions. The physician might pause and gently say "This news must be very hard to hear. How are you feeling?"

The physician also provides reassurance and support by, for example, informing the family of the availability and effectiveness of resources and interventions, giving the family a positive prognosis (if the rate and extent of improvement are known), reassuring the family of the physician's long-term follow-up and advocacy plan, educating the family about the disorder, and helping them mobilize their own strength and maintain their sense of competence and hope.

Suggesting Recommendations

Three general categories of recommendations include (1) direct interventions, (2) bypass strategies, and (3) nurturing strengths. Direct interventions are aimed at the problem and are intended to improve the situation or resolve the problem; these interventions are roughly classified as pharmacologic—for example, medical or physical (medications, physical therapy, biofeedback), or nonpharmacologic—for example, developmental-behavioral-emotional (speech therapy, special educational services, behavior modification, counseling). Recommendations may be aimed at the parent and family too—for example, individual, marital, or family therapy.

Bypass strategies are alternative strategies that bypass the problem per se; they enable the child to function and achieve goals by using other methods. For instance, a student with poor graphomotor skills (e.g., weak handwriting skills) would be taught to use a word processor for writing papers, would be allowed to give book reports in an oral (not written) format, and would be given extended time on timed (written) tests.

Nurturing strengths and interests means strengthening those strengths that the student already possesses; for example, a student with good verbal skills might be encouraged to join a debating team or would be placed in a learning environment based on frequent class discussions and small-group seminars.

Providing Resources

The physician might (1) recommend using federal laws to obtain a free school-based evaluation and appropriate spe-cial educational services for a child with mental retardation or (2) encourage parents to join the local chapter of CHADD (Children and Adults with Attention Deficit Disorder), the PTA (Parent Teacher Association), or a parent-support group, for example, Parents Without Partners.

Making Referrals

The physician might refer the child to a specialist for evaluation or management, for example, to a developmental-behavioral pediatrician, child psychiatrist, psychologist, or social worker.

The referral should be made in a supportive manner that does not imply the patient is "crazy" or that the physician is uninterested or wants to get rid of the patient or family. The physician should take time to explain the reason for referral to the family and decide who is best suited to follow up the child.

Providing Readings and Demystification

Educating and providing information about the child's or family's issues through explanations and suggested readings help the child and family understand the issues. The physician's explanations and interpretations are most helpful at this critical point of the child's evaluation. The interpretive process, known as demystifcation, greatly enhances the child's and parents' understanding of the problem and self-awareness, self-understanding, and coping ability. Demystification has several key components.

- The explanation is presented in a nonblaming, nonpathologic, and developmentally appropriate manner using nontechnical/nonmedical language and real-life examples to illustrate and clarify the phenomena.
- The issues are "normalized," for example, "I see many kids with these same issues."
- The issues are "externalized" or depersonalized, for example, "Let's talk about these attention difficulties" rather than "I want to talk about *your* attention problems."
- The issues are "reframed," that is, a negative perception is replaced with a neutral or positive one by clarifying the issues. For example, a child might be seen because he is perceived as rude and egocentric, constantly being punished and criticized, and consequently is developing a negative self-image. The physician might diagnose attention or activity problems and explain the child's marked impulsivity and insatiability as developmental difficulties of weak inhibition and delay of gratification and that the child is not intentionally being difficult. Another example is the adolescent who is seen as being oppositional and distant, but in reality he is acting in a developmentally appropriate manner as he tries to separate, individuate, and become more autonomous, even as the parent attempts to parent him like a younger child.
- A nonlabeling approach is utilized. Avoidance of labels such as ADD, major depressive disorder, or "difficult child" is critical, because they tend to be perjorative and exclusive (exclude contributing factors, complications, or compensatory strengths).

Descriptions should be based on the specific issues and not imply general pathology, incompetence, or shame, for example, "difficulty paying attention in learning situations that require sustained listening and rapid note-taking, such as long lectures" is a more helpful description than "ADD." The physician constructs a narrative profile of the child instead of using vague, general, simplistic labels. The profile includes the demystification, acknowledgment of the child's unique assets, the family's strengths and hard work, and any other relevant issues.

Summarizing

The physician provides a very brief summary of the salient aspects of the therapeutic-interpretive interview, which helps the family remember the important points.

The summary also conveys the impression of an organized, well-timed visit and avoids an abrupt ending, which appears unprofessional and leaves families feeling dissatisfied.

- The physician should tell the family he or she will answer their questions or address their final concerns; this greatly reduces their anxiety and uncertainties.
- The physician should not attempt to address a new concern or the "doorknob" question ("Oh, by the way, I'd also like to ask you about . . ."); instead he or she should arrange for a telephone call or another appointment to discuss the issue.
- The physician should avoid the temptation to socialize during the summary because it tends to diminish the intensity.
- Finally, follow-up appointments are scheduled and arrangements are made for handling unforeseen problems or for answering questions during the interval.

Follow-up Interview

The follow-up interview has six components: (1) starting with open-ended questions, (2) assessing the targeted goal, (3) if indicated, determining why things are not improving, (4) if indicated, addressing new problems, (5) providing anticipatory guidance, and (6) complimenting, summarizing, encouraging questions and discussion, and scheduling follow-up.

1. The physician first should obtain an overall, general picture of the child's status and start with a friendly greeting, for example, "It's good to see you again," and an open-ended question, for example, "How are things going?" This allows the family to settle down, relax, gather their thoughts, and bring up an issue that may be new and that they want to discuss first.
2. The physician should ask about changes (hopefully improvement) in targeted areas, for example, development, behavior, affect, family function, obtaining a school-based evaluation, or seeing a specialist.
3. If the situation has not improved or the family seems frustrated or disappointed, the physician might consider not only compliance (child, parents, school) but also whether the original diagnosis, perceptions, expectations of the family, and interventions were

accurate, timely, and appropriate. The physician might need to reconsider any or these factors and modify accordingly. The physician should not label a family "resistant," "oppositional," or "noncompliant."

4. If indicated, the physician should assess new problems with another cycle of diagnostic and therapeutic-interpretive interviews, which might be abbreviated because the physician has come to know the child and family.
5. The physician should provide anticipatory guidance for predictable developmental changes (the transition to early adolescence) and challenges (academic demands and social life in middle school).
6. The physician should always compliment the child and family for their hard work and continued hope, encourage them to continue to maintain strengths, summarize the meeting, give the family an opportunity to ask questions, and schedule another appointment.

POSTMEETING PHASE

Tasks of the Physician After Each Interview

The postmeeting phase has two components: (1) revising hypotheses and (2) dictating a chart note and letter.

1. The pediatrician should consider revising the original hypothesis and approach, if necessary, as more is learned about the family. The physician might want to change the focus, invite another member, try another interview strategy, or consider additional interventions, for example, medication, readings, or referral for the family or particular members. The physician should reflect on his or her own feelings about the family and share his or her thoughts and feelings with another experienced colleague if needed.
2. Many families appreciate and benefit from a brief summary letter (that may also serve as a chart note) that specifies the progress and the assignments, conveys hope, mentions ongoing concerns if necessary, and includes the next appointment time. In some cases, a separate chart note is necessary, which includes the pediatrician's own impressions, confidential information, and his or her plans for the next meeting.

A Brief Interview for Primary Care
(Table 66–8)

Developmental-behavioral and psychosocial problems constitute about 25% of presenting complaints in primary care (Dworkin, 1993). The primary care provider (PCP) is expected to at least detect and screen these problems, treat what he or she can, and refer what he or she cannot. Managed care is requiring the primary care provider to provide an initial assessment for many of these problems. Early detection and treatment of these problems does prevent later complications and increased severity, which are much more difficult and costly to treat.

Table 66–8 • Brief Interviews for Primary Care

I. Diagnostic interview
  A. Brief medical history (if needed)
  B. Brief family history
  C. Brief social history (questionnaire or interview)
  D. Brief parenting history (questionnaire or interview)
  E. Brief developmental-emotional screening/observation
  F. Problem-focused history, including onset, duration, and intensity of symptoms; developmentally appropriate expectations; affected domains of function
  G. "Trigger questions"
  H. $ABCB_1C_1$ model
  I. Review of past evaluations, treatments, and outcomes
II. Therapeutic interview
  A. Treat those problems within the expertise of the PCP and the time constraints of the office setting
  B. Referral
    1. Consultation
    2. Further diagnosis and treatment
    3. Collaborative management
  C. Follow-up
  D. Coordination of services
  E. Advocacy

The PCP can break these interviews into shorter visits and smaller time segments and still provide very good assessment and treatment. Most busy PCPs do not have the time to conduct an extensive interview, a task usually reserved for developmental-behavioral pediatricians. Many mild problems require only one slightly longer interview or two shorter interviews. Furthermore, the PCP usually has the advantage of knowing the child and the family through well-child visits and can therefore focus more directly and quickly on the presenting complaint. For both diagnosis and treatment, the PCP should always maintain a contextual approach (the child, the family, and if necessary, the community) within a biopsychosocial perspective. Ideally the PCP should plan two short visits and use the interval between visits to send out and review questionnaires.

The diagnostic interview should include a brief medical history only if necessary. The family and social histories may already be known to the PCP; if not, they should be briefly explored at this time or reviewed in the questionnaires. Past evaluations and interventions (and parents' understanding, acceptance, and compliance) should be briefly explored. These background questionnaires can be given to the parents on the first visit and sent to the pediatrician, who can then review them before the second meeting.

The parenting history (how the parents themselves were parented) is very useful for evaluating behavioral problems. The symptoms should be carefully described in terms of onset and duration, intensity, frequency, manifestations, and impact on various areas of function.

Trigger questions elicit important information in a time-efficient manner. "Tell me about Sarah's relationships with other children" and (if she plays sports) "How does she get along with the coaches?" For the child: "Tell me about your friends." "Do you have a best friend?" "What do you like to do together?" "Do your friends pressure you to do things you don't want to do?" "How are you getting along with your parent(s), brother(s), sister(s)?" "Do you belong to a gang? Have you thought about joining one?" (Green, 1994).

The *Diagnostic and Statistical Manual for Primary Care (DSM-PC): Child and Adolescent Version (DSM-PC*, 1996) is a very useful guide for the PCP. It covers a variety of behavioral and developmental problems at three stages of severity—normal variation, problem, and disorder—and describes the signs and symptoms as they may appear at different chronologic-developmental periods—infancy, early childhood, middle childhood, and adolescence. It also describes a host of environmental risk and protective factors that need to be taken into account within the biopsychosocial framework. Lastly, it provides a variety of diagnostic codes for reimbursement purposes.

A useful brief technique for assessing behavioral problems is the $ABCB_1C_1$ model:

- **A** is the Antecedent event, the situation or context in which the problematic behavior occurs. This may be a time of the day, a particular place, or the parents' communication style.
- **B** is the Behavior of the child; the physician should get a baseline measure of chronicity, frequency, and intensity of the behavior and mood.
- **C** is the Consequences of or the parents' reaction (behavior and mood) to the child's behavior.
- **B_1** is the child's Behavior in response to the parents' reaction.
- **C_1** is the parents' Reaction to the child's response.

This model provides a clear, concrete, dynamic real-life example of a specific parent-child interaction. The PCP can provide advice and support at various points of the interaction. See Table 66–8.

Consultation with colleagues and other specialists, starting with developmental-behavioral pediatricians, is very helpful and not costly.

Conclusion

The interview is the highlight of the doctor-patient interaction. Effective interviewing promotes good health and development and is satisfying to both the patient and physician. Using these interviewing skills will enable the primary care provider and the subspecialist to fulfill the most basic role of the pediatrician.

REFERENCES

American Academy of Pediatrics: Diagnostic and Statistical Manual for Primary Care: Child and Adolescent Version. Elk Grove Village, IL, 1996.
Bass LW, Cohen RL: Ostensible versus actual reasons for seeking pediatric attention: another look at the parental ticket of admission. Pediatrics 70:870, 1982.
Casey PH, Bradley RH: The impact of home environment on children's development: clinical relevance for the pediatrician. J Dev Behav Pediatr 3:146, 1982.
Cohen SE, Parmlee AH: Prediction of five-year Stanford Binet scores in preterm infants. Child Dev 54:58, 1983.
Coleman WL: Family-focused pediatrics: solution-oriented techniques for behavioral problems. Contemp Pediatr 14:121, 1997.
Coleman WL: The first interview with a family. *In* Coleman WL, Taylor EH (eds): Pediatr Clin North Am 42:119, 1995.

Coleman WL: Recurrent pain and Munchausen syndrome by proxy. *In* Levine MD, Carey WB, Crocker AC (eds): Developmental-Behavioral Pediatrics, 2nd ed. Philadelphia, WB Saunders, 1992, pp 339–349.

Coleman WL, Levine MD: Recurrent abdominal pain: the cost of the aches and the aches of the cost. Pediatr Rev 8:143, 1986.

Dworkin PH: Detection of behavioral, developmental, and psychosocial problems in pediatric primary care practice. Curr Opinion Pediatr 5:531, 1993.

Green M (ed): Bright Futures. Arlington VA, National Center for Education in Maternal and Child Health, 1994.

Green M: Sifting the clues to psychogenic illness. Contemp Pediatr 3:9, 1986.

Jellinek MS: Interviewing in pediatric outpatient practice. Curr Probl Pediatr 10:575, 1990.

Korsch BM, Gozzi EK, Vida F: Gaps in doctor-patient communication: doctor-patient interaction and patient satisfaction. Pediatrics 45:855, 1971.

Levine MD: The ANSER System. Cambridge, MA, Educators Publishing Service, 1996.

RECOMMENDED READING

Boyle WE, Hoekelman RA: The pediatric history. *In* Hoekelman RA (ed): Primary Pediatric Care, 2nd ed. St. Louis, Mosby, 1992, pp 56–66.

Lipkin M, Putnam SM, Lazare A (eds): The Medical Interview: Clinical Care, Education, and Research. New York, Springer-Verlag, 1995.

Morrison J: The First Interview. New York, Guilford Press, 1995.

Schmitt BD: Pediatric counseling. *In* Levine MD, Carey WB, Crocker AC (eds): Developmental-Behavioral Pediatrics, 2nd ed. Philadelphia, WB Saunders, 1992, pp 679–686.

67 Pediatric Assessment of Behavioral Adjustment and Behavioral Style

William B. Carey

Many pediatricians feel unsure about how best to evaluate the behavior of their patients. Instead of encouraging the use of screening checklists and the categorical pathology diagnostic model for assessing behavioral adjustment, this chapter recommends a primary reliance on interviewing of the parent directed toward clarifying the concern and obtaining a comprehensive behavioral profile. For determinations of temperament in routine care, a few interview questions are generally sufficient, but in case of parental concern, a standardized questionnaire will provide a fuller picture of the child's contribution to the interaction.

This chapter is concerned with suggestions on how the pediatrician in private or clinic practice can evaluate children's behavior competently without the aid of our allied disciplines. Techniques used by those specialists are discussed in later chapters.

Some terms should first be clarified. Elsewhere in this volume the point has been made that development and behavior are intertwined in the individual. Nevertheless, they can be assessed separately. *Development* refers to the evolution of capacities that is a reflection of the maturation of the central nervous system. The term *behavior* is intended to mean the content and style of the actions of the child in his or her relationships. The first part of this chapter discusses assessment of behavioral adjustment, which is the content of these actions. The second part deals with temperament, which is the style with which they are performed.

Behavioral Adjustment

THE CHALLENGE AND THE OBSTACLES

The proficient evaluation by the pediatrician of behavior in children is a complex challenge. Much is expected of him or her. Ideally every comprehensive pediatric evaluation and especially every investigation of a specific problem with possible developmental-behavioral components, such as headaches or scholastic difficulties, should include a clear picture of the child's behavioral adjustment pattern; the physical, developmental, temperamental, and environmental factors interacting with it; and a plan for possible alteration of these factors for the benefit of the child. Besides well-developed interviewing and counseling skills, this expectation presumes an understanding of whether specific behaviors are normal, and, if not normal, a judgment as to how severe they are, why they have developed, and what to do about them. These objectives represent a major shift for the practice of pediatrics that emerged only a century ago as the subdivision of medical science dealing with the nutritional and growth problems and physical diseases unique to childhood.

In rising to meet this challenge, the pediatrician is confronted with major obstacles:

1. Unclear presentation of concern by parents. Compared with most common physical illnesses, behavioral problems are likely to present themselves clinically in confusing, unorganized forms. The concern may be evident but its real focus may be obscure. The parent might simply ask the pediatrician for advice on discipline when the true distress is marital discord and the accompanying disputes over child-rearing. Another parent might request a different formula or complain about intestinal gas when the actual problem is excessive crying in the infant. The concern must be clarified before the diagnosis can begin.
2. Undefined parental expectations. A parent's mention of certain behavioral issues does not necessarily mean that he or she is asking for or expects the involvement of the pediatrician. On the other hand, the expectations of the parents may be unreasonable. A meeting of the minds must occur as to what the parents want and what the pediatrician can offer.
3. Skill and time required. As with any other area of clinical competence, evaluation of behavior requires training to achieve the necessary skill. Most pediatric residency programs expose trainees to an abundance of tertiary care of major illnesses but to a minimum of experience fostering the knowledge and skills of behavioral pediatrics. Graduates of these programs report an understandable feeling of inadequacy. Even the pediatrician with the requisite skills is confronted with many competing responsibilities during the available time with the patient, as well as with a reimbursement system that at present overvalues mechanical procedures and underpays for time spent in diagnostic interviewing and counseling.
4. Frequently confusing advice from mental health specialists. Conflicting theories about the origins of be-

havior problems and their management leave pediatricians confused. The techniques suggested by spokespersons of those disciplines may not be suitable for pediatric settings.

Confronted with these obstacles, some pediatricians feel tempted to avoid asking parents about behavioral issues or try to evade them when brought up. Some give standard prescription advice for the problem without fitting it to the needs of the particular child. Another alternative is to refer immediately to a mental health specialist all parents concerned about their children. The extent of this suboptimal performance is not easily determined, but it is probably not as great as has been estimated by the more severe critics (Costello, 1986; Horowitz et al, 1992; Lavigne et al, 1993; Simonian et al, 1991). This discussion first reviews the available classification systems and then describes the techniques for obtaining the data needed for classification.

DIAGNOSTIC CLASSIFICATION SYSTEMS

DSM-IV. The most widely known of the diagnostic systems for behavioral and emotional problems is the *Diagnostic and Statistical Manual of Mental Disorders,* 4th edition (*DSM-IV*) of the American Psychiatric Association (1994). This volume was preceded by several versions, starting with the *DSM-I* in 1952. The current formulation subdivides overall diagnoses into five components or axes: (1) clinical disorders, (2) personality disorders and mental retardation, (3) general medical conditions, (4) psychosocial and environmental problems, and (5) global assessment of functioning. In the last of these measures, the clinician indicates a general judgment from 1 (persistent danger to self or others) to 100 (superior functioning without any symptoms). Normality is not specifically defined but is assumed to be the lack of any of the conditions listed.

Because the *DSM* system has been virtually the only one available to physicians in this country for decades, many have assumed that it is the best possible. However, clinicians in pediatric care have increasingly become aware of its limitations.

1. The *DSM* system is primarily intended for adults and does not deal sufficiently with the variety of problems and concerns facing children, their parents, and the professionals trying to help them in primary care.
2. *DSM* diagnoses use the categorical "medical model," the diagnosis is either present or absent, a view that does not fit well with the primary care pediatrician's experience with the wide variation of children's adjustment along several dimensions of function.
3. The *DSM* system does not recognize normal variations of behavior. Temperament is not even mentioned. Many normal variations of temperament are overdiagnosed, as with the inattentive individual who is functioning normally but who is supposed to be given the "subthreshold" diagnosis of Attention-Deficit/Hyperactivity Disorder, Not Otherwise Specified.

DSM-PC. The American Academy of Pediatrics Task Force on Mental Health Coding for Children has developed and recently published the *Diagnostic and Statistical Manual for Primary Care: Child and Adolescent Version* (*DSM-PC*) (1996). The principal aim was to overcome all three limitations mentioned regarding the *DSM-IV* and its predecessors and "to help primary care clinicians better identify psychosocial factors affecting their patients so that they can provide interventions when appropriate, be reimbursed for those interventions, and identify and refer patients who require more sophisticated mental health care." This was an interdisciplinary effort in which psychiatrists and psychologists collaborated with pediatricians on an approximately equal footing.

The *DSM-PC* includes two principal parts, a listing of Environmental Situations that may affect children's behavior (e.g., caregiving changes, educational challenges) and a longer Child Manifestations Section of problems in 10 different areas (e.g., negative/antisocial behaviors, somatic and sleep behaviors). Within each of these 10 "behavioral clusters," the presentation of symptoms is subdivided into three levels: (1) developmental variations, by which is meant normal behavioral variations, ones that may nevertheless attract the concern of the clinician or the parent; (2) problems, which are behaviors serious enough to disrupt the child's social or scholastic functioning but are not severe enough to warrant a diagnosis of a mental disorder (like "the child who gets into fights intermittently in school or in the neighborhood"); and (3) disorders, as defined by the *DSM-IV*. The framers of the *DSM-PC* were required to incorporate the entire *DSM-IV* terminology unaltered as the standard inventory of behavioral diagnoses.

The *DSM-PC* is a big step forward toward designing a diagnostic system more appropriate for use by physicians for all sorts of behavioral concerns with children. Some of the major limitations of the parent DSM series have been eliminated. Many pediatricians will find it useful. However, there are still some significant limitations that must be overcome before it will achieve its maximum value:

1. Physical status. There should be a place to incorporate a consideration of the great variety of general physical and neurologic factors affecting behavior. The environment is not the only influence on it.
2. Temperament. The relegation of the formal presentation of temperament to two paragraphs in the preamble of the environmental situations section and scattered brief mention later betrays an insufficient recognition of its importance. Temperament variations are one of the three principal sources of behavioral concern that parents bring to pediatricians (the others being actual behavior problems and misperceptions of normality). Shyness and moodiness are mentioned in the *DSM-PC,* but most of those important traits like high intensity, unpredictability, high persistence, and sensitivity are not included. Through interactions with the environment, temperament participates in the formation of physical, developmental, and behavioral problems; it affects children's responses to physical illnesses and utilization of medical care; and it can alter the child's environment, with which he or she is interacting.
3. Development. The child's developmental status would be better listed as a component contributing to

the behavioral outcome rather than as simply another Child Manifestation.

4. Parent-child interactions. No suggestions are offered as to how to describe the parent-child interactions and the ways in which the Environmental Situations may be influencing the symptoms in the Child Manifestations.

5. Service needs. The *DSM-PC* has a useful section on determining the severity of the behavioral problem but no place to indicate the service needs of the child. The clinician who has evaluated the child should indicate what level of care is needed:

   a. Anticipatory guidance or brief educational counseling

   b. Reassurance or individualized counseling for bothersome normal variations

   c. Intervention counseling for mild to moderately severe situations or behavior problems, which need more time

   d. Referral counseling for major behavioral or emotional disorders

   The clinician generating the diagnosis is the person best qualified to make this determination about service needs. If he or she does not, that function will be left to others, such as health insurance companies.

6. Summary profile. The *DSM-PC* resembles the *DSM-IV* in presenting long lists of possible problems. Unlike the *DSM-IV* system with its five axes, however, the *DSM-PC* does not suggest a way to put all the findings together into a diagnostic profile. An example of how this could be done in a pediatric setting is to be found in Chapter 75 of this volume.

7. Omission of ratings of strengths. The *DSM-PC* system is still basically oriented toward the abnormal in that there is no opportunity for the clinician to make note of positive aspects of behavioral adjustment such as social competence, task performance, self-assurance, and general contentment.

8. Omissions of influences and problems. The list of possible problems is long but there are important gaps. For example, the powerful and pervasive environmental influence of television goes unmentioned. And colic, the most common behavior problem in the first few months of life, does not appear in either the index or the list of presenting complaints.

The developers of the *DSM-PC* acknowledge that this is a first attempt and that revisions will be inevitable. Its usefulness in its present state has not been critically reviewed.

ICD-10. The *International Statistical Classification of Diseases and Related Health Problems,* 10th revision (*ICD-10*) of the World Health Organization (1992) is, along with the DSM series, the other best-known diagnostic scheme. As the name implies, it also deals only with disorders. Those listed as having their onset in childhood and adolescence include hyperkinetic disorders, conduct disorders, mixed disorders of conduct and emotions, emotional disorders, disorders of social functioning, and tic disorders. Much effort was expended by the developers of this system and of the *DSM-IV* to make the two classification systems as convergent as possible. Nevertheless, some

significant differences can be found in criteria for diagnoses, as with the definitions of hyperkinesis.

DC:0-3. Another recent addition to the diagnostic procedures available to child health care practitioners is the *Diagnostic Classification: 0–3. Diagnostic Classification of Mental Health and Developmental Disorders of Infancy and Early Childhood* (*DC:0-3*), published by the National Center for Clinical Infant Programs (1994). It was offered as "a systematic, developmentally based approach to the classification of mental health and developmental difficulties in the first four years of life." Following the example of the DSM series, it offers the advantage of organizing the diagnosis into five axes: (1) the primary diagnosis, (2) the relationship classification, (3) physical, neurologic, and developmental disorders and conditions, (4) psychosocial stressors, and (5) functional emotional developmental level. The breadth of this approach is promising, but it has some drawbacks. The *DC:0-3* also fails to include temperament in any appropriate way. There is brief mention of it in the introduction, but it becomes entwined as part of the abnormality in the "regulatory disorders" diagnoses.

Comprehensive Child Assessment. Reasonable expectations for the performance of pediatricians and the actual conditions of pediatric practice call for a kind of diagnostic classification plan different from those described previously. In an effort to overcome all the defects in the systems mentioned, a comprehensive child assessment is offered here.

A good starting point in defining the areas of adjustment is to decide on what constitutes normality. In Chapter 8, Chess and Thomas described how hard it is to find a satisfactory definition of normality in children's behavior. They have proposed that social competence and task mastery be taken both as criteria for current normality and as goals of future achievement. Chess (personal communication, 1989) has also revised an earlier textbook definition of normality for inclusion here:

> As a working concept, keeping in mind its subjective nature, one may identify the following broad characteristics of normal children: They get along reasonably well with parents, sibs and friends; have few overt manifestations of behavior disturbance; use their apparent intellectual potentials to approximate capacity; are interested in and accomplish developmentally appropriate tasks; and are contented a reasonable proportion of the time. This description covers a wide range of temperamental and personality patterns. One should not arbitrarily consider certain children to be abnormal because their conduct is identified with types of behavior that do not conform to an abstraction.

Building on these guidelines, one can tentatively construct five general criteria for the assessment and rating of behavioral adjustment. There is no one definitive way to do this; the proposed scheme represents a consensus of current thinking. The criteria are suitable for pediatric use in that they include both positive and negative aspects of the major areas of adjustment and are relatively easily applied:

1. Relationships with people: parents, siblings, teachers, other adults, peers, and so on—social competence versus undersocialization (aggressiveness or withdrawal).

2. Task performance: work and play—achievement ver-

sus underachievement or excessive preoccupation with work or play.

3. Self-relations: self-assurance versus poor self-relations or overconcern for self. Included here are self-care, self-esteem, and self-regulation.
4. Internal status: reasonable contentment versus symptoms of distress in feelings, thoughts, and physical functions (e.g., sleep, eating).
5. Coping patterns: strategies typically used to deal with the problems confronted in daily life. Direct and appropriate engagement versus ineffective, maladaptive problem solving with overuse of "defense mechanisms" like denial, avoidance, or repression. This poorly studied aspect of a child's personality is probably derived from temperament, capacities, and experience, especially parental rearing practices (see Chapter 8).

Table 67–1 provides a possible plan for organizing information and judgments about a child's behavioral adjustment. The profile is separated into these five areas of adjustment, and each of them is subdivided into four levels of function from good to satisfactory to unsatisfactory to poor. Precise behavioral descriptions for placement along these four continua cannot be supplied for all children, although it would be helpful if that were possible. Criteria for these judgments depend on various circumstances such as age, sex, family, and cultural settings. Strengths are included as well as liabilities. Problems are considered as disruptions of various areas of function, not with regard to the presence or absence of "psychiatric" disorders. When these conclusions are incorporated into a comprehensive diagnostic formulation (see Chapter 75), they are accompanied by separate judgments regarding the child's physical health, neurologic status, developmental level, temperament, interaction with the environment, a summary, and a statement of service needs.

Child health profiles of this sort are rare in the medical and mental health literatures. Two others are the ABILITIES Index (Bailey et al, 1993) and the Child Health and Illness Profile (Starfield et al, 1993). Chapters 66 and 78 also describe behavioral assessment.

DIAGNOSTIC TECHNIQUES

The usual techniques for obtaining the data about children's behavior to be incorporated into whatever classification system is used are observations, questionnaires, and interviews. Observations of the child's behavior and of the parent-child interaction in the office setting can be highly illuminating to the process of diagnosis. However, these data are usually based on relatively brief contacts and might be atypical of the overall picture. Further observations reported by teachers and other caretakers can also be very helpful. The physician's own observations can confirm or raise doubts about the history but are seldom sufficient to replace the history as the basis of the diagnosis.

Questionnaires concerning the child's behavior can make a useful contribution to the diagnosis if they are descriptive and are used as part of the data-gathering process rather than by themselves as an oversimplified diagnostic mechanism.

Interviewing is the pediatrician's most powerful tool for the assessment of behavior in children. No other technique has the flexibility and subtlety of skillfully allowing the parent or patient to describe and express feelings about what is going on.

The two principal techniques for gathering diagnostic information about behavior in common usage today are (1) brief questionnaires for screening for psychopathology for the purpose of referral, and (2) a comprehensive pediatric assessment primarily by interview that allows and promotes pediatric management for most parental concerns about behavior.

Psychopathology Screening Method

A common view of the role of the pediatrician in behavioral matters is that pediatricians should screen for behavioral disturbances, as they do for developmental delay and various physical problems, so that they can refer the more troubled children to mental health specialists who are more proficient with these issues (Costello, 1986; Lavigne et al, 1993; Jellinek, Murphy, and Burns, 1986; Simonian et al, 1993). A dozen or more of these screening checklists are available. Among the best known are the Pediatric Symptom Checklist (Jellinek, Murphy, and Burns, 1986), the Eyberg Child Behavior Inventory (Eyberg and Ross, 1978), the Conners Parent Rating Scale (Goyette, Conners, and Ulrich, 1978), and the Child Behavior Checklist (Achenbach and Edelbrock, 1983).

The proposed advantages of these behavioral rating scales are as follows:

1. They gather information from the informants with the greatest experience with the child.
2. They include some behavior not likely to be observed by the clinician, such as sleep.
3. They are inexpensive and efficient.
4. Available normative data allow determinations of deviations.
5. They provide quantitative assessments concerning qualitative aspects of behavior.

Perhaps the most important use of such a screening scale by a pediatrician may be to facilitate communication between the physician and the parent or teacher, in that it indicates the physician's concern for behavioral issues and promotes discussion of them. However, despite their value in psychiatric research and practice, these questionnaires all have significant problems that interfere with their use in pediatric primary care.

1. The data produced are of little assistance in the identification and management of the common behavioral concerns parents bring to pediatricians, such as sibling quarrels and resistance to toilet-training (Perrin, Stein, and Drotar, 1991). Screening for major behavioral problems is only a small part of the appropriate mental health role of the pediatrician.
2. Although various claims are made for their psychometric qualifications, no proof has been offered that they detect important abnormalities any better than do a few appropriately phrased and directed interview questions (Stancin and Palermo, 1997). The accept-

Table 67–1 • Profile of Behavioral (and Emotional) Adjustment

Area of Adjustment	Adjustment Rating					Strengths	Problems
	Good: Better Than Average	*Satisfactory: Minimal Problems*	*Unsatisfactory: Mild to Moderate Problems*	*Poor: Major Problems*	*Insufficient Data or Not Applicable*		
Relations with Parents						Social competence: social skills, cooperation, affection, interest, honesty, sensitivity	Aggressiveness: opposition, defiance, rebellion, dishonesty, manipulation, violence, destructiveness, insensitivity, Withdrawal: overconformity, disinterest
Siblings							
Teachers							
Other adults							
Other children							
Medical caregivers							
Tasks Schoolwork						Task performance: achievement, skill development, mastery, interest	Underachievement: low achievement, low interest, school failure, truancy Excessive striving or preoccupation with work or play
Domestic							
Community							
Play-leisure							
Self-relations Self-regard						Self-assurance: autonomy, self-acceptance, self-esteem, self-care, self-reliance, self-direction, self-control, self-organization	Poor self-relations: low self-esteem, body image distortion, self-neglect, self-abuse, self-destructiveness, dependency Overconcern, overcontrol, overregulation, hypochondriasis
Self-care							
Self-regulation							
Internal status Feelings						Reasonable contentment: sense of well-being in feelings, thoughts, and physical function	Distress in feelings: anxiety, depression, fear, anger, guilt In thinking: reality distortions, phobias, obsessions, compulsions, delusions, posttraumatic stress reactions In physical function: eating, gastrointestinal, sleep, colic, tics, sex, pain
Thoughts							
Functions							
Coping patterns						Effective: appropriate engagement and direct action; support seeking	Ineffective: maladaptive problem solving; excess use of defense strategies: denial, avoidance, etc.

ability and efficiency of these scales in pediatric practice remains to be demonstrated.

3. With rare exceptions, the available scales rate only abnormalities and do not evaluate positive evidence of behavioral adjustment such as social competence or self-esteem.

4. They are highly impressionistic. An item like "talks too much" measures the caretaker's judgment of what constitutes an excess of talking as much as it does the actual quantity of the behavior in the child. Thus, the parents are exercising the diagnostic judgment that should be made by the clinician.

5. They usually give equal weight to ratings of problems of unequal significance, such as nose picking and fire setting.

6. They typically ask about the overall frequency of the behavior without regard for its varying significance in different settings, such as whether trouble paying attention is a problem with listening to safety rules or learning irregular verbs as well as with video games.

Critics in the mental health professions have complained that pediatricians are not doing a good job in this screening process and are failing to detect substantial numbers of problems present. These conclusions may be correct to some extent but they say little about the types and significance of problems being missed or the consequences of delay in detection. A more appropriate analysis of this situation (Horowitz et al, 1992) demonstrated "when using a classification system developed specifically for primary care settings, clinicians do identify a large number of children (with) psychosocial and developmental problems." Appropriately directed interviewing has been shown to produce a higher yield of the existing problems (Glascoe and Dworkin, 1994; Wissow, Roter, and Wilson, 1994).

Comprehensive Child Assessment Method

This chapter urges the view that pediatricians should make use of a comprehensive child health profile, as outlined earlier in this chapter, and that the best way to obtain the necessary data is by parent interview as supplemented with interview data from others, observations, and appropriate information from questionnaires.

Before undertaking the actual assessment of the behavioral adjustment, the clinician is well advised to take two preliminary steps: defining the concern and clarifying the goals (Fig. 67–1).

Define the Concern. The first step in the clinical assessment of behavioral adjustment is to clarify what areas of behavior arouse concern either from the caretakers or from the clinician. General parental concern is easily derived from a few introductory questions, such as "How are things going?" or "What sorts of things bother you at this point?" or "What kinds of problems are particularly troublesome now?" Queries more focused on behavior include "What is he/she like these days?" or "How is his/her behavior now?" or "How is he/she getting on with life these days?" or "How has he/she been treating you lately?" This part of the diagnostic process is neither difficult nor time-consuming. Any pediatrician can talk

with the parent or child about the general nature of outstanding problems in a very few minutes.

If concern about behavior either is expressed as the reason for the visit or comes up in the course of this initial inquiry, the interviewer should find out who has the concerns, what the concerns involve, where they come from, and why they emerge at this time. If, by contrast, at the outset of a general examination the caretaker (or patient) reports complete satisfaction with the child's status and progress in all areas, the questioning can be greatly abbreviated from what will now be described.

Clarify the Goals and Make an Agreement. Once the concern has been discovered, the next step is to determine whether and to what extent the family wishes to have the clinician help them with it. The clinician must clarify their objectives and set goals for management. For behavioral issues, the pediatrician does not simply take charge of the diagnostic and therapeutic procedure as when presented with physical illnesses like otitis media or pneumonia. For behavioral issues the process of evaluation and management is shared with the family, and an agreement must be established as to what the family expects and what the physician will provide (see Chapter 66). If the family does not want help, the physician can only express appropriate concern and monitor the problem, unless it is so severe that intervention on behalf of the child is mandatory.

When this agreement is reached, the process of diagnosis can continue: determining the behavioral profile and establishing the preliminary diagnostic impression and disposition.

Determine the Behavioral Profile. In the course of a standard history and physical examination, as supplemented by additional interviewing and office observations, the pediatrician can collect sufficient information to allow at least a preliminary clinical judgment on all five of the criteria previously mentioned and presented in Table 67–1.

There is no established set of questions to open and explore these areas. An inquiry regarding social competence might go, "How skillful is he/she at getting along with people?" or "How is he/she getting on with adults these days?" or "How socially mature does he/she seem for a child of his/her age?" or "How does he/she get along with other children?" or "What sorts of things happen between him/her and other people that do not seem right?"

The pediatrician can inquire as to task performance with questions such as these: "How are things going at school?" or "What does he/she do best/least well at school?" or "What does he/she like most/least about school?" or "To what extent is his/her performance up to his/her abilities?"

Self-assurance can be assessed by asking, "How does he/she seem to feel about himself/herself?" or "What is he/she most/least proud of?" or "How well does he/she take care of himself/herself?" or "How much trouble does he/she have controlling impulses?"

Regarding internal status one might ask, "How happy a child is he/she?" or "What sort of worries does he/she have?" or "What sort of physical complaints does he/she have that puzzle you?"

Coping strategies can be sampled by asking questions such as "How does he/she go about solving a tough prob-

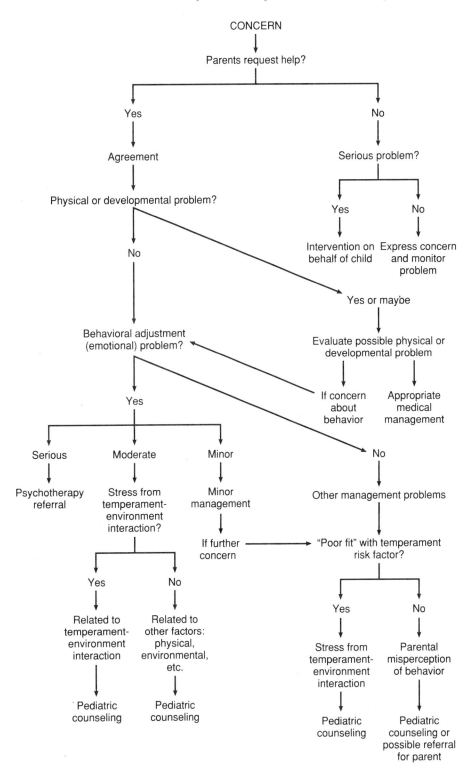

Figure 67–1. Algorithm for management of concerns about behavior.

lem?" or "What does he/she generally do when things are not going well for him/her?"

With the older child, the interview should also involve the patient directly. With adolescents the topics covered may be more specifically directed by the HEADSS approach: *H*ome, *E*ducation/employment, *A*ctivities, *D*rugs, *S*exuality, *S*uicide (see Chapter 6), but the results can still be contained in the suggested diagnostic profile.

Establish Preliminary Diagnostic Impression and Disposition. It should be possible at this point to categorize the problem and the concern about it into one of three levels: a minor problem, which can be dealt with adequately at the time (bothersome temperament or other normal variations or misperceptions of normality); a more complex issue requiring further attention from the primary care physician at that time or later (mild to moderately severe dysfunction in the child like colic or night waking); or a major disturbance needing the more advanced skills or greater time allotments provided by a mental health specialist (significant dysfunction in the child such as persistent antisocial behavior, declining school performance, or depression).

The objective of this diagnostic process is not only to screen for psychopathologic conditions, as some critics have suggested, but to develop a more complete picture of the child's status: successes as well as failures of all types and degrees. The specific tactics and amount of time required for an individual child vary from several questions in a few minutes to extensive interviewing for more than an hour. A second or third visit might be necessary to complete the evaluation, but a preliminary diagnostic impression can often be gained in several minutes by a skillful interviewer who knows the family.

Judgments as to whether the behavior described is a variation of normal, a temporary or isolated disruption, or a deviation requiring pediatric or psychiatric intervention depends on a knowledge of the range of normal behavior in the child's particular context, as is described in Chapters 2 through 6, and on the application of the criteria of satisfactory adjustment listed previously. The more numerous, severe, and chronic the behavioral symptoms, the greater the need the pediatrician has for seeking help from a mental health specialist. One cannot suggest a simple formula, such as a score on a behavior checklist, for defining indications for referral for concerns about behavior; much depends on the nature and extent of the symptoms, the skills of the pediatrician, and the quantity and quality of referral resources available. Further discussion of these matters is to be found in the chapters on interviewing (Chapter 66), counseling (Chapter 76), and referrals (Chapter 86).

SUMMARY

For the assessment of behavioral adjustment, some authors recommend the use of a checklist to screen for abnormalities needing referral to mental health specialists. This advice undervalues and underestimates the pediatrician's diagnostic and management skills. This chapter urges instead a comprehensive child assessment based primarily on descriptions of the child's behavior obtained by parental interview and comparisons of these data with some suggested criteria of adjustment. This improved evaluation puts the pediatrician in a better position to fulfill his or her expected role in dealing appropriately with parental behavioral concerns, most of which do not need such referral.

Behavioral Style or Temperament

Since temperament is defined and described by Chess and Thomas in Chapter 8, this section is limited to a discussion of the indications and techniques for temperament assessment.

INDICATIONS FOR ASSESSMENT

Routine Professional Care

Pediatricians can and should include a few screening questions about temperament in their periodic evaluations to look for evidence of stressful traits and concerns requiring further investigation. Although routine formal determinations of temperament of all children at certain regular times by pediatricians or schools might some day become an accepted practice, they are not now. No convincing case has been made for such detailed assessments if caregivers are generally satisfied with a child's current behavioral status and there are no discernable areas of malfunction in the child. Possible problems of compliance, uncertain value of the data, and misuse by inexperienced persons outweigh the potential advantages at present (Carey and McDevitt, 1995).

Nevertheless, the general education of parents and other caregivers about temperament is an important anticipatory guidance role for pediatricians. Because these discussions are not specific, they can be accomplished without a formal assessment. Several books are available for more extensive parent education (Carey and Jablow, 1997; Chess and Thomas, 1996; Kurcinka, 1998; Turecki and Tonner, 1989).

When Child Arouses Concerns

There are two principal indications for formal temperament determinations in children. In cases of behavioral adjustment deviations, it is helpful to determine the contribution of the child's temperament to the problem. Such information can provide help in explaining the magnitude and direction of the child's symptoms, and it assists the setting of realistic goals for any therapeutic intervention. With appropriate alteration of the management by caregivers, the reactive symptoms in the child should diminish or disappear. Meanwhile, the parents and other caregivers must learn to live in a more tolerant manner and be more flexible with the child's temperament, which is evidently less changeable (Carey and McDevitt, 1995).

The other principal situation for temperament determinations is when there is caregiver concern about the child's behavior or the parent-child interaction, but no definite behavioral adjustment problem is evident yet. If the child has a "difficult" temperament or one of the other "temperament risk factors" and these traits are causing a stressful "poor fit" (incompatible relationship) with the values and expectations of the parents or other caregivers, even without a secondary behavior disorder, it is important for the pediatrician to be fully aware of the child's participation in the problem. If the friction is coming from such a disharmonious interaction, the appropriate management consists of (1) recognition of the true nature of the dissonance, (2) a revision of the understanding and management by the caregivers, and (3) some suggestions to the parents and others on how to find relief from their own feelings of stress. Punitive discipline for the child or psychotherapy for the parent or child would be inappropriate. Figure 67–1 demonstrates these two uses of temperament data. Greater detail as to these techniques is available in several books (especially Carey and McDevitt, 1995; Chess and Thomas, 1986) (Fig. 67–2).

TECHNIQUES FOR TEMPERAMENT DETERMINATIONS

As mentioned in the first section of this chapter, there are three principal methods for obtaining data relating to

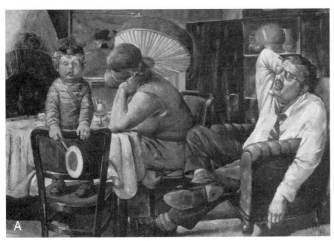
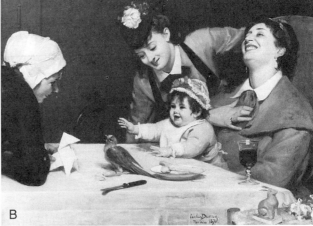

Figure 67–2. *A* and *B,* The varying impact of children's temperaments on their families. (*A,* Harald Duwe: Sonntagnachmittag. With permission of Hamburger Kunsthalle; *B,* Carolus-Duran. The Merrymakers. Founders Society Purchase, Robert H. Tannahill Foundation Fund. Photograph copyright The Detroit Institute of Arts, 1989.)

behavior: interviews, observations, and questionnaires. This is true for temperament as well as behavioral adjustment.

Interviews

The best-known interview technique for obtaining temperament data is the one devised over 40 years ago by the New York Longitudinal Study of Thomas, Chess, and colleagues (see Chapter 8). Although this interview was sufficient for the needs of their study, neither it nor any adaptation of it has found wide usage in research or clinical practice. Its flexibility makes it more sensitive to varying situations, but it also is less capable of standardization. Its length of 1 to 2 hours (plus another hour or more for dictation and rating) allows great richness of detail to be developed in behavioral descriptions but renders it impractical in any clinical and most research settings.

Nevertheless clinicians can, and often do, use these concepts in an abbreviated form in practical situations. A shortened interview of the clinician's own construction can yield usable data as long as he or she resists the temptation to generalize too readily from insufficiently comprehensive descriptions, such as just one or two instances of a trait. The interview approach, adapted to the particular needs of the occasion, is the most reasonable way to screen routinely for a "poor fit" or to obtain abbreviated temperament data when there is no need for a more detailed analysis (Carey and McDevitt, 1995).

Observations

Day care workers and teachers generally have extensive contact with their students, placing them in a good position to form sound judgments of individual children. Pediatricians should make use of their contributions. On the other hand, primary care clinicians usually witness only brief, sometimes atypical samples of behavior. There is still no standardized comprehensive observation technique for assessing temperament for clinical purposes. Various studies have devised methods for use with particular investigations,

but these are not easily applicable elsewhere. For example, Matheny (1980) developed an elaboration of the behavioral items on the Bayley development scale for ratings of temperament in the study of twins. This method requires trained observers and has not been applied clinically.

The Brazelton Neonatal Behavioral Assessment Scale (1973) is regarded by some as an appropriate way to determine "constitutional temperament." However, despite its considerable value for studying neonatal problems and for helping parents understand their newborns, one must recognize that newborn behavior is strongly affected by nongenetic prenatal and perinatal factors, is not very stable from one day to the next, and does not provide an adequate view of the primarily genetically determined temperamental characteristics that will emerge in the next few weeks. Comparison between newborn behavior, as measured by the Brazelton scale, and later temperamental traits has been hindered by these factors and by the fact that some of the newborn measures, such as muscle tone, are not temperament variables, and that none of the scale items or clusters is the same in both content and dimensions as the temperament characteristics of the New York Longitudinal Study.

Questionnaires

With the increased recognition of the theoretical and clinical importance of temperament and the lack of practical ways of measuring it accurately by interview or observations, a series of parent and teacher questionnaires has been developed. Table 67–2 lists most of the currently available scales, and Table 67–3 presents samples of items from one of them. Most are intended for completion by parents, but three of them are designed for ratings by teachers, including the Temperament Assessment Battery for Children by Martin. Table 67–2 does not include (1) scales based only on observations such as those by Matheny or Brazelton, (2) techniques possibly assessing temperament but ostensibly measuring something else, such as the Conners Parent and Teacher Rating Scales, (3) scales in foreign languages, (4) unpublished scales, and (5) the earlier scales intended

Table 67–2 • Questionnaires for Measuring Temperament:
I. Principal Questionnaires in English Using New York Longitudinal Study Categories

Age Span	Name of Test	Authors	No. Items	Retest Rel.†	Alpha Rel.†	Reference and Comments
1–4 months	Early Infancy Temperament Questionnaire (EITQ)	Medoff-Cooper, Carey, and McDevitt	76	0.69m	0.62m	J Dev Behav Pediatr 14:230, 1993
4–8 months	Infant Temperament Quest. (1970)	Carey	70	0.84m	0.47m	J Pediatr 77:188, 1970; replaced by revised version
	Infant Temperament Quest. (1978) (ITQ)	Carey and McDevitt	95	0.86t	0.83t	Pediatrics 61:735, 1978;* revised version
8–12 months	None					Use of ITQ possible.
1–3 years	Toddler Temperament Scale (TTS)	Fullard, McDevitt, and Carey	97	0.88t	0.85t	J Pediatr Psychol 9:205, 1984*
3–7 years	Parent Temperament Quest.	Thomas, Chess, and Korn	72	na	na	Thomas and Chess: Temperament and Development, Brunner/Mazel, 1977
	Teacher Temperament Quest.	Thomas, Chess, and Korn	64	na	na	Thomas and Chess: Temperament and Development, Brunner/Mazel, 1977
	Teacher Temperament Quest. (short form)	Keogh, Pullis, and Cadwell	23	0.69–0.88	na	J Ed Meas 29:323, 1982
	Behavioral Style Quest. (BSQ)	McDevitt and Carey	100	0.89t	0.84t	J Child Psychol Psychiatry 19:245, 1978*
	Temperament Assessment Battery for Children	Martin	48	0.53–0.81	0.6–0.9	Pro-Ed Publishers, 8700 Shoal Creek Blvd., Austin, TX 78757
8–12 years	Middle Childhood Temp. Quest. (MCTQ)	Hegvik, McDevitt, and Carey	99	0.87m	0.82m	J Dev Behav Pediatr 3:197, 1982*
12–18 years	None					
18–21 years	Early Adult Temp. Quest.	Thomas et al	140	na	0.82m	Ed Psychol Meas 42:593, 1982

*EITQ, ITQ, TTS, BSQ, and MCTQ may be obtained through one of the offices of Behavioral-Developmental Initiatives:
  1) 13802 North Scottsdale Road, Suite 104, Scottsdale, AZ 85254. Telephone: 1-800-405-2313.
  2) 1316 West Chester Pike, Suite 131, West Chester, PA 19382. Telephone: 1-800-BDI-8303.
†Retest reliability and alpha reliability (internal consistency) figures are given as median category (m) or total (t) values. na indicates that data are not available.

II. Principal Other Research Questionnaires in Order of Publication

Buss AH, Plomin R: A Temperament Theory of Personality Development. New York, John Wiley & Sons, 1975.
Garside RF, Birch H, Scott DM, et al: Dimensions of temperament in infant school children. J Child Psychol Psychiatry 16:219, 1975.
Bates J, Freeland C, Lounsbury M: Measurement of infant difficultness. Child Dev 50:794, 1979.
Rothbart MK: Measurement of temperament in infancy. Child Dev 52:569, 1981.
Lerner RM, Palermo M, Spiro A III, et al: Assessing the dimensions of temperamental individuality across the life span: The Dimensions of Temperament Survey (DOTS). Child Dev 53:149, 1982, revised 1986.
Goldsmith HH, Elliott TK, Jaco KL: Construction and initial validation of a new temperament questionnaire. Inf Beh & Dev 9:144, 1986.

Table 67–3 • Sample Items From Temperament Questionnaire

Middle Childhood Temperament Questionnaire (Hegvik, McDevitt, and Carey)

Using the scale below, please mark an "X" in the space that tells how often the child's recent and current behavior has been like the behavior described by each item:

Almost Never (1)	Rarely (2)	Variable; Usually Does Not (3)	Variable; Usually Does (4)	Frequently (5)		Almost Always (6)

1. Runs to get where he/she wants to go — Almost never ___:___:___:___:___:___ 1 2 3 4 5 6 Almost always

2. Avoids (stays away from, doesn't talk to) a new sitter on first meeting — Almost never ___:___:___:___:___:___ 1 2 3 4 5 6 Almost always

3. Easily excited by praise (laughs, claps, yells, etc.) — Almost never ___:___:___:___:___:___ 1 2 3 4 5 6 Almost always

4. Frowns or complains when asked by the parent to do a chore — Almost never ___:___:___:___:___:___ 1 2 3 4 5 6 Almost always

5. Notices (looks toward) minor changes in lighting (changes in shadows, turning on lights, etc.) — Almost never ___:___:___:___:___:___ 1 2 3 4 5 6 Almost always

6. Loses interest in a new toy or game the same day she/he gets it — Almost never ___:___:___:___:___:___ 1 2 3 4 5 6 Almost always

primarily for adults like those of Eysenck in 1956, Guilford and Zimmerman in 1956, Thorndike in 1963, and Strelau in 1972.

The questionnaires using the New York Longitudinal Study formulation have several advantages:

1. They are briefer and more efficient than comparable interview and observation techniques in that they require only 20 to 30 minutes for the caregiver to complete and about 10 to 15 minutes for the clinician or an assistant to score. They are low in cost and high in acceptability. Yet they are not excessively simple; all but one have 48 or more items, and most have 90 to 100.
2. They are based on clinically relevant theory. All nine characteristics, such as adaptability and mood, have been shown to be related to clinical problems.
3. They consist of specific behavioral descriptions (e.g., "The infant moves about much [kicks, grabs, squirms] during diapering and dressing") rather than parental perceptions or general impressions of the child's behavior (e.g., "Child is very energetic").
4. They are standardized as to norms for characteristics at various ages from 1 month through 12 years.
5. They have adequate psychometric characteristics as to retest reliability and internal consistency and also validity as far as it can be evaluated.

Some uncertainties persist about this set of questionnaires:

1. The question remains unresolved as to whether parents with less than a high school education can accurately respond to these scales. Parents with below average verbal skills may not be able to handle adequately the various shades of meaning, leading to distortions.
2. Parents in cultures or subcultures different from those of the standardization samples might understand the items in dissimilar ways, especially when translated. Restandardization is indicated in these situations (Carey and McDevitt 1995).
3. The issue of validity is not easily resolved. Behavioral scientists currently tend to speak of any parental judgments of temperament as "perceptions" and of their own data, no matter how brief and unrepresentative, as scientific "observations." It would be more appropriate to say that perceptions are general or hasty impressions and that ratings are a series of more carefully considered judgments of certain behavioral patterns in specific settings. Both parents and professionals can have perceptions and make ratings. The ideal test of the validity of the parental ratings on a temperament questionnaire would be a comparison with a comprehensive standardized observational rating scheme. As already mentioned, there is no appropriately matched one in existence now. However, every adequately designed test so far has demonstrated at least moderate validity of parental reports. Data from parents must be contemporaneous and relate to specific behavioral patterns rather than general impressions. Comparisons of parental and professional ratings must involve the same con-

tent and dimensions of behavior, a requirement overlooked in the few published reports claiming to discredit the validity of parental ratings (Carey, 1983). Clinical users of temperament questionnaires can, therefore, be reassured of at least a moderate degree of validity. Although distortions can occur, they can be minimized by the interviewing and observations that should always accompany the use of a questionnaire.

4. Several critical reviews of these and other psychometric properties of the existing questionnaires have been published by academic psychologists (see Carey and McDevitt, 1995). Although one can agree with them that all the scales have their shortcomings, these reviews suffer from a superficiality of analysis and the absence of a clinical perspective.

In situations of clinical concern about behavior, the best way to measure the contribution of the child's temperament to the interaction is by using one of the more sophisticated questionnaires (see Table 67–2) supplemented by observations and further history as needed. The briefer or more impressionistic questionnaires used by some in research and those presented in most popular books and articles for parents are not likely to be sufficiently objective and detailed for clinical use.

SUMMARY

Temperament or behavioral style determinations facilitate the diagnosis and management of most behavioral adjustment problems in children and can be helpful in counseling parents with other behavioral concerns. Parental questionnaires using their descriptions of the child's behavior, rather than their general perceptions of or reactions to it, have been found to serve these needs most effectively, but they are best supplemented by observations and interviewing. No convincing case has been made for routine formal temperament ratings of well children by either pediatricians or educators. Brief but carefully obtained interview data are generally sufficient for routine clinical management of children without significant problems.

REFERENCES

Achenbach TM, Edelbrock CS: Manual for the Child Behavior Checklist and Revised Child Behavioral Profile. Burlington, VT, University of Vermont, Department of Psychiatry, 1983.

American Academy of Pediatrics: Diagnostic and Statistical Manual for Primary Care: Child and Adolescent Version (DSM-PC). Elk Grove Village, IL, American Academy of Pediatrics, 1996.

American Psychiatric Association: Diagnostic and Statistical Manual of Mental Disorders, 4th ed (DSM-IV). Washington, DC, American Psychiatric Association, 1994.

Bailey DB, Simeonsson RJ, Buysse V, et al: Reliability of an Index of Child Characteristics. Dev Med Child Neurol 35:806, 1993.

Brazelton TB: Neonatal Behavioral Assessment Scale. Philadelphia, JB Lippincott, 1973.

Carey WB: Some pitfalls in infant temperament research. Infant Behav Dev 6:247, 1983.

Carey WB, Jablow M: Understanding Your Child's Temperament. New York, Macmillan, 1997.

Carey WB, McDevitt SC: Coping with Children's Temperament. New York, Basic Books, 1995.

Chess S, Thomas A: Temperament in Clinical Practice. New York, Guilford, 1986.

Chess S, Thomas A: Know Your Child. New York, Basic Books, 1987; Republished New Brunswick, NJ, Jason Aronson, 1996.

Costello EJ: Primary care pediatrics and child psychopathology: a review of diagnostic, treatment, and referral practices. Pediatrics 78:1044, 1986.

Eyberg SM, Ross AW: Assessment of child behavior problems: The validation of a new inventory. J Clin Child Psychol 7:113, 1978.

Glascoe FP, Dworkin PH: The role of parents in the detection of developmental and behavioral problems. Pediatrics 95:829, 1995.

Goyette CH, Conners CK, Ulrich RF: Normative data on revised Conners parent and teacher rating scales. J Abnormal Child Psychol 6:221, 1978.

Horowitz SM, Leaf PJ, Leventhal JM, et al: Identification and management of psychosocial and developmental problems in community-based, primary care pediatric practices. Pediatrics 89:480, 1992.

Jellinek MS, Murphy JM, Burns BJ: Brief psychosocial screening in outpatient pediatrics. J Pediatr 109:371, 1986.

Kurcinka MS: Raising your spirited child. New York, HarperCollins, 1991. Reissued 1998.

Lavigne JV, Binns HJ, Christoffel KK, et al: Behavior and emotional problems among preschool children in pediatric primary care: prevalence and pediatricians' recognition. Pediatrics 91:649, 1993.

Matheny AP Jr: Bayley's Infant Behavior Record: behavioral components and twin analyses. Child Dev 51:1157, 1980.

National Center for Clinical Infant Programs: Diagnostic Classification: 0–3. Diagnostic Classification of Mental Health and Developmental Disorders of Infancy and Early Childhood (DC:0-3) Arlington, VA, National Center for Clinical Infant Programs, 1994.

Perrin EC, Stein REK, Drotar D: Cautions using the Child Behavior Checklist: observations based on research about children with a chronic illness. J Ped Psychol 16:411, 1991.

Simonian SJ, Tarnowski KJ, Stancin T, et al: Disadvantaged children in pediatric primary care settings: II. Screening for behavior disturbance. J Clin Child Psychol 20:360, 1991.

Stancin T, Palermo: A review of behavioral screening practices in pediatric settings: do they pass the test? J Dev Behav Pediatr 18:183, 1997.

Starfield B, Bergner M, Ensminger M, et al: Adolescent health status measurement: development of the Child Health and Illness Profile. Pediatrics 91:430, 1993.

Turecki S, Tonner L: The Difficult Child (revised). New York, Bantam Books, 1989.

Wissow LS, Roter DL, Wilson MEH: Pediatrician interview style and mothers' disclosure of psychosocial issues. Pediatrics 93:289, 1994.

World Health Organization: International Statistical Classification of Diseases and Related Health Problems, 10th revision (ICD-10). Geneva, WHO, 1992.

68 Developmental Screening: Infants, Toddlers, and Preschoolers

James A. Blackman

 The early detection of developmental delays is an awesome responsibility for health care providers. Physicians are commonly in a position to serve as the first detectors of a developing nervous system that is somehow not meeting expectations. At the same time, clinicians must sort through parental concerns, differentiating between normal variation, dysfunction, and disability at the earliest possible age. This chapter integrates current knowledge of assessment techniques, enabling legislation, and early child development. In so doing, the author enables physicians to assemble a rational approach to the earliest possible detection (and intervention) so that the effects of developmental disabilities can be significantly lessened in the long run.

No aspect of care for children could be considered more basic and indispensable than monitoring growth and development. If optimizing the chances for a child's attainment of full potential is the cornerstone of pediatrics, then a systematic approach to assessing success or failure in this endeavor is mandatory. In this chapter, methods for incorporating developmental surveillance into routine care of young children are presented.

Rationale for Early Detection of Developmental Problems

In the past, some critics thought that the case for early intervention for developmental problems was weak and that enthusiastic claims of efficacy were largely unsubstantiated. However, accumulating evidence of the value of early intervention cannot be denied, particularly when the intervention is family focused, individually tailored, and directed toward global developmental needs (Guralnick, 1997). Thus, given the value of intervention for developmental problems, vigorous efforts to identify these problems as early as possible are justified. Besides the benefits of special services that a child can receive when problems are identified, parents appreciate knowing how their child is doing. Part C (formerly Part H) of the Individuals with Disabilities Education Act, a federal mandate to identify and treat developmental problems as early as possible, has stimulated better and more coordinated care for young children with or at risk for developmental disabilities. Communities are depending on pediatric care providers to find children in need of early intervention services and to refer them as early as is feasible. Screening is a useful, cost-effective technique for early detection when applied appropriately.

Specific Approaches to Screening

Although providers recognize that the physical, mental, and emotional development of children is a key component of pediatrics, the use of developmental screening tests has not become routine practice (Ambulatory Pediatrics Association, 1990). In fact the cost-effectiveness of such formal screening for every child has been questioned (Dworkin, 1989). In the average practice setting, the yield from most general developmental screening instruments, which are designed to detect severe intellectual or motor deficits, is low because the incidence of such problems is low. The detection of more subtle problems that may prove to be learning disabilities later on is not reliably possible during the preschool years (Blackman and Bretthauer, 1990; Corrigan et al, 1986). Thus there is an understandable reluctance to allocate professional time toward such activity. Yet experts agree that some form of developmental surveillance is imperative. Three approaches to this activity include informal screening, routine formal screening, and focused developmental screening.

INFORMAL SCREENING

Informal screening can be based on observing the child during a routine well-child check, asking parents if they have concerns about their child's development, or performing several developmental tasks appropriate for the child's age. Glascoe has developed the PEDS, a handy 5-minute questionnaire that alerts the health care provider to a parent's concerns about development or behavior (Table 68–1). Also, a list of developmental milestones can be included on health maintenance forms as reminders. The examiner relies primarily on parent reports rather than on direct observation. Although this approach has not been validated against routine formal screening, it might be practical and reasonable for low-risk populations, in that time and required materials are minimal. Supplementary information should be sought regarding concerns about hearing, feeding, behavior, and temperament. Such an informal approach is risky, however, especially for the less-experienced examiner. Several classic studies found pedia-

Table 68–1 • Selected Infant and Preschool Screening Tests and Parent Questionnaires

Name	Age Range	Time (min)	Source
Bayley Infant Neurodevelopmental Screener (BINS)	3–24 months	10–15	The Psychological Corporation P.O. Box 839954 San Antonio, TX 78238-3954 1-800-228-0752
Denver II	0–6 years	30–45	Denver Developmental Materials P.O. Box 6169 Denver, CO 80206 (303) 355-4729*
Batelle Developmental Inventory	0–8 years	30	Riverside Publishing Company 425 Spring Lake Drive Itasca, IL 60143-2079 1-800-323-9540
Parents' Evaluation of Developmental Status (PEDS)	0–8 years	<5	Ellsworth & Vandermeer Press 4405 Scenic Drive Nashville, TN 37204 (615) 386-0061 web: http://edge.net/≈evpress
Ages and Stages Questionnaire (ASQ)	4–48 months	10–15	Paul H. Brookes Publishing Co., Inc. P.O. Box 10624 Baltimore, MD 21285-0624 1-800-638-3775
Brigance Screens	0–7 years	10–15	Curriculum Associates P.O. Box 2001 N. Billerica, MA 01862-0901 1-800-225-0248
Early Screening Inventory-Revised	3–6 years	10–15	Rebus Inc. P.O. Box 4479 715 N. University Avenue Ann Arbor, MI 48106 1-800-435-3085
Early Language Milestone Scale (ELM)	0–3 years	1–3	PRO-ED 8700 Shoal Creek Boulevard Austin, TX 78758 1-800-897-3202
Clinical Adaptive Text–Clinical Linguistic and Auditory Milestone Scale (CAT-CLAMS)	0–3 years	10–20	See Capute and Accardo, 1996

*Denver Prescreening Developmental Questionnaire and Home Screening Questionnaire are also available from this source.

tricians to be quite inaccurate in their overall estimates of children's developmental status when they do not use specific criteria (Bierman et al, 1964; Korsch, Cobb, and Ashe, 1961). In the busy clinical setting, the examiner might not allocate sufficient time to assess developmental issues even in an informal way, or the focus of the visit might be an acute illness or the immediate concerns of parents. For children at risk because of biological or environmental factors, such an approach may be inappropriate, because formal assessment is usually indicated. Impression and intuition should be pursued, but they are not always dependable.

ROUTINE FORMAL SCREENING

Systematic developmental screening of all children with standardized instruments provides a safeguard for the busy clinical setting. Many clinicians in public and private settings have incorporated routine screening successfully into their practices. Oftentimes nurses or other well-trained personnel conduct the screening. The use of standardized parent prescreening questionnaires is one way to determine which children require formal evaluation, thus reducing

personnel costs. Although some level of developmental screening is obligatory, because of the low yield of positive results among low-risk populations, many practitioners have not found formal screening every child to be worthwhile. Therefore a third approach, focused screening, might be most practical.

FOCUSED DEVELOPMENTAL SCREENING

Because screening all children in a practice or clinic might be neither feasible nor practical, focused screening produces results that justify the effort. Children with conditions that have known high-risk levels, such as Down syndrome or meningomyelocele, do not need screening and can be referred for services immediately, but they should have ongoing surveillance by their general pediatrician. However, there are certain children who need screening because they have a higher than expected chance of developmental problems based on biological risk factors (Table 68–2).

In addition, environmental stresses (e.g., substance-abusing parents, lack of stable housing) increasingly have been shown to have major deleterious impact on develop-

Table 68–2 • Biological Risk Factors Warranting Systematic and Regular Developmental Screening

Prenatal or Perinatal	Postnatal
Birth weight less than 1000 g	Meningitis
Chronic lung disease of prematurity	Brain or spinal cord trauma
Apgar score of 0–3 at 5 minutes	Lead poisoning
ECMO therapy	Chronic serous otitis media
Hyperbilirubinemia requiring exchange transfusion	Seizure disorder
Grade III or IV intraperiventricular hemorrhage	Severe chronic illness (cystic fibrosis, cancer)
Periventricular leukomalacia	Child abuse or neglect
Neonatal seizures	
Documented systemic infection, congenital or acquired	
Intrauterine growth retardation	
Maternal phenylketonuria	
Maternal human immunodeficiency virus infection	
Maternal use of anticonvulsants	
Family history of childhood deafness or blindness	

ECMO = extracorporeal membrane oxygenation.

ment, especially when coupled with biological risks. Such risk criteria, available through the state agency responsible for administering Part C of the Individuals with Disabilities Education Act, can be used to target populations that warrant closer scrutiny, serial formal screening, or immediate, more comprehensive assessment depending on available resources. By using this paper screening (this process is sometimes called *child find*), the practitioner identifies a cohort that should be screened periodically, because many of these children eventually manifest developmental disabilities. If the community provides screening and assessment, there is no need to duplicate this service in an office or clinic, except to assist in identifying those children who should be referred for screening and follow-up.

Focused screening should also be targeted toward those children whose parents indicate concerns on prescreening questionnaires or in whom physicians, teachers, day care providers, or social workers suspect problems.

Available Techniques—Screening Instruments

Gesell, the American pioneer in child development testing, laid the groundwork for many screening tests used currently by establishing norms for gross motor, fine motor-adaptive, language, and personal-social functioning. Most general developmental screening tests do not address psychosocial or environmental issues. Thus there is not yet one perfect screening system that is both comprehensive and conveniently packaged. The Denver system attempts to approach this goal with prescreening parent questionnaires, a general developmental screening instrument, and an environmental screening form (Frankenburg and Thornton, 1989).

GENERAL DEVELOPMENTAL SCREENING INSTRUMENTS

Psychometric Properties

Many general developmental screening instruments have been constructed, most of them norm-referenced—that is,

they are based on expectations for attainment of developmental milestones at certain chronologic ages. For example, if a girl is unable to sit independently at an age when 90% of children are sitting, she fails that item. The Denver II and the Bayley Infant Neurodevelopmental Screener are examples of this approach. How good are screening tests at identifying children with problems but not overidentifying children who are slower than average but within normal limits? The answer involves the concepts of validity, reliability, sensitivity, and specificity (Stowers and Huber, 1987).

Validity refers to the ability of the instrument to assess what is intended to be assessed. For example, does the Denver II provide an accurate estimate of a child's developmental function at a given age?

A test is said to have good *reliability* if the results are the same if the test is given several times (test-retest reliability) or if the test is given by different examiners (interrater reliability). Reliable results depend on adequate instructions for the administration and interpretation of test items and proper training of those who perform the test.

Sensitivity and *specificity* are best understood by studying Figure 68–1. *Sensitivity* is defined as the ratio of a:a + c, or the proportion of truly developmentally delayed

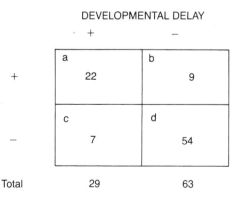

Figure 68–1. Sensitivity and specificity: relationship between presence (+) or absence (−) of developmental delay and pass (+) or failure (−) on a hypothetical screening test.

children correctly identified by the screening test. In the example in Figure 68–1, the sensitivity is 22:29, or 0.76. Ideally one would want a screening test to detect developmental delay in all cases. In this case, the test underidentifies a problem in about one of four cases (falsely negative). *Specificity* is the ratio of d:b + d, or the proportion of children not developmentally delayed who are correctly identified as not delayed by the screening test. In the example, the specificity is 54:63, or 0.86. This test indicates that a child might have a problem when he or she really does not in only 1.5 of 10 cases (falsely positive).

The levels of sensitivity and specificity that are acceptable depend on the desired characteristics. A highly sensitive test can increase the number of false positive results to an unacceptable level. Similarly attempts to increase specificity can increase the number of false negative results.

In addition to validity and reliability, screening tests must be analyzed according to other criteria. They should be *acceptable* to those who test, are tested, or receive resulting referrals. Conflicts between the screener and community service program can arise if the instrument is not thought to be valid. Indeed, there are many "home-grown" screening instruments that have not been validated. The tests should be relatively easy to teach, learn, and administer. Consideration of *cost* includes equipment, preparing and paying personnel, consequences of inaccurate results, and total cost versus benefits of early detection. The test must be *appropriate* for the age and culture of the child. General screening tests, such as the Denver II, are repeatedly criticized for their inability to predict school failure. Such tests were not designed to detect potential low-severity learning disabilities among preschool children. Thus the Denver II and screening tests like it are appropriate for very young children to detect major motor or cognitive deficits, but a different approach is needed for older children in screening for language, perceptual-motor, or sequencing difficulties.

Types of Screening Tests

1. *Parent-completed screening systems* are convenient first steps in systematic, formal screening. They provide a cost- and time-efficient method for gathering developmental information about a child. This approach is limited by the ability of the parent or caretaker to read, comprehend, and respond to the questions. Parent questionnaires are available that compare favorably with professional assessments of development (see Table 68–1). The Ages and Stages Questionnaires are available in both English and Spanish editions.

2. Some practitioners have used *check sheets* for each child's chart, which list developmental milestones in gross motor, fine motor-adaptive, communication, and personal-social function and their average ages of attainment. At each visit, the knowledgeable practitioner can observe or inquire about the child's current skills and determine whether they are appropriate for age. A convenient source for this information is the Revised Gesell and Armatruda Developmental

and Neurologic Examination (Knobloch, Stevens, and Malone, 1980).

3. Many developmental screening instruments requiring *direct examination of the child* have been developed over the years. Relatively few have been thoroughly evaluated for validity and reliability. The most widely used screening test in pediatric settings is the Denver II. No screening test is perfect, but critics point to its limited positive predictive value and overly high referral rate (Glascoe et al, 1992). Promising newer screening tests are the Batelle Developmental Inventory and the Bayley Infant Neurodevelopmental Screener (BINS). A list of selected developmental screening tools is found in Table 68–3 with their test properties, if available.

Cautions

A set of guidelines regarding developmental screening was developed under the direction of Zero to Three (formerly the National Center for Clinical Infant Programs) (see Table 68–3). Screening tests should not be used for diagnosis. For example, it is inappropriate to determine a "gross motor level" from a general developmental screening test or to label a child as developmentally delayed or mentally retarded based on a screening. The screening should be used on a pass-fail basis only. A failed developmental screening should lead to further assessment, just as an abnormal neonatal metabolic screening leads to expanded investigation. Failed screening can be due to acute illness, improper administration or scoring (e.g., failing to correct age for prematurity), a testing room that is too cold or too noisy, or a "bad day" for the child or examiner, as well as to true delay; therefore, concern but not conclusions should result from the screening process. It can take an extended period of observation and reassessment before certainty of diagnosis is achieved. Developmental screening is a simple and cost-effective process when expectations do not exceed its capabilities. Persons who administer screening tests should be trained well. It is often most cost-effective to have a nurse or health assistant perform the test.

Table 68–3 • Guidelines for Screening

- Screening instruments should be used only for their specified purpose.
- Developmental screening should take place on a recurrent or periodic basis.
- Developmental screening should be viewed as one path to more in-depth assessment.
- Multiple sources of information should be used in screening.
- Screening tools should be reliable and valid.
- Family members should be an integral part of the screening process.
- The more familiar and relevant the tasks and setting are, the more valid the screening results will be.
- Screening procedures must be culturally sensitive.
- Extensive and comprehensive training is needed by those who screen.

Adapted from Meisels SJ, Provence S: Screening and Assessment: Guidelines for Identifying Vulnerable Children and Their Families. Washington, DC, National Center for Clinical Infant Programs, 1989.

SCREENING TESTS FOR LANGUAGE, SOCIAL-EMOTIONAL-BEHAVIORAL DEVELOPMENT, AND FAMILY FUNCTIONING

Although language items are usually contained in more general developmental screening instruments, at times users have found a need to expand evaluation with a specific language screening, particularly for children older than 2 years of age. With younger children, it has been found that parental concern is a very reliable screen for problems, especially hearing deficits, which can be manifested by delays in receptive or expressive language, or both. Capute and Accardo (1996) have developed the Clinical Linguistic and Auditory Milestone Scale (CLAMS) for office screening of language development from birth to 36 months of age.

Behavior and socioemotional function is often intertwined with concerns about development. Studies have shown that parents report greater intensity and persistence of common behaviors, such as feeding problems, crying, and temper tantrums, among children with developmental disabilities (Blackman and Cobb, 1989). They also can confuse behavioral problems with underlying developmental dysfunction (Oberklaid, Dworkin, and Levine, 1979). Screening tools for infant-toddler socioemotional development that demonstrate reliability and validity are not yet available, although several promising products, such as the BABES (Finello and Poulsen, 1996) and NIAD (Bagnato et al, 1994), are currently under development and may prove useful in the health care setting. For older children, parents' reports of problems, systematically collected through a process such as the ANSER system (Levine, 1996), provide important dimensions of understanding that will aid in making correct referrals. Assessment of behavioral adjustment and temperament is discussed in Chapter 67.

Regarding *family function,* recognizing that the family is the constant in the child's life while the service systems and personnel within those systems fluctuate (Shelton and Stepanek, 1994), screening must include consideration of family and environmental issues. Escalona's (1982) description of the doubly vulnerable child suggests that a biologically compromised infant is at increased jeopardy of not fulfilling his or her developmental potential in an emotional, social, or physical environment that is not nourishing. Frankenburg and Coons (1986) have developed environmental screening instruments based on the Home Observation for Measurement of the Environment (HOME) (Caldwell and Bradley, 1979). When there are indications from general developmental screening tests that a child might not be reaching potential, identification of family strengths and needs must be a part of the evaluation that follows.

DEVELOPMENTAL SCREENING FOR SELECTED PRESCHOOLERS

General developmental screening instruments such as the Denver II are most effective in identifying young children with moderate to severe motor or cognitive deficits from any cause. They do not detect more subtle learning problems at early ages because the manifestations of these problems might not emerge until a child is several years old. As problems with attention, behavior, language, perceptual-motor skills, and memory become evident, such gross screening tests are not sufficiently sensitive to assess these dimensions. Unfortunately instruments to assess these dimensions in a format that is practical in most clinical settings are limited. The Early Screening Inventory was designed for preschool children and might prove superior to the Denver II for this population.

One system that was developed under the direction of Levine includes a series of combined neurodevelopmental, behavioral, and health assessments that generate a set of observations that can be helpful in planning health, education, and developmentally oriented services. For preschoolers there is the Pediatric Extended Examination at Three (PEET) and the Pediatric Evaluation of Educational Readiness (PEER) (see Chapter 69 for further details of this neurodevelopmental assessment system). Parent and teacher questionnaires designed to elicit pertinent information about a child's functional development and behavior in naturalistic settings augment the information obtained through direct observation and interviews. Although these procedures were standardized for Boston area populations, there have been few subsequent studies of their utility in various clinical settings or of their validity among other populations. One study evaluating the use of the PEER in a statewide high-risk infant follow-up program found its sensitivity to be 0.60 and its specificity to be 0.88 when compared with a battery of standardized psychometric tests. The authors concluded that the PEER could not be recommended as a routine screening instrument, but in individual cases in which there were concerns about potential learning difficulties, the PEER could be helpful in clarifying the nature of the concerns, in determining the most appropriate referrals for further evaluation, and, in some cases, in making recommendations about school placement, teaching strategies, and behavioral management techniques (Blackman and Bretthauer, 1990). The training required and the time necessary to administer these neurodevelopmental examinations also limit their use to motivated clinicians and problematic children.

Meisels (1987) has emphasized the distinction between developmental screening tests for preschoolers and school readiness tests. Developmental screening tests identify children who might need interventions or special education services *immediately,* whereas school readiness tests indicate whether a child has the prerequisite skills to succeed in a specific academic program. The screening tests listed in Table 68–1 generally assess developmental skills rather than academic readiness. Kindergarten readiness testing is conducted by most school systems, and most practitioners find it convenient to refer children and their parents to them for these services.

Referral for Diagnostic Evaluation

When a child fails screening, a referral to an appropriate diagnostic facility should follow. Most tertiary medical centers have the capability to respond. Other referral possibilities include state programs for children with special health care needs, early intervention programs, or pediatricians with special expertise in developmental assessments. It is important that the diagnostic evaluation be conducted from an interdisciplinary perspective so that the widest possible view of the child and family is obtained. When the assessment takes place in a nonmedical setting, the physical health component is in danger of being omitted. The referring physician should provide this part of the evaluation or insist that a medical consultant be a part of the evaluation team.

Practical Plan for Screening Infants, Toddlers, and Preschoolers

It is useful to separate procedures according to age (Fig. 68–2).

BIRTH TO 3 YEARS

If children have congenital or chronic conditions (such as spina bifida or cytomegalic inclusion disease) that are certain to be associated with cognitive, motor, language, or sensory impairments, they should be referred immediately for evaluation and services. Developmental screening is not appropriate for this group, although routine pediatric care should continue.

Children at high risk for developmental problems from biological factors (e.g., intracranial hemorrhage, birth asphyxia, or meningitis) or environmental factors (e.g., substance-abusing parents) should receive periodic developmental screening. If they fail screening, they should be referred to a multidisciplinary clinic for evaluation.

Parents of children at low risk should complete a developmental questionnaire at intervals. There are forms for this purpose, which usually correspond to well-child examination schedules. These questionnaires can be administered verbally and do not have to be in written form. If

potential problems are identified, full screening should be conducted.

3 TO 6 YEARS

Preschool children who have not been screened previously should first receive a general developmental screening, recognizing that only moderate to severe deficits will be detected. If there are concerns about less severe problems, such as language, perceptual-motor dysfunction, hyperactivity, or other problematic behaviors, the practitioner should use instruments such as the PEET or PEER, which were designed to address such concerns in a pediatric setting, or refer the child to other professionals or to a clinic that specializes in evaluations of preschool children. In some communities, the schools might deal with both developmental and school readiness issues. In this case, the practitioner would want to be sure that any health needs are included in programming. If attention deficits or hyperactivity is involved, a physician must take responsibility for assessing whether stimulant medication is indicated.

Training

Many of the developmental screening instruments come with detailed manuals. The Denver system has extensive training materials, including videotapes and proficiency tests, that are helpful in training personnel. Unless person who administer screening tests are adequately trained, the results will be suspect. If the practitioner desires to be involved in the initial screening of preschool children with learning and behavioral problems, further training is necessary. Several medical centers offer courses or minifellowships in assessment procedures. Even when the practitioner chooses not to conduct the assessments in the office or clinic, knowledge about goals and components of preschool evaluations can help in identifying which chil-

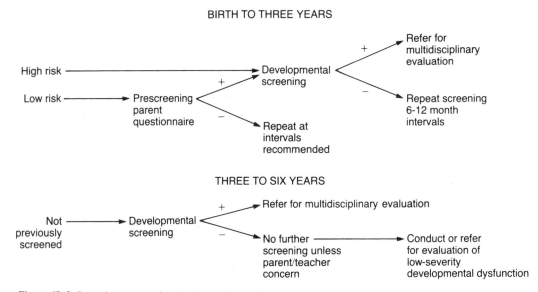

Figure 68–2. Screening as part of a developmental surveillance program.

dren would benefit from further assessment and in interpreting test results.

Conclusion

The concept of developmental screening is predicated on a strong belief in the efficacy of early identification and intervention. Although no perfect system of screening exists, there are tools that, if used in a systematic and coordinated approach to identification and service delivery, can get the job done well. The most difficult task in screening is to account for environmental and parenting factors, and more so to find supportive services when needs are identified. The role of the health care provider in early identification of developmental problems is to implement a system of developmental surveillance. For low-risk children, parent-completed developmental questionnaires or their equivalent should be used with all patients. When problems are identified, developmental screening should be conducted. For high-risk children, developmental screening should be conducted routinely. Ideally, all children who fail screening should receive a multidisciplinary developmental assessment. Screening preschool children for low-severity developmental dysfunction requires more extensive training and experience. Alternatively, preschool children can be referred outside the practice for evaluation of such concerns. For those who had insufficient training in developmental screening techniques and related skills, state coordinators of Part C of the Individuals with Disabilities Education Act (Early Intervention System) or medical school programs often offer continuing education opportunities.

Because most children are normal, developmental screening can be a frequent source of reassurance to parents.

REFERENCES

Ambulatory Pediatric Association: A statewide survey of pediatricians on early identification and early intervention services. Children with Disabilities: A Resource Guide. McLean, VA, Ambulatory Pediatric Association, 1990.

Bagnato SJ, Neisworth JT, Salvia J, et al: Neurobehavioral Indicators of Atypical Development. Research edition. 1994. Unpublished rating scale.

Bierman J, Conner A, Vaage M, et al: Pediatricians' assessments of the intelligence of two-year-olds and their mental test scores. Pediatrics 34:680, 1964.

Blackman JA, Bretthauer J: Examining high risk children for learning problems in the health care setting. Pediatrics 86:398, 1990.

Blackman JA, Cobb LS: A comparison of parents' perceptions of common behavior problems in developmentally at-risk and normal children. Child Health Care 18:108, 1989.

Caldwell BM, Bradley RH: Home Observation for Measurement of the Environment. Little Rock, University of Arkansas Press, 1979.

Capute AJ, Accardo PJ: The infant neurodevelopmental assessment: a clinical interpretive manual for CAT-CLAMS in the first two years of life, Part 1. Current Problems in Pediatrics, August, 1996.

Corrigan N, Stewart M, Scott M, et al: Predictive value of preschool surveillance in detecting learning difficulties. Arch Dis Child 74:517, 1986.

Dworkin P: British and American recommendations for developmental monitoring: the role of surveillance. Pediatrics 84:1000, 1989.

Escalona SK: Babies at double hazard: early development of infants at biologic and social risk. Pediatrics 70:670, 1982.

Finello KM, Poulsen MK. The Behavioral Assessment of Baby's Emotional and Social Style (BABES): a new screening tool for clinical use. Paper presented at the 10th International Conference on Infant Studies. Providence, RI, April 1996.

Frankenburg WK, Coons CE: Home Screening Questionnaire: its validity in assessing home environment. J Pediatr 108:624, 1986.

Frankenburg WK, Thornton SM: A child development program for a busy office practice. Contemp Pediatr 6(2):90, 1989.

Glascoe FP, Byrne KE, Ashford LG, et al: Accuracy of the Denver II: a major revision and restandardization of the Denver Developmental Screening Test. Pediatrics 89:91, 1992.

Guralnick MJ: The Effectiveness of Early Intervention. Baltimore, Paul H. Brookes Publishing, 1997.

Knobloch H, Stevens F, Malone AF: Manual of Developmental Diagnosis. Hagerstown, Harper & Row, 1980.

Korsch B, Cobb K, Ashe B: Pediatricians' appraisal of patients' intelligence. Pediatrics 27:990, 1961.

Levine MD: The ANSER System (Revised). Cambridge, MA, Educator's Publishing Service, 1996.

Meisels SJ: Uses and abuses of developmental screening and readiness testing. Young Child 42:5, 1987.

Oberklaid F, Dworkin PH, Levine MD: Developmental-behavioral dysfunction in preschool children: descriptive analysis of a pediatric consultative model. Am J Dis Child 133:1126, 1979.

Shelton TL, Stepanek JS: Family-Centered Care for Children Needing Specialized Health and Developmental Services. Bethesda, MD, Association for the Care of Children's Health, 1994.

Stowers S, Huber CJ: Developmental and screening tests. *In* King Thomas L, Hacker BJ (eds): A Therapist's Guide to Pediatric Assessment. Boston, Little, Brown, 1987.

69 Developmental Assessment of the School-Aged Child

Adrian D. Sandler • Olson Huff

 Within the field of pediatrics, there has been a reasonably sustained tradition of developmental assessment for infants and preschool-aged children. In this chapter, the author offers the same process in an uniquely different context, namely the developmental assessment of the school-aged child. Sometimes physicians believe (or want to believe) that schools are responsible for the development of the school-aged child. Yet increasingly there is an awareness that developmental delays in older youngsters often go undetected by schools. The current chapter examines the rationale for neurodevelopmental testing in school children, particularly those who are experiencing frustration in learning and keeping pace with academic expectations. In reading this chapter, a clinician can be helped to formulate an organized approach to monitoring the developmental function of school-aged children. Such an approach may involve good history taking or direct neurodevelopmental examination. What becomes clear is the danger and inappropriateness of neglecting developmental phenomenology once children arrive at school.

Primary care physicians who provide medical care for children must deal with increasingly complex problems, many of which are related to development and learning. More frequently than ever, children are coming to their doctors for help with learning difficulties, social and behavioral inadequacies, and disorders of attention, all of which may lead to poor school performance or even failure. For medical care providers to manage these children well, they must have knowledge of how their patients learn, remember, behave, and pay attention. Additionally, they must have the ability to provide relevant insight into how to manage such difficulties and be aware of the resources that will be useful to the child, family, and school for intervention. The following case illustrates these points.

EXAMPLE

Ron first presented to our center at the age of 5 years, 10 months. He was midway through kindergarten and events were not unfolding well for him. There were a number of distinct patterns of difficulties that seemed to best describe him to his teacher, his parents, and even his peers. He simply would not sit still. He was highly mobile with an intense need to hold, touch, or explore in some fashion, repeatedly, every object in his classroom that was not secured. He appeared to be clumsy, he tripped over his and others' feet, chewed his shirt collar, talked incessantly, and frequently interrupted the play or conversation of others. Even though he seemed to be quite bright, he had a great deal of trouble verbalizing common thoughts or ideas. He would often burst into tears with frustration because he could not communicate to others how he felt about himself or the happenings around him. And then, too, Ron would scream with provocation, throw toys, talk back to adults, and hit other children whenever he cared

to do so. He often battled with his parents about going to sleep at night and he frequently kicked the dog or pulled its tail.

Following a thorough assessment process, intervention was begun in a variety of ways. Gradually, improvement was noted. Ron began to gain more insight into his own nature as well. He was allowed, with parents' approval, to watch a limited amount of television. On one occasion, his father observed Ron watching a rerun of "I Love Lucy." When asked about that choice of programs, Ron answered: "It's the only time I know when someone else gets into more trouble than me!"

In this chapter, the questions raised by the difficulties that Ron and children like him encounter are addressed.

The Principles of Pediatric Developmental Assessment

Pediatricians have always assessed early child development. Monitoring a child's developmental progress in motor, cognitive, adaptive, language, and social function is at the very heart of pediatrics, and pediatricians are actively involved in screening, referral, care coordination, and advocacy. Child development does not end at the age of 5 years, so the question is how best to fulfill these responsibilities for the school-aged child.

There are many conceivable models for pediatric involvement in the assessment and management of children with school problems. They range from traditional screening for associated health problems, to the prescribing of medication for attentional problems, to a more extensive role as a diagnostician and long-term care coordinator. Should a pediatrician confine himself or herself to a routine physical and neurologic examination? Or should such a clinician make some direct observations of neurodevelopmental function? For those who choose the latter, what are the principles that underlie and support the distinctive role of the pediatrician in developmental assessment?

There is an extensive network of neurodevelopmental functions that converge and collaborate in increasingly sophisticated ways, enabling children to acquire and apply school-related skills. The skills combine in synchrony and with increasing automaticity, allowing children to keep pace with reading, writing, mathematics, and social demands. For example, reading relies heavily on phonologic awareness, phonologic short-term memory, and naming fluency (Kamhi and Catts, 1989). Writing, the most complex form of communication, requires a host of well-synchronized memory, language, and fine motor functions (Sandler et al, 1992). Neurodevelopmental functions may be grouped into eight broad constructs: attention, memory, language, temporal-sequential ordering, spatial ordering, neuromotor function, higher order cognition, and social cognition. There is rich interaction between a child's neurodevelopmental profile and genetic, environmental, experiential, educational, and cultural factors (see Chapters 52 and 53).

Children show rich diversity in their patterns of neurodevelopmental strengths and weaknesses, and wide variation does not necessarily represent pathology or abnormality. It is potentially dehumanizing and harmful to label children categorically, such as "learning disabled." The best prescription is likely to derive from detailed description: such specificity, rather than undue emphasis on categorical labels, allows for highly individualized management.

There are many opportunities to observe a child's performance on a variety of tasks and derive information that contributes to a descriptive assessment. Through repeated observation, astute classroom teachers are likely to know where the academic subskill breakdown points are occurring. Parents also have opportunities to make such observations. Many critical neurodevelopmental dysfunctions may be directly observable or at least partially evident in a child's history and in work samples. The assessment of a child with school problems should consist of the search for recurring themes; no one source of observations should be overinterpreted without other pieces of corroborating evidence, including those derived from standardized tests of intelligence and academic achievement. Most importantly, assessment should uncover a child's strengths and affinities in addition to relevant weaknesses or dysfunctions.

The Developmental History: Referral Concerns and Diagnostic Dilemmas

Physicians ask questions. This time-honored method of obtaining information, which leads to diagnosis and subsequent treatment of any disorder, is a critical portion of the evaluation strategy for a child who is not doing well in school. Even though many other forms of assessment are extremely valuable for determining the characteristics of the presenting difficulty, none will be as comprehensive or consistent as the history of the child's life, from conception to the present.

It is best to begin with an orderly and standard approach. The pediatrician should explain what the assessment is about and what will take place. He or she should seek to know the family and to appreciate their perception of what is now occurring with their child as well as what has transpired in the past. Listening for clues that suggest distance between family members or that describe support and ability to cope and engaging the family in conversation are valuable tactics, but the pediatrician should not ask questions that put either the parent or the child on the defensive.

We like to include both child and parent in the history portion of the assessment. We feel that is a valuable way to reassure the youngster that his or her concern is being considered correctly and fairly. However, the wish of the parents not to discuss sensitive issues with their child should be honored.

Children have stories. They possess a colorful and varied set of details and happenings, which require sorting out to learn their strengths and define their problems. To know them, understand their story, and detect the pattern that has brought them for assessment requires a great deal of curiosity and many questions. Thus, taking a history becomes the pivotal point in the evaluation for a learning disorder and requires attention to a child's and a parent's understanding, perception, and use of language. The story of those expressions and how they interact to produce meaning is the essence of learning and is the beginning point for the physician who must sort out the details. It is vital that the questioning and sorting stay true to the child's story and that key elements not be overlooked. This is well illustrated in the following vignette.

EXAMPLE

Norman is an 11-year-old boy who presented with a well-voiced complaint by all that he was hyperactive, unmotivated, and underachieving, and needed to be on medication. His story of overactivity began when he entered kindergarten. He was subsequently diagnosed as having attention-deficit hyperactivity disorder by his physician and was placed on methylphenidate. He did not do well and eventually entered a series of placements in group homes, child psychiatric units, and special school resources. A much later, in-depth evaluation of the events in his life (i.e., his "stories") at the time when he entered kindergarten was fascinating and illuminating. Several days before he was to begin kindergarten, he was sleeping in the bed with his adoptive grandmother. She died suddenly of a heart attack. He was convinced that he had killed her. A few weeks later, his mother, who previously had been severely affected by alcoholism, married an individual who turned out to be both alcoholic and abusive. She returned to alcoholism, and a cycle of intrafamily stress and abuse ensued. It was out of that set of circumstances that Norman presented to kindergarten with "hy-

peractive" behavior. The importance of knowing all of the story is evident.

To begin with, the physician must understand what it is that made the family, and of course the patient, come for the assessment in the first place. There are many reasons, or "presenting complaints," as voiced by those seeking advice. They include the following:

- Not keeping up with classmates
- Losing everything all the time
- Not being able to (or refusing to) follow directions, pay attention, or finish a task
- Not being able to carry thoughts or ideas to paper
- Not being able to read, write or spell well
- Struggling with mathematics
- Talking back, talking too loudly, acting up in class
- Being too shy or a loner or having few or no friends

These are but a few of the concerns that will ignite a cascade of responses in the clinician's mind. An interactive dialogue with child and parent will allow the clinician to sort, to "lump" some items and "split" others, to consider differential diagnoses, and to formulate hypotheses. The process will eventually lead to a diagnostic understanding and ultimately a plan for management.

To begin the sorting process, it is necessary to categorize the concerns. Ordinarily this will result in three separate sets, namely learning, attention, and behavior. Thus it is important to decide whether the problem is primarily one of learning, of attention, or of behavior. Each of these is separate enough from the other to be distinct, yet all share a remarkable amount of interrelated influence. To arrive at a diagnostic understanding that is clear and that truly "fits" the child's story requires that the examiner be aware of the division of complaints as well as their interrelated nature.

EXAMPLE

John is an almost 6-year-old boy who presented with deteriorating performance in kindergarten, appearing to be inattentive, preoccupied, or "overfocused," and having great difficulty completing simple tasks. The clinician, appreciating that these symptoms represented a change in behavior, asked his parents about other signs of stress. They volunteered that John had been seen recently by his doctor because of the need to urinate frequently, and also a problem of having to swallow repeatedly, neither of which was found to have organic etiology. A simple question to John, "Do you keep having to do things over and over again?" revealed a number of obsessions and compulsions, including obsessive counting of dots on the classroom ceiling. (John's drawings are shown in Fig. 69–3.)

The clinician or biographer must then help the child and his or her caregiver to elaborate and describe the details, and sort out those details to form a pattern. Once the pattern is developed, then more specific testing, assessments, or consultations may be obtained if necessary. Table 69–1 offers examples of questions that may help to elaborate upon the school-related presenting complaints and to describe a learning disorder. In asking such questions, it is generally helpful to move from the general to the specific

Table 69–1 • Examples of Common Presenting School-Related Concerns and the Kinds of Questions a Clinician May Ask to Clarify These Concerns

Concern	Possible Questions
Unable to carry thoughts or ideas to paper	What's the hardest thing about writing?
	Is it hard to remember how to make the letters?
	How is the child's spelling?
	Is writing always messy, difficulty with lines and spacing?
	Does the child's hand hurt when writing?
	Is it hard for the child to write quickly enough?
	Are there problems with organization and sequence of ideas?
Reading problems	What's the hardest thing about reading?
	Is it very hard to "sound out" words?
	How about sight words and flash cards?
	What's the child's spelling like?
	Does the child have trouble understanding what he or she read?
	How is the child's vocabulary?
	Does the child have trouble understanding oral instructions or stories?
Struggling in math	What is the child learning in math these days?
	Does the child have trouble understanding the math concepts?
	Are word problems especially hard?
	Does the child get lost or forget what he or she is doing in multistep problems?
	Does the child often make careless errors in math?

and from open-ended to more direct, closed-ended questions.

Table 69–2 suggests a framework for the history and provides a reminder of questions to ask that are valuable in determining antecedents of present concerns and the development of these concerns over time. In addition, there are critically important issues of family history and social history to explore. The clinician must balance the need for thorough history gathering with considerations of efficiency. In a typical consultation regarding a school problem, we usually allocate about 30 minutes to review questionnaires and complete the developmental history.

The Use of Questionnaires and Rating Scales in Developmental Assessment

When embarking on an assessment of a child with school problems that may encompass complex behavioral-developmental issues, questionnaires and rating scales are extremely helpful adjuncts. They promote efficiency by focusing the clinician on fruitful areas of enquiry. A review of questionnaires prior to the evaluation allows an opportunity to plan an evaluation to suit the needs of the child and family. Extensive information can be gathered regarding a wide range of concerns and potential influences, ranging from teratogenesis to tics, and this frees the pediatrician from having to wade through an extensive review of systems.

Parent-completed questionnaires have a number of other advantages. They give parents an opportunity to tell the doctor about their subjective experience of their child's problems. This is especially true with the open-ended questions, in which a parent may candidly use a phrase or metaphor to emphasize his or her concern, such as "He scares me," or "I blame myself." Such expressions become a focal point, and one that the clinician returns to after the assessment to help the parent feel empowered or to help alleviate guilt. Many parents seem to need the opportunity that a questionnaire allows to reflect on their concerns, and some prefer the less threatening medium of the questionnaire to state some of their concerns, which may be hard to talk about in face-to-face interview.

Systematic gathering of rating scales from parents and teachers can provide indispensable perspectives from different settings. Standardized rating scales of attention and behavior force respondents to rate specific component behaviors and aspects of performance rather than making global judgments. In this way, subjectivity is decreased. A comparison of different perspectives can be revealing, and a discrepancy between a child's behavior at home and at school, or indeed among different classes in school, can be an important issue to address. Rating scales can also be used to obtain a child's perspective, so that children as young as 8 or 9 years can be valuable participants.

There are many published questionnaires (Achenbach, 1991; Conners, 1985; Ullman, Sleator, and Sprague, 1984), and many more very useful questionnaires designed by individuals and practices to suit their particular needs.

Table 69–2 • Framework for the Systematic Gathering of Information for the Developmental History

Preconception and prenatal
    Parental age, education, health
    Pregnancy desired or unplanned
    Substance abuse, toxic exposures, and medical complications during
        the pregnancy
    Level of medical/social care; was prenatal care delayed?
    Genetic history; history of fetal demise
Perinatal
    Length of gestation; spontaneous onset of labor versus induced labor
    Characteristics of labor: prolonged? rapid?
    Medications used, if any
    Apgar scores
    Birth weight, head circumference, and general appearance
    Feeding, sleeping, spitting; state of alertness
    Consolable/irritable
Infancy
    Sleeping, eating, alerting
    Irritability and colic
    Weight gain
    Response to sound, touch; eye contact
Toddler
    Temperamental characteristics
    Motor development (sit, roll, crawl, walk)
    Language development
    Social development; imitation; object permanence; evidence of
        separation fears
Preschool age
    Sleep patterns
    Appetite/nutrition
    General health
    Adaptability to change; management of separation
    Response to stimulating environments
    Unusual sensory symptoms

The ANSER system constitutes a set of detailed parent and school questionnaires that are suitable for children of ages 3 through 15 years (Levine, 1980). They are comprehensive, detailed, and especially useful in eliciting information about a child's task performance. They include a student questionnaire to obtain the child's perspective (Rappaport et al, 1983). The Yale Children's Inventory is another broad-ranging questionnaire that has usefulness in evaluation of attentional and learning problems (Shaywitz et al, 1988).

Questionnaires should not be used as the sole source of information. There is always a need for clarification and exploration of parental concerns, elaboration of symptoms, and so on; however, they can assist the clinician in targeting the interview and assessment. The information in the questionnaires may be useful in "building a case" with multiple lines of evidence, attempting to validate examination findings with observations from home and school. Questionnaires can also be extremely helpful as a framework for report writing. The complexity of developmental assessment reminds us that we must be cautious and that incorrect formulations and treatments can be costly. Therefore, it is important to keep returning to the perspectives, opinions, questions, and metaphors (contained in the questionnaires) of those who know the child best.

Neurologic Examination and the Interpretation of Neurologic Soft Signs

A standard physical and neurologic examination is important to rule out disorders that may present with school problems (Kandt, 1984). It is essential to rule out hearing loss or poor visual acuity. Chromosomal disorders such as Turner syndrome and Klinefelter syndrome may present with learning difficulties. The physical features of fragile X syndrome may be quite subtle, especially in females, and it is important to consider this in the differential diagnosis of girls who struggle with mathematics and social skills. The unique role of the pediatrician is evident in the search for dysmorphic features, skin abnormalities, or goiter which may identify specific genetic or metabolic abnormalities.

The neurologic examination should discriminate between an isolated problem of learning and a more pervasive encephalopathy that is accompanied by mental retardation or cerebral palsy. The examination should also help to rule out the rare progressive encephalopathies. It should include vision and hearing screens, limited examination of cranial nerves, and determination of muscle tone, strength, coordination, and reflexes. In children with a history of staring spells, hyperventilation (by blowing a piece of tissue paper for 2 minutes) may occasionally reveal petit mal. It is important to measure head circumference, since even benign, familial macrocephaly may be associated with developmental problems (Sandler et al, 1997).

The interpretation of neurologic "soft signs" has been debated in the literature for decades (Touwen and Prechtl, 1970; Denckla and Rudel, 1978; Levine, 1987). The pivotal role such signs played in earlier formulations of learning and attention disorders is illustrated by the term *minimal brain dysfunction*. Some authors ascribed great significance to specific signs and even argued for specific anatomic localization. For example, difficulties with bilateral coordination were attributed to abnormalities of the corpus callosum, and mixed dominance was felt to be a powerful predictor of dyslexia. More recent accounts of learning disorders have placed less emphasis on these signs, and individual signs have been found to lack specificity or predictive value. Mirror movements, for example, are maturational, so that the majority of young school-aged children show some evidence of them. When these neurologic soft signs are considered in aggregate, however, they can be useful markers, in effect tipping off the examiner that neurologic factors are operating (Denckla, 1985). It is generally agreed that the presence of many soft signs (for any given age), raises the likelihood of "unusual wiring," with concomitant learning and attention disorders. Between one third and one half of children with learning problems demonstrate significant soft neuologic signs (Brown, Aylward, and Keogh, 1996). There are a few standardized procedures for eliciting neurologic soft signs, such as the examination procedure of Touwen (Touwen and Prechtl, 1970) and the PANESS (Denckla, 1985). The PEER, PEEX 2, and PEERAMID 2 (discussed later) also include systematic procedures to examine cerebral dominance and to elicit mirror movements, associated movements, dyskinesia, dysmetria, finger agnosia, dystonic posturing, proximal instability, and dysdiadochokinesia.

The Neurodevelopmental Examination: General Principles

Neurodevelopmental examination of the school-aged child can be helpful in generating a functional, descriptive profile of a child's cognitive and neurologic status. Such examinations are not designed to be a screening test for learning disabilities, but rather to clarify neurodevelopmental issues among children for whom concerns about learning have been raised. Such examinations are more comprehensive than a brief developmental screening test and may typically take 45 to 60 minutes to administer. The results can help to identify those areas of development that merit further and more specific evaluation and provide a pediatric neurodevelopmental perspective during multidisciplinary evaluations.

Neurodevelopmental examination should not be performed in isolation but should be supplemented by psychoeducational and other testing and historical information from many sources. School worksheets and writing samples can be revealing (Fig. 69–1). It is especially helpful to compare findings on neurodevelopmental examination with other test data, in this way seeking recurring themes that help to validate impressions of the child's strengths and weaknesses. For example, a 7-year-old first-grade student, referred for learning and attention problems, is found to have poor balance and coordination and also shows very weak figure copying skills. Psychological testing indicates solidly average verbal cognitive abilities but strikingly weak nonverbal abilities, with especially poor perceptual organization. Although academic skills at this age are

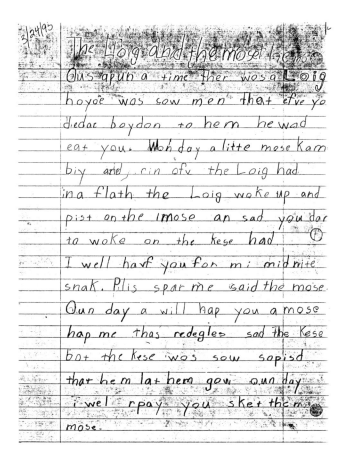

Figure 69–1. A writing sample entitled "The Lion and the Mouse" from a 9-year-old girl with average intelligence and a specific learning disability in reading and writing.

broadly consistent with full scale intelligence quotient (IQ) scores, the child has difficulty with quantitative and spatial concepts, and his writing skills are characterized by poor legibility, inconsistent letter formations, and lack of spatial organization on the page. A physical therapy evaluation showed overall gross motor skills at the 4- to 5-year age level, with striking deficits in proximal stability and motor planning. The constellation of findings fit together into a prevalent and well-recognized "subtype" of nonverbal or perceptual-motor learning disability.

Neurodevelopmental examination differs fundamentally from psychometric testing in that it does not generate a specific score or quotient. Although age equivalencies may be used to characterize a child's level of performance in specific developmental areas, neurodevelopmental examinations contribute to the development of a descriptive profile of a child's strengths, weaknesses, and learning style. Qualitative aspects are just as important as quantitative aspects of performance. For example, many children with language processing problems become increasingly anxious, withdrawn, or inattentive during tasks that place demands on language. Children may exhibit excessive performance anxiety, a finding that may have important therapeutic implications. Moreover, neurodevelopmental examination is an interactive and dynamic process, in which the examiner proceeds flexibly, sometimes modifying a task to assess how a child approaches the task. A clinician's alteration of a task in such a way as to allow a child to succeed, for example, by administering instructions more slowly, may have major implications for teaching that child.

The Pediatric Examination of Educational Readiness (PEER) (Levine and Schneider, 1988), Pediatric Early Elementary Examination (PEEX 2) (Levine and Sandler, 1996a), and Pediatric Examination of Educational Readiness At Middle Childhood (PEERAMID 2) (Levine and Sandler, 1996b) are a series of neurodevelopmental examinations developed by Levine and his colleagues and are in widespread use in North America. These are discussed in the next section. Other neurodevelopmental examinations for school-aged children include the PANESS (Denckla, 1985). Many other pediatricians use informal compilations of standardized tests, and some of these will be discussed later.

EXAMINING CHILDREN 4 THROUGH 15 YEARS OF AGE: PEER, PEEX 2, AND PEERAMID 2

The PEER, PEEX 2, and PEERAMID 2 are a family of neurodevelopmental examinations that allow the pediatrician to engage in structured play with children while deriving useful information about a child's learning and neurodevelopmental profile. The PEER spans ages 4 through 6 years, the PEEX 2 ages 6 through 9 years, and the PEERAMID 2 ages 9 through 15 years. Each examination takes approximately 1 hour to administer in its entirety, although many clinicians who are experienced in their use shorten and adapt the examinations. Parents are usually present during the administration. This provides security for the child and also gives parents an opportunity to observe their child's performance, which frequently enhances communication in subsequent conferences with the family.

The examinations consist of a series of tasks that are arranged sequentially to assess several broad areas of neurodevelopmental function: fine motor/graphomotor, language, gross motor, memory, and visual processing functions. (For the PEER, the arrangement of tasks is somewhat different, to take into account areas of function relevant to the kindergarten-aged child, including orientation/sensory processing, visual-fine motor integration, and preacademic learning.) In addition, there are "attention checkpoints" (which provide opportunities to make observations about a child's attention during task completion), notations of strategy usage and organization, minor neurologic indicators (soft signs), and the child's behavior and interactions during testing. The tasks are typically brief, interesting, and motivating for children. The entire examination is a positive experience for children, many of whom have been deprived of success in school, so that the encounter can be therapeutic. Frequently, the children who return for follow-up want to know, "When are we going to play more games?"

No task serves as a "pure" assessment of any single element of function. The Examination Manual provides a task analysis that uses clinical and empiric research data to clarify the specific processing and production elements that are important for successful completion of each task. The examiner assesses the child's performance on each task relative to normative data. For example, the 10-year-old child who cannot repeat a digit span of five digits forward has weak performance for her age. This finding suggests weak auditory short-term memory or attentional problems or both. Performance on different tasks and qualitative observations are considered as the examiner engages in a process of clinical hypothesis-testing. Weak performance on a number of tasks involving memory functions would suggest an underlying memory problem, whereas poorly sustained attention and inconsistent performance within tasks would suggest an attentional problem.

Despite their obvious clinical utility, there are limited published research data regarding these neurodevelopmental examinations and their usefulness. An exploratory study of the PEER identified four major factors, namely, perceptual-motor, gross motor, verbal-cognitive, and attention. Children's performance on the first two of these factors correlated with concurrent psychoeducational measures (Palmer et al, 1990). The validity of the PEEX was examined in both a clinical sample and a community sample (Levine et al, 1983). There were significant correlations between areas of concern on the PEEX and measures of intelligence and academic achievement. Preliminary studies of a prepublication version of the PEERAMID showed that many of the tasks distinguished between normal, school problem, and clinic-referred children (Levine et al, 1988). In addition, an empiric factor analysis demonstrated at least five factors measuring language, attention/memory, neuromotor control/minor neurologic indicators, visual perception, and automaticity/efficiency. More recent work investigated the construct and criterion-related validity of the PEERAMID with a clinic-referred sample (Sandler et al, 1993a). Construct validity was supported by a similar factor structure, and there were concurrent relationships with IQ and academic achievement. Also, the PEERAMID was shown to have clinical utility in terms of its discrimination among different types of writing disorder (Sandler et al, 1992).

NEURODEVELOPMENTAL INTERVIEW FOR OLDER ADOLESCENTS: STRANDS

Despite increasing recognition of learning disabilities in elementary school, there has been relatively little sensitivity to the spectrum of learning problems in the adolescent years. This is especially true in high school, where learning disabilities are sometimes overlooked, misunderstood, or neglected. Clinical experience and research evidence in the evaluation of adolescents suggest increasing ability among older adolescents to talk about their learning experiences and to reflect upon and describe their own cognitive processes. This increasing metacognitive sophistication is utilized in the Survey of Teenage Readiness and Neurodevelopmental Status (STRANDS), a multidimensional measure used by many pediatricians in the evaluation of high school students of ages 15 through 19 years. The STRANDS consists of a questionnaire and a structured interview, and takes about 1 hour to administer in full. The questionnaire is very broad in scope, eliciting information about a student's self-concept and academic and social functioning. The structured interview surveys domains of neurodevelopmental function thought to be of critical importance in adolescent learning, including attention, memory, language,

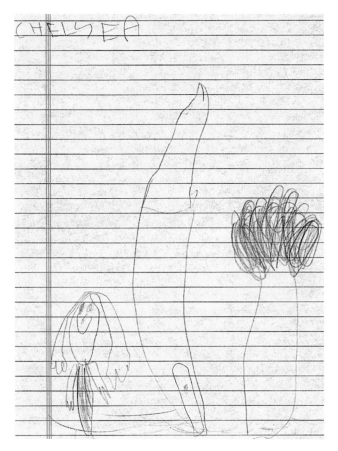

Figure 69–2. Visual-spatial problems are suggested by this disorganized and distorted drawing by a girl of age 6 years 9 months.

visual perception, efficiency, organization, and higher order cognition. Reliability, construct validity, and discriminant validity have been demonstrated (Sandler et al, 1993b). Moreover, adolescents typically enjoy a process in which their perceptions are taken seriously by an examiner. The STRANDS has the potential to provide information that can supplement or guide additional assessment and also plan educational programs to address self-perceptions of students. Many clinicians have also used the STRANDS as a tool for counseling high school students with academic difficulties.

The Drawings of School-Aged Children

Children create. They are filled with innovative and imaginative ways to express their various ideas and abilities. A useful portion of the assessment, children's drawings, taps into this creative process and provides yet another window through which portions of a youngster's learning, memory, and behavior can be seen. The Goodenough House-Tree-Person test is a standardized form of using children's drawings for developmental screening. This is easily expanded to determine a number of qualities and characteristics that are helpful in evaluating the school-aged child.

Fine motor skills, visual-motor and spatial abilities,

and impulse control and emotional status can be identified by observing and admiring children's drawings and by talking with them about their drawings. The use of drawings in the assessment will also help decrease anxiety and often engage the student at a level of more reliable performance. The following aspects of performance should be noted:

- Grasp of pencil or crayon; ease of hand and wrist movement
- Symmetry
- Line closure
- Accuracy of copying
- Distortion of shape
- Attention to detail (too little, too much)
- Expressions of mood such as joy, sadness, anger
- Persistence to task

Poorly structured drawings with inadequate or missing detail, distorted shapes, or random attempts at construction raise questions of the level of cognitive skill, visual-motor ability, and fine motor control, all of which may interfere with school performance. Drawings of this nature, as in Figure 69–2, should lead the examiner to evaluate more closely. A complete neurologic assessment, occupational therapy consultation, or cognitive testing may be needed. Pictures, such as in Figure 69–3, that strongly suggest mood disorders should lead the physician to address behavioral, emotional, or family unrest.

A word of caution is needed. Children's drawings are enjoyable to obtain and, for the most part, fun to produce. They may very well give important clues to the broader dimensions of the biology of brain function associated with presenting concerns. However, they should not be used as diagnostic tools. Their ability to reflect underlying brain dysfunction is quite plastic and their predictability for future events inconsistent. In the context of the entire assess-

Table 69–3 • Standardized Tests That May be Used in Pediatric Developmental Assessment of the School-Aged Child

Test	Age Range (Years)	Domains of Function
Peabody Picture Vocabulary Test	3–adult	Receptive vocabulary
Goodenough Draw-A-Person	3–15	Visual-motor integration
Gesell Figures	3–12	Visual-motor integration
Stanford-Binet Memory Test	2–adult	Auditory memory
Wide Range Achievement Test	5–adult	Reading, spelling, arithmetic
Durrell Test of Reading Comprehension	5–adult	Reading comprehension
Boder Word Recognition Inventory	5–adult	Decoding and spelling
Word Attack (Woodcock-Johnson)	6–adult	Phonology
Rapid Automatized Naming Test	5–adult	Fluency/automaticity
Block Design (WISC-III)	6–16	Nonverbal reasoning
Vocabulary (WISC-III)	6–16	Verbal reasoning
Kaufman Brief Intelligence Test	4–adult	Intelligence quotient

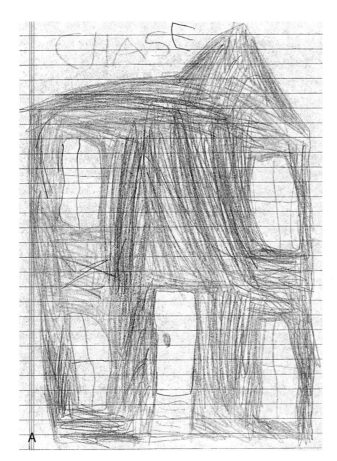

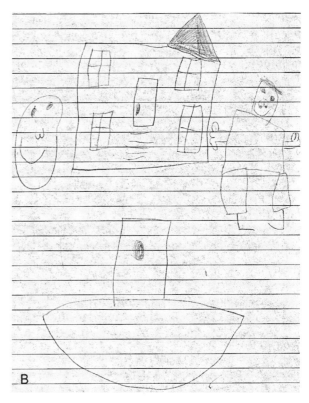

Figure 69–3. A bright, almost 6-year-old boy worked on drawing *A* for about 10 minutes. He was treated for obsessive-compulsive disorder with sertraline, and on follow-up, he completed drawing *B* in only 3 minutes.

ment, they have meaning; apart from it, their usefulness is reduced mainly to relieving the stress or anxiety associated with the visit. However obtained, drawings by children are yet another way of increasing information obtained from the assessment and adding more value to the concerns that the child who has difficulty learning brings to the interview.

The Pediatric Use of Standardized Tests

Many pediatricians use a variety of brief standardized tests, each one having limited scope, to compile information about a range of neurodevelopmental functions. There are many suitable tests, or subtests, from which to choose, and there are advantages to being familiar with many, to be able to choose among them with flexibility, according to the particular needs of the student. As with any test, standardization of administration is important for reliability and validity of the findings. Also, a high degree of familiarity with any such test allows the examiner to make useful, qualitative observations that augment "the score." Table 69–3 shows some of the more commonly used tests, the typical age ranges, and the domains of function that they measure.

Continuous Performance Tests

There is a long history of attempts to use performance on psychological tests to assess attention. For example, the subtests of the Wechsler Intelligence Scales for Children (WISC-III) that especially require focused attention (arithmetic, coding, and digit span) can be considered together as the "freedom from distractibility" factor. Continuous Performance Tests (CPTs) are now being widely used in the assessment of attentional problems. Most CPTs use letters or numbers presented on a screen at variable rates, and the child is asked to press a key or the space-bar when a target appears. The Gordon Diagnostic System is based on a 9-minute number sequence that requires a response each time the number 9 follows the number 1. The Conners CPT is a 14-minute letter sequence in which the child responds to any letter except X. The TOVA-CPT uses a 22-minute sequence in which the child responds when a square appears in a particular location. Over the past decade many studies have documented differences on CPTs between children with attention-deficit hyperactivity disorder (ADHD) and control groups. Accordingly, these tests are being used in the diagnosis of ADHD and also to monitor response to treatment. Clearly there are false positive and false negative results: it has been estimated that the probability of a "hit" (a positive CPT in a child with ADHD) is 0.73, while the probability of a "miss" (a negative CPT in a child who in fact has ADHD) is 0.27 (Baren and Swanson, 1996). Of course, calculations of sensitivity, specificity, and predictive value assume a "gold standard," which in the case of ADHD is not available. From a clinical standpoint, one of us has found the CPT to add valuable information in a proportion of evaluations. Also, it can be quite an efficient use of examination time to leave a child of 8 years or older working on a CPT for about 15 minutes while separately interviewing the parents about issues that may be difficult or impossible to discuss in the presence of the child.

Integrating, Prioritizing, and Communicating: The Interpretive Conference

During the assessment, most information gained is done so by the examiner; however, the usefulness of the information is limited unless interpreted to the child and family to whom it belongs. Information and understanding about the presented problem become powerful tools for action when they are incorporated into the family's strengths and their desire for change.

An interpretive conference is a continuing process of clarification for parents and also for the child that facilitates the recognition of reality and promotes adaptations to its demands. The objectives are to simplify (not complicate), to diminish false attributions and guilt (not induce guilt), to induce optimism and therapeutic energy (not deflate). It is a critical opportunity to make the family a part of the diagnostic-therapeutic process, to establish excellent rapport and alliance, and to provide practical advice.

There are many different kinds of interpretive conference, and many styles of conducting effective conferences. There may be occasions when two or more disciplines involved should relate the data, insights, and meaning of their portion of the assessment, and other times when the pediatrician alone provides interpretive feedback on behalf of other disciplines. It is important to encourage the family's questions, comments, and reactions. It is usually helpful to start with positive findings and strengths before describing specific areas of dysfunction. We mostly avoid "labels," although it may be necessary to introduce and explain diagnostic terms. It goes without saying that the conversation between the professionals and the family must be clear, must be related easily and without judgment, and must open the way to dialogue. One-way discussions are never apt to be productive nor pave the way for effective interventions. The physician should maintain good eye contact, use silence well, welcome expressions of grief, and watch for and solicit feedback.

Sensitive issues may surface during the interpretive conference that have not previously been revealed. Those attending must be aware of that possibility. This leads to the question of whether the child, who has been the focus of all the experience, should be present. Children should have the opportunity to know, from those who worked with them, what the evaluation showed. They will have an expectation about the examination and, in our experience, a very real desire to know "how they did." Usually, these needs can best be met with children and parents together, but sometimes it is necessary to have a separate, shorter conference with the child alone. It is important to

- Reassure them of their health (i.e., no "bad brains").
- Be honest about what has been learned.
- Enlist their cooperation in using the information for change.
- Use drawings and games to illustrate points to be made.

Families should be encouraged to keep notes during the conference, interrupt as desired, and use a tape recorder if they wish. When the conference is completed, the physician should send a summary including points addressed and recommendations made to the family. It may be helpful to follow this with a telephone call in 1 or 2 weeks to address unanswered questions and determine whether progress is being made. These steps will bring closure to the evaluation, open pathways for continued communication, and facilitate the transition to solution seeking. Usually, this means the beginning of intervention and flows into the next phase of the physician and team involvement, namely, management. Each professional should provide a written report or summary for the family to use, either for their own file or to assist in management (reports are also vitally important in the therapeutic process, but the specifics of effective report writing are beyond the scope of this chapter). Management will be significantly more effective as a result of the care taken and details addressed during the interpretive conference.

Practice Issues: Coding, Billing, and Managing Managed Care

Pediatricians and their patients have long struggled with the health insurance industry regarding issues of reimbursement for clinical services in developmental-behavioral pediatrics. Claims are denied because diagnoses such as ADHD are classified as mental health disorders or are simply not covered at all. Important and highly prevalent developmental diagnoses such as specific learning disability or developmental language disorder are considered "educational." Meanwhile, practitioners are forced to take financial losses or, when appropriate, to submit neurologic diagnoses such as hypotonia or static encephalopathy. The *Diagnostic and Statistical Manual for Primary Care: Child and Adolescent Version* (*DSM-PC*) may prove to be a valuable resource in the future regarding diagnostic codes of relevance to the primary care provider.

Pediatricians also need to be familiar with *Current Procedural Terminology* (*CPT*) codes that are useful in capturing some of the complexity of medical decision making, counseling, and coordination of care that is involved in assessing and managing children with school problems. The recent American Academy of Pediatrics publication (Rappo, 1997) as well as informal networking with colleagues and discussions with managed care organizations can be very valuable to the practitioner. There is extraordinary variability among payors in their "reasonable and customary" payments for specific *CPT* code payments, and extremely low discounted reimbursement is not unusual in a managed care environment. In capitated managed care, there are obvious financial disincentives for the primary care pediatrician to conduct developmental assessments or to refer children with school problems to colleagues with special expertise in this field.

Despite these hurdles, there are many successful models of community-based practice and growing numbers of pediatricians who provide exemplary service to school-aged children and their families. It can be done, it should be done, and we hope this chapter provides some guidance about how to do this exceptionally gratifying work well.

REFERENCES

Achenbach TM: Manual for the Child Behavior Checklist and 1991 Child Behavior Profile. Burlington, VT, University of Vermont Department of Psychiatry, 1991.

Baren M, Swanson JM: How not to diagnose ADHD. Contemp Pediatrics 13:53, 1996.

Brown FR, Aylward EH, Keogh BK: Diagnosis and Management of Learning Disabilities: An Interdisciplinary Lifespan Approach. San Diego, CA, Singular Publishing, 1996.

Conners CK: Conners Parent Symptom Questionnaire and Teacher Questionnaires. Psychopharmacol Bull 21:816, 1985.

Denckla MB, Rudel RG: Anomalies of motor development in hyperactive boys. Ann Neurol 3:231, 1978.

Denckla MB: Revised neurological examination for subtle signs (PA-NESS-R). Psychopharmacol Bull 21:733, 1985.

Kamhi A, Catts H: Reading Disabilities: A Developmental Language Perspective. Boston, MA, College-Hill, 1989.

Kandt RS: Neurologic examination of children with learning disorders. Pediatr Clin North Am 31:297, 1984.

Levine MD: Developmental Variation and Learning Disorders. Cambridge, MA, Educators Publishing Service, 1987, pp 469–473.

Levine MD: The ANSER System: Interpreter's Guide. Cambridge, MA, Educators Publishing Service, 1980.

Levine MD, Meltzer LJ, Busch B, et al: The pediatric early elementary examination: studies of a neurodevelopmental examination for 7- to 9-year-old children. Pediatrics 71:894, 1983.

Levine MD, Rappaport L, Fenton T, et al: Neurodevelopmental readiness for adolescence: studies of an assessment instrument for 9- to 14- year-old children. J Dev Behav Pediatr 9:181, 1988.

Levine MD, Sandler AD: The Pediatric Early Elementary Examination 2. Examiner's Manual. Cambridge, MA, Educators Publishing Service, 1996a.

Levine MD, Sandler AD: The Pediatric Examination of Educational Readiness at Middle Childhood 2. Examiner's Manual, Cambridge, MA, Educators Publishing Service, 1996b.

Levine MD, Schneider EA: The Pediatric Examination of Educational Readiness. Examiner's Manual. Cambridge, MA, Educators Publishing Service, 1988.

Palmer DJ, Garner PW, Lifschitz MH, et al: An exploratory study of the structure and validity of Pediatric Examination of Educational Readiness (PEER) factors. J Dev Behav Pediatr 11:317, 1990.

Rappaport L, Levine MD, et al: Children's descriptions of their developmental dysfunctions. Am J Dis Child 137:369, 1983.

Rappo P: Proper DSM-PC use expected to level the playing field. AAP News, April, 1997.

Sandler AD, Watson TE, Footo M, et al: Neurodevelopmental study of writing disorders in middle childhood. J Dev Behav Pediatr 13:17, 1992.

Sandler AD, Hooper SR, Levine MD, et al: The Pediatric Examination of Educational readiness at Middle Childhood (PEERAMID): factor structure and criterion-related validity in a clinic-referred sample of children and adolescents. Childrens Hosp Q 5:19, 1993a.

Sandler AD, Hooper SR, Scarborough AA, et al: Adolescents talking about thinking: preliminary findings of a self-report instrument for the assessment of cognition and learning. Diagnostique 19:361, 1993b.

Sandler AD, Knudsen MW, Brown TT, Christian RM: Neurodevelopmental dysfunction among non-referred children with idiopathic megalencephaly. J Pediatr 131:320, 1997.

Shaywitz SE, Shaywitz BA, Schnell C, et al: Concurrent and predictive validity of the Yale Children's Inventory: an instrument to assess children with attention deficits and learning disabilities. Pediatrics 81:562, 1988.

Touwen B, Prechtl H: The Neurological Examination of the Child with Minor Nervous Dysfunction. Clinics in Developmental Medicine, No. 38. London, UK, MacKeith Press, 1970.

Ullman R, Sleator E, Sprague R: A new rating scale for diagnosis and monitoring of ADD children (ACTeRS). Psychopharmacol Bull 29:160, 1984.

70 Intelligence: Concepts, Theories, and Controversies*

Helen Tager-Flusberg

Spearman's model emphasized the singular nature of intelligence, which he termed *g* for general intelligence.

For Hunt, intelligence could be best defined as speed of processing.

Wechsler called intelligence "the capacity of an individual to understand the world about him and his resourcefulness to cope with its challenges."

Intelligence quotient (IQ) correlates positively with whole brain volume and negatively with the rate of cortical glucose metabolism.

According to Gardner, there are seven relatively independent intelligences—linguistic, logical-mathematical, spatial, musical, bodily-kinesthetic, interpersonal, and intrapersonal.

For over 100 years, the concept of intelligence has been at the center of debate among psychologists and educators. Controversies continue to dominate discussions about how to define intelligence, whether there are numerous independent intelligences, how culture may play a role in defining different conceptions of intelligence and influence its development, as well as the genetic and neurobiological bases of intelligent skills. Although there is still no clear agreement on these issues, recent advances have provided important new directions in both our broad understanding of the concept of intelligence and its measurement.

Historical Views of Intelligence

Sir Francis Galton, a cousin of Charles Darwin, is generally credited with first developing a scientific and theoretical interest in intelligence. He viewed intelligence as a hereditary trait that was best conceptualized in terms of energy and sensitivity to stimuli (Galton, 1883). Galton set up a laboratory in which he developed measures of intelligence designed to tap into basic sensory and information processing mechanisms, such as reaction time and sensory discrimination tasks. His ideas and examples of his intelligence measures, as well as many new ones, were introduced in the United States by James McKean Cattell. One of Cattell's students, Clark Wissler (1901), later questioned the validity of these kinds of measures, however, because they did not correlate well with each other, and until very recently this approach to intelligence, based on sensory and perceptual tests, was essentially abandoned.

A different conception of intelligence motivated the work of Alfred Binet, who developed the first comprehensive intelligence test for children in response to his commission to identify a method for differentiating students who were suspected of being mentally retarded. Thus Binet's work grew out of practical and educational, rather than a basic scientific, concern about intelligence. Based on intuitions about what constituted academic intelligence, Binet and his collaborator Simon designed a battery of tests that tapped higher mental processes (including following directions, reasoning, memory, counting). This was highly reliable and showed substantial validity in predicting academic performance (Binet and Simon, 1916). The success of Binet's work on measuring intelligence is still evident today, as the content of most current comprehensive intelligence tests (e.g., the Stanford-Binet and the Wechsler scales) can be traced to his original ideas. These conventional intelligence tests also continue to play their most significant role in the identification and classification of mental retardation and in correlating with school performance across a wide range of children. At the same time, creators of intelligence tests generally acknowledge that scores on such tests reflect not only intellectual abilities, but also motivation and adaptive personality factors (Wechsler, 1950).

Defining Intelligence

From its beginnings with Galton and Binet, no unified definition of intelligence has guided researchers or theorists in this area. Only at the most general level of conceptualizing intelligence has any agreement emerged, according to Sternberg and Detterman (1986), who summarized the views held by a wide range of contemporary theorists. The main themes emphasized by these experts included the capacity to learn from experience and to adapt to the

*Preparation of this chapter was supported by grants from the National Institute of Child Health and Human Development (RO1 HD 33470) and the National Institute on Deafness and Other Communication Disorders (RO1 DC 01234).

Table 70–1 • Lexicon of Ability Terms

Term	Definition
Constitutional (innate)	
Aptitude	A natural ability. A tendency or capacity for learning. A talent. A combination of characteristics indicative of an individual's ability to learn or develop proficiencies.
Capability	Traits conducive to efficiency and ability. The capacity for specific use or development.
Capacity	Power to receive, hold, or store. Power to accommodate problems.
Ideation	The capacity to formulate abstractions or mental images.
Individual differences	Variation of potential among members of the human species
Intellect	The power of knowing. The capacity for rational knowledge.
Potential	An existing possibility. The power to develop into actuality.
Experiential (accomplished)	
Achievement	An accomplishment. The result of an endeavor. That which an individual has learned or mastered.
Competence	Demonstrated ability, experience, or training necessary for adequate performance. Fitness.
Knowledge	The range of an individual's acquired information and intellectual understanding.
Mastery	Possession of thorough understanding. Accomplished skill or technique.
Proficiency	Thorough competence derived through training and practice.
Qualification	Fitness for employment or engagement. Meeting with standards.
Understanding	A grasp of the meaning of, the nature of, the significance of, or an explanation of something.
Mixed	
Ability	Power, skill, or resource to accomplish an objective.
Adaptive behavior	Effectiveness of degree to which an individual meets standards of personal independence and social responsibility.
Attention	Alerting to or orienting toward. Focus on relevant information. Ability to sustain selective focus.
Cognition	The process of knowing, involving both awareness and judgment.
Comparison	Identifying relative features and values.
Comprehension	Mental grasp, apprehension, or full understanding.
Conceptualization	Mental operations of processing. Formulations or organization of observations or relationships.
Intelligence	The general capacity to use or exercise the intellect. "The capacity of an individual to understand the world about him and his resourcefulness to cope with its challenges" (D. Wechsler, 1975).
Problem solving	Means of resolving issues or seeking solution to a presented task.
Reasoning	The process of consecutive logical thinking. The drawing of inferences and conclusions.
Skill	Effective performance or execution of a task.
Thinking	Rational ordering. The processing of ideas. The internal conversation.

Data from Cushna B: Intelligence and its measurement. *In* Levine MD, Carey WB, Crocker AC (eds): Developmental-Behavioral Pediatrics, 2nd ed. Philadelphia, WB Saunders, 1992, pp 633–637.

environment and metacognitive abilities—understanding and controlling one's own problem solving, reasoning, or decision making. At the same time, more than two dozen additional attributes were mentioned (such as learning, reasoning, speed of processing, elementary attentional and perceptual abilities), but no consensus about their significance was reached.

Why is there no general agreement about how to define intelligence? Differences among theorists can be traced to several complex questions that can be raised in the way intelligence is conceptualized, both intuitively and empirically. First, should a definition of intelligence be limited to a construct that defines individual differences, or should it also reflect universal and relatively invariant human capacities? The majority of theorists focus their definition on individual differences, not including highly abstract and universal cognitive abilities, such the capacity to speak and comprehend complex grammatical sentences, as markers of intelligence. Second, should intelligence be conceptualized as a basic low-level capacity, as Galton did, or are higher-level capacities fundamental to its definition, as Binet argued? Third, to what extent should a definition of intelligence be limited to what is measured on intelligence tests? Limiting the definition in this way reduces intelligence to a construct that is isomorphic with academic performance. Broader conceptions of intelligence might incorporate developmental changes in knowledge and

thinking, cultural variation, and current ideas from the cognitive and neurosciences. Many terms are used by both researchers and theorists to refer to different types of ability, as shown in Table 70–1.

As various models of intelligence are reviewed in the next section, examples of how different approaches to these questions influence theories and definitions of intelligence will be more clearly illustrated.

Theoretical Models of Intelligence

Theories or models of intelligence can be classified into four main groupings: psychometric, computational, biological, and complex systems approaches.

PSYCHOMETRIC MODELS

Psychometric models of intelligence are generally concerned with the structure and organization of mental abilities. They focus on conceptions of intelligence that depend exclusively on the basis of intelligence tests as measures of individual differences, and the models are derived from statistical manipulations of scores obtained within and across IQ tests. Spearman (1927), who is credited with being the inventor of factor analysis, the major statistical

Table 70–2 • Concepts of Intelligence in Psychometric Models

Theorist	Concept	Definition
Spearman	*g*	General intelligence—a single factor that explains performance on all tests
	s	Specific factors that are involved on single tests of mental ability, e.g., arithmetic computation
Thurstone	Primary mental abilities	Seven factors which together define intelligence
	Verbal comprehension	Measured on vocabulary tests, e.g., defining the meaning of a word
	Verbal fluency	Ability to provide verbal responses in a limited time, e.g., say as many words as possible beginning with B in 1 minute.
	Inductive reasoning	Ability to solve analogy or completion tests, e.g., doctor: patient; teacher: [school; student; class]
	Spatial visualization	Measured on tests requiring mental rotation of pictures or letters
	Number	Arithmetic computations and problem-solving ability
	Memory	The ability to recall strings of words or pictures
	Perceptual speed	Measured on tests such as finding the difference between two highly similar pictures
Guilford	Structure of intellect	Three-dimensional model of intelligence composed of at least 120 factors
	Operations	Simple mental processes, e.g., cognition, memory, or evaluation
	Contents	Terms that appear in problems, e.g., words, numbers, sound, pictures
	Products	Kinds of responses required, e.g., single words or numbers, classes, relations
Cattell	Fluid intelligence	Requires understanding of abstract relations as in tests of inductive reasoning, analogies; or series completion tests
	Crystallized intelligence	Established knowledge as measured on vocabulary or information tests

method used by psychometric theories, initiated this approach (Table 70–2).

Spearman's model emphasized the singular nature of intelligence, which he termed *g* for general intelligence. Although individuals' scores across a number of subtests of an intelligence battery may differ, one still finds positive correlations across subtests. At a technical level, *g* represents the first principal component of a factor analysis of subtest scores, accounting for the common variance among the subtests. For Spearman, *g* was the essence of intelligence—a single attribute, which he thought of as a kind of mental energy. Despite years of debate and controversy about what *g* might represent, it is a statistical reality that is obtained from different populations with both high and low levels of intelligence. At the same time, *g* accounts for only a portion of the variance across subtests; the residual variance remaining on each subtest was termed *s* by Spearman, to represent additional specific factors of intelligence, such as spatial or verbal ability, but these were of only incidental interest to him.

Other researchers in the psychometric tradition criticized the reductionist approach to intelligence, represented by Spearman's emphasis on *g*. For Thurstone (1938), intelligence was best captured by a set of primary mental abilities, seven factors that included verbal comprehension, verbal fluency, inductive reasoning, spatial visualization, number, memory, and perceptual speed. The proliferation of primary factors of intelligence reached its peak in Guilford's (1967) model, which included 120 factors of the mind organized in a three-dimensional model of operations (mental processes, such as memory), contents (terms in a problem, such as words or numbers), and products (kinds of responses, such as single words or relations).

Cattell (1971) took an alternative psychometric approach, emphasizing the hierarchical structure of intelligence. In his model and others based on it (e.g., Vernon, 1971), general intelligence consists of two fundamental types of ability: fluid intelligence and crystallized intelligence. Fluid intelligence is defined as the understanding of abstract and sometimes novel relations that do not depend on particular content. It is best measured on analogy problems or series completion tasks. Crystallized intelligence reflects accumulated knowledge and well-established problem-solving procedures, as measured on tests of vocabulary or general information. In a hierarchical model, there may be further subdivisions within each of these main types of intelligence. This distinction between fluid and crystallized intelligence is now well-established, although the idea that tests of fluid intelligence may be purer measures of intelligence because they do not reflect social variables such as schooling or home environment (as argued by Jensen, 1980, for example) has been seriously challenged (Ceci, Baker-Sennett, and Bronfenbrenner, 1994).

Although psychometric models dominate the field of intelligence, they have not gone uncriticized. These models limit their definition of intelligence to what is measured on an intelligence test, and the emphasis is on the end product, or test scores, rather than on the mental processes that underlie performance on the tests. Ceci and colleagues (1994) point out that this approach cannot capture contextual influences on intelligence. In other words, the same skill operates with differential effectiveness as a function of the social or physical context, which cannot be captured in a static psychometric instrument. Finally, the reliance on statistical manipulation of test scores for deriving a model of intelligence is subject to methodologic debate and criticism, which means that the model is likely to change depending on which test and subtests are put into the analysis.

COMPUTATIONAL MODELS

What kinds of cognitive processes underlie intelligent behavior? This is the kind of question that motivates computational models, which focus on the information processing requirements of performance on tests of intelligence. These models draw on current research and theory in the cognitive sciences, extending beyond the intelligence test.

Hunt (1978) was the first to introduce a computational approach to intelligence. For Hunt, intelligence could best be defined as speed of processing. In support of his view, Hunt reported significant positive correlations between scores on intelligence tests and purer measures of processing speed, such as the time taken to match letters presented in different fonts, or in upper and lower case (e.g., A, a).

Sternberg (1982) analyzed the set of mental processes that were needed to perform on conventional intelligence tests into three basic components: encoding the problem, inferring and mapping relations among terms in the problem, and then applying them to new situations. He found that people who scored higher on intelligence tests took longer at the encoding or planning stage but less time on later stages in the computational process. While these kinds of models provide a useful approach to understanding the cognitive processes underlying intelligence, they do not say much about the structure and organization of intelligent abilities.

PHYSIOLOGIC MODELS

In recent years, with the explosion of research in the neurosciences, there has been a parallel growth of interest in exploring neurophysiologic correlates of intelligence (Vernon, 1993). These newer models have their roots in the ideas initially proposed by Galton and Spearman, but they did not have the means to investigate differences in the brains of individuals varying in intelligence. Current research on physiologic models rests on the assumption that there is some single general measure of intelligence, which is operationalized either as full-scale IQ score or as g.

For example, Jensen (1991) speculated that g represents a common underlying biological resource pool, specifically, the speed and oscillation of central nerve conductance. Some evidence for this comes from studies showing that full-scale IQ correlates significantly with speed of peripheral neural conduction (Vernon and Mori, 1992), as well as with cortical evoked potential measures (Matarazzo, 1994). Other studies have found that IQ correlates positively with whole brain volume (Willerman et al, 1991) and negatively with the rate of cortical glucose metabolism, as measured by positron emission tomography (Haier et al,

1988). This latter finding suggests that people with higher IQ scores may be using their brains more efficiently, as reflected in lower consumption of cortical glucose.

While these findings are intriguing, it is important to note that the magnitude of the correlations obtained between IQ and these various physiologic measures are relatively modest, generally accounting for less than one quarter of the variance. They also do not provide a theoretical model that might account for how and why brains of more intelligent people might be related to higher levels of g.

Deutsch (1998) recently speculated that g could be derived from both genetic and prenatal environmental factors that influence brain development. Such factors could have widespread effects on fetal brain maturation. To account for evidence of both general and specific abilities in intellectual functioning, Deutsch has proposed a dynamic systems approach to brain function and development. Individual neural networks subserve specific functions in problem solving, but the local interactions among these networks give rise to an emergent global structure that represents g. Deutsch's proposals have intuitive appeal and are solidly based on current models in computational neuroscience; it remains to be seen how they can be empirically tested.

COMPLEX SYSTEMS MODELS

The final set of models of intelligence to be considered here views intelligence as a complex system, rather than a single entity as captured by g. These kinds of models take a broader view of intelligence, not limiting it to what is captured on conventional intelligence tests. The models have greater intuitive appeal than the more objective psychometric models and are grounded in theories derived from cognitive science (Table 70–3).

The best known systems theory is Gardner's (1983) theory of multiple intelligences. Gardner based his theory primarily on neuropsychological evidence from adults suffering brain damage and individuals with exceptional talents, as well as evidence from developmental psychology and evolutionary biology. According to Gardner, there are seven relatively independent intelligences. These are linguistic, logical-mathematical, spatial, musical, bodily-kinesthetic, interpersonal, and intrapersonal intelligences. Each of these intelligences is a separate system of functioning,

Table 70–3 • Concepts of Intelligences in System Models

Theorist	Concept	Definition
Gardner	Linguistic intelligence	Related to all language-based performance, e.g., writing a poem, reading
	Logical-mathematic intelligence	Related to mathematic, arithmetic, and logical problem-solving abilities, e.g., balancing a checkbook
	Spatial intelligence	Related to visual-spatial problem solving, e.g., map reading
	Musical intelligence	Related to all musical performances, e.g., playing violin
	Bodily-kinesthetic intelligence	Related to all physical and athletic intelligence performance, e.g., playing basketball
	Interpersonal intelligence	Related to interactions with other people and interpreting others' behavior, motives, desires, and so on.
	Intrapersonal intelligence	Related to understanding ourselves, personal insight
Sternberg	Analytic intelligence	Solving problems using strategies that manipulate elements of the problem, e.g., comparing, evaluating
	Creative intelligence	Solving new kinds of problems that require novel solutions, e.g., designing, inventing
	Practical intelligence	Solving problems in everyday contexts by applying and using existing knowledge

although they can interact to produce intelligent behavior. Gardner criticizes conventional intelligence tests because they capture only the first three of these intelligence systems.

Sternberg (1985) has proposed a triarchic theory of intelligence composed of analytical or componential intelligence, which is tapped by intelligence tests; creative intelligence, which is concerned with combining experiences in novel ways; and practical intelligence, which is concerned with how to manipulate and adjust to the environment in everyday contexts. Sternberg emphasizes how these systems work together in dealing with different problems in a variety of contexts.

While many view the broader conceptions of intelligence that are manifest in these complex systems models as a real advance with important educational implications, others raise the concern that they may be too unconstrained, not allowing for rigorous empirical testing. Neisser and colleagues (1996), for example, suggest that some of the intelligences in Gardner's theory are more appropriately designated simply as special talents.

Intelligence and Cognitive Development

Across all the perspectives on intelligence that have been reviewed here, intelligence is primarily defined in terms of individual differences. No serious consideration is given to developmental changes in either the structural organization or processes involved in intellectual performance. One reason for this is that most models depend to a greater or lesser extent on IQ scores, which, because they are derived statistically as either a ratio or deviation score, do not vary with age. IQ scores as measures of individual differences are generally quite stable across the normal life span. At the same time, however, cognitive abilities clearly change and increase with age, as captured by the construct of mental age, or age-equivalent score. These changes in cognitive abilities have been the focus of research in the field of cognitive development, in which the internal psychological processes that underlie cognitive test performance are investigated. Such processes include the nature of mental representation, that is, the structure and organization of knowledge, which has been the focus of much of Piaget's research and theory. In addition, cognitive developmentalists address the issues of changes in processing capacity and efficiency (e.g., Case, 1985), the use of control processes such as planning, and the influence of social context (Vygotsky, 1962). A richer, more complex, and less quantitatively oriented view of intelligence would result from incorporating knowledge about developmental changes in cognitive abilities into conceptions of intelligence (Ceci et al, 1994).

Anderson (1992) proposed the first integrated view of intelligence, in which he incorporates both individual differences and developmental change in a unified model. He argues that intelligence encompasses both a low level capacity such as biological speed or efficiency and higher level knowledge-based systems. In his model, Anderson posits three types of mechanisms: (1) a basic processing mechanism that is low level and content free and does not

undergo developmental change; (2) two specific processors, one for verbal-propositional processing, and one for visual-spatial processing; and (3) a set of specialized modules that are complex mechanisms providing evolutionarily prescribed encapsulated information such as syntactic knowledge or the perception of a three-dimensional stable environment. There are individual differences in both the basic processing mechanism and the specific processors, but the specialized modules contain invariant universal information. Developmental changes are explained by changes in both the modules and the specific processors but are constrained by the basic processing mechanism.

Anderson (1992) has marshalled evidence for his model from a variety of sources, including normal and atypical developmental patterns and performance by adults on a range of experimental tasks as well as standard tests of intelligence. The strength of his theory lies in its attempt to encompass a broad definition of intelligence that draws on the psychometric, developmental, and cognitive traditions. Questions remain about how the three types of mechanisms interact and what might constitute a specialized module, but clearly the future of theories in the field of intelligence will need to take the comprehensive approach that his work exemplifies.

Factors Influencing Individual Differences in Intelligence

It is no longer useful to engage in a debate about whether genes or the environment exert the more significant influence on intelligence. There is now ample evidence supporting the important roles played by both, although there is still considerable discussion about how to best conceptualize the ways in which genes interact with specific aspects of the environment and variations in experience.

GENETIC FACTORS

Research on genetic influences relies exclusively on performance on intelligence tests, which are typically used in behavioral genetics studies to provide estimates of the heritability of g, or general intelligence. Heritability is a technical construct that refers to the percentage of variation of a particular trait, in this case g, among individuals within a population that is associated with purely genetic differences among those individuals.

Heritability estimates can be derived from studies of monozygotic twins, who have the identical genetic material, but who were reared apart and thus had not enjoyed shared environments or experiences. An alternative approach is to compare monozygotic twins with dizygotic twins, who share similar environments but on average have only half their genes in common. It is widely accepted that heritability estimates for general intelligence range between 0.45 and 0.75, suggesting that about 50% of the variance of IQ scores can be explained by genetic factors. One interesting finding is that heritability estimates increase with age, which is at first blush quite counterintuitive (Neisser et al, 1996). This may be because as children get older their transactions with the environment are increasingly influenced by their own characteristics that they bring to it, rather than by others such as parents.

Studies of genetic influences on intelligence have now moved beyond demonstrating their existence toward identifying some of the specific genes that may be responsible for its heritability, using the power of new molecular genetic technology. (Plomin et al, 1994). This research is complex and challenging because genetic influences on intelligence seem likely to involve multiple genes of varying effect size, which have been called quantitative trait loci, or QTL. Some progress in identifying QTL for intelligence is now being made by a number of different research groups (Plomin et al, 1994).

ENVIRONMENTAL FACTORS

From the moment of conception, phenotypes are influenced by the interactions between the genotype and a wide range of environmental effects. These can be divided into two categories: biological and social. It is well known that prenatal and postnatal exposures to poor nutrition, lead, and alcohol, for example, can have measurable effects on intelligence scores, as they influence brain development. Furthermore, perinatal factors, such as oxygen deprivation, are also associated with poorer cognitive outcome. Social-environmental influences on intelligence scores have also been widely documented. Thus, IQ scores are significantly correlated with family and home variables, social and parental occupational factors, schooling, and specific intervention programs, such as Head Start (see Neisser et al, 1996, for a review).

GENE-ENVIRONMENT INTERACTIONS

The Nature-Nurture debates are over for now, but differences remain among researchers in how they conceptualize the interactions between genetic and environmental influences on intelligence. Some emphasize a more biological perspective, arguing that the environment exerts its influence as a result of genetically determined factors; that is, the environment itself is genetically loaded (Scarr, 1992). Other more balanced interactionists may view biology as a set of genetically constrained cognitive potentials that are influenced and shaped as they develop in the context of specific experiences.

A more complex and ambitious interactionist model that has a clear developmental focus has been proposed by Bronfenbrenner and Ceci (1993), which they call a bioecologic view. They hold that intelligence is a multiple resource system that is only imperfectly gauged by intelligence tests. From the beginning, biology and experience are interwoven, but their relationship continually changes; with each change new possibilities are set in motion until even small changes may lead to cascading effects over the course of development. Environmental influences are specific to each type of cognitive resource or potential, both in timing of onset and in rate of development. The genetic influences may be limited to cognitive traits but could also include temperamental and motivational variables that exert an influence on measured intelligence (Ackerman & Heggestad, 1997).

Changes in Intelligence Scores Across Generations

One of the recurring themes in this chapter has been the relative weight given to conventional intelligence tests in our conceptions, theoretical models, and empiric research on intelligence. Despite the controversies that remain regarding the overreliance on intelligence tests, the fact remains that these tests are reliable and valid measures. In particular, research on the role of genetic and environmental variables on intelligence has depended exclusively on intelligence test scores, as discussed in the previous section.

Yet it is still not entirely clear what these tests actually measure. One of most intriguing findings in studies of IQ is the gradual increase in test scores that has taken place over the past several decades, not only in this country but in many nations around the world (Flynn, 1987). This increase, amounting to about three IQ points per decade, not only has been found on verbally loaded tests, but is especially apparent on nonverbal tests that tap primarily fluid intelligence, such as the Raven's Progressive Matrices. The so-called Flynn effect remains poorly understood, although a number of hypotheses have been proposed to explain why IQ scores are on the increase (Neisser et al, 1996). One possibility is that the increase in IQ reflects the increase in the complexity of our culture. A second proposal is that it reflects increases in nutritional status, which has also led to significant gains in height in many populations. Flynn (1987) and others speculate that abstract problem-solving ability has increased, rather than changes in *g*, or underlying processing efficiency, although this claim raises many questions about how intelligence has been conceptualized, even within the psychometric tradition.

Perhaps the most significant lesson to be learned from the Flynn effect is that intelligence, as measured by standard tests, does change over time; that IQ scores are not immutable either within an individual or across populations. Standard tests of intelligence remain the single best tool for predicting academic performance in children and in identifying learning disabilities or mental retardation. At the same time, there is a clear need to develop further instruments that will measure intelligence in a broader way and that can capture the dynamic developmental processes that underlie cognitive performance across many domains of functioning.

REFERENCES

Ackerman PL, Heggestad ED: Intelligence, personality, and interests: evidence for overlapping traits. Psychol Bull 121:219, 1997.

Anderson M: Intelligence and Development: A Cognitive Theory. Oxford, UK, Blackwell, 1992.

Binet A, Simon T; Kite ES (trans): The Development of Intelligence in Children. Baltimore, Williams and Wilkins, 1916.

Bronfenbrenner U, Ceci SJ: Heredity, environment, and the question "how"? A first approximation. *In* Plomin R, McLearn G (eds): Nature, Nurture, and Psychology. Washington, DC, American Psychological Association, 1993.

Case R: Intellectual Development: Birth to Adulthood. New York, Academic Press, 1985.

Cattell RB: Abilities: Their Structure, Growth, and Action. Boston, Houghton Mifflin, 1971.

Ceci SJ, Baker-Sennett JG, Bronfenbrenner U: Psychometric and everyday intelligence: synonyms, antonyms and anonyms. *In* Rutter M, Hay DF (eds): Development Through Life: A Handbook for Clinicians. Oxford, Blackwell, 1994.

Deutsch CK: Emergent properties of brain function and development. *In* Soraci S, McIlvane WJ (eds): Perspectives on Functional Processes in Intellectual Functioning. Norwood, NJ, Ablex, 1998.

Flynn JR: Massive IQ gains in fourteen nations: what IQ tests really measure. Psychol Bull 101:171, 1987.

Galton F: Inquiry Into Human Faculty and Its Development. London, Macmillan, 1883.

Gardner H: Frames of Mind: The Theory of Multiple Intelligences. New York, Basic Books, 1983.

Guilford JP: The Nature of Human Intelligence. New York, McGraw-Hill, 1967.

Haier RJ, Siegel B, Nuechterlein K, et al: Cortical glucose metabolic rate correlates with reasoning and attention studied with positron emission tomography. Intelligence 12:199, 1988.

Hunt EB: Mechanics of verbal ability. Psychol Rev. 85:109, 1978.

Jensen AR: Bias in Mental Testing. New York, Free Press, 1980.

Jensen AR: General mental ability: from psychometrics to biology. Diagnostique 16:134, 1991.

Matarazzo JD: Biological measures of intelligence. *In* Sternberg RJ, Ceci SJ, Horn J, et al (eds): Encyclopedia of Human Intelligence. New York: Macmillan, 1994.

Neisser U, et al: Intelligence: known and unknowns. Am Psychologist 51:77, 1996.

Plomin R, McLearn GE, Smith DL, et al: DNA markers associated with high versus low IQ: the IQ quantitative trait loci (QTL) project. Behav Genet 24:107, 1994.

Scarr S: Developmental theories for the 1990s: development and individual differences. Child Devel 63:1, 1992.

Spearman C: The Abilities of Man. New York, Macmillan, 1927.

Sternberg, RJ (ed): Handbook of Human Intelligence. New York, Cambridge University Press, 1982.

Sternberg RJ: Beyond IQ: A Triarchic Theory of Human Intelligence. New York, Cambridge University Press, 1985.

Sternberg RJ, Detterman, DK (eds): What is Intelligence? Contemporary Viewpoints on its Nature and Definition. Norwood, NJ, Ablex, 1986.

Thurstone LL: Primary Mental Abilities. Chicago, University of Chicago Press, 1938.

Vernon PE: The Structure of Human Abilities. London, Methuen, 1971.

Vernon PE (ed): Biological Approaches to the Study of Human Intelligence. Norwood, NJ, Ablex, 1993.

Vernon PE, Mori M: Intelligence, reaction times, and peripheral nerve conduction velocity. Intelligence 16:273, 1992.

Vygotsky L: Thought and Language. Cambridge, MA, MIT Press, 1962.

Wechsler D: Cognitive, connative, and non-intellective intelligence. Am Psychologist 5:78, 1950.

Willerman L, Schultz R, Rutledge J, Bigler E: In vivo brain size and intelligence. Intelligence 15:223, 1991.

Wissler C: The correlation of mental and physical tests. Psychol Rev Mon Suppl 3 (6), 1901.

71 Educational Assessment

Martha S. Reed

Commonly used educational tests include the Woodcock-Johnson Psychoeducational Battery–Revised, the Kaufman Test of Educational Achievement, the Peabody Individual Achievement Test–Revised, the Wechsler Individual Achievement Test, the Woodcock Reading Mastery Tests–Revised, the Test of Written Language–3, and the Key Math Diagnostic Test–Revised. However, sole use of these tests for diagnosis and instructional planning has serious drawbacks.

Curriculum-based assessment evaluates student performance and educational needs using those materials being employed for instruction. Tests may be designed by individual teachers, school systems, or developers of commercial instructional programs such as reading series.

Portfolio assessment involves evaluation of student performance and development through collected work samples.

Academic performance is the benchmark by which both student and school competence is measured, and almost every child of school age undergoes some type of formal academic testing in addition to regular class quizzes, tests, and examinations. There are six basic rationales for educational assessment: (1) measurement of group academic achievement level as an indicator of program effectiveness and teacher and school accountability; (2) measurement of individual achievement status and academic progress; (3) screening of children perceived to be at risk for learning problems; (4) determination of eligibility for special education services and placement decisions; (5) diagnosis of specific learning difficulties; and 6) instructional planning. Somewhat different testing procedures are employed for each purpose; however, all traditional practice typically involves some use of formal educational measures. Formal testing usually refers to the use of norm-referenced instruments with standardized procedures for administration and scoring. Formal tests fall into two broad categories: group administered and individually administered. Within each category are survey tests that assess academic achievement across several skill domains and those that are limited to a specific performance area, such as reading, writing, spelling, or mathematics. Table 71–1 lists many of the tests most frequently used, their age or grade ranges, and content coverage.

Accountability and academic progress are commonly measured by performance on group achievement tests, such as the California or Stanford Achievement Tests, that are administered at regular intervals, usually every 1 to 3 years. Achievement testing can also act as a screening mechanism for identification of students who are failing to make satisfactory academic progress and warrant further individual evaluation for eligibility and diagnostic purposes. Eligibility for special education services is determined by various formulas that indicate a significant discrepancy between learning aptitude, commonly defined as cognitive ability or intelligence quotient (IQ), and actual achievement. Eligibility criteria for special education services are set by individual states and vary widely. Some states use discrepancies based on age norms and others on grade level performance, and degrees of difference connoting a *significant* discrepancy differ, but all require individually administered, standardized measures of cognitive ability and academic achievement. The Wechsler Intelligence Scales (WPPSI-R, preschool; WISC-III, ages 6 to 16; and WAIS-R, adult) are the most frequently used measures of cognitive ability. Commonly used educational tests for this purpose include the Woodcock-Johnson Psychoeducational Battery–Revised, the Kaufman Test of Educational Achievement (K-TEA), the Peabody Individual Achievement Test–Revised (PIAT-R), the Wechsler Individual Achievement Test (WIAT), the Woodcock Reading Mastery Tests–Revised, the Test of Written Language–3, and the Key Math Diagnostic Arithmetic Test–Revised. Often, partly for the sake of efficiency, educational diagnosticians rely on these same individual, standardized tests for purposes of diagnosing the nature of specific learning problems and formulating instructional plans. Careful analysis of individual performance patterns can yield helpful diagnostic information. However, the sole use of these tests for diagnosis and instructional planning has serious drawbacks.

Weaknesses of Traditional Assessment Practices

Review of current literature reveals growing dissatisfaction with commonly used standardized methods of assessing academic progress and diagnosing learning problems (Algozzine and Ysseldyke, 1986; Goetz, Hall, and Fetsco, 1990; Hambleton and Jurgensen, 1990; Harvard Education Letter, 1988). School requirements for regular standardized group testing to measure group and individual achievement

Table 71–1 • Commonly Used Assessment Instruments

Test	Age (years) or Grade	Skill Areas
Group Achievement		
California Achievement Test	K–12	Word analysis, vocabulary, reading comprehension, spelling, language mechanics, language expression, mathematics computation, mathematics applications, science, social studies
Comprehensive Test of Basic Skills	K–12	Alphabet knowledge, word analysis, vocabulary, reading comprehension, language mechanics, language expression, spelling, mathematics computation, mathematics concepts and problem solving, science, social studies
Educational Records Bureau	K–12	Word analysis, vocabulary, reading comprehension, spelling, language mechanics, language expression, mathematics computation, mathematics problem solving
Iowa Test of Basic Skills	K–9	Word analysis, vocabulary, reading comprehension, language mechanics, spelling, mathematics computation, mathematics applications and concepts, science, social studies, listening
Metropolitan Achievement Test	K–12	Word recognition (analysis), vocabulary, reading comprehension, mathematics concepts and problem solving, mathematics computation, prewriting/composing/editing, spelling, listening, science, social studies, research and thinking
Stanford Achievement Tests (3 levels)	K–12	Sounds and letters, word analysis, word reading, vocabulary, reading comprehension, listening, language grammar and spelling, language mechanics, language expression, mathematics concepts and applications, mathematics computation, science, social studies, study skills
Tests of Achievement and Proficiency (upper level of Iowa)	9–12	Vocabulary, reading comprehension, written expression, mathematics, information processing, science, social studies
Test of General Educational Development (high school equivalence)	age 16 and up	Reading comprehension, writing, mathematics, science, social studies

Other examples include the PSAT (Pre-Scholastic Aptitude Test), grades 9–10, SAT (Scholastic Aptitude Test), grades 11–12 for college entrance, ACT (American College Testing), grades 11–12 for college entrance, and GRE (Graduate Record Examination), graduate school entrance. These tests typically cover vocabulary, verbal reasoning (analogies), reading comprehension, mathematics computation, and mathematics problem solving.

Test	Age (years) or Grade	Skill Areas
Individual Achievement		
Diagnostic Achievement Battery–2	age 6–14	Story comprehension, characteristics, synonyms, grammatic completion, word identification, reading comprehension, writing mechanics, spelling, written composition, mathematics reasoning, mathematics computation
Diagnostic Achievement Test for Adolescents–2	age 12–19	Receptive and expressive vocabulary, receptive and expressive grammar, word identification, reading comprehension, mathematics computation, mathematics problem solving, spelling, written composition
Kaufman Test of Educational Achievement	age 6–8 or 1–12	Word identification, reading comprehension, spelling, mathematics computation, mathematics problem solving
Peabody Individual Achievement Test–Revised	age 5–18	Word identification, reading comprehension, spelling, mathematics, general information, written expression
Scholastic Abilities Test for Adults	age 16 and up	Verbal reasoning, nonverbal reasoning, quantitative reasoning, vocabulary, reading comprehension, mathematics computation, mathematics problem solving, spelling, writing mechanics, written composition
Wechsler Individual Achievement Test	age 5–19 or K–12	Word identification, reading comprehension, spelling, written composition, mathematics computation, mathematic application, listening comprehension, oral expression
Wide Range Achievement Test–3	age 5 and up	Word identification, spelling, mathematics computation
Woodcock-Johnson Psychoeducational Battery–Revised (Achievement Scale)	age 5 and up or K–12	Word identification, reading comprehension, mathematics calculation, mathematics applications, dictation, writing samples, science, social studies, humanities, word attack, vocabulary, quantitative concepts, proofing, writing fluency

levels may have serious counterproductive effects. Such testing practices may contribute to or reinforce equating test scores with ability and overemphasize competition and student comparison. Students and also parents may interpret low scores as meaning poor ability. This misconception coupled with perceived failure to keep pace in the academic race frequently results in misplaced attributions of lack of effort, declining self-esteem, and diminished student motivation for learning, ultimately placing a student at risk for school dropout and more serious social conse-

quences such as substance abuse and delinquency. Policies dictating evaluation of teaching accountability and student eligibility for special education services perpetuate the emphasis on categorization and quantification. This concern with numbers tends to augment the dangers of the labeling process and dependence on scores as a measure of ability or need. Labels can become self-fulfilling prophecies constraining the perceptions, expectations, and efforts of teachers, parents, and even students. Furthermore, labels are only gross generalities that imply a common disorder but

Table 71–1 • Commonly Used Assessment Instruments *Continued*

Test	Age (years) or Grade	Skill Areas
Domain Specific: Reading		
Formal Reading Inventory—silent and oral	age 6–19	Oral reading accuracy, oral reading comprehension, silent reading comprehension
Gates-MacGinitie Reading Tests (group or individual)—silent	K–12	Reading vocabulary, comprehension
Gates-McKillop-Horowitz Reading Diagnostic Tests—oral	1–6	Sight word recognition—timed, word identification—untimed, word attack: syllabication, sound blending, phonetics, letter identification, auditory discrimination, spelling, writing
Gray Oral Reading Test–3	age 7–19	Reading accuracy, reading comprehension
Nelson-Denny Reading Tests—silent	9–college	Reading vocabulary, reading comprehension
Slosson Oral Reading Test–Revised	age 5 and up or K–12	Word identification
Test of Reading Comprehension–Revised—silent	age 7–18	General vocabulary, syntactic similarities, comprehension, sentence sequencing, mathematics vocabulary, social studies vocabulary, science vocabulary, reading directions
Test of Early Reading Ability–2	age 3–9	Construction of meaning: awareness of print, knowledge of vocabulary relationships, discourse comprehension; knowledge of alphabet: letter naming, oral reading (letter-sound associations); conventions of written language: book handling, response to convention of print, proofreading
Watson-Glaser Critical Thinking Appraisal—silent	9–college	Inferential comprehension, deductive comprehension, evaluating arguments, drawing conclusions
Woodcock-Johnson Reading Mastery Tests–Revised—oral and silent	age 5 and up	Visual-auditory learning, letter and word identification, word comprehension, passage comprehension
Domain Specific: Writing and Spelling		
Test of Early Written Language–2	age 3–10	Transcription (copying); conventions of print: paragraphs, capitalization/punctuation, spelling, proofing; communication (writing notes, lists); creative expression; record keeping
Test of Written Language–3	age 7–18	Vocabulary, spelling, style, logical sentences, sentence combining, contextual conventions, contextual language, story construction
Test of Written Spelling–3	age 6–18	Rule governed words, irregular words
Writing Process Test	age 8–18	Written composition: development, purpose, audience, vocabulary, style, support, organization; fluency: sentence structure, grammar/usage, capitalization/punctuation, spelling
Domain Specific: Mathematics		
Key Math Diagnostic Arithmetic Test–Revised	K–8	Basic concepts: numeration, rational numbers, geometry; operations: addition, subtraction, multiplication, division, mental computation; applications: measurement, money, time, estimation, interpretation of data, problem solving
Sequential Assessment of Mathematics Inventories	K–8	Mathematics language, measurement, ordination, geometric concept, number and notation, mathematical applications, computation, word problems
Stanford Diagnostic Mathematics Test–3	2–12	Number identification, numeration, computation, applications
Test of Early Mathematics Ability–2	age 3–9	Concepts of relative magnitude; counting; knowledge of conventions (reading and writing numbers); number facts; calculation (written and mental); base-10 concepts (place value and money)
Test of Mathematics Abilities–2	age 8–18 or 3–12	Attitude toward math, vocabulary, computation, general information, story problems

subsume a wide variation in abilities, behaviors, and dysfunctions that require widely different interventions (Levine and Jordan, 1987).

Tests used to produce the labels, even those purporting to be diagnostic, contain inherent inadequacies involving content, scoring, and sensitivity. Content problems include format and skill coverage. The same techniques and task formats are used for assessing students at all grade levels, thereby failing to reflect the changes in performance expectations that occur as children progress through the grades. Yet these changes can have a profound impact on learning and academic success. Test items are highly structured and present little demand for independent generation, elaboration, organization, and integration of information. Items tend to be short and place minimal demands on sustained attention, information processing and storage

capacity, and retrieval memory. Memory demands are further reduced by the frequent use of multiple-choice formats.

Skill coverage often inadequately reflects the curriculum to which the student has been exposed and thus can yield both false negative and false positive results. A study conducted by Jenkins and Pany (1978) vividly showed how reading test scores can vary according to the test and reading series used. Freeman and colleagues (1982) found striking differences in the mathematics content covered by commonly used standardized achievement tests and concluded that "because of the profound variety in content taught in schools and content tested, significant mismatches between the content of classroom instruction and the content of a standardized test are likely" (p 50). Furthermore, tests that do not reflect the curriculum provide little information about the student's learning ability; a student cannot have failed what he or she has not been taught. In addition to lack of curriculum responsiveness, skill coverage is frequently spotty, inadequate, or both. Tests also tend to assess skills in isolation and not within the context of actual use. A student might perform adequately when attention is directed to a single element but be unable to recall and manipulate multiple elements simultaneously, such as required in written expression.

The scoring methods of standardized tests present another area of difficulty. Test scores are based on performance accuracy and the number of items completed, and might not reflect actual conceptual understanding or skill acquisition. Another problem arises from the increasing use of cluster or composite scores. A cluster or composite score lumps performance on subtests measuring specific skills into a broad domain score and thus may mask significant strengths and weaknesses in subskills. Knowledge of specific skill discrepancies not only is important in evaluating a student's eligibility for special education assistance but also is critical information for planning an appropriate intervention. Finally, the criteria for scoring in some cases are questionable. One widely disputed example is evaluating vocabulary in written expression by the use of words of seven or more letters, thereby excluding a number of sophisticated but shorter words.

Some issues concerning test sensitivity have already been touched upon: lack of responsiveness to school curriculum, to instructional goals and techniques, and to changing processing and performance demands. Also mentioned are the limited item pool for valid and reliable diagnosis and the weakness of most tests in evaluating or even eliciting use of planning and performance strategies. Test formats can be insensitive to or penalize individual learning styles. A creative, divergent thinker has little opportunity to demonstrate these abilities on short-answer or multiple-choice questions. Most diagnostic tests are untimed and thus fail to reflect rate of processing and production. Finally, a one-shot performance in a quiet, one-to-one setting can differ significantly from daily production in a classroom environment.

Alternative Evaluation Techniques

Criterion-referenced tests, curriculum-based assessment and measurement, and portfolio assessment are more recently developed methods for evaluating student performance that eliminate some, but not all, of the shortcomings of standardized achievement tests.

Criterion-referenced tests, which may be norm-referenced and commercially produced or locally developed by teachers and school systems, are designed to assess mastery of skills in very specific, well-defined domains. The term *criterion* applies to the specific skill or behavior being tested, such as addition with regrouping. Student performance is usually reported as the percent of items answered correctly, and frequently a cutoff score is established to denote mastery. Criterion-referenced tests typically include multiple items sampling the same skill and thus provide more reliable and useful information for purposes of diagnosis and instructional planning. Locally developed tests

also are more directly reflective of the curriculum being taught. Nevertheless, there are no rules governing how many test items are sufficient to measure a skill, requiring common cutoff scores across domains, or designating common standards for judging mastery. Thus, interpretation is subject to wide variability.

Curriculum-based assessment evaluates student performance and educational needs using those materials being employed for instruction (Fuchs and Fuchs, 1990). Tests may be designed by individual teachers, school systems, or developers of commercial instructional programs such as reading series. Curriculum-based assessment, being directly tied to what is being taught, can assist instructional planning in the regular classroom by indicating deficiencies on materials already covered and readiness for subsequent instruction. Nevertheless, the focus is on short-term goals and may fail to represent long-term teaching objectives, more global integration of skills and conceptual understanding, or general student progress. Also, performance indicators cannot be generalized from one set of materials to another, which can cause problems if a student changes schools or if a system adopts a new curriculum series or textbook.

Curriculum-based measurement, a variant of curriculum-based assessment, focuses on long-term instructional goals. Tests are designed to reflect the end objective, and the same test (or equivalent form) is administered at regular intervals throughout the year. Student performance is graphed to determine the amount and adequacy of progress. At the same time, student responses are analyzed to determine instructional needs. Although curriculum-based measurement is sensitive to classroom instruction, can indicate student progress toward long-term goals, and is less susceptible to content and administration variability than curriculum-based assessment, it also has short-comings. Like curriculum-based assessment, evaluation results are not readily generalized. Furthermore, there are no established guidelines regarding the subcomponents or subskills of long-term objectives that should be measured, the format for assessing them, or the rate of progress deemed satisfactory. Rate of student progress may also be highly unstable depending on the variation in the difficulty of steps toward the final goal and student variables at the different administration intervals.

Portfolio assessment is the most recent newcomer to the field of educational evaluation. Portfolio assessment involves evaluation of student performance and development through collected work samples. Decisions about what to include in portfolios are usually made by students and teachers in collaboration. In addition to reflecting "real world" performance (what is required in the classroom) and assisting in integrating assessment and instruction, a goal of portfolio assessment is to encourage students' critical thinking and self-evaluation. As yet, however, portfolio assessment is in its infancy, and there are many unanswered questions regarding its utility. The content of portfolios will differ from one subject area to another, and each tends to be evaluated in and of itself without comparison, thus preventing identification of performance patterns across the curriculum. There are no set criteria for what should be included in a portfolio, how frequently materials should be collected, what domains (skills) should be included in evaluating student performance, scoring procedures, or what constitutes satisfactory progress. The creation and evaluation of portfolios remains highly subjective, reducing the reliability and validity of interpretation, limiting generalization, and seriously confounding decision making for purposes of placement, making comparisons between students, and judging achievement levels. Even when given considerable training in methods of appraisal, raters have tended to yield highly variable evaluations of portfolios (Salvia and Ysseldyke, 1995). Finally, portfolio assessment is extremely time-consuming, especially without established guidelines for performance evaluation; although not as much an issue for teachers of self-contained classes, it places an unrealistic burden on those content-area teachers who may serve as many as 100 to 150 students per day.

Developmental, Process-Oriented Assessment: An Integrated Perspective

Learning is a complex, evolving, cumulative, and interactive process. Each child brings to school his or her own innate capabilities, temperament, and prior experiences, which continue to evolve as they act on and are acted upon by curriculum materials, different teaching styles, changing educational demands, and experiences beyond the school walls. Figure 71–1 illustrates this interactive model of learning. In addition to direct testing, a comprehensive educational evaluation needs to include examination of the student's background, educational history, daily work samples, and the school environment. Educational assessment that will lead to effective instructional planning and

management and make the goal of successful inclusion in the regular education program a reality for students with varying patterns of learning is a multifaceted process requiring integration of information from several sources. The result should be a descriptive profile of learning strengths and weaknesses from which a detailed program of intervention can be generated.

Family and developmental history may provide useful information regarding several parameters that can have an impact on learning, and the child's pediatrician can be a valuable member of the evaluation team. A review of school history and observations obtained from past and present teachers can yield extremely valuable diagnostic information, especially when direct observation of the child in the classroom is unfeasible: Does the child exhibit particular patterns of performance over time and across subject areas? Are the problems long-standing? When did they begin to emerge? Under what circumstances do they occur?

The student is another valuable source of information. Self-ratings and descriptions of abilities in subject areas, modes of processing and expressing information, teaching techniques and materials that facilitate or impede learning, methods of studying, athletic and social skills, and general areas of interest can yield clues to preferred learning styles, learning difficulties, organizational skills, and metacognitive awareness. Structured student interviews (Alley, Deshler, and Warner, 1981; Levine, 1988, 1994; Wiener, 1986) are a helpful addition to a diagnostic educational evaluation. Even simple comments made in response to questions about school or to particular test items can be diagnostically revealing.

A fine-tuned, direct examination of academic functioning is a four-dimensional process that (1) assesses specific skill acquisition and application; (2) reflects the developmental aspect of learning and changing demands on neurodevelopmental processing abilities imposed by the curriculum, teaching methods, task formats, and educational environment; (3) includes observation and analysis of behavior, error patterns, and performance strategies; and (4) incorporates student interests, affinities, and processing strengths as well as weaknesses. Tasks and materials used in the evaluation should be similar to those used in the classroom.

Assessment Parameters and Interpretation of Performance

Table 71–2 defines the basic parameters of educational assessment. Evaluation of each parameter is discussed within an evolving educational timetable, an adaptation of the stages of reading described by Chall (1983).

Stage 1 (kindergarten to first half of grade 2) is a period of skill acquisition. Emphasis is on learning the tools or codes of reading, writing, and mathematics. Learning is a bottom-up process in which content meaning is of relatively little importance. Language is redundant, vocabulary simplistic, and little new conceptual or content knowledge is imparted. The focus of assessment is on the mechanics of reading, writing, and mathematics.

In reading, emphasis is given to evaluation of decoding skills: symbol identification, knowledge and application

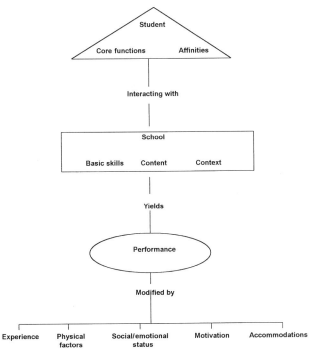

Figure 71–1. Inclusionary, interactive model of student performance.

Table 71–2 • Parameters of Educational Assessment

Reading	Writing	Mathematics	Listening	Study Skills
Word Recognition Automatic sight recognition of high-frequency words as wholes; application of word analysis skills; vocabulary **Word Analysis** Knowledge of phonology (sound-symbol associations) and morphology (structural elements: suffixes, prefixes, syllables); rule application; sound segmentation and resynthesis; vocabulary ***Oral Reading*** Rate, fluency, and expression; finger pointing and keeping place; accuracy and error patterns (e.g., omissions, substitutions); application of word analysis skills; semantic and syntactic awareness of errors; comprehension ***Silent Reading*** Rate; finger pointing; summarization (accuracy, comprehensiveness, saliency, organization, expressive fluency); response to questions (grasp of main ideas, recall of detail, inferential reasoning, vocabulary); narrative versus expository content; length of passage	***Spelling*** Recognition (multiple choice) versus retrieval (dictation); rule application; application of word analysis skills (see under Reading); error patterns (e.g., phonetically correct or incorrect, letter omissions, transpositions, impossible letter combinations) ***Alphabet Writing*** Knowledge of letter sequence and formations (manuscript and cursive); automaticity; reversals ***Copying*** Visual-motor integration with reduced memory: rate; accuracy (omissions, additions); spatial organization; legibility; handwriting; proofreading ***Sentence Dictation*** Memory of content; spelling; application of writing mechanics; handwriting; proofreading; awareness of semantic and syntactic integrity ***Proofreading*** Recognition and correction of errors in spelling and writing mechanics: punctuation, capitalization, word usage, syntax, sentence structure; rule knowledge and application ***Written Summary*** Recall and organization of salient information; spelling; mechanics; handwriting; proofreading; rate of production; synchrony of subskills ***Composition*** Ideational fluency, elaboration and organization; vocabulary; spelling; writing mechanics; syntactic maturity; usage; proofreading; rate of production; synchrony of subskills ***Handwriting*** Pencil grasp, pressure and control; motor planning; fluency; rate; legibility; automaticity	***Basic Concepts*** Symbol recognition; counting; one-to-one correspondence; symbol quantity associations; number sequencing; forming numbers; reversals; number vocabulary; clock time; money value ***Mathematical Facts*** Automaticity and accuracy of recall; use of concrete counting strategies ***Basic Computation*** Addition, subtraction, multiplication, and division with whole numbers, decimals, and fractions; knowledge of correct algorithms; understanding of place value and regrouping; sequencing of steps; computational accuracy and counting strategies; alignment; attention to signs; legibility; self-monitoring ***Advanced Computation*** Understanding of fraction-decimal-percent equivalence; solving equations for unknowns; computation with signed numbers; geometric functions and proofs; square roots; trigonometric functions; understanding of technical vocabulary; abstract, nonverbal reasoning ***Word Problems*** Understanding of language; identification of salient information, correct operations, and sequence of steps; equation construction; computation accuracy; self-monitoring; estimation skills; appreciation of quantitative relationships; logical reasoning, flexibility, alternative strategies	Comprehension and recall of orally presented information: sentence repetition; following directions; summarization; response to questions (see under Silent Reading)	Note taking; underlining; paraphrasing and summarizing; test preparation and taking; planning work and setting priorities; memory and performance strategies; self-monitoring and metacognition

of letter-sound associations, and sight word recognition. Pervasive deficits can denote an underlying weakness in association memory. Problems that are specific to appreciation and discrimination of letter-sound associations are suggestive of language difficulties, and examination of early language development could provide clarification. Confusions of letters that are similar in general form (b, d, p, and q; m and w; n, h, and u) are not uncommon. In most cases, these confusions do not represent a visual-perceptual problem and more usually reflect lack of visual attention, impulsiveness, weak spatial appreciation, or perhaps weakness in retrieval memory. Visual discrimination can easily be assessed by placing an array of the confused letters before the child and asking him or her to identify similarity or difference.

Most reading is oral, and the focus is on decoding accuracy. Typically at this stage, children rely heavily on sight recognition in reading, and errors tend to be substitutions based on whole word configuration or prominent visual elements. Therefore it is advisable to assess phonic knowledge separately. Frequent loss of place, however, may reflect problems with visual attention, spatial awareness, or sequencing. At this stage, reading tends to be slow and hesitant, but a noticeable lack of expression may signal underlying language difficulties. Reading comprehension is relatively undemanding. Words and sentences are simple and repetitive, the subject matter is familiar to daily experience, and texts tend to be highly illustrated. Comprehension commonly is measured by the ability to respond to specific questions. Problems may reflect weaknesses in receptive language, retrieval memory, or active working memory. Weak decoding skills can compromise comprehension because so much attention and effort must be expended on the reading process that there is little available to process meaning. Although not customarily included at this stage, unaided retelling of reading passages can give an indication of expressive language, recall, and sequencing abilities. In analyzing a child's reading performance at this level, it is important to be familiar with the teaching methods and curriculum being used in the classroom, since this will have a significant bearing on the word analysis skills and sight vocabulary the child has acquired.

Listening skills, only sporadically included in a standard educational assessment battery, are critical to successful performance in the classroom. Rate of delivery, length, complexity of language, and volume of information are all important factors affecting the child's ability to process and retain oral information. Having the child repeat sentences of varying length and syntactic complexity provides indication of short-term retention capacity. Analysis of errors can show a child's semantic appreciation and knowledge of syntax. Asking the child to execute pencil and paper commands of increasing length and complexity yields information about processing of meaning. Assessment of listening comprehension is also a valuable supplement to evaluation of reading comprehension by distinguishing to what degree comprehension is affected by the process of reading decoding. Varying the length of the listening passage gives additional information regarding receptive language abilities, active working memory capacity, and the amount of information that can be retained and recalled.

Spelling demands, relatively limited at this level, consist largely of writing letters, single words, and short sentences from dictation. Spelling performance should be analyzed for memory of letter formations, appreciation of letter-sound associations, and accuracy in revisualizing letter sequence.

Written composition is not emphasized at this stage, although some instruction is provided in basic elements of writing mechanics: capitalization, end punctuation, and use of complete sentences. Copying and handwriting skills are given highest priority. In view of the value placed on copying and neatness of writing, assessment of pencil grasp, pencil control, and the ability to execute letter formations is very important. Correction of a dysfunctional pencil grasp is easier and more likely to be accepted in the early stages than after the child has firmly established a faulty grip. The importance of pencil grip becomes much more critical when cursive writing is introduced and writing assignments become more lengthy. Attention should also be given to regularity and efficiency in forming letters. It is important to distinguish between the child's ability to copy letters and the ability to write them from memory. Letter reversals, while still common, may signal weakness in visual-spatial memory, inattention to visual detail, or both. Copying should include near- and far-point tasks, and care should be taken to determine whether the child is able to read the material. Spacing, use of lines, letter formations, and content accuracy are important elements to examine in evaluating visual-motor integration, spatial awareness, memory, and attention capacities.

Development of mathematics computation skills and understanding quantity take place at a concrete level. Evaluation should encompass basic concepts as outlined in Table 71–2, addition and subtraction without regrouping, and solving simple word problems. Most children rely on some type of counting strategy for computation, and the accuracy and degree of abstractness of such strategies should be noted: concrete objects, marks on paper, a number line, finger counting, representative dots on numbers, and counting strategies with numbers greater than 10. Trouble with word problems that is not related to reading ability can reflect language difficulties, poor appreciation of quantity, or both. Examination of the child's performance on other language-based tasks can provide clarification.

Stage 2 (second half of grade 2 through grade 4) is a period of continuing acquisition of the basic tools of learning and of practice and consolidation of what has already been learned.

Assessment of reading and decoding abilities should include words that must be learned by sight and those that adhere to regular phonetic and morphologic rules. Analysis of error patterns can provide indication of weakness in phonologic and morphologic knowledge and rule application. Substitutions based on whole word similarity, omissions of internal elements or word endings, or both can reflect impulsiveness, overreliance on sight recognition, and weak visual attention to detail. Painful sounding-out of simple, high-frequency words is suggestive of deficits in visual recognition memory. Problems with sound segmentation and resynthesis can signal weakness in active working memory (the beginning is forgotten by the time the end is reached). Omissions of parts of words in the sounding process can indicate problems with sequencing. Reading nonsense words is an effective technique to assess mastery of word analysis skills independent of meaningful context or any specific curriculum.

Oral reading, in addition to being analyzed for patterns of decoding errors, should be evaluated for fluency and phrasing. Irregular phrasing, inattention to punctuation, or failure to recognize reading errors that do not make sense may be symptomatic of underlying language problems. Use of finger pointing or reduced accuracy in oral reading of connected discourse in comparison with identification of words in isolation can reflect erratic attention, poor visual scanning, or both. Conversely, greater accuracy in reading connected text can signal strong language abilities and strategic use of contextual cues. Vocabulary and subject matter remain similar to daily experience. Responses to comprehension questions, however, can reflect differences between recall of facts and inferential reasoning. Unaided retelling should be evaluated for saliency and selective attention, recall of information, sequencing and organization, and expressive language.

Silent reading is introduced during this period. Silent reading speed can give additional evidence of decoding efficiency. Subvocalization is not unusual at the beginning of this stage, but if still present by the end of fourth grade, it can suggest problems with attention or the need for auditory input to convey meaning. Silent reading comprehension, like oral comprehension, should be assessed through both unaided retelling and specific questions. If a child struggles with passage comprehension, reducing the length of the material can aid in distinguishing between language comprehension problems and limited storage and retrieval capacity.

Evaluation of listening skills, as already described in the section on stage 1, should continue to be included.

Writing requirements undergo greater change during this period. Cursive is introduced and imposes additional demands on fine motor control and fluency, motor planning, motor memory, and visual retrieval memory. A dysfunctional pencil grip becomes a great barrier to cursive writing speed and ease of production. Contrasting the child's ability to produce lower case letters in isolation with connected writing can assist in distinguishing between problems with memory of letter formations and motor planning. In evaluating copying, particular attention should be paid to rate and chunking strategies, as well as to accuracy. Spelling requires knowledge and application of more advanced word analysis skills, more complex segmentation of multisyllable words, and a greater revisualization capacity. Spelling errors should be analyzed for overreliance on phonetic spelling, frequency of visual approximations that are dysphonetic, impossible letter combinations, and lack of appreciation of common letter patterns. Contrasting performance on multiple-choice spelling tasks with spelling dictation is useful in distinguishing between recognition and retrieval memory abilities.

More emphasis is placed on rules of writing mechanics and written composition. Spelling and knowledge of mechanics (punctuation, capitalization, sentence structure, and word usage) should be examined both in isolation and in the context of written composition. A significant deterioration of writing skills in composition may be indicative of problems with managing multiple simultaneous memory demands. Composition at this stage is primarily narrative in style, and content should be evaluated for ideational fluency and organization.

Mathematics also encompasses a growth in the complexity of demands. Regrouping is introduced. Prior to the need for regrouping, working problems left to right has no effect on the answer, but unless detected and corrected, it will produce a serious impediment to further progress. Regrouping also presents multiple-step problems necessitating active working memory, sequencing, spatial organization, and fine motor accuracy. Place value, the conceptual underpinning of regrouping, is especially difficult for children to grasp. Often, children learn the procedural steps for regrouping through rote memorization without ever acquiring a clear understanding of place value. Confusion, however, can have far-reaching consequences as students move on in multiplication and division, fractions, decimals, percentage, and negative integers. The introduction of multiplication and division toward the end of stage 2 presents multiple-step problems of increased complexity. Furthermore, the multiplication tables, which are less amenable to concrete counting strategies, place an added stress on memory capacities. Performance in computation should be examined for faulty algorithms, confusion in the sequence of steps, fact and counting strategy inaccuracies, and attention weakness (lack of recognition of change in sign or operational inconsistencies). Word problems now need to receive greater emphasis in the assessment of mathematic abilities. If difficulties are present, first consideration should be given to the child's reading ability. Paraphrasing is a means of assessing language comprehension. Use of incorrect operations can signal problems with language, appreciation of quantity, or both. Inability to distinguish salient information can reflect weakness in receptive language, selective attention, impulsiveness, or all of these elements. Some children, although they can compute prewritten number problems, do not know how to set up equations by themselves, an indication of incomplete conceptual understanding or possibly poor spatial awareness. Multiple-choice problems provide a useful means of assessing concept understanding and quantitative appreciation in a child who exhibits problems with recall of facts, computation deficiencies, or expressive language. Estimation tasks can yield further information regarding quantitative conceptualization.

Self-monitoring of performance takes on more importance, and observations should be made regarding whether the child spontaneously checks his or her work.

Stage 3 (grades 5 through 8) is a period when academic demands change dramatically, and students with an array of mild learning dysfunctions often become overwhelmed and falter for the first time. Learning increasingly becomes a top-down process, in which the tools acquired during the early elementary years are applied for the purpose of acquiring new knowledge. The volume of material to be processed and expressed takes an enormous surge, and the tools of reading, writing, and mathematics need to have become well automatized and easily retrieved if the child is to keep up with productivity demands. Organization and study skills also become critical. Changing classes requires management of materials, class schedules, multiple assignments, and differing teacher expectations. The increased volume of homework necessitates planning and setting priorities nightly and over longer periods.

Reading becomes the avenue for most learning across the curriculum. Assessment should include automatic recognition of high-frequency words in addition to decoding of textbook vocabulary. Oral reading plays a less important role in the classroom but can be included for clarification if the student exhibits problems with silent reading rate or comprehension. The active engagement of oral reading can help focus attention, and the auditory input may facilitate comprehension. Subvocalization during silent reading can provide further evidence that auditory input is helpful.

The two most significant changes in reading occur in the volume and the nature of the content. With the increased amount of reading, rate of silent reading becomes an extremely important aspect to evaluate. Content switches from narrative to exposition, removing plot structure that may have aided comprehension and recall. New vocabulary, concepts, and information are presented so that experiential knowledge is a less effective comprehension and mnemonic aid. When problems with comprehension in content area subjects surface, it is important to assess a student's fund of knowledge on the topic. Insufficient prior knowledge has been found to be a major barrier to comprehension, especially in secondary school and college (Aaron and Baker, 1991; Chapman, 1993). The increased volume and density of new material can strain processing, storage, and retrieval capacities. Language structures become more complex, and redundancy is minimal. Children with subtle language or attention problems, or both, can have difficulty determining saliency of information. In the assessment of comprehension, it becomes more important to include summarization of reading passages; problems with selective attention, salience determination, and organization might not be evident in responses to specific questions. Assessing summarizing skills also provides a window into a student's expressive language facility. Difficulty answering questions may signal weakness in convergent memory (recall of factual detail) and, possibly, superficial processing.

Written output emerges as the primary mode through which learning is evaluated, and any impediment to effective written expression can have devastating effects on academic success. There is the need for automatic retrieval of letter formations, basic spellings, and the rules governing mechanics. All of these factors have to be integrated simultaneously and synchronized with motor and ideational fluency. Writing skills should be evaluated both in isolation and within the context of written expression. A breakdown in application of skills in composition is often evidence of problems with simultaneous recall and integration. Since a test setting is not conducive to creativity, a more valid indication of ideational and verbal fluency might be obtained from a preassigned writing task and examination of a collection of work samples. Within the context of the evaluation, having the student write a summary of a reading passage can provide indication of selective attention, organization, and application of writing mechanics. Constricted written ideation should be compared with oral expression to determine the impact of the writing process or the

presence of generalized expressive language deficiencies. Proofreading skills rise in importance at this level and warrant examination. Research has shown that teacher grading is more often based on appearance and technical accuracy of written expression than on ideational content. Since it is very difficult for a student to proofread his or her own work, especially immediately after writing, it might be more informative to give the student an "anonymous" writing sample to correct.

Automaticity and integration become keys to success in mathematics as well. Complex multiplication, long division, and computation with decimals and fractions all require that basic facts be quickly and accurately retrieved, and a simple timed test of fact recall can provide helpful information. The student must also recall and apply several procedures in the correct sequence, placing a heavy demand on active working and sequential memory. These multistep problems require correct alignment, and performance should be analyzed for visual-spatial attention and effects of fine motor problems. The introduction of fractions, decimals, and percentage necessitates a more complex conceptual understanding of computation processes, number equivalence, and place value: rote memorization of computation procedures is no longer sufficient for success. Word problems, like other reading material, become more lengthy and complex. Paraphrasing, estimation, and explanation of solutions are valuable techniques for assessing language comprehension, conceptual understanding, selective attention, and appreciation of quantity.

Study skills take on major importance and warrant inclusion in the assessment process. Much valuable information can be obtained through interviewing the student regarding study habits and strategies for report writing and test preparation. Direct assessment techniques include underlining, taking notes, outlining or summarizing a content area reading passage, and taking notes from or summarizing a listening passage. Examination of class notebooks will provide further indication of note taking and organization skills.

Stage 4 (grade 9 and beyond) is an ongoing period when previously learned skills must be used for a variety of purposes. Emphasis is on interpretation and manipulation of information. All subjects present increasing use of specialized vocabulary, and reading performance should be analyzed for word knowledge, use of context cues, and appreciation of word derivations and morphology for purposes of decoding and understanding. Evaluation of prior knowledge on a topic is essential. In addition, assessment of reading comprehension should include analysis and interpretation of different textual formats and critical evaluation of intent and bias. Reading no longer simply involves direct exposition of fact, and comprehension problems can reflect weaknesses in higher-order reasoning and in advanced linguistic appreciation (language pragmatics and figurative expression). Awareness of content organization structures, such as definition and examples, cause and effect, comparison and contrast, and temporal sequence, is a valuable addition in assessing reading comprehension skills.

Listening skills take on added importance, as a great deal of classroom instruction occurs via a lecture format. Sustained and selective attention, rapid processing, appreciation of language pragmatics, interpretation of intent, and evaluation of saliency must be executed simultaneously and translated into some form of note taking. Examination of class notes can give some indication of how effectively the student is able to manage these rapid, simultaneous demands. Within the testing process, a passage that is read or tape-recorded could be used to assess note-taking and clarify the point at which the breakdown occurs. Additionally, having the student orally summarize or dictate notes can elucidate the impact of the process of writing. Insufficient background knowledge can also have a profound impact on listening and note-taking proficiency.

Written expression becomes paramount for academic success. Writing must be used for a variety of purposes and includes different textual formats. Ideational fluency, elaboration, easy retrieval of vocabulary, and appreciation of language usage are essential. Longer writing assignments demand greater planning and organization, both of content and of time. In addition, research projects introduce new writing mechanics. A comprehensive examination of the varied and complex writing skills required for successful academic performance cannot be realistically conducted within a clinical testing session. Examination of classwork and a preassigned structured writing task, supplemented by a brief writing exercise and structured interview such as those developed by Levine (1994), Warden and Hutchinson (1992), and Wiener (1986), are more efficient and informative methods of assessing writing abilities.

Success in mathematics is heavily dependent on abstract, logical reasoning; appreciation of quantitative and spatial relationships; understanding of concepts of equivalence and proportion; and cumulative, sequential memory. It also poses a challenge for language and rapid assimilation of technical vocabulary. Geometry provides a prime example. New symbols and their meaning must be learned, placing added strain on association memory. Although signed integers require much closer attention to visual detail, basic computation skills become less critical, as access to a calculator, even during tests, is increasingly permissible. Flexible problem-solving and estimation abilities are more important aspects to evaluate. Presenting problems that have no single answer, and asking the student to estimate answers and describe his or her thought process, can provide a more effective means of assessing logical reasoning and quantitative appreciation.

Foreign language is a new addition to the curriculum. Examination of the student's history in acquisition of speech, reading, spelling, and writing skills can provide valuable insights into the nature of difficulties in learning a second language. Early difficulties in one or more of these areas, particularly phonologic skills and grammatical understanding, or generalized weakness in memory abilities, although surmounted in one's native language from constant exposure and practice, are likely to resurface and have a negative impact on learning a second language, which is taught and practiced only briefly each day. The possibility of native language interference in foreign language learning should also be explored, especially if the sound codes, prosody, and grammatical structures are dramatically different.

Efficient study skills, planning, organizational strategies, and metacognitive evaluation of one's learning and performance become even more essential. A student interview might be the most effective means of assessment, and several structured formats for this purpose have been developed (Alley, Deshler, and Warner, 1981; Levine, 1988; Wiener, 1986).

Educational Management of Learning Difficulties

Educational management of learning difficulties likewise requires a multifaceted process. To be effective and ensure successful inclusion of affected students in regular education programs, it must involve the collaborative efforts of student, parents, teachers, and often the pediatrician, especially if medication is involved. Since inconsistency, confusion, lack of communication, and disorganization often are primary problems interfering with a child's ability to meet school expectations, it is essential that these same problems not compromise the management efforts.

The descriptive performance profile developed from an integrated analysis of all the evaluation data should generate a detailed, multidimensional plan of management. A range of special education services is available for students who qualify: material and performance accommodations, consultation in the regular classroom, varying amounts of small group and individual instruction in a resource room, self-contained special class placement, specialized therapies, or a combination. Alternatives to public school services include private school programs, tutors, and therapists. Educational management typically involves some combination of direct remediation of specific skill deficits, instruction in study skills, the employment of bypass strategies, and classroom accommodations. Selection of the modes and amount of intervention depends on the student's eligibility for special education services, the severity and pervasiveness of the problem, prior remedial attempts and responsiveness, the age of the student, and patterns of learning strength and weakness. For the younger child or the child who has received no prior remedial instruction, or in cases in which the deficit is very circumscribed and skill-specific, direct remediation is usually the first course of action. Even in these cases, however, the child will benefit from some classroom modifications that will allow successful participation without risk of humiliation. For the older student who has already received remedial work, or in cases in which the learning dysfunction is so severe or pervasive that it impedes acquisition of new knowledge in several subject areas, more emphasis is given to bypass strategies that provide continued access to new concepts and information. Whether the focus is on direct remediation, accommodations, or a combination, the first step should be student demystification (explaining to the student his or her specific learning patterns). A child who understands his or her learning strengths and weaknesses will be more receptive to intervention efforts, be able to help in the process, and be able to use them to better advantage. Other general principles and techniques of remediation and accommodation that facilitate effective management follow.

PRINCIPLES OF REMEDIAL INTERVENTION

1. Intervention should begin at the point of breakdown in the learning process, thus the need for careful analysis of error patterns, student understanding of processes and underlying concepts, and performance strategies being employed. For example, the student who is good at mathematic computation but is having trouble identifying the operations necessary to solve word problems might be asked to select from a group of word problems all those that require multiplication or be asked to write word problems that involve a specified operation.

2. Methods and materials that utilize preferred learning styles, processing strengths, and interest affinities are more apt to be accepted, result in improvement, and promote maintenance and generalization of instruction. Visual learners and students with language or attention problems might grasp new concepts more effectively through graphic representation, models, demonstration, and manipulative materials. Topical magazines, comic books, television and film scripts, technical manuals, and other highly motivational material often provide a more meaningful medium for instruction in basic skills.

3. To be effective, intervention efforts need to be directly relevant to classroom demands. Skills taught in isolation without application and practice within the context of regular use are less likely to be used, maintained, and generalized.

4. Intervention efforts need to be coordinated between remedial-tutorial and regular classroom instruction so that skills and strategies are applied consistently and practiced across all subject areas. This will require close, regular contact and consultation among all teachers, tutors, and therapists. Parents also should be kept abreast of intervention goals and be involved in their support at home.

5. Teaching techniques that involve active participation by the student promote greater understanding and retention of skills and concepts and, at the same time, provide a means of monitoring mastery. Cooperative small-group learning activities, group problem-solving and critical thinking exercises, and opportunities for the student to explain or teach skills are examples.

Table 71–3 • Classroom Accommodations

Accommodation Parameter	Example
Physical arrangement: Alteration of seating and classroom furnishings to reduce distractions and facilitate student performance	Preferential seating: near to teacher, near to board, away from doors, windows, and noisy areas
	Reduce amount of bulletin board and classroom display
	Study carrel, single desk versus table
Rate adjustment: Additional time to process information, complete tasks, and demonstrate knowledge	Slowed rate of presentation with repetitions and summaries
	Extended time for tests
	Long response time to answer questions in class
Volume adjustment: Smaller amounts of information to be processed or produced	Highlighted textbooks
	Selective sampling of task items (every odd number)
	Shorter reports
Complexity adjustment: Reduced number of details, simplified language, more concrete examples and fewer abstract ideas	Simpler versions of textbooks
	Using shorter sentences and simple vocabulary to deliver information and give directions
	Illustrating concepts with examples from everyday experience
Staging: Tasks broken down into a sequence of steps or smaller segments	Previewing material prior to reading
	Answering questions while reading rather than at the end
	Writing reports in a series of steps so as to concentrate on one subcomponent at a time (ideas, planning, drafting, revising, editing for mechanics, rewriting, proofing)
Prioritizing: Emphasis only on selected components of a task	Not grading for spelling and mechanics when demonstration of knowledge is important
	Setting up the equation for solving a problem without having to perform the calculation
Format change: a. Presentation of information in modes that facilitate understanding b. Production of information in modes that facilitate demonstration of competence	Augmenting verbal delivery with visual materials (pictures, diagrams, demonstrations, video and films)
	Replacing a written report with oral presentation, graphic depiction, demonstration model
	Giving open-book and take-home tests to offset memory problems
	Allowing students to write in test booklets to replace bubblesheets
Evaluation modification: Different systems for assessing performance	Grading in stages, first for content then for mechanics
	Giving partial credit for self-correction
	Grading on display of progress toward goal, not on absolute mastery
Curriculum alternatives: Change in course requirements or sequence	Substituting literature in translation and history of a country for foreign language
	Deferring advanced mathematics courses
	Altering the sequence of science or math courses
Material supports: Devices that facilitate learning and demonstration of ability	Tape-recorded texts, reading scanners, calculators, word processors, taped lectures, notetakers, scribes, printouts of class notes

Including the student as a partner in developing the intervention plan will promote greater insight, investment, compliance, and feeling of self-worth.

6. Modeling skills, providing guided practice, and giving immediate, *constructive* feedback have been shown to increase learning. The focus of instruction should begin with what the student is already doing correctly.

7. Preteaching activities to connect new learning with prior instruction, to clarify learning objectives, and to ensure that students have a sufficient knowledge base for comprehension, building new skills, and formulating new concepts have been shown to have a significant impact on facilitating successful learning.

8. Study skills need direct teaching. All students will benefit from instruction in note-taking, planning time and setting priorities, organizing workload, critical thinking, test-taking skills, mnemonic aids, metacognitive strategies, and self-monitoring of learning.

9. Game formats can make skill drill more tolerable. Board games, flashcard games, games with dice and playing cards, word games such as Scrabble and Hangman, and computer software provide multiple possibilities (Mercer and Mercer, 1993).

10. Use of affinities and special interests can improve remediation efforts. A student is likely to become more engaged and exert greater effort and persistence when the subject matter of instructional materials holds a high personal interest.

TECHNIQUES OF ACCOMMODATION

First priority should be given to seeking ways through which the child can experience success and avoid humiliation in front of peers. Specific talents should be exploited. Accommodations and bypass strategies should be used discretely so as to prevent public notice and discrimination. They may be arranged through a private agreement between student and teacher. Often, however, these same accommodations can benefit all students at one time or another and might easily be made available to everyone upon individual request. For example, tape-recorded notes and lectures can help the student who is slow in processing information or has difficulty with sustained attention and also aid students who have to miss class for some reason.

Table 71–3 outlines basic categories of classroom accommodations and bypass strategies (Levine, 1994).

Provision of bypass strategies and accommodations should not be given freely as a matter of course but carries a cost that ensures student accountability and demonstrates respect for student integrity. If a student does fewer problems, the problems should carry heavier weight. Quality can substitute for quantity. A shorter written report might carry increased demands for graphic illustration as an accompanying model. More reading and references might be the payment for shortening the required length of a research paper. Flow charts might substitute for written explana-

tions. Reduction in the amount of reading might carry a cost of extra time spent on drill practice in word identification.

Conclusion

Learning problems do not necessarily begin with entry into school, nor do they end when the first hurdle is surmounted. Educational assessment should be viewed as an ongoing process through which a child's academic progress is closely monitored and interventions are implemented and adjusted to allow successful inclusion in regular education and enable the child to meet evolving academic expectations.

REFERENCES

Aaron PG, Baker C: Reading Disabilities in College and High School: Diagnosis and Management. Parkton, MD, York Press, 1991.

Algozzine B, Ysseldyke J: The future of the I.d. field: Screening and diagnosis. J Learning Disable 19(7):394, 1986.

Alley GR, Deshler DD, Warner MM: The Bayesian Screening Procedure for Identification of Learning Disabled Adolescents: Administration, Scoring and Interpretation. Monograph #10. University of Kansas, Institute for Research in Learning Disabilities, 1981.

Chall JS: Stages of Reading Development. New York, McGraw-Hill, 1983.

Chapman A (ed): Making Sense. Teaching Critical Reading Across the Curriculum. New York, College Board Publications, 1993.

Freeman DJ, Kuhs TM, Knappen LB, Porter AC: A closer look at standardized tests. Arithmetic Teachers 29(7):50, 1982.

Fuchs S, Fuchs D: Curriculum-based assessment. *In* Reynolds CR, Kamphaus RW (eds): Handbook of Psychological and Educational Assessment of Children: Intelligence and Achievement. New York, Guilford Press, 1990.

Goetz ET, Hall RJ, Fetsco TG: Implications of cognitive psychology for assessment of academic skill. *In* Reynolds CR, Kamphaus RW (eds): Handbook of Psychological and Educational Assessment of Children: Intelligence and Achievement. New York, Guilford Press, 1990.

Hambleton RK, Jurgensen C: Criterion-referenced assessment of school achievement. *In* Reynolds CR, Kamphaus RW (eds): Handbook of Psychological and Educational Assessment of Children: Intelligence and Achievement. New York, Guilford Press, 1990.

Harvard Education Letter: Testing: is there a right answer? 4:1, 1988.

Jenkins JR, Pany D: Standardized achievement tests: how useful for special education? Except Child 44:448, 1978.

Levine MD: Educational Care: A System for Understanding and Helping Children with Learning Problems at Home and in School. Cambridge, MA, Educators Publishing Service, 1994.

Levine MD: Survey of Teenage Readiness and Neurodevelopmental Status: STRANDS. Chapel Hill, NC, Clinical Center for the Study of Development and Learning, 1988.

Levine MD, Jordan NC: Learning disorders: assessment and management strategies. Contemp Pediatr 5:31, 1987.

Levine MD, Reed MS: Developmental Variation and Learning Disorders, 2nd ed. Cambridge, MA, Educators Publishing Service, 1998.

Mercer CD, Mercer AR: Teaching Students with Learning Problems, 4th ed. New York, Macmillan Publishing Company, 1993.

Salvia J, Ysseldyke JE: Assessment, 6th ed. Boston, Houghton Mifflin Company, 1995.

Swanson HL: Handbook on the Assessment of Learning Disabilities: Theory, Research, and Practice. Austin, TX, PRO-ED, 1991.

Warden MR, Hutchinson TA: Writing Process Test. Chicago, IL, Riverside Publishing Company, 1992.

Wiener J: Alternatives in the assessment of the LD adolescent: a learning strategies approach. Learn Disabil Focus 1:97, 1986.

72 *Psychological Testing*

Karen Levine

 Norm-referenced comparisons look at a child's performance in relation to that of other children who share a set of characteristics, usually age or grade. Intelligence tests, developmental screening tests, and personality tests are generally norm-referenced. Alternatively, criterion-referenced tests compare a child's performance to a specific, externally determined standard or progression. Achievement tests, for example, may be designed to measure whether a child has mastered a specific body of knowledge.

Many of the traditionally used language and intelligence tests in the United States have Spanish equivalents. Clearly this adaptation will not always be possible. Often, omitting testing is the best option.

The domains typically assessed on intelligence tests include different forms of memory (short-term and long-term, visual, auditory), aspects of language development, problem solving, spatial ability, and numeric reasoning.

Infant testing is extremely valuable as a route to intervention but not as a predictor of later intelligence quotient (IQ) scores.

Standardized psychological testing is a traditional tool of psychologists and educators, used for the purpose of measuring a broad range of human attributes. These include intelligence, learning profile, personality, and behavior. There are perhaps two main reasons why psychological testing has a somewhat negative perception by many non-psychologists: (1) Perhaps because of the "spirituality" of human attributes, the very attempt at their measurement can be perceived as futile at best, and as cold or inhumane at worst. How can we really quantify something as elusive and personal as, for example, "personality," and why would we even want to? (2) Psychological tests are generally very limited, concrete, and specific in what they are able to measure validly, yet they are often given great weight in their interpretation and impact. There are many different conceptualizations of intelligence, not all of which lend themselves to testing (Kai and Pellegrino, 1985). The purposes and the misuses of psychological testing are discussed subsequently.

Standardized testing has been used for a broad range of purposes. One of the original purposes was to determine eligibility for regular public school attendance. Alfred Binet was asked by the French government to develop a scale to determine which children would benefit from regular schooling and which should be placed in a specialized program (Binet and Simon, 1905). Determining eligibility for a variety of types of educational and social services continues to be a common function of psychological testing. Types of services include special education services, services for "gifted and talented" children, public funding for support for people with disabilities, mental health support services, and psychiatric hospitalization. Another common use of psychological testing is to enhance understanding of confusing or unusual developmental patterns or behavior, especially to formulate recommendations about educational or programmatic approaches best suited to a child's learning and emotional style. Additionally, a frequent use of testing is to measure the impact of various service-based interventions such as educational programs or medical treatments (e.g., removal of a brain tumor; administration of psychotropic medication).

Standardized psychological testing has many limitations. Just as a specific blood measurement tests only for a specific type of problem, each psychological test assesses only one sort of psychological dimension. Ethical and practical problems arise when results from a test are interpreted as implying something that the test does not validly assess. There have been many instances of this sort of "test abuse." For example, adults who achieve a standardized intelligence quotient (IQ) score above the number 70 (e.g., 71) are generally deemed ineligible for the array of support services for people with mental retardation, even though their everyday needs may be as substantial or more so than somebody with an IQ score of, for example, 69. Although overall IQ score generally correlates with a need for support services, it does not precisely predict this need. Other factors such as motor, behavioral, and psychiatric issues also affect level of functioning and need for support. The psychological test result, the IQ score, is often interpreted as implying level of functioning, which is not what is being measured.

Another situation in which test scores have been broadly misinterpreted as implying more than is valid is that of the educational implications of test scores of children from other than middle class white American cultural backgrounds. These children often have erroneously low scores on IQ tests (Jenson, 1980) because such measures are generally somewhat reliant on culture-specific knowledge. Their scores have been interpreted as reflecting an innate quality that denotes capacity or potential, rather than a combination of an innate quality and cultural experience. There have been several attempts to create "culture-free" intelligence tests following the studies by Kamin (1976) and others (e.g., the Leiter International Performance Scale).

Principles of Psychological Testing

The quantification of relatively difficult-to-measure attributes is a science that has evolved substantially over the past 95 years since Binet developed the first intelligence test. This science relies on several mathematic principles, including sampling, referencing, validity, and reliability.

SAMPLING

Because it is not possible to observe and record all of a child's behavior, assessment of any attribute, including intelligence, involves developing a systematic and interpretable method of "sampling" that behavior, just as a poll provides a sampling of people's opinions. There are many general techniques for sampling, including the following: observational measures such as recording what a child is doing or saying over the course of a specific interval; parent interview methods asking about a child's typical behaviors or abilities across specific circumstances; and activity-based sampling. This last approach is the one typically used in most individually administered psychological studies. Specifically, the child is asked to perform a variety of tasks measuring different types of abilities. The tasks have been determined through research to relate to a child's ability to perform a range of other related activities. The child's performance on these tasks is then considered representative of the child's abilities in specific areas. Thus the child's abilities are sampled through performance on a set of tasks that are well studied and determined to reflect a variety of known skills.

VALIDITY

Validity refers to the extent to which the test reflects what it is supposed to be testing. If one is claiming to measure mathematic ability, then the test one proposes must actually measure mathematic ability. Clearly validity is a vital component of any test. There are several ways of assessing whether tests measure what they are meant to measure.

"Face validity" refers to what a test "seems like" it measures, to the layperson. Hence "face validity" actually refers to the *perception* of validity. When this is high, that is, when a test "seems like" it would measure what it purportedly measures, this can give a test more credibility than it deserves. Teen magazines and "pop" psychology books often have personality or intelligence quizzes that appear to relate to some construct such as "ambitious personality type" although they have no support for actually measuring anything about a person other than how the person answers those specific questions. On the other hand, low face validity can arouse incredulity in response to what may be a quite valid test. For example, the high correlation

of the Fegan Test of Infant Intelligence, based on infant gaze behavior, with later intelligence test scores has received little popular attention, perhaps because of the intuitive impression that infant gaze does not seem like it could relate to something as complex as subsequent intelligence.

Predictive validity is important for most tests. This refers to whether the test is able to accurately predict future performance. Tests that affect program eligibility clearly must show high correlation with later program performance. Scholastic aptitude test (SAT) scores are used in college entrance decisions as they correlate with, or predict, college performance. The higher the predictive validity, the more useful a test is in determining eligibility.

Concurrent validity refers to whether performance on a test correlates with performance on other tasks or other tests purported to measure the same attributes. There are many methods of assessing this. Content validity is one form of concurrent validity that is subjectively assessed by examining whether the content of the test relates to the domain that is being assessed. Relatedly, construct validity, which refers to whether the items on a test that relate to a specific psychological construct are indeed correlated, can be measured statistically through factor analysis. For example, if one is developing sets of items to measure memory, including long-term and short-term visual memory, the items measuring short-term memory should covary within subjects, as should the items measuring long-term memory. Further, items measuring long-term visual memory should correlate with the child's performance on other tests established to measure long-term visual memory and should not correlate as highly with tests established to measure other constructs (e.g., long-term verbal memory). This last method, correlating items on one test with established measures of similar and different constructs, is called *criterion-related* validity.

RELIABILITY

Reliability refers to the extent to which test results are repeatable. Clearly if results vary significantly with each administration, one is not measuring a stable attribute, which is usually the intent of the tester. If one wishes to measure intelligence, or reading ability, or memory skills, one must devise a test that produces consistent results over several administrations to ensure that one is assessing a steady characteristic. Reliability over time is generally called *test-retest reliability*. The relationship between items within a test is often measured though what is called *split half* reliability, whereby the items are randomly divided in half and the scores on the two halves are correlated across many children.

Many factors influence test scores besides the key factor one is trying to measure. These may include the setting, the child's mood at that moment, the time of day, the child's previous experience or lack of experience with similar tasks, and the administration style of the psychologist. Statistically, the degree of reliability of a test can be calculated, and the lower the degree of reliability, the greater the impact of other factors. That is, when test results vary dramatically from test to retest and within the test across similar items, the test has low reliability and a large *standard error of measurement*. Every test has a standard error of measurement, which is the range of scores within which the child's performance is likely to fall, were the test administered multiple times. Traditionally this range is reported as part of a child's score, to remind the reader that the score reflects an approximation and to inform those using the test how accurate or inaccurate the test results are likely to be. This is generally reported as a score with a plus-or-minus ($+/-$) range. For example, a test report may contain the sentence "Johnny obtained a score of 67 $+/-$ 4." Test manuals contain statistical tables regarding the standard error of measurement for each score obtained within each age group.

NORM-REFERENCED AND CRITERION-REFERENCED TESTS

Once behavior has been selected to be sampled, the child's performance must be compared to some reference point to determine how the child is doing along the attribute being measured. There are two ways of doing this: norm-referenced comparisons and criterion-referenced tests. Norm-referenced comparisons compare a child's performance to the performance of other children who share a set of characteristics, usually age or grade. Sometimes the child will be compared to children who share more than one characteristic, for example, age, ethnic background, gender. In interpreting results, it is important to indicate and discuss the norming group. Intelligence tests, developmental screening tests, and personality tests are generally norm-referenced.

Alternatively, criterion-referenced tests compare the child's performance to a specific, externally determined standard or progression. Achievement tests, for example, may be designed to measure whether a child has mastered a specific body of knowledge. Tests that assess where on a set progression of stages a child is performing are also criterion-referenced.

Ethical Issues of Psychological Testing

Psychological testing involves working closely with an individual child, using complex standardized materials, interpreting results accurately, and obtaining highly personal information for appropriate use. Acknowledging each of these factors, a variety of regulations govern test administration and also the profession of psychology.

CONFIDENTIALITY

Because psychological testing reveals highly personal and private information, and also information that is subject to misuse, as discussed earlier, there are strictly enforced laws around issues of use and confidentiality. Psychological test results of children are confidential and can be accessed only by written permission of parents or guardians (Buckley Amendment: The Family Educational Rights and Privacy Act of 1974). Psychologists are bound by various regulations of their profession regarding this confidentiality. Further, psychologists are also obligated to provide appro-

priate, clearly comprehensible, verbal and written explanation of test results to the parents or guardians. Parents may also give permission for the information to be distributed to others involved in the child's care (e.g., teachers, doctors, therapists, and agencies). Even in situations in which these other parties referred the child for the testing, and perhaps paid for it, they cannot obtain the results without parental permission.

TEST ADMINISTRATION AND FEEDBACK

Tests are closely regulated in terms of who can administer them. The test distributors limit sales to qualified professionals and require proof of licensure for purchase of some test instruments. The test manuals delineate guidelines for administration that must be closely followed to ensure the reliability and validity claimed by the test. To be qualified to administer tests independently, psychologists must have completed appropriate training and supervision in the field of child assessment. In this way, proper administration and interpretation of findings are most likely. The psychologist must also be trained in working with families, inasmuch as providing feedback regarding testing results is often a sensitive and deeply personal activity. Some psychologists are primarily trained to administer tests, and they work with other psychologists who are trained in family work and can provide the feedback effectively.

SPECIAL POPULATIONS

There are several populations for whom traditional standardized testing may not be valid. These include infants, individuals with developmental disabilities, individuals with sensory impairments (e.g., visual or hearing), and individuals from cultures different from those of the norming sample.

Several standardized tests can be administered to infants (e.g., Bayley Scales of Infant Development; Mullen Scales); however, babies' behavior and cooperation level over time vary greatly, and the test must be administered by a psychologist who is experienced with babies and able to interpret whether the results are valid. Careful observation by a clinician specializing in infants can often yield information that may be more appropriate than the standardized test results.

Individuals from cultures different from those of the norming sample should be tested only with great caution and reservation. Whenever possible these individuals should be tested by a psychologist from the same culture, and when possible, using instruments norm-referenced on other children from that culture. Many of the traditionally used language and intelligence tests in the United States have Spanish equivalents, for example. Clearly this adaptation will not always be possible. Often, omitting testing is the best option. However, when it is deemed that some sort of testing will be in the child's best interest for a specific reason, such as access to a program, then test results should be interpreted very cautiously and combined with extensive observations, parent and teacher interviews, and evaluation of progress over time.

Many individuals with developmental disabilities cannot be validly assessed using standardized measures.

For example, individuals who are nonverbal cannot be evaluated using tests involving language. Individuals who have significant motor difficulties cannot be assessed using tasks involving motor skills. Individuals with motor as well as communication issues present an even greater challenge. Significant sensory difficulties and significant attentional difficulties also affect valid assessment.

There are some specific assessment measures designed for certain populations. These contain items that do not rely on systems that are affected by the specific disability and also generally are norm referenced on groups of individuals with the same disability. The Hiskey-Nebraska is one such test, an intelligence test for children who are hearing impaired. This test contains many subtests from traditional instruments, adapted for children with hearing limitations. For example, the "Digit Span" subtest included on most traditional intelligence tests is presented with small plastic numerals; the child looks at the numerals, looks away, and then selects the numerals from an array. The French Pictorial Test of Intelligence is another intelligence test designed for children who are nonverbal and also who may have significant motor problems. The child uses eye gaze (or points) to select from a series of groups of four choices. Some of the subtests involve receptive language. That is, the child must answer a question by selecting from the array. Other subtests are purely nonverbal, involving picture matching and picture memory.

Purposes of Psychological Testing

When requesting or interpreting psychological testing, it is important to keep in mind the purpose of the testing. This will maximize the utility of the results. Testing to address specific questions that are clear in the minds of those involved with the child will usually yield the most useful results. Following are some specific questions that can be addressed through psychological testing.

TESTING TO UNDERSTAND A PROBLEM A CHILD IS HAVING

The most common reason for testing is to develop further understanding about a problem a child is having. The young child may be late to achieve an expected milestone such as language, and the parents or pediatrician may refer for psychological testing to determine why language is late, if other developmental processes are also delayed, and what sorts of interventions may be helpful. A young child may be showing behavioral differences, such as extreme shyness or anger or lack of sociability, and the parents or pediatrician may refer to a psychologist. The school-aged child may be experiencing difficulty with a specific subject, or with all school subjects, or showing attentional or behavioral difficulties at school. The psychologist then, through a combination of psychological testing, observation, and parent and teacher interview, can develop a further understanding of why the child is showing the particular difficulty and work with the family to formulate a plan of intervention. Psychological testing results can highlight the child's learning profile of strengths and weaknesses and, in combination with the other information, can help develop

a thorough understanding of the child. Sometimes the psychologist will determine that other specialists are needed, such as a psychiatrist, developmental pediatrician, speech and language therapist, or occupational therapist, to develop a full understanding of the child's overall strengths and difficulties.

Overview of Specific Tests

There are a variety of types of standardized psychological tests. Intelligence tests measure intellectual capacity of some sort. Achievement tests measure what the child already knows in specific areas. Tests to assess emotional and behavioral issues in childhood include projective tests, observational measures, and parent interviews. The reader is referred to a number of other chapters that provide related material. See Chapter 67 for tests on behavioral adjustment and temperament, Chapter 68 on preschool developmental screening, Chapter 69 on developmental assessment of school-aged children, Chapter 70 on intelligence, and Chapter 71 on educational testing. Following is a brief overview of a variety of tests. For more detailed comprehensive discussions and evaluations of individual tests please see *Children's Psychological Testing* (Woodrich, 1997) or *Assessment of Children* (Sattler, 1988) and the *Twelfth Mental Measurement Yearbook* (Conoley and Impara, 1995).

INTELLIGENCE TESTS

Intelligence tests are generally divided into several subtests, each measuring different domains of the large set of skills we group together and call intelligence. Some domains typically assessed on intelligence tests include different forms of memory (short-term and long-term, visual, and auditory), aspects of language development, aspects of problem solving, spatial ability, and numeric reasoning. Intelligence test results, when interpreted carefully, can provide very useful information regarding how a child learns best and what kind of learning is most difficult. Specific patterns of scores indicate particular types of problems, such as a learning disability or an attentional problem. As children grow older, scores on intelligence tests tend to be increasingly stable, perhaps because factors such as attention, cooperation, and motivation become less variable. Scores of young children must be interpreted with caution, and scores of infants should never be interpreted as predictive of later intelligence.

In general, an IQ score below 70 that is felt to be validly obtained on an appropriate intelligence test, in conjunction with significant needs in adaptive skills at a commensurate level, suggests mental retardation. An uneven profile, with some scores at age level or above and other scores significantly below age level, suggests a learning disability.

INFANT TESTS

Because assessment of infants is more an art than a science, results must be interpreted with great caution. Infant testing can be very useful in identifying infants showing developmental challenges and in determining eligibility for services such as Early Intervention. Infant assessment can also lead to early detection of some developmental disabilities, such as autism, that can often be significantly ameliorated by intensive early help. However, infant tests for typically developing children do not correlate with later measures of intelligence until 1 1/2 to 2 years of age.

Infant tests are often in the form of observational checklists such as the Denver Developmental Test or the Hawaii Early Learning Profile. The Bayley Scales of Infant Development is the most widely used standardized, individually administered test. Administration of this test, unlike the checklists, requires substantial training and supervision.

PRESCHOOL INTELLIGENCE TESTS

Preschool-aged children are referred for psychological testing for four primary concerns: (1) kindergarten readiness, (2) language delays, (3) global delays, and (4) attentional or behavioral difficulties. Preschool test instruments typically measure the child's abilities across several areas, including expressive and receptive language, visual-spatial processing, fine motor skills, visual-motor integration, memory, general knowledge, and preacademic skills (e.g., knowledge of letters and numbers). By preschool age, many children are able to attend and follow directions sufficiently to obtain reliable comprehensive test results across a broad set of learning areas, whereas some children, especially children with communication, attentional, and developmental problems, are not. Children's performance and skills at this age are also highly dependent on familial situation and experiences, as many children in this age range have had little or no exposure to school. However, careful psychological assessment of children can be very helpful in determining specific types of problems (e.g., language processing problems), as well as attentional difficulties.

There are several frequently used and well-standardized preschool tests. These include the Stanford-Binet Intelligence Scale, the revised Wechsler Preschool Primary Scale of Intelligence (WPPSI-R), the McCarthy Scales of Children's Abilities, and the Kaufman Assessment Battery for Children. Each of these tests has verbal and nonverbal subtests. The specific nature of the nonverbal tasks vary somewhat across tests, but all contain measures of visual processing as well as visual-motor integration. All of these tests except the WPPSI-R also have measures of visual memory. Each of them has measures of vocabulary and

of language processing. The Stanford-Binet Scale has the advantage of continuing on through adulthood and so can be used to follow individuals over a lifetime. The WPPSI-R is the preschool form of the Wechsler scales, which also has school-aged (WISC-R) and adult (WAIS) forms. The Kaufman Assessment Battery for Children has an advantage in that it is very fast paced with a very easy to administer "easel" format. The tasks are novel and tend to be interesting for children who may have difficulty engaging in more traditional tests such as the WPPSI-R.

Each of these instruments requires significant proficiency in attentional capacity and language ability, even for many of the nonverbal subtests, to understand what is required. There are some tests normed for this age range that are more self-explanatory and visually based and hence useful for children with significant language impairments, nonverbal children, children who are highly self-directed (e.g., children with autism or behavioral challenges), or children who speak languages other than English or the language of the evaluator. The Merrill-Palmer Scale of Mental Tests has a broad array of interesting and appealing visual materials, most of which are self-explanatory. A problem with this set of instruments is that they are not well norm-referenced. They can be very helpful in developing further understanding of a child's learning profile, however. For example, a young child with autism may not understand what is required in the more traditional tests but may be very drawn to the colors and shapes on the Merrill-Palmer test and may understand intuitively how to assemble the puzzles presented by the materials. Hypotheses regarding a child's rate of processing and learning strategies, and, with repeated administration, information regarding a child's learning curve can be generated from observing the child as he or she completes these tasks (Table 72–1).

SCHOOL-AGE INTELLIGENCE TESTS

The Wechsler Intelligence Scale for Children is the most commonly used school-age intelligence test. It provides a screening of children's abilities and processing skills across a wide range of verbal and nonverbal domains. When a child is having academic problems, this test provides a beginning exploration of the source of the problems. Sometimes the information is sufficient to delineate a learning disability. For example, a child who receives a nonverbal score significantly above average and a verbal score significantly below average likely has some form of language-

Table 72–1 • Preschool and Elementary School Tests

Test	Recent Norms	Includes Achievement	Broad Range of Skills Assessed	Low Language and Attention Demands
Stanford-Binet IV	X		X	
McCarthy Scales of Children's Abilities	X		X	
Kaufman Assessment Battery for Children	X	X	X	
Wechsler Tests (WPPSI-R, WISC-III)	X	X	X	
Merrill Palmer Scale				X
Differential Abilities Scale	X		X	X
Leiter International Performance Scale				X
Hiskey-Nebraska			X	X

based learning disability. Detailed neuropsychological testing can further pinpoint the specific nature of the child's learning disability and the child's strengths and weaknesses. There are many such measures for this age range that assess very specific aspects of processing and learning (see Chapter 73).

TESTS OF ADAPTIVE FUNCTIONING

It can often be very helpful to obtain information about a child's level of independent functioning in areas such as self-care and dressing in younger children and community and social functioning in older ones. While this information is helpful in assessing any child, it can be particularly valuable when evaluating children for whom traditional tests are not valid. The Vineland Adaptive Behavior Scales is a comprehensive and thorough set of interview measures for this purpose. There are parent and teacher versions, which are also available in Spanish.

PERSONALITY TESTING

Personality tests are designed to measure various aspects of children's emotions and behavior. Children who are exhibiting behavioral difficulties, such as getting in trouble frequently, having emotional difficulties, or appearing depressed or even suicidal, or children who have been through specific trauma such as losing a parent may be referred for projective testing to develop a further understanding of their way of understanding their social and emotional world. While in some instances the psychologist can simply directly ask the child questions regarding his or her emotional world (e.g., "What makes you sad?"), most children have sufficient defenses in place such that direct questioning will not yield as comprehensive information as a combination of interview, interactive play, and personality testing.

There are several forms of personality tests. For young children, parents are often given scales to fill out that yield information regarding behavior in relationship to other children of the same age. The Achenbach Child Behavior Checklist is one such form. This test is scored along various factors such as depression or impassivity. The Conners Parent and Teacher rating scales are similar and especially used to assess attentional problems.

Projective tests are personality tests in which the child responds to ambiguous stimuli designed to evoke a range of responses around specific themes. Projective tests are often in the form of pictures, including photographs of children in everyday situations, or line drawings. Some projective tests are in the form of sentence completions (e.g., "Sometimes I wish I could _____"). In the projective test called the Tasks of Emotional Development, as a way to evaluate the child's self esteem, the child is shown a picture of a child of the same sex looking in a mirror and asked what the child in the picture is thinking and feeling and what he or she will do next. The manual includes typical responses and implications of various responses.

Some personality measures involve the child's responding to a list of questions. These have been normed on various groups of children who have specific diagnoses. The Minnesota Multiphasic Personality Inventory is a common self-report measure.

Conclusion

To summarize, psychological testing provides a tool to gain understanding of children's intellectual and emotional functioning. Psychological testing should be only one part of an assessment process. Observing and interacting with the child and gathering information from those who know the child across different settings (e.g., family, teachers) are also vital components of the process. Psychological tests should be interpreted cautiously, with interpretation closely bound to what the test validly measures.

REFERENCES

Binet A, Simon T: New methods for the diagnosis of the intellectual level of subnormals. Ann Psychol 11:191, 1905.

Conoley JC, Impara JC: The Twelfth Mental Measurement Yearbook. Lincoln, University of Nebraska Press, 1995.

Jenson AR: Bias in Mental Testing. New York, MacMillan, 1980.

Kai IR, Pelligrino JW: Human Intelligence: Perspectives and Prospects. New York, Freeman, 1985.

Kamin LJ: Heredity, intelligence, politics, and psychology. *In* Block NJ, Dworkin G (eds): The I. Q. Controversy. New York, Pantheon, 1976.

Sattler JM: Assessment of Children. San Diego, CA, Jerome M. Sattler, 1988.

Woodrich DL: Children's Psychological Testing: A Guide for Nonpsychologists, 3rd ed. Baltimore, Brookes, 1997.

73 Neuropsychological Assessment of Children

Stephen R. Hooper • Camille T. Fine •
Michael G. Tramontana

A thorough neuropsychological assessment can contribute to the identification of the specific underlying dimensions of learning dysfunction.

The primary intent of a fixed-battery approach is to measure a comprehensive array of brain functions using an invariant set of validated test procedures.

Historically there has been little evidence of specificity with respect to the type or pattern of brain dysfunction associated with different forms of child psychopathology.

Child neuropsychology is a discipline that combines aspects of psychology, pediatrics, and neurology to study brain-behavior relations through systematic assessment of behavior. As noted in the previous edition of this text, this field has proliferated in recent years, owing to factors such as federal legislation, continued advances in medical care, and an ever-increasing knowledge base with respect to brain development and related functions. For example, the recent reauthorization of the Individuals with Disabilities Education Act Amendments of 1997 has continued to support greater public awareness of learning disabilities, traumatic brain injury, and other neurologic and neurodevelopmentally based disorders. Awareness of special education legislation also has motivated parents to become more informed consumers and stronger advocates for comprehensive assessment and intervention for their children. Similarly, advances in medical care have contributed to an increased prevalence of children surviving a variety of childhood illnesses and trauma. This increased prevalence, in turn, has created a greater need for careful and detailed assessments of the extent, pattern, and developmental significance of possible neuropsychological sequelae in survivors of these injuries and illnesses.

In this chapter, we provide an overview of child neuropsychological assessment and compare it with other types of assessment. We also discuss several of the more popular approaches to child neuropsychological assessment, with additional emphasis being placed on recent advances in assessment technology and conceptualization. Finally, recent findings with respect to selected clinical applications are described.

Child Neuropsychological Assessment and Its Relationship to Other Types of Assessment

The measures that constitute a neuropsychological assessment are selected, designed, or adapted to facilitate the conceptualization of a child's performance in terms of what is known or hypothesized about brain-behavior relation-

ships. Although the components of the basic psychological examination typically include measures of intelligence, achievement, and personality functioning designed to assess cognitive abilities and social-emotional characteristics, a psychological examination generally does not attempt to relate findings to neurologic features or neurodevelopmental issues. Although similar tests can be used in both psychological and neuropsychological examinations, there are major differences in how these test procedures are applied and how their results are interpreted. Further, basic psychological testing typically is not designed to describe the child's functional strengths and weaknesses as clearly and distinctly as can be done in neuropsychological testing.

In contrast to the traditional psychological examination, the classic pediatric neurologic examination does attempt to make inferences about brain function from a child's behavior and performance. Although this examination varies with the age of the child, the core components of a pediatric neurologic examination include a determination of (1) station and gait, (2) sensory-motor functions, (3) reflex integrity, (4) general physical development, and (5) mental status. Similar to the neuropsychological assessment, the pediatric examination can provide evidence for generalized versus focal central nervous system dysfunction; however, the basic pediatric neurologic examination best represents a screening of the integrity of the central nervous system. The general absence of standardization and quantification with precise normative data tends to make it less sensitive to more subtle deficits, particularly with respect to higher cognitive functioning.

Current Approaches in Child Neuropsychological Assessment

FIXED-BATTERY APPROACHES

The primary intent of a fixed-battery approach is to measure a comprehensive array of brain functions using an invariant set of validated test procedures. Consequently, not all of the tasks will be pertinent to the chief presenting questions or complaints regarding the individual patient.

However, the comprehensive nature of a fixed-battery approach typically ensures that specific referral questions can be addressed in an adequate manner, provided that the battery has been designed to tap a broad range of human capabilities. Given the fixed nature of the questions, the time involved in administration may be unnecessarily lengthened in certain situations, but the use of a fixed-battery approach does provide a consistent framework for evaluating findings across different children. To date, batteries such as the Halstead-Reitan Neuropsychological Battery (HRNB) and the Luria-Nebraska Neuropsychological Battery (LNNB) have represented the most commonly used methods in this category of neuropsychological assessment. More recently, the Neuropsychological Investigation for Children (NEPSY) was also developed and will provide child neuropsychologists with another fixed-battery option for conducting child neuropsychological assessments.

Halstead-Reitan Neuropsychological Battery

Two versions of the HRNB exist for use with children. These are the Reitan-Indiana Neuropsychological Test Battery for Children (ages 5 to 8 years) and the Halstead-Reitan Neuropsychological Battery for Older Children (ages 9 to 14 years). The latter version of the HRNB is a downward extension of the adult version of the battery, with most of the adult tests simply being shortened for this version. Similarly, the HRNB for younger children consists of modified versions of the tests in the older children's battery. The appropriate Wechsler intelligence scale and a standardized test of academic achievement typically accompany each version of the HRNB.

A child's results on the HRNB are evaluated in terms of *level of performance, pattern of performance, right-left differences*, and *pathognomonic signs*. Inferences regarding brain dysfunction are based on findings across each of these methods of analysis. The results are also used to generate a profile of specific strengths and weaknesses for each child. To that end, a number of investigators have recently undertaken factor analyses of the children's versions of the HRNB. When an expanded sample of motor, psychomotor, and visual-spatial tests was employed, factor analysis resulted in five correlated factors: simple motor skill, complex visual-spatial relations, simple spatial motor operations, motor steadiness, and speeded motor sequencing (Francis et al, 1992). Such results provide evidence for the discriminant validity of an expanded HRNB. When the underlying factor structure of the Reitan-Indiana Neuropsychological Battery is examined, a four-factor solution has been deemed the most heuristic. These factors included speed of operation, tactile-motor integration, attention, and visual-spatial memory (Krug, Dean, and Anderson, 1995).

The HRNB has been found to distinguish brain dysfunction in an accurate manner. Although attempts to localize brain injury in children using the HRNB have not been as successful, it can be quite useful in delineating the effects of localizing injuries. It also has been shown to identify children with learning disabilities and to distinguish different subtypes of learning disability on the basis of differential patterns of performance (Hooper and Willis, 1989). There are some areas of function that are weakly assessed with the HRNB (e.g., attention, language, mem-

ory), but it clearly has been a dominant approach in child neuropsychological assessment for several decades.

Luria-Nebraska Neuropsychological Battery

Golden and colleagues (Golden, 1981) developed two versions of the LNNB based on the theory of Luria (1973): the Luria-Nebraska Neuropsychological Battery (ages 13 years through adult) and the Luria-Nebraska Neuropsychological Battery—Children's Revision (ages 8 through 12 years). As with the HRNB, the younger children's version of the LNNB is a downward extension of the adult version of the battery, with both versions organized around 11 summary scales: motor, rhythm, tactile, visual, receptive speech, expressive speech, writing, reading, arithmetic, memory, and intellectual processes. Both versions are supplemented by three second-order scales: pathognomonic (consisting of the items in the battery that provide the best discrimination of brain damage), and the left sensory-motor and right sensory-motor scales (based on items from the motor and tactile scales performed with the contralateral hand).

Each item in the battery is scored on a three-point system (0 to 2), with higher scores being indicative of dysfunction or impairment. Item scores are summed within each scale, with each total converted to a *T*-score (mean = 50, standard deviation = 10). In addition to inspection of the overall profile, interpretation is based on a careful analysis of performance on the individual items in the battery. In contrast to the HRNB, the test items on the LNNB are more basic and geared toward assessing the specific cognitive underpinnings of their respective summary scale. This feature of the LNNB allows for the incorporation of a more qualitative analysis of an individual's performance.

Generally, the LNNB appears to discriminate brain dysfunction in children about as well as the HRNB does, and, at least for general classification purposes, the two batteries yield highly comparable results. It has been found to yield a correct classification rate of 79% for children with brain damage and of 89% for typically developing children, with an overall hit-rate of 85%. It also has been found to discriminate effectively between children with learning disabilities and typically developing children, but its discriminative power tends to be limited to the expressive speech, writing, and reading scales once intelligence quotient (IQ) is statistically controlled for. Further, the LNNB appears to be less sensitive to factors underlying mathematics deficits than reading or spelling deficits in children with learning disabilities. It provides a better appraisal of language abilities and memory than the HRNB, but, similar to the HRNB, it lacks a specific assessment of attention. Moreover, the children's revision has been criticized for its omission of items sensitive to frontal lobe dysfunction.

The NEPSY

"NEPSY" is not a true acronym in that each letter does not stand for a word; rather, it represents "NEuroPSYchological" Investigation for Children. The NEPSY represents a new neuropsychological battery that recently became available to child neuropsychologists and other child psychologists (Korkman, Kirk, and Kemp, 1997). It was designed to be used with children from ages 2 1/2 through 12 years. The NEPSY comprehensively assesses discrete functions via 37 subtests within five broad constructs: attention and executive functions, language, sensory-motor, visual-spatial, and memory and learning. The NEPSY holds the distinction for being one of the best normed and standardized sets of neuropsychological procedures that has been available to date, and it has been used with children with acquired injuries as well as children manifesting a variety of neurodevelopmental disorders. Scoring of the NEPSY permits a clear quantitative analysis of the child across the various domains, but it also provides detailed qualitative observations that also have been normed for children in this age range. This latter feature should prove useful for increasing understanding of neurologic soft signs in children.

In addition to the test development features, the NEPSY is embedded in Luria's (1973) theoretical framework for brain functioning. Thus test results may be used simply to describe a child's pattern of strengths and weaknesses; or they may be interpreted for primary and secondary deficiencies consistent with Luria's principles of syndrome analysis. Further, the design of the test does not require that an examiner administer the entire set of procedures, and selected subtests or subtests within a specific domain can be selected depending on the clinical or research questions being presented. Another distinct advantage of the NEPSY is that it was designed for young children, for whom there has been a relative dearth of neuropsychological measures; however, the ultimate utility of the NEPSY will be examined as it is put to the test of day-to-day clinical and research practice.

ECLECTIC BATTERY APPROACHES

Investigators using the eclectic approach to neuropsychological assessment attempt to preserve the quantitative nature of testing by selecting standardized tests that measure a broad range of neurocognitive functions. Although there is at least an implicit outline of the relevant neurodevelopmental constructs that should be assessed (e.g., motor, sensory-perceptual, attention, language, memory, executive function), any of a variety of available tests may be selected to quantify the extent of deficit or dysfunction within each area. For example, selective and sustained attention can be assessed via continuous performance tests administered by various computerized formats (e.g., the Gordon Diagnostic System, Test of Variables of Attention, Conners' Continuous Performance Test); moreover, there are even models that can guide the development of an eclectic battery in a selected domain of interest (e.g., attention) (Barkley, 1997). In general, the psychometric properties of individual tests (e.g., adequacy of norms) and their complementarity when embedded in a battery typically are important factors guiding specific test selection. Interpretive concerns can be raised, however, given the different normative bases from which quantitative information is generated and compared.

OTHER APPROACHES

Other approaches to neuropsychological assessment include qualitative approaches (Luria, 1973) and the Boston Process Approach (Milberg, Hebben, and Kaplan, 1986); however, space does not permit a fuller discussion of these methods. A major concern with these approaches has been the lack of sufficient validation research on which to judge their adequacy. For example, the absence of standardization in qualitative approaches is incompatible with conducting independent appraisals of reliability and validity. Moreover, most neuropsychologists would regard standardization and quantification as hallmarks of neuropsychological assessment and would view qualitative approaches as more aligned with methods in behavioral neurology. In practice, there probably are relatively few neuropsychologists who are purists with respect to one approach or another, and a melding of approaches probably is quite common. This makes good sense, since the different perspectives can be combined in a complementary fashion in an effort to maximize both the breadth and the depth of assessment for an individual child.

Selected Applications

Historically, the primary goal of child neuropsychological assessment was to aid in the detection of brain dysfunction for the purpose of differential diagnosis. More recently, this has evolved to encompass a broader range of clinical applications. These include (1) identifying the behavioral effects of known brain injury, (2) identifying the specific underlying dimensions of dysfunction in specific disorders or injuries, (3) using assessment data to help construct treatment strategies, (4) providing information with respect to the child's prognosis and risk for certain developmental outcomes, and (5) conducting follow-up assessments in an effort to chart functional change over the course of development and disease process and in response to particular interventions. The exact nature and relative importance of these different applications of neuropsychological assessment depend, in part, on the particular clinical population under consideration. We consider here important applications of neuropsychological testing in four distinct yet interrelated clinical populations of children typically encountered by developmental-behavioral pediatricians: those with learning disabilities, psychiatric disorders, systemic illness, and neurologic disorders.

LEARNING DISABILITIES

The area of learning disabilities has constituted an important subject of neuropsychological investigation. The explicit presumption of central nervous system dysfunction in current definitions of learning disability, and the widening recognition that the term "learning disability" is a generic one representing a heterogeneous group of disorders, have served to underscore the important role of neuropsychological assessment in this population. A thorough neuropsychological assessment can contribute to the identification of specific underlying dimensions of learning dysfunction and can assist in the development of specific educational intervention plans. Work in learning disabilities addressing the child's adaptive capacity in the real-life context of school has taken an exemplary lead in relating neuropsychological findings to day-to-day aspects of an individual's life. Much remains to be learned, but major advances have been achieved in the area of syndrome definition and subtype analysis (e.g., Morris et al, in press), the identification of developmental precursors of reading disabilities (Share and Stanovich, 1995), possible neuroanatomic and neurophysiologic factors (Hynd and Semrud-Clikeman, 1989), and treatment strategies (Lyon and Moats, 1997). Specific neuropsychologically based theories also have surfaced (e.g., Nonverbal Learning Disabilities [Rourke, 1989]; Balance Model for Dyslexia [Bakker, 1994]), and these should fuel additional progress in the area of learning disabilities.

PSYCHIATRIC DISORDERS

There is a strong trend in the literature to suggest that children with brain dysfunction are at an increased risk for experiencing psychiatric disorders. This relationship appears to apply to children with documented brain damage as well as to those with soft neurologic signs. Further, the association between brain dysfunction and psychiatric disorders appears stronger than associations between physical disabilities and psychiatric disorders. Moreover, this risk is compounded by factors such as psychosocial adversity and any preexisting tendencies toward behavioral or emotional disturbance, particularly in persons who are acutely brain injured. This increased risk applies not only during the immediate aftermath of a brain insult but also to the child's long-term behavioral adjustment.

Conversely, among children with psychiatric disorders, there is a relatively high rate of neuropsychological dysfunction. This rate remains excessively high even when cases of known brain damage are excluded. The presence of neuropsychological deficits in children with psychiatric disorders has been found to be associated with more extensive behavior problems among younger boys, regardless of factors such as IQ, socioeconomic status, or whether the deficits could be linked specifically to a history of brain injury. Thus the presence of neuropsychological deficits in childhood appears to point toward limitations in adaptive capacity and to the potential for increased psychiatric morbidity (Hooper and Tramontana, 1997).

Historically, there has been little evidence of specificity with respect to the type or pattern of brain dysfunction associated with different forms of child psychopathology, as the available evidence suggested more of a nonspecific, indirect relationship between brain dysfunction and psychopathology in childhood (Hooper and Tramontana, 1997). With the evolution of more sophisticated neuropsychological and neuroimaging techniques, however, researchers in this area have begun to make more complex linkages between cerebral anomalies and dysfunctional behavior. For instance, Asarnow and coworkers (1994) assert that children with schizophrenia have reduced information-processing capacity and speculate about specific reasons for this (e.g., the component processes of information processing are part of a network that includes the frontal lobe and thalamus in interaction with the reticular activating

system). Similarly, in children with bipolar affective disorder, initial neuroimaging findings are suggestive of the presence of enlarged ventricular volumes, bilaterally, as well as white matter abnormalities (Botteron et al, 1995); however, specific neuropsychological correlates have yet to be discovered.

SYSTEMIC ILLNESS

A variety of systemic illnesses can affect the developing nervous system. Such illnesses might involve defects in specific organ systems, metabolic disorders, autoimmune disorders, or infections. As advances in medical care contribute to significant increases in the survival rates of children with serious illnesses, ongoing neuropsychological assessment should be of assistance in the monitoring of the continuing development and functioning of these children. It also may suggest the need for other kinds of intervention (e.g., special education).

Children infected with the human immunodeficiency virus (HIV), for example, or those with full-blown acquired immunodeficiency syndrome (AIDS) can vary widely in their neurologic, neuropsychological, and neurodevelopmental outcomes. Papola, Alvarez, and Cohen (1994) observed that 54% of their sample of children and adolescents with vertically infected HIV functioned within the borderline to mentally retarded range of intelligence. About 84% of their sample exhibited some form of developmental language impairment, 63% received special educational services, and about 25% were diagnosed with attention-deficit hyperactivity disorder. Further, approximately 16% of the sample manifested emotional difficulties severe enough to warrant psychiatric diagnoses. Whitt and associates (1993) examined the neuropsychological functioning in males with hemophilia who were HIV-infected. They measured six domains of neuropsychological functioning and found no differences between HIV-seropositive and HIV-seronegative groups. A high incidence of subtle neuropsychological deficits was detected on motor performance, attention, and speeded visual processing within both the infected and the uninfected groups. They concluded that it was premature to attribute early, subtle neuropsychological deficits in seropositive children with hemophilia to the central nervous system effects of HIV. These findings continued to be present at a 2-year follow-up point (Hooper et al, 1997). When neuroanatomic abnormalities are present, however, other investigators have found linkages to neuropsychological deficits. For example, Brouwers and colleagues (1995) found significant correlations among computed tomographic (CT) brain scan abnormalities and neuropsychological functioning, as well as an association between calcifications and neurocognitive deterioration independent of degree of brain atrophy. These correlations were significantly stronger in vertically infected patients than in infusion-infected patients.

Another example comes from recent investigations of children with phenylketonuria. Children whose plasma phenylalanine levels were elevated as minimally as three to five times normal (previously considered safe) demonstrated impaired prefrontal cortical functioning when required to hold information on-line (i.e., working memory) and inhibit prepotent responses (Diamond, 1994). Diamond and Herzberg (1996) also found that such moderately elevated levels of plasma phenylalanine contributed to adverse effects on dopamine neurons in the retina and those projecting to the prefrontal cortex. This, in turn, leads to deficits in contrast sensitivity and prefrontal cortical dysfunction.

NEUROLOGIC DISORDERS

As with the pediatric systemic illnesses, there are a variety of pediatric neurologic disorders that may require a careful neuropsychological assessment. These include genetic disorders, structural abnormalities of the brain, and traumatic brain injuries. Neuropathologic processes such as anoxic episodes, viral and bacterial encephalitis, toxicity, metabolic disorders, demyelinating diseases, and neuromuscular disorders also represent pediatric neurologic disorders in which a neuropsychological assessment could prove useful. In addition, although tumors and cerebrovascular accidents occur less frequently in children, a thorough neuropsychological evaluation can yield useful clinical information in these instances, particularly from a treatment-monitoring perspective.

Although the nature of most neurologic disorders does not lend itself to the delineation of specific neuropsychological profiles, several disorders are, in fact, characterized by distinct profiles. Individuals with Turner syndrome (Rovet, 1993), for instance, tend to present with a profile consistent with the nonverbal learning disabilities syndrome. Children with hydrocephalus also have been found to have depressed nonverbal abilities (Brookshire et al, 1995). Specifically, although their overall performance has been found to fall within normal limits, they have demonstrated compromised efficiency in processing complex or novel nonverbal stimuli (Donders, Rourke, and Canady, 1991).

Despite these findings, the effects of most insults to the immature nervous system are only beginning to be understood. Moreover, the precise effects of brain involvement depend on a complex interaction of factors such as the type of injury, individual variables, and environmental variables. The variability among children with neurologic disorders certainly underscores the importance of careful and thorough assessment of the individual child. The precise and quantified nature of neuropsychological test results can provide an invaluable adjunct in evaluating the child's neurologic status and neurodevelopmental progress.

Clinical Vignettes

Although it is beyond the scope of this chapter to provide much in the way of clinical descriptions for discussion, two examples are presented to illustrate the value of a neuropsychological assessment in pediatric practice. In each instance, the neuropsychological evaluation contributed to increased clinical understanding of the child, provided additional suggestions for treatment planning and implementation, and assisted in ongoing neurodevelopmental monitoring efforts.

EXAMPLE: MILD TRAUMATIC BRAIN INJURY

Robert is a 7-year-old boy who sustained what appeared to be a mild closed-head injury following a motor vehicle accident in which he was an unbelted passenger. The accident occurred during the Spring of his first-grade year. Robert incurred a brief loss of consciousness (approximately 5 minutes) but was awake prior to going to the hospital emergency room. Neurodiagnostic procedures were unremarkable, and his general neurologic status was deemed satisfactory. He was sent home to be followed by his family pediatrician. No premorbid difficulties were apparent in his history. Subsequent to the accident Robert began to experience attentional difficulties, increased irritability, and frequent memory problems; however, school ended for the year and these difficulties seemed to subside. Upon entry into second grade, however, Robert again experienced learning difficulties, with specific problems being reported in his attention, memory, and organization. His pediatrician referred him for a comprehensive neuropsychological evaluation. This showed evidence of subtle frontal lobe dysfunction that was contributing to all of these difficulties and more likely than not related to his closed-head injury. In addition, issues pertinent to recovery from such an injury were discussed with his parents and teachers, and a multimodal intervention was instituted. Robert's progress continued to be monitored via regular appraisals of his attention, memory, and related executive functions, in tandem with his pediatric management, and over the course of the next 6 months many of these difficulties began to resolve.

EXAMPLE: NONVERBAL LEARNING DISABILITY

Rebecca is a 9-year-old girl who was referred to her pediatrician because of ongoing problems with selected aspects of learning, with particular concerns being raised in respect to her social functioning. Specifically, Rebecca was encountering problems understanding basic mathematic facts, experiencing difficulties with most mathematic calculations, and manifesting social skill deficits. Her developmental history was relatively unremarkable, although she had always been described as socially withdrawn and isolated. She also experienced initial problems learning to read, although this apparently had resolved over the previous 2 years. A neuropsychological evaluation showed a significant clustering of findings suggestive of right hemisphere dysfunction. This included an array of visual-perceptual difficulties, problems with visual attention and visual organization, and deficient visual memory. She also evidenced left-sided sensory-motor deficits. In contrast, she demonstrated nicely developed language abilities, although her language pragmatics were poor; good verbal memory and learning capabilities; and intact auditory attention. By obtaining this detailed constellation of abilities, the pediatrician was able to work with the family in devising strategies to address the initial referral concerns. In addition, educational suggestions could be provided for the school with respect to meeting her strengths and weaknesses in a more productive fashion. One of the treatment strategies, for example, was to provide Rebecca with social skills training wherein she could develop her verbal mediation and problem-solving strategies. She was then no longer dependent on her weak nonverbal abilities for interpretation of social cues and related paralinguistic aspects of social communication. Further, these findings also placed Rebecca at risk for social-emotional difficulties (i.e., internalizing types of problems), and she now is being monitored for these concerns on a routine basis by her pediatrician.

REFERENCES

Asarnow RF, Asamen J, Granholm E, et al: Cognitive/neuropsychological studies of children with a schizophrenic disorder. Schizophrenia Bull 20:647, 1994.

Bakker DJ: Dyslexia and the ecological brain. J Clin Exp Neuropsychol 16:734, 1994.

Barkley RA: Behavioral inhibition, sustaining attention, and executive functions: Constructing a unifying theory of ADHD. Psych Bull 121:65, 1997.

Botteron KN, Vannier MW, Geller B, et al: Preliminary study of magnetic resonance imaging characteristics in 8- to 16-year-olds with mania. J Am Acad Child Adolesc Psychiatry 34:742, 1995.

Brookshire BL, Fletcher JM, Bohan TP, et al: Verbal and nonverbal skill discrepancies in children with hydrocephalus: a five-year longitudinal follow-up. J Pediatr Psychol 20:785, 1995.

Brouwers P, DeCarli C, Civitello L, et al: Correlation between computed tomographic brain scan abnormalities and neuropsychological function in children with symptomatic human immunodeficiency virus disease. Arch Neurol 52:39, 1995.

Diamond A: Phenylalanine levels of 6–10 mg/dl may not be as benign as once thought. Acta Paediatrica 407:89, 1994.

Diamond A, Herzberg C: Impaired sensitivity to visual contrast in children treated early and continuously for phenylketonuria. Brain 119:523, 1996.

Donders J, Rourke BP, Canady AI: Neuropsychological functioning in hydrocephalic children. J Clin Exp Neuropsychol 13:607, 1991.

Francis DJ, Fletcher JM, Rourke BP, York MJ: A five-factor model for motor, psychomotor, and visual-spatial tests used in the neuropsychological assessment of children. J Clin Exp Neuropsychol 14:625, 1992.

Golden CJ: The Luria-Nebraska Children's Battery: theory and formulation. *In* Hynd GW, Obrzut JE (eds): Neuropsychological Assessment and the School-Age Child: Issues and Procedures. New York, Grune & Stratton, 1981, p 277.

Hooper SR, Tramontana MG: Advances in the neuropsychological bases of child and adolescent psychopathology: proposed models, findings, and ongoing issues. *In* Ollendick TH, Prinz RJ (eds): Advances in Clinical Child Psychology, Vol 19. New York, Plenum Publishing Corporation, 1997, p 133.

Hooper SR, Whitt JK, Tennison MB, et al: HIV-infected children with hemophilia: one and two year follow-up of neuropsychological functioning. Pediatric AIDS and HIV infection. Fetus to Adolescent 8:91, 1997.

Hooper SR, Willis WG: Learning Disability Subtyping: Neuropsychological Foundations, Conceptual Models, and Issues in Clinical Differentiation. New York, Springer-Verlag, 1989.

Hynd GW, Semrud-Clikeman M: Dyslexia and brain morphology. Psychol Bull 106:447, 1989.

Korkman M, Kirk U, Kemp S: NEPSY. San Antonio, The Psychological Corporation, 1997.

Krug D, Dean RS, Anderson JL: Factor analysis of the Halstead-Reitan Test Battery for Older Children. Int J Neurosci 83:131, 1995.

Luria AR: The Working Brain: An Introduction to Neuropsychology. New York, Basic Books, 1973.

Lyon GR, Moats LC: Critical conceptual and methodological consideration in reading intervention. J Learn Disabil 30:578, 1997.

Milberg WP, Hebben N, Kaplan E: The Boston Process Approach to neuropsychological assessment. *In* Grant I, Adams KM (eds): Neuropsychological Assessment of Neuropsychiatric Disorders. New York, Oxford University Press, 1986, p 65.

Morris RD, Stuebing KK, Fletcher JM, et al: Subtypes of reading disability: coherent variability around a phonological core. J Educ Psychol. In press.

Papola P, Alverez M, Cohen HJ: Developmental and service needs of school-age children with human immunodeficiency virus infection: a descriptive study. Pediatrics 94:914, 1994.

Rourke BP: Nonverbal learning disabilities: the syndrome and the model. New York, The Guilford Press, 1989.

Rovet JF: The psychoeducational characteristics of children with Turner syndrome. J Learn Disabil 26:333, 1993.

Share DL, Stanovich KE: Cognitive processes in early reading development: a model of acquisition and individual differences. Issues Educ 1:1, 1995.

Whitt JK, Hooper SR, Tennison MB, et al: Neuropsychologic functioning of human immunodeficiency virus-infected children with hemophilia. J Pediatrics 122:52, 1993.

74 Diagnostic Studies of the Central Nervous System

David K. Urion

Three monks walked along a road and saw a banner flapping in the breeze. "That flag is moving," said the first. "You are wrong," said the second, "it is the wind that is moving." "You are both wrong," said the third, "it is your mind that is moving."

Zen Koan of the Rinzai sect

Neurology as a clinical discipline is still within its semiotic phase of development: it is still centered around the recognition and interpretation of signs. Despite this orientation, certain test procedures have evolved that aid the practitioner in the interpretation of the clinical picture the child presents. This chapter is devoted to a discussion of these testing procedures and their appropriate uses.

One may divide neurologic tests into two sorts: referential and inferential (Table 74–1). *Referential* tests allow the clinician to examine parts of the nervous system directly, usually in the clinical pathology laboratory. Examination of the cerebrospinal fluid (CSF) and its cellular and protein constituents, and biopsies of muscle, nerve, skin, and conjunctivae are examples of referential tests of the nervous system. Postmortem examination of the brain may also be considered a referential examination technique, but by its nature is of cold comfort to the patient, family, and clinician.

Inferential examination techniques use varying modalities to examine the nervous system through its physiologic or anatomic properties and thus allow the clinician to *infer* the validity of a differential diagnostic point. Inferential techniques may be divided into two types: *physiologic*, or functional, techniques, and *anatomic*, or structural, techniques. Examples of physiologic inferential techniques include electroencephalography, quantitative electroencephalography, electromyography and nerve conduction studies, evoked potential studies, single photon emission computed tomography, positron emission tomography, and magnetic resonance spectroscopy. Anatomic inferential examination techniques include cranial ultrasonography, computed tomography (CT), angiography, magnetic resonance imaging (MRI), and magnetic resonance angiography (MRA).

This division of inferential diagnostic techniques is somewhat artificial. Most "physiologic" techniques allow one to make inferences regarding both structure and function, just as most "anatomic" techniques allow one to speculate about structural as well as functional processes. Nonetheless, this division is useful in clinical practice because each technique has a paramount strategic advantage in one or another diagnostic milieu.

General Principles

When attempting to order a differential diagnostic process into likely and unlikely possibilities, history and examination are the critical parameters. Although the diagnostic techniques discussed subsequently will, on occasion, provide the answer to a poorly formed diagnostic question by a gratifyingly pathognomonic finding, "fishing expeditions" are to be avoided. It is more useful to generate a set of hypotheses and then investigate those conjectures with a series of diagnostic techniques. The goal is for one hypothesis to emerge as the most parsimonious explanation for the findings.

The examination techniques should be chosen so that some critical aspect of a hypothesis may be tested. If one considered Tay-Sachs disease the leading possibility, then immediate measurement of hexosaminidase A is indicated. Most situations are murkier.

The first general principle is to use a series of tests, one from each of the three domains described (referential, inferential-physiologic, inferential-anatomic), to confirm or deny the leading hypothesis. The generation of those leading hypotheses requires knowledge and discussion of which

Table 74–1 • Diagnostic Methods

Referential Methods	Inferential Methods
Cerebrospinal fluid examination	Physiologic
Biopsy	Electroencephalography
Skin	Evoked potential studies
Muscle	Electromyelography and nerve
Nerve	conduction studies
Conjunctivae	Single photon emission computed
Urine profiles	tomography
Plasma/serum profiles	Positron emission tomography
White blood cell studies	Magnetic resonance spectroscopy
	Anatomic
	Ultrasonography
	Computed tomography
	Magnetic resonance imaging
	Magnetic resonance angiography
	Conventional angiography

particular neurologic disorders produce a pattern of dysfunction compatible with the patient's history and presentation. Although that consideration is beyond the scope of this chapter and is discussed elsewhere in this text (see Chapter 27), a paradigm can be offered to guide the generation of a reasonable differential diagnosis.

Kolodny (unpublished data, 1986) proposed a decision tree for approaching the patient with significant developmental delay and suspected neurologic disease. This paradigm has been modified (Weiner, Levitt, and Urion, in press) and is presented in Figures 74–1 and 74–2. It uses points from the history and examination that are readily available to the clinician. It has advantages over other paradigms in that it does not require a decision regarding age at onset (see Bresnan, 1986), which in our recent experience at the Children's Hospital in Boston has been a troublesome consideration.

The first decision point concerns the child's overall appearance. Although it is sometimes difficult in a young infant to decide whether certain physical features are dysmorphic or familial, in practice this decision can usually be made. In the *nondysmorphic* child, the next important decision regards the localization of the bulk of clinical signs. In simple practice, the hallmark of *gray matter* disorders is the presence of seizures and loss of milestones early in the course of the process. In *white matter* disorders, spasticity is the cardinal early sign, with seizures and loss of milestones usually occurring quite late in these disorders. *Peripheral* nervous system disease in the child usually presents as ataxia and areflexia. The decision regarding visceromegaly is made on the basis of general physical examination, whereas microcephaly is readily established with a tape measure and head circumference chart.

For the child with dysmorphic features, *pattern recognition* becomes an important tool. Certain features, collected together, represent recognizable syndromes. Examples of such pictures include Cornelia de Lange syndrome or the fetal alcohol syndrome. Discussion of recognized patterns of human malformation is not feasible in this section, but reference is made to Chapter 25.

In other instances, notable features include a large forehead, prominent brows, a broad nose, and full lips,

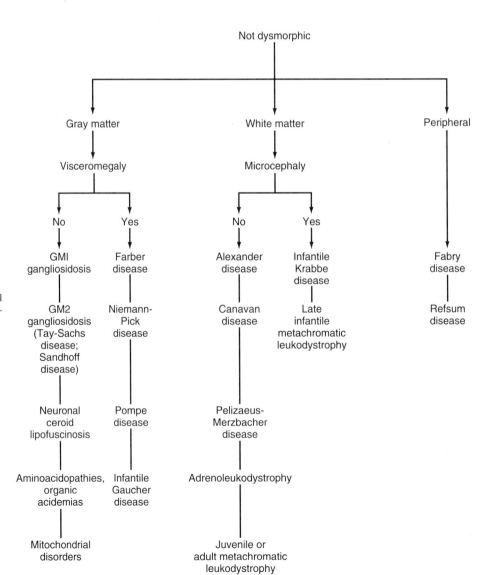

Figure 74–1. Algorithm for differential diagnoses of white matter and gray matter disease.

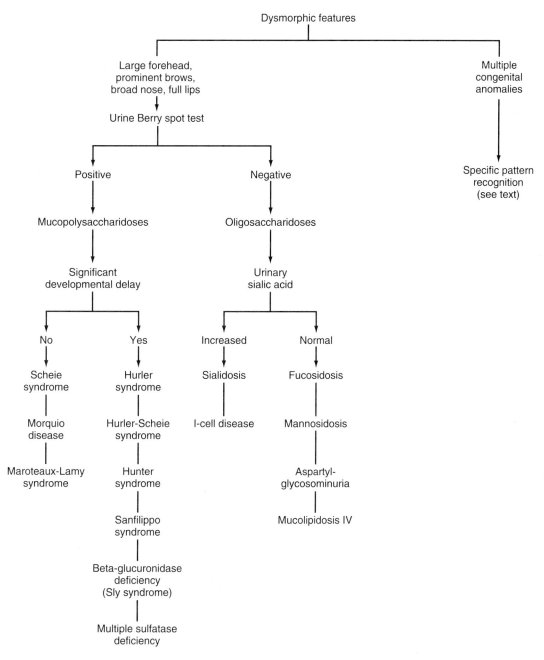

Figure 74–2. Algorithm for differential diagnoses for a child with dysmorphic features, such as Cornelia de Lange syndrome.

previously referred to as a "coarse facies." For such a child, the Berry urine spot test is the first decision point. Those children with a positive test result have one of the mucopolysaccharidoses; they can be further divided on the basis of their overall developmental history (the presence or absence of significant mental and developmental retardation). Those dysmorphic children with negative Berry urine spot test results have one of the oligosaccharidoses, which can be further subdivided on the basis of urinary sialic acid excretion.

This paradigm may be considered the second general diagnostic principle. By using it and some simple findings from physical examination and the laboratory tests, one can reduce the differential diagnosis into a manageable number of possibilities. The paradigm should not be viewed as anything other than an introductory schema by which one might approach thorny clinical problems with a certain pattern of priority.

EXAMPLE

A 35-month-old boy is brought to the office for evaluation of irritability and developmental delay. The boy's mother, a 27-year-old primigravida, had had an uncomplicated pregnancy, labor, and delivery. His parents are nonconsanguineous, and neither is Jewish and both are of mixed Western European ancestry. The boy sat at age 6 months, walked at 17 months, never ran, and has recently begun stumbling. His first words emerged shortly after his first birthday, and he spoke in phrases by 2 years of age. Of late, however, his parents note that he has become somewhat difficult to understand and drools. Review of his history does not suggest seizures. Examination demonstrates a nondysmorphic young boy whose head circumference is at the 10th percentile. Old records suggest it was at the 50th percentile at birth and throughout the 1st year of life. When the child is suspended under the arms, his legs scissor. Deep tendon reflexes are absent in the legs, although the parents report that the last pediatrician had no difficulty obtaining them at the 2-year visit. Both great toes go up when the soles are stroked.

Using the paradigm from Figures 74–1 and 74–2, one can note the absence of dysmorphic features, the presence of spasticity, and a loss of motor milestones without a history of seizures. This strongly suggests a white matter disease. This is buttressed by the developing dysarthria and apparent late-onset peripheral neuropathy (drooling and poor articulation, and absent reflexes, respectively). Furthermore, one can note the presence of microcephaly. Thus, the differential diagnosis can be narrowed to two probabilities: infantile Krabbe disease and late infantile metachromatic leukodystrophy. Before embarking on enzymatic diagnostic tests, however, one would be well advised to check this differential diagnosis by the application of the first general diagnostic principle.

The suspicion of white matter disease given this picture is quite high, and the consideration of gray matter disease is not warranted. The head circumference data are, however, potentially "soft," since old records for well-child examinations are fraught with inconsistent recordings of head circumference. Thus, a series of referential and inferential tests would help confirm or deny the leading clinical possibilities.

White matter disorders are usually associated with an elevation of CSF protein without increased CSF cell count, and therefore CSF examination would be the referential test of choice. The inferential physiologic test of choice would be electromyography and nerve conduction studies, since most white matter diseases are accompanied by a peripheral neuropathy. This was suspected on the basis of clinical examination, and confirmation of this suspicion would validate the proposed differential diagnosis. The inferential anatomic test of choice would be MRI. Most white matter disorders demonstrate striking abnormalities on MRI, given that technique's great sensitivity to altered water content in tissue. In addition, four of the five nonmicrocephalic white matter disorders (Canavan disease, Alexander disease, Pelizaeus-Merzbacher disease, and adrenoleukodystrophy) have characteristic if not pathognomonic appearances on MRI. Use of the test would therefore help to determine the validity of the original path through the diagnostic schema (i.e., toward a differential diagnosis between Krabbe disease and metachromatic leukodystrophy).

For the child in question, use of this approach yielded the following results: increased CSF protein content, delayed nerve conduction velocities, and abnormal signal intensity in a nonspecific pattern on T2-weighted images of brain MRI. This argues strongly for the process being either infantile Krabbe disease or late infantile

metachromatic leukodystrophy. The final step in the diagnostic procedure would be tests for blood levels of galactosyl-ceramidase (altered in Krabbe disease) and arylsulfatase A (altered in metachromatic leukodystrophy).

By combining the first and second general principles, an ordered approach to selecting laboratory evaluations may be undertaken.

Referential Methods

CEREBROSPINAL FLUID EXAMINATION

Cerebrospinal fluid for examination is usually obtained with a lumbar puncture. Contraindications for lumbar puncture in children are few: Posterior fossa mass, acute lead intoxication, Reye disease, and brain abscess are viewed as absolute contraindications because of the propensity of these situations to produce a "pressure cone" on lumbar puncture and thus lead to transtentorial or transmagnum herniation.

Measurement of CSF pressure is a useful, and usually neglected, maneuver. The CSF pressure is commonly elevated in meningeal disorders, including meningitis. Routine examination for cell count, protein, glucose, and microorganisms is well reviewed elsewhere (Barringer, 1970; Cole, 1969). Evaluation of CSF content of pyruvate and lactate has proved useful in the diagnosis of mitochondrial disorders (Jordan et al, 1983).

BIOPSIES

Tissue samples that provide direct morphologic data regarding the nervous system are an increasingly useful part of the clinician's armamentarium.

Skin biopsy is of particular use in the diagnosis of diseases that produce intraneuronal inclusion material, such as neuraxonal dystrophy or neuronal ceroid lipofuscinosis (Carpenter, Karpati, and Andermann, 1972). Skin biopsy specimens contain high concentrations of small nerve twiglets and sweat gland duct cells, which are useful because of the pathognomonic changes they demonstrate in certain conditions. Although light microscopy may provide some information, electron microscopy is more often the modality that provides the greatest insight into structural alterations. Methodologies for optimal technical conditions under which skin is obtained, preserved, and examined are reviewed elsewhere (Carpenter and Karpati, 1981).

Muscle biopsy is the referential test of choice for the evaluation of suspected myopathies, muscular dystrophies, and mitochondropathies. Structural evaluation, with both light and electron microscopy, may yield pathognomonic features diagnostic of certain myopathic processes, including nemaline rod myopathy, central core disease, and the mitochondrial encephalomyopathies. In other instances, such as the muscular dystrophies, structural abnormalities may be consistent with, but not diagnostic of, the suspected disorder. Molecular diagnostic techniques, evaluating cellular DNA or dystrophin content, may then prove useful (Kunkel et al, 1986). The reader is referred to Dubowitz and Brook (1973) for a complete discussion of muscle biopsy. Finally, biochemical evaluation of muscle tissue for electron transport chain abnormalities is available in certain centers.

Nerve biopsy, separate from the examination of small nerve elements in skin biopsy, is of use in suspected peripheral neuropathies in childhood. The sural nerve, a pure sensory nerve accessed on the dorsal aspect of the foot, is usually the nerve of choice for biopsy. Structural analysis, including light and electron microscopy, is the usual diagnostic method. Teased fiber analysis, first used in the evaluation of adult peripheral neuropathies, is now coming into use in pediatric neurology (Gibbels et al, 1985).

Conjunctival biopsy is used for essentially the same indications as skin biopsy. For the clinician, the choice between skin and conjunctival biopsy is based on the expertise of the local reference laboratory. That is, one should obtain the sort of biopsy specimen one's pathologist likes to examine.

Quantitative assays for the levels of specific enzymes, amino acids, organic acids, and urea cycle intermediary metabolites are of clear use in the diagnosis of specific metabolic disorders. Tissues sampled include plasma, serum, white blood cells harvested from blood, and urine. The most efficient use of these diagnostic modalities is to select a small number of assays for determination rather than an "enzyme panel."

Inferential Methods

PHYSIOLOGIC METHODS

Electroencephalography. Electroencephalography has a long history in pediatric neurology practice, elegantly reviewed by Holmes (1987). It is of great use in the diagnosis of seizure disorders and may be of some use in the evaluation of encephalopathic states. The clinician should be aware of the reference laboratory's familiarity and comfort with pediatric patients; electroencephalographic technical production and interpretation are notably operator dependent. Quantitative electroencephalography is a technique whereby electrical signals undergo complex analysis aided by computer; it may be particularly useful in finding deep seizure foci and subtle background changes associated with encephalopathy.

Evoked Potentials. The methods of somatosensory, visual, and auditory evoked potentials are in general applicable to children. The reader is referred to the excellent review monograph of Spehlmann (1985).

Single Photon Emission Computed Tomography and Positron Emission Tomography. Both of these scans are tomographically presented maps of cerebral function with radionuclide-labeled probes that allow measurement of blood flow, oxygen utilization, glucose metabolism, or specific ligand binding on a regional basis. Although these techniques are currently research tools in most institutions, examples from the adult literature suggest that once certain technical barriers are overcome, they will provide neurochemical data that could illuminate poorly understood disorders the etiologies of which have been obscure to date (e.g., developmental language disorders, Gilles de la Tourette syndrome, dystonia musculorum deformans).

Magnetic Resonance Spectroscopy. Magnetic resonance spectroscopy is a technique for looking at regional metabolism of the central nervous system, by examining tissue content for elements of energy transformation (adenosine triphosphate, adenosine diphosphate, adenosine monophosphate, and inorganic phosphate). It has proved particularly useful in evaluation of basal ganglia disorders and following the progression of brain tumors.

ANATOMIC METHODS

Ultrasonography. Cranial ultrasonography is the brain imaging screening technique of choice for fetuses and newborns (Hill and Volpe, 1989; Volpe, 1987). The window provided by the anterior fontanel provides the opportunity for excellent imaging without reconstruction in the sagittal, coronal, and horizontal planes. Periosteal and parameningeal regions are poorly imaged because of the angle with respect to the transducer, as well as the echogenic properties of bone. Thus, cranial ultrasonography will image ventricular diameter, major malformations and dysgeneses, and intraparenchymal hemorrhages quite well, whereas subarachnoid and subdural fluid collections are poorly imaged.

Computed Tomography. CT is the imaging screening maneuver of choice for children older than 10 months of age (Barnes, Urion, and Share, 1990). It has the capacity to determine structural relationships in the horizontal plane directly and, with some difficulty, in the coronal plane as well. Sagittal views are produced through reformatting.

Limitations of CT scanning include relatively poor imaging of the white matter when compared with MRI and poor delineation of brainstem and cerebellar features. Bone can be simultaneously imaged, in contrast to MRI. Blood and blood-containing structures are well visualized on CT scans, and delineation is improved with intravenous administration of contrast media. The reader is referred to the monograph of Barnes, Urion, and Share (1990) for an exhaustive review of neuroimaging in pediatric practice.

Magnetic Resonance Imaging. Magnetic resonance as an imaging modality can provide better delineation of white matter, brainstem, and cerebellar structures, as well as primary imaging of the spinal cord. It can image the central nervous system in sagittal presentation and horizontal presentations directly, thus providing valuable information regarding suspected midline pathology.

REFERENCES

Barnes PB, Urion DK, Share K: Clinical principles of pediatric neuroradiology and MR imaging. *In* Wolper R, Barnes PB, Strand RD (eds): M.R. in Pediatric Neuroradiology. St. Louis, CV Mosby, 1990.

Barringer R: A simplified procedure for spinal fluid cytology. Arch Neurol 22:305, 1970.

Bresnan MJ: Degenerative disorders. *In* Weiner H, Levitt L, Bresnan MJ (eds): Pediatric Neurology for the House Officer, 2nd ed. Baltimore, Williams & Wilkins, 1986.

Carpenter S, Karpati G: Sweat gland duct cells in Lafora body disease: diagnosis by skin biopsy. Neurology 31:1564, 1981.

Carpenter S, Karpati G, Andermann F: Specific involvement of muscle, nerve, and skin in late infantile and juvenile amaurotic idiocy. Neurology 22:170, 1972.

Cole M: Examination of the CSF. *In* Toole J (ed): Special Techniques for Neurologic Diagnosis. Philadelphia, FA Davis, 1969.

Dubowitz V, Brook MH: Muscle Biopsy: A Modern Approach. Philadelphia, WB Saunders, 1973.

Gibbels E, et al: Severe polyneuropathy in Tangier disease mimicking syringomyelia or leprosy: clinical, biochemical, electrophysiological, and morphological evaluation. J Neurol 232:283, 1985.

Hill A, Volpe JJ: Fetal Neurology. New York, Raven Press, 1989.

Holmes GH: Diagnosis and Management of Seizures in Children. Philadelphia, WB Saunders, 1987.

Jordan GW, et al: CSF lactate in diseases of the CNS. Arch Intern Med 143:85, 1983.

Kunkel LM, et al: Analysis of deletions in DNA in patients with Becker and Duchenne muscular dystrophy. Nature 322:73, 1986.

Spehlmann R: Evoked Potential Primer. Stoneham, MA, Butterworth, 1985.

Volpe JJ: Neurology of the Newborn, 2nd ed. Philadelphia, WB Saunders, 1987.

Weiner H, Levitt L, Urion DK: Pediatric Neurology for the House Officer, 4th ed. Baltimore, Williams & Wilkins, in press.

75 Comprehensive Formulation of Assessment

William B. Carey • Melvin D. Levine

 Before proceeding from the diagnostic phase to management of the problems or issues, the clinician has to bring together a wide range of information: environmental and biological, developmental and behavioral, strengths and liabilities, major and minor, historical and observed. This chapter suggests a way to include all of these elements in an organized presentation that will enhance understanding of the child and the situation by avoiding oversimplified labels and that will lead to optimal management.

As the process of assessment nears completion, the clinician arranges and weighs evidence from various sources to compile a diagnostic formulation, one that will evolve into a therapeutic plan. The preceding chapters in this book have explored a wide range of biological and psychosocial factors influencing children's development and behavior. There has been extensive review of the many possible symptomatic manifestations of these factors, along with consideration of assessment techniques by which they may be evaluated. Only a comprehensive formulation that integrates pertinent information from these multiple sources will effectively coordinate the clinician's plan of management while facilitating discussions about the child with the family and allowing for effective communication with colleagues and referral resources. One approach to such a formulation is delineated here. (Some others were mentioned in Chapter 67.)

Deficiencies Commonly Encountered in Present Diagnostic Practice

Diagnostic reasoning commonly employed in clinical practice today may be susceptible to problems of oversimplification of various sorts and to a tendency to view the child too narrowly. Perhaps the most common weakness in current diagnostic practice is the use of the child's worst problem as the main or only diagnosis. To refer to a child as "CP," "asthmatic," "ADD," or "drug abuser" may identify the most troublesome focus of parental and professional concern and even may be a useful form of mental shorthand for the clinician. However, such labels fail to consider the important array of relevant strengths and weaknesses of the child and his or her milieu. Since all children with a specific condition, such as asthma, are not the same, a false sense of homogeneity may be conveyed through inappropriate use of labels. Furthermore, certain particularly meaningless and perhaps misleading labels are often used as summary statements about children. "Hyperactivity" is a prime example of this practice; the term is poorly defined and means different things to different persons (Carey and McDevitt, 1995). "Emotionally disturbed"

is another diagnosis that is too vague to convey a specific meaning and is potentially harmful to parents and children.

Another diagnostic distortion occurs when examiners put their own main interest or area of expertise first and give little or no attention to other aspects of the child. To the allergist, the child's hypersensitivities may be taken as his or her most pressing or only problem. To the family therapist, family dynamics are of paramount and sometimes exclusive significance. Although various aspects of the child and his or her situation may contribute to a comprehensive diagnostic formulation, no single facet should be mistaken as constituting an adequate account of the total child.

The problem-oriented approach has its supporters, who maintain that documenting specific clinical concerns clearly ensures that they will be remembered and dealt with adequately. One cannot quarrel with that goal. However, the message of this chapter is that unless all pertinent weaknesses and strengths of the child and his or her situation are assembled into a single formulation, there is a real danger that some complication or critical redeeming aspects of a child will be overlooked.

The inadequacies for pediatric practice of the currently available psychiatric diagnostic schemes are explored in Chapter 67. Unfortunately the new *Diagnostic and Statistical Manual for Primary Care: Child and Adolescent Version (DSM-PC)* presents only lists of "environmental situations" and "child manifestations" and does not offer any scheme for constructing a comprehensive formulation comparable to the one proposed in this chapter.

Elements of a Comprehensive Formulation of the Assessment

Having strongly urged a comprehensive formulation, one must acknowledge that it is difficult, and perhaps impossible, to present a single scheme on which all potential users can agree. The following are some basic elements of one articulated diagnostic profile (Table 75–1).

For purposes of diagnostic formulation, it seems reasonable to suggest a three-part separation of the status of the child into physical health, development, and behavior. A complete assessment must also include an evaluation of

Table 75–1 • Comprehensive Formulation of Assessment

STATUS OF CHILD

A. Physical Health

Area	Significant Strength(s)	Significant Deficit(s)	Service Need(s)
General physical health—organic			
Physical health—functional			
Physical maturation			
Nutrition and growth			
Neurologic status: sensory, motor, reflexes, coordination			

B. Developmental Function

Area	Significant Strength(s)	Significant Deficit(s)	Service Need(s)
Language ability			
Skill/knowledge acquisition			
School/preschool performance capacity			
Motor function: gross and fine			
Attention and organization			
Social cognition			

C. Behavior and Emotions (Affect)

Area	Significant Strength(s)	Significant Deficit(s)	Service Need(s)
I. Temperament: behavioral style traits and clusters			
II. Behavioral adjustment: content and performance—general			
Interpersonal relations			
Task performance: school, work, play			
Self-relations: esteem, care, regulation			
Internal status: thinking, feeling, functional somatic status			
Coping style and ability			

ENVIRONMENTAL TRANSACTIONS

Area	Significant Strength(s)	Significant Deficit(s)	Service Need(s)
Input 1: parental care patterns			
Input 2: sociocultural influences			
Input 3: other factors in environment—nonhuman			
Outcome 1: effects of child on parents and other caregivers			
Outcome 2: concerns of caregivers			
Other inputs and outcomes			

SUMMARY OF FINDINGS:

PLANS:
 To meet needs:
 For follow-up:

the child's transactions with the environment. Thus, four general domains require assessment.

STATUS OF THE CHILD

Physical Health

An appraisal of the physical health describes the child's organic and functional condition and includes organic illness and malfunction or handicaps of various organ systems (such as the skin and respiratory and cardiovascular systems) as well as nutritional status, growth and physical maturation, and such problems as malnourishment, obesity, disturbances of growth or bodily development, and evidence of substance abuse. Some of these conditions and their impacts are discussed in Part IV of this book.

The neurologic status subsumes sensory and motor function, reflexes, and coordination. Problems in this area might include sensory loss, including vision and hearing, "cerebral palsy," convulsive disorders, "soft signs" (minor neurologic indicators), or motor incoordination. These findings and the biological influences affecting them are considered extensively in Part III of this book.

Developmental Function

The section of the diagnostic formulation on capacities includes the various elements of development and their current level and degree of appropriateness for age. Included are a child's gross motor function, fine motor skills, language proficiency, spatial orientation, temporal-sequential organization, higher-order conceptual abilities, and various aspects of social perception and skills (see Chapter 53). The child's level of academic performance skills and age-appropriate task performance capacities are also documented. The current status of the child's attention and organizational ability should be taken into account. These latter characteristics are hard to classify and thus are also found in this comprehensive formulation under *temperament*. This section of the formulation is where one includes neurodevelopmental variations and disorders of learning.

The diagnostician should undertake a careful search for developmental strengths, special talents, and content affinities. It is these highly individualized abilities that can serve as a critical support system for self-esteem and motivation. In particular, the clinician needs to uncover strengths that are not being encouraged, a child's assets that are being neglected by parents and the school. Such abilities need ongoing nurturance.

Instead of seeking to characterize a child's overall cognitive ability with a numeral (such as an intelligence quotient [IQ] score), it is far more beneficial to focus on a child's profile of strengths and weaknesses. There is growing recognition that there exist many forms of intelligence (Gardner, 1983). An astute clinician should uncover and describe a child's unique areas of intellectual competency.

Assessment of these various capacities is discussed elsewhere, particularly in the other chapters of this section.

Behavior and Emotions (Affect)

The child's temperament or behavioral style should be considered and evaluated independently of his or her be-havioral performance or adjustment. The various dimensions of temperament and the clinical clusters derived from them have been described fully in Chapter 8, and indications and techniques for their assessment are discussed in Chapter 67.

As already noted, a quandary arises in regard to the placement of attention, considered to be an aspect of cognitive function and of temperament. There may be similarities or differences in the various components of attention required for specific learning tasks and those involved in a child's overall interaction with his or her social environment. For the present, the characteristic can tentatively appear under both headings, attention being more of an aspect of cognition, while persistence at tasks is more a part of temperament or behavioral style.

The assessment of behavioral performance or adjustment, as described especially in Chapters 54, 66, and 67, deals with the following:

1. The child's relations with persons—the degree of social competence or undersocialization
2. Performance of tasks, especially schoolwork, and play—the extent of task mastery or underachievement; actual performance of tasks should be rated here and differentiated from the capacity to perform them, which is an aspect of development
3. Self-relations—whether self-assured or troubled with problems in self-relations: self-neglect, poor self-esteem, and inadequate or excessive self-regulation
4. Internal status: other thoughts, feelings, and physiologic function—a sense of well-being versus disturbed feelings (anxiety, depression), disturbed thinking (phobias, obsessions), or physiologic dysfunctions (sleep disorder, pains)
5. A final part of this section is an appraisal of the child's adaptive or coping style and abilities (see Chapter 8)

Motivation is an important dimension of behavior, but since it is estimated only with great difficulty by the primary care clinician, it is not included as a component of this comprehensive profile. It may be possible to estimate it from other components of behavioral adjustment.

ENVIRONMENTAL TRANSACTIONS

The interaction of the child with his or her environment should reflect both the ways in which the environment is affecting the child and how the child is altering his or her milieu. These environmental factors are covered in Part II of this volume.

Parents

Parental care consists of parental attitudes including expectations (How realistic and how supportive are they?), parental feelings (What is the amount of attachment or detachment and of affection or anger and rejection?), and the actual management of the child (What is the amount and quality of physical care, stimulation, affection, guidance, and socialization given to the child?).

Mrazek and colleagues (1995) suggested a Parenting Risk Scale, which is an overall judgement of parenting divided into three levels of function: (1) adequate parenting, by which is meant either average or exceptional parenting; (2) concerns about parenting, which describes the situation with some degree of problems like intense marital conflict or parental emotional problems, but not serious enough for immediate intervention beyond close follow-up; and (3) parenting difficulties, which includes serious problems like punitive parenting and neglect.

The key dimensions of parenting used by Mrazek and colleagues in arriving at the general judgement of its adequacy are (1) emotional availability, or degree of warmth; (2) control, or degree of flexibility and permission; (3) parental psychosocial status: the freedom from (or presence of) overt disorder in the parents; (4) knowledge base: the parents' understanding of emotional and physical development as well as basic child care principles; and (5) commitment: an adequate prioritization of child care responsibilities (see also Chapters 7, 11, and 16).

Sociocultural Milieu

The sociocultural situation describes the impact of siblings, other family members, peer group, neighborhood influences, television, school, and health care practices. Which are helpful and which are not?

It is important to take into consideration the cultural background of a child and his or her family. A clinician should describe and respect behaviors, values, and attitudes that are a product of an individual's national or ethnic background. Bilingual children, including those born in other countries, should be thought about in terms of their adjustment to any divergent cultural demands and their success in forging an identity that bridges the two cultures.

Assessments of the general sociocultural situation should include a review of a variety of extrafamilial factors: quality of the community, adequacy of educational services, parental employment status, housing, economic conditions, quality of health care, interactions with the legal system, and other issues. The available psychiatric diagnostic schemes *(DSM-IV, ICD-10, DC:0-3)* as well as the *DSM-PC* (see Chapter 67) have all presented lists of environmental situations to consider in diagnosis, but all suggest ratings only of problems, without offering the clinician opportunities to make note of the positive features in the child's environment.

Nonhuman Environment

An appraisal of the nonhuman environment rates the degree of suitability or hazard in housing, pets, environmental substances, disease exposure, climatic conditions, and so forth.

The impact of the child on his or her surroundings is a highly important part of the interaction that is frequently either ignored or not explicitly included in diagnostic formulations. One rates here the degree of pleasure or displeasure and satisfaction or dissatisfaction experienced by parents, teachers, and others who regularly encounter the child. It should include a statement about the aspects of the child that are most bothersome and that have led to clinical attention.

SUMMARY OF FINDINGS

At the end of the comprehensive diagnostic formulation it is appropriate to summarize the various details in a single statement or two.

EXAMPLE

This 8-month-old male infant is physically, neurologically, and developmentally normal and has a relatively easy temperament, but he has become very demanding of his mother's attention. He cries repeatedly and prolongedly and his mother feels obliged to pick him up and comfort him whenever he cries. The mother has become angry about the infant's demands and thinks that there is something wrong with him. The reason seems to be that the authoritarian grandmother persuaded the mother that the infant should not be allowed to cry because of his umbilical hernia.

Sometimes clinical syndromes emerge from certain combinations of findings. Many of these are described in Part V of this book. For example, the so-called vulnerable child syndrome (see Chapter 33) characterizes the child who is physically and developmentally normal but has a particular pattern of behavioral maladjustment related to the continuation of inappropriate parental concern and handling following recovery from a worrisome early illness. The summary is the section in which such syndromes could be mentioned.

PLANS FOR SERVICE NEEDS

Finally, it is desirable to select from the list of findings in the comprehensive diagnostic formulation those areas calling for action on the part of the clinician. Not all of the suspected or definite problems need be dealt with. For example, if parents are coping well with a child with a difficult temperament, intervention is not indicated, as it would be if there were parental-child conflict because of the problem. Similarly, a pediatrician generally should not attempt to influence the course of a parental divorce but should help the family understand and cope with its impact on the child. The service needs for the demanding infant in the example would include sufficient examination to reassure the clinician and the family that there is no physical problem with the child other than the umbilical hernia, suggestions to the mother about revision of her handling of the baby, and help for the mother in evaluating more critically the advice received from her own mother.

Having thus defined appropriate service needs, the clinician can proceed to implement them, which is the process of management described in Part VII of this book. Plans for follow-up complete the formulation.

Unfortunately, the recently published *DSM-PC*, although including a section on estimation of the severity of the clinical problem, does not suggest a way to formulate, prioritize, and execute the needs for clinical services (see Chapter 67).

Advantages of a Comprehensive Formulation

The advantages in the use of the comprehensive diagnostic formulation can be found in practice, research, and education.

In practice one gains the assurance in making a complex diagnosis that a broad range of pertinent factors is considered so that relevant issues are unlikely to be omitted. This wide view of the child enhances the clinician's diagnostic reasoning, his or her discussions with the patient and family, and his or her communications with other professionals. One can reasonably argue that such a comprehensive evaluation is not necessary in the immediate management of acute minor illnesses such as otitis media or gastroenteritis. However, if professional contacts extend into well-child care or involvement with chronic physical problems, a broader evaluation becomes very helpful. With concerns in the area of development and behavior, this is a necessity, not a luxury. Plans for management of problems in the latter areas stand a far better chance of meeting the child's needs if they are based on a truly comprehensive, empiric assessment rather than on incomplete data or stereotypical diagnostic labels.

In carrying out research, the use of this model of formulation encourages more precise definition of subjects, thus allowing studies to become more interpretable and more significant. For example, as already mentioned, investigations referring to patients simply as "hyperactive" or "ADHD" without any further clarification of their overall function are of little value. In whose view is the child excessively active or inattentive, and how was that determined? Will not the study outcomes be affected by how a child rates in each of the four components of the comprehensive formulation (physical and neurologic status, development, temperament and behavioral adjustment, and interactions)? There are serious dangers in attempting to study a child or a cohort identified by only a single symptom.

In medical education, the use of this approach to assessment would encourage both teachers and students to think of children in terms of their true complexity and avoid overly facile diagnoses based on inadequate information or narrow observer bias.

Problems in Formulation

One must acknowledge that although primary care clinicians need to reason comprehensively, this admirable goal is not easily achieved. In the first place, the various professional persons dealing with the child's development and behavior may not agree that any one particular profile of the child's status is an acceptable one. Various settings and points of view may argue for modifications of contents and subdivisions. For example, the advocates of neurology and psychiatry may plead for an expansion of their spheres of interest. One should not object to this as long as the other elements of the formulation are retained and considered in the final diagnosis and service plan.

Another problem is the lack of standardized criteria for diagnostic ratings in some areas, particularly behavioral adjustment. One can agree that this topic deals primarily with the child's relationship to others, to tasks, and to himself or herself, and so on, but the dividing line between normal and abnormal is broad and variable.

How is the clinician to arrive at a comprehensive diagnostic formulation if there is a major area of missing data, as with the pediatrician evaluating a problem of school adjustment without specific data about information processing skills? Clearly he or she must refrain from proposing a final diagnosis until such assessments are available. On the other hand, the same information may be largely superfluous in other situations, as in the case of helping the child and surviving parent deal with the death of the other parent. All the areas of the formulation should be borne in mind, but clinical data in each are sought only to the extent appropriate for competent management of the child.

Finally, a major problem in the use of this sort of diagnostic profile is its implementation, that is, in persuading oneself and others to give up old habits of abbreviated and distorted conceptualizations and to think comprehensively.

REFERENCES

Carey WB, McDevitt SC: Coping with Children's Temperament. A Guide for Professionals. New York, Basic Books, 1995.
Gardner G: Frames of Mind. New York, Basic Books. 1983.
Mrazek DA, Mrazek P, Klinnert M: Clinical assessment of parenting. J Am Acad Child Adolesc Psychiatry 34:272, 1995.

BIBLIOGRAPHY

Levine MD, Brooks R, Shonkoff JP: A Pediatric Approach to Learning Disorders. New York, John Wiley & Sons, 1980.
Rose JA: Pediatric interview manual. Unpublished manuscript, 1962.
Talbot NB, Howell MC: Social and behavioral causes and consequences of disease among children. *In* Talbot NB, Kagan J, Eisenberg L (eds): Behavioral Science in Pediatric Medicine. Philadelphia, WB Saunders, 1971.

PART VII

The Enhancement of Development and Adaptation

76 Pediatric Counseling

Barton D. Schmitt

 Counseling is the clinician's most consistently effective management technique for developmental-behavioral issues. Pediatricians can help families to improve or resolve most of the behavioral problems they encounter by a combination of a basic knowledge of the field and skillful interviewing followed by individualized counseling. This chapter provides a comprehensive review of the essential components of this process and how to acquire them. As this competence increases, the practitioner is likely to deal more appropriately with parental concerns and to avoid excessive use of medication and referrals.

Behavior problems are very common in childhood. Periodically, all children have behavioral symptoms. Ten percent to 15% of children develop behavioral problems that interfere with life adjustment. Physicians caring for children are called on to provide counseling about behavior and development many times each day.

A definition of pediatric counseling is found in Table 76–1. The fact that the pediatrician works with basically healthy families has a significant impact on the nature of counseling. In many cases the pediatrician's role consists of delineating and clarifying problem behavior patterns and trying to change them through active advice. Frequently this requires only one or two visits. Usually such efforts are successful and highly efficient. The primary care physician has an advantage over many other counselors in knowing how the family operates and having their trust because of his or her previously established efficacy with physical

illnesses. Families who do not respond to pediatric counseling can be referred for psychotherapy at a later time. The sensitive pediatrician often can detect more seriously disturbed families and refer them after the first visit.

In this chapter, several types of pediatric counseling that fall within the primary care domain are reviewed. The behavior problems selected as examples are commonplace ones, and the counseling methods discussed can be integrated into the practicing pediatrician's office time frame. Levels of intervention are covered in approximate order of increasing complexity and time requirements. Generally the pediatrician acts at the lowest level of intervention that is effective for the issue with which he or she is dealing. Pediatricians are in a unique position to be eclectic. Most problems require a combination of treatment approaches (e.g., education, reassurance, advice, and advocacy). Although every pediatrician provides some counseling, individual interest and training vary greatly. Each physician should participate in this aspect of health care only to the degree to which he or she feels comfortable.

Once a meaningful alliance has been established, specific techniques of counseling can be employed. Most pediatricians tend not to adopt any stereotyped or consistent approach. The nature of the problems, the family's coping style, and the likelihood of a child's or parent's benefiting from various approaches are among the factors that need to be taken into consideration. Some general modalities of counseling are covered in the following sections and are summarized in Table 76–2.

Releasing Painful Feelings

Some parents and patients are in acute emotional distress when they visit their physician. They are preoccupied with

Table 76–1 • The Pediatric Counselor's Orientation (Relative to That of the Psychotherapist)

Works mainly with stable children and parents
Focuses more on the present
Focuses more on behavior than on thoughts or feelings
Focuses more on minor variations in behavior and development
Requires less extensive evaluations
Leads the interview more (provides less total listening time)
Uses more action-oriented, direct, specific approaches
Uses more empirical approaches (if an approach works, one does not need to know the theory behind it)
Uses more behavior modification
Relies more on education, reassurance, specific advice, and environmental intervention
Provides briefer follow-up visits (20 or 30 minutes)
Provides fewer visits (two to three for most problems; six maximum)
Sets a shorter time frame for results (usually 3 months)

Table 76–2 • Types of Pediatric Counseling

Releasing painful feelings—first deal with pressing emotional issues
Education—supplying needed general information
Reassurance—specific information that counteracts fears
Clarifying the problem and its cause—providing parents with a clearer perspective about the child's problems
Approval of the parents' approach—helping parents to use their own resources
Specific advice—suggestions about altered parental handling of specific problems
Environmental intervention—suggestions about other changes in the child's environment
Extended counseling—more visits for more complicated issues

painful issues. Until these painful feelings find an outlet, the parent probably will not be able to relate an accurate medical history or interpret medical advice. Also any counseling that requires thinking (e.g., behavior modification) may be less successful until compelling emotional issues are dealt with.

The process of releasing painful feelings may be called *ventilation*, a term that has numerous implications. The angry parent may need to ventilate about having to deal with their child's encopresis. The frightened patient may need to express fears (e.g., a hyperventilation attack). The mourning patient may need to grieve about the loss (e.g., sudden death of a parent). A patient who has been attacked (e.g., a rape victim) may need to pour out feelings about what has happened.

For the process of ventilation to occur, the setting must be relaxed and private. The patient or parent is encouraged to talk. Usually ventilation begins spontaneously. The process can also be initiated by openers such as "You look angry (worried or sad). Why don't you tell me what's troubling you?" The repetition of emotionally laden words that the parent has used will help to continue the process (e.g., "You felt put down"). The essential response to ventilation is noncritical listening. Any censure removes the invitation to talk freely. Even if the parent's feelings seem excessive, the physician must express agreement that the situation is "unfortunate." The parent or child does not want to hear that "It could be worse" or "Be grateful that (such and such) didn't happen." The success of ventilation depends on the patient's perception that he or she has expressed personal anguish to someone who really understands. As a distressed parent or child expresses deep feelings, there may be a recovery of composure and emotional equilibrium.

Providing Education

Education involves the presentation of facts or medical opinions to a parent or child. Education is undertaken mainly to impart information, but it also plays a critical role in reducing anxiety, dispelling misconception, and fostering feelings of effectiveness on the part of a parent or child.

Requested Education. Education may be particularly effective when it has been asked for. In these instances the timing of the education is optimal. Adolescents com-

monly have questions about acne, sexually transmitted diseases, the prevention of pregnancy, tattoos, and smoking. These topics obviously deserve thoughtful answers. A family may ask a physician about the pros and cons of getting a dog. The physician can remind them that most children under 3 years of age cannot be taught to treat a dog appropriately and risk being bitten. If parents wish to have a dog during this developmental period, they can be advised not to leave their child alone with the dog at any time.

The difficult situation of having to give parents bad news about the health of their child is covered in various chapters about specific situations, such as the birth of a child with Down syndrome (Chapter 24).

Anticipatory Guidance. Anticipatory guidance (or preventive counseling) is the advice pediatricians provide to avoid problems that could occur in the future. Topics such as nutrition, accident prevention, behavior management, developmental stimulation, sex education, and general health education all may be covered during every visit. Most expectant parents have many questions that can be discussed with their pediatrician several weeks prior to delivery. The most frequent concerns include arguments for and against breast-feeding and circumcision, hospital policies about rooming-in and the father's presence in the delivery room, separation problems with siblings during the mother's confinement, ways of decreasing sibling rivalry, and essential baby equipment.

Printed or Audiovisual Approaches. Comprehensive education of the parents can be very time-consuming for the physician. More efficient methods are available. Printed materials include information sheets written by the physician, health pamphlets, or books. Not only do information sheets save the physician's time, they also give the father (or other family members who were not present during the office visit) the opportunity to read what the physician recommends. In addition, these handouts can provide more information than most physicians have the time to give and they help to prevent recall problems for the mother. Some offices also have audio cassettes or video cassettes that are available in the waiting room to impart information. These aids may cover specific age groups (e.g., newborn care) or chronic diseases (e.g., asthma). These educational aids can supplement individualized discussion with the family.

Providing Reassurance

Reassurance can be defined as a special kind of education that counteracts fears. Reassurance relieves or removes unnecessary anxiety, especially regarding one's physical or emotional health. Reassurance is the physician's most commonly used type of counseling. Reassurance is very therapeutic. Parents need some reassurance during almost every office visit. Reassurance is more likely to be effective if the following guidelines are followed. (See also Chapter 31 in regard to the management of minor illnesses.)

Precede by Data Collection. To be effective, reassurance must be properly timed. It should never be too hasty or offered too early. In patients with emotional concerns, a careful history should be elicited. Reassurance based on meager data is likely to be unconvincing to the parent. Only after the parent or child believes that the physician has explored the problem adequately and understands it, will the reassurance be acceptable. (See Chapter 66 on interviewing.)

Be Specific. The most effective reassurance is specific and focused. The targeted concern or worry is identified by listening carefully. For example, a parent may be afraid primarily of a brain tumor in a child with recurrent headaches, appendicitis in a child with recurrent abdominal pains, or a heart attack in a child with chest pains. Once the precise overriding fear is identified, the physician can carefully investigate that specific concern and offer reassurance when the fear is unfounded. Blanket reassurance (e.g., "There's nothing to worry about," "Everything will be just fine," or other extravagant promises) leads the parent to suspect the physician of being somewhat dishonest or insensitive and dilutes the value of any specific advice.

Be Honest. What the physician tells the parents must be honest. If the physician is caught in one lie, the balance of his or her reassurance will be thrown into question. On the other hand, the physician need not reveal everything he or she is thinking. Any nonessential data that would be anxiety producing can be withheld (e.g., the differential diagnosis).

Be Brief. Reassurance should be offered in as few words as possible. When reassurance is tenuous, the physician may be tempted to prolong the discussion of those aspects of the case that are reassuring. Most parents sense that the physician is hiding his or her real feelings and worries behind a long speech.

Universalize the Problem. Physicians can offer great comfort to parents and children by commenting on the universality of their problems (when appropriate). Statements such as "Do you know any 2-year olds who don't have tantrums?" or "That argument goes on in every home where there's a 16-year-old" can alleviate much anxiety.

Provide Nonverbal Reassurance. Nonverbal messages often communicate more to the parent than the physician's words. The physician can show concern for the patient without expressing alarm. For example, a physician can examine a patient's heart without wearing a worried facial expression. If a parent relates a history of symptoms that have frightened him or her to a physician who remains calm, he or she will often conclude, "If this doesn't upset my doctor, I guess everything is going to be all right." Most parents and children believe body language more than words or logic.

Examples of Reassurance. Parents of infants need reassurance that their child's red face and grunting with bowel movements do not mean that the child is constipated. Head rolling and body rocking in infants do not represent an emotional problem but are methods of making a transition into sleep. Thumb-sucking in young children is comforting but does not mean that insecurity is present. This example is also a reminder that reassurance is age dependent and that after age 5 or 6, thumb-sucking should be discouraged because it can cause malocclusion of the permanent teeth. Although the parents of young infants should be reassured about postural abnormalities of the legs and feet (e.g., toeing-in or bowlegs), the physician must be careful not to raise false hopes about the rapidity

of the self-correction. The parents can be reassured that the correction will be complete but that it will not begin until the child starts to walk and then will take approximately 12 months or longer of walking before the child's legs and feet will begin to look straight.

School-aged children who are reacting to a divorce need reassurance that visitation with both parents will continue, that their parents still love them, and that their school and friends will not change. Children with a history of retentive soiling need reassurance that their bowel movements will be pain free if they take a stool softener and that they do not need to hold back the bowel movements to protect themselves from pain. Adolescent patients are concerned often about rapid growth and body change. They need reassurance that their particular somatotype, genital size, breast size, and other body parts are normal.

Clarifying the Problem and Its Cause

Listening. To be effective at counseling, one needs a complete and accurate picture of a problem. A common error in giving advice is offering it too quickly. The parents and child should be listened to if one wishes to understand their worlds. Any conclusions about whether parents are reasonable or unreasonable should be delayed until they have been allowed to describe their unique situation. Listening in itself is therapeutic; it conveys respect and encourages independent decision making. (See also Chapter 66 on interviewing.)

Minimal Psychosocial Database. Children with one or two behavior symptoms (e.g., thumb-sucking or nightmares) can be treated by offering direct advice if the physician observes a happy child and a positive parent-child interaction. An expeditious approach usually can also be taken with families whom the physician knows from long experience to be stable. In these cases only three additional questions need to be asked. First, "Does he (or she) have any other behavior problems?" Second, "Why do you think he (or she) is acting this way?" Third, "What have you already tried?" In this way, the physician will not prescribe advice that has already failed. In children with multiple symptoms (e.g., multiple discipline problems) or complex problems (e.g., encopresis), a complete psychosocial database should be collected before advice is offered. (See Chapters 66, 67, and 75.)

Clarification of Problems. Clarification involves identification of the problem and an explanation of its possible causes and effects. The objective of clarification is to help parents understand their child's behavior. The physician must carefully review with the parents the behavior patterns they want changed. The parents have the final word about the selection of target behaviors. The physician can state, "If I understand you correctly, you are most concerned about . . ." Pediatricians, however, may not have enough time to allow parents to work out their own understanding of the cause of their child's problems. Once the physician understands the situation, he or she may explain it in general terms. In some cases the parents are either too strict or too lenient. Sometimes the central issue is a vicious cycle or power struggle (e.g., pressure brings resistance; constant criticism leads to giving up and depression). The parents should be given credit if their analysis of the problem seems correct. Once the physician has presented an interpretation to the parents, he or she can ask whether it makes sense to them.

Reducing Parental Guilt Regarding the Cause. The parents of children with emotional problems usually take them personally and feel somewhat responsible. Once the parent-child relationship has been examined and parents have been advised to change what they are doing, this guilt is inevitable.

Guilt can be reduced in several ways. The physician will do best by keeping a no-fault attitude during counseling. The guilt can be universalized (e.g., "Everyone tries that."). The physician can absolve the parents (e.g., "I can easily understand why you tried that."). The blame can be shared with schools, relatives, siblings, and other etiologic factors (e.g., "Your actions were just one of the reasons behind this problem."). The parents can be reminded that the harm was not intentional. Also the parents' errors can be relegated to the past (e.g., "That was long ago and much has happened since then."). Mainly the physician can show empathy and emphasize, "All parents make some mistakes, and that is part of being an involved parent." Positive aspects of the parent-child relationship can be underscored. Sometimes problems stem from parental leniency and overindulgence, and the physician can state, "You love him too much." or "You tried too hard." One can end with the viewpoint that "The main need now is to look ahead rather than behind. Don't be too hard on yourselves."

Approving the Parents' Approach to Treatment

A definite trend in the delivery of health services is self-care. Parents are being encouraged to become active participants in their family's health service. Just as parents learn how to manage their child's coughs and colds by themselves, the common sense they possess about human behavior should also be supported. The physician is in a position to foster independent decision making. Not only is this approach sound economically, it also enhances the parental sense of competency. Inexperienced new parents are often overanxious and insecure. They need to be temporarily dependent on their physicians. Bringing such parents to a level of independent problem solving and self-care is a gradual but achievable process.

Reinforce the Parents' Strategies. After clarification of a problem, parents may formulate their own treatment plan. Others can be encouraged to problem-solve. The physician can ask, "Now that you understand the problem, what are your options?" He or she can endorse their plans (if they are reasonable) and encourage them to adhere to them. Often parents seek the physician's approval to do what they wanted to do anyway (e.g., using the pacifier). In this way independent thought is encouraged and the parents' self-confidence is strengthened. The physician constantly operates on the premise that a wide variation of workable approaches exists for most problems and that the selection of a strategy must take into account the

parents' lifestyle, culture, and value system. Since the parents will have to live with the consequences of the plan, they should be encouraged to arrive at final management decisions themselves. If the parent's plans are unlikely to be successful, however, the physician should discuss his or her reservations with them.

Approval of Parenting. Parents can be complimented regarding their parenting skills during every visit. Mentioning that a child is courteous, patient, brave, or cooperative or shows other desirable personality traits in the office setting helps the parents believe they are doing a good job. Parents of children with emotional problems are usually on the defensive and need to hear that the physician knows they love their child.

Avoid Criticism. Criticism of parents has several unfortunate side effects. First, it engenders guilt. Many parents normally blame themselves for causing their child's symptoms (e.g., by losing their temper and yelling), and the physician should alleviate rather than accentuate such self-accusation. Second, parents who are criticized may become angry at the physician, and his or her medical advice then may be followed poorly. Even harmful approaches usually can be changed without confrontation by stating diplomatically, "Recently we have found that a different approach works better."

Providing Specific Advice for Management

The physician should make specific recommendations for the relief of symptoms. Advice is indicated whenever a simple behavioral problem exists for which the parents are unable to devise an approach. The direct giving of advice is the mainstay of brief counseling. Suggestions about childrearing are among the most common types of advice offered. Standard advice can be given for symptoms with a clear etiology. More individualized advice must be prescribed for problems with a differential diagnosis of several etiologic subtypes. Practical, clear-cut instructions are more likely to be successful. Pediatricians should have treatment packages (consisting of one to 10 pieces of advice) for all common parental complaints. In emotionally healthy persons, one does not need to worry about symptom substitution. The physician should restrict advice to his or her areas of expertise and should avoid giving speculative advice in areas in which he or she is not trained or experienced, no matter what they may be. Examples of specific advice geared to the age of the child are presented in Chapters 2 to 6.

The following is a specific and very familiar advice-giving scenario: Negativism is a normal healthy phase seen in most children between 2 and 3 years of age. The perspective that this phase is an important declaration of independence needs to be shared with parents. To the child, "No" means "Do I have to?" It should not be confused with disrespect. If the parent can keep a sense of humor about this phase, it will only last 6 to 12 months. Second, the child should not be punished for saying "No." Third, the parents should try to minimize their directives and rules; they should avoid unnecessary demands and keep safety as their main priority during this time. Fourth, they should give the child extra choices and alternatives to increase his or her sense of freedom. Examples are letting him or her choose the book he or she wants to read, the toys that go into the bathtub, and the fruit he or she wants for a snack. The physician can ask which ear the child wants looked at first. The more quickly the child gains a feeling that he or she is a decision maker, the more quickly this phase will pass. Fifth, the child should not be given choices when no choice exists. Taking a bath and going to bed are not negotiable. Sixth, when a request must be made, the child can be given a 5-minute warning to help with the transition. The parent must avoid the two extremes of punishing the child or giving in to all the child's "No's." Helping children learn to cope with illnesses (see Part IV) and various social stressors (see Part II) are covered earlier in this volume.

Gain the Parents' Acceptance of the Advice. The physician needs feedback from the parents about the advice that has been suggested. To avoid confusion, he or she can ask the parents to repeat the substance of what has been said. He or she can say, "Please review for me what our new plan is." If misunderstandings are present, they can be resolved before action is taken. To avoid noncompliance with advice, the physician must also ask whether this particular advice is acceptable to the parents. He or she can ask, "Does that seem reasonable to you?" or "How do you feel about that approach?" If the parents seem unconvinced, the physician must decide whether to persuade them to accept this particular advice or to suggest another option.

Write Down Advice for the Parents. The physician should jot down the main suggestions that the parents have agreed on and give it to them as they leave, making a copy for his or her own records. Another option is to provide a parent handout on this subject. Exceptions to the generic advice can always be pencilled in. In this way the physician can be assured that the plan will not be undermined by forgetfulness. Parents usually appreciate this added demonstration of concern.

Follow-Up Visits. If advice is given, the results of the advice should be learned. Advice should be followed by at least one visit or phone call. This is in contrast to prior techniques of reassurance and education in which follow-up visits may be optional. If more than two follow-up visits are needed, probably the physician needs to acquire a more complete psychosocial database and a more precise concept of the etiology. The physician can ask the parent to keep a written record (diary or calender) between visits. This provides material for discussion. The second visit should be scheduled approximately 1 week after the first. The problem identified should remain the focus of follow-up visits. One can assess progress on the basis of symptom elimination, symptom improvement, a lack of change, worsening of symptoms, or the occurrence of a new symptom. The physician can then refine and recalibrate the treatment plan with the parents' contribution. The parents should be congratulated about any success they have had. If the treatment plan fails after several visits and the problem is sufficiently severe, a family meeting may help, or the family can be referred to a mental health resource.

Parental Adherence to the Treatment Plan. Counseling does not become effective until the parent accepts the diagnosis and carries out the therapeutic recommendations (i.e., adherence or compliance). Treatment nonadherence takes many forms, including missed appointments, not implementing advice, not giving medications, and "doctor shopping." Adherence is improved by including the parents in goal selection and treatment planning, explaining the reason for each treatment, clarifying misconceptions, simplifying the treatment regimen, linking medication-taking with daily routines, and providing written instructions. Excellent physician-parent communication and rapport also enhances compliance.

Pitfalls. A common pitfall in giving advice is rigidity on the part of the physician. The gap between the physician's request of the parents and the behavior that the parents are willing or able to provide should be kept to a minimum. If the physician's expectations are too high, he or she will lose the family to follow-up. Advice should always be presented as a consideration rather than a requirement or order.

Two examples of areas in which physicians commonly give advice that is in conflict with parents' inclinations are the child's sleeping in the parents' room and weaning. Some mothers (especially those who are breast-feeding) prefer to have their infants sleep in a cradle in the parents' bedroom until they reach an age at which nighttime feedings are unnecessary (i.e., 3 or 4 months of age). No proven harm comes from this approach. Although many physicians expect the infant to be weaned from breast or bottle by 1 year of age, many parents wish to continue breast- or bottle-feeding to 2 years of age. If the infant feeds from the breast or bottle only three or four times a day, also eats solid foods, does not carry a bottle around during the day or go to sleep with it at night, and is otherwise developing normally, the physician need not challenge the parents' position in this matter.

Providing Environmental Intervention

Environmental intervention consists of recommendations for specific changes in the patient's physical or extrafamilial environments. These recommendations attempt to reduce factors that are contributing to the patient's problems or to mobilize persons outside the family unit who can help. Environmental intervention is a part of many treatment plans. The physician becomes effective in this sphere after he or she acquires a thorough knowledge of the community's resources. Often a social worker can provide advice when he or she is uncertain about available help for a specific problem. Usually the school system and other agencies respond positively to the physician's suggestions.

In simple problems, environmental manipulation may be curative (e.g., a night-light for the child who fears the dark). In children with multifactorial problems, it may offer temporary improvement while counseling paves the way to more permanent solutions (e.g., school attendance for school phobia). Environmental interventions on behalf of the patient at home, in the school, and in the community are best illustrated by the following specific examples.

Home Recommendations. Home recommendations

can be used to change the home environment. For discipline problems, a time-out room can be designated and prepared. A quiet place can be provided for study. For sleep problems, the infant can be moved to a separate room or the adolescent can be permitted to decide about his or her own bedtime. Chores or allowances can be increased or reduced, depending on circumstances. The television set might be disconnected temporarily to encourage studying or conversation.

School Recommendations. The following recommendations can be implemented to improve the child's school environment. Nursery school or Head Start may be indicated for the child who is overprotected or understimulated. Children with a learning disability require remedial classes or tutoring after school. (See Chapter 79.) High-school students may be enlisted as tutors for younger children. For the student who develops physical symptoms of anxiety while at school (e.g., abdominal pain), the physician may request that the school nurse permit the child to rest periodically in the nurse's office for 15 minutes rather than sending the child home. For some anxious children, the physician may need to request a temporary shower excuse or gym excuse. Most children with problems can receive considerable support from their teachers if the pediatrician keeps them informed as to the child's special needs (e.g., extra bathroom privileges).

Community Recommendations. The general advice for "full activity on doctor's orders" is especially beneficial for the depressed or overprotected child. Children with socialization or peer avoidance problems need more peer contact time. The possibility of joining clubs, teams, or other recreational outlets should be explored. A summer camp program serves a similar purpose, but the camp counselors must be prepared to deal with homesickness. Special camps exist for many children with chronic diseases or handicaps. Infants with developmental delays due to environmental deprivation might be enrolled in stimulation programs.

Mobilizing a Support System. Physicians understand the value of support systems and can help mothers mobilize these. Taking care of a newborn during the first 3 months of life often requires at least two adults. The extended family may need to be enlisted if the mother has not done so. It is crucial that a relative or friend help care for siblings and assist the mother in obtaining naps, so that she will not be excessively fatigued. Sometimes a support system exists but needs to be consolidated. The father should be invited to come to a health supervision visit during the 1st year of life (as should a grandparent if one lives in the home), so that he will know that his child's pediatrician values his input and also so that he will be more accepting of the physician's telephone advice in future acute illnesses.

When no support group is available, the physician and public health nurse may temporarily provide a support system for the mother. Volunteers also may be helpful, especially mothers who have successfully managed a similar problem in their own child (e.g., colic, breast-feeding, breath-holding, or attention deficits). A physician may decide to keep a card file of the names and the phone numbers of successful mothers who are willing to provide such support and teaching. For the family in a serious crisis,

temporary placement of the children with a relative, friend, or even foster home may need to be considered.

Implementation of Environmental Intervention. In order of increasing time commitment, environmental change can be initiated by having the parents do everything, making a telephone call oneself, writing a letter, or attending a conference. Having the parents explore the possibilities in their neighborhood and then coming up with a plan constitutes the easiest approach (e.g., finding an extracurricular activity for their child). If a parent-teacher conference is the recommendation, clearly the parents can carry out this plan without the physician's further input. Telephone calls by the physician to other agencies or professionals can have an important impact (e.g., calling the psychiatrist when a child with bipolar disorder is expelled from school). More commonly the physician makes phone calls to relatives (e.g., calling grandparents for support or calling the father if he is unreasonable about child custody or when the disciplinary approaches of the father and mother are highly inconsistent). A brief letter takes little more time than a telephone call. Often the physician writes the teacher, principal, school nurse, counselor, social worker, or several of these persons regarding school recommendations. He or she may need to phone a camp director to gain special permission to allow a child with a handicap to attend camp. Scheduling a special conference in his or her office may be the only way of dealing with an alcoholic father who is having a devastating impact on his son. Occasionally the physician will need to attend a school staff meeting (e.g., when a patient has frequent seizures in school).

Extended Counseling

In brief counseling, specific advice or options are offered for one or two behavioral symptoms. Good results are expected with one or two follow-up visits. Direct advice can be given after a minimal psychosocial database has been obtained. Every pediatrician should provide brief counseling and advice.

By contrast, extended counseling requires longer visits and more extensive contacts. Extended counseling is needed for children with multiple or complicated symptoms and should be preceded by the obtaining of a more complete psychosocial database. Extended pediatric counseling may require three to six visits (or more).

Two examples of extended counseling that are common in practice of pediatrics are psychosomatic counseling and discipline counseling. Pediatricians must be fully trained to evaluate and treat children who have any symptom that might stem from psychological causes as well as organic ones (e.g., recurrent headaches, abdominal pains, and syncope). No other professional has the background to assess these complaints efficiently and completely. The main barrier to successful treatment is changing the family's focus from organic to nonorganic. Gaining the parents' confidence in a new diagnosis is usually the critical step for dealing with any psychosomatic symptom. Table 76–3 lists an approach helpful for these problems.

Skills in discipline counseling or child management counseling are a prerequisite to the enjoyment of pediatric

Table 76–3 • Steps in Psychosomatic
Evaluation and Counseling

1. Elicit a complete history.
2. Perform a meticulous physical examination.
3. Order sufficient laboratory tests to convince yourself of the child's physical health.
4. Tell the parents the diagnosis after the evaluation is complete.
5. Clarify that the child is in excellent physical health.
6. Explain that emotions can cause physical symptoms.
7. Tell the parents the reasons why the symptom is not the result of physical disease.
8. Reassure the parents about any specific diagnosis they fear.
9. Clarify for the parents that this condition occurs in normal children and in normal homes.
10. Reassure the parents that you can effectively treat this condition.
11. Encourage normal activities, especially full school attendance.
12. Have the child spend more time with age-mates.

practice. Childrearing problems are mentioned during at least one half of office visits. The steps in discipline counseling are listed in Table 76–4. A pediatrician can learn these skills by reading books for parents and taking appropriate courses.

Three additional areas in which counseling is most commonly requested center around divorce, school problems, and adolescence. Involvement in this additional counseling should be considered optional for the busy practicing pediatrician. It will usually require additional skills and training. The physician who elects to engage in these areas of expanded counseling must set attainable therapeutic goals regarding what will and will not be attempted. Although the physician will use some behavior modification and advice, most extended counseling entails active listening, family meetings, clarification, and support.

One error in extended counseling is taking on a patient who clearly needs long-term psychotherapy. A variation on this error is to remain involved with a case despite a lack of progress. Children with serious emotional problems should be referred to a mental health setting (see Chapter 77). Major education problems require the collaboration of an educational specialist. Multiproblem families should be referred to a social worker. If progress has not been accomplished by the fifth or sixth session of extended counseling, referral usually is indicated.

The Logistics and Economics of Counseling

Although some may believe that it is unrealistic for the pediatrician to become involved with time-consuming be-

Table 76–4 • Steps in Discipline Counseling

1. Teach the basic principles of behavior modification.
2. List the types of problem behavior.
3. Help the parent assign priorities to the problems.
4. Devise a treatment plan or consequence for each target behavior.
5. Demonstrate appropriate responses in the office.
6. Praise the child for adaptive behavior.
7. Write down the treatment plan.
8. Provide follow-up visits.

havioral problems, he or she is very well suited for this role. Most primary physicians are efficient. If the physician is the child's regular doctor, he or she has two advantages: he or she knows the family well and the evaluation can be done in much less time. In addition, the parents already trust his or her advice. The physician can attain the same results that it would take an unknown counselor much longer to achieve. This section reviews some aspects of office organization that may improve the physician's efficiency in counseling.

Counseling: Whom to Include. The counseling time spent with the child compared with that spent with the parents increases with age. Children younger than 5 years of age theoretically can be treated by working exclusively with the parents (ideally both of them). The child can be left with a sitter while the parents meet with the physician. Benefits of leaving the child with a sitter are that the child does not disrupt the adult conversation and also is not exposed to negative comments about himself or herself. Disadvantages are that the physician does not get a true picture of the child's behavior and does not have an opportunity to demonstrate appropriate responses to it. The youngster definitely needs to come in if he or she needs to overcome a problem that requires special motivation (e.g., thumb-sucking or encopresis). In general, I like the child present at any age so that he or she can be made a little more accountable for change. By school age, the parent and children often are seen together and therefore share the counseling time equally. If the adolescent has a personal problem, the parents may not be seen at all. If the difficulty is largely a family communication problem, the parents and adolescent come together during part of the visit, leaving some private time for the adolescent to meet with the physician. For parents who need individualized counseling, the presence of a part-time social worker in the physician's office is very helpful (e.g., for marital problems).

Data in Advance. The initial evaluation visit proceeds much more efficiently if the family or adolescent has completed a behavioral screening or descriptive questionnaire in advance (see Chapter 67). After scanning the results, the physician can focus the discussion on the main problem areas. More specific information is also helpful. Parents of a child with a bedwetting problem may be asked for several bladder capacity measurements. Other important information to have the parents collect before being seen are a food intake diary for obesity, a school report for school problems, a pain diary for recurrent pains, and a sleep diary for sleep disorders. The results of previous laboratory or radiologic studies should be known. If time is short, this information may be gained by phone. The consulting physician should send a report to the referring professional or agency following his or her evaluation so that communication is optimal and environmental intervention is maximized.

Scheduling Appointments. The initial evaluation commonly requires 45 to 60 minutes. A common error is to set aside inadequate time or to try to carry out an abbreviated evaluation during a visit for another purpose. If behavioral or psychosomatic problems are detected during a health supervision or acute illness visit, the patient should be rescheduled for a longer visit at a later time.

Follow-up visits can usually be 20 to 30 minutes long, depending on the problem. Parents should be given an exact date and time for follow-up. Telling them simply to come back if advice does not work out is not sufficient. If physicians agree that otitis media requires follow-up, they should readily see that a treatment plan for discipline problems or encopresis also needs to be monitored. Some physicians prefer to use the 5 PM to 6 PM time for initial evaluations because their office staff has left and their overhead is thus reduced. However, others find themselves more tired and less sensitive at that hour.

Fees for Counseling. Many physicians charge inadequately for the counseling they provide, and this may be one of the reasons they become disillusioned about dealing with psychosocial issues. Pediatricians must keep in mind that their productivity with counseling may be higher than that of any mental health professional. They should charge a reasonable amount for this time, for example, $3 per minute. An initial 45- to 60-minute evaluation would generate a CPT code of 99204 (approximately $180). A follow-up visit of 15 to 30 minutes is a 99212 ($66) code and 30 to 45 minutes is a 99213 ($92) code. The fees and the estimated total number of visits should be discussed with the family before the initial evaluation is scheduled. This can be done by the physician if the subject comes up during a health supervision visit or by the office assistant who schedules long appointments. If the parents cannot afford to pay the physician for the amount of time he or she spends with them, they might be referred to a mental health clinic or another center with a sliding fee scale. If families are being seen in a prepaid health maintenance organization, such counseling fees can more readily be absorbed.

Conclusion

Counseling is an inescapable, intrinsic part of pediatric care. Parents often seek out physicians who feel comfortable dealing with both physical and emotional issues. Optimal pediatric care requires competent counseling skills. Full enjoyment of a pediatric practice is enhanced through a knowledge of behavior modification principles (see also Chapter 78) and childrearing counseling techniques. Without such skills, physicians may turn excessively to psychotropic drugs and psychiatric referrals. Through clinical experience, seminars at medical meetings or local colleges, reading books and magazines for parents (see list at end of chapter), and discussion groups, pediatricians can upgrade their counseling skills to match their competency in treating physical illness.

REFERENCES

American Academy of Pediatrics: Diagnostic and Statistical Manual for Primary Care (DSM-PC): Child and Adolescent Version. Elk Grove Village IL, AAP, 1996.
Bergman AS: Pediatricians as counselors: the relationship as treatment. Pediatrics 73:730, 1984.
Coleman WL, Howard BJ: Family-focused behavioral pediatrics: clinical techniques for primary care. Pediatric Rev 16:448, 1995.
Dworkin PH: Detection of behavioral, developmental, and psychosocial problems in primary care practice. Curr Opin Pediatr 5:531, 1993.
Green M: No child is an island: contextual pediatrics and the "new" health supervision. Pediatr Clin North Am 42:79, 1995.
Green M: Behavioral and developmental components of child health promotion: how can they be accomplished? Pediatr Rev 8:133, 1986.
Hickson G, Altemeir W, O'Connor S: Concerns of mothers seeking care in private pediatric offices: Opportunities for expanding services. Pediatrics 72:619, 1983.
McCune Y, Richardson M, Powell J: Psychosocial health issues in pediatric practices: parents' knowledge and concerns. Pediatrics 74:183, 1984.
Morgan ER, Winter RJ: Teaching communication skills: an essential part of residency training. Arch Pediatr Adolesc Med 150:638, 1996.
Schmitt BD, Brayden RM, Kempe A: Parent handouts: cornerstone of a health education program. Contemp Peds 14:120, 1996.

BOOKS FOR PARENTS ON CHILDREARING

Brazelton TB: Touchpoints: Your Child's Emotional and Behavioral Development. Reading, MA, Addison-Wesley Publishers, 1992.
Chess S, Thomas A: Know Your Child. New York, Basic Books, 1987. Republished, New Brunswick, NJ, Jason Aronson, 1996.
Christopherson ER: Little People: Guidelines for Common Sense Child Rearing. Kansas City, Westport Publishers, 1988.
Dinkmeyer D, McKay GD: Parenting Young Children. Circle Pines, MN, American Guidance Service, 1989.
Heins M, Seiden AM: Child Care, Parent Care. Garden City, NY, Doubleday, 1987.
Popkin M: Active Parenting. San Francisco, Harper & Row, 1987.
Schmitt BD: Your Child's Health: A Pediatric Guide for Parents. 2nd ed. New York, Bantam Books, 1991.

77 *Psychotherapy With Children*

Stuart Goldman • William Beardslee

 The essential elements in child psychotherapy are (1) presentation of a problem, (2) a careful multidimensional assessment, (3) establishment of a defined treatment plan, and (4) monitoring progress over time. All of this occurs in a context of an experiential relationship that involves trust.

A comprehensive theory underlying the etiology of emotional and behavioral disorders is lacking. Nonetheless, the evidence for carefully evaluated psychotherapeutic studies with children is generally positive.

The field of psychotherapy with children encompasses a wide array of services and approaches, although they all share certain common elements. These include the recognition of distress, accurate diagnostic assessment, and the application of an intervention designed to remove or ameliorate the problem. The breadth of these approaches can challenge even the most astute practitioners within the field. Referring primary physicians are often overwhelmed as they try to help families find the most appropriate services. Although a detailed description of each psychotherapeutic approach is well beyond the scope of this chapter, we offer an overview and critique that will aid the referring physician in navigating successfully through these complicated waters. We focus on the common elements across different schools of psychotherapy and confine ourselves primarily to outpatient approaches.

Child psychotherapy itself is a relatively recent phenomenon that has essentially been limited to the 20th century. It started as a child guidance movement associated with the juvenile courts in the early 1900s. Child psychotherapy then evolved over the years, as clinicians of different disciplines, in different settings, refined the practice into the wide array of services currently available. Despite its almost 100-year history, it is only in the last 2 decades that rigorous outcome studies (Fonagy and Target, 1996; Shirk and Russell, 1992; Weisz et al, 1995) have appeared in the literature. There are many reasons for this (Shirk and Russell, 1992; Target and Fonagy, 1997), but chief among them is the lack of a comprehensive theory underlying either the etiology or the treatment of emotional and behavioral disorders. This has been compounded by different disciplines' training their practicioners in somewhat different ways, driven by the skill of clinicians rather than by empiric evidence. Until recently, clinicians, based on their theoretical framework, would often postulate an elaborate etiology and then proceed with an highly individualized treatment for a given case. This made comparing cases managed by different clinicians in different settings so difficult that rigorous clinical outcome studies were nearly impossible to carry out. Only with the advent of a descriptive diagnostic approach *(DSM-III, DSM-IV)* and prescribed interventions has outcome research been able to

systematically proceed. The lack of a comprehensive etiologic theory continues to challenge researchers. It complicates all aspects of intervention, from diagnosis through treatment, and on to outcome measures. Nonetheless, as with adults, the evidence for carefully evaluated psychotherapeutic studies with children is generally positive (Shirk and Russell, 1992) and there is considerable optimism that with rigorous evaluation the exact mechanisms of psychotherapy will be better understood.

Essential Elements

Although there are many schools of psychotherapy, all share certain elements. The first is the presentation for evaluation of a problem that is compromising the child or family. If the family, child, or system is not in some distress, rarely is there the motivation needed to engage in treatment. The second is a careful, multidimensional assessment that specifies the nature of the problem and the treatment goals. The third is the establishment of a defined treatment plan along which to proceed. The fourth is the monitoring of progress over time to ensure that the agreed-upon goals are being met and to revise the plan as needed.

Each of these elements must be in the context of an experiential relationship that involves significant amounts of trust. This trusting relationship, coupled with an agreed-upon set of problems and a plan for addressing them, defines the therapeutic alliance. The therapeutic alliance (whose core elements are relationship, problems, plan) is both with the child and with the family. Many treatments fail secondary to problems in the establishment of the three core elements. Treatment rarely proceeds well unless the child and family are voluntarily supporting it.

Beyond these generalities, the specifics of different types of interventions can vary considerably from therapeutic approach to therapeutic approach (e.g., psychodynamic, cognitive, behavioral, family) and even from practitioner to practitioner within a specific school. Systematic evaluation within each school or approach to examine the nature and consistency of the treatment or treatment integrity (Shirk and Russell, 1992) is one of the greatest contemporary challenges to the field as it strives to demonstrate outcome efficacy.

Assessment

Rigorous, integrated, multidimensional assessment that embraces the biopsychosocial model is the foundation of all contemporary psychotherapies. A concentric model of assessment, with the child at the center surrounded by successive layers of family, peers, school, community, and culture, provides the scaffolding for comprehensive understanding. Viewing the child without the surrounding contexts is far too restricted a perspective for most clinical circumstances. As one proceeds, each layer's elements of strength as well as weakness should be considered. Therapies that "fit" and build upon a system's strengths to help compensate or correct for a system's weaknesses and that try to understand how the different factors interact as a system are far more likely to succeed.

A challenging limitation for many clinicians is posed by the limits of the observing clinical lens. Observations are dependent both on the context of the observation and on the orientation of the therapists. Problems presenting in the office may be different from those observed in the classroom, and family therapists tend to see family problems, behavioral therapists tend to see behavioral ones, psychoanalysts see psychodynamic ones, and so on.

EXAMPLE, PART I

A 16-year-old boy named Sam was referred for evaluation because of escalating behaviors, including poor school performance, staying out all night, and suspected substance abuse. More detailed history reveals attention-deficit hyperactivity disorder (ADHD) dating back to his early school years, a parental history of depression, and recent marital separation of his parents. Sam complained that everything would be all right if he just could live with his dad. His dad has made it clear that he had to show that he could contain his behaviors before he could live with him, since he worked long hours and could not be there to supervise him. While most practitioners would agree about the ADHD and probable oppositional defiant disorder diagnosis, the behaviorist might postulate that the undesirable behaviors are being inadvertently rewarded, the family therapist might feel that the boy's behavior is an expression of the underlying difficulties between the mother and father, and the psychoanalyst might argue that the boy unconsciously, despite his protests, does not want to leave his mother to live with his father and that the behavior effectively sabotages any change. The thoughtful psychotherapist would attempt to integrate each of these into a complex, multidimensional treatment plan. The ADHD would be treated with a combination of medication, educational planning, and behavioral techniques. A more careful assessment for both an adjustment disorder and depression would be undertaken with individual treatment as indicated. Finally there would be family work of some type to address managing the disruptive behaviors and the other possible family contributors. In this integrated approach, the multidimensional treatment is tailored to each of the clinical needs at hand with specific goals and rationale for each.

The referring physician can play a critical role ensuring that the whole patient is being seen and that the prescription "fits" the child and family as well as possible.

DIMENSIONS OF ASSESSMENT

While challenging, assessment in a three-dimensional matrix offers the clearest picture of the child and his or her world. The first dimension is a descriptive one obtained by careful, history-taking in each of the spheres in which the child functions, including family, school, peers, and within himself or herself (inner life). The first three categories of family, school, and peers are relatively self-explanatory. The fourth category "within self" means how the child feels about himself or herself and how the child deals with these feelings. It would also include elements of fantasy life or imagination and conscience. The second dimension is one that considers time, since we all live in the present, past, and future to differing degrees. A temporal dimension relating past and present experiences along with future expectations can often bring new clarity to a puzzling situation. As an illustration: A child who is possibly feeling suicidal but is making detailed plans for summer vacation is much less likely to be at risk for self-destructive behavior than a child who just shrugs his shoulders when asked about summer plans. The final dimension of assessment is one that considers multiple clinical vantage points. This covers the many systems of understanding, including developmental, biological, cognitive-behavioral, psychodynamic, educational, cultural, and family, which help inform us about our patients. Although some considers the child in each of these dimensions, a full evaluation in each dimension is rarely indicated. This complex three-dimensional evaluation provides a picture that offers far greater clarity than that of a more narrow vantage point. The multidimensional formulation of the situation serves as the road map along which treatment is planned, carried out, and measured.

EXAMPLE, PART II

A more detailed evaluation reveals that Sam has chronically had trouble controlling his behavior, with periods of marked difficulty and relative calm. He states that he hated the "troublemaker" side of himself when he was younger but now it is okay since "That is just the way I am, I guess that I am used to it." He averts his eyes when saying this. When asked about having a "really good time" he states that 2 years ago the family went to Disney World, but he is silent when asked about more recent experiences.

Both of his parents agree that they have never known exactly what to do with Sam and that there have been many disagreements about discipline in the past and that they still regularly disagree. There appears to be a split, with the father insisting that he will "grow out of it" and the mother's eyes tearing up when asked what the future will bring.

A multidimensional analysis finds the following: Biologically there is Sam's long-standing ADHD and possibly depression. Psychologically, the sense of himself as a "troublemaker" distresses him, even though he states otherwise, and he needs attention to help him correct his self-image (improve his self-esteem). Socially his parents need help. His parents need to stop fighting over Sam and to resolve the differences of opinion as a family, collaborating on a consistent behavioral plan. With this more detailed assessment, the treatment plan can be more specifically fleshed out and implemented. This plan would include a biological intervention of medication, a psychological intervention to help Sam with his self-esteem, and a social plan for family or parent work to help manage his acting out.

Treatment Plan

ALLIANCE

Upon completion of a detailed assessment, the psychotherapist enters the critical phase of negotiating a treatment alliance with both the child and the family. The treatment or therapeutic alliance is built upon several principles: (1) There must be the positive, trusting relationship that Rosenfeld (1994) and others describe as vital to the therapeutic process. (2) There is the often underacknowledged psychoeducational approach needed to inform the child and family of the nature of the problem, its typical course, and the treatment options available. It is hard for children and their parents to collaborate optimally if they are not fully informed and do not fully understand the plan. (3) There needs to be identification of the problem, setting of treatment goals, and agreeing upon the modality (e.g., individual, family, behavioral) of the psychotherapeutic work. Lazare and colleagues (1975) described a request model for the initial evaluative sessions ("How do you think that I can be most helpful to you and your family?") that underscores the collaborative nature of the work and often facilitates the negotiation by stimulating active discussion of the therapeutic options and processes. A parent's unspoken sense of responsibility, the perceived stigma of seeing a therapist, or the pain of acknowledging the disorder can make negotiating the treatment plan formidable. These ongoing discussions provide a context to help the family understand the difficulties, to accept the treatment plan that best addresses the disorder, and to establish the therapeutic relationship. The psychotherapist's allying himself or herself with the parents' wish for the best for their child, or with a hope for relief in either the parent or child, will overcome most initial patient and family reluctance. Reviewing the treatment plan with the primary physician and enlisting his or her support for the treatment plan can also be critical.

Failure to negotiate successfully the initial treatment alliance or to update it as the treatment evolves is a common cause of treatment disruption or failure. Fractures in the treatment alliance can occur between the child and therapist, therapist and family, or therapist and referring physician (if there are unresolved differences of opinion) at many points during the therapy. Ongoing communication and review between all parties is the most effective way to prevent these mishaps.

INTERVENTIONS

Clinical interventions for a child and family follow logically from the detailed biopsychosocial assessment. Historically this process has been heavily influenced by the clinical orientation of the therapist. Many past treatment decisions have reflected decision making informed by allegiance to a theory rather than a choice informed by clinical efficacy studies or by a comprehensive treatment plan. Today's state-of-the-art clinical interventions (1) are grounded in multidimensional assessment, (2) clearly specify the goals of treatment prior to the initiation of the plan, (3) match the treatment modality to the problem based on efficacy studies, (4) rely on integrated multimodal treatment to act synergistically, and (5) monitor progress toward the specified goals, with "in flight" corrections as needed. At present effective treatments are available for almost the entire spectrum of psychiatric disorders, ranging from adjustment disorders or tics on the milder end of the spectrum, through depressive disorders and psychosis on the most severe end. Matching the assessment and treatment to the disorder has become refined to the point that detailed practice guidelines are now available for many disorders. The cornerstone for much of this progress has come from reliable intervention studies.

Outcome Studies

Outcome studies in child psychotherapy have been appearing in the literature for over 4 decades. Reports have ranged from "no indisputable evidence of success" (Hendren, 1993) to the meta-studies of Weisz and colleagues (1995) and Kazdin (1995), each of whom found that about three fourths of the children in all studies are measurably better off after a course of treatment regardless of which treatment was used.

We have identified three broad sets of challenges that have been obstacles for outcome researchers as they attempt to undertake and then implement the findings of careful studies into clinical practice. Understanding these challenges helps to contextualize the challenge that each clinician faces as he or she tries to proceed with the optimal plan. The first challenge is that of undertaking studies in a field that has yet to develop a comprehensive etiologic framework. This lack of framework is in part due to the limits of our current knowledge and in part due to the multiple sets of etiologic factors that are integral to the genesis of almost all psychiatric disorders. Anything but a drastically reductionistic framework will always be plagued with the problem of multiple concurrent etiologies that are nearly impossible to untangle.

The second challenge is to correct the earlier flaws in study design. Weisz and colleagues (1995) and others have described the characteristics of reliable studies, specifying first the identification and selection of an appropriate study group. They emphasize the consistent application of a set of standardized techniques by a well-trained group of clinicians, followed with appropriate monitoring of clinical progress over time.

The third set of challenges has been around implementing research findings into clinical practice. Several authors (Weisz et al, 1995; Hoagwood et al, 1995) pointed out that many clinicians are skeptical about embracing laboratory findings in clinical practice for a wide variety of reasons. Most often they believe that research, by design, fails to capture the complexity, richness, and unpredictability of the lives of their patients and their families and thus oversimplifies what is really needed.

Despite all these challenges, on many fronts, researchers have consistently found that the size of therapeutic effect in almost all studies, when appropriately undertaken, is in the medium to large range (Shirk and Russell, 1992). The next section reviews the current state of clinical interventions and the studies of efficacy within each approach to date.

Clinical Interventions

PSYCHODYNAMIC PSYCHOTHERAPY

Psychodynamic psychotherapy has its roots in the writings of Sigmund Freud. It has evolved into many subschools of theory, all sharing certain elements. Each psychodynamically informed system of understanding patients has four critical components. The first is that we are all historical beings with our current functioning dependent on our past histories. The second centers on the understanding of the role of relationships and emotional states as primary determinants of our well-being. The third is the belief that there are conscious and unconscious components to our functioning and that one can only truly understand a patient when one has some grasp of all the components. The fourth and final one is that all the subschools emphasize the curative role of the patient/therapist relationship. This role occurs in the therapeutically constructed patient/doctor relationship based on past experiences (transference) and to a lesser degree on the present "real" relationship. This relationship is believed to be critical for a patient to develop the capacity for self-reflection or insight, two of psychodynamic psychotherapy's major curative elements. Psychodynamic psychotherapy most often occurs as a dialogue but may be carried out through play, especially with younger children.

Broadly put, psychodynamic therapists fall into two at times overlapping schools. The first major school includes the Drive and Ego psychotherapists, who focus on the processing of unwanted, unpleasant, or unacceptable, emotionally charged experiences. They believe that all people are subject to low or modest levels of conflict or distress that arise from the gap between our wishes or desires and our capacity to gratify them. The tension created by this gap is countered by a set of protective conscious or unconscious maneuvers, described as defenses, which allow one to maintain a reasonable level of equilibrium. When the experiences are too intense or the defenses are not up to the task, significant disequilibrium occurs and symptoms or diseases emerge. Drive theorists place a stronger emphasis on the wishes, and Ego theorists focus on the defenses and their vicissitudes as well as on general personal competences. The emergence and therapeutic analysis of the present relationship with the therapist that is based on an earlier primary relationship is known as transference. The transference provides the framework for the verbalization of emotions and experiences, which helps to re-equilibrate the troubled emotional states that may have either blocked or distorted healthy functioning. This triad of conflict resolution, emotional discharge, and the development of more mature defenses are the principal processes through which traditional psychodynamic psychotherapy in this school is believed to work.

The second major grouping of psychodynamic therapies focuses on the individual's experience of relationships and are described as the Object Relations and Self Psychology schools. These practitioners hypothesize that appropriate interpersonal experiences early in life lead to the internalization of healthy, secure interpersonal relationships (object relations) or a healthy sense of self. When one has experiences that do not fit one's needs, either because of the failures of the primary caretaker or because of a mismatch between the child and the caretaker, a deficiency occurs. This deficit leads to significant relationship problems with others, an impaired sense of self, or often both. In these theorists' eyes, this hypothesized experiential failure accounts for many of the difficulties described by patients of all sorts, especially those with character disorders. They believe that in the early caretaking relationship there is an optimal developmental balance between too much frustration on one side and too much indulgence on the other. Problems can arise from failures on either side. The central role of the psychotherapeutic relationship is to experientially replace or repair these early relationship failures with more appropriate interpersonal experiences. The corrective emotional experiences of therapy provide new internal representations of relationships, leading to an improved sense of self, which allows for better functioning of the individual patient.

The intense nature of the relationship necessary for the majority of psychoanalytically oriented work, coupled with the psychoanalytically posited normal resistance to change, dictates a therapeutic time frame that is usually on the longer side. Most treatments are scheduled for at least once a week and generally last over a year, depending on the scope of change needed and the patient's reluctance to change.

EXAMPLE

Ben was a 6-year-old boy who presented with the complaint that he had "no friends" and that he was increasingly oppositional at home and in school. Ben was a highly precocious boy whose academic prowess awed many people. He was encouraged to read scientific books, particularly in the area of astronomy. He had little free time and no playmates. His dramatic talent was often shown off by his parents and at times by the school. The first time he was seen, his mother sent him off to the distant cafeteria, by himself. When I, somewhat taken aback, asked if that was typical, she replied "Why not, he can read." While he enjoyed the attention and his specialness, he would complain afterwards that he would "just like to play." Shortly after the therapy began we started a storybook that he dictated while I wrote. The book was about a boy who could do magic; the only trouble was no one appreciated it, and he was so lonely that he went to live in outer space. Over the next months, the story evolved. The boy found many new friends in space, in the context of the psychotherapy, most of whom were only fleetingly interested in his magic; they just wanted to play. He began to have play dates on the outside, and his parents began to treat him more age-appropriately. As his symptoms resolved, the storybook boy returned to earth as the therapy was drawing to a close. He left the therapy with a pass card that he designed, which could instantly transport him back to therapy (outer space) if he ever got stuck again.

Psychodynamic psychotherapy has a long and honorable history and has been widely and successfully used in child guidance clinics for many years. Despite this outcome, studies in psychodynamically oriented psychotherapy have been plagued with design difficulties. Uncontrolled studies or case reports have been the rule, and there has often been "poor definition of disorders and treatment procedures." To date, no large, well-controlled prospective studies of children treated with psychodynamic psychotherapy have appeared in the literature, although smaller well-designed studies (Target and Fonagy, 1997) have been published.

At present there are a number of published reports of chart reviews, the most extensive being the one by Fonagy and Target (1996). In their chart review of more than 700 child cases they found rates of improvement in children diagnosed with the emotional disorders of anxiety or depression to be 72%, provided that they remained in treatment for at least 6 months. In children with behavioral disorders (such as those with ADHD or conduct disorder), they found overall rates of improvement of under 50%, although those who stayed in treatment for over 6 months did appreciably better. Syndrome-specific rates ranged from 56% for oppositional defiant disorder to 36% for ADHD, to a low of 23% in children with conduct disorder. About one third of the children terminated treatment within 1 year. In those children who continued treatment beyond 1 year, 69% were no longer diagnosable at termination.

While this study suggests that children with certain disorders are responsive to this type of treatment, it is clear that treatments of longer than 6 months (emotional) or 1 year (behavioral) were needed to demonstrate a significant effect. Younger children (under 11 years of age) and those with certain subsets of disorders (simple phobias, oppositional defiant disorder) did relatively well, and others (conduct disorder) did worse. This is in contrast to other studies (Hendren, 1993) that reported that there were no demonstrable positive outcome findings in psychodynamically oriented psychotherapy. Clearly, more work is needed to bring outcome research for this modality of treatment up to the next level, particularly because of the widespread popularity of this therapeutic approach. Beyond the issues of controls, outcome measures, and soon that many interventions wrestle with, the challenge of treatment integrity (standardized and reproducible) remains a daunting one for psychodynamically oriented researchers.

BEHAVIOR THERAPY

Behavioral therapy has become increasingly popular over the last several decades and is used in individual, parent, and family contexts. Based on the work of Skinner and others, it is by far the most thoroughly evaluated of the psychotherapies (Southam-Gerow et al, 1997). It relies on the basic principle that rewards or punishments, when regularly applied, will change the frequency of any behavior. Practitioners focus on the specification of a target behavior and then carefully record the antecedents to and consequences of that behavior. Interventions consist of the setting up of a formal observational system that notes the behavior and then regular application of either positive or negative contingencies (although most favor positive). Observations of unintentional reinforcement within the family or more extended system are also made and altered to shape the desired behavior. There is a high level of mandated collaboration between the therapist and the child or family. Active involvement of the school or other major home contacts is also often indicated.

EXAMPLE

Sally was a 9-year-old who had always been on the shy side. While this had made life a bit more challenging, the family had always found ways of helping her cope. After Christmas vacation she missed a few days of school with the flu. Her return to school was marked by a dramatic relapse of the terrible headaches she had had while ill. At the time of consultation, Sally had been home for more than 3 weeks. Her mother was on leave from her job, staying home with Sally, and the school was considering a tutor. After a careful medical evaluation, it was suggested that home was "too inviting" for Sally and that she should begin to spend time, in increasing amounts, in school. At first this was mostly in the school nurse's office with a fairly rapid planned phasing back into the classroom. There were rewards scheduled for each increment in her time spent in class. Her mother remained on leave for the first few days "just in case." The plan sputtered slowly forward. Shortly after her mother returned to her work, Sally was able to spend full days in class.

Failures occur in two basic ways from the behavioral therapist's perspective. The first occurs when either there is some breakdown in the alliance or the family is unable to comply with the plan. Most often this is a breakdown in the consistency with which the parents or school is able to implement the plan. The second is when the analysis of the behavior is inaccurate or incomplete and the prescribed plan is faulty. In these instances, even when the plan is consistently carried out, the results will not be satisfactory and one must redesign the plan.

Outcome studies in behavior therapy have repeatedly shown that these techniques can be successfully applied to a wide range of problems (Wiesz et al, 1995). These have included tics, trichotillomania, sleep and elimination disorders, phobias, some disruptive behavior disorders, and eating disorders. These have in common a highly specific target symptom in which changes in the intensity and number of symptoms can be measured. There have been less clear results with the anxiety or depressive disorders.

Commentators from outside the behavioral school have criticized the monodimensional approach that behaviorists apply to observed behaviors without regard to the patient's underlying experiences or mental processes. Some have wondered whether symptomatic relief without regard to hypothesized underlying mechanisms would result in symptom substitution. To date this has not been shown. Most behavioral practitioners couple behavioral techniques with cognitive techniques, called cognitive-behavioral therapy (CBT).

COGNITIVE THERAPY

Cognitive therapies have been blossoming at a dramatic rate over the past 2 decades. Generally they have been incorporated into a broader cognitive-behavioral approach, as noted. The cognitive component focuses on two types of breakdown in cognitive functioning, cognitive distortion and cognitive deficiency (Kendall and MacDonald, 1993). Cognitive distortions focus on a primary failure in information processing. These include major distortions of experiences, distortions regarding the intentions of others, or distortions in the perspective of self. They have been associated with internalizing disorders such as anxiety and depression. Cognitive deficiencies are associated with the breakdown of planning so that actions appear that have not "benefited from forethought" (Kendall and McDonald, 1993). Not surprisingly they are also associated with the externalizing disorders such as impulsiveness or inattention. Aggressive antisocial problems are posited to stem from a combination of both types of cognitive difficulties. Cognitive therapists address these problems by analyzing the difficulty and then developing more adaptive and appropriate patterns of information processing that counter the distortions or repair the deficiencies using a variety of techniques.

COGNITIVE-BEHAVIORAL THERAPY

Most clinicians and researchers combine elements of behavioral and cognitive approaches into CBT. The cornerstone of CBT is the identification and description of a specific problem; therapy then involves improving how one goes about problem solving. Southam-Gerow and colleagues (1997) elaborated the strategies of CBT as (1) affective education and the recognition of affect and somatic states, (2) relaxation training, (3) social problem solving, (4) cognitive restructuring and attribution retraining, (5) contingent reinforcement, (6) modeling and (7) role playing. There are components of increased awareness from strategy 1, alterations in how one thinks and understands things (strategies 3 and 4), improved problem solving (strategies 3, 4, 6, and 7) and practicing with rewards (strategies 5 and 7). Relaxation training cuts across several of these descriptors and is a useful skill unto itself. Many of the CBT interventions have been systemized into treatment manuals with training and training certification for practitioners. This approach provides for far more consistency and treatment integrity than many of the other psychotherapies, making successful outcome studies far more likely since they address common study flaws.

Outcome studies in CBT have run the gamut, with a general trend showing significant short-term improvement, especially with well-defined problems (Weisz et al, 1995). The efficacy of CBT with situations such as tics and elimination problems has appeared in the literature for years. In the last decades, more complex disorders have been systematically studied. Anxiety disorders have been shown to be responsive in both the short and the long term (Kendall and Southam-Gerow, 1996). March and colleagues (1994) described an intervention for children with obsessive compulsive disorder combining CBT with medication that is quite promising. Successful treatment of depressive disorders in adults has spawned CBT treatments for adolescents. Short-term results have been positive but not well maintained at longer-term follow-up (Southam-Gerow et al, 1997). Further study of the longer-term problems with recidivism with these disorders is needed.

Outcome studies of the subset of externalizing disorders in children, including oppositional defiant disorder and conduct disorder, have shown mixed results to date. Generally speaking, there have been significant short-term gains that are not well maintained over longer time periods. More specifically, CBT with aggressive children helps them gain greater control, particularly in the clinical environment. Maintenance of these gains over time and application of these newly acquired sets of skills to outside contexts has been questioned. Most clinicians working with children who have conduct disorder advocate a multisystemic treatment approach for this highly challenging population.

ADHD has been studied extensively using CBT-based interventions. It would appear that the seemingly excellent match between the child's deficits and the types of interventions offered by CBT would make ADHD an ideal candidate for study. To date, however, the results have been modest, with some improvement in selective symptoms but no marked improvement overall. Researchers have offered many explanations, but the search continues to explain these unexpected findings and to find the right combination of CBT techniques to successfully treat ADHD.

PSYCHOEDUCATIONAL PSYCHOTHERAPY

Psychoeducational psychotherapy builds on a subset of the premises underlying all of the cognitive approaches to intervention. It centers around the idea that flawed or limited thinking about a disorder will make matters worse and that improving and broadening the understanding or thinking about a disorder will make it better. It has been described and applied in a variety of contexts (Beardslee et al, 1996) and is practiced by a wide range of clinicians both within and outside of the formal mental health field. It is time-limited, generally requiring three to 15 visits, and often relies on detailed didactic presentations about an illness as its cornerstone. Its general goals are to improve coping or adaptation to a disorder or to anticipate problems and offer preventive strategies. Most typically it begins with a detailed and thoughtful description of the disorder, its treatment, and probable course, which is designed to broaden and deepen the child's or families' understanding of the disorder. Psychoeducational interventions attempt to identify and alter faulty beliefs and to provide more appropriate information about the problem. It also often includes components of behavioral treatment and supportive therapy, although the degree to which any components are added beyond the educational part is variable.

Outcome studies tend to be unavailable except for

those studies that have been manual driven. Manual-based psychotherapies rely on a detailed definition of the specifics of a psychotherapeutic intervention. This makes them more a mode of structuring an intervention than subscription to a specific therapeutic school. They all have relatively high treatment integrity, making them more ideal approaches for studying outcome. The variety of manual-driven therapies ranges from adaptations of Klerman's interpersonal psychotherapy for adolescents (Southam-Gerow et al, 1997) to Beardslee and colleaques' preventive intervention with the children of seriously depressed parents (1996). They tend to be designed to recruit a homogeneous population, require intense intervention training for practitioners, offer specific techniques, and be highly structured and monitored; These features are all likely to optimize outcome results, according to Weisz and associates (1995). Cognitive psychoeducational approaches are among the most widely used approaches with parents. Illustrating this with children are the manual-based treatments of adolescent depression (Mufson and Fairbanks, 1996) and preventive interventions (Beardslee et al, 1996), both of which have demonstrated solid outcome results.

As an example, more specifically, Beardslee and associates (1996) addressed whether overall adaptive functioning and symptom levels could be reduced in a preventive intervention for youngsters at risk because of parental depression. They demonstrated that use of a manual-driven approach, which linked the presentation material to the family's life, could improve functioning and decrease symptom levels in these children. This approach offers considerable promise for the future in terms of the focus of psychotherapy.

PARENT PSYCHOTHERAPY OR GUIDANCE

Parent therapy or guidance, like manual-based therapy, is really an approach rather than a theoretical orientation. It continues to define the general locus of the problem as being within the child but sees the parents as having a major impact on the child's progress. It defines the parent's role as an active collaborator with the therapist. It sees the time outside of the therapy sessions as an opportunity for parents to amplify the work of the therapy and empowers the parents to feel that they are a part of the cure. Parent psychotherapy may entail elements of support, guidance, psychoeducation, and cognitive-behavioral techniques. It is generally time-limited and is practiced by a wide variety of mental health care professionals as well as others. Charismatic writers have written a large number of highly popular self-help books that are widely available.

Supportive parent work focuses on helping parents through a stressful period, whether in response to a developmental crisis or to environmental pressure. The therapist offers a relationship in which the parents can ventilate and review their feelings, sorting them out to develop perspective or to diminish the impact of misfortunes. Parent guidance typically includes educational and cognitive-behavioral components geared to improving the parent's problem-solving skills. More descriptive components of parent guidance were noted earlier.

Outcome studies in parent psychotherapy tend to be embedded in the outcome studies of specific theory-driven psychotherapies. In specific instances with specific problems—pica, enuresis, and mild behavioral problems, among others—parent guidance has been shown to be effective as a component of the core therapy.

FAMILY PSYCHOTHERAPY

Family therapists focus on families as the locus of change. They see the problem either as family based or as individually based but with a major family component as a modifier for the individual's problem. While there are a wide range of approaches and schools of family therapy, which at times practitioners advocate almost religiously, they all share certain common goals. These goals are to promote or restore growth to individuals and their families, to overcome obstacles or losses to the family, and to provide more flexibility and fulfillment in relationships, especially within the family. They all frame psychotherapy as occurring in the context of conversation or communication between family members. They see family functioning as more than just a sum of its individual parts; they see a family as a unique, dynamic entity of its own. Within families they see major potential for growth enhancement or symptom reinforcement, depending on a family's functioning.

All schools of family therapy are built to some degree on general systems theory (Sargent, 1997). This states that any system is more than a sum or its parts, that any change in the system will change all parts of the system, and that a change in any part of the system will change the system as a whole. This bidirectional frame leads to the commonly held family therapist's viewpoint that all interactions are circular and continuous. Taken the next step, this calls into question most linear models of causality for disorders when taken from a systems theory perspective (Tomm, 1983). From these points of departure there is a branching off into many different schools of family therapy, each with its own, often elaborate, theoretical framework. The schools of family psychotherapy include structural, strategic, cognitive-behavioral, psychodynamic, and narrative.

Structural family therapy focuses upon identifying, analyzing, and then changing the organization or structure within the family. The organization of the family is reflected in their patterns of relating and centers on identifying roles within the family and boundaries between family members. Dysfunctional or inappropriate roles or boundaries that are too close (enmeshment) or too distant (disengaged) become the targets of change. The interactive family format is then used to alter roles or restore boundaries to effect change.

Strategic family therapy focuses on the maladaptive patterns of behavior or communication within a family that have arisen in response to the family's failed strategies at problem solving. Practitioners within this school often challenge the family with prescribed tasks that will disrupt the old patterns of problem solving and allow new, more effective, patterns or behaviors to emerge within the family system.

Psychodynamic family therapists believe that family dysfunction occurs in the context of individual conflicts or experiences from the parents' own past. They believe that parents get stuck visiting their failures or unresolved experiences from the past on their current family. Intervention occurs as parents gain insight into their past experience, working on their own past conflicts and recognizing old patterns of relating. These corrections to their past experiences, particularly when they occur in a family context, allow them to resolve the distortions or dysfunctions in their current relationships and improve family functioning.

Narrative family therapists believe that failures in a family stem from troubles in the composite story that they have constructed about their experiences. Family dysfunction occurs as the story or narrative that the family tells no longer fits the context of their current lives. Therapeutic growth proceeds as the therapist facilitates the family's construction of new and more adaptive stories (cognitive models) that better meet their current needs.

Cognitive-behavioral family therapists focus on the problem solving or skill training that builds on the learning theory framework that underlies all of cognitive-behavioral work. Their work is primarily in the here-and-now and uses contingent reinforcement, cognitive reframing, prescribed tasks, and homework assignments, among other techniques. Psychoeducational family work, often used with families with a chronically ill member, is an important subset of this school.

EXAMPLE

Joe, a 17-year-old and the youngest of three brothers, was referred for evaluation because of a serious decline in his grades and escalating acting out. Two previous attempts at individual work had failed. He met criteria for oppositional defiant disorder but there were no other diagnosable problems. The therapy began with some individual sessions with Joe and parent guidance. The therapy never really took hold and neither Joe nor his family could comply with the treatment program. A major episode of Joe's acting out was precipitated by the parent's taking an action, against the therapist's strong protests, that appeared to sabotage the limited gains Joe had made. At this point the therapist changed tactics, re-examining the situation from a family perspective. It appeared that the mother was quite depressed at the thought of her youngest and favorite son getting ready to go off to college. The whole family agreed that if Joe's behavior continued he "might not even graduate from high school." Joe's rebellious acting out was recast as an act of sensitivity and kindness to his mother so that she would not be upset as he grew up and got ready to leave home. His misbehavior and his parents' mismanagement were prescribed as a caring way for the family to meet one another's pressing needs and that they should not change, at least for now. Joe left the office in a rage and his parents looked bewildered, shrugging their shoulders on their way out. Joe's behavior dramatically changed over the next weeks although he complained bitterly that the therapist was "out to lunch."

Outcome studies in family therapy have had to wrestle with the dilemmas faced by all the individual therapies, including diagnostic grouping, diversity in approach, treatment integrity, and monitoring outcome. Additionally they have had to wrestle with an epistemology that questions the validity of linear models of causality (Tomm, 1983). Despite these obstacles, family therapy has been shown to be effective in several areas, although primarily with adolescents and young adults. Family therapy with schizophrenic patients has been shown to reduce relapse by 50% to 80% (Diamond et al, 1996). Similarly it has been shown to reduce recidivism and to decrease treatment attrition rates in adolescent substance abusers. Family therapy has also been shown to be helpful in weight maintenance for patients with anorexia nervosa (Russell et al, 1987). As part of a multimodal approach to conduct disorders it has been helpful, particularly with treatment compliance and reducing recidivism. It has not been shown to help children with ADHD. Results with depression and anxiety disorders in children and adolescents have been promising but not consistent to date.

GROUP PSYCHOTHERAPY

Many types of group therapy for children and adolescents have been used. Most of today's group therapies build on the pioneering work of Slavson and Schiffer (1975) and use many of their principles. Group therapies have the advantage of simulating certain elements of real-world experience with peers and family that cannot be created in an individual office setting. Group therapy allows the child to develop social skills with peers through modeling and practice. It provides a context to develop relationships and support and to share pressing elements within each member's life. The sense of catharsis one has in a group of people sharing their experiences and knowing that one is not alone in one's troubles are also believed to be therapeutic.

Successful group therapy depends, in large part, on the composition of the group, and care must be taken to select the group such that developmental levels, types of problems, defensive structures, and personal skills are taken into consideration. Patients who are unable to relate (psychosis, developmental disorders), have conduct disorder, or are suicidal generally are not well suited to group therapy. On the other side, children with certain anxiety disorders, poor social skills, decreased self-esteem, and isolation are good candidates. Children with a set of common individual or family problems, such as a medical problem or living in a substance abusing family, are also good candidates. Groups fall into several main categories: activity-centered, interpersonal, cognitive-behavioral, and topic-centered.

Activity-centered groups are often excellent for withdrawn, isolated, anxious patients who use the context of the activity to develop relationships. Interpersonal groups rely on many psychoanalytically informed principles focusing on conflicts, desires, and defenses. They may be play- or discussion-based and have been useful for gaining insight into one's self. Cognitive-behavior groups rely on learning theory, often using interpersonal contingencies to help members develop more appropriate social skills and behaviors. Specialized groups that focus on a select topic are more homogeneous and often rapidly promote the development of supportive relationship and offer a place for catharsis. Groups centering around divorce, abuse, chronic illness, eating disorders, and familial substance abuse, among many others, have been reported.

Outcome studies for group therapies have suffered

the same design challenges that we described earlier. Most of the reports in the literature refer to adult groups or a mixture of child and adult group therapies (Kymissis, 1996). Findings have generally shown that group treatment is appreciably better than no treatment for a wide variety of troubles. To date, a well-matched controlled study of group versus individual or family treatment has not appeared in the literature. Specific indications for group treatment tend to be organized either around social skills problems or around a defined topic. The elaboration of more specific set of indications and the appropriately matched techniques remains for the future.

MILIEU PSYCHOTHERAPY

Milieu therapy is used on both an inpatient and an outpatient basis. We do not review inpatient treatments here, but hospitals, residential schools, and day programs offer psychotherapeutic interventions that generally include the modalities described earlier as well as a therapeutic living space or milieu. Based on the work of Aichorn and others with delinquent children, milieu therapy relies on the intensity of the experiential and treatment components, coupled with removing the child from a dysfunctional or inadequate environment, for its strength. Given the disruptive nature of the intervention, along with its cost, it is generally reserved for the most seriously ill children who have failed to be adequately helped by outpatient treatment or are at risk for harming themselves or others. The synergy between the multimodality treatment inherent in this approach and the continuous corrective experiences of an extended milieu are hypothesized to be the essence of the experience.

Outcome studies with this population of children are extremely hard to undertake. In addition to the usual challenges, the majority of the children have multisystem difficulties that are difficult to quantify and control for. This, coupled with the protective nature of the clinical problems neccesitating such an approach, makes an untreated control group nearly impossible to establish. Although anecdotal reports abound, controlled studies of outcome and of cost-effectiveness are yet to be reported in the literature for milieu therapy.

Treatment Planning

With the diversity of the therapeutic interventions described, many practitioners feel perplexed about recommending or choosing a particular approach. A detailed review of treatment planning, syndrome by syndrome, is beyond our scope, but some guidelines for the practitioner emerge from the literature. Many of these are incorporated into the Practice Guidelines recently published by the American Academy of Child and Adolescent Psychiatry.

Generally speaking, disorders in children and adolescents can be divided into four broad categories: reactive, externalizing (acting out), internalizing (mood), or multisystem. The presence of a diagnosable disorder is usually the entry point into the mental health system but is not sufficient to recommend treatment. Children and families should be engaged in treatment when the disorder does, or is highly likely to, cause significant dysfunction. It is

the combination of symptom clusters and dysfunction that is the indication for treatment. Before proceeding with treatment, one should, as noted earlier, conduct a detailed assessment from the biopsychosocial vantage point. This also should include a review of the role of the systems surrounding the child, including the family, peers, and school, as they contribute either positively or negatively to the situation. It is vitally important to understand these from a developmental and cultural perspective. The needs of children, the rates of disorders, and the impact of environmental events (e.g., divorce, illness) all vary with the age, sex, and developmental level of the child, and they cannot be fully understood without a cultural context. From this assessment comes a detailed formulation of the difficulties and a treatment plan. This plan serves as a road map for all future interventions.

The reactive disorders include problems with adjustment or adaptation to any of life's events. They range from new-school years, modest illnesses, and familial discord on the milder end to divorce, death, abuse, and severe illness on the more severe end. Intervention for this group of disorders should be targeted at facilitating the mastering and working through of the event, addressing the challenges at hand. At some point there is follow-up to assess the new adjustment or adaptation. Disorders in which the dysfunction persists, particularly but not limited to when the stressors have ended, may move on into one of the other remaining three categories.

Supportive, shorter-term counseling or therapy is the cornerstone of all interventions for this group and may be carried out in individual, group, or familial format. The choice of format should reflect an evaluation of who or what group is being affected and what resources are available for the individual or family and within the health care system. The intervention generally provides a context for verbalization of the events, serving a cathartic function as well as providing cognitive-behavioral and psychoeducational components to broaden the patient's understanding and develop more appropriate coping skills. Short-term, symptom-targeted psychopharmacologic intervention may employed as an adjunct therapy. Re-evaluation, in this context, focuses on the resolution of the life events and the degree of adaptation or resiliency that the child and family have attained. These children generally do well if the life events are containable and they have the support at home. If the events continue or worsen or when the degree of adaptation is limited by either the child or family, often significant symptoms will persist that necessitate further intervention.

Externalizing disorders are the cluster of situations that have disruptive, difficult behaviors at the heart of the symptom list. This group, sometimes called the disruptive behavior disorders, includes ADHD, oppositional defiant disorder, and conduct disorder. Most of these children could be characterized by an "act first, think later" approach that often compromises their individual and social functioning. Their action-oriented style is well suited for action-oriented (cognitive-behavioral) rather than reflective (psychodynamic) approaches. With younger children (under 8 or 9 years of age) the majority of the work is done with parents or teachers or in a family context. With older children, who have greater cognitive capacities, individual work is often quite helpful. This would include the development of alternative problem-solving strategies, reframing the way they view things, and techniques or strategies that help them slow down.

A typical treatment approach would start with a careful and descriptive assessment of their functioning, often employing standardized checklists or a formal behavioral record. The cognitive-behavioral treatment then proceeds, building on this record with the child, family, and often school. Targeted pharmacotherapy has also been an integral part of the interventions for ADHD but has been far less successful in the other disruptive behavioral disorders.

Many of these children have self-esteem problems often thought to be secondary to the negative response of others to their behaviors. For these children, additional interventions in either individual psychotherapy or a group may be quite helpful, with self-esteem as a clear target. Supportive family therapy, in challenging cases, may also have a useful role. Persistent and uncontrollable behaviors may, in some instances, mandate an environmental (milieu) treatment that provides the comprehensive, intensive care that this small subset of externalizing patients needs.

As noted earlier and following this approach, outcome studies with this group have been highly positive for oppositional defiant disorder, and they have been mixed, although in the balance mildly positive, for ADHD and conduct disorders.

Internalizing disorders center around mood difficulties, typically depression and anxiety. These are children whose biggest problem is that they feel bad, although they may act out in response to their sense of despair or in fear. Historically these have been the children targeted for individual, psychodynamic psychotherapy. Most clinicians and families believe that this form of psychotherapy works well, but well-controlled prospective outcome studies have not appeared in the literature. Chart review–based studies, as noted earlier, do support the effectiveness of this type of intervention when therapy is carried out over the longer term (6 months to years).

Individual psychotherapy today, as in the past, remains the cornerstone of treatment for this group of children. More recently, the utilization of cognitive behavioral interventions has been growing rapidly. For certain anxiety disorders, particularly phobias and separation problems, the treatment of choice has been cognitive-behavioral. More recently, March and associates (1994), working with obsessive-compulsive disorder, and Southam-Gerow and associates (1997), working with depressed adolescents, have had favorable results as well. At this point the treatment of choice for obsessive-compulsive disorder is behavioral (with medication), while the optimal treatments for depression in children and adolescents continues to evolve.

In the last decade, pharmacologic treatment for depressive and anxiety disorders has been increasingly studied. Although the results have not always been clear, there is a strong suggestion that for seriously depressed or anxious children, medications should be considered as part of the core treatment modalities for this group.

For many of these children, their difficulties extend well out into the environment around them to their families, friends, and school. Family therapy may be helpful to the child and family, offering support, education, and specific intervention strategies. It may also prove preventive as it has for the children of families with depressed adults (Beardslee et al, 1996) and in reducing recidivism in schizophrenia (Diamond et al, 1996).

The recurrent nature of the depressive and anxiety disorders makes careful re-evaluation and monitoring particularly important. A target for all interventions should include decreasing the long-term impact of these recurring disorders.

Multisystem disorders are, as implied in the name, disorders that affect multiple areas of the child's functioning. They include the developmental disorders, psychosis, and the more severe personality disorders. Generally speaking they respond more favorably to the action-oriented approaches that target the many deficits that these children and their families must attend to. Cognitive behavioral strategies, family-based interventions, and attention to the milieu have been the mainstays of those interventions that have had the most favorable outcomes. Many of these children have tremendous social difficulties, and group psychotherapy to address these has also been helpful for some. Each of these disorders may have comorbid conditions, each of which needs attention. Pharmacotherapy of these disorders generally is used as an adjunct to target certain behaviors or comorbid symptomology. The exception is for the psychotic disorders, for which it is part of the primary strategy.

Supportive psychotherapy may be helpful for these children to adjust to the challenging lives that most of them are faced with. There have been no clear successes reported with this population when treated with insight-oriented therapy. For patients who do not respond to multimodal outpatient interventions or in families who cannot manage these children any longer, residential or day programs are indicated.

Future Directions

We expect that future work in child psychotherapy will take two major directions. In the more immediate future, studies of outcome will help us refine therapeutic techniques and define the parameters that allow one to form the best "fit" between disorder and type of therapy. We expect that manual-driven therapies, with a more standardized approach, will become more widespread in their use. Substantial efforts are underway in these areas, and the early fruits of these labors are appearing in the literature. Continued refinement of these efforts will lead to a more defined set of interventions. Whether clinicians will employ them has been questioned by some (Hoagwood et al, 1995; Wiesz et al, 1995), but at least the data will be available for clinicians and patients to make a more informed decision. The key challenge will be developing treatments that combine these psychotherapeutic approaches with pharmacotherapy that can be integrated into a school and neighborhood system. We believe that a greater awareness of culture in terms of etiology and understanding as well as treatment will also become increasingly important.

In the longer term, the quest for the knowledge base that will enable us to make an etiologic diagnosis will come to the fore. It is clear by this point that this will not take the linear and monodimensional form that is possible in some fields of medicine. The model will be more complex, much like that for the etiology of heart disease. For some patients, there will be an overwhelming genetic or environmental factor that accounts for the development of the disease. For most patients, there will be a complex interrelationship between genetic vulnerability and environmental or experiential factors. We expect that there will be some multidimensional matrix of understanding that will include biological, social, and psychological domains that will allow us to identify the underlying factors and design a treatment plan of psychotherapy that addresses each of them optimally. We expect that the majority of future treatment plans will continue to be multidimensional, as they are today. They will continue to include an experiential relationship with the child, a collaborative relationship with the parents, and monitoring over time to ensure quality. As we refine our ability to understand and successfully target specific disorders, we are confident that treatment outcomes will continue to improve.

BIBLIOGRAPHY

Beardslee WR, et al: Response of families to two preventive intervention strategies: long-term differences and attitude change. J Am Acad Child Adolesc Psychiatry 35:774–782, 1996.

Diamond GS, Serrano AC, Dickey MS, et al: Current status of family-based outcome and process research, J Am Acad Child Adolesc Psychiatry 35:6–16, 1996.

Fonagy P, Target M: Predictors of outcome in child psychoanalysis: a retrospective study of 763 cases at the Anna Freud Centre. J Am Psychoanal Assoc 44:27–77, 1996.

Hendren RL: Adolescent psychotherapy research: a practical review. Am J Psychother 47:334–343, 1993.

Hoagwood K; et al: Introduction to the special section: efficacy and effectiveness in studies of child and adolescent psychotherapy. J Consult Clin Psychol 63:683–687, 1995.

Kazdin AE: Bridging child, adolescent and adult psychotherapy: directions for research. Psychother Research 5:258–277, 1995.

Kendall PC, MacDonald JP: Cognition in the psychopathology of youth and implications for treatment. *In* Dobson KS, Kendall, PC (eds): Psychopathology and Cognition. San Diego, Academic Press, 1993, pp 387–432.

Kendall PC, Southam-Gerow MA: Long-term follow-up of a cognitive-behavioral therapy for anxiety disordered youth. J Consult Clin Psychol 64:724–730, 1996.

Kymissis P: Group psychotherapy. Psychotherapy Child Adolescent Clin North Am 1:173–184, 1997.

Lazare A, Eisenthal S, Wasserman L: The customer approach to patienthood. Arch Gen Psychiatry 32:553–558, 1975.

March JS, Mulle K, Herbel B: Behavioral psychotherapy for children and adolescents with obsessive-compulsive disorder: an open trial of a new protocol-driven treatment package. J Am Acad Child Adolesc Psychiatry 33:333–341, 1994.

Mufson L, Fairbanks J: Interpersonal psychotherapy for depressed adolescent depression: a 1-year naturalistic follow-up study. J Am Acad Child Adolesc Psychiatry 35:1145–1155, 1996.

Rosenfeld AA: Resolved: the therapist-patient relationship is the crucial factor to change in child psychotherapy. J Am Acad Child Adolesc Psychiatry 33:1047–1053, 1994.

Russell GFM, et al: An evaluation of family therapy in Anorexia Nervosa and Bulimia Nervosa. Arch Gen Psychiatry 44:1047–1057, 1987.

Sargent J: Family therapy in child and adolescent psychiatry. Child Adolesc Psychiatr Clin N Am 6:151–171, 1997.

Shirk SR, Russell RL: A reevaluation of estimates of child therapy effectiveness. J Am Acad Child Adolesc Psychiatry 31:703–709, 1992.

Slavson SR, Schiffer M: Group Psychotherapies for Children: A Textbook. Madison, CT, International Universities Press, 1975.

Southam-Gerow MA, et al: Cognitive behavioral therapy with children and adolescents. Child Adolesc Psychiatr Clin N Am 6:111–136, 1997.

Target M, Fonagy P: Research on intensive psychotherapy with children and adolescents. Child Adolesc Psychiatr Clin N Am 6:39–53, 1997.

Tomm L: The old hat doesn't fit. Family Therapy Networker 7:39–41, 1983.

Weisz JR, et al: Child and adolescent psychotherapy outcomes in experiments versus clinics: why the disparity? J Abnorm Child Psychol 23:83–106, 1995.

78 Child Behavior Management

John M. Parrish

One of the greatest challenges confronting pediatricians in the developmental-behavioral area is actually helping parents to bring about appropriate changes in their children's behavior. Many doctors and parents are familiar only with spanking and time out but are not well informed about other possible interventions. This chapter urges the practitioner to think of behavior in terms of antecedents and consequences and to employ the full range of techniques known to be effective, such as differential reinforcement and instructional training. The basic elements of an effective child behavior management program are described.

The practicing pediatrician is frequently challenged to detect, diagnose, manage, and prevent troubling behaviors evinced by children and youth. Recent advances in behavioral health care practices, predicated largely on the principles and procedures of applied behavior analysis, can inform the pediatrician's effort to evaluate and counsel about behavioral concerns. This chapter provides an overview of these principles and an introduction to selected assessment and management procedures based on them, as a means of providing the pediatrician with a practical framework within which to identify and address prevalent behavioral concerns. The mechanisms and methods described herein pertain chiefly to operant conditioning (i.e., behavior modification) and are not to be confused with child and family therapy, or the myriad alternative approaches to counseling, described in Chapters 76 and 77 and elsewhere.

Principles and Procedures of Child Behavior Management

Based on a burgeoning area of clinical investigation centered on the development of practical procedures, *applied behavior analysis* focuses on human behavior (i.e., what people do and say) and the biological and environmental influences on such behavior (Miller, 1980). Assessment and management protocols based on the principles of applied behavior analysis have often proved to be effective, feasible, and cost-beneficial as a means of ameliorating innumerable behavioral excesses and deficits, including, but not limited to, academic underachievement, variations of activity level, physical and verbal aggression, attentional variations, disruptive behavior, enuresis, encopresis, feeding difficulties, hair-pulling, impulsivity, inappropriate play, lack of community survival skills, lack of self-help or social skills, noncompliance, parent-child conflict, poor peer relationships, property destruction, recurrent pain, self-injurious behavior, sleep problems, and throwing tantrums (Van Houten and Axelrod, 1993). Applied behavior analysis can be used alone or in combination with many compatible therapies, such as implementing cognitive-behavioral interventions or a tandem intervention involving both behavior therapy and a trial of medication. Variation is observed in response to most, if not all, interventions, including those presented in this chapter (see Chapter 8 regarding individual differences).

A fundamental assumption underlying applied behavior analysis is that behavior is a function of its *antecedents* and *consequences*, including those related to biological determinants and concomitants. Antecedents are those events or contextual factors that precede or coincide with a behavior (Smith and Iwata, 1997). Consequences are those events or contextual factors that occur subsequent to the behavior and may or may not be related causally to it (Martin and Pear, 1996). Based on the preponderant evidence, applied behavior analysts contend that behavior is typically learned, rather than being a manifestation of intrapsychic drives, impulses, motives, conflicts, or traits (Catania, 1984). Effective management requires (1) accurate identification of biological and environmental variables that instigate and maintain problem behavior and (2) alteration of these variables to facilitate learning of alternative *prosocial behaviors* (i.e., socially acceptable behaviors) that serve functions equivalent to those of the problem behavior (Carr, 1988). It depends significantly on an appreciation of the following fundamental processes.

Positive Reinforcement. *Positive reinforcement* is a process whereby consequences following a behavior result in an increase in that behavior over time (Martin and Pear, 1996). For example, allowing a child to view her preferred videotape if and only if the child accepts her prescribed medication may increase the probability that she accepts the medication in the future. The consequences are referred to as *positive reinforcers*, which may include preferred social exchanges, activities, objects, or edibles. Table 78–1 presents examples of common positive reinforcers. Such reinforcers are of limitless variety. They are defined as reinforcers solely on the basis of their effects on a given child's behavior, not upon their appearance, common appeal, presumed quality, or assumed value. A common mistake is to assume that positive reinforcers are universal or remain constant in value. In fact, positive reinforcers vary widely in type and value across children, and with each child over time. Another frequent error is the contention

Table 78–1 • Examples of Positive Reinforcers

Social reinforcers
    Affection (e.g., hug, kiss, pat on back, smile)
    Allowing child to have her way
    Arranging for demonstration by child of a mastered skill or preferred
        activity
    Casual conversation
    Descriptive praise
    Offering assistance upon child's request
    Physical proximity
Activity reinforcers
    Assembling model
    Drawing, painting
    Going to a birthday party
    Playing games
    Reading storybooks
    Singing
    Talking on telephone
    Visiting grandparents
Manipulatable reinforcers
    Bicycle
    Computer
    Crayons
    Magazine
    Money
    Musical instrument
    Toys
Edible reinforcers
    Carrots
    Celery
    Cookies
    Dry cereal
    Fruit
    Ice cream
    Juice
    Raisins

Adapted from Parrish J: Behavior management: Promoting adaptive behavior. *In* Batshaw M (ed): Children with Disabilities, 4th ed. Baltimore, Paul H. Brookes Publishing Co., 1997. P.O. Box 10624, Baltimore, MD 21285-0624.

that some children do not have any positive reinforcers. Every alert child, without exception, has preferences. These preferences can be identified by asking or observing the child, asking others familiar with the child, and by structuring systematic reinforcer assessments.

It is important to select positive reinforcers consistent with the child's chronologic age. For instance, an adolescent may be provided *age-appropriate* opportunities to listen to music, look at age-appropriate magazines, or enjoy private time with peers. Selection of *natural positive reinforcers*, that is, those items or activities that are likely to be available routinely to the child, is essential to behavior change. For example, when the child plays by the rules, a preferred game is continued. Or, when teaching a child to say "juice," juice is provided as a reinforcer, rather than some arbitrary reinforcer, such as a toy.

At least seven factors influence the *effectiveness* of an item or event as a positive reinforcer.

1. One key factor is that the item or event be accessible to the child on a *contingent* basis; that is, if and only if the child exhibits a desired behavior *targeted* (i.e., pinpointed) for increase. Inconsistent delivery of a positive reinforcer may slow learning of prosocial behavior. For example, if father were to offer a child an allowance whether or not the child completed

home chores, the child would be less likely to learn that payment depends on satisfactory work completion.

2. Another important factor is the child's degree of *deprivation* in regard to the item or event. For an item or event to be effective, the child must experience some level of deprivation specific to that item or event immediately prior to its delivery. Offering a child access to a game that the child has not played thus far that day is more likely to be effective as a reinforcer than offering the child an opportunity to repeat a game already played several times that day.

3. A third critical factor is the degree of *immediacy* of reinforcer delivery. Typically, immediate reinforcement is more effective than delayed reinforcement. Delayed reinforcement is usually not as effective because unwanted behaviors that occur soon after the desired behavior occurs, but before reinforcer delivery, may also be reinforced. Also, the child may find it difficult to discern the *contingency in effect*, that is, the relationship between the child's behavior and the positive reinforcement delivered as a consequence of it.

4. The *amount* of reinforcement provided is important. If the child receives too much of a reinforcer, satiation can occur; that is, the child may have had so much of a given reinforcer that the child no longer wants it. On such occasions, the reinforcing effect of an item or event is diminished or temporarily lost. The amount of positive reinforcement provided should be proportional to the effort required of the child to behave appropriately. At the onset of a protocol designed to strengthen the child's adaptive behavior, larger amounts of reinforcement may be needed to establish a new behavior because more initial effort by the child is required.

5. Another factor has to do with the *schedule of reinforcement*. Positive reinforcement can be provided after a set number of desired responses have occurred (e.g., in the case of *ratio schedules*) or after passage of a certain amount of time relative to the child's performance (e.g., with *interval schedules*). Ratio schedules are generally appropriate when the behavior being reinforced has a definite beginning and ending. For example, the child receives mother's approval every other time he obeys her request. Interval schedules are more suitable when behaviors are continuous or of extended duration. For instance, the child receives a sticker for playing appropriately with a peer for 2 minutes. Positive reinforcement can be dispensed on a continuous or intermittent basis. *Continuous reinforcement* is often necessary to develop new behaviors. However, *satiation* needs to be avoided. Once a behavior occurs more routinely, *intermittent reinforcement* may be enough to maintain it.

6. The *quality* of the positive reinforcer is also relevant. The child is more likely to demonstrate a behavior when the reinforcer that is available contingent on its occurrence is highly valued by the child. The *value* of a given reinforcer is always relative to other available reinforcers.

7. Another consideration is the *novelty* of the reinforcer. Positive reinforcers are typically more effective when they are first introduced. Presenting new reinforcers periodically, and otherwise varying reinforcers administered previously, better ensures that the child does not get too much of any reinforcer and that the child is more likely to be desirous of a given reinforcer when it is provided.

Although positive reinforcement procedures can be skillfully designed and implemented to promote the child's prosocial behavior, in everyday life the process of positive reinforcement may also increase inappropriate behavior unintentionally if it is misdirected or is applied inconsistently. For instance, a parent who attends to a child's persistent whining and eventually "gives in" to the child's demands may inadvertently increase the likelihood of "whiny" behavior by the child in the future. It is commonly understood that children behave inappropriately at times to garner attention or to gain access to a preferred activity or object. Any occurrence of positive reinforcement, when administered incorrectly, can have negative side effects (Table 78–2).

Planned Ignoring (Extinction). If the child has previously received positive reinforcement of misbehavior, the child's poor conduct will continue, or possibly intensify. In these situations, a procedure termed *planned ignoring* has been demonstrated to be effective, over time, in decreasing problem behavior (Kazdin, 1989). Planned ignoring is based on the process of *extinction* (Lerman and Iwata, 1996). Extinction is achieved via consistent withholding of positive reinforcement (e.g., adult attention) of nondangerous, nondestructive problem behavior (e.g., nagging, whining, crying, complaining, noise-making, talking back). For example, mother responds to the child's persistent whining by continuing to read mother's preferred book, while ostensibly ignoring the child's escalating demands. Consistent ignoring of nondangerous, nondestructive behavior will usually result in a decrease in these annoying behaviors over time.

The desired effects of planned ignoring are seldom immediate, however. Planned ignoring often sparks a temporary increase in the frequency, duration, and intensity of the problem behavior before a reduction occurs. For instance, when mother first ignores the child's whining, the child's whining is likely to escalate, and the child may even have a tantrum or throw objects. Such a flare-up, although often construed to be a setback, is actually an indication that previously dispensed reinforcement is the basis for the problem behavior, and that planned ignoring is likely to be an effective intervention over time, if it is

administered consistently. The competent behavior manager allows the "bursts" to subside before providing any positive reinforcement. During the process of extinction, the child is likely to test periodically whether positive reinforcement is again available contingent on the problem behavior. When this occurs, if the competent behavior manager continues to ignore the behavior, a rapid and sustained decrease in the problem behavior typically ensues.

Many parents find it difficult to ignore a child's misbehavior consistently. Parents may confuse planned ignoring with "doing nothing," especially when they adopt the outlook that the conscientious parent must not allow a child's misbehavior, however minor, to go unchecked. These parents may often be heard to issue statements of disapproval, such as "no," "don't," and "stop." Unfortunately, such statements are likely to exacerbate the disruptive behavior they are intended to curtail.

Negative Reinforcement. *Negative reinforcement* is the process whereby avoidance, cessation, or removal of an *aversive stimulus* contingent on the occurrence of another behavior results in an increase in the frequency of that behavior in the future (Iwata, 1987). Consider, for example, the situation in which a teacher consistently requires any student who does not complete assigned seatwork accurately and on time during morning work periods to participate in a remedial study period scheduled each schoolday afternoon. The students may learn that satisfactory completion of assigned seatwork serves to avoid study hall. In this manner, effective work completion is reinforced negatively via the avoidance of study hall.

Examples of negative reinforcement are prevalent in everyday settings. In fact, human behavior is often motivated by avoidance of or escape from unwanted situations. For instance, a child may learn over time to wear a sweater to avoid or escape from being cold. Negative reinforcement is often confused with punishment because both of these processes revolve around an aversive event. However, negative reinforcement and punishment are very distinct phenomena, and their specific effects could not be more disparate. The key difference is whether the process increases or decreases the behavior it follows. If the behavior increases in frequency, reinforcement (whether positive or negative) has occurred. If the behavior decreases in frequency, punishment has occurred.

In parallel with positive reinforcement, negative reinforcement may function to increase unacceptable as well as acceptable behavior. For instance, when a parent "gives in" to a child's persistent demands for a toy in a public place, the child thereby receives positive reinforcement for being "bossy," and the parent receives negative reinforcement when the child's "bossy" behavior and the parent's feelings of public humiliation subside. As a result, the child is more likely to escalate defiantly when the parent initially denies the child's inappropriate request, and the parent is more likely to "give in" if and when the child's escalating behavior causes a sufficient disturbance.

Similarly, negative reinforcement is at work when a parent responds to a child's demanding behavior with threats, yelling, or spanking, and the child conforms to the parent's wishes. As a result of this negative reinforcement, the parent is more likely to rely on these *coercive* interven-

Table 78–2 • Fundamental Processes of Behavior Change

Effect on Behavior	Presentation of Stimuli	Withdrawal of Stimuli
Increase in frequency	Positive reinforcement	Negative reinforcement
Decrease in frequency	Punishment	Extinction or punishment

tions in the future when the child's behavior becomes troubling (Patterson, 1982). Hence, the process of negative reinforcement can have both gainful and deleterious effects and must be managed judiciously, or it will worsen problem behavior on the part of the child, the care provider, or both.

Punishment. *Punishment* is a process whereby a penalty is imposed or a positive reinforcer is withdrawn contingent on the occurrence of a behavior, resulting in a decrease in the future probability of that behavior (Martin and Pear, 1996). For instance, issuance of a verbal reprimand in response to misbehavior may result in a decrease in that behavior over time and thereby be a punisher. Likewise, removal of a privilege when an infraction occurs may result in a similar decrease in problem behavior. In everyday language, punishment typically is understood as doing something "mean" or "hurtful" to someone who made a mistake or did something "bad." Such an action may or may not involve the process of punishment, however. A seemingly unpleasant event to one person may not be a punisher to another, and the same event that is a positive reinforcer for one person may be another person's punisher. Any generalization regarding what is a punisher or a reinforcer is unwise. It is more astute to define an event or action on the basis of its impact on the behavior it follows.

Use of punishment of any sort is controversial. Skillful professionals aim to avoid or to minimize use of punishment procedures. Many tactics predicated on positive reinforcement strategies, when implemented competently, are effective. Punishment may engender negative side effects (e.g., counter-coercive behavior and conflictual relationships). Punishment procedures can be misapplied and cause harm. At best, punishment procedures reduce problem behaviors. On occasion they enable the child to learn what not to do. However, they typically provide relatively little direct instruction in regard to what the child is to do instead of the unwanted behavior (Matson and DiLorenzo, 1984).

Responsible professionals either do not use punishment procedures at all or use them infrequently while exercising considerable caution. Positive reinforcement strategies are almost always used first. Rare exceptions arise when the child's behavior puts the child or others at severe imminent risk for harm, and immediate suppression of the challenging behavior is warranted. If punishment procedures are practiced, the pediatrician must remain cognizant of and fully sensitive to the rights and welfare of the child, including the child's right to effective treatment (Van Houten et al, 1988).

Intervention options that include punishment strategies are usually selected only when positive reinforcement strategies have proven to be ineffective across multiple applications over an extended time period. When punishment procedures are adopted, they are best implemented in conjunction with positive reinforcement strategies, thereby providing differential (i.e, discriminably different) consequences for appropriate versus inappropriate behavior. Emphasis is placed on the child's acquisition of pivotal adaptive skills, especially those equivalent in function to the aberrant behaviors undergoing treatment, and promoting the child's full inclusion in *positive behavioral support services* (Koegel, Koegel, and Dunlap, 1996). Discontinuation criteria must be in effect prior to any application of punishment. Every effort should be expended to fade the use of punishment when the child's high-risk behavior abates.

Stimulus Control. Over time, as the individual's learning proceeds, specific stimuli acquire properties that serve to control the individual's behavior. For instance, children learn to behave differently as a function of the presence of a parent versus the presence of their peer group, or as a function of being in the classroom versus being on the playground. Specific cues in each situation, termed *discriminative stimuli*, signal that reinforcement is available to the individual if and when situationally appropriate behavior is demonstrated by that individual. Other cues, referred to as *S-deltas*, indicate that reinforcement is not available in the situation, such as when a street sign indicates a "dead end" to a bicycle-riding child who simply wants to exit the neighborhood. Yet other cues signal that an aversive event may be in the offing, such as when a child with a reputation of being a "bully" joins a competitive game. Much of our behavior is controlled, at least partially, by stimuli that enable us to discriminate the probability of reinforcement and punishment.

Such stimuli in the child's immediate environment influence the child's behavior to such an extent that the behavior is typically *situation-specific* (i.e., is said to be *under stimulus control*). For example, children often behave differently at home than they do when they are visiting a friend or attending school or church. Effective behavior management incorporates an understanding of immediate stimulus control into each planned intervention and aims to adapt stimuli in situations in which problem behavior is most probable. For instance, with two boys who have a history of frequently fighting with one another during a competitive game, a concerted effort is made to present opportunities for each of them to accrue positive reinforcement via cooperation, such as being teammates rather than opponents during organized sports. In this way, stimuli and situations are arranged so as to elicit appropriate behavior while suppressing inappropriate behavior.

Setting Events and Establishing Operations. Behavior analysts increasingly recognize that influences other than those that occur immediately before or after the target behavior are important determinants of that behavior. Events that are more complex or temporally distant often influence current behavior. For example, complex concurrent factors, including physiologic variables such as deprivation, satiation, fatigue, infections, discomfort, and pain, may influence how the child responds. Other complex concurrent factors include the presence or absence of particular people (e.g., the child's parent, teacher, best friend), the amount of space available, access to alternative or preferred activities, and level of task difficulty or preference.

In addition to concurrent factors, historical events may influence the child's current behavior. For instance, a child's scuffle with a peer at the neighborhood playground may be related to a conflict with mother the day before, a history of having been teased by that peer, or having been admonished by the teacher at school earlier that day. Such prior events are no longer present as immediate stimuli, yet they may nonetheless contribute to current states of arousal and may compound the influence of current triggering events, such as an inadvertent bump or shove on the playground. Hitherto more the province of psychotherapy than applied behavior analysis, the identification of previous or concurrent influences, referred to as *setting events* or *establishing operations*, is increasingly considered to be important to the selection and use of competent behavior management strategies.

Summary of Fundamental Processes. Environmental influences on child behavior are largely a function of the processes of *positive reinforcement, extinction, negative reinforcement, punishment, stimulus control*, and *setting events* (or *establishing operations*). The skillful pediatrician who practices as a behavior analyst seeks to ascertain how these processes serve to maintain and to alter each target behavior in question. Based on a systematic analysis of these processes, individually tailored interventions are then designed, implemented, and refined until the desired behavioral changes occur. Table 78–2 presents a graphic display of the relationships among the processes of positive reinforcement, extinction, negative reinforcement, and punishment.

Selected Instructional Procedures To Increase Adaptive Behavior

Differential Reinforcement. In most cases, the child presents several inappropriate behaviors that warrant intervention, as well as a number of appropriate behaviors that require ongoing positive reinforcement. Given this, positive reinforcement and planned ignoring are often used in combination through a process termed *differential reinforcement*. The primary goal of differential reinforcement is to reinforce acceptable behavior while concurrently withholding reinforcement for unacceptable behavior. For example, mother responds affirmatively to the child's request when the child issues the request beginning with a "please," while mother ignores any request that does not include this polite expression. Table 78–3 presents the principal variants of differential reinforcement.

Differential reinforcement is preferred typically over planned ignoring because it is more effective for teaching

the child that specific behaviors are appropriate and others are not. The efficacy of differential reinforcement hinges both on the consistency of its administration and on the nonavailability of positive reinforcement for troubling behavior. For instance, if the child's antics result in positive reinforcement in the form of sibling laughter and attention, then the parent's efforts to ignore the child's disruptive behavior may be ineffective. Consistent application of differential reinforcement by multiple individuals across diverse settings is usually necessary for enduring behavior change.

Instructional and Imitation Training. With many children, it is enough to merely "show and tell," followed by consistent use of differential reinforcement, when teaching new behaviors. During *instructional training*, the teacher (e.g., the parent, the pediatrician) simply describes the behavior the child is to demonstrate, requests that the child perform the described action, gives the child an appropriate, supervised opportunity to initiate and complete the directed activity, and provides positive reinforcement upon satisfactory completion of the task by the child. During *imitation training*, the teacher demonstrates for the child what the child is to do, asks the child to imitate the demonstrated action, gives the child an opportunity to do so, and provides the child with positive reinforcement when the child's imitation results in completion of the demonstrated skill. Imitation training typically requires less verbal skill and is often used with young children or with older children whose receptive vocabulary is delayed or deficient. As the child learns how to follow directions and how to imitate observed appropriate behavior, then the child can be guided efficiently to learn academic and social skills that prevent or replace aberrant behavior.

Compliance Training. Before some children can benefit from instructional and imitation training, they first need to learn how to follow simple instructions (Forehand and Long, 1996; Forehand and McMahon, 1981). When a child learns how to follow directions and to complete requested actions independently, cooperative learning is facilitated. In fact, routine instruction following has been found to prevent or significantly reduce the occurrence of problem behaviors, even in the absence of interventions

Table 78–3 • Variants of Differential Reinforcement

Variant	Goal	Illustration
DRO (Differential Reinforcement of Other Behavior)	Nonoccurrence of targeted behavior during observation interval	Child permitted to play game as long as child does not violate rules of game (breaking rules is target behavior)
DRA (Differential Reinforcement of Appropriate Behavior)	Increased frequency of targeted appropriate behavior in absence of targeted problem behavior	Child earns privilege contingent upon satisfactory completion of assigned homework without complaining (homework completion is targeted appropriate behavior; complaining is targeted inappropriate behavior)
DRI (Differential Reinforcement of Incompatible Behavior)	Increased rate of a targeted appropriate behavior that is incompatible with a targeted problem behavior	Child is called upon when child's hand is raised; child's requests for attention ignored when child's hand is not raised
DRL (Differential Reinforcement of Low Rate Behavior)	Occurrence of problem behavior at acceptably low rates	Child is granted privilege contingent upon low rates of talking back

Adapted from Parrish J: Behavior management: Promoting adaptive behavior. *In* Batshaw M (ed): Children with Disabilities, 4th ed. Baltimore, Paul H. Brookes Publishing Co., 1997. P.O. Box 10624, Baltimore, MD 21285-0624.

designed to ameliorate problem behaviors (Parrish et al, 1986). During *compliance training*, the teacher (e.g., parent or other caregiver) orients the child to attend to her or him, and then issues a developmentally appropriate "do" request. A *"do" request* is a statement that specifies an action (e.g., "take your vitamins"). The teacher issues the "do" request with a firm yet matter-of-fact tone of voice. The teacher then gives the child an opportunity to follow through, while the teacher waits quietly. The duration of the wait is determined by the complexity of the requested action. The teacher is to avoid nagging, lecturing, threatening, yelling, or apologizing for the request. If and when the child complies with the request, the teacher provides praise and other social reinforcers (e.g., a hug), and perhaps a tangible reinforcer (e.g., a raisin) as well.

If the child does not comply, the teacher simply restates the request, using the same words and tone of voice as before. The only procedural shift is that the teacher then pairs the repetition of the verbal request with a gesture, such as pointing to the vitamins. The teacher again waits quietly. If the child complies with the first repetition of the request, the teacher provides social, but not tangible, reinforcement. If the child again does not comply, the teacher uses *full* or *partial graduated guidance* to assist the child to complete the requested action. During full graduated guidance, the teacher keeps her hands in full contact with the child's hands, arms, or shoulders throughout the planned activity, and provides descriptive praise whenever the child cooperatively completes the task. During partial graduated guidance, the teacher uses minimal physical contact paired with praise so long as the child proceeds to complete the desired activity independently. The teacher does less and less as the child's learning progresses, adjusting her level of guidance to match the child's skill and motivation to participate competently. Once the child reliably completes the desired skill sequence with minimal physical guidance, the teacher simply *shadows* the child, by keeping her hands within an inch of the child's hand as the child completes the activity or task. Verbal requests, gestural hints, and physical prompts are faded gradually as the child demonstrates independent task completion consistently.

Building Momentum. When typical methods of teaching a young child to follow instructions are ineffective, it may be helpful to identify requests to which the child has complied frequently in the past. Such requests are termed *high-p* (i.e., high probability) requests. Once high-p requests are identified, the teacher issues a few of them in quick succession, prior to issuing a *low-p* request to which the child has seldom complied. For instance, the child often refuses to complete oral reading assignments. Upon request, however, the child frequently agrees to color, play a computer game, and sharpen pencils. Being aware of this, the parent strives to build *behavioral momentum* with the child when redirecting her to engage in reading. The parent first requests that the child participate in a sequence of the preferred activities, acknowledging the child's compliance with each request to color, and so on. Then, the parent firmly yet matter-of-factly asks the child to complete her oral reading assignment for the evening. For more information about building behavioral momentum

as a means of promoting compliance, the interested reader is referred to the work by Mace and associates (1990).

Shaping. In some instances, the desired behavior may not yet be in the child's repertoire or may occur infrequently. More is required than straightforward instruction, demonstrating the wanted behavior (i.e., *modeling*), standard compliance training, or building behavioral momentum, while providing differential reinforcement for acceptable versus unacceptable behavior. Often the child exhibits troubling behavior merely because she or he has not learned how to behave appropriately. Through a systematic procedure termed *shaping*, new prosocial behaviors can be acquired by the child. Gradual development of a new behavior is facilitated by reinforcing small improvements in the child's repertoire. The child receives positive reinforcement as each step of the targeted skill is demonstrated. As steps are performed in proper sequence with increasing consistency, delivery of positive reinforcement is faded.

For example, in teaching a child of preschool age to hold a pencil, the parent may provide the child a preferred treat paired with praise when the child merely touches an oversized pencil. Once the child routinely touches the pencil, positive reinforcement is delivered if and only if the child grasps the pencil. When such grasping occurs on a consistent basis, positive reinforcement is given only if the child both grasps the pencil and places its point on a piece of paper. Later, the child receives positive reinforcement only upon making a mark on the paper with the pencil, and so forth. This procedure of providing positive reinforcement for *successive approximations* to the target behavior continues until the desired sequence of skills is demonstrated independently by the child.

Often shaping is enhanced through use of *graduated guidance* and *guided compliance*. Graduated refers to providing only that level of assistance necessary for the child to complete a task competently. Graduated guidance centers on using *prompts* (e.g., verbal, gestural, manual, visual, or auditory cues) that direct the child to participate in a targeted activity (e.g., dressing, eating, sharing, waiting, toileting). Guided compliance involves the use of graduated guidance in the context of compliance training, as described earlier. For more detailed information about graduated guidance and guided compliance, including the use of prompts, *forward and backward chaining* of newly acquired skills, and full to partial guidance to shadowing, the interested reader is referred to the work by Foxx (1982b).

Fading Prompts and Positive Reinforcement. Long-term use of prompts and positive reinforcement is time- and labor-intensive and may engender the child's excessive dependency on external cues. Via *fading*, a process whereby prompts and positive reinforcers are withdrawn slowly, the child learns to continue participation in a targeted activity while becoming less reliant on systematic cues and consequences. For instance, the parent may initially remind the child every school night to organize his or her books and complete homework assignments. Once the assignments are completed satisfactorily, the parent offers to join in the child's preferred play activity. As the child increasingly initiates this process independently, the parent issues fewer and fewer reminders. As the child competently completes homework assignments more and more consistently, the parent joins in the child's subsequent play less and less frequently. Over time, prompts and positive reinforcers are no longer necessary. The parent simply provides periodic praise contingent on the child's satisfactory completion of homework. Fading increases the probability that desired behaviors will occur spontaneously and in situations other than those in which training occurred. Fading can be achieved by delaying the use of prompts as well as decreasing the frequency of their use. Fading can also be accomplished by decreasing the frequency and amount of reinforcement provided following a target behavior, or by requiring several occurrences of a target behavior before positive reinforcement is provided.

Selected Punishment Procedures for Decreasing Challenging Behavior

Punishment by Contingent Aversive Stimulation. *Punishment by contingent stimulation* (e.g., spraying water mist; introducing lemon juice, aromatic ammonia, mouthwash; applying mild faradic shock; engaging in contingent exercise [e.g., additional calisthenics]; spanking; and excessive repetition of the undesirable behavior) upon occurrence of a severe challenging behavior is seldom, if ever, indicated. These punishment procedures are considered to be especially aversive, intrusive, and potentially harmful if misapplied. Although spanking, for example, is a prevalent parental practice, it seldom if ever is the intervention of choice. Professional experts are entrusted to identify, recommend, and promote the use of alternative disciplinary tactics that are more likely to be effective than these punishment tactics, and less likely to cause harm if used inappropriately or excessively.

Statements of Disapproval. The most ubiquitous variant of punishment by contingent aversive stimulation is a *negative verbal statement*. Adults and children alike often issue warnings, threats, or reprimands following misbehavior. Such statements have inconsistent effects. Sometimes such remarks suppress ongoing misbehavior immediately, or prevent its occurrence altogether. On other occasions, such statements function as positive reinforcers as sources of *negative attention* (which is not to be confused with negative reinforcement). For example, a parent who issues a preponderance of "don't" requests (e.g., "no," "don't," and "stop") instead of "do" requests is more likely over time to inflame the escalation of a child's misbehavior than to redirect the child away from such behavior. The way by which verbal disapprovals are issued may partially determine their efficacy. *Private reprimands* delivered softly may be more effective than loud reprimands expressed in the presence of others.

Punishment by Contingent Withdrawal. In the context of planning a systematic behavior management program, *punishment by contingent withdrawal* is a more prevalent, reliable selection than punishment by contingent aversive stimulation. The former often involves administration of *exclusionary time out* (e.g., quiet time in a hallway) and *nonexclusionary time out* (e.g., response cost, contingent observation), among other interventions.

Time In and Time Out. *Time out* is removal from *time in*. To maximize the impact of time out, one must orchestrate time in. Time in for a given child is said to occur when the child is participating in an activity preferred at that time by that child. Time in is in effect when the child gets what she or he wants when she or he wants it. Time in is often conducive to the child's learning and motivation to cooperate. During time in, the child is likely to approach and then engage in an activity, given that it is preferred. Through participation in the activity, the child is likely to acquire new skills or to practice skills already acquired.

Time in is an essential prerequisite for the effectiveness of most, if not all, instructional strategies. Time in can be arranged by attending carefully to the child's preferences and by ensuring that these preferences are accessible when the child is engaged in appropriate behavior. Time in is typically characterized by enabling the child to select from an array of preferred options. The child is provided social reinforcement (e.g., praise) or tangibles (e.g., access to a preferred object or activity) frequently as a consequence of acceptable behavior, or successive approximations to it. Demands placed on the child are kept to a minimum.

Exclusionary and Nonexclusionary Time Out. Time out is a procedure whereby positive reinforcement is withdrawn for a predetermined amount of time following an occurrence of problem behavior. Time out usually occurs in two formats: (1) exclusionary time out and (2) nonexclusionary time out. Exclusionary time out occurs when the child who misbehaves is removed from time in for a defined time interval. Nonexclusionary time out is said to occur when the child is allowed to remain at the site of the infraction, but is not allowed to engage in any preferred activities for a prespecified period of time. Exclusionary time out requires the child to be removed from positive reinforcers, while nonexclusionary time out requires that these reinforcers be removed from the child. For instance, the former may involve sending the child to his room for 5 minutes. The latter may entail loss of a privilege, such as rollerskating, for the remainder of the day.

When Time Out Makes Sense and When It Does Not. Application of time out makes sense if the predetermined serious yet low-rate problem behavior it is designed to alter is maintained by positive reinforcement (e.g., social, tangible, edible reinforcers) available during time in. For example, a child's destructive tantrums may have been reinforced either by social attention (e.g., a verbal reprimand or a statement intended to soothe) or by "giving in" (e.g., giving the child a snack). In such situations, time out from positive reinforcement may be effective. However, if the problem behavior functions to avoid or escape from an unwanted or demanding activity (e.g., brushing teeth), then time out is unlikely to be effective. Time out is often even contraindicated, and seldom is warranted as the first-order intervention.

Parameters of Effective Exclusionary Time Out. Exclusionary time out works best with children 2 to 6 years of age (Forehand and McMahon, 1981). It is more likely to be effective when (1) the child has frequent access to time in; (2) the use of time out is restricted to infrequent dangerous or destructive behaviors maintained by positive social reinforcement; (3) time out is administered immediately and only when targeted inappropriate behavior occurs; (4) the child and involved adults have practiced a simulated time out procedure prior to actual use; (5) the location of time out is safe, amenable to ongoing observation of the child, and in a place where the child can serve time out while being minimally disruptive to others; (6) one, and only one, warning is issued to the child that time out will be effected if a labeled misbehavior occurs or persists; (7) the duration of time out is preset and brief; (8) during time out, verbal exchanges and the child's access to positive reinforcement are kept to a minimum; (9) upon completion of time out, the child is returned immediately to the situation wherein the problem behavior warranting time out occurred, and the child is given an opportunity to demonstrate alternative prosocial behavior; and (10) a record of incidents warranting time out, the child's behavior during time out, and the impact of time out on the subsequent rate of the child's targeted challenging behavior is maintained.

Frequently the misbehaving child refuses to serve time out. The child may ignore or protest the directive to serve time out, or may attempt to negotiate around the instruction. The child's unacceptable behavior may escalate as a means of avoiding or escaping from time out. On such occasions, the adult caregiver provides that minimal physical guidance necessary to escort the child safely and quickly to the chosen site of time out. Nagging, lecturing, threatening, yelling, and wrestling are not recommended.

The duration of time out is optimally brief. One to 5 minutes is typically sufficient. When practicable, it is helpful to set a kitchen timer or a watch to beep when the predetermined time out interval is exhausted. Reliance on a beep generated by a device may serve to direct the child's attention more to the awaited signal than to the actions (including the attention) of the adult care provider. If the child leaves the location of time out before time out is over, the child is quietly and gently escorted back to the time out area, without explanation or admonishment. Usually the child is required to achieve a brief interval of being relatively calm before the child is informed that time out is over.

When time out is completed, it is important to return the child to time in, with a focus on the situation that was at hand when the child's misbehavior warranted time out. It is best to avoid further discussion, scolding, nagging, threatening, or reminding related to the infraction. Rather, in the event the misbehavior occurred in the context of an adult instruction for the child to engage in a task or activity, the instruction is simply repeated. Whatever may be the focus of time in, the adult caregiver assigns a premium to acknowledging the child's alternative acceptable behavior as interactions proceed.

If exclusionary time out is administered effectively, it sends a helpful message to the young child that an unacceptable behavior has occurred. Disadvantages of exclusionary time out include (1) risk that child is provided positive reinforcement for inappropriate behavior during its implementation, by way of adult attention; (2) delaying or allowing escape from completion of a task or activity as time out is served; (3) disruption of ongoing activities; (4) possible occurrence of dangerous or destructive behavior by the child during time out; and (5) difficulties in effecting time out, especially in public places. Exclusionary time out is a restrictive procedure that is effortful and intrusive. It does not directly assist the child to acquire and demonstrate alternative adaptive skills. Its use should be kept to a minimum and its effects should be monitored carefully.

Nonexclusionary Time Out. Nonexclusionary time out can be achieved using several different tactics, including response cost; star, point, or token systems; contingent observation; and use of time in symbols.

1. *Response cost* occurs when the child demonstrates a targeted inappropriate behavior and either a positive reinforcer is withdrawn or a penalty is imposed as a result. The child must first be receiving positive reinforcement. The more the child values this reinforcement, the more effective response cost will be. The *privilege* to be revoked or the *penalty* to be applied is best defined in advance of each targeted problem episode and is administered consistently without extensive explanation.

2. Response cost is often achieved through *star, point,* or *token systems* in which positive reinforcement is provided contingent on appropriate behavior and withheld (or withdrawn) for inappropriate behavior (Kazdin, 1977). Any balance of earned currency remaining subsequent to the subtraction of imposed fines can be exchanged for *back-up reinforcers,* such as preferred activities and treats, which are typically selected by the child from a menu of positive reinforcement options. *Fines* are typically small in value to increase the probability that the child earns more currency than she or he loses.

   Use of response cost may result in child avoidance of or aggression toward the adult care provider, or escalation of *counter-control behaviors* on the part of the child (e.g., tantrums, property destruction) when response cost is effected. In such instances, the adult aims to attend to what the child does well, provides positive reinforcement for desired behavior, and does not "give in" to the child's demands. Usually response cost procedures are easy to implement and often yield rapid and sizeable decreases in challenging behavior. For more detailed information regarding structured economies, the interested reader is referred to work by Christophersen (1994) and Kazdin (1977).

3. During the procedure of *contingent observation,* at the point of an infraction during a social interaction, the offending child is asked to sit on the sidelines while continuing to observe the ongoing activity from which she or he was withdrawn. The child's participation in time in is disrupted temporarily. Yet the child can observe alternative, more acceptable behaviors as demonstrated by peers and adult supervisors. Contingent observation thereby affords the unruly child an opportunity to learn adaptive behaviors via *positive modeling* by others and subsequent imitation by the child of observed skills. Contingent observation is especially useful as a means of teaching social skills, such as sharing and taking turns. However, contingent observation is contraindicated when inappropriate behavior on the part of others continues after the child is withdrawn from the interaction. Observation of inappropriate behavior, such as fighting among peers, may be more reinforcing for the child than participating in it.

4. Another method of nonexclusionary time out involves use of a *time in symbol*, such as a ribbon, sticker, or button pin. Initially, the child is given one of these to be worn at the wrist or on clothing. With the time in symbol in place, the child receives positive reinforcement contingent on appropriate behavior. The child's appropriate behavior is described, and mention is made that the child is wearing the time in symbol. This consistent pairing of the symbol with delivery of positive reinforcement establishes the time in symbol as being a discriminative stimulus that positive reinforcement is available for acceptable behavior. Over time the child comes to understand that wearing the time in symbol is a prerequisite for delivery of positive reinforcement. Subsequently, the adult caregiver can effect a nonexclusionary time out simply by removing the time in symbol whenever the child misbehaves. The time in symbol is withdrawn for a brief interval. During this period, the child's participation in preferred activities is discontinued. At the conclusion of time out, the time in symbol is restored and the adult supervisor resumes providing positive reinforcement contingent on acceptable behavior.

Use of a ribbon, sticker, or button pin in this manner can be implemented effectively with groups of children. Inappropriate peer reinforcement can be diminished by removing the ribbon, sticker, or button pin of any student who reinforces another student's inappropriate behavior. Sequences of inappropriate behavior can be interrupted early by announcing the first occurrence of a problem behavior, such as "Judy, you're using Sally's notebook," and removing the time in symbol from the misbehaving child. The presence versus absence of the time in symbol is readily discriminable by most children and by caregivers as well, and reminds the latter to reinforce the child's appropriate behavior. Time in symbols can be worn in public settings, facilitating the consistent application of nonexclusionary time out across multiple venues. The disadvantages of using a ribbon, sticker, or button pin are the same as those associated with response cost and contingent observation. For more information regarding the use of a time in symbol, the interested reader is referred to the work by Foxx (1982a).

Overcorrection. Another disciplinary method with an even more educative emphasis, which is neither a form of exclusionary nor of nonexclusionary time out, is overcorrection. *Overcorrection* involves (1) *restitution*, which is immediate restoration of any remediable damages caused by the child's misbehavior and then improving upon the condition of those things disturbed (i.e., overcorrection), and (2) *positive practice*, which requires the child to demonstrate repeatedly a relevant prosocial alternative to the problem behavior. For example, if the child spills milk on the kitchen floor as she pours milk into her bowl of cereal, the child is first guided gently to mop up the spilled milk and then a larger area of the floor than that area covered by the milk, and then is guided to practice how to pour milk into a bowl. Overcorrection is an effective educative procedure that is often implemented to strengthen the child's adaptive skills (e.g., toileting). Overcorrection is most likely to work when it is applied immediately after the misbehavior, when both restitution and positive practice are functionally related to the problem behavior, and when the child's positive reinforcers are withheld until overcorrection is completed. If more than minimal physical guidance is required for the child to engage in overcorrection, then another disciplinary tactic (e.g., response cost) is indicated.

Use of Punishment. Use of punishment, even in tandem with positive reinforcement, is debatable (Matson and DiLorenzo, 1984). Punishment strategies should be implemented only after efforts to optimize the impact of positive reinforcement strategies have failed to ameliorate a child's challenging behavior. For example, structuring quality time for the parent and child as an opportunity to pinpoint what the child enjoys and does well is often the first-order management tactic, rather than the use of exclusionary time out. Before any punishment procedure is introduced, including exclusionary time out, care must be taken to review the rationale for it with the child's parents or legal guardians, other care providers, and with the child when practicable. Each of these individuals should be informed of the side effects of punishment.

Once the advantages and disadvantages of using punishment are understood, and informed consent or assent has been obtained, the application of punishment should be problem-specific and monitored continuously, and its practice and effects should be recorded carefully. The effectiveness of a punishment-mediated intervention is a function of (1) its immediacy and intensity, (2) its schedule of occurrence, (3) the availability from others of positive reinforcement for the punished response, (4) the timing of punishment in the sequence of events resulting in the target problem behavior, and (5) the delivery of positive reinforcement for alternative appropriate behavior.

Behavioral Diagnosis and Treatment: A Practical Plan for Pediatricians

Steps typically required for the competent design and implementation of an effective behavior management program include *differential diagnosis, treatment planning, intervention, programming for generalization* and *fading intervention*, and *follow-up assessment and care.* These steps are defined briefly in Table 78–4. (See also Chapter 67 on pediatric assessment of behavior.)

Differential Diagnosis. The first step after receiving the parental complaint is to define the problem or problems. Several pertinent screening measures are available (Stancin and Palermo, 1997). More in-depth assessment techniques include semistructured clinical interviews with key informants (e.g., parents, teachers, child), administration and scoring of questionnaires and rating scales (Reynolds and Kamphaus, 1990), and direct observation of the child's target behaviors during interactions with selected individuals and environmental conditions (Kelley, 1990; Miller, 1980). During the diagnostic interview, the assessor first

Table 78–4 • Typical Components of a Child Behavior Management Program

Differential Diagnosis	Define the problem. Record review; interview with child and family, teachers, other care providers; scoring and interpretation of completed rating scales and questionnaires; direct observation of targeted behavior (when practicable); descriptive and functional analysis (to be conducted by consulting behavior analyst).
Treatment Planning	Negotiate general goals and target specific behavior(s) for treatment. Select specific techniques appropriate for objectives. Design of skill- and problem-specific protocol(s) based on key assessment findings. Each protocol defines what is to be done, how, by whom, when. Each protocol includes information regarding "do's" and "don't's," how to assess progress, expected effects and side effects, common pitfalls, and cautionary notes.
Intervention	Provision of education and training to child and adult care providers regarding safe, feasible, and effective administration of protocol(s) prior to routine implementation. Continuous collection of outcome data to determine extent of progress toward treatment goals. Revision or discontinuation of protocol(s) as may be indicated.
Programming for Generalization	Use of combination of methods to ensure desired behavioral changes occur across people, behaviors, settings, and over time.
Fading Intervention	Gradual withdrawal of systematic contingencies, once desired behavior change occurs consistently.
Follow-up Assessment and Care	Ongoing surveillance of child and family, with remedial interventions provided if and when warranted.

Adapted from Parrish J: Behavior management: Promoting adaptive behavior. *In* Batshaw M (ed): Children with Disabilities, 4th ed. Baltimore, Paul H. Brookes Publishing Co., 1997. P.O. Box 10624, Baltimore, MD 21285-0624.

obtains an overall evaluation of the child's strengths and problem behaviors. Checklists are often incorporated into the interview. The examiner then selects measures focused on a specific problem (e.g., aggression) or a specific diagnosis (e.g., attention-deficit hyperactivity disorder) or creates individually tailored assessment tools. More detailed assessments of the behaviors of greatest concern are completed (Table 78–5).

Informants are assisted to render operational definitions of the chief complaints. For example, the child may

Table 78–5 • Sample Outline for Behavioral Assessment

   I. Background information
      A. Child/family identifying data
      B. Reason(s) for referral
      C. Referral source
      D. Person(s) present for interview
  II. Checklist of common problem behaviors
 III. Detailed analyses of priority concerns
      A. Definition of problem behavior
      B. Estimated frequency and duration
      C. Onset
      D. Trend
      E. Settings
      F. Antecedents
      G. Consequences
      H. Previous management strategies
      I. Findings based on direct observations
      J. Management goals
      K. Initial monitoring plan
      L. Initial management plan
 IV. Other relevant information
      A. Prior professional contacts to resolve reported concerns
      B. Medical information
      C. School information
      D. Child's strengths
      E. Child's reinforcers
  V. Caretaker information
      A. Caretakers' daily routine
      B. Potential obstacles to delivery of indicated services
 VI. Other information
 VII. Initial impressions
VIII. Initial recommendations
  IX. Case disposition

be described initially as being "stubborn." A more useful formulation would be to convert this adjective into a set of action examples, such as "he refuses to do his homework." The informants are then asked to describe the frequency, duration, and/or intensity of each of the principal behaviors of concern. Based on an understanding that the child's behavior is situation-specific (see preceding section regarding stimulus control), the interviewer asks where and under what conditions each behavior does or does not occur.

Upon ascertaining the setting of the target behaviors, the pediatrician then seeks to pinpoint the specific environmental conditions (i.e., variables or factors) that precipitate or maintain the problem behavior. Common antecedents and consequences associated with the occurrence of the targeted aberrant behavior are defined. Additional relevant information is obtained, including brief descriptions of previous efforts to teach or manage the target behaviors, prior professional contacts to resolve reported concerns, pertinent developmental and medical history, current medications and dosage levels, present school placement and academic status, daily family and individual routines, and present obstacles to participation in indicated services.

Emphasis is given to an understanding and appreciation of child and family strengths, enabling selection and design of interventions that build on these assets. The child's preferred objects, activities, events, and treats are identified in preparation for development of *contingency management programs* (i.e., behavior protocols) centered on positive reinforcement processes. A focus on the child's endearing qualities and what the child does well serves to orient involved adult care providers to use positive reinforcement as a means of supporting the child.

The pediatrician who practices as a behavior analyst seeks opportunities to obtain data collected by parents and teachers based on their direct observations of the child's behavior during daily routines. For more information regarding alternative methods of direct observation, the interested reader is referred to work by Miller (1980) and Kelley (1990). When feasible, the pediatrician also observes available videotapes of the child's behavior at home and at school to ascertain specific factors that potentiate or exacerbate targeted behaviors in everyday situations. When practicable, the pediatrician structures a series of direct observations that is conducted during clinic visits, or prescribes a series for completion by others in everyday field settings.

Many common parental complaints put before the pediatrician are relatively simple to manage. However, pediatricians are increasingly reporting that more and more complaints are complex and difficult to resolve within the confines of a busy practice. In such cases, the pediatrician may consider referring the child and family for consultation visits with an expert in applied behavior analysis. Such experts increasingly employ the methods of *descriptive* and *functional analysis*. A descriptive analysis involves the observation of the child's behavior during routine activities that are often associated with either a very high or very low rate of the targeted behaviors. The goal is to assess child behavior during the routine conduct of each pinpointed activity, while providing typical antecedents and consequences. For example, specific findings may implicate the role of adult or peer attention, access to tangible reinforcers, or avoidance of or escape from demands contingent on the occurrence of problem behavior.

Based on these data, the consulting applied behavior analyst develops hypotheses regarding how identified antecedents elicit (i.e., precipitate) or particular consequences maintain the targeted behaviors. In the context of a functional analysis, these hypotheses are tested by the behavior analyst in well-controlled conditions under which the hypothesized variables (e.g., attention) are manipulated systematically to determine their impact on the targeted behaviors. Findings derived from the descriptive and functional analyses culminate in precise differential diagnoses that directly dictate highly focused management strategies that can be implemented by the child's parents and teachers, with the help of the pediatrician or consulting behavior analyst. Based on the findings of the functional analysis, the family, pediatrician, and (when applicable) the consulting behavior analyst select interventions designed to *match* (i.e., directly address) the variables demonstrated to be the ongoing basis of the challenging behaviors.

Treatment Planning and Intervention. Throughout the initial assessment process, the pediatrician consults with the child and family to discuss whether intervention is indicated and, if so, what its focus and goals could be. Every effort is made to integrate the child's and family's perspectives and preferences into the planning of the behavior management protocol. Either directly or via the services of selected experts, the pediatrician provides the child and family with whatever education, training, and consultation is needed to make informed decisions in regard to the goals and priorities of the treatment plan. (See also Chapter 76 regarding pediatric counseling.)

Factors typically considered when prioritizing among several target behaviors are (1) the availability of effective treatments, (2) the relative severity of each presenting problem, (3) the amount of effort and skill required of the child and adult care providers to implement the recommended intervention protocols, and (4) the preferences of the child and care providers regarding the initial focus of treatment. Behaviors manageable solely through positive reinforcement strategies and other positive behavioral supports, or dangerous or destructive behaviors that place the child or others at imminent risk, are frequently selected first.

Once the child and family identify their treatment goals and priorities, the pediatrician develops or oversees the development of individually tailored intervention plans that emphasize specific action steps framed as "do's" and "don'ts." Emphasis is given to assisting the child to acquire and demonstrate prosocial behaviors that serve a function equivalent to that of the problem behaviors. For example, a child with a history of fighting as a means of avoiding an aversive work assignment may be taught how to ask for help with difficult tasks. If the prosocial behavior becomes a more effective means of obtaining positive or negative reinforcement than the problem behavior, then the child will select the prosocial options more and more frequently.

The pediatrician provides the child and family with systematic instruction regarding how to implement the recommended interventions. The interventions frequently involve *direct learning trials* with the child, *parent education and training*, and *teacher and staff consultation*. Focused treatments are aimed at the child's and family's strengths as well as skill deficits, more so than at the child's diagnosis per se. During parent education and teacher consultation sessions, the pediatrician recommends *problem-specific, procedure-driven protocols* designed to enable these pivotal care providers to effect recommended interventions in home, school, and community settings. The interested reader is referred to Christophersen (1994) for several examples of effective, feasible, replicable, and cost-beneficial protocols that summarize the most important "do's" and "don'ts."

The pediatrician usually begins by describing the procedures to be implemented, along with a rationale for their use. Predicted effects and possible side effects are discussed. Typical challenges and pitfalls are anticipated. Training is provided in regard to specific child behavior management skills (i.e., competencies). *Competency-based training* is optimal when it is systematic and data-driven. Such training usually consists of the following steps: (1) identification and prioritization of target skills; (2) analysis of each skill into specific steps to be taught; (3) determination of each learner's level of proficiency prior to training (i.e., establishing a baseline); and (4) provision of systematic training through verbal description, modeling, and supervised practice. Evaluation of the learner's skill acquisition continues, with remedial instruction offered as indicated.

The child and parents are often asked to complete homework assignments designed to encourage their implementation and practice of recommended interventions. When feasible, parents, teachers, and even the child receive consultation in regard to how to observe and record the child's target behaviors, so as to monitor the quality and impact of the interventions put into effect. As necessary, intervention protocols are revised to maximize gains in treatment. Parent education and training sessions continue until the following criteria are met: (1) the caregivers demonstrate on a routine basis the competent administration of the recommended interventions and (2) the child's behavior exhibits stable and sufficient improvement. Progress is often facilitated by enabling the caregivers to engage in parallel reading of "how to" books and articles on child behavior management (Baker et al, 1976; Blechman, 1985; Christophersen, 1988; Garber, Garber, and Spizman, 1987), or by referring interested parents to selected lectures or workshops on effective parenting.

Promoting Generalization of Desired Behavioral Changes. A child's behavior is typically situation-specific, that is, it changes somewhat from one situation to the next. If a behavior is consistently reinforced either positively or negatively in a particular situation, it is likely to increase in frequency especially in that situation. Through a process termed *stimulus generalization*, it also may increase in highly similar situations. Generalization occurs across behaviors as well as across situations. Changing one behavior usually causes changes in other related behaviors via a process called *response generalization*. For instance, provision of high rates of positive reinforcement, whether provided contingently or not in the context of a child's compliance with adult requests, may also result in substantial reductions in challenging behaviors, such as aggression, disruption, and property destruction.

When the focus of intervention is highly specific to particular target behaviors and settings, the effects may not endure or generalize to new behaviors and situations. Skillful behavior managers employ a variety of tactics to ensure that desired outcomes persist and spread across multiple behaviors and settings (Stokes and Baer, 1977).

1. One tactic involves the sequential introduction of the effective intervention to each behavior and setting where change is targeted to occur. For example, an intervention focused on teaching the child of preschool age to share with other children may require use of positive reinforcement in the context of the child's cooperative play with several peers across in-home, daycare, and other community settings.

2. Another tactic is to set "behavior traps" through which the targeted appropriate behavior is brought under the control of everyday events and consequences. For instance, initially it may be necessary for the adult care provider to praise the child each time the child shares. However, as the child learns how to initiate sharing more and more frequently, the child's peers are likely to become more cooperative and will share more and more themselves. Such cooperation and reciprocal sharing may be enough to sustain (i.e., "trap") the child's sharing behavior in the absence of continued praise by the adult.

3. A third tactic is to provide the child several opportunities to observe and practice recently acquired skills across slightly modified situations. For example, if the child is learning how to ask appropriate questions, the child is given an opportunity to ask questions with many different people in different contexts. This continues until the child can routinely ask appropriate questions without assistance or structured reinforcement.

4. Generalization may also be enhanced by training "loosely"; that is, by purposefully teaching a behavior through designed imprecision in poorly controlled settings. For instance, the child who is learning to ask appropriate questions is encouraged to interact in

varying contexts (e.g., home, school, neighborhood) with people who vary along multiple dimensions (e.g., age, sex, status) and who randomly answer the posed question squarely, respond to the question obliquely, alter the question and then respond, ask for clarification, or ignore the question altogether. In this way, the child's question-asking skills are more likely to generalize across people and settings.

5. When assisting a child to learn a new skill, it is important that the contingencies in effect (i.e., the relationships between what the child does and what happens as a result) are clear and applied consistently. When the goal is to sustain and generalize an already acquired skill, use of relatively unclear and inconsistent contingencies is often recommended. Contingencies are arranged so that the child cannot easily determine whether they are in effect. As a result, the child is more likely to behave appropriately across situations to maximize positive reinforcement while minimizing punishment. For example, mother may aim to manage three of the child's challenging behaviors (e.g., disorganizing a room, shouting, and fighting) by periodically putting contingencies in effect for only one of these behaviors, and by noting its occurrence throughout the day. The child is not informed which behavior "counts." By the end of the day, if the rate of the occurrence of the targeted behavior is below a preset criterion frequency, the child earns a privilege.

6. To enhance continuance and transfer of appropriate behavior, it is often advisable to use the same materials under the same conditions during the training of the behavior as the child will use and encounter in everyday contexts. For instance, when teaching a child how to self-inject medication via a needle, it is best to use during training the same equipment, supplies, and procedures as the child is likely to use everyday thereafter once training is completed.

7. Teaching the child to direct and manage his or her own behavior is another proven method of promoting generalization. This often requires teaching the child choice-making and problem-solving skills. Concurrent with learning how to make sound decisions and to resolve problems, the child can learn how to establish performance criteria for self-evaluation and self-reinforcement, and how to obtain the privilege or other positive reinforcers earned. Many children can learn how to complete assigned home chores using posted reminders and other self-instructions and self-reinforcement.

The aforementioned methods of generalization can be employed in isolation or combination. They are not mutually exclusive.

Fading the Interventions. When intervention goals are achieved, structured contingencies are usually removed gradually (i.e., are faded). Gradual reductions in structure and consistency increase the likelihood that desired changes will persist. Sudden withdrawal of systematic antecedents and consequences may result in a setback. Gradual withdrawal of positive reinforcement can be orchestrated by altering the amount and timing of reinforcement. For example, the child may earn a point or token for completion of homework every third day, rather than every day. Gradual withdrawal of systematic positive reinforcement prepares the child for everyday situations in which behavioral consequences are not systematic, may be delayed, or may not be available at all. In fact, maintenance of acquired skills and appropriate behavior is furthered if consequences are progressively delayed, and are provided more and more intermittently.

Follow-Up Assessment and Aftercare. Skill-specific and problem-specific interventions that are applied competently over time frequently lead to significant improvements in the child's behavior. However, sustained follow-up assessment and care are often warranted, given that the child's learned behavior and the environments influencing it continuously change. Revisions to previously recommended assessment and intervention protocols are frequently indicated. The effectiveness of earlier interventions may diminish over time or new behaviors of concern may emerge. A common misperception about behavior management is that a permanent "cure" or "fix" can be attained if the optimal assessment and intervention protocols are implemented. It is often true that treatment goals can be achieved. However, once a behavior is in a child's repertoire, it can seldom be eliminated altogether. At most, the behavior can be managed with competently revised protocols under the specific conditions that precipitate its recurrence. The astute pediatrician will, therefore, routinely develop and implement a plan for continuing care. Periodic assessments and "booster" sessions with the child and family are frequently conducted. Between such sessions, the pediatrician remains accessible to the child and family to "trouble shoot" as needed.

When to Refer. It may be advisable to refer the child and family to a child behavior specialist if and when one or more of the following conditions is evident: (1) The child's behavioral concerns are multiple in number, of long-standing duration, of moderate to high levels of severity, and complicated by family-systems issues such as parental separation or divorce or parental psychopathology. (2) The pediatrician is not familiar with or does not possess problem-specific and procedure-specific protocols pertinent to the principal concerns. (3) The pediatrician does not have sufficient time in the context of a busy practice to provide the needed counseling and consultation. (4) Competent child behavioral specialists who will collaborate with the pediatrician effectively are accessible and affordable.

Continuing Education. The pediatrician interested in learning more about the assessment and management of child behavior may be well advised to attend local grand rounds, institutes, and workshops that center on advances in current best practices in developmental-behavioral pediatrics, applied behavior analysis, or child behavior therapy. Some academic medical centers sponsor collaborative office rounds to provide pediatricians in community practice an opportunity to present and discuss difficult cases with experts in developmental-behavioral pediatrics and child psychiatry. Several introductory textbooks are readily available on special order, including those by Martin and Pear (1996), Miller (1980), and Miltenberger (1997). The principal professional society for applied behavior analysts is the Association for Behavior Analysis (tele: (616)387-8341), headquartered at 213 West Hall, Western Michigan University, Kalamazoo, Michigan 49008-5052. This association maintains a membership directory and may be able to assist with the location of qualified behavior analysts in local practice.

Conclusion

Skillful child behavior management requires an understanding of environmental as well as biological processes. Processes such as positive reinforcement, extinction, negative reinforcement, punishment, stimulus control, setting events, and establishing operations are key determinants of the child's behavioral repertoire. Based on a rigorous assessment of the child's behavior and its antecedents and consequences, selected intervention procedures can be adapted to address the specific needs of each child, including but not limited to differential reinforcement, instructional and imitation training, compliance training, building behavioral momentum, shaping, prompting, punishment by contingent withdrawal (e.g., exclusionary time out, response cost, contingent observation), and overcorrection. The basic elements of an effective child behavior management program include differential diagnosis, treatment planning, intervention, programming for generalization, fading intervention, and follow-up assessment and care.

In the context of office visits for well-child health supervision or for management of minor acute illness, the pediatrician has an opportunity to examine for and detect early indicators of behavioral concerns. Often competent anticipatory guidance or problem-centered counseling in regard to these concerns can prevent their further exacerbation. Such guidance and counseling is more likely to be effective if the pediatrician conducts a focused behavioral assessment of the chief complaints and systematically implements individually tailored interventions based on the key assessment findings. When presenting behavioral concerns are multiple in number, of moderate to high severity, or of long duration, the busy pediatrician may be well-advised to refer the child and family to a behavior specialist.

REFERENCES

Baker B, Brightman A, Heifetz L et al: Behavior Problems. Champaign, IL, Research Press, 1976.
Blechman E: Solving Child Behavior Problems at Home and School. Champaign, IL, Research Press, 1985.
Carr E: Functional equivalence as a mechanism of response generalization. In Horner R, Koegel R, Dunlap G (eds): Generalization and Maintenance: Life-Style Changes in Applied Settings. Baltimore, Paul H. Brookes Publishing Co, 1988.
Catania A: Learning, 2nd ed. Englewood Cliffs, NJ, Prentice-Hall, 1984.
Christophersen E: Pediatric Compliance: A Guide for the Primary Care Physician. New York, Plenum Press, 1994.
Christophersen E: Little People: Guidelines for Common Sense Child Rearing, 3rd ed. Kansas City, Westport Publishers, 1988.
Forehand R, Long N: Parenting the Strong-Willed Child. Chicago, Contemporary Books, 1996.
Forehand R, McMahon R: Helping the Noncompliant Child: A Clinician's Guide to Parent Training. New York, Guilford Press, 1981.
Foxx R: Decreasing Behaviors of Severely Retarded and Autistic Persons. Champaign, IL, Research Press, 1982a.

Foxx R: Increasing Behaviors of Severely Retarded and Autistic Persons. Champaign, IL, Research Press, 1982b.

Garber S, Garber M, Spizman R: Good Behavior. New York, Villard Books, 1987.

Iwata B: Negative reinforcement in applied behavior analysis: An emerging technology. J Appl Behav Anal 20:361, 1987.

Kazdin A: Behavior Modification in Applied Settings, 2nd ed. Homewood, IL, The Dorsey Press, 1989.

Kazdin A: The Token Economy. New York, Plenum Press, 1977.

Kelley, M: School-Home Notes: Promoting Children's Classroom Success. New York, The Guilford Press, 1990.

Koegel L, Koegel R, Dunlap G: Positive Behavioral Support: Including People with Difficult Behavior in the Community. Baltimore, Paul H. Brookes Publishing Co, 1996.

Lerman D, Iwata B: Developing a technology for the use of operant extinction in clinical settings: An examination of basic and applied research. J Appl Behav Anal 29:345, 1996.

Mace C, Lalli J, Shea M et al: The momentum of human behavior in a natural setting. J Appl Behav Anal 24:163, 1990.

Martin G, Pear J: Behavior Modification: What It Is and How to Do It, 5th ed. Upper Saddle River, NJ, Prentice Hall, 1996.

Matson J, DiLorenzo T: Punishment and Its Alternatives: A New Perspective for Behavior Modification. New York, Springer Publishing Co, 1984.

Miller L: Principles of Everyday Behavior Analysis, 2nd ed. Monterey, CA, Brooks/Cole Publishing Co, 1980.

Miltenberger R: Behavior Modification: Principles and Procedures. New York, Brookes/Cole Publishing, 1997.

Parrish J, Cataldo M, Kolko D, et al: Experimental analysis of response covariation among compliant and inappropriate behaviors. J Appl Behav Anal 19:241, 1986.

Patterson G: Coercive Family Process. Eugene, OR, Castalia Press, 1982.

Patterson G, Reid J, Dishion T: Antisocial Boys. Eugene, OR, Castalia Press, 1992.

Reynolds C, Kamphaus R: Handbook of Psychological and Educational Assessment of Children: Personality, Behavior, and Context. New York, The Guilford Press, 1990.

Smith R, Iwata B: Antecedent influences on behavior disorders. J Appl Behav Anal 30:343, 1997.

Stancin T, Palermo T: A Review of Behavioral Screening Practices in Pediatric Settings: Do They Pass the Test? J Dev Behav Ped 18(3):183, 1997.

Stokes T, Baer D: An implicit technology of generalization. J Appl Behav Anal 10:349, 1977.

Van Houten R, Axelrod S (eds): Behavior Analysis and Treatment. New York, Plenum Press, 1993.

Van Houten R, Axelrod S, Bailey J, Favell J, Foxx R, Iwata B, Lovaas I: The right to effective behavioral treatment. J Appl Behav Anal 21:381, 1988.

79 Special Education Services for Children With Disabilities

Susan E. Craig

 Current best practices in special education offer a host of services that build the capacity of natural environments to serve all children. These include consultation to classroom staff, collaborative planning, coteaching, supervision of paraprofessional personnel, cross-training, and modeling.

Parents sometimes question the results of school-based assessments. They may feel that the school is founding its conclusions more on the availability of services than on a commitment to their child's well-being. In these cases, parents or the school may request an outside evaluation, paid for with school district funds.

From its inception, special education has been intricately connected to the medical profession. Traditionally, physicians, not educators, have diagnosed the disabilities that made children eligible for special education services. Although their role is more clearly defined in the case of children in established risk categories, such as Down syndrome or cerebral palsy, physicians are also called on to determine the presence of more subtle anomalies, such as attention-deficit disorder. Families often ask physicians for advice about the best placement for their child with learning disabilities or sensory integration problems. The close relationship between medical and educational needs in young children suggests that physicians and special education practitioners work together in planning and implementing required interventions.

Therefore it is critical for physicians to have a thorough understanding of the laws that govern the provision of special education services, as well as an appreciation of their goals. Shared assumptions about the nature of disability, as well as appropriate responses to it, are the basis for coordinated services to children with disabilities and their families.

EXAMPLE

Our school district holds quarterly round-table discussions about children who have various types of disabilities. All of the pediatricians in town are invited, as well as the child's family, teachers, therapists, and anyone else the family or school wants to invite. It is something like grand rounds. Together we tease out where educational support is necessary as opposed to situations that are strictly medical. As a physician, I find that these sessions have given me a better understanding of what special education is all about. The teachers tell me they get a lot out of the clinical information I can give them. Families are just glad to have us all in one room, because it cuts down on mixed messages and conflicting information.

Traditionally disability has been defined within the narrow parameters of the normal curve. Children whose performance on tests of developmental milestones was one to two standard deviations below average were considered "delayed." Time and repetition were considered keys to helping these children catch up. Children with even greater deviation from the norm (low-incidence disabilities) were considered uneducable, and thus best cared for within institutions.

Greater understanding of the brain and learning theories that acknowledge human diversity have changed the paradigm of disability to reflect a greater complexity. No longer considered a unidimensional characteristic, disability is now recognized as handicapping only to the degree that the child's ecological systems fail to compensate for or accommodate to it. The "cure" model has been replaced with the accommodation model.

As a result, society's response to persons with disabilities has changed radically. These changes are evident in the federal legislation that establishes eligibility for special education, in best practices that emphasize inclusion and family-centered services, and in efficacy studies that define child outcomes in terms of accommodation and participation rather than remediation.

It is important that physicians understand these changes and how they affect their responsibilities to children with disabilities, the families of these children, and professionals who support them (Fig. 79–1).

EXAMPLE

It really annoys me when professionals refer to children with Down syndrome as if they were all alike. The children I've taught with Down syndrome have all been very different. Patsy could read and did quite well on paper-and-pencil tasks, whereas Patrick is a more concrete learner. He understands concepts better when I present them through hands-on activities and real-life experiences. And Nathan, well, he's pretty busy — needs to be moving around all the time. His daily schedule has to include lots of school jobs and social interaction. That's why reports that state "child has Down syndrome, there-

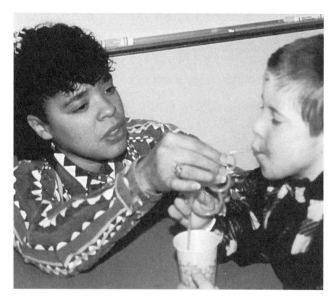

Figure 79–1. Functional accommodations make daily routines accessible to all children.

fore needs special education" do me no good. It's like saying "child is overweight, therefore needs physical exercise." What I need as an educator are realistic expectations and viable accommodations.

Federal Legislation

Five federal laws drive special education and other support services for children with disabilities and high-risk populations. The Individuals with Disabilities Education Act (IDEA), Americans with Disabilities Act (ADA), and Section 504 of the Rehabilitation Act of 1973 establish the right of children with disabilities to a free appropriate public school education, and access to other natural childhood settings. Federally funded Head Start and Title 1 provide compensatory programs for young children whose home environment increases their risk for academic failure.

INDIVIDUALS WITH DISABILITIES EDUCATION ACT

The IDEA reasserts the educational rights of children with disabilities originally established by Public Law 94-142 in 1975.

Reauthorized in 1997 as PL 105-17, this legislation requires each community to provide a free appropriate educational program for students with disabilities with age-appropriate peers in the "least restrictive environment." No student can be denied access to an education, preferably within a natural setting. While the definition of "least restrictive environment" varies by child, the IDEA clearly establishes the right of all children to be educated among peers, in the public schools.

Part B and Part C of the IDEA set policy for services to young children with disabilities and their families. Part B mandates services for children 3 to 21 years of age. Part C provides discretionary funding to the states to serve

infants and toddlers from birth to 3 years. The IDEA stresses the need for interagency collaboration and decentralized family-centered services. It also reflects a shift in both our understanding of disability and the appropriate response to it.

The ADA (1990) and Section 504 of the Rehabilitation Act of 1973 protect the educational rights of children with disabilities as well, but go a step further as they also protect the civil right to necessary accommodations in natural settings.

AMERICANS WITH DISABILITIES

The ADA secures the rights of children with disabilities in public *and* private settings. This is particularly important in providing services to children under the age of 5 years, since programs for these children are often privately funded. Refusing to admit children with disabilities is prohibited unless "undue burden" or "direct threat" can be demonstrated. This has affected both public and private child care and preschool settings.

SECTION 504 OF THE REHABILITATION ACT OF 1973

In recent years, advocates for the rights of children with disabilities have challenged the traditional service delivery models used in special education, calling them segregating and restrictive. Some have gone so far as to challenge their legality, citing the Supreme Court's decision in *Brown vs. The Board of Education* (1954), which prohibited "separate but equal" education programs for students grouped by race. As a result, schools are now required to appoint 504 officers who are responsible for protecting the civil rights of children who require educational accommodations and other special education services.

HEAD START AND TITLE 1

Both Head Start and Title 1 were established in 1965 as part of the "Great Society." Head Start's overall goal is the development of social competence in preschool-aged children from low-income families. Ninety-five percent of the children attending Head Start programs are from families with income below the federal poverty line. Comprehensive services including health, education, parent involvement, and social services are provided in an effort to prepare children for successful participation in public school kindergarten and first grade. Current Head Start regulations support the inclusion of children with disabilities and coordination of services with other early childhood and elementary school programs (US Department of Health and Human Services, 1993). Many communities have access to "Early Start" funding for children from birth to 3 years of age. These programs are also expected to serve families below the federal poverty line. Guidelines require acceptance of infants and toddlers with disabilities.

Title 1 funds have traditionally provided remedial services to children from low-income families. The law's reauthorization in 1995 encourages the use of Title 1 funds to provide additional classroom support for all children.

However, schools tend to limit this support to children not identified as having a disability.

Shifts in the Definition of Disability

Policies toward educating children with disabilities have shifted the focus of intervention from individual to environmental deficits. Since physicians are often the first to diagnose a child's disability, they must understand these changes and be able to prepare families for the kinds of support they can expect from public funds and what financial responsibility the family will retain.

Physicians are responsible for helping families appreciate the ecological nature of disability and the role special education plays in building the capacity of schools to educate children who have them. This requires a thorough understanding of the nature of disability in children and developmentally appropriate responses to it (Fig. 79–2).

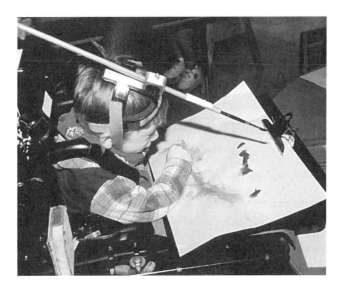

Figure 79–3. Accommodations that increase access to classroom events are the goal of special education services.

TRADITIONAL ASSUMPTIONS

Drawing on stage theories of child development, traditional disability models assumed that all children pass through a set of developmental milestones in a similar manner at similar times. Children with disabilities were referred to as "delayed" and the goal of special education was to help them "catch up," the assumption being that with enough remedial work, their performance could approximate the standardized expectations of the normal curve. Within this paradigm, intervention focused on curing or fixing the individual. Mainstreaming, or a return to natural settings, occurred in direct proportion to the child's ability to align his or her development with that of "typical" peers, that is, to be "normal" (Fig. 79–3).

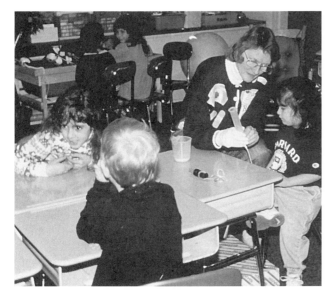

Figure 79–2. G-tube feedings can be easily attended to within the natural routines of school.

EXAMPLE

One of the most shocking experiences of my professional life occurred at a team meeting about a little 7-year-old boy named Kevin. In addition to being severely retarded and having multiple disabilities, Kevin had had a stroke, resulting in partial paralysis on his left side.

Kevin's school district was happy to place him in first grade, making the necessary accommodations to have him participate with children throughout the day. The problem was his physical therapist: she insisted that he be pulled out of the classroom for therapy, because (and this is a direct quote) "It's still possible that he might walk independently with enough treatment."

To me it was immoral. Why not help him participate in life as fully as possible, rather than fueling the false hope of a perfect child?

CURRENT THINKING

Ecological models of child development present a multidimensional understanding of the interplay between characteristics of the child's internal and external systems that influence growth and potential (Bronfenbrenner, 1979). Within this context, the impact of disability is contingent on the capacity of micro- and macro-level environments to create access and opportunities for successful participation. Emphasis is on system change. The definition of intervention extends to environments as well as individuals. Inclusion, or participation in natural settings, is considered a child's birth right. Adults responsible for the child's care and education are charged with making it happen.

For physicians this means working with families to understand the role of therapy and special education in helping their children participate as much as possible in age-appropriate activities and routines. To do so effectively, physicians must actively contribute to the interagency collaboration called for by Part C of the IDEA. Working with other community professionals, they can help families gain access to local school and child care programs, while at the same time helping staff accommodate the special needs of children with disabilities.

ELIGIBILITY

Traditionally children were referred to special education through a process that was initiated by parents or professionals concerned about a lack of developmental or educational progress. These children often had developmental disabilities that placed them at risk for educational failure. Others were suspected of having a specific learning disability because of prolonged difficulty in learning to read.

With the introduction of early intervention services (ages birth to 3 years), the scope of special education broadened to include children who were at risk for delayed development or academic failure due to social or environmental factors. These children qualified for services as a way of preventing future failure, not because they had a disability known to have an effect on learning.

This interpretation of risk provided special education programming to populations of children formerly served by compensatory programs such as Head Start. It also challenged the medical and educational communities to be proactive on issues related to the certain preventable causes of developmental delays in children, such as poverty and poor prenatal care.

Research conducted in the 1980s stressed the impact that accommodating environments could have on the physical, social, and cognitive development of at-risk infants and toddlers (IHDP, 1990). Environmental factors such as poverty, violence, and drug-addicted parents are now included in the list of possible causes of childhood developmental disability.

As a result, school districts began the arduous task of modifying classroom environments to accommodate an increasingly heterogeneous group of students (NASBE, 1992; Putnam, Spiegal, and Bruininks, 1995). Evidence of "prereferral" planning became a requirement prior to special education services. Only when these environmental changes failed to improve student participation could clinical assessments be introduced.

This change in the referral process reflects a shift in the assumptions that inform special education service delivery. Disabilities are no longer defined as strictly physical or mental anomalies. Environmental factors also play a role. Intervention needs to include not only changes in children, but also changes in the environments around them. Accommodations that foster participation and functional independence have replaced standardization of performance as special education's criterion for success.

EXAMPLE

Jorge was referred to the public school kindergarten from Early Intervention. At 5 years old he was nonverbal and still unable to walk by himself. Having recently been weaned from g-tube feedings, he continued to need assistance in all areas of self-care. He was not yet toilet trained.

Special education staff worked with the kindergarten teacher and teaching assistant to make classroom accom-

modations that would allow Jorge to participate. These included special seating, frequent opportunities for weight bearing and range of motion exercises, and picture boards for communication. By the end of kindergarten, Jorge was walking around the building, supported only by an adult's finger. He had learned to anticipate familiar routines and seemed genuinely glad to see familiar playmates.

When Jorge started third grade, he was using sounds to indicate preferences and respond to his name. He was toilet trained, independently mobile, and able to feed himself. Participation in accommodating school environments was helping him become functionally independent.

Physicians need to understand that recognition of the role environment plays in determining the impact of a disabling condition results in service delivery models that are less intrusive, less clinical, and more indirect than those traditionally associated with special education. Programs that integrate accommodations and support into classroom curriculum have replaced substantially separate classrooms and "pull-out therapies" as indicators of quality. Families may need the support of the family physician in understanding the benefits of an integrated approach, especially if the false hope of "cure" has been held up to them as the goal of therapy or special education.

Special Education: A Process, Not a Place

Despite legislative mandates to the contrary, special education has traditionally emphasized evaluation and placement, rather than an agreed-upon plan for helping children participate to the greatest extent possible in the natural routines of their families and age groups. Placement discussions typically substituted for the more difficult task of accommodating natural settings.

EXAMPLE

When I started working in special education, it was like a placement service. The evaluation indicated a learning disability: put the student in a resource room. Evidence of mental retardation? Must need the Life Skills self-contained program.

No one ever asked how those placements would benefit the student or whether accommodations to the regular classroom were more appropriate. The conversation went from diagnosis to placement. It was like a life sentence. The greater the disability, the more restrictive the placement. The message was really "come back when you're cured."

This was due in part to a continued allegiance to the medical model, as well as persistent myths about service delivery that defy efficacy research as well as developmental theory (Bruder, 1997). These myths include a belief that more is better, that all children benefit from a standard number of treatments per week, and that contact with specialized staff is of more benefit to a child with disabilities than participation in her family, school, and community.

MORE IS BETTER

Within traditional definitions of disability, it is often difficult to determine how much therapy or special education support is enough, since the goal of "normalcy" or success on standardized measures of achievement is seldom achieved. As a result, children are seldom discharged, and direct services such as occupational therapy are recommended well past the time that they are developmentally appropriate. Rather than building the capacity of students to participate in natural routines, this type of service delivery promotes the learned helplessness and dependence often observed in special education "lifers" (Grimes, 1981). Families can be caught in the denial fueled by this type of service delivery, limiting their ability to plan for their children's social integration and functional independence.

Physicians can help families work with school personnel to set realistic goals for their children with disabilities. This includes an understanding of the limits of direct intervention, as well as an appreciation of developmentally appropriate alternatives. Physicians can also help children understand their own profiles of strengths and liabilities, so that they can be actively involved in identifying beneficial accommodations.

EXAMPLE

Special education used to be like the "white elephant in the living room." No one ever talked to children about their own disabilities. We just tip-toed around them, pretending they weren't there: "You're no different than the other kids in your room; so what if you're pulled for Occupational Therapy, Speech, Resource Room?" We thought we could cure them before they noticed! How foolish!

2x30 PARADIGM

The purpose of special education has always been to augment regular education so that all children could receive an appropriate education. The intent was never to supplant regular education or to provide fully for the medical treatment of children with disabilities. However, in the absence of a clearly defined model of school-based services to children with disabilities, the link between regular and special education got lost. This is particularly apparent in how therapies are provided.

Occupational therapists, physical therapists, speech pathologists, and other related service providers working in public schools often have little or no training in how their expertise relates to the educational process. Many receive their preparation in programs affiliated with hospitals or medical schools. Their course of study is clinically driven, with emphasis on identification of deficits in normal functioning.

As a result, they often replicate the clinical model in schools. Children are "pulled out" for treatment following a standardized model of two 30-minute treatments (2x30 paradigm) of recommended services per week. The purpose

of therapy is seldom discussed. Rather, parents, teachers, and therapists assume that if a child has a certain type of disability or exhibits certain deficits, therapy will help.

This decision-making process violates the criteria of the IDEA legislation, which establishes school-based therapy as an integral part of the educational process, not an ancillary medical one. All therapeutic interventions in schools must somehow relate to children's successful participation in educational activities and routines.

In this educationally driven model, the classroom and school activities provide the criteria to determine what interventions are needed. Therapists, working with parents and classroom staff, identify needed and appropriate skills that the child can learn in the educational environment, as well as requisite accommodations. They then work with other staff to implement necessary interventions.

Physicians may need to help families understand the difference between educational and medical needs for therapy. Therapies that respond to educational needs are the responsibility of the school system. Therapies that respond to clinically determined medical needs are the responsibility of the family.

SPECIALISTS KNOW BEST

Traditionally, special education has favored direct intervention with children, usually in a small group or individualized setting. Recently the appropriateness of this type of service delivery has been questioned in terms of both its efficacy (Karnish, Bruder, and Rainforth, 1995) and its insensitivity to varying cultural expectations of the adult-child relationship (Weston et al, 1997).

In terms of efficacy, direct service models limit intervention to times when the therapist or special educator is available. Little or no energy is put into building the capacity of the environment to serve the child in their absence. Efficacy is also compromised by the fact that the benefits of direct service are seldom generalized into natural settings.

Cultural issues arise when the structure of the intervention contradicts cultural norms. For example, asking children from Southeast Asian cultures to make eye contact or children from Hispanic cultures to initiate turn-taking sequences with adults violates expectations of the adult-child relationship in these cultures. They are, however, frequently listed as target objectives on individualized education plans (IEPs) for children from diverse ethnic backgrounds.

Current best practices in special education complement the direct service model with a host of indirect services that minimize the need for generalization, while at the same time building the capacity of natural environments to serve all children. These include (1) consultation to classroom staff; (2) collaborative planning; (3) coteaching; (4) supervision of paraprofessional personnel; (5) cross-training; and (6) modeling.

Team teaching rather than whole-group instruction characterizes inclusive classrooms. Teams include a special education teacher and one or more therapists as well as the classroom teacher. Some teams also include paraprofessional staff. Working together, teams help children with disabilities gain access to classroom activities and participate in them as fully as possible. In some classrooms, this means a therapist and a teacher coteaching a lesson using alternative methods. In others, it means taking a child through range-of-motion exercises on a mat as the class listens to a story; or showing a child how to use an augmentative communication system to take part in a classroom discussion. Target objectives are addressed throughout the day but within a classroom that offers opportunities for incidental learning and peer interaction, which are unavailable in a more segregated approach.

This type of integrated service delivery provides children with more consistent daily routines while at the same time providing sufficient variation in service delivery to accommodate cultural differences. It is a disservice to both families and children when their integration is judged to represent an effort by special education to control costs or resolve staffing problems.

EXAMPLE

Whenever I think about inclusion, I remember working with a 1st-grade teacher who was determined to teach one of the children in her classroom how to read. Lawrence has Down syndrome and uses sign language to communicate. So that's the language she used to teach him to read. When the other children used their voices, Lawrence used his fingers; and by the end of the 1st grade he had read all three preprimers. That's what inclusion is all about.

It is important for physicians to understand special education's need for flexibility in programming for individual children. Hospital recommendations for specified units of treatment or placements in segregated settings, although not legally binding, restrict the school's ability to tailor services to the child's age and cultural background. Recommendations for specific accommodations or target objectives are much more useful and more in keeping with the federal policies that govern special education service delivery.

TEAM-BASED INTERVENTION

Special education service delivery has always involved a team process. Since 1975, legislation has mandated that teams of parents and professionals meet to develop IEPs and monitor their implementation.

Traditionally, these teams had a multidisciplinary structure, often meeting in hospital- or center-based programs. Professionals from various disciplines evaluated the child's performance across developmental domains. Discipline-bound goals and objectives were developed with little or no effort made to integrate them into a larger context.

As special education services moved into public schools, an interdisciplinary team structure replaced the multidisciplinary one. While continuing to emphasize discipline-specific goals and objectives, this team structure recognized the need to integrate services into the public school context. Team members continued to function from individual disciplines, but some effort was made to interpret clinical findings according to educational impact.

By 1986, two separate policy shifts toward children with disabilities resulted in further changes in the special education team structure. The first was the downward ex-

tension of services to infants and toddlers with disabilities. The 1986 Amendments to the IDEA moved away from the deficit interpretation of disability, focusing instead on the systemic nature of its impact. Early intervention was defined as a system of support for families as they adjusted to the special needs of their child with disabilities. Individualized Family Service Plans (IFSPs) centered on building family resources, rather than "curing" the child's deficits. Phrases like *consensual decision making* and *role release* found their way into the literature, as professionals struggled to integrate their skills into informal family and child care settings.

At the same time, the inclusion movement took hold in public schools. A Carnegie Report published in 1980 challenged the way society dealt with people with disabilities (Gliedman and Roth, 1980). The home school movement questioned the placement of children with disabilities in segregated schools away from their communities (Brown et al, 1989). School reform replaced child study teams with teacher assistance teams, moving away from an emphasis on student deficits to a greater appreciation for variations in learning styles and intelligences (Will, 1986).

For special educators, these events were a wake-up call. Service delivery systems that isolated children with disabilities and did nothing to make classroom environments accessible to them were questioned at both the moral and professional level (Stainback and Stainback, 1992). In much the same way as early intervention professionals tried to build systems of support around infants and toddlers with disabilities and their families, school-based special educators embarked on the arduous task of building the capacity of regular classrooms to accommodate the educational needs of all children.

Early intervention's emphasis on family-focused or family-centered services also affected special education service delivery. The legitimacy of a family's definition of the disability, as well as variations in their understanding of intervention, was established.

As a result, transdisciplinary teams, characterized by shared priorities and integrated service delivery, replaced more discipline-bound models. These teams have a different purpose and involve more complicated decision making and implementation planning than more traditional models. The intent of these teams is to arrive at a shared set of student goals that can be achieved through the combined resources of all team members.

EXAMPLE

Marta was a beautiful little girl whose mother was from the United States and whose father was Lebanese. She was born in Beirut, during a period of frequent bombings. At 3 months of age, while taking refuge in a bomb shelter, she spiked a fever. According to her mother, she was never the same afterwards.

When she entered the public schools in the United States, she was 7 years old, with multiple disabilities and severe retardation. Her mother and father, though not living together, had joint custody. Marta was placed in a regular 2nd grade with special education support and a full-time teaching assistant.

Marta's mother was very satisfied with this placement. Her father on the other hand was appalled. In his

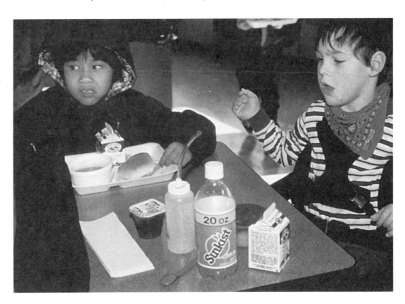

Figure 79–4. Addressing functional skills in natural settings reduces the need for generalization and encourages independence.

country, children like Marta were cared for at home, away from the curiosity of other children. He felt it was irresponsible to leave her in this placement and kept her with him whenever possible. What looked like neglect from our point of view was concern from his. It took many meetings over many months to find an intervention plan that satisfied both parents.

Reaching agreement is a difficult process that requires team members to release their own bias and preferred ways of doing things to achieve a common goal: student success on an agreed-upon priority. It requires members to blur professional boundaries to develop interventions and strategies. Each participant seeks to promote the child's functional independence and participation in age appropriate activities and routines.

Transdisciplinary teams require greater diagnostic skill than other team models. Members are required to discern differential etiologies in symptoms that appear similar. They must also be able to train one another to extend accommodations and address target objectives in natural environments throughout the day. In so doing they encourage a developmentally appropriate approach to children by limiting the number of adults they are required to interact with and maintaining the continuity of daily routines.

In many ways, this transdisciplinary approach resembles the rehabilitation model of adult services. Emphasis on mastery of developmental milestones is replaced with the priority of accommodating environments to facilitate participation in natural settings. Emphasis on discipline-bound splinter skills is replaced with quality-of-life issues such as friendship, social competency, and functional independence. Emphasis on clinical precision is replaced with systemic change: building the capacity of natural environments to respond to the needs of children with disabilities (Fig. 79–4).

Natural Assessment

CLINICAL ASSESSMENT

Clinical assessments continue to play a role in determining a child's eligibility for special education services, as well as in developing implementation plans. Current special education practice, however, encourages an analysis of both quantitative and qualitative aspects of the child's clinical performance in determining program recommendations. This reflects current interest in the metacognitive processes of children with disabilities, as well as a recognition of the systemic nature of children's performance.

Clinical assessments traditionally use discipline-bound measures of the child's cognitive, language, affective, and motor development. Results of these independent evaluations are used to establish eligibility for special education services. For children suspected of having a learning disability, they serve as the basis for establishing a discrepancy between the child's potential and actual performance on academic tasks.

A shortcoming of this type of assessment is that it assumes a degree of differentiation not typical of the development of young children (Foley, 1986). It therefore has limited usefulness in identifying how a delay in one developmental domain may or may not affect the child's performance in another. Efforts to assess children's performance in a more developmentally appropriate manner include arena assessments and ecological analysis.

ARENA ASSESSMENTS

The structure of arena assessment allows a group of professionals to simultaneously observe the child performing a series of functional tasks. The primary benefit of the arena assessment is that it makes it possible for the professional team to observe when a deficit in one system is compensated for by other strengths and, conversely, its impact when no compensatory resources are available.

Observation of the "points of intersection" by transdisciplinary teams facilitates a more precise evaluation of the child's actual functioning than is possible using traditional models. Additional benefits of arena assessment include the use of a familiar examiner, a high degree of involvement by parents, and the opportunity for team members to work cooperatively in developing both accommodations and intervention plans.

ECOLOGICAL ANALYSIS

Clinical assessments of children's performance on developmental milestones now constitute only a portion of the child's profile. Equally important are ecological assessments of the child's compensatory resources and environment. In other words, identification of deficits in one developmental domain is no longer sufficient cause for special education services. The impact of the deficit on the child's educational functioning must also be documented.

EXAMPLE

Sometimes it's really hard to draw the line between deficits in some splinter skills and the presence of a real educational disability. I mean, there are some highly educated, successful people who can't skip, or have trouble with the "sh" sound. I remember being called in to do a physical therapy evaluation on a 13-year-old girl who had just made All Star on her junior high field hockey team. She had also scored slightly below the norm on part of a physical fitness examination. Her mom wanted the school system to provide her with special education services to correct this "deficit." It took a long time to convince the parent that her daughter had more than compensated for her weakness in this one area, and since it was not interfering with her successful participation in school sports, it did not warrant a special education referral.

Ecological assessment uses structured observation and task analysis to make classroom environments accessible and productive for all students. The combined skills of the transdisciplinary team are used to identify naturally occurring opportunities to work on target objectives, as well as necessary accommodations to ensure student participation and success (Table 79–1).

For many students with disabilities, the content of curriculum is the most accessible aspect of the classroom ecology. Other "embedded" characteristics of the combined cognitive infrastructure are more difficult: discourse rules, expectations of behavior, shifts in emphasis. Using ecological assessments, special educators and speech pathologists articulate these hidden characteristics of the classroom for students whose cognitive or perceptual characteristics blind them to their existence. Accommodations can then be made that allow these students to participate.

Table 79–1 • Ecological Assessment of a Natural Site: School Cafeteria Line

Activity	Potential IEP Objectives
Locating the menu	Attending, discrimination
Choosing the kind of sandwich	Choice-making
Ordering the sandwich	Language, communication skills
Paying for the sandwich	Matching, money skills, fine motor
Eating the sandwich	Feeding, social skills, ADL
Cleaning up	ADL, fine motor
Leaving	Mobility

ADL = activities of daily living; IEP = individualized education plan. Copyright 1994. AGH Associates, Inc. Reprinted with permission.

Ecological assessment also identifies alternative input/output systems for students who are not fluent in reading and writing. For example, children with fine motor problems can be taught to use keyboarding and predictive software for written expression; students who cannot read fluently can use voiced software to review content and complete assignments. These types of environmental accommodations encourage grade level instruction in regular classrooms for students with disabilities. Pitfalls of more traditional special education programming, such as watered-down curriculum and learned helplessness, are replaced with strategies to develop functional independence and success.

OUTSIDE EVALUATIONS

Parents sometimes question the results of school-based assessments. They may feel that the school is founding its conclusions more on the availability of services than on a commitment to their child's well-being. Schools may decide they need more data to establish the etiology of a child's problems. In these cases, parents or the school may request an outside evaluation, paid for with school district funds.

Although school-based teams are not bound by recommendations of an outside evaluator, they are often helpful in program development. They offer additional accommodations or different target objectives to help the child reach the goals of increased participation or greater functional independence.

It is important for physicians and other outside evaluators to recognize the legal limits of school-based services to children with disabilities, as well as their role in helping families separate educationally relevant issues from strictly medical concerns. Special education funds are intended to help children with disabilities acquire an appropriate education. They are not intended to cover other therapeutic needs the child may have.

Special education is also charged with providing services in the least restrictive environment, with age-appropriate peers. Interventions in natural settings are required prior to any discussion of more restrictive placements, such as self-contained classrooms or private placements. In any case, no one on the team, including the outside evaluator, can recommend placement or services until there is agreement on accommodations, goals, and objectives.

When outside evaluators, school personnel, and parents work together cooperatively, the result is always better services for children. Conversely, when they work outside the team process, a breakdown in services and the advent of adversarial relationships with families are the most likely outcomes.

Individualized Planning

Individualized planning is the hallmark of all special education service delivery. Across age groups, the goal of such planning is to ensure the successful participation of children with disabilities in age-appropriate activities and routines. For infants and toddlers, planning revolves around the child's role in the family. School participation is at the center of planning for older children, while transition into the world of work is emphasized in planning for adolescents.

DEVELOPING THE INDIVIDUALIZED FAMILY SERVICE PLAN

The IFSP is a blueprint of support for the family of an infant or toddler with disabilities or risks. Developed by the family and representatives of various community agencies available to offer support (e.g., child care, visiting nurses, respite care providers, early intervention programs), IFSPs list the kinds of services needed to integrate a young child with disabilities into the family's daily life. Because of the great variation in resources that families bring to the care of the child, each IFSP is unique in the types of supports recommended.

DEVELOPING THE INDIVIDUALIZED EDUCATION PLAN

The IEP is developed by the transdisciplinary team that supports the child with disabilities in a school or preschool setting. The child's parents and teacher are always members of this team, as well as other professionals who can contribute to the child's successful participation in classroom activities. The IEP includes a profile of the student as a learner, as well as a description of the types of environmental support he or she requires to learn.

Current practice recommends the development of a single set of IEP goals and objectives for each school year. These are formulated through a team discussion of student priorities in one or more of the following domains: cognition, community/social awareness, activities of daily living, vocational, leisure, and mobility. Focusing on these areas allows individual team members to move outside the narrow confines of their discipline and think about the child's overall functioning. Parents welcome the structure of the domains, since it provides them with a context to express concerns and priorities that may not be immediately apparent to school personnel.

Objectives are not limited to intervention by one team member or to a restricted number of activities. Rather they are integrated into classroom activities and routines throughout the day and can be addressed by whoever is supporting the child in the natural setting. IEP objectives are written in measurable fashion, with a set criterion for success, such as, "will demonstrate sufficient balance to complete gross motor activities such as skipping as indicated on 4/4 trials across 30 days." A child's lack of progress is attributed to a choice of the wrong target objectives or environmental accommodations, or both. In this case, the team reconvenes to make necessary changes in the IEP (Table 79–2).

Transition Planning

Transition planning is one of the most important services provided by special education. Although transition planning should occur as the child moves from grade level to grade level, it is most critical when a child moves between programs with different funding sources, for example, the transition from early intervention to public preschool, or when adolescents move from school-based services into job placements and community housing.

Physicians have an important role in supporting families and team decisions during these trying periods. As children move into preschool programs, families may need help in appreciating the changing needs of their child and in identifying age-appropriate services that reflect the child's needs for autonomy and self-determination. Strategies that are appropriate to infants and toddlers, such as frequent home visits and close relationships between parents and early interventionists, are less appropriate for preschool children, whose interest should be directed toward peers and activities outside the home. Physicians can assist families by placing transition issues within an age-appropriate context.

EXAMPLE

Our school held focus groups for families to discuss transition issues. We all worked together to identify the concerns we had as our children moved into preschool, kindergarten, and the middle school. It didn't seem to matter whether our children had disabilities or not. Our concerns were the same: how to form relationships with professionals at the next level, how to strike a balance between keeping our children safe and encouraging them to try new things, how to keep communication flowing.

The transition into the workforce and community housing emphasizes whole-life planning focused on future trends and opportunities rather than a restricted number of school-based goals and objectives. Interagency collaboration is a critical component of this transition, as well as working with the student and family to establish priorities for socialization, friendship, employment, and housing. Physicians can help parents see their children as "young adults" with similar needs for self-determination and independence as their teenaged counterparts, regardless of their developmental disability.

Controversies in the Field

The primary controversy in special education is disagreement about the nature of disability and appropriate responses to it. Despite the significant gains achieved by those lobbying for the right of children with disabilities to actively participate in their own childhood, resistance to their full inclusion continues. This is apparent in the controversy over the release of children with disabilities to the care and instruction of regular education staff, as well as controversies over the role of related service providers and what constitutes successful intervention.

INCLUSION VERSUS CONTINUUM OF SERVICES

Some advocates for children with disabilities question the ability of regular classrooms to meet the needs of these students. Particularly vocal in this regard are members of the deaf community, the National Learning Disabilities

Table 79–2 • Sample Individualized Educational Plans

Traditional IEP for Jake

Service	Setting	Personnel	Frequency
Reading	Resource room	LD Teacher	5 × 60/week/group
OT	Therapy room	OTR	2 × 30/week/individual
Speech	Therapy room	Speech pathologist	2 × 30/week/group

Goal 1: To improve reading skills
    Objective 1: Jake will demonstrate the ability to recognize beginning Dolch sight words, as indicated on 5/5 trials across 30 days.
    Objective 2: Jake will demonstrate the ability to use consonant sounds in oral reading, as indicated on 5/5 trials across 30 days.
    Objective 3: Jake will demonstrate the ability to answer literal comprehension questions presented in a "yes/no" format as indicated by 90% accuracy on 5 reading tests within 1 month's time. Tests will be at the preprimer level.
Goal 2: To increase tone
    Objective 1: Jake will demonstrate the ability to keep his mouth shut and not drool, as indicated by 5/5 observations of seatwork across 30 days.
    Objective 2: Jake will demonstrate an ability to sit in an upright position, without slouching for 25 minute intervals, as indicated by 5/5 observations of seatwork across 30 days.
Goal 3: To improve articulation
    Objective 1: Jake will pronounce the final "s" on the plural of familiar words, as indicated by success on 5/5/trials across 30 days.
    Objective 2: Jake will project his voice and pause between words when speaking to peers and adults, as indicated by success on 5/5 trials across 30 days.
    Objective 3: Jake will correctly pronounce the "th" sound when it appears in sight words, as indicated by success on 5/5 trials across 30 days.

Integrated IEP for Jake

Domain	Setting	Personnel	Frequency
Cognitive	Third grade	Classroom staff	Ongoing
		Resource room staff	20 min/day
		Speech pathologist	20 min/week, then monitor as needed
Mobility	Third grade	Classroom staff	Ongoing monitor/wkly; change as needed
		OT staff	

Goal 1: Jake will participate in classroom language-based activities.
    Objective 1: Jake will demonstrate the ability to recognize beginning Dolch sight words, as indicated on 5/5 trials across 30 days.
    Objective 2: Jake will demonstrate the ability to use consonant sounds in oral reading, as indicated on 5/5 trials across 30 days.
    Objective 3: Jake will demonstrate the ability to answer literal comprehension questions presented in a "yes/no" format as indicated by 90% accuracy on 5 reading tests within 1 month's time. Tests will be at the preprimer level.
    Objective 4: Jake will pronounce the final "s" on the plural of familiar words, as indicated by success on 5/5 trials across 30 days.
    Objective 5: Jake will project his voice and pause between words when speaking to peers and adults, as indicated by success on 5/5 trials across 30 days.
    Objective 6: Jake will correctly pronounce the "th" sound when it appears in sight words, as indicated by success on 5/5 trials across 30 days.
Goal 2: Jake will independently participate in classroom routines.
    Objective 1: Jake will demonstrate an understanding of what comes next in a routine by using environmental cues to transition from one activity to another, as indicated on 10/10 observations across 30 days.
    Objective 2: Jake will demonstrate an ability to sit in an upright position, without slouching for 25-minute intervals, as indicated by 5/5 observations of seatwork across 30 days.
    Objective 3: Jake will demonstrate an ability to monitor his own physical state by signing up for a 5-minute break every 30 minutes, as indicated by 10/10 observations across 30 days.

Key

Term	Meaning
IEP	Individualized educational plan; refers to the annual educational plan developed by parents and school staff for each student with a disability that interferes with his or her educational progress.
OT	Occupational therapy
Resource room	Classroom staffed by certified special education teachers, paraprofessionals. In a traditional service delivery model, children with disabilities are assigned to this type of instructional environment for small group work and/or one-on-one instruction.
LD Teacher	Teacher with special training in the instruction of children with learning disabilities
OTR	Registered occupational therapist
5 × 60/week/group	Student receives service described in five 1-hour long blocks each week. Services are provided in a small group of children with similar needs.
2 × 30/week/individual	Student receives service described in two half-hour long blocks each week. Services are provided individually.
Seatwork	Paper-and-pencil tasks, silent reading, and tabletop activities done in the classroom.
Classroom staff	Both regular and special education teachers, as well as paraprofessional staff working in the classroom that the student with disabilities attends
Ongoing	The continual use of recommended accommodations for each student, as well as targeting specified goals and objectives throughout the school day
Monitor	A scheduled review of student's progress with other team members

Modified from Craig SE, Haggart AG: Integrated Therapies. Hampton, NH, AGH Associates, Inc., 1994. Copyright 1994. Reprinted with permission.

Association (NLDA), and those concerned with the risks posed by children with severe emotional disorders (Villa et al, 1996). Proponents of this position equate special education with placement options and believe that a continuum of services ranging from substantially separate self-contained settings to full inclusion in regular classrooms is necessary to ensure that children receive the support they need (CASE, 1997).

Critics argue that this type of service delivery denies children with disabilities access to curriculum options available to other children, often relegating them to lives of "permanent practice." The model is further challenged by special education's failure to provide methods substantially different from those used in regular classrooms (Roach, 1995).

Resolution of this issue lies in the creation of school communities that allow children with different needs to learn together, in this way protecting each child's right to an education in the least restrictive environment. When all of the resources of a school are available to provide for the educational needs of all children, a "goodness of fit" between resources and need can be continually negotiated. The accommodations and individualized instruction required by children with disabilities can take place in any age-appropriate environment.

Physicians can help families stay focused on the overall development of their children with disabilities, reminding them of the need children have for consistent attachment figures, predictable routines, opportunities for friendship, and self-competence. Decisions about placement can then be shaped by a concern for the whole child, rather than acquisition of specific skills. Physicians' support in this process can be invaluable to families as they struggle to balance their children's right to childhood with the inflated demands of a culture driven by perfection.

Related Services

The provision of related services is another area of special education riddled with controversy. Factors that contribute to this include the IDEA's restriction of all therapy services to those that can influence the child's educational progress, as well as clinicians' frequent inexperience with schools and school-based services. Preschool and elementary curriculum is centered on fine and gross motor development, language acquisition, and social skills. The role of related services is not to supplant curriculum, as, for example, when children are seen by occupational therapists for handwriting or keyboarding. Rather, therapists have the responsibility to make the necessary accommodations to allow children with disabilities access to and participation in classroom activities and routines. In this way, school-based therapists are similar to therapists working in a rehabilitation setting. They use their skills to help children become as functionally independent as possible. Accommodation, not curing, is the goal. Physicians can play an important role in helping families distinguish between the medical need their child may have for various therapies, and the type of support they require to benefit from an appropriate education.

Special Education Outcomes

Finally, determining realistic outcomes for special education continues to be problematic. This is due in part to traditional expectations of cure or elimination of the disabling condition as indicated by federally mandated triennial evaluations to determine eligibility for services.

Lack of specificity as to the actual interventions that comprise special education services further exacerbates measurement of its effect. Past emphasis on placement limited the identification of those program features that are beneficial to children as opposed to those that have little or no effect.

An accurate assessment of the impact of special education requires an analysis of outcome measures that extends beyond the limits of developmental milestones. Global measures of child success, such as greater participation and increased functional independence, need to be considered.

Physicians can assist in this process by working with families and schools to develop whole-life plans for their patients with disabilities. Their participation in this process can help teams focus on interventions that result in improved quality of life, rather than acquisition of discrete developmental achievements that may or may not result in increased functional independence and greater participation in daily activities and routines.

Conclusion

The last 25 years has seen major changes in special education. Shifts in assumptions about the nature of disability, coupled with social policies supporting the rights of children with disabilities to an education in the least restrictive environment, have resulted in decentralized service delivery that emphasizes accommodations to natural settings. Children who in the past may have been placed in institutions or center-based private programs now attend public schools with their sisters and brothers and peers.

As a result, the role of professionals caring for these children has expanded. Interagency collaboration, cross-training, and family support are now part of special education services for children with disabilities. For physicians, these changes mean a commitment to team membership, a willingness to promote goals of participation and functional independence, and a vision of the whole child within the contexts of family, school, and community.

REFERENCES

Bronfenbrenner U: The Ecology of Human Development. Cambridge, MA, Harvard University Press, 1979.

Brown v. Board of Education, 347 US 483, 1954.

Brown L, Long E, Udvari-Solner A, Davis L, VanDeventer P, Ahlgren C, Johnson F, Gruenewald L, Jorgensen J: The home school: why students with severe intellectual disabilities must attend the schools of their brothers, sisters, friends, and neighbors. J Assoc Persons with Severe Handicaps 14:1, 1989.

Bruder M: The effectiveness of specific educational/developmental curricula for children with established disabilities. *In* Guralnick M (ed): The Effectiveness of Early Intervention. Baltimore, Paul H. Brookes, 1997.

CASE (Council of Administrators of Special Education, Policy and Legislative Committee): Delivery of services to students with disabilities. CASE Newsletter 39:1, 1997.

Foley G: The Transdisciplinary Approach (videotape). Lawrence, KS, Learner Managed Designs, 1986.

Gliedman J, Roth W: The Unexpected Minority. New York, Harcourt, Brace & Jovanovich, 1980.

Grimes L: Learned helplessness and attribution theory: redefining children's learning problems. J Learn Disabil 4:91, 1981.

IHDP (Infant Health and Development Program): Enhancing the outcomes of low birthweight and premature infants. JAMA 263:3035, 1990.

Karnish K, Bruder M, Rainforth B: A comparison of physical therapy in two school-based treatment contexts. Phys Occup Ther Pediatrics 15(4):1, 1995.

NABSE Study Group on Special Education: Winners All: A Call for Inclusive Schools. Alexandria VA, National Association of State Boards of Education, 1992.

Putnam JW, Speigal AN, Bruininks A: Future directions in education and the inclusion of students with disabilities: a delphi investigation. Exceptional Children 61:553, 1995.

Roach V: Winning ways: Creating Inclusive Schools, Classrooms, and Communities. Alexandria, VA, National Association of State Boards of Education, 1995.

Stainback S, Stainback W: Curriculum Considerations for Inclusive Classrooms: Facilitating Learning for All Children. Baltimore, Paul H. Brookes, 1992.

U.S. Department of Health and Human Services: Creating a 21st Century Head Start: Final Report of the Advisory Committee on Head Start Quality and Expansion. Washington, DC, US Government Printing Office, 1993.

Villa R, Thousand J, Meyers H, Nevin A: Teacher and administrator perceptions of heterogeneous education. Exceptional Children 63:29, 1996.

Weston DR, Ivins B, Heffron MC, Sweet N: Formulating the centrality of relationships in EI: an organizational perspective. Infants Young Children 9(3):1, 1997.

Will M: Educating children with learning problems: a shared responsibility. Exceptional Children 52:411, 1986.

80 Early Intervention Services

Donna Spiker • Kathleen Hebbeler

 Early intervention services are special services for children in their early years either with known developmental disabilities or with substantial biomedical or psychosocial risk factors for abnormal development (e.g., prematurity or parental neglect). This chapter describes the supporting legislation, the varying interdisciplinary components found in such programs, and the importance of participation by parents. The efficacy of these procedures in enhancing development has been defined by research. The pediatric role is described as surveillance, referral, interdisciplinary collaboration, ongoing pediatric care responsive to the needs of the child and family, and advocacy.

Need for Early Intervention

Early intervention refers to a variety of programs and services aimed at the prevention and remediation of developmental difficulties, delays, and disorders for infants, toddlers, and preschoolers up until school age, or approximately the first 5 years of life. Such services are provided by professionals and paraprofessionals from a variety of disciplines, including persons with training in early childhood special education, developmental and clinical psychology, speech pathology and communication disorders, physical and occupational therapy, child psychiatry, social work, and nursing.*

The need for early intervention is widely recognized for particular categories of young children, including (1) children with known disabilities (developmental delays; conditions with a high likelihood for mental retardation, such as Down syndrome; autism; sensory and neuromotor impairments), (2) children with biomedical risk factors (e.g., low birth weight, prematurity, medically fragile conditions, infection with human immunodeficiency virus), and (3) children with psychosocial risk factors (e.g., parental neglect or abuse, parental substance abuse, parental mental retardation, conditions associated with extreme poverty, very young parental age).

Many young children who receive early intervention have a combination of biomedical and environmental risk conditions. Furthermore, research conducted over the past 30 years has found that young children with multiple risk factors and their families are particularly in need of early intervention services (Sameroff, 1993).

Brief History of Early Intervention

The current field of early intervention services has evolved from a rich historical tradition of research and social policy

extending back over 100 years. The early writings of Darwin and others laid the groundwork for an appreciation of infancy and the preschool years as an important developmental period. In the United States, the concept of early education of young children outside the family took form with nursery schools for normally developing children early in the 20th century. The enormous proliferation of programs for young children to achieve a particular social purpose, however, began in the 1960s. The Head Start program, an important part of the War on Poverty, was created to improve the early development of preschoolers from low-income families (Zigler and Valentine, 1979). Head Start and other programs like it provided preschool-aged children with several hours a day of enriched experiences aimed at the goal of long-range improvements in academic achievement. Studies had shown that children from low-income families often performed poorly in school, with school failure seen as perpetuating the cycle of poverty. Programs like Head Start were developed in an era of great hope and drew heavily from the rapidly expanding knowledge base about infants and young children, showing them to be highly competent and capable of benefiting from properly structured early experiences.

The initial enthusiasm about early intervention focused on the potential for improving the developmental outcomes of young children living in poverty. However, there was also growing interest in helping infants with disabilities, such as Down syndrome or blindness. A decline in institutionalization resulted in increasing interest and need for programs to assist families who were raising their child with a disability at home.

In 1968, Congress created the Handicapped Children's Early Education Program, which over the next few decades would fund the development and testing of hundreds of program models for providing early intervention to children with disabilities from birth to 8 years of age. The earliest early intervention programs for children with Down syndrome, for example, were experimental studies conducted at universities. These programs had a comprehensive focus on all areas of development, with a special focus on language and communication development. These programs typically consisted of a home visiting component

---

*The phrase *early intervention* has historically been used to refer to services for children younger than school age, that is, children from birth to age 5 years. The primary federal law governing early intervention uses the term to refer exclusively to programs for infants and toddlers, from birth to age 3 years, and describes services for 3- to 5-year-olds as *special education and related services*. In this chapter, the term *early intervention* is used to refer to the broader age range except where the federal law is explicitly discussed, and then the term is used the way the law defines it.

to teach parents how to stimulate their infant's development, and center-based programs for children in the preschool years. The earliest studies of these programs indicated that the programs enhanced the rate of acquisition of basic developmental milestones.

Over the next few decades, programs for young children with disabilities proliferated. The federal government came to play an increasingly important role in facilitating and ultimately mandating these programs. In 1975, the passage of a federal law known as Public Law 94-142, the Education of All Handicapped Children Act, established society's commitment to school-aged children with disabilities by guaranteeing them the right to a free and appropriate public education. In addition to mandating that states educate all school-aged children with disabilities, PL 94-142 provided incentives to states to develop programs to provide services through the public schools for children 3 to 5 years of age.

This important piece of legislation was amended several times in the next 10 years, and with each amendment, the incentives for states to serve children younger than 6 years old were strengthened. Meanwhile, programs to provide early intervention services for infants and toddlers were being created around the country. These programs were operated by a variety of public and private agencies and were often not coordinated even in the same community. States had no single agency responsible for overseeing early intervention, and it was not uncommon for three to seven state agencies to be involved in delivering services.

Legislation Governing Early Intervention

The most important amendment to the Education of the Handicapped Act (which has since been renamed the Individuals with Disabilities Education Act, or IDEA) for children from birth through age 5 years with disabilities occurred in 1986. Public Law (PL) 99-457 stipulated that states must provide services to all 3- to 5-year-olds with disabilities by 1991–1992 to receive any federal special education funding. The law made education agencies responsible for serving these children. Part H (now Part C) of PL 99-457 created a new program to address the needs of infants and toddlers with disabilities. Part H provided funds to states to develop and implement a statewide, comprehensive, coordinated, multidisciplinary, interagency early intervention program. The purpose of Part H was to (1) enhance the development of infants and toddlers with disabilities and minimize their potential for developmental delay, (2) reduce the educational costs to society, including public schools, by minimizing the need for special education and related services after infants and toddlers with disabilities reach school age, (3) minimize the likelihood of institutionalization of individuals with disabilities and maximize the potential for their independent living in society, and (4) enhance the capacity of families to meet the special needs of their infants and toddlers with disabilities (PL 99-457, 1986, Sec. 671). Federal law has a strong family orientation that encompasses the resources, priorities, and concerns of the families of eligible children as they relate to the needs of the child.

One of the concerns that guided congressional deliberations on Part H was the need for flexibility in state implementation. Congress recognized that only a few states had statewide programs that served children from birth to age 3 years. Congress also realized that the federal government did not have all the answers regarding what worked (or all the money to fund them) and did not want to dictate procedures, given the great variation among states' policies, organizational structures, and so on. Congress specified basic minimum concepts and components but provided for state discretion in determining the exact population to be served, and each state was left to develop its own structures and to determine what would be best for its residents. Consequently, the provision of early intervention services varies considerably from state to state.

Several of the Part H requirements are especially relevant to community pediatricians. The law requires that states develop their own definition of developmental delay, which must be based on appropriate diagnostic procedures and cover five areas of development (cognitive, physical, communication, adaptive, and emotional and social development). Part H requires that states provide services to all infants and toddlers with developmental delay and establishes conditions that carry a high probability of resulting in delay (e.g., Down syndrome). States may choose to serve those who are at risk, but only a few states have chosen to do so. Furthermore, owing to fiscal concerns, some states that have been serving at-risk children are reevaluating whether to continue serving this group of children. Because eligibility requirements vary from state to state, it is imperative that physicians acquaint themselves with the precise eligibility requirements for early intervention services in the state in which they practice.

Part H requires that early intervention programs conduct timely and comprehensive multidisciplinary evaluations of each infant or toddler with disabilities. Assessments of the needs of families to appropriately assist in the development of the child are also to be conducted. Part H requires that an individualized family service plan (IFSP) be developed by a multidisciplinary team (which must include a parent or guardian) for each child and family enrolled in an early intervention program. The IFSP is a process as well as a product, in that it is intended to provide a way for families and professionals to work together as a team to identify formal and informal resources to help families meet their chosen goals. When appropriate, the child's physician should be included as a member of the IFSP team, either through direct participation in team deliberations or through contributing information and recommendations for the other team members to use in designing a plan of services. The resulting written document specifies multiple aspects of early intervention services for a child and family. The IFSP includes the identification of the child and family needs, which are determined from a comprehensive multidisciplinary evaluation; the types, frequency, and location of services to be provided; the identity of the service providers and of a service coordinator who is responsible for making sure that the plan is implemented; and outcomes and goals.

Part H contains three components designed to assist in identifying and enrolling all children eligible for early intervention.

1. All states are required to develop a public awareness program to inform the general public and in particular primary referral sources, such as physicians or child care providers, about the availability of early intervention services in the community.
2. A comprehensive "child find" system must be established to ensure that every eligible child is located and served. The child find system is to include a system for making referrals to appropriate agencies and to provide for participation by primary referral sources.
3. Each state must also maintain a central directory that includes public and private early intervention services, resources and experts in the state, research and demonstration projects being conducted in the state, and professional and other groups that provide services to eligible children and their families. These directories can be valuable resources for persons trying to locate early intervention services.

Part H provided states several planning years (with extensions in subsequent amendments) to establish statewide coordinated systems of services. All 50 states have passed through the planning years and are in full implementation. Full implementation means that states must provide early intervention services to all infants and toddlers who meet the state-established eligibility criteria.

Varying Components of Early Intervention Programs

As discussed, early intervention programs encompass a large variety of different services. Table 80–1 shows the types of services that can be provided.

These services can be delivered in a variety of settings, most typically in the child's home or a center. At an early intervention center–based program, service providers work with groups of children with special needs and possibly their families. Center-based programs are sometimes

Table 80–1 • Possible Early Intervention Services

Assistive technology services
Audiology
Family training, counseling, and support
Health services
Medical services for diagnosis and evaluation
Nursing services
Nutrition services
Occupational therapy
Physical therapy
Psychological services
Service coordination services
Special instruction for the child
Speech-language pathology
Transportation
Vision services

preferred over home-based programs for toddlers and preschoolers with disabilities because they provide opportunities for the child to socialize with other children (Fig. 80–1). These centers are located in a variety of physical settings including schools, hospitals, churches, and private buildings. Therapy services may also be delivered in the home or in more traditional medical settings such as hospitals, clinics, and offices. Many children and families use a combination of settings, with a typical example being in the home and at a center.

The frequency of early intervention service delivery varies across program models and individual families. A recent survey of 65 early intervention programs found the typical length of an early intervention session to be 1 to 2 hours (73%), with the next most typical lengths being 30 minutes (14%), half day (8%), and full day (3%). Services were most commonly provided 1 to 2 days per week (66%), although some programs offered services as frequently as 3 to 5 days per week and others as infrequently as once a month.

A fundamental assumption shared within the early intervention field and codified in PL 99-457 is that effective

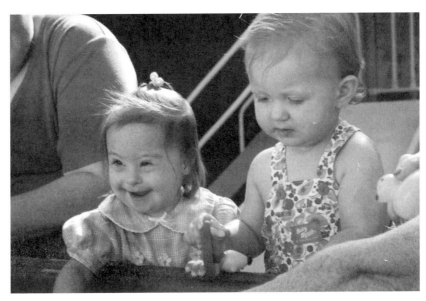

Figure 80–1. Play and peer interactions are an integral part of programming.

early intervention requires an interdisciplinary collaboration. Early intervention encompasses a vast array of services because the problems of young children with specific disabilities or vulnerabilities are diverse. The many disciplines and theoretical models include medicine, education, social service, child care, speech and language pathology, occupational and physical therapy, nursing, respite care, public health, and psychology (Meisels and Shonkoff, 1990). The professionals working with an individual child and family function as a team, of which there are several kinds. A transdisciplinary team is considered the best practice; however, it may be the least frequently found. It is made up of professionals from several disciplines as well as the family. One of the defining features of the transdisciplinary team is that its members work across disciplinary boundaries to plan and provide integrated services. Family members are integral to it and can be involved at whatever level they choose with regard to decision making for themselves and their child. The service plan is developed jointly by all team members, but the responsibility for carrying out the plan rests with the family and one team member.

High-quality early intervention services should also be "normalized" to the maximum extent appropriate to encourage conditions of everyday living that are as close as possible to those of society at large. For young children, this means helping them in a way that allows the family and consequently the child to have as normal a family life as possible. It could mean providing services in community-based settings such as a child care center rather than in medical facilities such as hospitals, or it could mean providing opportunities for interaction with children without disabilities. This principle means that the least intrusive and most normal strategies resulting in effective intervention are being used (Buysse and Bailey, 1993).

Table 80–2 summarizes critical dimensions along which early intervention services vary.

Role of Parents in Early Intervention Programs

Persons concerned with developing early intervention services have had a strong and persistent interest in the involvement of parents in the early intervention enterprise. The earliest perspectives sought to engage parents as teachers or therapists of their young children, in the belief that an involved didactic role for parents would lead to optimal development in children. Views about parents' roles are beginning to change, reflecting transactional, ecological models and a growing appreciation for the variability among families. Perhaps more than any other feature of the early intervention enterprise, views about the role of parents have changed the most over the past 35 years, and, many would argue, for the better.

It is widely recognized that one of the most far-reaching and challenging aspects of early intervention is its strong philosophical commitment to a family focus in all aspects of implementation. Whereas issues of parent involvement and "empowerment" have been a central feature of the early intervention field since its beginnings, the family focus of PL 99-457 is much broader. It involves concepts of partnerships and true collaboration between

Table 80–2 • Dimensions and Characteristics of Early Intervention Services

Nature of service
  Child therapy or stimulation
  Consultation services
  Family training, support, or counseling
  Child care
  Service coordination; linkages to existing community services
Provider of service
  Professional therapist (speech, occupational, physical)
  Early childhood special educator/infant specialist
  Social worker
  Nurse
  Psychologist
  Other professional (e.g., child psychiatrist)
  Paraprofessional
  Parent
Location of service
  Home
  Specialized center or school program
  Community child care center/family day care home
  Hospital clinic or specialized clinic
Entity providing service
  Public (e.g., public health, developmental disabilities, school systems)
  Private (e.g., Easter Seals, United Cerebral Palsy, small unaffiliated programs)
  Individual practitioners
Format of service
  Individual
  Group with other children with disabilities
  Group with other children without disabilities
  Group with a mixture of children with and without disabilities
Intensity of service
  Hours per session
  Number of days per week or month
Duration of service
  Over months or years
Use of curriculum models
  Variety of developmentally based curricula
  Variety of parent education, training, or support models
Strategies and models of parent involvement
  Parent training and education models
  Parent-child interaction models; relationship-oriented models
  Parent social support models

families and early intervention professionals (Fig. 80–2). Guralnick's (1989) review of research on parent involvement in early intervention suggests that efforts should be "designed to build and strengthen the abilities of families to confidently and competently nurture the development of their child." The language of Part H reflects a belief that family functioning and child development are inextricably intertwined, with parent support being a prominent goal of early intervention.

Providing genuine family support has been and continues to be a significant issue in the early intervention field. Perspectives from parents of children with disabilities have been the subject of many empiric research studies and essays. Prominent early interventionists have argued that the family must be the proposed center of the early intervention enterprise, and the goal is to support the family so that the family can support the child over time. This viewpoint acknowledges that the family support aspects of early intervention provide the first step in helping the family to meet the special needs of their child in the community, and to enable them to remain capable and

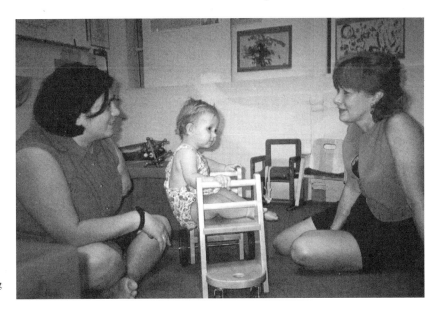

Figure 80–2. Parents and professionals working together is an essential feature.

resourceful over the child's entire childhood. Thus, participation in early intervention benefits the family unit by enhancing their knowledge, resources, and ability to care for their child with a disability.

Part of the impetus for the family focus of Part H was the difficult experiences of families with infants or toddlers with disabilities or developmental delays. Often, entry into the early intervention service delivery system was not easy for these families. Common complaints were that the system was fragmented and often dehumanizing. The initial period during which parents begin to suspect that their infant or toddler has a developmental problem is particularly stressful. Anecdotally, many parents complain that their community pediatrician, frequently the first professional whom families approach with their concerns, was not helpful because the pediatrician did not take their concerns seriously. Families want pediatricians to make prompt and appropriate referrals for assessments, to inform them about the availability of early intervention, and then to support their efforts to obtain services.

Much of the research and conceptual work about families of children with disabilities has had a negative, pessimistic perspective, focusing on families' burdens and stresses (financial, time, emotional) associated with having a child with a disability. However, more recent research indicates that mothers with and without disabled infants did not necessarily differ in mean levels of maternal depression or feelings of parenting competence. Moreover, in families with an infant with a disability, the perceived caregiving difficulty often predicts maternal depression, and support from the spouse is a more important factor for the mother's psychological well-being (see reviews in Guralnick, 1997). These results highlight the currently accepted view that many interacting factors contribute to positive family adjustment and functioning. A consensus emerging in the early intervention field is that families of infants and toddlers with developmental disabilities are as varied as families are generally. They have different strengths and difficulties, and all families do not have the same needs.

A variety of models of parent involvement exist in early intervention programs. Generally, the models focus on one or more of the following:

- Training parents as teachers of their children
- Facilitating positive parent-infant interactions
- Providing social support for parents and families
- Providing ancillary family services aimed at strengthening overall family functioning (e.g., facilitating access to financial assistance, job training, access to child care)

Research has begun to conceptualize family needs and resources and to assess changes in needs and resources related to program participation (Table 80–3). Using this model of informational, instrumental, emotional, and financial needs, recent research indicates that families vary in the types of needs they express and in the priorities placed on different needs (Bailey, Blasco, and Simeonsson, 1992). Parents expressed the greatest need for information, for selected areas of financial support, and for opportunities to meet other parents who have children with disabilities.

Table 80–3 • Family Needs Related to
Early Intervention Participation

Information about the child's condition: health, development, assessment results
Help in identifying appropriate services for the child: early intervention, medical care
Help with basic child care services
Help in interacting with the child: play and instructional activities and materials
Help in maintaining confidence in parenting a child who is different: support from other parents, stress management, counseling advocacy activities
Financial assistance for caring for child and meeting service needs: respite services, special equipment
Assistance to help siblings deal with the child's disability

Adapted from Bailey DB Jr, Blascoe PM, Simeonsson RJ: Needs expressed by mothers and fathers of young children with disabilities. Am J Ment Retard 97:1–10, 1992.

The goal of many early intervention services is to address family needs and support their ability to care for and enhance the development of their child. Family support services have been reported to have a variety of positive effects on families, including (1) enhanced commitment to care for the child at home, rather than in out-of-home placements, (2) reduced stress, (3) increased respite from daily caregiving demands, leading to improved parental ability to care for the home, pursue recreation, and seek employment, (4) improved overall quality of life of the family, and (5) improved skills to meet the child's habilitative needs (see reviews in Guralnick, 1997; Meisels and Shonkoff, 1990; Zeanah, 1993). The Part H legislation fundamentally changed early intervention by requiring early intervention professionals to work with parents as partners in planning the most appropriate services for them and their child.

Comprehensive Assessment: A Critical Early Intervention Service

Developmental assessment of young children is necessary for three related purposes: (1) to determine initial eligibility for early intervention services, (2) to determine functioning in major developmental areas (cognitive development; physical development, including vision and hearing; communication development [speech and language]; social and emotional development; self-help skill development) in order to plan the needed services, to establish the program goals outcomes, and to monitor progress, and (3) for use in program evaluation activities.

There are many infant evaluation measures; some are norm-referenced, and others are criterion-referenced. These measures are used to assess developmental milestones or attainments and to yield scores or age equivalents for development overall or for specific areas of development (e.g., cognitive, receptive language, expressive language, fine motor). The concept of developmental milestones has been central to screening and evaluation of health programs for infants and children. Developmental milestones have also served as the basis for deriving items for standardized measures of child development, producing normative information for skill attainment.

Most early intervention practitioners and program evaluators tend to conceptualize child assessment broadly. Multiple domains of development are measured to ensure sensitivity to the variable rates of growth shown across different domains by infants with disabilities. Attention is given to areas other than cognitive development, particularly social competence and adaptive functioning. Some of the newer approaches toward assessment, commonly associated with the infant mental health perspective, examine the infant in the context of relationships with parents and significant caregivers (Zeanah, 1993),* paying particular attention to the infant's social interaction behaviors, quality of engagement with objects and people, and temper-

---

*Several excellent comprehensive volumes about the recent advances in developmental screening and assessment are available from The Zero to Three National Center for Infants, Toddlers and Families, 734 15th Avenue NW, 10th Floor, Washington, DC 20005-1013.

amental characteristics such as activity level, attention span, and reactivity to stimuli (see Meisels and Shonkoff, 1990; Zeanah, 1993; and Chapters 67 and 68.)

Early Intervention Efficacy Research—How Effective Is It?

As discussed previously, early intervention had its origins in studies of programs for low-income children and their families in the 1960s. The first studies were based on the theoretical and empiric discussions in the child development field about the nature-nurture debate and the ability to modify and enhance environmental stimulation and thereby improve intelligence. By the late 1960s, there was a parallel movement for children with known developmental disabilities, and early experimental programs for children with Down syndrome, for example, began to appear (see Spiker and Hopmann, 1997, for a review). For both children in poverty and those with known disabilities, many studies were small in scale and experimental in design, with a narrow range of child outcomes. Some large-scale early intervention studies were initiated after the implementation of Head Start, when early intervention emerged as a national social policy issue. The key question of this period was "does early intervention work?" in terms of promoting child developmental outcomes.

In the past 10 to 15 years, numerous review articles and texts have been devoted to summarizing the empiric work concerning the efficacy of early intervention for infants and preschoolers with disabilities and at risk for developmental difficulties (Guralnick, 1997; Meisels and Shonkoff, 1990). A recently published book edited by Guralnick (1997) contains a comprehensive review of the vast literature about the effectiveness of early intervention. Generally, the three categories of infants and preschoolers mentioned earlier have been considered in research on early intervention. Much of this research has focused on how early intervention services enhance optimal cognitive, social, emotional, and motor development and adaptive behavior in the child.

Although many unanswered questions about the effectiveness of early intervention remain, there is a coherent and consistent body of literature to document the effectiveness and value of early intervention programs (Guralnick, 1997). In several review articles, meta-analytic techniques have been used to compare and summarize results across many studies of children from disadvantaged backgrounds and of those with known disabilities (see reviews in Meisels and Shonkoff, 1990). Farran (1990), summarizing efficacy studies and these meta-analyses, noted that there appears to be a 6 to 7 IQ point difference or improvement with early intervention participation, but effects are not long lasting. Others have noted that small sample sizes have been the rule, limiting statistical power to detect differences. Some reviews have focused on specific disability groups. For example, reviews of early intervention results for infants and preschoolers with Down syndrome have concluded that there are significant but modest improvements in the rate of early development, and such reviews have routinely noted the rather wide individual variation among infants and young children with Down syndrome (Spiker and Hopmann, 1997).

Programs for Environmentally At-Risk Preschoolers

The federal commitment to developing preschool programs to enhance school readiness for children living in poverty emerged in the 1960s as part of the War on Poverty. Some of the programs were model preschool programs developed within university settings, based on the explosion of basic research of the era that documented the learning capacities of infants and young children and the benefits of properly structured early experiences to enhance development. A federal initiative for low-income children and their families, the Head Start program, began during this period. Children enter Head Start at age 3 or 4 years, and the services generally include an early childhood center–based program, various health services, parent education, and family support activities. Federal data from 1994 indicate that approximately 700,000 children are served in Head Start. The goals of Head Start are to provide a comprehensive preschool for the children and to promote parent education.

Haskins' (1989) conducted a comprehensive review, which focused exclusively on model preschool programs (i.e., developed and implemented in controlled environments such as within university communities) and Head Start programs for children living in poverty. He reached four major conclusions:

1. Both model programs and Head Start programs produced significant effects on intellectual and socioemotional development.
2. There is a decline in these gains over a few years for both types of programs.
3. For variables such as reduction in special education placement and grade retention, model programs and Head Start programs yield strong and modest positive effects, respectively.
4. There are modest long-term effects for model programs on such life success or adaptive measures as teen pregnancy, juvenile delinquency, welfare participation, and employment (but no evidence of these for Head Start), suggesting possible "sleeper" effects, particularly for social competence outcomes.

The programs reviewed were predominantly for children ages 3 to 5 years, so there are unanswered questions about possible effects if programs had begun earlier.* Evaluations of the Head Start programs have a number of methodologic limitations because of problems with comparison groups used, lack of random assignment, and a wide range of program quality, from quite poor to quite good. Policy makers and researchers interested in Head Start programs have generally agreed that the higher quality programs lead to more optimal outcomes in the children.*

Programs for Low–Birth Weight, Premature Infants and Preschoolers

There has been a recent proliferation of programs and intervention studies conducted with medically fragile, low-birth weight, premature infants and their families (Achenbach et al, 1993; Gross, Spiker, and Haynes, 1997; Palmer et al, 1988; Piper et al, 1986). Many of these investigations have included large samples and rigorous study designs. For example, the Infant Health and Development Program (IHDP), a multisite study of the effectiveness of a comprehensive early intervention, used a randomized clinical trial model with 985 low–birth weight, premature infants and their families, studied from birth to age 3 years (Gross, Spiker, and Haynes, 1997). The impetus for this and other studies came from concerns in the medical community and the early intervention field about the potential for significant developmental morbidity of infants being saved by modern neonatal technology. With the rapid and remarkable advances in neonatology over the past 30 years, there has been a considerable improvement in infant mortality rate for very premature and low–birth weight infants. Yet these surviving infants, particularly those born the most prematurely, with the lightest birth weights, and who are small for gestational age, are particularly vulnerable to a host of developmental, behavioral, and health problems and are at risk for significant disability (Friedman and Sigman, 1992; McCarton et al, 1996).

Results from the IHDP indicated that a comprehensive early intervention program implemented over the first 3 years of life led to significant improvements at age 3 years in cognitive ability and reductions in behavioral problems, with no increased risk of health problems associated with a group care component of the intervention. The positive effects on cognitive performance, although statistically significant, were greater for the heavier birth weight infants (those weighing more than 2000 g at birth) (McCormick et al, 1993). Small positive effects of the intervention program were also reported for the quality of the home environment and mother-child interactions (Gross, Spiker, and Haynes, 1997). The IHDP data also showed that the more intensive the participation in the intervention, the more positive the benefits.

The IHDP intervention ended at age 3 years, and follow-up assessments at ages 5 and 8 years showed a diminution of positive effects on cognitive performance (Brooks-Gunn et al, 1994; McCarton et al, 1997). The IHDP intervention was withdrawn at age 3 years, and the gradual disappearance of positive effects over time suggests the continuing need for high-quality stimulation and

---

*Recently, the initiation of programs for children younger than age 3 years, called Early Head Start, has begun, and a national evaluation study of Early Head Start is underway.

---

*Several excellent volumes on policy issues, efficacy research, and implementation issues regarding home visiting programs, programs for low–birth weight infants, long-term outcomes of early childhood programs, effects of welfare reform, as well as school-linked services for older children are published in a series called *The Future of Children*, available from The David and Lucile Packard Foundation, 300 Second Street, Suite 102, Los Altos, CA 94200.

intervention over the remaining preschool and early school years.

Other less intensive interventions of shorter duration for low–birth weight infants have been shown to have positive effects on the development of this population, some of the effects still being apparent at age 9 years (Achenbach et al, 1993). There is still much to be learned about the exact timing, intensity, and duration of interventions in the early years. Generally, programs that are begun earlier, with greater intensity and longer duration, tend to result in more substantial benefits.

There has also been considerable interest in evaluations of physical therapy and sensory integration therapies for infants with cerebral palsy and other neuromotor difficulties; frequently, these infants are born prematurely, of low birth weight, and/or with a variety of birth complications. Literature reviewed by Harris (1997) suggests modest improvements in neuromotor functioning for these therapies, but there are still a number of unresolved issues about the types of infants who benefit most, the intensity and type of therapy used, and the interaction of therapy with other interventions. For more severely affected infants, the evidence that physical therapy results in significant improvements in range of motion, muscle tone, and strength is not convincing. Harris (1997) suggests having therapy goals that aim to assist parents and caregivers in learning techniques for positioning and handling that result in greater ease in caregiving. In a well-designed randomized clinical trial examining the effects of physical therapy with a group of high-risk infants, Piper and colleagues (1986) compared a group who received physical therapy with a group who received an infant stimulation program that used the Learning Games curriculum from the IHDP. More significant developmental progress was shown for the group who received the comprehensive developmental stimulation curriculum.

Critical Issues in Early Intervention Efficacy Research

Past research has documented the wide variability among infants and young children with disabilities and supports the view that there are complex interactions between biological and environmental factors, which, in turn, influence intervention effectiveness. For instance, in the IHDP, the program had stronger positive effects on cognitive outcomes for the heavier-born than the lighter-born premature infants; for the white and educationally more advantaged group, the intervention appeared not to be necessary (Brooks-Gunn et al, 1992). Likewise, in a longitudinal study of infants and their families in 29 community-based programs in Massachusetts and New Hampshire conducted by Shonkoff and associates (1992), the strongest predictor of developmental change was the severity of the infant's disability at study entry, with the most severely disabled infants making the least progress. Results from other studies indicate that earlier age at entry into intervention services did not predict greater developmental progress in very low–birth weight, premature, medically fragile infants (White and Boyce, 1993). Because earlier age of entry into early intervention services is often confounded with

severity of the infant's disability, there are still unanswered questions about the "earlier is better" notion. Taken together, these studies highlight the need for continued study of the relationships between infant characteristics and types of interventions.

As the early intervention field has matured over the past several decades, research about efficacy has become more differentiated and refined. Rather than asking simply whether early intervention is effective, researchers are asking what kinds of interventions are effective for which children and types of families and for what child and family outcomes. Specific planned variations that are being examined include the following critical elements of early intervention experiences: (1) the intensity of the intervention, (2) the age at which the intervention begins, and (3) variations in program components related to parent involvement. There is a need for more well-designed research of early intervention treatments, using the established controlled randomized clinical trial methodology, which has been proven to be feasible in earlier studies (Spiker et al, 1991).

Referred to as "second generation research" (Guralnick, 1997), the most recent efforts to study the effectiveness of early intervention are characterized by several important new developments, including (1) greater *specificity* in linking child and family characteristics, program factors, and outcomes; (2) improved *scientific quality* by examining different levels or forms of intervention and by including rigorous clinical trial designs, larger sample sizes, and better and more frequent measurements; and (3) conceptual and empiric models that include *developmental, transactional,* and *ecological* perspectives. These current perspectives raise more complicated questions about the effects of early intervention and have led to an acceptance of the complex interplay of child, parent, family ecology, and community factors that interact with the early intervention service delivery system and influence outcomes for children and their families.

Role of the Pediatrician in Early Intervention

Community pediatricians are frequently the first professionals to whom parents come for information, advice, and support about the developmental concerns they have about their young children. As such, this group of professionals is in a unique position to give parents the information and support they need. First and Palfrey (1994) have highlighted the important role of the community pediatrician in identifying the at-risk infant as early as possible. They urge that these practitioners engage in ongoing surveillance rather than viewing their role as providing one-time screening. Furthermore, these authors urge physicians to serve as advocates for children with developmental delays and their families, working to ensure that services are available in their local communities and maintaining open and ongoing communication with locals schools and community agencies who serve young children.

To follow these recommendations, pediatricians need to become aware of the various early intervention services available in their local communities and with procedures

Table 80–4 • Pediatricians and Early Intervention: Assisting and Supporting Families

---

When a parent expresses a concern about the development or behavior of their infant or young child, take the concerns seriously. All children should have routine developmental surveillance.

Refer the family promptly for a more complete developmental assessment to identify the nature of the possible developmental problem.

Take great care in how a diagnosis of a developmental disability or the possibility of a developmental disability is communicated to parents. Information should be given in a sensitive and caring manner.

Make a prompt referral to early intervention services and encourage the family's participation in these services. A prompt referral gives parents hope and reduces their anxiety about their child.

Present any statements about long-term prognosis carefully. Parents should be informed that information about prognoses is based on data for groups of children, and long-term predictions about individual children are much less certain.

On subsequent medical visits, ask questions about the child's early intervention services and the child's progress as a way of expressing encouragement of the family's efforts on behalf of their child.

---

for assisting families in obtaining appropriate and timely assessments of their children and referral to the available services. Many communities have an interagency early intervention organization, with which pediatricians should become familiar and in which they may want to participate. Additionally, many communities have parent resource centers that provide information and support for families. To become familiar with all early intervention and family support services in their local area, pediatricians can contact the local school district or any individual early intervention program.

Table 80–4 identifies some ways in which community pediatricians can inform and support families who are in need of referrals to early intervention services. These suggestions acknowledge that community pediatricians are critical professionals in families' lives. Because of the developmental surveillance role they play with infants and young children, pediatricians need to be well informed and supportive about early intervention services.

Table 80–4 identifies six key issues for the community pediatrician. First, the pediatrician has a unique opportunity to listen with an open and sensitive attitude to parents' worries and questions about their child's development and behavior. When parents express a concern about the development or behavior of their infant or young child, the concerns should be taken seriously. Routine developmental surveillance should always be performed.

Second, when parents express a concern about the development or behavior of their infant or young child, the pediatrician should refer the family promptly for a more complete developmental assessment to identify the nature of the possible problem. The pediatrician can assure the parents that a thorough assessment is an important first step to determining whether a problem exists.

Third, if the pediatrician is the person to convey to parents a diagnosis of a developmental disability or the possibility of a developmental disability, she or he needs to take great care in how information is presented to parents. Many parents have noted that they remember for a very long time how they are given diagnoses of develop-

mental disorders in their children; the exact words used, the tone of voice, the amount of time taken with them by their physician, and the manner in which a physician shows concern for how parents receive this news are all critical features from the parents' perspective.

Fourth, pediatricians should be knowledgeable about the early intervention services in their communities and should refer parents to them promptly. While acknowledging the child's disability, the pediatrician can also give parents hope and reduce their anxiety by referring them to and encouraging their participation in early intervention. The pediatrician is in a unique position to support the hope that parents have for their child's future.

Fifth, the pediatrician needs to be especially careful about any statements about long-term prognosis because such comments are remembered by parents, often forever. Because the data available about the long-term prognosis of various developmental disabilities are derived from data for groups of children, it is important to communicate to parents that predictions about individual children are much less certain. The reality is that many predictions about future development are guesses, and parents are often better served by messages that provide hope rather than hopelessness.

Sixth, once the family has been referred to early intervention, on subsequent medical visits, the pediatrician needs to ask questions about how the early intervention program is going. The physician's interest and encouragement of the family's efforts are important. The pediatrician can support the activities and efforts of the early intervention professionals who are working with the family by staying informed about the services being provided and the child's progress.

REFERENCES

Achenbach TM, Howell CT, Aoki MF, Rauh VA: Nine-year outcome of the Vermont Intervention Program for low birth weight infants. Pediatrics 91:45–55, 1993.

Bailey DB Jr, Blasco PM, Simeonsson RJ: Needs expressed by mothers and fathers of young children with disabilities. Am J Ment Retard 97:1–10, 1992.

Brooks-Gunn J, Gross RT, Kraemer HC, et al: Enhancing the cognitive outcomes of low birth weight, premature infants: for whom is intervention most effective? Pediatrics 89:1209–1215, 1992.

Brooks-Gunn J, McCarton CM, Casey PH, et al: Early intervention in low-birth-weight premature infants: results through age 5 from the Infant Health and Development Program. JAMA 272:1257–1262, 1994.

Buysse V, Bailey DB: Behavioral and developmental outcomes in young children with disabilities in integrated and segregated settings: a review of comparative studies. J Special Education 26(4):434–461, 1993.

Farran DC: Effects of intervention with disadvantaged and disabled children: a decade review. *In* Meisels SJ, Shonkoff JP (eds): Handbook of Early Childhood Intervention. Cambridge, Cambridge University Press, 1990.

First LR, Palfrey JS: The infant or young child with developmental delay. N Engl J Med 330:478–483, 1994.

Friedman SL, Sigman MD (eds): The Psychological Development of Low-Birthweight Children: Annual Advances in Applied Developmental Psychology, Vol 6. Norwood, NJ, Ablex, 1992.

Gross RT, Spiker D, Haynes C (eds): Helping Low Birthweight, Premature Babies: The Infant Health and Development Program. Stanford, CA, Stanford University Press, 1997.

Guralnick MJ (ed): The Effectiveness of Early Intervention. Baltimore, Paul H. Brookes, 1997.

Guralnick MJ: Recent developments in early intervention efficacy research: implications for family involvement in P.L. 99-457. Top Early Child Special Ed 9:1–17, 1989.

Harris S: The effectiveness of early intervention for children with cerebral palsy and related motor disabilities. *In* Guralnick MJ (ed): The Effectiveness of Early Intervention. Baltimore, Paul H. Brookes, 1997, pp 327–347.

Haskins R: Beyond metaphor: the efficacy of early childhood intervention. Am Psychol 44:274–282, 1989.

McCarton CM, Brooks-Gunn J, Wallace IF, et al: Results at age 8 of early intervention for low-birth-weight infants: the Infant Health and Development Program. JAMA 277:126–132, 1997.

McCarton CM, Wallace IF, Divon M, Vaughan HG Jr: Cognitive and neurologic development of the premature, small for gestational age infant through age 6: comparison by birth weight and gestational age. Pediatrics 98:1167–1178, 1996.

McCormick MC, McCarton C, Tonascia J, Brooks-Gunn J: Early educational intervention for very low birth weight infants: results from the Infant Health and Development Program. J Pediatr 123:527–533, 1993.

Meisels SJ, Shonkoff JP (eds): Handbook of Early Intervention. New York, Wiley, 1990.

Palmer FB, Shapiro BK, Wachtel RC, et al: The effects of physical therapy on cerebral palsy: a controlled trial in infants with spastic diplegia. N Engl J Med 318:803–808, 1988.

Piper MC, Kunos VI, Willis DM, et al: Early physical therapy effects on the high-risk infant: a randomized controlled trial. Pediatrics 78:216–224, 1986.

Sameroff AJ: Models of development and developmental risk. *In* Zeanah CH (ed): Handbook of Infant Mental Health. New York, Guilford Press, 1993, pp 3–13.

Shonkoff JP, Hauser-Cram P, Krauss MW, Upshur CC: Development of infants with disabilities and their families: implications for theory and service delivery. Monogr Soc Res Child Dev 57:1–167(6, Serial No. 230), 1992.

Spiker D, Hopmann MR: The effectiveness of early intervention for children with Down syndrome. *In* Guralnick MJ (ed): The Effectiveness of Early Intervention. Baltimore, Paul H. Brookes, 1997, pp 271–305.

Spiker D, Kraemer HC, Scott DT, Gross RT: Design issues in a randomized clinical trial of a behavioral intervention: insights from the Infant Health and Development Program. J Dev Behav Pediatr 12:386–393, 1991.

White KR, Boyce GC (eds): Comparative evaluations of early intervention alternatives (special issue). Early Ed Dev 4, 1993.

Zeanah CH (ed): Handbook of Infant Mental Health. New York, Guilford Press, 1993.

Zigler E, Valentine J (eds): Project Head Start: A Legacy of the War on Poverty. New York, Free Press, 1979.

81 The Arts Therapies

Donna Madden Chadwick

The early history of the arts is intimately associated with healing.

Arts therapists are highly trained clinical specialists, valued by treatment teams for their unique ability to combine psychotherapy with the creative process.

Arts therapies embody natural childhood behavior, a fail-safe context, creative expression, nonverbal qualities, improvisation, and aesthetic reception.

Several studies report the notable success of music therapy for young girls with Rett syndrome.

The Arts Therapies

Creative expression has been essential to human nature since the beginning of time, and the use of the arts against illness is as old as humankind itself. Early history of the arts is intimately associated with healing. Rituals employing a combination of music, visual arts, images, and dance to restore the health of an ailing individual are still used in various traditions as they were countless centuries ago. Art has always been included in humane treatment movements.

In all cultures, infants begin life soothed by lullabies, rocked in parents' arms. This fundamental experience inaugurates an instinctual connectedness to the arts. Everyone can relate in some way to dance, drama, song, and painting, because these art forms pervade religious, social, entertainment, and recreational domains. Professionally, these creative media become powerful diagnostic and treatment tools in the hands of skilled clinicians.

The first half of the 20th century brought recognition of the arts' treatment potential and inclusion of various arts into rehabilitation practices of the longer established disciplines of occupational therapy, physical therapy, and psychology.

Self-definition and strong professional identity propelled the formation of national associations for each art discipline. Research journals were published. By the 1970s, each organization had established academic training curricula. Universities granting degrees in art, dance and movement, and music therapy now number over 100 in the United States. Independent testing boards currently administer national credentialing examinations.

Undergraduate and graduate degree programs feature advanced art concentration, physiology, and emphasis on psychology. Intensive study of development, personality, group process, and population-specific intervention prepare the student for a rigorous apprenticeship-model internship. Psychodrama certification requires institute attendance.

Arts therapists are highly trained clinical specialists, valued by treatment teams for their unique ability to combine psychotherapy with the creative process. Creative arts therapists meet criteria as psychotherapists and should not be characterized as adjunctive or auxiliary (Zwerling, 1989).

Today, physicians and arts therapists interact as colleagues and collaborate on such efforts as the International Arts-Medicine Association and *International Journal of Arts Medicine*. A common expectation is that advanced neuroscience technology will allow validation of previously held intuitive beliefs about the healing capacities of the arts (Lippin, 1991).

The Arts as a Clinical Tool

Arts therapies are incomparable modalities, both because of their inherent nature and because of their unique application in clinical practice. They provide experiences that are available in no other intervention.

Although each discipline has its own manner of assessment and determining the desired outcome of treatment, they share certain salient features that make the arts different from all other therapies.

1. Natural childhood behavior: Children thrive in the arts because they incorporate the familiar, enjoyable acts of drawing, pretending, moving the body, singing, and exploring interesting instruments. Uninhibited expressions emerge easily through these intrinsically inviting channels.
2. Fail-safe context: In arts therapy, the child functions in a safe haven. All judgment is suspended and failure is prevented. The child is supported as he or she self-explores, takes risks, and assumes power.
3. Creative process: The essence of the therapy lies in creative expression and the relationships that develop as a result of them. Artistic acts can be satisfying and transformative. They access and nourish the "well" part of the child. The pride of creation is innately vitalizing and ignites self-esteem.
4. Nonverbal quality: Use of one's body, instruments, or art media can stand alone and "speak for itself." The art form is a metaphor, a surrogate voice. This gives the child a valid new avenue of communication free from verbal vulnerability.

5. Improvisation: Therapists use no rigid formulas. Rather, they apply art to mirror the child's emotional state continuously and spontaneously. The treatment is entirely child-centered and constantly evolving; the clinical relationship exists within the present moment of the art.

6. Aesthetic reception: Experience in beauty invests in the heart of the child. Identifying with the arts develops the capacity to be deeply moved, more balanced, and fully humanized.

Target Populations

Referral for treatment in arts therapy is on a child-by-child basis, but young persons who are partial to the arts are generally thought to have potential for most successful outcomes. Some client groups, characterized by diagnosis, are particularly good candidates for creative arts therapy.

EARLY INTERVENTION

Early identification of children who have special needs is imperative. As well as being cost-effective, it increases the probability that these children will achieve their fullest potential.

Often the profile of impaired infants and toddlers includes passivity caused by motor, sensory, and communication deficits that act as barriers to participation in the environment. In turn, underparticipation limits skill acquisition. The importance of active learning on young children's cognitive and social development has been established. Manipulating materials, engaging in activities, and interacting with others constitute active participation (Rosenberg et al, 1992).

A characteristic aspect of art experiences is personal involvement (Kreitler and Kreitler, 1972), and arts therapy makes a critical contribution by inciting interest in engaging with the external world. Within the context of the family, dance therapy uses movement and props to establish relationships and stimulate motor milestones. Music therapy employs a full complement of irresistable multisensory objects and activities. Imitating and expanding on the child's slightest expression, the clinician creates "arts contagion" by engulfing the child in sound, movement, tactile stimulation, and visual attraction. The special child responds much as a typical child would, by seeking involvement with the interesting presentations. His or her efforts are immediately reinforced by pleasant sensory feedback and the cognitive realization of cause and effect.

This high motivation to explore and interact externally generates momentum and generalizes to other experiences, developing a pattern of active learning.

THE CHILD WITH DEVELOPMENTAL DELAY

Art contributes to overall development by providing the conduit for responding to experience and expressing the change that occurs at every developmental stage (Ferrara, 1991). Able to address the cognitive, physical, social-emotional, and communication domains at any given juncture, arts therapies are so flexible that they seem "all-purpose" for the individual with developmental disabilities.

It is precisely this pliability that allows for a broad scope of application. The clinician is able to assess and address the needs of the child, no matter how diverse.

Treatment might focus on simple learning readiness goals such as attention span and eye contact or may strengthen more advanced areas. Working individually or with small groups of children, the therapist gives hands-on experiences that promote gross and fine motor skills, arouse feelings of self-worth, and stimulate communication.

When a creative art therapy is found to be particularly effective with a given child, other staff personnel may occasionally join in cotreatment for the purpose of acquiring and sharing techniques. This collaboration is often between physical therapy and dance and movement therapy or speech-language pathology and music therapy. For instance, the dance therapist and physical therapist may work together on sensory integration for a youngster diagnosed with pervasive developmental disorder, or on mobility with a teenager who has cerebral palsy. Music therapy encourages children without language to communicate and has developed a significant place in the treatment of mental disability in children (Aldridge, Gustorff, and Neugebauer, 1995).

Chief among music therapy approaches effective with children who have developmental delay is creative music therapy. Also known as the Nordoff-Robbins method, it features piano improvisation and musical interresponsiveness as a basis for development of the child's expressive freedom. Immersion in the beauty of creative music therapy taps artistic intelligence and awakens the child's aesthetic appreciation (Fig. 81–1).

These values are often overlooked in children with developmental disabilities. But attraction to aesthetics, and in some cases their achievement through arts, can be as strong as in any human being. Artwork by some persons with mental retardation is described as having beautiful purity of pictorial style, created with intuitive awareness (Arnheim, 1994). Many persons with developmental delay love to show off their accomplishments by performing. Although never an end in itself, public performance can be a goal of treatment because of the self-discipline and social benefit it provides.

EXAMPLE

Blind, nonverbal, and profoundly multiply disabled, Lauren was cognitively untestable. Yet music therapy proved her intelligence by uncovering a staggering memory, interpretive sensitivity, taste, and humor. With confidence and self-esteem, she now sings accurate lyric approximations of repertoire from opera to jazz. She performs annually with other differently abled musicians and enjoys music as the foundation of her community interaction. Doctors report that music therapy has improved respiration and countered gastroesophageal reflux and the constant threat of pneumonia. Lauren's mother, who often participates in sessions at home, says, "Music therapy has made a dramatic contribution to the physical and emotional quality of both our lives. In a lifetime of thera-

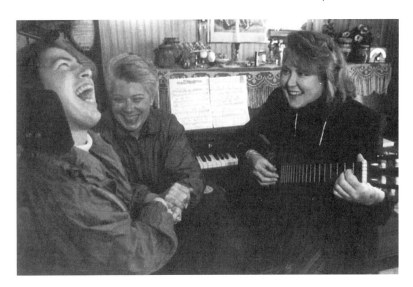

Figure 81–1. Mother and daughter share exhilaration during music therapy. (Photo copyright Joanne Ciccarello, 1997.)

pies, it is the single most important treatment my daughter receives."

Of particular importance is the social value of arts participation. It can become the common denominator in peer interactions throughout a special child's life. Very Special Arts recognizes and celebrates the significance of artistic endeavors to persons who have disabilities. Although not formally allied with the arts therapies, the organization is mentioned here because their programs, available in each of the 50 states, promote creative experiences for children and adults with disabilities. Involvement in Very Special Arts for the adult with developmental delay is never a substitute for arts therapies, but it offers some degree of continuity after arts therapies in individual education programs have ceased. The arts can be a lifelong basis for social experience and community association.

RETT SYNDROME

From infancy, most girls diagnosed with Rett syndrome find music captivating even if they eschew other activities. Music therapy treats the whole child and is strongly recommended by many physicians, as it was by Professor Andreas Rett, who discovered this disorder (Allan, 1989). There may be a physical basis for its effectiveness. The limbic system, particularly the hypothalamus, registers music as pleasurable. Pleasure evokes feelings, and feelings generate an impulse to open action. Emotion and motivation are essential manifestations of limbic function. Music animates the girl internally. It is an agent of arousal that starts in motion a cycle of excitement and action.

The most universal and clearly identifiable feature of Rett syndrome is hand stereotypies, in which neurologically driven rhythmic movements such as wringing, clapping, washing, and squeezing present at midline or mouth level. These involuntary patterns are so pervasive that they prevent functional hand use. One major objective in music therapy for patients with Rett syndrome is managing hand use and promoting active contact with the environment. Using live vibrotactile music in close proximity, the clinician attempts to influence the energy of the child and thus modify the stereotypies in either of two completely different ways:

1. To relax the child to a degree that enables her to separate and then to some extent functionally use her hands
2. To excite the child to a degree that allows her to override the stereotypies and use her hands to reach out (to an irresistible instrument or person)

Several studies report success of music therapy with young children with Rett syndrome (Hadsell and Coleman, 1988; Wesecky, 1986; Wigram, 1991). Hand use such as touching, tapping, grasping, and maintaining contact with an instrument dramatically increased in two girls after a period of music therapy (Wylie, 1996). A second and equally important goal of music therapy is establishing an affective connection, through which life experience can be reflected. These girls, who are so rhythmic, so audiominded, and so emotional, function on that deep level of consciousness where music also has its roots. Through music therapy, the girls' inner desires and abilities can be captured (Lindberg, 1991).

THE CHILD IN EMOTIONAL DISTRESS

The child in emotional distress may have exhausted his or her tolerance for verbal communication or may be confused and entirely unwilling or unable to express himself or herself, while harboring intense and unbearable subconscious feelings. Creative arts therapies are highly appropriate regardless of the source of distress. The child is naturally attracted to the art medium, which serves as a point of contact and mutuality. Here, the arts support the child's coping efforts and provide channels through which fear, anger, sadness, and loneliness can be expressed (Rollins, 1993). The child is free to "act out" in ways unacceptable in other settings—by wildly banging a drum, screaming, constructing and then destroying a clay figure, or bodily letting go. Masterful guidance by the clinician establishes a trusting relationship that provides a vehicle to catharsis.

Perceived as "fun," the arts overcome the vulnerable

child's conscious resistance and give him or her natural tools for expressing any mood. Nonverbal and symbolic, they tap directly into primary emotional processes.

Art therapy may enable the child to put on paper unspeakable feelings of sexual violation; psychodrama may allow the child to act out his or her own feelings under the guise of "playing a part." The inherent form and structure of the arts contributes to containing these volatile experiences. This "ordering" promotes internal self-organization and influences impulse control. There is a delicate balance between improvisational freedom and the child's gaining self-control.

One's movements, artwork, and music improvisation are metaphors of one's inner life. They are surrogate voices that give form to deeply held thoughts. Acts of creation in these media arouse and release potent perceptions that the therapist can immediately address in treatment.

In situations in which words seem to escalate discord and divide people even further, arts therapies afford a different and creative approach. The arts are used in crisis intervention as well as conflict resolution. Trauma also warrants new models of healing emotional wounds. Art therapy was applied to children who survived the 1994 Los Angeles earthquake (Roje, 1995), and music therapy helped survivors of the Oklahoma City bombing (Borczon, 1995).

HOSPITALIZATION

The hospitalized child experiences serious psychological and physical stress. The arts therapist is his or her ally, a nonthreatening person who not only does not cause pain but may even alleviate it. Music is effective as a noninvasive method of pain management, used to distract pediatric patients during procedures such as intravenous starts and venipunctures (Malone, 1996).

Many therapists invite family members to join the patient and participate in group sessions. This shared time "away" from the illness provides respite from fear and anxiety, while all participants are swept into the process of creating. Moving, drawing, or singing allows them to simply experience pleasure together, and returns the comforting feeling of unity known by the family before the hospital admission. Individual sessions often center on assisting the child to comprehend and cope with the experience, externalizing concerns, and alleviating psychic pain (Prager, 1993).

Accessing Services

Under PL 105-17, known as the Individuals with Disabilities Education Act (IDEA), a physician or family member can refer a child to the local school administration for assessment by a creative arts therapist. The assessment is then considered by a team composed of pertinent educators, therapists, and the parents as they design the individual educational plan (IEP), which is the blueprint for the next year's detailed education and treatment program. Creative arts therapies are mandated as essential services in an increasing number of IEPs. When art, dance and movement, or music therapy is called for in the IEP, it is funded by the community in which the family resides.

In some states such as Massachusetts and California, creative arts therapists are sanctioned as Licensed Mental Health Counselors or Marriage and Family Counselors. As such, they are eligible to receive insurance reimbursement from the HMO industry and Blue Cross and Blue Shield. If a family wishes to contract the services of a creative arts therapist on a private basis, they will find the cost to be similar to that for other clinical disciplines, such as speech pathology or physical therapy.

> Creative arts therapies are mandated as essential services in an increasing number of IEPs.

RESOURCES

Arts therapists are employed by hospitals, mental health agencies, community clinics and centers, and private and public schools. Increasingly, individuals are operating private clinical practices, which provide client assessment, treatment, and consulting services.

The national association for each creative arts therapy compiles an annually updated directory that contains the geographic location and clinical specialty of its credentialed members. The association can supply a referral to practitioners in any community. A list of resources can be found following the references.

REFERENCES

Aldridge D, Gustorff D, Neugebauer L: A preliminary study of creative music therapy in the treatment of children with developmental delay. Arts Psychother 22(3):189, 1995.

Allan I: Rett Syndrome: A View on Care and Management. Clinton, MD, International Rett Syndrome Association, 1989.

Arnheim R: Artistry in retardation. Arts Psychother 21(5):329, 1994.

Borczon R: Remembering Oklahoma City. Natl Assoc Music Ther Notes Summer Issue:1, 1995.

Ferrara N: Art as a reflection of child development. Am J Art Ther 30:44, 1991.

Hadsell N, Coleman K: Rett syndrome: a challenge for music therapists. Music Ther Perspect 5:52, 1988.

Kreitler H, Kreitler S: Psychology of the Arts. Durham, NC, Duke University Press, 1972.

Lindberg B: Understanding Rett Syndrome. Toronto, Canada, Hogrefe and Huber Publishers, 1991.

Lippin R: A message from the president of International Arts Medicine Association. Int J Arts Med 1(1):4, 1991.

Malone AB: The effects of live music on the distress of pediatric patients receiving intravenous starts, venipunctures, injections, and heel sticks. J Music Ther 33(1):19, 1996.

Prager A: The art therapist's role in working with hospitalized children. Am J Art Ther 32(8/93):2, 1993.

Roje J: LA '94 earthquake in the eyes of children: art therapy with elementary school children who were victims of disaster. Art Ther J Am Art Ther Assoc 12(4):237, 1995.

Rollins J: Medical students as facilitators of the arts for children in hospitals. Int J Arts Med 2(1):7, 1993.

Rosenberg S, Clark M, Filer J, et al: Facilitating active learner participation. J Early Intervention 16(3):262, 1992.

Wesecky A: Music therapy for children with Rett syndrome. Am J Med Genet 24:253, 1986.

Wigram T: Music therapy for a girl with Rett's syndrome: balancing structure and freedom. *In* Bruscia K (ed): Case Studies in Music Therapy, Phoenixville, PA, Barcelona Publishers, 1991, p 39.

Wylie ME: A case study to promote hand use in children with Rett syndrome. Music Ther Perspect 14(2):83, 1996.

Zwerling I: The creative arts therapies as "real therapies." Am J Dance Ther 11(1):19, 1989.

Resources: National Associations

American Art Therapy Association
1202 Allanson Road
Mundelein, IL 60060
(847)949-6064
www.arttherapy.org

American Dance Therapy Association
Suite 108
2000 Century Plaza
Columbia, MD 21044
(410)997-4040

American Association of Group Psychotherapy and Psychodrama
301 North Harrison Street, Suite 508
Princeton, NJ 08540
(609)452-1339
www.asgpp.org

In 1998, the AAMT and NAMT unified to form one organization:
American Music Therapy Association
8455 Colesville Rd., Suite 1000
Silver Spring, MD 20910
(301)589-3300
www.musictherapy.org

82 Pediatric Psychopharmacology

Martin Baren

 Psychopharmacology has become an increasingly prominent component of the developmental-behavioral pediatric curriculum. The use of drugs to improve behavior, affect, and learning during childhood has become widespread. There are a multitude of advantages and disadvantages inherent in this form of treatment. This chapter, written by a pediatrician, provides a uniquely pediatric approach to psychopharmacology. It describes what is known, what is suspected, and what remains a mystery when it comes to the pharmacology of behavior and development. What emerges is a conservative and careful set of guidelines for the pediatric use of these brain-altering potions.

The treatment of childhood behavioral, emotional, and psychological disorders with medication is a new and burgeoning growth industry. Over the past 30 years or more, as more definitive diagnostic studies have identified and further defined and refined the various disorders, clinicians have tried to keep therapeutic approaches (including the use of psychotropic medications) abreast with the diagnostic categories.

In the 1960s and 1970s, the use of psychostimulants on "hyperactive" children was beginning to focus on the use of medication for child and adolescent behavioral problems; since then, the number of diagnostic categories and drugs that are used has grown at a rapidly increasing pace (Towbin, 1995).

As more children and adolescents continue to be given diagnoses of these types of disorders, it is likely that the use of psychotropic medication will continue to increase. It is also probable that the number of different and newer drugs used in this population will grow at the same rate or even faster. This chapter looks at diagnostic categories that are thought to be amenable to treatment with psychotropic medication and at the increasing number of drugs being used to meet these needs. The most important point to establish, however, is whether good matches of drug and diagnosis are being made or whether a "square" medication is being fit into a "round" diagnosis.

The first step in establishing diagnostic and therapeutic ground rules for treatment is to arrive at the correct diagnosis. Not only is it important to establish the correct diagnosis, but also it is important to determine the severity and the amount of impairment for this group of diagnoses.

One of the major problems encountered in dealing with mental, behavioral, emotional, and psychological disorders is the fact that the "gold standard" for establishing a diagnosis is always the history, which often needs to be obtained from many sources. Thus, in many cases, a correct diagnosis is not reached because of an imperfect diagnostic process. This is often seen in the most common behavioral disorder of childhood—attention-deficit hyperactivity disorder (ADHD). Many children and adolescents are underdiagnosed and overdiagnosed; therefore, can we surmise that

an imperfect medical intervention might well follow an imperfect diagnosis? The answer is yes.

Another fact to consider concerning the diagnostic process is that clinicians usually rely on sets of criteria as set forth in the various editions of the *Diagnostic and Statistical Manual of Mental Disorders (DSM)* (American Psychiatric Association, 1994). Often, the criteria for the diagnosis of various disorders change through each edition of the manual. Thus, a child or adolescent's diagnosis might be made or missed according to the set of criteria invoked at that particular time, and many clinicians use either all criteria or no criteria at all to establish a diagnosis. Can medical mismanagement be far behind? Finally, many workers in this field do not recognize the validity of the *DSM*-generated criteria, and medical therapy is thus often generated on the basis of experience, a feel for some disorder, or not much evidence at all. This situation often makes it difficult to evaluate the efficacy of the treatment among various groups of disorders and patients when there is no level playing field of diagnosis.

Once a diagnosis *is* established, a whole host of interventions might be indicated for a proper therapeutic approach. In treating children and adolescents, there are at least three major areas of concern: (1) behavioral and emotional care for a child and his or her family, (2) the school situation, and (3) medication therapy. In addition to these therapeutic modalities, other needs must be met, including addressing physical problems, disorders of the special senses, and dietary and nutritional concerns.

Another important and often ignored dictum is the establishment of the amount of impairment that the particular disorder is causing the child or adolescent before a therapeutic plan is implemented. For example, a child with ADHD might do perfectly well with only educational and behavioral interventions instead of psychostimulant medical therapy, or perhaps a child has disorders that cause no social or academic concerns.

Clinicians must also consider whether medical therapy is even effective for most of the diagnostic categories that are being treated. The use of psychotropic medications for children and adolescents has not been well documented with well-controlled studies for the most part, except perhaps in the area of ADHD and perhaps some depressive disorders, tic disorders, and, to some degree, some child and adolescent psychoses and obsessive-compulsive disorders (OCDs) (Famularo and Kinscherff, 1992; Walkup, 1995). Thus, it is often difficult to formulate a therapeutic regimen that is based on solid evidence of efficacy. Because of this, the use of these medications for many children and adolescents is often based on studies in adult patients, clinical experience, case reports, open "studies," anecdotal experiences culled from medical peers, or other unsubstantiated sources.

Whenever a course of treatment with psychotropic drugs is indicated, the results of efficacy should be discussed with the parents or guardians and, when appropriate, the patients. In the case of medication that has been approved only for adults but that has been used and reported as being somewhat successful in children, there is a so-called community standard of practice dilemma. Even if a drug has been approved by the Food and Drug Administration for established and safe usage for specific age groups, it does not limit the prescribing of this drug for only these indications (Towbin, 1995). Thus, this often makes it much easier to transfer accepted and proven results in adults to trial and error in children and adolescents. This practice is widely used and, in many cases, has led to some excellent results. However, the physician who does the prescribing must be fully aware of the background of this particular medical intervention.

As part of this picture of pediatric pharmacology, there is a question of whether medications should be used in combination for many disorders. "Polypharmacy" or combined "psychopharmacology" has become an acceptable route to take for many of the disorders that are being treated. This is true for diagnostic entities that have shown a proven response to certain medications as well as those disorders that have not been shown to be responsive to any one medication, let alone a combination of such medical trials. In many cases, there are fairly good results from this type of approach (such as in ADHD with concomitant depression, anxiety, or tic disorders, or in children and adolescents with other comorbid diagnoses such as OCD or aggressive behavior). In many cases, however, these combinations do not meet specific therapeutic goals, are poorly conceived, present undesirable side effects, or even interfere with or increase the absorption of each other. In some cases, the physician prescriber is not even aware of the danger or adverse conditions engendered by such therapy.

Another recent trend has been not only the use of multiple medications in children or adolescents but also the rapid change from one combination to another as in treating some types of infections with antibiotics. In most such cases, the polypharmacy was instituted without a good understanding of the diagnostic disorders being treated, the usual response of these patients to various medications, the goals of treatment, and the lack of utilization of other interventions. This practice has seemed to have caught on solidly in both the literature (usually in uncontrolled studies or case reports) and clinical practice. Even though some children and adolescents do need more than one drug to help them overcome their problems, especially if they have more than one diagnosis, clinicians must still be very careful of the time honored doctrine to "do no harm."

Once a physician decides on the medical interventions to be tried, the goals of therapy should be clearly defined to the patient or parent and should be fully understood by the physician himself or herself. The physician must develop a clear-cut picture of behavior to be affected with the medication as well as possible side effects and adverse responses and then effectively communicate this to the parents and patients.

Every child or adolescent who is given psychopharmacologic therapy should have not only a complete diagnostic investigation but also a thorough medical, and when indicated, laboratory evaluation. The patient and his or her family should also be assured that the professional who is prescribing the medication is fully aware of not only the positive results to be hoped for but also any negative or adverse responses to be aware of. Thus, the following dicta should always be observed:

1. No matter who the physician is, if the disorder, the needs of the patient, and the positive or negative merits of the medication are not fully understood, the patient should be referred to someone who is more familiar with the essentials.
2. Similarly, a physician who is quite knowledgeable in the tenets of psychopharmacology in children and adolescents but who is unfamiliar with the physical or laboratory necessities to be used with such interventions should not administer this drug.

With these two criteria in mind, no medication in this group should be prescribed without the physician's total knowledge of the patient's condition and the particular medication. No medication should be prescribed without the patient's undergoing a complete physical examination and providing a medical history, and without laboratory investigations, when applicable.

Finally, the issue of informed consent must be considered. Before any psychotropic medication is prescribed, a parent or guardian should be fully informed of the objectives of therapy as far as symptoms are concerned and of the adverse effects of the medications. The information should include details about the medication itself, known efficacy in previous scientific studies and clinical experience, common and most observed side effects and risks, what should and should not occur, problems with interactions with other medications, and how to follow up the course of treatment with the physician. This information should be presented to the parents or caretakers (as well as the patients when applicable) in written form. Finally, signed documentation that the patient was informed of possible special risks involved in some conditions should be included in the patient's chart (such as in the case of the use of stimulants in children with tic disorders or with various combination of drugs such as clonidine and methylphenidate).

As the course of treatment evolves, communication with the patient's family, the patient himself or herself when appropriate, teachers and other school personnel, and other professionals such as mental health workers is essential. Follow-up visits vary according to the severity of the problem or the particular practice of the prescribing physician. These visits must include ongoing appropriate physical examinations including height and weight, blood pressure, heart rate, hearing and vision, appropriate laboratory tests, and electrocardiograms where necessary. Every child or adolescent who is taking any psychotropic medication must be physically examined at least two to three times a year. Educational histories and evaluations should also be carefully followed up in order to more appropriately deal with the total needs of the patient. Telephone conversations, rating scales, and other exchanges of information about the patient are indispensable to the appropriate total care package that must evolve. A prescription alone never suffices and may be the biggest cause of the lack of a better understanding of what value psychotropic medications actually do have in this age group.

Current Conditions for Which Medication Is Used

1. Psychotropic medication is used in the following fairly well-documented disorders: ADHD, tic disorders including Tourette disorder, major depressive disorder, some psychotic disorders, and OCD.
2. Disorders in which medication is often used but in which efficacy is still not well established include dysthymic disorders, other mood disorders including mania and bipolar disorder, conduct disorder, anxiety, and aggressive disorders.
3. Disorders in which medication is used despite poor documentation concerning efficacy include oppositional defiant disorders, phobias, panic disorders, and pervasive disorders including autism (Famularo and Kinscherff, 1992).

The medical therapy of the aforementioned disorders is discussed herein with the understanding that the diagnostic evaluation, medical and laboratory (when indicated) examinations, and other appropriate interventions have been initiated. For instance, the child with ADHD should have in place a program that includes educational interventions and circumventions and the use of behavioral and psychological modalities, with a total approach to the particular disorder having been discussed with the patient and family. This chapter deals only with the current medical approach to each diagnostic entity. For each entity, medications that are considered to be efficacious are discussed, as are medications for which efficacy is uncertain.

Fairly Well Documented Conditions

ATTENTION-DEFICIT HYPERACTIVITY DISORDER

ADHD is the most common behavioral disorder of childhood and engenders the most controversy as to diagnosis and management. This section highlights the medical management of ADHD (see Chapter 52).

To start, the clinician must be certain that he or she is dealing with a bona fide diagnosis that has been documented by extensive history and neurodevelopmental evaluation and other diagnostic modalities that are well documented as necessary for a complete and valid diagnosis (Baren, 1994). After arriving at the diagnosis (for which the gold standard of diagnosis is still behavioral rather than by laboratory or high-technology means), the clinician must ensure that the various signs and symptoms shown by the patient are being caused by ADHD and not by another disorder such as learning or language disabilities, anxiety, or depression or by other problems. Finally, the clinician must establish whether other types of disorders might be present (comorbid diagnoses) that alter or interfere with any medical therapy prescribed.

When the clinician is ready to treat ADHD, he or she must be certain to use the multimodal model that is agreed on by most authorities; this model includes educational, behavioral, psychological, and other interventions, sometimes before medication is suggested (Levine, 1992).

When all the aforementioned situations have been addressed and a course of psychopharmacology is to be undertaken, there are some important points to consider concerning the efficacy of the medical treatment of ADHD. Just what does medication accomplish or not accomplish? The most common and effective medications used for ADHD are the psychostimulants (see Stimulant Medications Used for Attention-Deficit Hyperactivity Disorder) (Cantwell, 1995). There are many secondary and tertiary drugs that are used and that are not as effective, but they might be considered in the case of an adverse response, comorbid diagnoses, or other negative effects of the stimulants. However, stimulant medications are effective for at least the short-term treatment of ADHD in 60% to 90% of patients (DuPaul and Stoner, 1994).

When using these medications, improvements can be expected in symptoms and signs such as overactivity, inattention, impulsivity, compliance, hostility (and perhaps aggression), social interaction, and academic productivity, including handwriting. Clinicians should not expect a prediction of response by any neurologic, physiologic, or biochemical markers; nor should improvement in academic skills (such as reading, spelling, and mathematics) be expected, except in performance (which entails listening, completing assignments, organization, study skills, and following directions) (Swanson, McBurnett, and Wigal, 1993).

Psychostimulant medication produces stimulation of the central nervous system in areas that control impulses, attention, and self-regulation of behavior. Effects of the medication are probably related to the increased availability of the neurotransmitters dopamine and noradrenaline by either increased production or decreased absorption at the synapses.

Stimulant Medications Used for Attention-Deficit Hyperactivity Disorder (Table 82–1)

Stimulant medications used for ADHD include the following:

- Methylphenidate (Ritalin)
- Dextroamphetamine sulfate (Dexedrine, Dextrostat)
- Dextroamphetamine saccharate and sulfate, amphetamine aspartate, and amphetamine sulfate (Adderall)
- Methamphetamine (Desoxyn)
- Pemoline (Cylert)*

This group of medications is the standard bearer for ADHD therapy. Methylphenidate is the most widely used

---

*No longer considered a first-line drug because of an unfavorable side effect profile.

Table 82–1 • Psychostimulants

Medications	Methylphenidate (Ritalin)
	Amphetamines—dextroamphetamine sulfate (Dexedrine, Dextrostat); dextroamphetamine saccharate and sulfate, amphetamine aspartate and sulfate (Adderall); methamphetamine (Desoxyn)
	Pemoline (Cylert)—considered to be a second-line drug because of reports of cases of liver failure
How supplied	Ritalin: 5-, 10-, 20-mg tablets: sustained release 20-mg tablets (SR 20)
	Dexedrine: 5-mg tablets; 5-, 10-, 15-mg spansules
	Dextrostat: 5- and 10-mg tablets
	Adderall: 5-, 10-, 20-, and 30-mg tablets
	Desoxyn: Gradumets (sustained release—5-, 10-, 15-mg tablets)
	Cylert: 18.75-, 37.5-, 75-mg tablets; chewable tablets 37.5 mg
Mode of action	Increased release of dopamine and norepinephrine by preventing reuptake into presynaptic nerve endings and probably stimulating direct production as well. Methylphenidate may have more of a dopaminergic effect than amphetamines, which may be more noradrenergic.
Side effects	Most common: anorexia, weight loss, insomnia (? from rebound), rebound when wearing off, abdominal pain, headaches, nausea.
	Less common: tachycardia, blood pressure elevation, nervousness, skin rashes, hives, dizziness, lower complete blood count and platelet counts, abnormal liver function (Cylert), fever, arthralgia.
	Rare: psychotic symptoms, hair loss, growth suppression.
Adverse reaction	Usually resulting from overdose or improper choice: irritability, lethargy, mood change and depression, sleepiness, sadness, crying.
	Tic situation: Many children with attention deficits have associated tic disorders. Stimulants may cause them to emerge or worsen, but do not cause the tics. Tics are not considered a contraindication for stimulant therapy at this time.
Dosage	Always start with lowest dosage and give once a day with or after meals. Then slowly increase as reports are received about efficacy or problems. Short-acting forms are usually given twice daily, but third and fourth doses are often needed. Always start with short-acting to better titrate. Usual dose of Ritalin is 0.3 to 0.5 mg/kg/dose with a daily dose not usually exceeding 2 mg/kg. Amphetamines are usually thought to be 25%–30% more potent than methylphenidate, so 10 mg of methylphenidate will usually be equivalent to 7.5 mg of amphetamines.
Length of action	Ritalin: approx. 4 hr; SR 20: 6–8 hr
	Dexedrine: 4–5 hr; spansule: 6–10 hr
	Adderall: 4–6 hr; Cylert: 6–8 hr
Comments	Do blood counts at least yearly with Cylert. Also do baseline and ongoing liver function tests. Do not have medication chewed; no withdrawal problems. Do not give amphetamines with orange juice. Be careful in depressed or anxious patients.
Drug interaction	Occasional increase of heart rate with nasal decongestants. May increase blood level of tricyclic antidepressants, some anticonvulsants, and anticoagulants. Dexedrine inhibits adrenergic blockers. Lithium slightly inhibits action of amphetamines.

drug, but each of the aforementioned medications has been relatively successful. In planning a therapeutic approach, it should be noted that there is much variability in the response of individuals to each of these medications. If one of the stimulants does not produce a desired therapeutic effect, each of the others should be tried before giving up.

Methylphenidate and dextroamphetamine sulfate are the drugs that are probably best to use for a therapeutic trial, simply because they come in a shorter-acting form for which the response time is approximately 4 hours. Thus, it is easier to regulate the initial response in most patients rather than to use a medication with a longer half-life. Adderall has a bit longer half-life and produces a 5- to 6-hour effect. Pemoline and methamphetamine come only in longer-acting forms and thus may be very successful in some situations, especially for older patients, but they are harder to titrate when starting therapy.

Other Medications for ADHD

When the stimulants do not work or have adverse effects, there are many other medications belonging to various different groups that have been used. Some of the indications for nonstimulant treatment include poor response or adverse reactions, side effects that are difficult to live with,

the presence of comorbid conditions such as depression, anxiety, aggressive behavior, and tics, and the possibility of abuse by the patient or family. The duration of therapy and dosing problems should also be considered.

Tricyclic Antidepressants (Table 82–2)

Imipramine (Tofranil), desipramine (Norpramin), and nortriptyline (Pamelor) are the drugs that have the most noradrenergic properties in this group. They have been shown to be fairly successful for patients with ADHD who cannot take stimulants for various reasons (Green, 1995). This group might also be helpful for the patient with ADHD and tic disorders in which the tics are exacerbated by the stimulant and the use of several medications is undesirable (Spencer et al, 1993). The tricyclics seem to work fairly well for the impulsivity and hyperactivity of ADHD, but not as much for inattention (Wender, 1988). They are usually thought to be less effective overall than the stimulants. Another issue that makes this group strictly a second line of attack is the side effect profile, especially their cardiovascular and anticholinergic properties. Desipramine has shown the greatest efficacy for ADHD in this group, but recently nortriptyline has also been shown to produce good results.

Table 82–2 • Tricyclic Antidepressants

Medications	Imipramine (Tofranil)—10-, 25-, 50-mg tablets; PM cap: 25, 100, 125, 150 mg Desipramine (Norpramin)—10-, 25-, 50-, 75-, 100-, 150-mg tablets Nortriptyline (Pamelor)—10-, 25-, 50-, 75-mg caps, solution Amitriptyline (Elavil)—10-, 25-, 50-, 75-, 100-, 150-mg tablets Clomipramine (Anafranil) (mostly used for OCD)—25-, 50-, 75-mg caps
Mode of action	Imipramine and desipramine block reuptake of noradrenalin; nortriptyline has noradrenergic as well as other cholinergic effects; amitriptyline is both noradrenergic as well as serotonergic; clomipramine is primarily serotonergic.
Side effects	There are many possible adverse reactions listed in the *Physician's Desk Reference*. The most common ones seen in children include nervousness, sleepiness, dry mouth, and mild gastrointestinal disturbances including constipation. There can also be weight gain or loss, irritability, nightmares, anxiety, seizures, syncope, and dizziness. With higher doses, ECG changes may be seen. The major problems are in conduction system with increases in the PR, QRS, and QT$_c$ intervals. Also increased heart rate and blood pressure might be present. Several cases of sudden cardiac death have been seen in young children taking desipramine and it is thought that this probably does represent a slightly increased risk in children younger than age 12 years. Other side effects include rashes, trouble urinating, and blurred vision. Clomipramine may cause the same profile of side effects, but it also shows a risk of 1/1000 for seizures.
Withdrawal	Flulike syndrome with headaches, other aches and pains, gastrointestinal symptoms, nervousness, malaise.
Dosage	Start with smaller doses of 10 or 25 mg daily, given at bedtime and slowly increase every 5 to 7 days up to total daily dose of 2.5 mg/kg (nortriptyline 1.5 mg/kg) or when clinical improvement is seen. Doses of 2.5 to 5.0 mg/kg have been used by some workers, but possible toxicity occurs at higher doses. As doses increase, blood levels and ECGs should be done at each level. Clomipramine should start with divided doses with meals. Start with 25 mg and increase to 100 mg or 3 mg/kg (whichever dose is smaller) and finally give entire dose at bedtime. Other tricyclic antidepressants are usually given twice daily to children and adolescents.
Comments	Smaller doses of imipramine, nortriptyline and desipramine needed for ADHD symptoms, effects seen sooner. Upper limit of 0.45 seconds for QT$_c$, especially with desipramine. Routine CBC and liver function tests.
Drug interaction	May block effect of clonidine. Be careful using with anticholinergics or sympathomimetics. Do not use with thyroid medications. May increase psychostimulant levels and vice versa. Watch with antiasthmatic drugs. Avoid sunlight. Avoid use with MAO inhibitors.

OCD = obsessive-compulsive disorder; ECG = electrocardiogram; CBC = complete blood count; MAO = monoamine oxidase.

Alpha-2 Adrenergic Agonists (Table 82–3)

Clonidine (Catapres) and guanfacine (Tenex) are alpha-2 adrenergic agonists. Clonidine has been the most used drug in this group for ADHD (Hunt, Capper, and O'Connell, 1990). This drug helps hyperarousal, impulsivity, and aggressiveness by cutting down noradrenergic output, but it does not have much of an effect on inattention. This group of drugs also might be helpful in patients with comorbid tic disorders. Many physicians use clonidine along with a psychostimulant to increase the effect in the hyperactive impulsive behavior and perhaps help lower the dose of stimulant medication. Other patients may be given clonidine to help with the sleep problems that many ADHD patients have, especially when on stimulant medications. However, the combined use of stimulants and clonidine is under scrutiny since a report of at least six cases of sudden cardiac death (Swanson et al, 1995) in patients who were on this combination.

Other Antidepressants (Table 82–4)

Bupropion (Wellbutrin), which is not related to the tricyclics, exhibits dopaminergic as well as serotonergic and some weak noradrenergic activity. Several small studies have shown positive effects for ADHD in children. However, because of the side effect profile and scarcity of controlled studies, this drug is still considered to be second or third line (Popper, 1995a).

Venlafaxine (Effexor) inhibits the uptake of serotonin and norepinephrine and has a slight effect on dopamine.

Table 82–3 • Alpha-2 Adrenergic Agonists

Medications	Clonidine (Catapres)—0.1-, 0.2-, 0.3-mg tablets; 0.1–0.3 mg transdermal patch Guanfacine (Tenex)—1-, 2-mg tablets
Mode of action	Stimulates alpha-2 adrenoreceptors, resulting in reduced sympathetic outflow.
Side effects	Mainly drowsiness; also dry mouth, hypotension, depression, constipation, headache, vascular changes, skin reaction to patch.
Withdrawal	Stop slowly to prevent sudden increase in blood pressure and other side effects.
Dosage	Clonidine: 3–7 μg/kg/d in three doses. Start with 0.025–0.05 mg at bedtime and increase slowly. Guanfacine: longer acting than clonidine, therefore two doses/d. Start with 0.5 mg/d and may increase after 1 week to 1 mg. Do not use more than 2–3 mg/d.
Drug interaction	Increased sedation when given with other central nervous system depressants. Tricyclic antidepressants reduce clonidine levels.

Table 82–4 • Antidepressants

Buproprion (Wellbutrin)—75- and 100-mg tablets	
Chemically unrelated to tricyclics or tetracyclics. An aminoketone with effects on serotonin uptake as well as dopamine and to some extent norepinephrine.	
Side effects	Seizures in 4/1000 patients. Other common side effects include agitation, dry mouth, constipation, insomnia, rashes, headache, nausea, vomiting, tremors, sweating, anxiety, weight loss.
Dosage	Use t.i.d. with maximum dosage of 450 mg/d. Start with 75 mg b.i.d. Optimal dose in children, 3–7 mg/kg/d (100–250 mg/d).
Comment	Used for attention deficits in older children and adolescents. Not well established for depression.
Drug interaction	Not well established. Do not use in patients with eating disorders (seizure risk).
Venlafaxine (Effexor)—25-, 37.5-, 50-, 75-, 100-mg tablets	
Selectively inhibits reuptake of norepinephrine as well as serotonin and weakly affects dopamine reuptake—an amphetamine analogue.	
Side effects	Sleepiness, nausea, dizziness, dry mouth, sustained increase in diastolic blood pressure, headache, insomnia, and many other less frequent effects such as sweating and constipation.
Dosage	Initial dose in children: 12.5 mg b.i.d.–t.i.d. with food. Optimal dose in children not established. In adolescents: 1–3 mg/kg/d up to 150–200 mg/d.
Drug interaction	Not well established except with MAO inhibitors
Trazodone (Desyrel)—50-, 100-, 150-, 300-mg tablets	
Questionably inhibits serotonin uptake.	
Side effects	Dry mouth, dizziness, drowsiness, fatigue, and orthostatic hypotension. Nervousness and many others in smaller numbers.
Dosage	No accepted doses for children, but range is probably 2–5 mg/kg/d. Take after meals. Start with 150 mg/d in divided doses. Do not exceed 400 mg/d.
Comments	Often gives response in first week. Has been used for aggression, disruptive behavior, and insomnia in children.

t.i.d. = three times a day; b.i.d. = twice daily; MAO = monoamine oxidase.

Table 82–5 • Antidepressants—Serotonin-Reuptake Inhibitors

Medications	Fluoxetine (Prozac)
	Sertraline (Zoloft)
	Paroxetine (Paxil)
	Fluvoxamine (Luvox)
How supplied	Fluoxetine: 10-, 20-mg pulvules; oral solution 20 mg/5 mL
	Sertraline: 50-, 100-mg tablets (scored)
	Paroxetine: 10-, 20-, 30-, 40-mg tablets
	Fluvoxamine: 50-, 100-mg tablets (scored)
Mode of action	Inhibition of CNS neuronal serotonin uptake. Fluvoxamine is chemically unrelated to other serotonin reuptake inhibitors.
Side effects	Nausea, headache, weight loss or gain, anxiety, nervousness, dizziness, insomnia or somnolence, fatigue, sweating, tremors, diarrhea, dry mouth, rash. There are many other less common (such as male sexual dysfunction), listed in the *Physician's Desk Reference*.
	Toxic serotonin syndrome is usually due to high doses or interaction with other drugs such as TCAs, lithium, MAO inhibitors, and others. Symptoms vary from mild to major and include mood swings, neurologic symptoms, vegetative problems, and many others affecting mostly all organ systems. Mood changes, myoclonus, shivering, and tremors are early signs, and fatalities have occurred.
	Fluoxetine and other serotonin reuptake inhibitors have also produced prefrontal symptom aggravation including hyperactivity, impulsivity, inattention, and rages. There have also been reports of an "amotivational syndrome," with apathy and indifference.
Dosage	Fluoxetine: Start with 10 mg; up to 0.5 to 1.0 mg/kg/d. Give once in morning; may take 4 weeks to achieve effect.
	Sertraline: Start with 25 mg b.i.d.; may increase to 100–200 mg/d (1.5–3.0 mg/kg/d). Steady state achieved in 1 week. Give in morning.
	Paroxetine: Start with 10 mg and slowly increase to 0.2–0.6 mg/kg/d. Give in morning.
	Fluvoxamine: For OCD, 25 mg to start and increase by 25 mg every 3 to 4 days to maximum of 200 mg/d in adolescents. Give b.i.d.
Drug interaction	Contraindicated with MAO inhibitors. May increase level of other antidepressants up to three times the norm. Watch with lithium. For other possible interactions, see *Physician's Desk Reference*.
Comment	Publicity has suggested that fluoxetine may cause suicidal thoughts, but this is very rare if it occurs at all.

CNS = central nervous system; TCA = tricyclic antidepressants; MAO = monoamine oxidase; b.i.d. = twice a day; OCD = obsessive-compulsive disorder.

There are no studies showing efficacy in children and adolescents for ADHD, but the novel neurotransmitter profile of this medication may make it a useful addition, especially for older patients in this group with comorbid depression and ADHD (Kutcher, 1996a).

Serotonin-Reuptake Inhibitors (Table 82–5)

Serotonin-reuptake inhibitors have not been proven to be efficacious for ADHD symptomatology, but they may be a valid addition to the stimulants for comorbid depression and ADHD. Serotonin-reuptake inhibitors include fluoxetine (Prozac), sertraline (Zoloft), paroxetine (Paxil), and fluvoxamine (Luvox).

Augmentation of stimulant medication with paroxetine has been shown to be helpful for comorbid anxiety, depression, and occasional oppositional behavior in selected cases. However, the emergence of adverse symptoms such as impulsivity, hyperactivity, and excitability sometimes seen in patients taking these medications should be carefully monitored. There is also the possibility of the "serotonin syndrome," which includes major signs and symptoms such as amotivational behavior, mood changes, myoclonus, tremors, and many other potential serious problems (Radomski, Dursen, and Revley, 1995; Riddle et al, 1990/1991).

Monoamine Oxidase Inhibitors

Because of the possibility of serious adverse effects, the monoamine oxidase inhibitors (MAOIs) are rarely used in children or adolescents. However, there are some ongoing studies using the MAOI meclobemide (not available in the United States at this time) in several foreign countries, especially Germany, which show some success with ADHD symptoms. This drug shows fewer side effects than the usual MAOI with no dietary restrictions (Trott et al, 1992).

Neuroleptics (Table 82–6)

The neuroleptics were used much more frequently in the 1970s for ADHD. Because of the potential for serious side effects in most of these drugs, as well as the lack of efficacy for cognitive and attentional improvement, they are rarely, if ever, used, except when comorbid psychotic, pervasive, aggressive, or tic disorders are present. Thioridazine has been noted to be especially successful in mentally retarded patients and is often helpful for the treatment of young children with aggressive and impulsive behavior when the stimulant medications cause major adverse effects.

Recently there has been a push in some circles to treat ADHD with some of the atypical neuroleptics such as risperidone because of the decrease in extrapyramidal signs and symptoms. At this time, there is no good evidence for efficacy, but perhaps they could be used in certain populations of patients with ADHD with comorbid conditions such as aggressiveness, psychoses, or mental retardation.

Antianxiety Medications

There is no evidence that treatment with the benzodiazepines is effective for ADHD symptoms. However, there have been some reports citing some efficacy with the use of buspirone, a nonbenzodiazepine anxiolytic, which has some dopaminergic effect (Balon, 1990).

Other Medications and Polypharmacy

There have been many attempts to treat ADHD symptoms with various other drugs such as fenfluramine, lithium, and anticonvulsants (carbamazepine, valproic acid, and diphenylhydantoin). There is no good reason at the present time to use any of these medications for ADHD, except in the

---

Table 82–6 • Neuroleptics/Antipsychotics

Medications	Typical (dopamine receptor antagonists)
	Phenothiazines
	High potency: trifluoroperazine (Stelazine), periphenazine (Trilafon), fluphenazine (Prolixin)
	Low potency: chlorpromazine (Thorazine), thioridazine (Mellaril), mesoridazine (Serentil)
	Thioxanthenes (high potency)
	Thiothixene (Navane)
	Butyrophenones (high potency)
	Haloperidol (Haldol)
	Indolones (low potency)
	Molindone (Moban)
	Atypical (dopamine and especially D_4 and serotonin receptor antagonists)
	Dibenzodiazepine
	Clozapine (Clozaril)
	Benzisoxazole
	Risperidone (Risperdal)
How supplied	Consult individual medication
Mode of action	Atypical antipsychotics have higher affinity for D_4 as well as serotonin receptors and thus lack extrapyramidal effects and are less likely to develop tardive dyskinesia.
Side effects	There are numerous minor and more serious side effects of this group of medications. Because of the multiple drugs available with differential toxicity profiles, it is more efficacious to consult individual drug listings for a complete list of possible adverse effects.
Dosage	Dosage varies according to medication used as well as condition being treated (e.g., tic versus psychoses). Thus, it is important to consult literature about individual drugs to be certain to stay within safe limits.
Drug interaction	These vary considerably within the various classes of drugs in this group. Again, individualization is necessary.

case of serious comorbidity in which well-accepted therapy has been unsuccessful. Because of the large number of ADHD patients who exhibit other disorders, polypharmacy or combined psychopharmacology has become a more common practice. Usually this might be frowned upon. However, in some cases, drugs from various other classes might increase the efficacy of usual treatments such as the stimulants and perhaps decrease dosage as necessary. Finally, great care must be used in all of these cases to be certain that proved medical approaches are used, especially in children and adolescents.

Questionable Attention Disorders and Responses to Medication

There is a group of children, adolescents, and even adults who do not qualify for a diagnosis of ADHD, but who, for one reason or another, are placed on stimulant medication. Some of these patients actually seem to respond to the medication either in the area of poor impulse control or inattention and distractibility.

There may be several good reasons for this phenomenon. However, one of them is not the oft-heard saying that a positive response to stimulant medication confirms the diagnosis of ADHD; most people would seem to at least pay attention better with these drugs. However, this does not mean that they have a neurologic disorder causing the inattention. The seemingly positive response does not meet the true criteria for a therapeutic improvement, which consist of an increase in academic performance, memory, and true cognitive changes, rather than a seemingly increased attention span.

This situation of improvement is most often seen with inattention and not hyperactive and impulsive behavior. The diagnosis and response to medication is much harder to evaluate for true inattention than it is for hyperactive and impulsive behavior. Some of the more common reasons for the improvements include the following:

1. Diagnostic criteria for ADHD are often cumbersome to use and not specific enough. Therefore, some children and adolescents may not actually be diagnosed with a disorder of attention when they truly do have this problem and would respond to stimulant treatment.
2. Age and sex differences must be considered. This is especially seen in very young as well as adolescent patients and also in girls—who may have a true disorder of attention and distractibility and not meet the published criteria for a diagnosis. Therefore, these patients respond in a therapeutic manner without a true diagnosis having been made.
3. Information gathered from parents and teachers may not be correct or often may be biased, leading to improper diagnostic consideration—both overdiagnosis and underdiagnosis.
4. A "positive" response to medical treatment is a measure of some other phenomenon and does not reflect a valid therapeutic situation in terms of inattention.
5. Pediatricians and other primary care physicians often do not see the same types of patients as are seen in psychiatric settings. This has an effect on both diagnosis and treatment.

There are no easy solutions to this dilemma, but some of the following suggestions might apply:

1. Using better diagnostic criteria and gaining a more concise idea of the problem
2. Making better and more complex evaluations before medication is started
3. Looking at the whole patient rather than only a "criteria list"
4. Using double-blind placebo-controlled medical assessments, measuring true cognitive and performance changes
5. Remembering that people are easily fooled; placebos very often work at least 35% of the time for a short while or perhaps even longer

TIC DISORDERS

Tic disorders vary from a simple transient motor or phonic tic to complex recurrent and chronic tics and finally to the extreme of Tourette syndrome. The decision to treat a tic disorder medically depends on many factors, the most important of which is the impairment that is being caused.

Alpha-2 Adrenergic Agonists

Clonidine (Catapres) and guanfacine hydrochloride (Tenex) are often the first drugs prescribed for tic disorders because of their lower side effect profile. However, there are very few good studies that prove their efficacy, and it is estimated that only around 25% to 30% of patients show a satisfactory response (Chappell, Leckman, and Riddle, 1995). Guanfacine has a better side effect profile than clonidine and perhaps is longer acting, but it has been less well studied.

Neuroleptics

Typical neuroleptics include haloperidol (Haldol) and pimozide (Orap), both butyrophenones, and fluphenazine (Prolixin), a phenothiazine. These drugs have shown a greater efficacy for tic disorders. However, because of fairly significant side effects, they must be monitored carefully and the dose must be kept as low as possible.

Atypical neuroleptics include risperidone (Risperdal), clozapine (Clozaril), and olanzapine (Zyprexa). These drugs are just being introduced for tic disorders, and controlled studies are being done. Clozapine is not as promising as risperidone because of its side effect profile. Risperidone may turn out to be used more than the typical neuroleptics because there is a lower associated rate of tardive dyskinesia and other extrapyramidal symptoms.

Although there have been no controlled studies on sulpiride and tiapride, they have been used in England and other European countries with some success and fewer side effects.

Clonazepam

Clonazepam (Klonopin) is one of the diazepam group and has been used successfully for tic disorders, including Tourette disorder. The side effect profile is lower for this drug, although the efficacy has not been proven in large well-controlled studies.

Other Medications

Many other attempts for the control of tic disorders have been made, but none of them have proven that the result is as good as with the aforementioned medications. These include the serotonin-reuptake inhibitors, some of the antidepressants such as desipramine and imipramine, and nonneuroleptic antidopaminergic agents such as tetrabenazine (Nitoman).

TIC DISORDERS ASSOCIATED WITH COMORBID CONDITIONS

The most common problem faced by clinicians in the area of comorbidity with tic disorders is the association with ADHD. In the past, it was common practice for many clinicians to avoid the use of stimulant medication in a patient with tics. However, in recent years, it has been evident that stimulants do not increase the occurrence of tics in more than 30% to 40% of patients and in some cases actually decrease the number and severity of tics in patients with ADHD (Gadow et al, 1995). In the case of this combination of disorders, it is a generally accepted practice to use the combination of one of the psychostimulants along with one of the anti-tic medications. It was common practice to use clonidine and a stimulant until recently, when this combination was put under surveillance because of a possible association with cardiac deaths. The combination of stimulants and neuroleptics or clonazepam is apparently an acceptable approach to this dilemma.

Another route that has been taken is the use of one of the tricyclic medications such as imipramine, desipramine, or nortriptyline instead of the stimulants for the ADHD, with the hope that the tics would be less likely to emerge (Wilens et al, 1993). However, there are some drawbacks to this situation, given the possibility of cardiac side effects of the tricyclics (especially desipramine), as well as the question of the comparative efficacy of these medications compared to the stimulants for the signs and symptoms of ADHD, especially inattention. This subject remains a difficult one in many patients, especially because there are often other disorders to consider such as OCD, anxiety, depression, and oppositional defiant disorder as well as conduct disorder. Thus, many other medications may be thrown into the therapeutic mix before an acceptable endpoint is reached.

There is increasing use of combinations of several drugs for the treatment of Tourette syndrome alone. This might include clonidine, a neuroleptic, and clonazepam. Even in the absence of comorbid disorders, this is an approach that might also be successful in terms of enabling the amount of each individual drug to be decreased. However, as mentioned earlier, the recent increase in polypharmacy in children or adolescents must continue to be carefully evaluated and monitored.

As with other behavioral and neurologic disorders, it is important to use the other approaches to treatment such as behavioral therapy. The ones most commonly used for tic disorders include habit reversal training (HRT), self-monitoring, and relaxation training. It is not clear whether large numbers of children or adolescents will respond to these approaches.

MAJOR DEPRESSIVE DISORDER

Until recently it was uncommon for children and adolescents to undergo treatment for depression, let alone for clinicians to make such a diagnosis in these groups. However, in the past 20 years or so, the existence of childhood depression has been fairly well established (Carlson and Cantwell, 1980).

However, proof of the efficacy of antidepressant medication for the child and adolescent population lags behind the establishment of diagnostic criteria. It is still a far from settled situation (Kye and Ryan, 1995). It is fairly well agreed that the tricyclics are not especially effective in this area. With the advent of the serotonin-reuptake inhibitors, a more optimistic outlook has emerged, although there is still not a solid body of evidence for the effectiveness of medical therapy for this disorder.

Despite the absence of good evidence for the efficacy of psychopharmacologic therapy in childhood and adolescent depression, most clinicians embark on a course of medical therapy in children and adolescents with major depression, which often carries through to other depressive disorders including dysthymia. Other interventions such as psychotherapy are also used.

Tricyclic Antidepressants (see Table 82–2)

Tricyclic antidepressants used in the treatment of major depressive disorder include the following:

- Imipramine (Tofranil)—relatively noradrenergic
- Nortriptyline (Pamelor)—noradrenergic as well as acting on other catecholamines
- Desipramine (Norpramin)—also noradrenergic
- Amitriptyline (Elavil)—more serotonergic than the aforementioned drugs and possibly more helpful for anxiety as well as depression
- Clomipramine (Anafranil)—a serotonergic drug that is used, for the most part, for OCD

The tricyclic antidepressants do have a long track record as far as treatment of depression in children and adolescents, as well as of other disorders such as anxiety, enuresis, phobias, and ADHD. As suggested, however, the safety situation has come into more focus recently, especially for desipramine, which has been associated with sudden cardiac deaths in four children. The effect of this drug on the QT_c, PR, and QRS intervals may be associated with some of the problems seen in this group of children, although it is not totally agreed on that desipramine was the actual inciting agent in the cardiac problems reported.

Because of the lack of proven efficacy of the tricyclic antidepressants for major depression in childhood and adolescence (Popper, 1995b), and taking into consideration the possible (although rare) cardiovascular implications, it has become common practice for the first-line agent to be considered for this disorder to be one of the serotonin-reuptake inhibitors.

Serotonin-Reuptake Inhibitors (see Table 82–5)

There are now four drugs in this class in current use:

- Fluoxetine (Prozac)

- Sertraline (Zoloft)
- Paroxetine (Paxil)
- Fluvoxamine (Luvox)

This group of drugs is growing in popularity for the treatment of childhood and adolescent depression. There is more information available on fluoxetine, but sertraline has become used more often recently because of the possibility of a lesser chance of side effects in children because of the shorter half-life and less sedation, as well as its better track record when used with other drugs. Because of this shorter half-life, a steady state is reached more quickly. Paroxetine is the most serotonin-specific drug in this group, reaching a steady state in about 10 days. Fluvoxamine has not been used in children to any great extent and is more often used for the treatment of OCD.

Other Antidepressants (see Table 82–4)

Bupropion (Wellbutrin) is in the aminoketone class and is unrelated to either tricyclic or tetracyclic drugs. This medication has an effect mainly on serotonin, but it also affects dopamine and, to a mild extent, norepinephrine. There are no solid reports on the treatment of depression in children, but bupropion has been found to be useful in some studies for the treatment of ADHD.

Venlafaxine (Effexor) selectively inhibits the uptake of norepinephrine as well as serotonin and is an amphetamine analogue. There are no data for its use in the treatment of depression in children.

Nefazodone (Serzone) is unrelated to serotonin-reuptake inhibitors or tricyclic antidepressants. It inhibits the reuptake of serotonin and norepinephrine, but its efficacy in children younger than 18 years has not been proven.

Tetracyclic Antidepressants

Maprotiline (Ludiomil) is noradrenergic and has some minimal dopaminergic and serotonergic effects. It has not been approved for use in children younger than 18 years.

Monoamine Oxidase Inhibitors

MAOIs are not usually used for the treatment of children and adolescents because of their side effect profile as well as the dietary restrictions that are necessary. There are two types:

- MAOI-$_A$ (noradrenergic and serotonergic)
- MAOI-$_B$ (more dopaminergic)

Meclobemide is in the MAOI-$_A$ group and has been used in some foreign countries for depression as well as ADHD. There are no well-documented, controlled studies completed at the present time, however.

Trazodone

Trazodone (Desyrel) is a serotonergic drug that is unrelated to other antidepressants. It has been helpful to some degree in aggressive disorders, but again its use is not established in children younger than 18 years.

Supplementation of Antidepressant Medication

Occasionally, there is augmentation of some of these medications with drugs such as lithium or L-thyroxine (Table 82–7). This situation has not been studied extensively in children or adolescents.

PSYCHOTIC DISORDERS

Psychotic disorders are actually a heterogeneous group of conditions with multiple causes, including schizophrenia (see Chapter 64). Most children and adolescents do not have schizophrenia, but most psychoses share similar symptomatology. Because of the diverse diagnostic and therapeutic situations that occur under this umbrella, it is rare that a developmental-behavioral pediatrician will have the training or experience necessary to either diagnose or treat this group of disorders.

Because of this situation, the use of antipsychotic medication in children and adolescents is usually foreign to most practitioners, except perhaps for the nonpsychiatric usage such as in movement disorders, aggression, anxiety disorders, and perhaps pervasive disorders. Thus, it is important to stress that the diagnosis and treatment of psychotic disorders is most often best left to the professionals well trained in this area, which usually means child and adolescent psychiatrists. Therefore, this section includes a review of the psychotherapeutic agents commonly used for psychotic disorders, with the caveat that the prescription of such drugs is a delicate task that should be handled by experts.

The differential diagnosis of psychotic disorders is often difficult, and there is much overlapping of symptomatology with other behavioral and emotional problems in childhood and adolescence. In addition to this often difficult diagnostic situation, it is not uncommon, especially in adolescence, to see one of the psychoses as a comorbid condition with other disorders of childhood and adolescence. It is also not unlikely that a child who is given the diagnosis of a rather common psychiatric disorder, such as ADHD, later in life manifests signs and symptoms of a psychotic disorder.

The final preamble to the discussion of psychopharmacologic agents goes back to the important aspect of who is undergoing treatment. This group of patients presents a totally different set of needs and situations than do adults with similar disorders. School and learning problems, unique social situations, and a special physical and medical environment all must be considered. Thus, every child and adolescent who is referred for diagnostic and therapeutic interventions should have a total approach to the management of these disorders. This includes close attention to developmental issues, educational and vocational management, psychosocial therapy including social skills training, and family therapy and education. Medication alone is never a proper approach to the care of children and adolescents with any developmental, behavioral, or psychosocial disorder including psychoses.

Medical Management of Any Psychiatric Disorder

A referral to a psychiatrist includes the whole child—not just the psyche or central nervous system. Thus, no child

Table 82–7 • Mood Stabilizers

Lithium	
	Lithium carbonate tablets: 300 mg; 150-, 300-, 600-mg caps
How supplied	Lithobid—slow release, 300 mg
	Eskalith—lithium carbonate caps, 300 mg; caps, 300 mg
	Lithane—lithium carbonate, 300-mg scored tablets
Mode of action	Alters sodium transport in nerve and muscle cells and effects shift of intraneuronal metabolism of catecholamines; blocks GABA turnover
Side effects	Most common: diarrhea, nausea, vomiting, numbness, weight gain, thirst, abdominal pain, frequent urination, tremors, weakness.
	Others less common: blurred vision, low thyroid function, seizures, renal problems (see *Physician's Desk Reference*).
Dosage	Must follow serum level. Start with 12–30 mg/kg/d in two doses. Increase until serum level is 0.6 to 1.2 mEq/L. If no response in 8 weeks, it will not work.
Caution	Do laboratory work (CBC, SMA 20, U/A, thyroid function) as baseline and frequently thereafter. Follow serum levels closely for first few weeks and obtain 10 to 14 hours after last dose.
Drug interaction	Antiinflammatory medications may increase levels. Combined use of Haldol and lithium is contraindicated. Be careful with diuretics.
Carbamazepine (Tegretol)	
	This is an iminostilbene anticonvulsant drug; chemical structure is like that of imipramine.
How supplied	200-mg tablets; 100-mg chewable tablets; suspension, 100 mg/tsp
Mode of action	Suppresses temporal lobe and limbic system; noradrenergic reuptake blockage of increased GABA activity.
Side effects	Common: sleepiness, dizziness, clumsiness, nausea, diplopia.
	Others: bone marrow depression, rashes.
Dosage	Under 12: 100 mg b.i.d. and increase slowly to 400–800 mg/d
	Over 12: 200 mg b.i.d. and increase slowly to 1000 mg/d
	Use blood levels—usual therapeutic range 5–15 mg/mL
Drug interaction	Tricyclic antidepressants, erythromycin, fluoxetine, lithium.
Caution	CBC baseline and frequently thereafter. Also liver and thyroid function tests.
Valproic acid (Depakote)	
How supplied	125, 250, 500 mg
Mode of action	Anticonvulsant drug—main action may be due to increased production of GABA.
Side effects	Sedation, nausea, weight gain, possible bone marrow toxicity and liver failure, thinning of hair, anorexia, abdominal pain, rash, and many other less common side effects.
Dosage	Initial dose 15 mg/kg/d and increase to maximum of 50–60 mg/kg/d (t.i.d.). Usually 125 mg b.i.d. (child) and 250 mg b.i.d. (adolescents). Monitor plasma levels, which should be 50–125 mg/mL.
Drug interaction	Valproic acid may cause various problems when used with carbamazepine or many of the benzodiazepine anxiolytic drugs.
Caution	Carefully monitor hepatic and renal function as well as blood counts.

CBC = complete blood count; U/A = urinalysis; b.i.d., twice daily; t.i.d., three times a day.

should be initiated into a course of medication without a complete physical examination by the prescribing physician, along with any additional laboratory or other procedures indicated for the particular drug.

MEDICATIONS FOR PSYCHOSIS

The most successful group of drugs for psychotic disorders in adults is the neuroleptics. However, there is not much evidence for the efficacy of this group of agents in children. Adolescents are more likely to show responses similar to adult patterns (Lohr and Birmaher, 1995).

The neuroleptics are effective in 60% to 75% of adults, but much less of a response is seen in adolescents and especially in children. The side effect profile (e.g., extrapyramidal signs and tardive dyskinesia) is also important to take into consideration when treating this group of patients. This group of drugs is currently divided into the typical and atypical neuroleptics, with the latter group being even more poorly understood in the child and adolescent population, although the side effect profile of the latter agents may turn out to suggest a better therapeutic situation for children and adolescents.

Typical Neuroleptics

The following drugs are usually linked to dopamine T_2 receptors, and some affect many other receptors (names in parentheses are trade names):

Phenothiazines
    Chlorpromazine (Thorazine)
    Thioridazine (Mellaril)
    Mesoridazine (Serentil)
    Fluphenazine (Prolixin, Permitil)
    Perphenazine (Trilafon)
    Trifluoperazine (Stelazine)
Thioxanthenes
    Thiothixene (Navane)
Butyrophenones
    Haloperidol (Haldol)
Dibenzoxathines
    Loxapine (Loxitane)

Dihydroindolones
    Molindone (Moban)

Atypical Neuroleptics

Atypical neuroleptics differ from the typical neuroleptics in several ways. These drugs not only have a blocking effect on DA_2 receptors but also block serotonin $5HT_2$ receptors, thus setting up an interaction of the noradrenergic and dopaminergic systems. Because of this effect, these agents seem not only to decrease the positive signs and symptoms of schizophrenia, such as delirium and hallucinations, but also to deal with some of the negative symptoms, such as flat affect, social withdrawal, poor motivation, and poor attention (Kopala et al, 1996). Another important difference is the low incidence of extrapyramidal side effects, including tardive dyskinesia, as well as less cognitive blunting. There are a number of small studies and reports regarding the efficacy of these medications in children and adolescents, but clinicians must still proceed with caution. This group includes risperidone and clozapine.

Risperidone

Risperidone (Risperdal) may be useful in some schizophrenic patients, especially those resistant to other drugs, along with children with tic disorders and perhaps aggressive children, especially those with pervasive disorders such as autism.

Clozapine (Clozaril)

Clozapine (Clozaril) has the same profile and is similar to risperidone both chemically and therapeutically, except it possesses both D_1 and D_2 receptor activity as well as serotonin receptor activity. However, because of the severity of side effects (e.g., bone marrow depression, electroencephalographic changes, seizure risk), Clozaril is currently not recommended for adolescents and certainly not for children in most cases. Many more studies on the efficacy and side effect profiles of this medication must be completed before it can be used further in the pediatric age group.

Olanzapine

Olanzapine (Zyprexa) has receptor affinities similar to those of risperidone and clozapine with some differences in the ratio of serotonergic-dopaminergic effects. It also has a good profile on the negative symptoms of psychoses. There are no good studies in children or adolescents.

Other Medications Used for Psychotic Disorders

For the most part, there is not much evidence that drugs other than the neuroleptics are successfully used in psychotic disorders. However, occasionally medications in the benzodiazepine group have been used in highly agitated patients along with the neuroleptics. Some of the neuroleptics are used in other disorders as well.

OBSESSIVE-COMPULSIVE DISORDER

OCD is not an uncommon disorder in children and adolescents (see Chapter 64). It is estimated that possibly one in 200 young people suffer from this disorder (March, Leonard, and Swedo, 1995). There is a rich neurobiological background that includes genetic, traumatic, neoplastic, and infectious etiologies for this disorder. A final common pathway of dysfunction with serotonergic regulation seems to be an accepted role in this disorder.

The treatment of OCD involves diagnostic specificity as well as the identification of many comorbid disorders that often accompany OCD, including Tourette syndrome, ADHD, depression, panic disorders, and general anxiety disorder. Thus, this is one diagnosis that often necessitates some form of polypharmacy because of the multiplicity of problems that are present.

As with other diagnostic entities discussed in this chapter, a combination of behavior therapy along with pharmacotherapy is the most effective modality. Approaches such as cognitive-behavioral psychotherapy and HRT are often used in conjunction with psychopharmacologic approaches. Many children and adolescents with OCD are not given a chance at cognitive behavior therapy, and medications are used immediately. Because of the evidence that OCD is chronic, despite treatment, it is thought that bimodal therapy is probably more effective than either alone, although a complete remission is not usually the norm. The medical approach to OCD follows.

Clomipramine

Clomipramine is a tricyclic antidepressant with almost exclusive serotonergic action and very little or no noradrenergic effects. It was first studied and approved for use with adults and has since been approved for use in adolescents and children down to the age of 8 years. The side effects profile with clomipramine is not a major problem, although like all tricyclic antidepressants, there is an increased potential for cardiac toxicity. Thus, many clinicians prefer to start therapy with one of the serotonin-reuptake inhibitors.

Serotonin-Reuptake Inhibitors

Serotonin-reuptake inhibitors have not been studied extensively in OCD, either in adults or in children and adolescents. However, open studies and clinical trials have shown fairly good efficacy, especially for fluoxetine. Paroxetine has not been studied as well as some of the other drugs in this group but will probably show similar effects. Fluvoxamine is being marketed specifically as an antiobsessional drug and shows promise in adults, and it has recently been approved for this use in children and adolescents. All of these medications show a better side effect profile than clomipramine, especially in the case of sertraline and fluvoxamine, which are probably better tolerated by children and adults.

Benzodiazepines

The most often used medication for OCD in this group of patients has been clonazepam. This drug has serotonergic as well as other neurotransmitter effects and has been used for OCD increasingly in the past few years. One well-designed, controlled study revealed an equal response of clonazepam and clomipramine in reducing OCD symptoms, with the former showing a more rapid response (Hewlitt, Vinogradov, and Agras, 1992). This medication has been used more frequently in recent years, especially when the other mainstays have been unsuccessful. Studies using various other benzodiazepines have not shown as much efficacy as clonazepam.

Combination Therapy

In many patients with refractory OCD, it has become common to use several medications to try to control the symptoms. This includes augmentation with such agents as neuroleptics, lithium, clonidine, and antidepressants. This approach is especially helpful when comorbid disorders such as psychoses, anxiety, or depression or tics are present. ADHD is not uncommon, and stimulant medication would be used in this case. Another increasingly common practice is to use two different types of serotonergic agents together—such as fluoxetine and clomipramine. (Clinicians must watch carefully for symptoms of "serotonin syndrome," however.)

Despite the efficacy of medical therapy for OCD, however, the results of such treatment are still not as satisfactory as they could be. It is important to carefully consider this disorder when considering the differential diagnosis of child and adolescent behavioral problems. It is also important to remember that there is a high rate of tic and Tourette disorders with OCD in childhood and that the signs and symptoms may vary quite a bit from adult OCD, with compulsion being more common than obsession.

Conditions in Which Medication Usage Is Not Well Established and/or Documented

DYSTHYMIC DISORDER

The discussion of a psychopharmacologic approach to dysthymic disorder mirrors the situation established for major depressive disorders—with two important points to consider:

1. The diagnostic specificity of dysthymia is far from being clarified by current standards.
2. This diagnosis is often mixed and confused with many other childhood and adolescent behavioral and emotional disorders.

Thus, it is difficult to distinguish dysthymia from anxiety, school problems, oppositional defiant disorder, attentional disorders, and OCD, to name a few diagnostic categories. Children are often seen with signs and symptoms of mood disorders, which are secondary to other problems such as learning disabilities. Thus, it is often difficult to specifically diagnose dysthymia as an entity.

As far as therapy is concerned, antidepressant medications have a rather spotty efficacy record for major depressive disorder, which is more specifically diagnostically

defined than dysthymia. Therefore, the use of medication to treat this disorder is on shaky ground. For example, a boy with oppositional defiant disorder who was told he could not have his way may seem to show severe signs of depression, but the signs rapidly clear up when the inciting event passes.

Therefore, the use of medication specifically for dysthymia should be carefully weighed, taking into consideration all of the aforementioned caveats. If it is fairly well established that there is a true mood disorder present that cannot be ameliorated by a behavioral or psychological approach or by the defusing of a primary inciting situation, medication would be indicated.

The drugs that are used in these cases are usually the same as those used for major depressive disorder. However, because this diagnosis is often less concrete than major depressive disorder, and because there are usually some cross-diagnostic situations, choice of therapeutic agents should be limited to drugs with the most true efficacy and the best side effect profile. In this case, the clinician is most likely to use one of the serotonin-reuptake inhibitors and not go "medication surfing" as is done with some of the other disorders.

MANIA

There is very little current research available concerning the treatment of mania and bipolar disorders in children and adolescents, although there has been quite an increase in the presentation of these disorders in the past several years (Botteron and Geller, 1995). It is thought that because of the neurologic differences, children and adolescents probably have a different response to therapy than adults as well as a more difficult differential diagnostic pattern. Thus, many children with aggressive ADHD, psychoses, and conduct and other disorders might mistakenly be diagnosed as manic or hypomanic. In the same vein, however, some children with true mania might be missed if this diagnosis is not considered as a possible cause of their behavioral manifestations.

This disorder may be precipitated by other medications such as tricyclic antidepressants, steroids, and even serotonin-reuptake inhibitors at times. Thus, treatment should not be instituted without taking other drug therapy into consideration.

Lithium

Lithium is still the mainstay treatment for mania in adults and has been used in children for many years. However, corroboration of efficacy is still minimal. In many children with aggressive disorders but without a clear-cut diagnosis of mania, lithium has been reported to be helpful. The combination of lithium and other medications, especially the psychostimulants in children with a combination of ADHD and possible mania, has been helpful. Before deciding to treat with lithium, it is imperative that the clinician follow the guidelines as far as pretreatment evaluations and therapeutic levels are concerned.

Anticonvulsants

Valproate

Recent studies have shown valproate (Depakote) to be fairly compatible to lithium in treatment of mania in children and adolescents. This medication has also been shown to be helpful when depression is present as well as with aggressive disorders (Papatheodorou, 1996).

Carbamazepine

Carbamazepine (Tegretol) is also considered as a reasonable alternative to lithium in adults, but there are no established studies of efficacy in children. Side effects of this medication must be watched carefully and include, among many others, neutropenia and aplastic anemia, and the drug must be monitored very carefully.

Other Agents

Other agents such as clonidine, clonazepam, and calcium channel blockers have been used in adults with mania with mixed results. There are no studies of efficacy in children or adolescents, however.

CONDUCT DISORDER (AND OTHER AGGRESSIVE STATES)

There are many causes for aggressive states in children and adolescents (see Chapter 49). These include psychosocial, emotional, physical, posttraumatic, and presumed neurobiological and personality disorders. Specific diagnostic categories that fall into this group include ADHD, conduct disorder, oppositional defiant disorder, episodic discontrol, and intermittent explosive disorders. This section discusses aggressive behavior in general, although the diagnostic prototype would be considered to be conduct disorder, which has received much of the therapeutic attention (Stoewe, Kruess, and Leilo, 1995).

Medications used for this group of disorders cross diagnostic lines in that many of the signs and symptoms are fairly nonspecific. However, earlier concern regarding the often helter-skelter approach to the use of multiple drugs without evidence of efficacy is no more evident in this group than it is in any childhood disorders. The lack of diagnostic specificity in aggressive states should be very strongly considered before a therapeutic plan is contemplated. Because treatment often spans diagnostic categories, clinicians must be very careful in their evaluation before medication is begun. In this section, the medications discussed would be considered for the treatment of conduct disorder as a prototype as well as the many other causes of childhood aggressive states, especially because conduct disorder is usually not the only disorder operating.

Medications for Conduct Disorder and Aggression

Many psychopharmacologic agents have been used for the treatment of outwardly exhibited childhood and adolescent aggression. There are no specific medications for aggression itself, but the drugs that are most commonly used are discussed in this section.

Psychostimulants

Psychostimulants have long been associated with excellent results in the amelioration of explosive and hyperactive behavior, especially in ADHD. They have also been considered for many years to be effective for aggressive symptoms, although it has become evident that many patients who exhibit aggression have comorbid diagnoses such as conduct disorder and oppositional defiant disorder, so that it is difficult to measure the true response to these agents for the aggressive symptoms alone. It is likely that an aggressive child will show a fairly decent clinical response to these medications based on improved self-control, without any lowering of the specific aggressive feelings. Thus, the patient would only *appear* to be less aggressive for that period of time.

Alpha-2 Adrenergic Agonists

The two most commonly used alpha-2 adrenergic agonists used are clonidine and guanfacine. There have been very few controlled studies showing a high efficacy rate for aggression with these medications, but some of the open studies and clinical trials have shown some promise. On the other hand, there is suspicion that some of the positive therapeutic results may be totally due to sedative effects. In my experience, use of these agents resulted in about a 30% improvement in child and adolescent aggressive and oppositional behavior. These medications may be especially helpful with comorbid disorders such as Tourette syndrome, mania, explosive disorders, impulsivity in ADHD, and perhaps anxiety disorders.

Lithium

Lithium has been used in children and adolescents with aggressive behavior apart from its usual use as a mood stabilizer in manic states. Lithium might be more effective for explosive rages than in chronic aggressive states, although it is also used for impulsivity and emotional lability. Many children with ADHD and aggression have undergone treatment with a psychostimulant and lithium with a fairly good response.

Neuroleptics

There is a long history of the use of neuroleptics for aggressive behavior in children and adolescents. Even though the medical trials often involve children with psychotic and pervasive disorders, the current practice includes prescribing for aggressive states across many diagnostic categories. The most widely used and established drugs in this class include haloperidol, thioridazine, and chlorpromazine. These drugs have long been approved for young children; however, because of their dangerous side effect profiles, these medications have been used less in recent years, except perhaps for thioridazine, which has less effect on the dopaminergic system and thus is likely to cause fewer extrapyramidal symptoms.

The newer neuroleptic agents such as risperidone and clozapine have recently been used for aggressive symptoms, but there is no good evidence of efficacy, except in some preliminary studies of the use of risperidone in autistic children. This agent might prove to be helpful in this particular area because of a lower incidence of extrapyramidal symptoms.

Another medication in this group is molindone, which has been used in aggressive hospitalized children, but this drug is not in common use for this group of patients. There are other newer atypical neuroleptics that may be used in the future. This group of medications might be considered more specifically in aggressive patients with psychoses, mental retardation, and organic brain dysfunction.

Antidepressants

Many children with aggressive disorders are also given the diagnosis of depression. Therefore, the medical treatment of depressive disorders has been thought to be a possible aid in the amelioration of aggressive symptoms. However, because the tricyclic antidepressants have not been proven to be efficacious for depressive symptoms, it would follow that they would not work well in aggressive disorders. This has been proven to be true in the case of the tricyclic antidepressants (Ambrosini et al, 1993). In the case of the serotonin-reuptake inhibitors, there is also very little solid evidence for the therapeutic efficacy for either the depression or aggressive states. However, when a patient shows severe anger, irritability, or depressive symptoms along with aggression, the use of one of the serotonin-reuptake inhibitors might be indicated. Clinicians should also watch carefully for the impulsive and aggressive symptoms that might be a *result* of therapy with this group of medications.

Several other antidepressants have been used for aggression, and one that has shown some promise is trazodone (Desyrel), which is one of the more serotonergic drugs in this class. Open clinical trials have shown some promise in this area.

Anticonvulsants

Many different anticonvulsants have been used in the management of behavioral disturbances in children. The first wave included phenobarbital and the phenytoins, neither of which is considered to be useful at the present time. The most recent drugs in this class that have been used include carbamazepine and valproic acid (Zobieta and Alessi, 1992). These agents are also used for the treatment of manic disorders in adults, and their efficacy in aggressive situations in children and adolescents may be somewhat related to this effect, as well as in the possible amelioration of rage or temper outbursts as part of a seizure type disorder.

Despite the use of these two agents for conduct disorder and aggressive behaviors in children and adolescents, however, there are no well-controlled studies showing efficacy in these patients for either agent. Aggressive, explosive, or rage outbursts are said to respond to carbamazepine. However, a recent double-blind placebo-controlled study (Cueva et al, 1996) showed no effect for this drug for a variety of aggressive behaviors. Thus, clinicians must be careful before embarking on a course of any of these medications for childhood aggressive disorders.

Antianxiety Agents (Table 82–8)

Antianxiety agents that have been used include the benzodiazepines and buspirone. For the most part, the benzodiazepines have not been proven to be effective, with the possible exception of use in children and adolescents with severe anxiety who exhibit rages or outbursts secondary to generalized anxiety disorders. The use of buspirone has been growing somewhat recently, with reports of efficacy in explosive outbursts and rages as well as in some autistic children. The advantages of buspirone over the diazepines include lessened tolerance and fewer addictive problems.

Beta-Blockers (Table 82–9)

Beta-blockers have been shown to control aggression in patients with mental retardation, organic brain syndrome, posttraumatic stress disorders, and other neurologic problems. At least one study in children without impairments has shown some promise in this area (Connor, 1993). However, because of the major caution necessary with the use of these drugs, especially for the cardiovascular system, as well as the problems of use of other medications along with this group, great care should be taken before deciding upon this group of agents. The most commonly used drugs in this group are propranolol, nadolol, atenolol, and metoprolol.

ANXIETY DISORDERS

Anxiety disorders are more common in children and adolescents than most physicians realize (see Chapter 62). Anxiety disorders often coexist with many other disorders such as ADHD, depression, OCD, and Tourette syndrome, and they may even mimic the symptoms of these conditions. However, the pharmacologic management of anxiety is far from being a settled affair, and there are only a few studies available to support the efficacy of medication for anxiety in children and adolescents (Bernstein and Perwien, 1995). As with all other childhood and adolescent behavioral and emotional disorders, it is important to present a broad array of interventions to the family and patient, especially including the use of psychological and behavioral therapies.

Antianxiety Medication

Antianxiety medications include benzodiazepines (diazepam [Valium], which is not often used in children because of the risk of dependence; alprazolam [Xanax]; clonazepam [Klonopin]; and lorazepam [Ativan]) and buspirone (BuSpar).

Because of the lack of good studies to support the efficacy of these medications in children and adolescents as well as the potential for tolerance, abuse, and dependency, they should not be used over long periods of time and, if used, should be monitored by an experienced clinician, usually a child psychiatrist.

Buspirone, however, is a newer anxiolytic agent that is relatively under-studied, but some studies do show promising results. Several promising attributes of this drug include the absence of impairment of cognition and a minimal risk of abuse (Kutcher, 1996b).

Table 82–8 • Antianxiety Drugs

Benzodiazepines	
Diazepam (Valium)—2-, 5-, 10-mg tablets; injectable (short acting, not often used in children, risk of dependence)	
Aprazolam (Xanax)—0.25-, 0.5-, 1-, 2-mg tablets (short acting, use t.i.d.)	
Lorazepam (Ativan)—0.5-, 1-, 2-mg tablets (short acting, use t.i.d.)	
Clonazepam (Klonopin)—0.5-, 1-, 2-mg tablets (long acting, b.i.d.–t.i.d.)	
Mode of action	Act as GABA receptors (to inhibit neurotransmitters), limbic system, hypothalamus and other neuroregulating systems.
Side effects	Drowsiness, headaches, nausea, agitation, coordination loss, slurred speech, tremors. There are many other adverse reactions seen with these drugs, some of which are quite serious, including bone marrow depression. Consult side effect profile of each medication if used.
Other concerns	Risk of dependence, abuse; withdraw slowly to avoid gastrointestinal, flulike, sleep, muscular symptoms. Also may cause depression, delirium, and other serious problems.
Dosage	Varies according to medication, age of child, and disorder being treated. Consult individual literature concerning each drug and consult studies performed on children and adolescents because of the novelty of the use of this group in this age group.
Drug interaction	Other CNS depressants, alcohol, tricyclic antidepressants, various anticonvulsants, analgesics, antihistamines, antipsychotics.
Buspirone (BuSpar)—5-, 10-mg tablets	
Mode of action	An azaspirodecanedione unrelated to benzodiazepines and barbiturates. Has high affinity for serotonin inhibitors, moderate affinity for D_2 dopamine receptors, noradrenergics systems.
Side effects	Dizziness, nausea, abdominal pain, headache, nervousness, paresthesias, syncope, excitement, insomnia, and many other less common
Dosage	0.2–0.5 mg/kg/d. Use 5–10 mg t.i.d. up to 30–60 mg/d maximum. May take up to 2 weeks for effect and 4–6 weeks for maximum efficacy.
	Low risk of dependency and abuse, less withdrawal likelihood, much safer than benzodiazepines.
	Drug interaction rare.

t.i.d. = three times a day; GABA = gamma aminobutyric acid; CNS = central nervous system.

Antidepressants

There is a long history of the use of the tricyclic antidepressant in anxious children or adolescents, because anxiety and depression often coexist. However, because the response to tricyclic antidepressants in depression is not very robust, not much can be expected in the way of help for the anxiety symptoms. Multiple studies have shown some positive effects in the treatment of separation anxiety as well as of panic disorder with some of these agents. However, there is still not a good body of evidence to support their use in most cases. There is also no approval for the use of most of these drugs for children and adolescents for anxiety.

Recently, the serotonin-reuptake inhibitor group of antidepressants has also been used for children and adolescents with anxiety disorders. The most studied of this group in children has been fluoxetine, and there are some promising reports, especially in cases of separation anxiety. As with the previously mentioned agents, much work needs to be done in this area before these drugs can be used safely to treat anxiety in children.

Other Medications

Various other agents such as the beta-blockers and MAO inhibitors have been used in adults with anxiety disorders as well as in sparse trials in children. There is as yet no evidence of efficacy or safety for their use in children.

Like for the many other disorders in this group, the results of the medical treatment of anxiety in children and adolescents are far from solid at this time. Extreme care and very well informed decision making are as important here as in all of the other diagnostic categories included in this chapter—perhaps even more so because of the limited information available.

Conditions in Which There Is Very Little Documentation of Efficacy

PERVASIVE DEVELOPMENTAL DISORDERS

Pervasive developmental disorders include various diagnostic categories such as autism, pervasive developmental disorder–not otherwise specified, and Rett and Asperger disorders. The behavioral problems associated with this group that would possibly lend themselves to pharmacologic interventions include aggressive and violent behaviors, rages, irritability, hyperactivity, rituals, and impulsivity. It becomes evident, then, that the target symptoms of any treatment plan will necessarily include behaviors seen in many other diagnostic categories and that there are not

Table 82–9 • Beta-Blockers

Medications	Propranolol
	Nadolol
	Atenolol
	Metoprolol
	The most common medication used in children is propranolol (Inderal) supplied in 10-, 20-, 40-, 60-, 80-mg tablets
Mode of action	Beta-adrenergic receptor blocker, which lowers the effects of CNS catecholamines and decreases GABA turnover. Affects B_1 and B_2 receptors and crosses blood-brain barrier.
Side effects	Common: bradycardia, hypotension, dizziness. Serious: wheezing, sadness, hallucinations, diabetes, thyroid, and cardiac problems. Check drug information before using.
Withdrawal	Increased blood pressure, chest pain, tachycardia, emotional disturbances.
Dosage	Start with 0.8 mg/kg/d (t.i.d.) and slowly increase over 2 weeks to maximum of 4 mg/kg/d. Monitor pulse for bradycardia before each dose.
Drug interaction	There are many special concerns about interaction with a large number of other medications as well as with various medical conditions such as thyroid disorder and diabetes. Consult drug literature before and during usage.

CNS = central nervous system; GABA = gamma aminobutyric acid; t.i.d. = three times a day.

going to be specific therapeutic modalities for these children and adolescents. At present, there are no specifically approved medications for the treatment of pervasive developmental disorders because of the overlap of symptoms among many other developmental and behavioral disorders (Cook and Leventhal, 1995). The most common symptoms targeted for therapy are usually in the aggressive category; thus the list of medications to be considered mirror those discussed in Medications for Conduct Disorders and Aggression.

Psychostimulants

Many children and adolescents show signs and symptoms similar to those of ADHD. Psychostimulants are often used—with some success—to ameliorate the hyperactive and impulsive behavior that may be seen in these patients. Thus, drugs such as methylphenidate and the amphetamines have been used to treat these symptoms fairly successfully in children and adolescents, and they are worth trying in many instances.

Neuroleptics

Neuroleptics have a long history of use in pervasive developmental disorders. The agents that have been used until recently have been the so-called typical neuroleptics, which include haloperidol, trifluoperazine, pimozide, and thioridazine. All of these medications have been noted to diminish signs and symptoms of pervasive disorders, especially those of the positive type. The major problem with this group, however, remains the danger of the side effects of

tardive dyskinesia and extrapyramidal symptoms, especially when used for long periods of time.

Recently, some of the newer atypical neuroleptics have been used for these disorders. Because of the lesser risk of extrapyramidal symptoms in this group as well as the response of many of the negative symptoms of pervasive disorders, these drugs may become important therapeutic agents in the future. The drugs in this class include clonazepam and risperidone. The former is not used much for children and adolescents because of the side effects, including hematologic problems. Risperidone is being studied for aggressive behaviors in autistic patients, and some of the early results seem positive.

Antidepressants

None of the tricyclic antidepressants have been especially effective for pervasive developmental disorders, with the exception of clomipramine. The potent serotonergic effect of this drug seems to be especially helpful in the presence of symptoms such as rituals, anxiety, and aggression (Gordon et al, 1993). However, because of the cardiac effects and other possibly disturbing side effects often seen with this drug, it is more common to use the other serotonin-reuptake inhibitors such as fluoxetine, sertraline, paroxetine, and especially fluvoxamine, which seem to work well for the ritualistic behavior of some children and adolescents with autistic symptoms.

Alpha-2 Adrenergic Agonists

Alpha-2 adrenergic agonists include clonidine and guanfacine. These drugs primarily act on aggression, over-arousal, and impulsivity. There are few studies to support the efficacy of this group of medications for use in pervasive developmental disorders.

Anticonvulsants

The anticonvulsant medications most often used for pervasive developmental disorders are carbamazepine and valproic acid. These medications may exert their therapeutic effect by decreasing the occurrence of seizures in autistic patients as well as their possible amelioration of aggressive behavior. (See Medications for Conduct Disorder and Aggression.)

Antianxiety Drugs

In general, antianxiety drugs are of little value for pervasive developmental disorders. Case reports and open trials have shown little or no efficacy for either the benzodiazepines or buspirone.

Other Agents

Many other drugs have been tried for pervasive developmental disorders, including lithium and some beta-adrenergic agents such as propranolol and nadolol. Again, these medications are nonspecific and are used essentially for their possible antiaggressive effect.

One medication that was previously thought to have

specific therapeutic effects in the treatment of autism is naltrexone (Trexan), which is an opiate antagonist. Most recent studies have shown limited efficacy, however, except for the possible reduction of hyperactive symptoms.

Finally, there was quite a bit of interest in the use of fenfluramine (Pondimin), a sympathomimetic amine, several years ago. Recent studies have not born out this optimism, however, although this drug might have limited success in hyperactive and impulsive behavior in these disorders (Leventhal et al, 1993).

OPPOSITIONAL DEFIANT DISORDER

Most authors include oppositional defiant disorder under the same diagnostic umbrella as conduct disorder as one of the disruptive disorders of childhood. This is the manner in which these two categories is presented in *DSM-IV.* However, there are some important differences between these two entities, especially in the case of management with pharmacologic agents.

Almost every criterion for conduct disorder includes some type of aggressive behavior, and even though there are no clear-cut specific target behaviors that would call for a specific drug or drugs, many of the behavioral manifestations of conduct disorder fit to some degree under the umbrella of the aggressive disorders and thus can lend themselves to the pharmacologic approach of those entities. However, in the case of oppositional defiant disorder, there are two major differences noted in *DSM-IV:*

1. Most of the criteria listed are not what would really be termed aggressive, but perhaps would be more fittingly referred to as annoying or irritating, as well as perhaps disruptive.
2. A very important aspect of this disorder is the fact that, in the majority of cases, the target behavior occurs most often in the company of family or familiar figures. This means that many of these children show signs and symptoms of the disorder only for a limited time on most days. Thus, any pharmacologic therapeutic approach would be overkill for a large portion of the patient's waking time.

Therefore, is it proper to consider the use of medications, some of which can be potent and often replete with serious side effect profiles, for a "disorder" (1) that is poorly understood as to etiology, (2) that often may simply represent a variant type of personality or the result of family turmoil, and (3) that often exists for a very short period of time each day? I believe that, in most cases, the answer is definitely "no."

It is common for children and adolescents with oppositional defiant disorder to also have other comorbid disorders. In many cases, such as with ADHD, there are excellent track records for pharmacotherapy for the coexisting problems. Short of this, it does not seem prudent to medicate the patients, often with a multitude of drugs in rapid-fire succession for a set of symptoms and signs that are often much more efficaciously approached by solid behavioral interventions.

Certainly, if other conditions are present, they should be treated if possible. If oppositional defiant disorder behavior becomes more severe and pervasive, medications discussed for aggressive behaviors may be tried. However, before embarking on a trial of psychopharmacology, the physician must be certain of exactly what it is that he or she is trying to accomplish. The simple fact is that most patients with oppositional defiant disorder simply cannot be improved unless we are able to develop a suitable procedure for a "personality transplant."

PHOBIAS AND PANIC DISORDERS

Phobias are usually considered under the general group of anxiety disorders. The most common phobia seen in developmental and behavioral pediatric practice is school phobia, which has been renamed as part of separation anxiety disorder. Many children with fears and phobias should be managed with counseling and psychological therapy, but medical intervention is sometimes indicated in recalcitrant cases. The two phobic disorders that occasionally require medical therapy include school and social phobias.

The agents most often used are in the benzodiazepine anxiolytic group. The longer-acting clonazepam may be more efficacious, especially given the tolerance and dependency possibilities of this group of drugs (Biederman, 1987). The other groups of medications showing occasional promise for these disorders include the tricyclic antidepressants, such as imipramine, and possibly the serotonin-reuptake inhibitors, such as paroxetine. However, specific therapeutic efficacy for these agents is still far from proven.

Panic attacks are also considered as being included in the general purview of anxiety disorders. There has been some evidence that clonazepam has been effective in some of the studies in children and adolescents with panic attacks. Some patients have also been shown to respond to treatment with one of the tricyclic antidepressants (e.g., imipramine). However, the overall response rate of children and adolescents for this problem continues to be less than robust.

REFERENCES

Ambrosini P, Biauch M, Rabinovich H, et al: Anti-depressants in children and adolescents. I. Affective disorders. J Am Acad Child Adolesc Psychiatry 32:1, 1993.

American Psychiatric Association: Diagnostic and Statistical Manual of Mental Disorders, ed 4. Washington, DC, American Psychiatric Association, 1994.

Balon R: Buspirone for attention deficit disorder? (Letter to editor). J Clin Psychopharmacol 10:77, 1990.

Baren M: ADHD: do we finally have it right? Contemp Pediatr 11(11):96, 1994.

Bernstein MD, Perwien AR: Anxiety disorders. Child Adolesc Psychiatr Clin N Am 4(2):305, 1995.

Biederman J: Clonazepam in the treatment of prepubertal children with panic-like symptoms. J Clin Psychiatry 48:38, 1987.

Botteron KN, Geller B: Pharmacologic treatment of childhood and adolescent mania. Child Adolesc Psychiatr Clin N Am 4(2):283, 1995.

Cantwell D: Attention deficit disorder: a review of the past 10 years. J Am Acad Child Adolesc Psychiatry 35(8):978, 1995.

Carlson GA, Cantwell DP: Unmasking masked depression in children and adolescents. Am J Psychiatry 137:445, 1980.

Chappell PB, Leckman JF, Riddle MA: The pharmacologic treatment of tic disorders. Child Adolesc Psychiatr Clin N Am 4(1):197–204, 1995.

Connor D: Beta-blockers for aggression: a review of the pediatric experience. J Child Adolesc Psychopharmacol 3:99, 1993.

Cook EH, Leventhal BL: Autistic disorder and other pervasive developmental disorders. Child Adolesc Psychiatr Clin N Am 4(2):381, 1995.

Cueva JE, Overall JE, Small AM, et al: Carbamazepine in aggressive children with conduct disorder. J Am Acad Child Adolesc Psychiatry 35(4):480, 1996.

DuPaul GJ, Stoner G: ADHD in the Schools: Assessment and Intervention Strategies. New York, Guilford Press, 1994, p 62.

Famularo R, Kinscherff R: Pediatric psychopharmacology. *In* Levine MD, Carey WB, Crocker AC (eds): Developmental-Behavioral Pediatrics, 2nd ed. Philadelphia, WB Saunders, 1992, p 740.

Gadow KD, Sverd J, Sprafkin J, et al: Efficacy of methylphenidate for attention-deficit/hyperactivity disorder in children with tic disorder. Arch Gen Psychiatry 52:444, 1995.

Gordon C, State R, Nelson J, et al: A double-blind comparison of clomipramine, desipramine, and placebo in the treatment of autistic disorder. Arch Gen Psychiatry 50:441, 1993.

Green WH: The treatment of attention deficit–hyperactivity disorder with nonstimulant medications. Child Adolesc Psychiatr Clin N Am 4(1):169, 1995.

Hewlett WA, Vinogradov S, Agras WS: Clomipramine, clonazepam, and clonidine treatment of obsessive-compulsive disorder. J Clin Psychopharmacol 12(6):420, 1992.

Hunt R, Capper L, O'Connell B: Clonidine in child and adolescent psychiatry. J Child Adolesc Psychopharmacol 1:87, 1990.

Hunt RD, Lau S, Ryu J: Alternative therapies for ADHD. *In* Greenhill LL, Osman BB (eds): Ritalin: Theory and Patient Management. New York, Mary Ann Liebert, 1991, p 75.

Kopala LC: Risperidone for child and adolescent schizophrenia. Child Adolesc Psychopharmacol News 1(2):1, 1996.

Kutcher S: Venlafaxine—mini review. Child Adolesc Psychopharmacol News 1(4):1, 1996a.

Kutcher S: Buspirone for generalized anxiety disorder in children and adolescents. Child Adolesc Psychopharmacol News 1(1):1, 1996b.

Kye C, Ryan N: Pharmacologic treatment of child and adolescent depression. Child Adolesc Psychiatr Clin N Am 4(2):261, 1995.

Leventhal B, Cook E, Morford M, et al: Fenfluramine: clinical and neurochemical effects in children with autism. J Neuropsychiatry Clin Neurosci 5(307), 1993.

Levine MD: Attentional variation and dysfunction. *In* Levine MD, Carey WB, Crocker AC (eds): Developmental-Behavioral Pediatrics, 2nd ed. Philadelphia, WB Saunders, 1992, p 468.

Lohr D, Birmaher B: Psychotic disorders. Child Adolesc Psychiatr Clin N Am 4(1):237, 1995.

March JS, Leonard HL, Swedo SE: Pharmacotherapy of obsessive-compulsive disorder. Child Adolesc Psychiatr Clin N Am 4(1):217, 1995.

Papatheodorou G: A review of valproate in acute adolescent mania. Child Adolesc Psychopharmacol News 1(1):10, 1996.

Popper CW: Balancing knowledge and judgement. Child Adolesc Psychiatr Clin N Am 4(2):492, 1995a.

Popper CW: A clinician looks at new developments in child and adolescent psychopharmacology. Child Adolesc Psychiatr Clin N Am 4(2):485, 1995b.

Radomski JW, Dursen SM, Revley MA: Toxic serotonin syndrome "TSS": an update and review of diagnostic criteria (abstract 84). J Psychopharmacol Suppl A 21, 1995.

Riddle MA, Krug RA, Hardin MT, et al: Behavioral side effects of fluoxetine in children and adolescents. J Child Adolesc Psychopharmacol 1:193, 1990/1991.

Spencer T, Biederman J, Kerman K, et al: Desipramine treatment of children with attention-deficit/hyperactivity disorder and tic disorder or Tourette's syndrome. J Am Acad Child Adolesc Psychiatry 32:211, 1993.

Stoewe JR, Kruess MJP, Leilo DF: Psychopharmacology of aggressive states and features of conduct disorder. Child Adolesc Psychiatr Clin N Am 4(2):359, 1995.

Swanson JM, Flockhart D, Urdea BA, et al: Efficacy and side effects of clonidine in the treatment of children with ADHD. J Child Adolesc Psychopharmacol 5:301, 1995.

Swanson JM, McBurnett K, Wigal T: Effect of stimulant medication on children with attention deficit disorder: a "review of reviews." Exceptional Children 60(2):154, 1993.

Towbin KE: Evaluation, establishing the treatment alliance, and informed consent. Child Adolesc Psychiatr Clin N Am 4(1):1, 1995.

Trott GE, Friese HJ, Menzel M, et al: Use of meclobemide in children with attention-deficit/hyperactivity disorder. Psychopharmacology (Berl) 106:S134, 1992.

Walkup JT: Clinical decision making in child and adolescent psychopharmacology. Child Adolesc Psychiatr Clin N Am 4(1):23, 1995.

Wender PH: Attention-deficit/hyperactivity disorder. *In* Howell JG (ed): Modern Perspectives in Clinical Psychiatry. New York, Brunner/Mazel, 1988, p 149.

Wilens TE, Biederman J, Geist DE, et al: Nortryptyline in the treatment of ADHD: a chart review of 58 cases. J Am Acad Child Adolesc Psychiatry 32:270, 1993.

Zobieta J, Alessi N: Acute and chronic administration of trazadone in the treatment of disruptive behavior disorders in children. J Clin Psychopharmacol 12:3346, 1992.

83 The Emergency Department Management of Behavioral Crises

Marjorie S. Hardy • Ann R. Ernst • Ken L. Cheyne

 Behavioral difficulties are most commonly thought of as chronic conditions that demand long-term management. However, the clinician must also have expertise in handling the more acute behavioral crisis. In this chapter, two distinct forms of behavioral urgent care are delineated. First there are the emergencies brought on by maladaptive behaviors, the potentially self-destructive life events that often represent the extreme exacerbation of symptoms or the ultimate manifestation of risk factors. Second is the situation in which a true medical crisis has significant developmental-behavioral implications. In both instances, careful assessment, prompt management, and appropriate long-term follow-up are essential. Although we do not advocate the design and construction of behavioral intensive care units, it is certainly the case that the clinician who deals with developmental-behavioral problems must be responsive to the unsettling acute crisis.

Physicians working with children in crisis are often placed in the position of playing multiple roles: medical care provider, comforter, educator, and decision maker. There is one role, however, that has received little attention, either in the literature or in medical school training programs: that of mental health provider. The physician and other medical care providers are often the first and only conduit for immediate and long-term psychological care for children and their families. A survey of 44 large children's hospitals in the United States revealed that 72% did not have Child Life program workers available, even for consultation (Krebel, Clayton, and Graham, 1996). At hospitals where psychologists, psychiatrists, and Child Life program workers are available for consultation, they often work only during the day, despite the fact that more patient contacts are made during the evenings (Krebel, Clayton, and Graham, 1996). Thus, physicians and nurses must be prepared to deal with both obvious psychiatric emergencies and less obvious ones.

It is usually clear what delineates a psychiatric emergency from a medical emergency. Typical psychiatric emergencies include substance abuse, panic attacks, conversion disorder, depressive disorders, and suicide. However, children and their families with medical emergencies are often in need of immediate psychological services as a result of the trauma they have suffered.

EXAMPLE, PART I

The pungent odor of smoke radiated from the hair of Ben, who had suffered smoke inhalation, and drifted out of the emergency department examination room. Ben was quiet and withdrawn, too passive for a 6-year-old. He had been rescued from the fire in the middle of the night. He wanted his mother, who had not yet arrived at the hospital. He wanted his siblings, who had escaped without injury. He also was being needled for an arterial blood gas

analysis and carboxyhemoglobin level. A chest radiograph was obtained. He had been snatched from his home filled with black suffocating air and been taken to a hospital where strangers were invading the privacy of his body. After emergency medical care was completed, the mother arrived to provide the comfort he needed. She also needed some time to recount her witness of the crisis and to prepare for meeting the immediate needs of Ben and her other children.

In this example, it might be easy to overlook the psychological needs of Ben and his family while focusing on their more immediate medical needs. This oversight, however, could have long-term negative sequelae. Although prevalence data are unavailable for children, it has been suggested that children who experience natural disasters, domestic violence, abuse, neglect, gunshot injury, the death of a loved one, or chronic illness are at risk for developing posttraumatic stress disorder (PTSD) (Kronenberger and Meyer, 1996). For these children, the future may hold nightmares, agitation, disorganized behavior, and emotional numbness (see Chapter 19). This disorder and its symptoms, however, can often be avoided when preventive services are given immediately after the event. Thus, the prevention or amelioration of immediate and future symptoms falls into the hands of frontline physicians. Fortunately for Ben, various professionals in the hospital attended to his psychological needs as well as to his medical needs:

EXAMPLE, PART II

While in the hospital, Ben made pictures of his memory of the experience, which were copied and presented along with a thank-you note dictated to the firefighter who rescued him. He dictated a story about being in a fire, which he later shared with his classmates. He developed a safety plan and had the family rehearse escape routes after moving to the family's new home.

Before leaving the hospital, Ben was given information geared to his level to understand his laboratory studies and radiographs. It seemed important to deal not only with the fire but also with the subsequent events. After discharge, Ben was followed up for possible neurologic dysfunction secondary to hypoxia. None developed.

The situations in which behavioral management may become necessary are broad. They include cases in which children are assaulted, traumatically injured, or involved in natural disasters (e.g., a hurricane). Other emergencies include those in which children hurt themselves, either deliberately or accidentally. Children may also experience crisis secondary to specific medical conditions (e.g., noncompliance) or psychiatric emergencies (e.g., panic attacks). Finally, the emotional needs of children cannot be overlooked when they have witnessed or learned of the death of others. This chapter presents several vignettes that describe actual and typical pediatric emergency department crises. The examples in this chapter illustrate the wide array of situations in which physicians may find themselves having to respond to a child's and family's emotional needs. Both medical emergencies with a psychological component and psychiatric emergencies are included. Management of each crisis and suggestions for handling similar behavioral emergencies are included. The suggestions may be applied broadly across any number of behavioral emergencies, although treatment should be tailored to a child's and family's individual needs.

Psychological Management of Medical Emergencies

Typically, the medical management of physical injuries in children overrides their psychological needs. In any emergency, the immediate goal is to administer aid and sustain life. After the crisis is over, however, the child or family may be left physically healed but psychologically traumatized. This section discusses the psychological needs and interventions for children who have been assaulted, accidentally injured, or noncompliant in their treatment regimen. However, *any* incident that results in emergency department treatment may eventually lead to behavioral and emotional difficulties.

CHILDREN AS VICTIMS OF ASSAULT

EXAMPLE

Natalie, an eighth-grader, was talking with a friend in the school hallway when she was confronted by a group of girls who accused her of spreading rumors. They pushed her into a locker, banging her head. Natalie reported that she thought she "blacked out" for a moment. At the emergency department, Natalie complained of headache. A bump, 3 cm in diameter, appeared on the posterior aspect of her skull.

The emergency department staff assessed vital signs, completed a neurologic examination, and ordered a computed tomography scan. When the results were reported to be within normal limits, acetaminophen was recom-

mended for the headache. A follow-up physician's office visit was scheduled within 3 days with instructions to call sooner if problems arose.

The mental health consultant was called to the scene and met with Natalie and her parents; an authorization to share the information with the school was obtained, the school counselor was contacted, and the parents were encouraged to discuss with their lawyer their desire to press charges. Referral information for ongoing counseling services was provided. A plan for school reentry was developed in conjunction with the school counselor.

Increasingly, children are becoming the victims of assault at the hands of other children, adults, and even their parents. Other children are witnesses to violence (see Chapters 17 and 51). Much has been written to address the issue of sexual and physical abuse (see, for example, Knutson and DeVet, 1995); the focus here is on children who have been victims of general assault. Bullying, for example, affects 15% to 20% of students and is becoming more frequent and taking on more serious forms as students bring weapons to school (Batsche, 1994). To address the emotional needs of the victims of bullies, several suggestions are offered.

First, physicians and nurses are urged to consider and treat the assault seriously, regardless of the perpetrator. Too often, fights between children and adolescents are considered less serious than fights between adults or between adults and children. Children, however, can be capable of inflicting serious harm on one another, particularly when there is an imbalance of power or size. Just as a physician may involve the legal system when adults assault one another, so should legal action be considered when the individuals involved are children or adolescents. With releases to share information obtained, the school counselor should be notified of the situation. A bully who is allowed to continue bullying other children may, in time, become an adult who assaults other adults.

Second, the physician is urged to consider the unique situation in which a child is placed. Being the victim of assault by more powerful peers often leaves a child feeling inferior, weak, and out of control. Therefore, the physician is encouraged to give the child some sense of control over the situation. For example, the child could be included in the discussion of pressing charges against the assailant. Also, if there is opportunity, the child should be allowed to assert control during his or her treatment as well. The type of control the child is allowed to assert, however, should be carefully monitored. Telling the child, "I will give you a shot in your arm when you are ready" may result in a child's being overwhelmed with the decision of *when* to experience more pain, whereas asking a child, "Where do you want the shot—in your arm or your leg?" allows the child to assert control without controlling the situation.

Third, the child may be referred for outpatient counseling. The long-term impact of bullying on children includes school avoidance, withdrawal, dangerous behaviors (especially, carrying a weapon to school to defend oneself), and declines in academic performance (Batsche, 1994). Furthermore, victims of bullying typically come in two "sizes": the passive, anxious, insecure victims and the hot-tempered, restless, provocative victims (Batsche, 1994). Both types of children may benefit from counseling in order to teach them more effective ways of asserting themselves.

ACCIDENTAL INJURIES AND THEIR SEQUELAE

Oftentimes, children are the victims not of the wrath of others, but of misfortune, accident, or lack of supervision. Children may accidentally ingest substances, fall off their bicycles, be involved in car accidents, fall into swimming pools, get too close to a fire, and so on. In these cases, the injuries are often treated without consideration of the possible emotional impact on the children.

EXAMPLE, PART I

Andrea, a 4-year-old girl, was visiting relatives when she attempted to pet their German shepherd, which was unaccustomed to young children. The animal growled, pounced, and bit Andrea's chin, shoulder, and hand. The child and parents were tearful and trembling on arrival at the emergency department. There, initial wound hygiene and inspection for possible chest trauma or major vascular injury occurred. The surgeon on call arrived clothed in green scrubs, and it was determined that surgery under general anesthesia was required.

In most cases, such a scenario is straightforward and no psychological intervention appears necessary by the medical care personnel. But accidents such as this can be traumatic for children. While in the hospital, Andrea played out scenes and talked to others about the initial incident. For several days after the hospital stay, she woke fretfully with nightmares of a "green monster."

Are Andrea's behaviors typical? Why is she dreaming about "green monsters" instead of dogs? Consultation with a pediatric psychologist on staff at the hospital revealed the source of her anxieties:

EXAMPLE, PART II

At the suggestion of the therapist, the surgeon met with the child at her postoperative outpatient visit. The surgeon showed Andrea pictures of his children and a set of green scrubs. Thereafter the child's nightmares subsided. Andrea continued to display mild distress and to seek adult comfort on seeing large dogs. Her parents praised her for her wariness, but they reinforced her verbalization of feelings rather than her being tearful or clinging. At Christmas, the family sent the surgeon homemade cookies with a family portrait including a smiling Andrea and a cocker spaniel puppy.

In this case, the role of the on-call surgeon extended beyond the operating room. Through no fault of his own, he was the source of Andrea's anxiety, no doubt because of her heightened arousal while in the emergency department. Because of the psychological intervention, any future visits to the hospital or emergency department will not be as terrifying for Andrea and her family as they could be had the intervention not taken place.

When children with traumatic accidental injuries are seen at emergency departments, they are often in a state of heightened arousal. This state of arousal can make normal events and stimuli frightening, and it can make frightening events and stimuli terrifying. Emergency department personnel should be aware of this state in the children and try to minimize excessive stimulation. Thus, quiet rooms, dimmer lights, and "normal" clothing can all help the child remain somewhat calmer. These suggestions are relevant to the inpatient setting as well.

Personnel should also be aware of the heightened state of arousal in parents of injured children. The response of parents to a child's injuries and distress can have a significant impact on the child's reported level of anxiety and concomitant disruptive behaviors. Most physicians can recall parents crying and holding their children and saying to them, "I'm so sorry" or "You'll be okay." It is not surprising that if a parent is distressed, the child may become more distressed. What is not so obvious, however, is the counterintuitive finding that parents who provide reassurance, empathy, and apologies to children may actually heighten their children's distress by cueing and reinforcing their fears. What, then, is a parent to do? Research suggests that distraction before a procedure and coaching of coping techniques (e.g., "Take a deep breath; think about grandma's house") during any actual procedures may serve to diminish distress in an anxious child (Varni et al, 1995). Thus, physicians and nurses may find that by first calming parents, explaining to them the impact of their behavior on their child, and coaching them on more adaptive ways to interact in the current situation, the child may be less distressed.

As in the case of assault presented earlier, allowing children some control over the medical situation may be reparative in the aftermath of an injury that was uncontrollable.

EXAMPLE

Ronald, a 6-year-old boy, was sleepwalking when he collided with the aquarium. He was not asleep when the pediatric psychologist arrived at the emergency department. A pediatrician and nurse were attempting to extricate glass splinters from his body. Ronald was not helping; he was alternately yelling and sobbing.

The pediatric psychologist told Ronald what had happened, what needed to be done, and what choices Ronald had. Thereafter, Ronald chose self-management over leather restraints or general anesthesia, and he chose to have his father observe his bravery. With Ronald thus given "control" over the situation, treatment was administered.

With respect to accidental injuries, medical personnel are reminded that traumatic experiences can have long-lasting impact on the adjustment of the child. A child who nearly drowns may develop a phobia for water; a child who is in an automobile accident may become frightened to get into a car. To avoid such long-term sequelae, children need the opportunity to "work out" the trauma they have experienced. In Andrea's case, for example, she talked to people about the experience and played out scenes. Ben, who was involved in the house fire, drew pictures relating to the incident. Just as adults need the opportunity to talk about traumatic experiences, so do children need the opportunity to work out and replay the events they have experienced. Thus, if children attempt to talk about what happened to them, they should be encouraged to do so and not be told, "Hush, don't think about it." Furthermore, given the potential long term impact of the experience, the family should be encouraged to consult with a psychiatrist or a psychologist on staff or to seek outside counseling following their return home. Sometimes the traumatic experience can have recurring consequences, which can be successfully managed.

EXAMPLE

Mike, a 3-year-old boy, swallowed a quarter. When rushed to the emergency department, he was surprisingly asymptomatic, although he reported it was painful to swallow. The Heimlich maneuver had been attempted without success. An x-ray confirmed a coin was lodged in the esophagus. Although removal was successful, the patient became phobic about eating any solid foods. Subsequent pediatric psychology consultation worked with Mike and his family on relaxation and desensitization procedures and behavior modification with regard to trying new foods. The food phobia disappeared.

Two years later, Mike appeared at his physician's office saying he felt he couldn't breathe. While being interviewed by the physician, who recalled the quarter incident, Mike revealed that an older cousin had stuffed newspapers in his mouth. Mental health services again were initiated. Cognitive therapy procedures went well as Mike recalled the relaxation techniques he had learned earlier. A family session was also held to deal with reducing symptoms of posttraumatic stress reaction and the family's issue of how to deal with the misconduct of the extended family member. Mike was asymptomatic within 5 days. Further outpatient therapy was of brief duration.

CHRONIC ILLNESS AND NONCOMPLIANCE

Managing chronic illnesses is not new to pediatricians (see Chapter 34). Sometimes, children with chronic illnesses experience immediate worsening of their illnesses (e.g., a child with sickle cell disease experiences a pain crisis). The information presented earlier about managing pain and distress in the Accidental Injuries section may be helpful in this situation. Children with asthma often are seen with frightening and potentially life-threatening respiratory crises. (For information on management of the emotional needs of asthmatic children in crisis, see Creer and Bender, 1995.) For some of these children, their medical needs are brought on simply through the physiologic process of their illness and can be managed medically. For other children, their own behavior plays a role in their crises and, as such, should be addressed as well.

EXAMPLE, PART I

Jill, a 14-year-old girl with poorly controlled insulin-dependent diabetes mellitus (IDDM) of 8 years' duration, is seen in the emergency department following an episode of drinking a half-bottle of whiskey approximately 4 hours earlier. Jill was mildly intoxicated, but still conversant.

She had experienced six episodes of vomiting within the past 2 hours. Her father reported that lately Jill has been injecting her insulin and then refusing to eat her meals. Jill and her mother often end up in screaming matches over her eating habits.

Compliance (sometimes referred to as adherence) with medical regimen has long been a concern of physicians, psychologists, parents, and other caregivers. Compliance is an issue in a number of pediatric illnesses, including asthma and diabetes, and in any illness that requires a child (or parent) to monitor his or her status, to take prescribed medications, or to adhere to a behavioral regimen (e.g., exercise). Children who do not comply with treatment sometimes "strike a nerve" with physicians. It can be frustrating to provide care for children who do not take care of themselves.

Understanding why children do not comply with regimens is the first key to helping these children help themselves, and the reasons are many. Some children are cognitively incapable of handling the responsibility of taking care of their medical needs, in which case the parents need to increase their involvement. Other children use noncompliance to express their anger or as a form of rebellion. For example, one child who had received a heart transplant several years earlier stopped taking her posttransplant medication whenever her mother disciplined her, because she believed that her mother would "get into trouble" (medical neglect) if she became ill. In this case, immaturity and anger played roles in her behavior. Other children fail to comply because of the side effects, both physical and psychological, of the treatment. Children with diabetes may resent not being able to eat sweets, and children who must take steroids may refuse to do so because of the weight gain. Finally, and possibly underlying all of the other issues, children often do not have the foresight that adults have, so they are less cognizant of the possible consequences of their noncompliance. When the heart-transplant patient was asked what would happen if her body rejected the heart because she did not take her medication, she replied, "I'd just get a new one."

Besides patient variables, other researchers have found physician variables to have an impact on compliance. For example, parental satisfaction with medical care, friendliness, warmth, empathy, support, continued contact, convenience of medical care, and adequate communication among the doctor, patient, and family members have all been implicated in studies of compliance (LaGreca and Schuman, 1995). Knowing these factors may influence compliance, physicians may assess their own possible role in the immediate situation.

Interventions to improve compliance with medical regimens typically require a referral to a mental health provider or liaison with such providers in the hospital. Oftentimes, providing individual and family social support, behavioral incentive programs, or self-monitoring can be effective in helping these children and their families.

Actions that a physician or nurse may immediately take include educating the patient and families. Perhaps the child does not understand what needs to be done, despite the parent's belief to the contrary. Perhaps the parents do not understand what must be done as well. Page and colleagues (1981) found that health care providers of children with diabetes made an average of seven recommendations to parents. Parents recalled, on average, only two, and some of the recalled recommendations were not even the ones made by the health care providers. Thus, giving written instructions and recommendations is suggested to decrease the need to rely on parents' and patient's memory.

Along the lines of education, providers may also want to make sure that patients and their families understand the consequences of noncompliance. Because children and adolescents may not appreciate the long-term complications of noncompliance, providing them with such information may be useful. When the heart recipient patient reported, "I'd just get a new [heart]," she was informed that this may not be possible.

The pediatrician may want to encourage the child to either increase his or her responsibility for self-care, in the cases of adolescents who are "rebelling" from their parents, or decrease responsibility, in the case of the child who is too young to care for his or her own medical needs. Also, having the parents post reminders for the children in various places (e.g., the bathroom mirror) may minimize confrontation between the parent and child while making the child aware of what must done. Finally, encouraging self-monitoring and frequent visits or calls to the physician's office may serve as reminders as well.

EXAMPLE, PART II

Medical assessment of Jill in the emergency department included assessing vital signs, measuring blood glucose and alcohol levels, and giving intravenous fluids and insulin to ensure adequate hydration and stabilization of blood glucose. Careful monitoring was provided to ensure normalization of blood sugar. Mental health intervention included individual and family assessment of stressors, depression, substance abuse, and feelings regarding Jill's diabetes. A contract regarding rules, chores, and privileges with rewards and consequences was established. The contract was developed with input from Jill, her parents, and physician. Reeducation was provided on diabetes and its management. Information was also provided regarding the effects of alcohol on Jill's diabetes.

Ongoing therapy was scheduled. Autonomous functioning and family stress reduction were advanced by having Jill spend four postdischarge weekends with a favorite aunt, who was also a registered nurse. Jill maintained weekly medical appointments and called in to the physician's nurse on a regular basis to report her blood sugar levels. Communication was exchanged between her therapist and physician after appropriate releases had been signed before hospital discharge. After 6 weeks, Jill was self-managing her diabetic regimen, had stopped drinking, and agreed to continue to work with the therapist and her parents to improve communication.

Psychiatric Disorders

Children in the midst of a psychiatric emergency often first come to the attention of physicians and nurses. Even though a psychiatric consultation is typically warranted, the medical care providers are often an integral part of the treatment plan and initiation. In this section, two cases are presented, one in which the child has apparently attempted suicide and another in which the child is excessively angry and possibly violent. Although these cases demonstrate the two broad bands of psychological disorders in children—internalizing problems (e.g., anxiety, depression) and externalizing problems (e.g., aggression, defiance)—they are not exhaustive of the wide range of psychiatric difficulties with which physicians come into contact. Medical care providers are often the first to confront children who are experiencing panic attacks, school refusal, psychotic disorders, pregnancy, and eating problems, among other difficulties.

WHEN A CHILD ATTEMPTS SUICIDE

Nothing is more alarming or concerning than a child or adolescent who believes that life is not worth maintaining (see Chapter 64). The rate of suicides among young people is increasing rapidly. The underlying disorder that leads to the feelings accompanying suicidal ideation and attempts is not always depression; children with behavioral problems (including substance abuse), anxiety, and social rejection are also at increased risk for suicide.

EXAMPLE, PART I

Rachel, a 13-year-old girl, was seen at the emergency department with her parents the day after having a friend stay overnight. Twelve hours before her arrival at the hospital, Rachel ingested thirty 500-mg acetaminophen tablets in the bathroom of her home. Her friend also ingested numerous acetaminophen tablets at the same time. Both went to bed and fell asleep within 1 hour of the ingestion; however, Rachel awoke 4 hours after the ingestion with nausea and vomiting. She vomited approximately eight times over the next 4 to 6 hours. She was not certain whether there were any pill fragments in the emesis. Approximately 11 hours after the ingestion, Rachel's parents learned of the ingestion from her friend's parents and brought her to the emergency department.

Rachel's parents, who both appeared at the emergency department, had been divorced for 1 year, and both were involved in new relationships. Rachel, an eighth-grader in middle school, was passing all subjects with B's and C's. During the interview, she reported that she was sexually active with her 15-year-old boyfriend. She acknowledged she smoked cigarettes and had used both marijuana and alcohol recently.

Is Rachel depressed? In cases of suicidal attempt, this is the initial hypothesis that a medical care provider may entertain. Certainly, suicidal ideation is present in more than one fourth of children with depression (Stark, Rouse, and Livingston, 1991). But that leaves three fourths of depressed youngsters who are not suicidal. What factors separate the two? In other words, what emotional and cognitive variables predict suicidal behavior? Research suggests that suicidal ideation is frequently accompanied by feelings of hopelessness, low self-esteem, and unbearable psychological pain (Leenaars and Wenckstern, 1991; Pataki and Carlson, 1990). Other risk factors include life stresses (ranging from the anticipation of punishment to the death of a parent); poor coping skills; family environments marked by poor boundaries, inflexibility, stress, and parental psychopathology; recent suicide attempts or completions in the child's family or school environment; lack of perceived support; substance use; and poor impulse control. In addition, children who attempt suicide are often "repeat attempters," have threatened suicide in the past, are preoccupied with death, and may leave a suicide note (Kronenberger and Meyer, 1996). Therefore, it is these characteristics that should be assessed if a physician is concerned about the potential of suicide, independent of the presence of other depressive features. In addition, one should not hesitate to ask children if they are considering suicide—asking will not "give them the idea" and may avert a tragedy. It is important that the child be interviewed with respect to his or her feelings toward suicide and other emotional turmoil; oftentimes, parents are unaware of their child's internal state. There are several standardized interviews and scales that may be administered to a child who is suspected of being depressed or suicidal, although an informal interview with a warm and empathic professional may better uncover the desired information.

Once the physician is certain that the child is feeling suicidal, the physician's course of action is crucial. The reaction to the child's attempt should be carefully monitored. Anger toward the child or dismissal of the attempt could be detrimental. A 7-year-old child seen in an outpatient setting reported that she had tried to kill herself by pushing a pillow down on her face. Even though it might be easy to dismiss such an attempt because of its lack of lethality, her underlying desire to kill herself and her feelings of anxiety and depression could not be denied. The child who makes what appears to be a half-hearted or nonlethal attempt may be the child who succeeds next time, given the opportunity and means. Equally important is the physician's role with the parents. Parents often react with disbelief or anger toward their child when a suicidal attempt is made. These same parents may say, "Go ahead—kill yourself! You still won't get. . . ." The medical care provider can and should play the role of calming the parents and helping them to realize the seriousness of the situation.

At this point, the physician must decide whether to discharge the (medically stable) patient, admit the patient to the general hospital for observation, or secure commitment to a psychiatric unit or hospital. These decisions should be made in consultation with a mental health provider and should address the current status of the child and the stability and coping resources of the family. If the physician feels comfortable releasing the patient, believing that the child is no longer suicidal and will be safe until counseling can begin within the next few days, a suicide contract with the patient may be drawn before discharge. In such a contract, the patient signs a statement agreeing not to kill himself or herself. If the child refuses to sign such a contract, it should be taken as a message that the child does not feel safe to go home. If the physician is unsure of the child's safety, it is best to be cautious; involuntarily hospitalizing a nonsuicidal patient is far less concerning than releasing a suicidal patient. Once the patient is in therapy, the underlying causes of the suicidal attempt may be addressed (perhaps necessitating substance abuse counseling, family counseling, or medication), and treatment begun.

EXAMPLE, PART II

The emergency department physician ascertained that Rachel was medically stable by assessing her vital signs. Acetaminophen toxicity, liver function, renal function, pregnancy status, and the possibility of coingestants were assessed, with serum chemistries, urinalysis, and urine drug screen including substances of abuse. Activated charcoal was administered to aid with acetaminophen elimination. Preparation was made to begin Mucomyst if indicated. Rachel was admitted to an observation bed to monitor for toxicity and to solidify a behavioral intervention plan to prevent recurrence.

Mental health interventions included interviewing for symptoms of depression and other mental disorders, crisis counseling to the family, and assessment of parental strengths and weaknesses to determine management strategies for this adolescent at discharge. Social, family, and school histories were obtained to determine other stressors and family history of mental disorders. Information was elicited on recent behaviors at school, with peers, and at home with emphasis on recent behavioral changes. Releases were obtained from the patient to discuss the pregnancy and drug test results (state law required the patient's consent to discuss these findings with anyone, even parents). A tentative treatment plan with input from all parties involved, including the attending physician, was developed. Revisions were made after information was obtained from standardized psychological tests. Releases to exchange information with the school were obtained, and individual and family counseling continued after discharge, with the school counselor providing liaison services in that setting. Substance abuse education also was scheduled. Before the patient's discharge, a gynecologic evaluation was scheduled to provide information on responsible sexual decision making, pregnancy prevention, and sexually transmitted disease prevention, including prevention of human immunodeficiency virus infection. All of these measures were agreed upon by the patient and family.

THE AGGRESSIVE CHILD

Behavioral problems are common among young children, with prevalence estimates for clinically significant levels ranging from 2% to 16% of boys and 2% to 9% of girls (American Psychiatric Association, 1994). The behaviors range from relatively minor oppositional and defiant behavior to more serious forms of misbehavior and aggression, such as fighting, setting fires, abusing animals, and breaking the law (see Chapter 49).

Such behaviors are less common in girls, although adolescent girls with behavioral problems often have substance use problems, promiscuity, and minor violations of the law.

EXAMPLE, PART I

Richard, a 14-year-old boy, was brought to the emergency department by his mother and a local law enforcement officer. Richard had become angry at his mother when she told him that he could not leave the house after dinner. He had then immediately begun swearing at his mother, knocked a lamp off an end table, and put his fist through a door. His mother became frightened and called the police. Richard had always had a "short fuse" but had not become so physically destructive in the past.

Disruptive behavior disorders typically begin early in a child's life. The 5-year-old child who angrily defies his parents is at risk for becoming the 15-year-old adolescent who drops out of school, uses substances, breaks the law, and is aggressive toward his peers. That is not to say, by any means, that any oppositional behavior in a child is a sure sign that the child is likely to become delinquent. In fact, most oppositional defiant children do not develop conduct disorder later in life. However, retrospective studies of adolescents with conduct disorder do reveal that nearly all had met the criteria for oppositional defiant disorder earlier in their lives (Loeber, Lahey, and Thomas, 1991). To distinguish between the typical and "normal" opposition of a young child and more serious forms of the disorder, the duration, frequency, and intensity of the behaviors should be considered. Such behaviors include anger, defiance, losing one's temper, blaming others for misbehavior, and vengeful, annoying, or provocative behavior. Because parents often dismiss such behaviors as typical, it is important that physicians routinely assess behavioral and emotional functioning of their patients. Likewise, physicians should evaluate the parents' typical means of handling these behaviors and suggest educational counseling if the child is at risk. In the case of behavior disorders, the adage "an ounce of prevention is worth a pound of cure" often holds true.

Medical care providers should also gather other pertinent information once they have reason to believe a child may have a disruptive behavior problem. An assessment of the family environment is especially important, given that the parents of children with behavior problems are often excessively punitive and inconsistent in their discipline of their child. They have also been found to show a higher rate of depression, substance abuse, and criminal behaviors. The mechanism by which these family factors influence behavior problems in the child is unknown, although there is most likely some interaction by the time the child manifests difficulties. For example, a child who kicks and screams to get his way receives positive reinforcement for the behavior when parents reward him with acquiescence, whereas the parents' behavior is negatively reinforced by the temporary peace acquiescence buys. It is important to obtain detailed information on how the parent handles the child's misbehavior (and how the child "handles" the parent).

Once it has been established that the child is exhibiting significant behavioral difficulties, the physician may offer advice on parenting. Parents sometimes forget to reward their children for good behaviors, focusing instead exclusively on negative behavior. Parents may also not be aware of alternatives to harsh discipline or they may use such nonviolent techniques as "time out" incorrectly and thus ineffectively. Some physicians may not feel comfortable providing such advice to parents. Alternatively, the physician may make a referral for counseling, encouraging the entire family to become involved. Sometimes, community groups and churches offer parenting classes that provide support and educate participants on basic parenting skills, a forum that sometimes reduces defensiveness and resistance in parents.

The aforementioned suggestions are not meant to imply that once parents change their approach to their misbehaving child, their child will suddenly, or even shortly, begin behaving. The child has had several years to learn these behaviors, and it will take time and attention from a mental health provider to "unlearn" them. A referral to counseling may lead to a program designed to help children manage their anger, develop social skills, and problem solve in social situations.

Finally, the physician may want to consider medication in severe cases. However, results of controlled studies of the effectiveness of medication for behavior problems have been equivocal. The exception to these findings is when the behavioral problems co-occur with either depression or attention deficits (see Chapter 82), in which case medication can be beneficial. In general, however, medication is most effective when used in conjunction with behavior modification and family therapy.

EXAMPLE, PART II

Richard's medical care included wound hygiene, a radiograph to rule out a fracture, suturing of the lacerations, and tetanus prophylaxis after records revealed no recent tetanus immunization. Richard said he had been angry with his parents, who refused to let him leave to visit friends. He denied substance abuse or suicidal ideation. Family assessment revealed increasing family conflict owing to diminishing grades and economic stressors because the father had been laid off his job. Immediate intervention arranged for a time out cooling-off procedure when Richard's temper escalated. Richard and family agreed to a referral for ongoing counseling dealing with adolescent development, anger management, and conflict resolution.

Conclusion

The vignettes and suggestions offered in this chapter are not intended as "recipes" for the treatment of all patients, because both medical and psychological care should be implemented on an individual basis. General guidelines for medical care providers or allied health care professionals fulfilling the role of behavioral counselor are as follows:

1. Obtain accurate information as to the crisis situation: what happened, where it happened, who was involved, and who came to the emergency department or clinician's office. Keep detailed records of the information obtained.
2. Assess how the crisis and its aftermath are being perceived by those involved. Encourage discussion of the experience.
3. Assess coping strategies of the child and family, as well as the current resources available to support the child.
4. Determine whether further behavioral intervention is indicated. The emergency department physician should notify the primary care physician. Obtain consent to proceed.
5. Develop a specific plan. Determine where and by whom the plan will be implemented. Proceed with the treatment, revising the plan when changes are indicated.

6. Obtain consents so liaisons with appropriate schools and agencies can be initiated.
7. Document contacts with notes in the patient's hospital chart or confidential office file.
8. Summarize services when crisis contacts are completed.
9. Throughout treatment, if further care is not coordinated by the child's own physician, keep the primary health care provider informed of the patient's status.
10. Advise the patient and family of the procedures necessary to reinitiate contact if needed in the future.

Training in crisis intervention is available throughout the world through organizations such as International Critical Incident Stress Foundation, Inc., and the American Red Cross. Some communities have trained and developed a cadre of mental health professionals on call for local disasters or family crises, such as accident, fire, and suicide. Many school districts have developed crisis intervention teams consisting of professionals from within the school system and from the community to address behavioral emergencies within the school setting. These teams provide support following the death of teachers, the death of students, violence within the school setting, and numerous other crises that affect students.

Further research on the outcome of behavioral emergency care is needed. The health care reform movement and consumer advocacy will be additional factors that determine whether the "stitch in time" for the soul, as well as the suture for the skin, is effective crisis management.

REFERENCES

American Psychiatric Association: Diagnostic and Statistical Manual of Mental Disorders, 4th ed. Washington, DC: American Psychiatric Association, 1994.
Batsche GM: Bullies and their victims: understanding a pervasive problem. School Psych Rev 23(2):165–175, 1994.
Creer TL, Bender BG: Pediatric asthma. *In* Roberts MC (ed): Handbook of Pediatric Psychology. New York, Guilford Press, 1995, pp 219–240.
Knutson JF, DeVet KA: Physical abuse, sexual abuse, and neglect. *In* Roberts MC (ed): Handbook of Pediatric Psychology. New York, Guilford Press, 1995, pp 589–616.
Krebel MS, Clayton C, Graham C: Child life programs in the pediatric emergency department. Pediatr Emerg Care 12(1):13–15, 1996.
Kronenberger WG, Meyer RG: The Child Clinician's Handbook. Boston, Allyn & Bacon, 1996.
LaGreca AM, Schuman WB: Adherence to prescribed medial regimens. *In* Roberts MC (ed): Handbook of Pediatric Psychology. New York, Guilford Press, 1995, pp 55–83.
Leenaars, AA, Wenckstern S: Suicide in the school-age child and adolescent. *In* Leenaars AA (ed): Life span perspectives of suicide. New York, Plenum, 1991, pp 95–107.
Loeber R, Lahey BB, Thomas C: Diagnostic conundrum of oppositional-defiant disorder and conduct disorder. J Abnorm Psychol 11:379–390, 1991.
Page P, Verstraetek DG, Robb JR, et al: Patient recall of self-care recommendations in diabetes. Diabetes Care 4:96–98, 1981.
Pataki CS, Carlson GA: Major depression in childhood. *In* Hersen M, Last CG (eds): Handbook of Child and Adult Psychopathology. New York, Pergamon Press, 1991, pp 35–50.
Stark KD, Rouse LW, Livingston R: Treatment of depression during childhood and adolescence: cognitive-behavioral procedures for the individual and family. *In* Kendall PC (ed): Child and Adolescent Therapy: Cognitive-Behavioral Procedures. New York, Guilford Press, 1991, pp 165–206.
Varni JW, Blount RL, Waldron, SA, et al: Management of pain and distress. *In* Roberts MC (ed): Handbook of Pediatric Psychology. New York, Guilford Press, 1995, pp 105–123.

84 Alternative Therapies

Ronald L. Lindsay

 Clinicians are confronted incessantly with "miraculous cures," new and seductive treatments that promise the elimination of undesirable symptoms in the widest range of developmental-behavioral conditions. Commonly pediatricians learn of these quick fixes from parents who are understandably attracted to them. Many such interventions benefit from potent placebo effects. Unfortunately, these therapies are not without their side effects. Among other things, they may delay appropriate and definitive treatment. This chapter examines a group of alternatives that have come to be known as *alternative therapies*. Their claims, their evaluations, and their actual efficacy are considered. This review should help clinicians be more responsive as such possibilities for treatment are considered seriously by families.

Severe neurologic disabilities such as mental retardation, cerebral palsy, and autism share a number of common factors with relatively milder developmental and behavioral problems such as learning and attentional difficulties. These common factors include difficulty of diagnosis, the need for therapy or habilitation over a period of many years (if not throughout a lifetime), and the limited and varying prospects of improvement, much less "cure." These factors result in the emergence of novel therapies that offer families hope (often false) for a "cure" at a time when they are extremely vulnerable. These approaches claim to be less dangerous, invasive, and costly, while being more natural and effective. Parents of children with developmental and behavioral problems tend to view these therapies as reasonable alternatives to approaches that are widely accepted by professionals specializing in the care of children with developmental and behavioral problems. Hence this chapter uses the term *alternative therapies*. Other authors label such therapies *controversial, unproven, nonstandard, other,* and *quackery*; these names reflect both the views of the authors and the nature of the therapies.

There is a clear differentiation between the therapeutic approaches that are accepted by professionals from many disciplines (as discussed in this textbook) and the alternative therapies discussed in this chapter. These differences have been extensively defined (Cohen, 1986; Golden, 1984; Silver, 1995; Sprague and Werry, 1971; Starrett, 1996) and are outlined in Table 84–1.

The purpose of this chapter is to discuss an approach to alternative therapies for the developmental and behavioral problems of childhood. The chapter begins with a differentiation between accepted and alternative therapies. A description of why parents seek out alternative therapies includes a section on how physicians should discuss alternative therapies with parents and children. Finally, individual alternative therapies are outlined and discussed.

Parent Vulnerability

Parents who have the best interests of their children in mind are under considerable psychological and emotional distress when considering the various forms of evaluation and treatment for their children with developmental and behavioral problems. Parents are aware that their child has a problem that they are unable to handle by themselves. When seeking help, parents are confronted by a variety of opinions of what to do. Both lay people and professionals, who may or may not be knowledgeable about the nature of developmental and behavioral problems, offer a multitude of often contradictory or exclusive opinions. It is both challenging and anxiety-provoking for parents to determine the best course for their child.

In many areas of the country, adequate educational, psychological, and medical services either are unavailable or vary considerably in quality, depending on the level of public support or interest. Many primary care physicians do not have adequate knowledge of developmental and behavioral problems. They may not be as familiar with the array of educational and social services available in their community or state. Conversely, nonmedical professionals working with children with developmental and behavioral problems may be unaware of possible medical etiologies for these problems or otherwise resistant to referring children to physicians. At times there is an almost adversarial role between the diverse professionals who are supposed to be working together for the best interests of the child.

Parents are often "kept in the dark" during evaluations for developmental and behavioral problems. This occurs in both the medical and psychoeducational realms. As a result, parents have little choice but to assume a passive role. They are often not included in the evaluation process, save for a cursory history. Often their first opportunity for involvement occurs when they are asked for their permission to initiate educational or medical interventions at the end of an evaluation process. Such a sequence of events can alienate the parents and drive them toward alternative therapies. An unfavorable prognosis, the message that standard therapies are expensive and time-consuming, the inability to guarantee success, and the prospect of slow or minimal improvement can also influence parents to become frustrated and seek the "quick fix" offered by the proponents of alternative therapies.

Table 84–1 • Differences Between Accepted and Alternative Therapies

Accepted Therapies	Alternative Therapies
The theories on which these therapies are based are consistent with scientific knowledge and can be tested by hypothesis-driven studies to confirm or refute the effectiveness of the therapy.	The theories on which these therapies are based are novel and are not completely consistent with scientific knowledge.
Therapies are targeted for specific problems with indications and contraindications.	Therapies are presented as being effective for a broad range of problems.
The therapy is accepted and widely used by profesionals.	Treatments are presented as "natural," based on exercises, or manipulation of the diet or body.
Therapies can be incorporated into a multimodal approach.	Therapies are used in an isolated way.
The initial medium of presentation is a peer-reviewed scientific journal.	The initial medium of presentation is often, but not always, in a medium other than a peer-reviewed scientific journal.
Therapies are proposed to and are accepted by (which can take years) traditional medical, educational, and psychological professionals.	Therapies are proposed to the public before any research results are available; preliminary research has not been replicated; or proposed therapy goes beyond what research data support.
Controlled studies can be replicated by independent researchers. These studies use objective criteria such as uniformity of subjects, standard doses, objective, verifiable dependent measures, control group, placebo and double-blind design.	Controlled studies that do not support the use of the treatment are discounted as being improperly performed or biased because of the unwillingness of the medical establishment to accept novel ideas.
Professional organizations issue policy statements rejecting therapies that are without evidence of effectiveness or are deemed harmful. Textbooks and professional reviews support therapies that have documented effectiveness.	Lay organizations develop and support the use of the treatment, proselytize new members, and become socially active in attempting to develop special interest legislation and regulations.

Parents encounter alternative therapies through many sources. For example, they can come into contact with other parents at school or in support groups who have embraced alternative therapies. Some groups advocating alternative therapies take on the form of social movements, in which antiprofessionalism and criticism of physicians can emerge. Parents are bombarded by a wide array of magazine articles, parenting manuals, self-help books, and other media. It is hard for parents to tell which of such claims are scientifically based. To further complicate matters, the media will tout both scientifically sound and unsound forms of therapy. Scientifically based research articles can be misquoted and individual findings overemphasized or paraphrased to such an extent that their conclusions are different from the author's intent. Sensational accounts of novel but unproven forms of therapy, or "exposés" highlighting the "dangerous" aspects of standard therapies, are a common feature on newscasts, news magazines, and talk shows. Even when a well-researched and professionally reported feature is presented on national television, attempts by the local media to put their own "spin" on the report can lead to confusion when an unproven therapy is given "equal time." The lack of constraints on the advertising of therapies in the media and a general level of cynicism toward and distrust of standard medical care also contribute to the general public confusion over therapeutic choices. To combat this, physicians who care for children with developmental and behavioral problems should make themselves available to the media to provide clear, understandable, and accurate advice to parents.

The Internet is the latest addition to the Babel of information confronting parents. Both accepted and alternative therapies are discussed on the Internet. Frequently, parents are able to discover information about both forms of therapies before physicians are. It is imperative for physicians to become familiar with the Internet to keep up with their more technologically astute patients and families.

How Physicians Can Approach the Subject of Alternative Therapies

Each physician should develop an approach to dealing with parents' questions about alternative therapies. This should begin with the demystification of the diagnostic process, the diagnosis, and the proposed (accepted and effective) forms of therapy. Parents generally welcome an invitation to participate in a family-centered evaluation process. A discussion of the findings that is developmentally appropriate and not condescending can assist in fostering the involvement of children and their families in the therapeutic process. Physicians should approach these discussions with the parents (and the child if he or she is old enough) in a sympathetic and forthright manner. An accurate and detailed description of the child's strengths and weaknesses can enhance both the discussion and acceptance of the prescription of interventions (medical, psychological, and educational) that are recommended. The goals of therapy and the expectations of progress for the child must be realistic. Interdisciplinary teams that are family centered are ideal for diagnostic evaluations and intervention. However, owing to the changing health care environment that places limits on the interdisciplinary process, less formal arrangements between physicians and other professionals are becoming more common.

The physician needs to be aware of the array and quality of services for children with developmental and behavioral problems in the community. The physician should also take an active role in advocating at the local, state, and national levels to maintain and expand services for children. The first priority of every physician is to ensure that every child, regardless of disability, has access to those medical and educational services needed to achieve his or her potential. Physicians have an obligation to lend their expertise to community-based service organizations. Physicians should participate in support groups for families of children with developmental and behavioral problems, not to control these groups, but to advocate for proven and effective forms of intervention.

If parents bring up questions about alternative therapeutic approaches, their questions should be discussed in an open and nonconfrontational manner. Care must be taken to listen to the concerns of the parents. The parents' interest in such alternative approaches may be a reflection of confusion about the diagnosis or therapy, frustration over a perceived lack of progress in standard approaches, or a sense of hopelessness. Discussions about alternative therapies should not become emotionally charged. Parents should not be made to feel foolish or defensive. Neither should physicians become defensive when such questions arise.

Asking parents about where they received the information about the alternative therapy is a useful first step in the discussion. If the source of misleading information is a relative or family friend, then the physician can discuss the child's problems with the relative or friend. If the information comes from school personnel or other professionals, then a discussion should be initiated with them directly (with the parents' permission), rather than placing the parents in the middle of the discussion of conflicting advice (Silver, 1986). If the alternative therapy is one that is unfamiliar to the physician, then he or she should be willing to review the available information about the alternative therapy and determine the basis for its claims. Often the information is based on testimonials or excerpts from books.

EXAMPLE

A mother of two children under treatment for attention and learning problems contacted her developmental-behavioral pediatrician. She told the doctor about a new combination of products that she had read about as an alternative to psychostimulant therapy. The doctor asked the mother to send a copy of the information packet for further review before forming a judgment on the therapy.

A few days later an information packet arrived in the mail. The therapy was described as a "100% natural supplement" consisting of three parts: (1) a delicious liquid form of colloidal minerals (over 60 in every 32-ounce bottle) that were extracted from plants, (2) an antioxidant ("OPC") derived from a grape-seed extract that in combination with Ginkgo biloba and other herbs has "a very positive impact on one's health," and (3) a multienzyme capsule. The capsule was to be taken with every meal and significant snack. Elimination of as much sugar as possible from the diet was also recommended.

A newsletter article was included in the packet of information. Claims were made of "hundreds and perhaps many thousands of cases later, parents are hearing glowing reports" about their children. The author did admit that there was no "certified statistical evidence to support this conclusion other than anecdotal."

After researching textbooks and the Internet, the doctor called the mother to inform her that no scientific information about the specific antioxidant could be found. The mother was also informed that the information provided about the colloidal minerals and multienzymes was too

vague to be researched with regard to possible positive or harmful effects. Therefore, the doctor could not confirm or deny that the treatment was either effective or harmful. The doctor recommended caution, given the uncertain nature of the proposed therapy. The mother agreed with the recommendation. She then updated the doctor about her children's progress in school and asked specific questions about school-based services.

Parents should be given a clear and understandable explanation of why a standard therapy is effective while the alternative therapy is unlikely to be of benefit. Parents can be provided with written material such as medical reviews or position statements from the American Academy of Pediatrics or other professional organizations (see Appendix). The implications of alternative therapies such as potential toxicity or harm, expense, stress, and loss of time and energy due to the diversion from standard therapies should be discussed.

Parents have a right to choose any therapy for their children that does not produce harm. Physicians and other professionals are not required to participate in the alternative therapy and should not indulge in the rationalization that an alternative therapy "could not hurt and might help." An alternative therapy that in and of itself may be relatively harmless can deflect the parent and child from pursuing forms of intervention with proven effectiveness. If parents and physicians disagree about a choice of therapy to the extent that termination of the therapeutic relationship is contemplated, then the physician is obligated to provide care until another physician can assume the care of the child. Physicians should be willing to renew the therapeutic relationship if the family wishes to return for care.

Dietary and Nutritional Therapies

One of the most popular and persistent myths about alternative therapies is found in the plethora of food, food allergy, and food additive explanations for the chemical abnormalities presumed to underlie various developmental and behavioral problems (Accardo and Lindsay, 1994). Over time, these three explanations have been combined, resulting in recommendations to restrict sugar, additives, and preservatives from children's diets to improve or prevent developmental and behavioral problems. Considerable efforts have been made to refute these myths and shed the light of scientific reason on the array of anecdotal "evidence," personal testimony, and pseudoscientific assertions of the role of micronutrients, food additives, and sweeteners on behavior. Reviews of the objective evidence about dietary therapies can be presented to parents who seek such therapies (Wolraich, 1996).

SUGAR AND ARTIFICIAL SWEETENERS

During the past quarter century, sugar has been implicated in a variety of developmental and behavioral problems, especially hyperactivity. Excess intake of refined sugars in the diet has been postulated to result in a rise in blood sugar after ingestion, reflex hypoglycemia several hours after ingestion, and an allergic response (Wender, 1991).

Parents often attempt to restrict their children's sugar intake and substitute artificially sweetened foods and drinks. As aspartame is currently the most widely used artificial sweetener, concern has been raised about possible adverse effects. The warning labels on products containing aspartame, which are intended for persons with phenylketonuria, does little to calm parental fears for children who do not have phenylketonuria. There has been some speculation that the metabolic products of aspartame may be responsible for behavioral changes. In the case of phenylalanine, it has been suggested that increased levels in the blood and brain alter monoamine neurotransmitter synthesis (Fernstrom, 1991).

Wolraich and associates (1994), in a double-blind controlled study of preschool children and school-aged children described by their parents as sensitive to sugar, found that neither dietary sucrose nor aspartame affects children's behavior or cognitive function, even when intake exceeds typical dietary levels. A meta-analysis of 23 studies on the effect of sugar did not find any significant behavioral or cognitive effects (Wolraich, Wilson, and White, 1995). Shaywitz and associates (1994) demonstrated that consumption of aspartame at greater than 10 times usual levels had no effect on the cognitive or behavioral status of children with attention deficits. In addition, aspartame did not appear to affect urinary excretion rates of monoamines and metabolites.

FOOD ALLERGY

Food allergies have been implicated in developmental and behavioral disorders owing to empiric observations by pediatricians and allergists that children with allergies have a higher rate of learning difficulties. Rapp (1986) identified certain foods or food groups that children may be allergic to such as milk, chocolate, eggs, wheat, corn, peanuts, and pork. Rapp recommends that parents try a specific elimination diet until they identify a specific food allergy. Rapp does not believe that allergy skin testing can always detect the foods that cause problems. Crook (Crook and Stevens, 1987) has written extensively on the relationship between allergies, which he called the "allergic-tension-fatigue syndrome," and developmental and behavioral disorders. No clinical or research studies have confirmed his theories or treatment program.

FOOD ADDITIVES: THE FEINGOLD DIET

Feingold (1975) claimed that certain children have a genetic predisposition to react adversely to salicylates and food additives that is not allergic in nature. He claimed that, when treated with a diet that eliminates these substances, 50% of hyperactive children and children with learning disabilities would achieve a "full response," while 75% can be removed from drug management, "even if full response to other symptoms is not achieved" (p. 71). The response to his book was enthusiastic, resulting in a number of uncontrolled studies. Soon thereafter, well-designed studies were conducted that used standardized measures to define the study population, double-blind conditions with placebo controls, and a sufficient number of subjects. These studies were extensively reviewed by Wender (1986), who

reported that there was little (at best only 1%) effect of food coloring and other additives on the behavior of hyperactive children. Because the Feingold diet is not harmful if supplemental vitamin C is provided, it has been suggested that no harm may result if the diet is tried while other aspects of treatment are continued (Wender, 1986). Golden (1984) cautions that such dietary therapy is not without costs (both monetary and time commitment), may result in stress, and can deflect the family from other forms of therapy that ultimately may be more effective.

A recent study by Rowe and Rowe (1994) reopened the issue of food additives. In a double-blind placebo-controlled study of children referred for suspected hyperactivity (no formal diagnosis was made), 24 of 34 subjects responded adversely to tartrazine (a synthetic food color) compared with 2 of 20 control subjects. The adverse responses were dose related, unlike what would be expected in a usual allergic response. The study was limited by the use of two behavior rating scales completed by the parents. The results of this study point out the need for further study to substantiate these results.

ORTHOMOLECULAR TREATMENTS

Deficiencies in a number of nutrients have been postulated to be responsible for a number of developmental and behavioral problems. Although these theories were initially proposed over 30 years ago, new combinations of these treatments involving trace elements, vitamins, and antioxidants continue to enter the arena of alternative therapies.

Pauling (1968) initially proposed that schizophrenia may be the result of low vitamin concentrations in the brain. He also proposed that the common cold could be treated with vitamin C therapy (Pauling, 1970). These theories were soon disproven, but the megavitamin approach resurfaced for the treatment of learning and attentional problems (Cott, 1971, 1985). Evidence soon accumulated that megavitamin therapy was both ineffective and potentially dangerous. As early as 1976, the American Academy of Pediatrics published a specific warning about the dangers of and lack of validity to this approach. Despite this warning, some individuals continue to propose and use this approach. Continued objective studies of this approach (Haslam, 1992) have shown that "positive behavioral responses, particularly those associated with ADHD [attention-deficit hyperactivity disorder] were more apparent during placebo as compared to vitamin therapy. A behavioral observer documented 25% more disruptive behavior during vitamin therapy compared to placebo (p<.01)." Haslam also revealed a significant elevation of serum transaminase levels in 42% of the subjects and significant increases in serum bilirubin levels. He concluded that megavitamin therapy not only was ineffective but should be avoided because of potential hepatotoxicity.

Trace elements have also been implicated in developmental and behavioral problems. There are several centers that use hair and fingernail samples to determine the level of trace elements and recommend therapy.

Antioxidant therapy is the latest addition to this class of therapies. One such antioxidant is Pycnogenol, which is a commercial mixture of bioflavonoids derived from the bark of the French Maritime pine tree. A Medline review of the medical literature in 1998 revealed only six scientific studies on Pycnogenol. None of these studies used human subjects, much less examined anything remotely connected to developmental and behavioral problems in children. The Internet site for Pycnogenol references one of these articles (Cheshier et al, 1996) as evidence of a double-blind study's proving Pycnogenol's effectiveness. This study examined immune dysfunction in normal mice and mice fed ethanol or infected with retrovirus.

A lay monograph touting Pycnogenol as a treatment for attention-deficit disorder reported that this therapy was neither a "drug" nor an "herbal" remedy. It is "composed of forty-plus compounds" and is "relatively new to health care professionals in North America." The monograph recommends the use of Pycnogenol along with supplemental beta carotene, ester C, vitamin E, zinc gluconate, selenium, and bioflavonoids. No scientific references are provided, only testimonials. The only side effect listed is increased firmness of stools; however, the monograph includes excerpts from the package inserts of three psychostimulants, with the warning: "Were you fully aware of all the 'warnings,' 'drug dependency risk,' 'precautions,' and 'adverse reactions' related to their [psychostimulant] use?"

Lay groups also advocate the use of other forms of antioxidant therapy (see case example).

Neurophysiologic Therapies

Neurophysiologic therapies purport to improve functioning of the central nervous system by stimulating specific sensory inputs or exercising specific motor patterns. These methods include patterning (the Doman-Delacato method), sensory integration, various visual techniques, and auditory integration.

DOMAN-DELACATO METHOD

"Patterning" for brain damage and other disorders was initially developed by Doman and Delacato at the Institutes for the Achievement of Human Potential in Philadelphia. This method is based on the theory that movement patterns of lower vertebrates are present within humans. Failure to pass properly through a certain sequence of developmental stages (motor, language, and sensory) reflects poor neurologic organization (Doman and Delacato, 1968). Treatment consists of taking a child back to basic movements, such as crawling like a human or an amphibian. These patterning exercises are administered in a home program that exerts enormous time demands on parents and volunteers. Beginning in 1968, several professional organizations have issued policy statements regarding this form of therapy. In 1982, the American Academy of Pediatrics (AAP) reissued its policy statement concluding that "patterning treatment offers no special merit, that the claims of its advocates are unproven, and the demands on families are so great that in some cases there is harm in its use."

SENSORY INTEGRATION THERAPY

Sensory integration therapy, as initially proposed by Ayers (1972), who was an occupational therapist, holds that disordered sensory integration underlies a vast array of developmental and behavioral problems She developed two tests to assess vestibular dysfunction. The Southern California Postrotatory Nystagmus Test (SCPRNT) examines the presence and duration of postrotatory nystagmus after the child is spun. The Southern California Sensory Integration Tests (SCSIT) evaluate various motor functions, right-left orientation, spatial orientation, space, balance, kinesthesia, proprioception, and visual-perceptual functions. A remediation program, designed to improve integration of primitive reflexes and equilibrium reactions, is supposed to improve academic functioning.

The American Academy of Pediatrics (1985) maintains that this therapy is not beneficial for children with learning disabilities. The official position of the American Association of Occupational Therapists (1981) is as follows: "The educationally related (occupational therapy) service is in the purposeful use of activities to increase the functional performance of independent living skills" of the student.

CEREBELLAR-VESTIBULAR DYSFUNCTION

A variation of sensory integration therapy is the approach of Levinson (1980), who proposed that the vestibular and vestibular-cerebellar systems contribute to learning disabilities. Frank and Levinson (1976) used caloric testing to evaluate vestibular function as well as passing stimuli across the subject's visual field at varying speed to determine the speed ("blurring speed") at which words could not be recognized. The most objective sign of vestibular dysfunction, however, is nystagmus. Caloric testing does not measure nystagmus, and "blurring speed" is considered to be a form of visual stimulation. Some of the symptoms associated with developmental disabilities, such as poor coordination, balance, and spatial orientation, can mimic the symptoms of a vestibular disorder.

The proposed treatment of these problems is the use of anti–motion sickness medications such as meclizine (Antivert), cyclizine (Marezine), dimenhydrinate (Dramamine), and diphenhydramine (Benedryl). Other forms of medications and special education have been recommended in later publications.

A study by Polatajko (1985) examining vestibular function in children with learning disabilities found no significant differences in the intensity of vestibular responsiveness or in the prevalence of cerebellar dysfunction between children with and those without learning disabilities. Her findings did not support the theories of Frank and Levinson nor those of Ayers.

AUDITORY PROCESSING TRAINING

Two approaches to auditory processing training proposed by French physicians as treatment for learning disabilities and ADHD were reviewed by Silver (1995). The first approach is Auditory Integration Training based on the theory of Guy Bernard that some students have unusual responses (often uncomfortable) to sound in the normal range of hearing, hyperacute or hypoacute hearing, or perceived distortion of sound. Testing and therapy are performed using a device (Audiokinetron) that not only determines the frequencies to which a person is hyperacute or hypoacute but also can desensitize the person by playing music that amplifies or filters out selected frequencies. The second approach is the Listening Training Program of Alfred Tomatis, based on the theory that some children turn off or lose the ability to hear sounds within the normal spectrum. Again, filtered music and sounds are used to "help the ear focus on the sounds it hears."

VISUAL THERAPIES

It is obvious that some children have difficulty reading because of treatable forms of visual difficulty such as myopia. Although pediatricians can identify the majority of children with reduced visual acuity, farsightedness may not be identified by routine screening. It is critical that refractive errors, strabismus, and tracking difficulties be ruled out by proper examination. However, it is not surprising that dyslexia has been attributed to more "subtle" ocular or visual abnormalities.

There has been a conflict between pediatric ophthalmologists and optometrists concerning the effectiveness of optometric visual training. This therapy is supposed to change visual functions such as convergence, accommodation, ocular mobility, and binocular fusion through the use of eye exercises. The optometric literature generally supports such an approach, while the ophthalmologic literature challenges the studies that claim success. Irlen (1983) proposed that dyslexia could be due to "scotopic sensitivity syndrome." This results in photophobia, eye strain, poor visual resolution, impaired depth perception, and reduced span or sustaining of focus. Treatment of this "syndrome" involves a trial-and-error approach using 54 tinted lenses to discover which color lens can filter out distracting light, thus allowing the dyslexic child to read. A low-cost variation of this therapy, which continues to be advocated by some individuals, substitutes colored plastic sheets that are then placed over reading material.

The Committee on Children with Disabilities of American Academy of Pediatrics, the American Academy of Ophthalmology, and the American Association for Pediatric Ophthalmology and Strabismus issued two joint statements (1984 and 1992) strongly supporting the need for early diagnosis and educational remediation of dyslexia and related learning disabilities. These statements pointed out that the claims of improved reading and learning through these visual methods are typically based on poorly controlled studies that rely on anecdotal information or testimony. The 1992 statement concluded: "There is no known eye or visual cause for dyslexia and learning difficulties, and no effective visual management. Multidisciplinary evaluation and management must be based on proven procedures demonstrated by valid research."

Other Alternative Interventions

CHIROPRACTIC: CRANIAL MANIPULATION

The latest group to join in the array of alternative therapies are chiropractors. They claim to be able to cure learning problems through cranial manipulation or "applied kinesiology." "Damage" to the sphenoid and temporal bones in the child's skull is purportedly reversed by massaging these skull bones into their "correct position." There are no data to support this theory.

FACILITATED COMMUNICATION

Facilitated communication (FC) is a technique that is reported to allow nonspeaking children, such as children with autism, to communicate. It is a "method of training people in the use of augmentative communication aids which involves the communication partner, or facilitator, providing physical assistance to the aid users to help them overcome physical and emotional problems in using their aid" (Batt, 1992). This form of therapy was developed in Australia by Crossley in the 1970s and was introduced in the United States by Biklen in 1990. The facilitator guides the nonspeaking child's hand, wrist, elbow, or shoulder to letters on a keyboard or nonelectronic system.

This form of therapy was reviewed by Hostler (1996), who outlined independent research efforts to demonstrate the efficacy of FC. These studies have shown that when the nonspeaking child and the facilitator are shown different stimuli, the only labels generated through FC were for stimuli shown to the facilitator, regardless of what the subject saw (Wheeler et al, 1993). In a compilation of controlled evaluations of FC, 316 of 334 subjects in 43 studies failed to demonstrate communication with FC (Rimland, 1993).

Hostler concluded that FC "is not consistent with the developmental theories of language and communication, especially when it espouses that the facilitator and not a family member is the preferred communication partner. Objective research studies have satisfactorily demonstrated that FC is not an effective intervention for children with severe communication disorders. Most FC must be recognized as facilitator communication." She also noted the "dark side" of FC, in which a series of alleged sexual abuse cases were brought against parents after FC was initiated.

Conclusion

The spectrum of developmental and behavioral disorders shares common factors that can result in the emergence of novel therapies. Such alternative therapies are clearly differentiated from approaches that are accepted by professionals from many disciplines. Alternative therapies share many features, including theoretical constructs that are not completely consistent with scientific knowledge, claims of effectiveness for a broad range of developmental and behavioral problems, being presented as "natural," and often being used in isolation. Alternative therapies can be subdivided into a number of classes: dietary and nutritional therapies, neurophysiologic therapies, and other therapies.

Physicians should be aware of the array and quality of services that are available for children with developmental and behavioral problems in the community. The first priority of every physician is to ensure that every child, regardless of disability, has access to those medical and educational services needed to achieve his or her potential. Parents should be given a clear and understandable explanation of why standard therapies for developmental and behavioral problems are effective while alternative therapies are unlikely to be of benefit. In this way, physicians can protect and guide families to scientifically proven approaches to therapy for developmental and behavioral problems.

APPENDIX

Position Statements

American Academy of Cerebral Palsy, American Academy of Neurology, American Academy of Pediatrics, American Academy of Physical Medicine and Rehabilitation, American Congress of Rehabilitation Medicine, American Academy of Orthopedics, Canadian Association for Children with Learning Disabilities, Canadian Rehabilitation Council for the Disabled, and National Association for Retarded Children (USA): The Doman-Delacato treatment of neurologically handicapped children. Neurology 18:1214, 1968.

American Academy of Pediatrics, American Association for Pediatric Ophthalmology and Strabismus, American Academy of Ophthalmology: Learning disabilities, dyslexia and vision. Pediatrics 90:124, 1992.

American Academy of Pediatrics: The Doman-Delacato treatment of neurologically handicapped children: a policy statement from the American Academy of Pediatrics. Pediatrics 70:810, 1982.

American Academy of Pediatrics, Committee on Nutrition: Megavitamin therapy for childhood psychoses and learning disabilities. Pediatrics 58:910, 1976.

American Academy of Pediatrics, Committee on Children with Disabilities: School-aged children with motor disabilities. Pediatrics 76:648, 1985.

American Academy of Pediatrics, Committee on Children with Disabilities, Ad Hoc Working Group of the American Association for Pediatric Ophthalmology and Strabismus, American Academy of Ophthalmology: Learning disabilities, dyslexia and vision. Pediatrics 74:150, 1984.

American Association of Occupational Therapists: The role of occupational therapy as an education-related service. Official position paper. Am J Occup Ther 35:811, 1981.

Consensus Conference, National Institute of Allergy, and National Institute of Child Health and Human Development: Defined diets and childhood hyperactivity. JAMA 248:290, 1982.

REFERENCES

Accardo PJ, Lindsay RL: Nutrition and behavior: the legend continues. Pediatrics 93:127, 1994.

Ayers AJ: Sensory Integration and Learning Disorders. Los Angeles: Western Psychological Services, 1972.

Batt M, cited in Cummins RA, Prior MP: Autism and assisted communication: a response to Biklen. Harvard Educ Rev 62:228, 1992.

Cheshier JE, Ardestani-Kaboudanian S, Liang B, et al: Immunomodulation by Pycnogenol in retrovirus-infected or ethanol-fed mice. Life Sci 58(5):PL87, 1996.

Cohen MW: Controversies continue in the treatment of learning disabilities and attention deficit disorder [editorial]. Am J Dis Child 140:986, 1986.

Cott A: Orthomolecular approach to the treatment of learning disabilities. Schizophrenia 3:95, 1971.

Cott A: Help for Your Learning Disabled Child: The Orthomolecular Treatment. New York, Times Books, 1985.

Crook WG, Steven L: Solving the Puzzle of your Hard-to-Raise Child. Jackson, TN, Professional Books, 1987.

Doman G and Delacato C: Doman Delacato philosophy. Hum Potential 1:113, 1968.

Feingold B: Why Your Child Is Hyperactive. New York, Random House, 1975.

Fernstrom JD: Central nervous system effects of aspartame. In Kretchmer N, Hollenbeck CB (eds): Sugars and Sweeteners. Boca Raton, FL, CRC Press, 1991.

Frank J, Levinson HN: Compensatory mechanisms in C-V dysfunction, dysmetric dyslexia, and dyspraxia. Acad Ther 12:133–149, 1976.

Golden GS: Controversial therapies. Ped Clin North Am 31:459, 1984.

Haslam RH: Is there a role for megavitamin therapy in the treatment of attention deficit hyperactivity disorder? Adv Neurol 58:303, 1992.

Hostler SL: Facilitated communication [commentary]. Pediatrics 97(4):584, 1986.

Irlen H: Successful treatment of learning disabilities. Presented at the 91st Convention of the American Psychological Association, Anaheim, CA, August, 1983.

Levinson HN: A Solution to the Riddle of Dyslexia. New York, Springer-Verlag, 1980.

Pauling L: Orthomolecular psychiatry. Science 160:265, 1968.

Pauling L: Vitamin C and the Common Cold. San Francisco, W.H. Freeman and Company, 1970.

Polatajko HJ: A critical look at vestibular dysfunction in learning-disabled children. Dev Med Child Neurol 27:283, 1985.

Rapp DJ: The Impossible Child in School and at Home. Buffalo, NY, Life Sciences Press, 1986.

Rimland B: F/C update: critical PBS program adds to controversy. Autism Res Rev Int 7(4):7, 1993.

Rowe KS, Rowe KJ: Synthetic food coloring and behavior: a dose response effect in a double-blind, placebo-controlled, repeat measures study. J Pediatr 125:691, 1994.

Shaywitz BA, Sullivan CM, Anderson GM, et al: Aspartame, behavior, and cognitive function in children with attention deficit disorder. Pediatrics 93:70, 1994.

Silver LB: Controversial approach to treating learning disabilities and attention deficit disorder [Review]. Am J Dis Child 14:1045–1052, 1986.

Silver LB: Controversial therapies. J Child Neurol 10(Supp 1):S96, 1995.

Sprague RL, Werry JS: Methodology of psychopharmacological studies with the retarded. Int Rev Res Ment Retard 5:147, 1971.

Starrett AL: Nonstandard therapies in developmental disabilities. In Capute AJ, Accardo PJ (eds); Neurodevelopmental Disabilities in Infancy and Childhood, Vol. II: The Spectrum of Developmental Disabilities, 2nd ed. Baltimore, Paul H. Brookes, 1996, pp 593–608.

Wender EH: The food additive–free diet in the treatment of behavior disorders: A review. J Dev Behav Pediatr 7:35–42, 1986.

Wender E: Review of research on the relationship of nutritive sweeteners and behavior. In Diet and Behavior. Washington, DC, National Center for Nutrition and Dietetics, 1991, pp 65–80.

Wheeler D, Jacobson J, Paglieri RA, et al: An experimental assessment of facilitated communication. Mental Retardation 31:49, 1993.

Wolraich ML: Diet and behavior: what the research shows. Contem Ped 13(12):29, 1996.

Wolraich ML, Lindgren SD, Stumbo PJ, et al: Effects of diets high in sucrose or aspartame on the behavior and cognitive performance of children. N Engl J Med 330(5):301, 1994.

Wolraich ML, Wilson DB, White JW: The effect of sugar on behavior or cognition in children: A meta-analysis. JAMA 274:1617–1621, 1995.

85 Pediatric Self-Regulation

Dale Sussman • Timothy Culbert

 Within developmental-behavioral pediatrics there is a constant need to seek new therapeutic approaches to the functional problems of children and adolescents. In this chapter, Drs. Sussman and Culbert look at various forms of self-regulation aimed at facilitating "a child's natural, developmental drive for mastery and autonomy." Hypnosis, biofeedback, and other forms of self-regulation are surveyed and applied to specific clinical conditions. The examples used in this chapter ring responsive chords and encourage us to maintain open minds as new avenues of intervention are presented.

Self-regulation skills give children the means to help themselves with common biobehavioral problems. Self-regulation techniques are described as strategies that identify and cultivate the innate ability of pediatric patients to achieve a desired level of health and wellness. Through the use of hypnosis, biofeedback, and other self-regulation modalities, children of all ages and abilities learn to participate actively in the regulation and resolution of many medical, behavioral, and psychophysiologic problems encountered in childhood. Table 85–1 lists self-regulation strategies used with pediatric patients.

Self-regulation treatment strategies facilitate a child's natural, developmental drive for mastery and autonomy. Learning self-regulation empowers patients to focus their minds in a way that positively affects their bodies. Self-regulation skills include the voluntary modulation of selected physiologic functions, directed use of mental imagery, self-monitoring, positive self-talk, and enhanced awareness of mind-body connections. Through the use of self-regulation, children are encouraged to acknowledge and take "ownership" of their problem. Furthermore, they must be invested in the program and motivated to want to change specific symptoms.

Behavioral modification, environmental manipulations, and psychopharmacologic interventions are important and proven treatment strategies that approach biobehavioral problems from an external standpoint. Through the use of self-regulation strategies, children and adolescents develop an internal sense of control of their problem. They feel less helpless, and they become active participants in their care.

In the past 15 to 20 years, self-regulation techniques have been widely used and increasingly appreciated as valid and effective treatments for a wide variety of biobe-

havioral problems (Culbert, Reaney, and Kohen, 1994). The literature documenting the efficacy and cost effectiveness of self-regulation techniques as the sole treatment or as an adjunct to mainstay medical therapy for a variety of medical and behavioral problems continues to grow. Children should always receive the appropriate medical therapy in addition to self-regulation strategies. This is especially true when self-regulation techniques are used in children with chronic diseases such as asthma, seizure disorders, juvenile rheumatoid arthritis, sickle cell anemia, and malignancies. Table 85–2 identifies pediatric disorders responsive to self-regulation techniques.

Definitions, Myths, and Misconceptions

Strategies that emphasize and cultivate self-regulation skills have been termed *cyberphysiologic*. The prefix *cyber* is derived form the Greek *kybernan* meaning to steer or to take the helm (Olness, 1991). Children are encouraged to "be the boss of their bodies" and are expected to participate actively in the treatment process. When pediatric patients are taught a cyberphysiologic skill or skills, the therapist serves as a coach and facilitator. The patient helps to determine which type of self-regulation strategy will fit best for his or her personalized treatment plan. Children of all ages are expected to participate in daily self-monitoring of symptoms and are responsible for daily practice of the skills that they have been taught.

The intimate connection between the mind and body is discussed in a developmentally appropriate manner so that the pediatric patient gains an appreciation of the physiologic responses of the body in relation to different feelings and situations. The impact of thoughts and emotions on certain symptoms (e.g., headaches, shortness of breath, and muscle tension) and overt behaviors (e.g., aggression, crying, and withdrawal) is explored with each child. The idea that a change in thinking and feeling can result in a change in a physiologic process is interesting and exciting for many children.

Studies over the past 30 years have clearly documented the ability of adults and children to modulate vol-

Table 85–1 • Pediatric Self-Regulation Techniques

Self-hypnosis
Biofeedback
Diaphragmatic breathing
Progressive muscle relaxation
Autogenics
Cognitive-behavioral therapy

Table 85–2 • Pediatric Problems Responsive to Self-Regulation Techniques

Chronic/recurrent pain	Tics and Tourette syndrome
Recurrent abdominal pain, headaches	Pruritus
	Warts
Acute pain	Attention disorders
Medical procedures	Learning disorders
Trauma	Seizure disorders
Burns	Impulse control problems
Anxiety and stress disorders	Anger management
Obsessive-compulsive disorder	Disruptive behavior
Trichotillomania	Feeding and swallowing problems
Disorders of elimination	
Enuresis	Dysphagia
Encopresis	Cyclic vomiting
Sleep disorders	Anorexia
Autonomic nervous system dysregulation	Bulimia
	Chronic illness
Raynaud	Asthma
Reflex sympathetic dystrophy	Juvenile rheumatoid arthritis
Hypertension	Sickle cell anemia
Neuromuscular rehabilitation	Malignancies
Habit disorders	Diabetes mellitus
Thumb-sucking	Dysfluencies
Bruxism	
Habit cough	
Nail biting	

untarily a number of physiologic processes, many of which were previously thought to be exclusively under autonomic control. Experts in the fields of hypnosis and biofeedback have noted children's superior self-regulatory abilities. For example, as a group, children appear to be more hypnotically susceptible than adults (Olness and Kohen, 1996). Biofeedback clinicians have pointed out that despite certain developmental challenges, children make excellent biofeedback subjects (Attansio et al, 1985). They note that, as compared with adult subjects,

- Children are more enthusiastic.
- Children learn more quickly.
- Children are less skeptical about self-control procedures.
- Children have more confidence in special abilities.
- Children have more psychophysiologic lability.
- Children enjoy practice sessions.
- Children are more reliable at symptom monitoring.

However, not all children are good candidates for self-regulation training. For example, children with attention difficulties, depression, or cognitive impairment may not respond optimally to self-regulation techniques.

A child's age, developmental strengths and weaknesses, and natural talents and interests are all taken into account when crafting a self-regulation treatment plan. Most children are able to learn several self-regulation strategies and achieve good symptom control within four to six 30-minute sessions (Kohen et al, 1984).

When a child is referred for self-regulation training, it is important to identify treatable organic disease. In one group of 80 children with behavioral symptoms who were referred specifically for hypnotherapy, 20 of those children were found to have an undiagnosed medical problem that accounted for their symptoms (Olness, 1987).

BIOFEEDBACK

Biofeedback is the use of electronic or electromechanical equipment (usually computer based) to measure and then feed back information about physiologic processes. The goal of biofeedback is to help patients become aware of their ability to control physiologic changes in their bodies so that they can learn to control these changes in their everyday lives without the biofeedback equipment. Goals of biofeedback treatment commonly include improvement of the pediatric patient's ability to discern and cultivate lowered levels of sympathetic nervous system arousal and a subjective sense of "relaxation." Patients are coached in a variety of techniques, including the awareness and control of breathing, the discrimination and modulation of muscle tension levels, and the modulation of peripheral temperature.

Biofeedback equipment can be used to measure a number of physiologic parameters, either one at a time or in combination. These include muscle activity (electromyography), peripheral temperature (thermography), heart rate (photoplethysmography), breathing (pneumography), electrical brain activity (electroencephalography), and sweat gland response (electrodermal activity). Studies have clearly demonstrated children's ability to control a variety of physiologic responses, including finger temperature, breathing rate and rhythm, and electrical brain wave activity. Research has also indicated consistent and dramatic changes in parameters such as heart rate and electrodermal activity associated with children's use of specific types of mental imagery (Lee and Olness, 1996).

Computerized biofeedback equipment with game-display type formats is culturally in tune with present-day youth and offers an attractive and engaging treatment vehicle. Biofeedback display formats that are set up as games offer intrinsically motivating elements that can enhance patient engagement in the treatment process. Patients can be coached to achieve desired therapeutic outcomes (e.g., decreased muscle tension, slow diaphragmatic breathing) through participation in games that challenge them and that hold their attention using high-quality graphics and audio. In one such game, children are encouraged to tense and relax muscle groups in order to control their spaceship and avoid oncoming asteroids. In another game, children are rewarded for increasing hand temperature (through relaxation) by viewing a beautiful butterfly in flight; when a preset temperature is achieved, the butterfly lands on the flower. Another relaxation training game called Pachyderm is depicted in Figure 85–1.

SELF-HYPNOSIS

Hypnosis is an altered state of awareness within which an individual experiences heightened suggestibility. During everyday activities, children move readily in and out of hypnotic states. Fantasy, imagery, and intensely focused or absorbed attention are common experiences and reflect natural developmental tendencies for children. Hypnotherapy, or self-hypnosis, refers to the use of hypnosis by an individual to achieve a personal goal. Self-hypnosis is usually associated with a sensation of relaxation, well-being, and enhanced self-control.

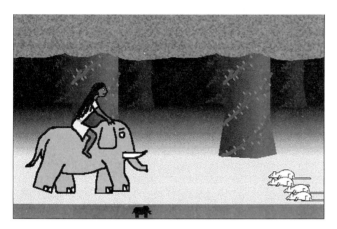

Figure 85–1. This picture is taken from a biofeedback game display called Pachyderm by Creative MultiMedia and Marketing. This is a PC-based software package that runs under "Windows" and is compatible with various brands of biofeedback hardware devices. The pediatric patient takes on the identity of the animated elephant character and is "challenged" to walk through the jungle without becoming scared. The patient is attached to one or more EMG sensors, which measure muscle tension values. As the elephant encounters stressful stimuli in the form of mice and snakes, the players are coached on remaining calm and in control of their reactions as demonstrated by low, stable EMG readings. If the players are successful in staying relaxed, they are rewarded at the end of the jungle trail by being united with the mother and father elephant characters, and the game sequence ends. (Courtesy of Creative MultiMedia, Inc., Houston, TX.)

The goal of hypnotherapy is always to teach the patient an attitude of hope in the context of mastery. The patient learns to be an active participant in his or her own behalf, to focus on creating a solution rather than on enduring a problem, and to discover and use resources for inner control as much as possible (Olness and Kohen, 1996).

There are a number of common myths and misperceptions about hypnosis. Hypnosis is not a sleeplike state. Individuals in hypnotic states cannot be forced to do things against their will. In fact, there is usually heightened awareness of physical sensations and increased self-control while in a hypnotic trance. Pediatric practitioners believe that all hypnosis is self-hypnosis, and, therefore, the therapist can facilitate and influence but not "control" those experiences for pediatric patients.

Self-hypnosis has a wide variety of valuable applications. It is highly personalized for each child, with particular consideration given to his or her developmental status. Some children demonstrate greater hypnotizability than others do, with hypnotic responsivity increasing markedly in middle childhood. Hypnotherapy facilitates children's innate creative and imaginative skills to construct helpful solutions to their problems. Pediatric patients describe various mental images, with some preferring visual and others creating more auditory images. Individual differences might also include olfactory or kinesthetic imaginative preferences. Through the use of carefully selected and developmentally appropriate language, the practitioner encourages children's imaginative abilities to explore and create unique ways to help themselves (Kohen and Olness, 1993).

COGNITIVE-BEHAVIORAL THERAPY

Cognitive-behavioral therapy is a therapeutic technique that emphasizes a person's awareness of internal positive and negative self talk patterns and behavioral habits, and it helps that person to develop effective problem-solving strategies. Children are coached in the self-directed development of positive coping strategies and in enhanced perceptions of self-efficacy. They are encouraged to identify problematic situations and to respond with acceptable adaptive behavior. Cognitive-behavioral therapy can be beneficial with impulse control problems, anxiety, and acute and chronic pain (Kendall, 1991).

DIAPHRAGMATIC BREATHING

Breathing control is a seemingly simple skill, but one with extremely powerful and widespread applications (Schwartz, 1995). Diaphragmatic breathing, also called "belly breathing," is useful for many different pediatric problems, including sleep disturbance, panic and performance anxiety symptoms, somatic complaints including headache and recurrent abdominal pain, anger management, chronic conditions such as asthma, and disorders related to autonomic nervous system dysregulation. It can be particularly helpful for children undergoing painful medical procedures such as venipuncture, bone marrow aspiration, or laceration repair (Kuttner, 1989). The basic technique involves coaching children in the development of a relaxed, rhythmic breathing pattern that results in a controlled, deep state of relaxation. Often, encouraging younger children to blow bubbles facilitates their use of "belly breathing." Figure 85–2 provides a basic description of diaphragmatic breathing (Kajander, 1997). A child's depiction of "belly breathing" is illustrated in Figure 85–3.

AUTOGENICS AND PROGRESSIVE MUSCLE RELAXATION

Other self-guided techniques cultivate states of decreased muscle tension, lower sympathetic nervous system arousal,

---

Put your hand gently over your belly button

Imagine you have a balloon underneath your belly button that you blow up when you breathe

Breathe slowly in through your nose and pull air deep into your lungs - feel your belly expand - like a balloon blowing up - breathe in (inhale) SLOWLY - (to the count of 3 or 4)

Keep your shoulders loose and relaxed while breathing in

Breathe out through your open mouth - feel your belly go back in like a balloon deflating - breathe out (exhale) SLOWLY - (to the count of 6 to 8)

Practice in front of a mirror to see if you are breathing correctly

Remember - the more you practice - the better you get!!

Figure 85–2. Belly breathing instructions. (Adapted from Kajander R: The Pediatric Self-Regulation Series Monographs: Diaphragmatic Breathing. Minneapolis, Just Imagine, Inc., 1997.)

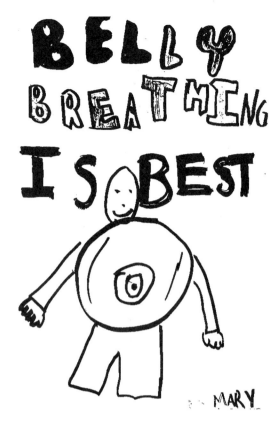

Figure 85–3. A picture by an 11-year-old girl with attention difficulties and anxiety who learned belly breathing to help herself with sleep initiation.

Clinical Applications

NOCTURNAL ENURESIS

Self-regulation techniques can be very useful in treating disorders of elimination, such as enuresis and encopresis, in children. Self-hypnosis has been well described as a helpful strategy for children with primary nocturnal enuresis (Olness, 1975). Conditioning alarms, which are considered to be biofeedback devices, can also be very effective.

In the following example, Laura achieved 100% dryness after only one meeting. Usually, pediatric patients are introduced to self-hypnosis on the initial visit. Over the next three to four follow-up appointments, they review and practice their skills, and, typically, they achieve increasing dryness. Although some children become dry after only one visit, many children require at least four to six visits before resolving their problem. The urinary system and the mind-body connections depicted in Figure 85–4 were drawn by a 10-year-old girl at a follow-up visit for nocturnal enuresis.

EXAMPLE

Laura was a 9 1/2-year-old girl who wet the bed almost every night. She had been given the diagnosis of primary nocturnal enuresis, and treatment had been unsuccessful over the past few years. Laura had taken imipramine and DDAVP for this problem but achieved no long-term success. She had used an alarm system, but the alarm was used inconsistently and awakened everyone in the house

and facilitate the subjective sense of relaxation and comfort. Progressive muscle relaxation is a technique in which the client is taught to alternately tighten and then relax specific muscle groups throughout the body and to improve the ability to discriminate and control areas of muscle tension (Jacobson, 1977).

Autogenics training teaches the use of a number of self-administered, repetitive suggestions involving a person's awareness and experience of sensations of warmth, heaviness, and relaxation throughout various regions of the body (Linden, 1990). Progressive muscle relaxation and autogenics may be beneficial in the treatment of sleep onset problems, headaches, and anxiety-related symptoms in children.

INTEGRATED STRATEGIES

Self-regulation strategies are commonly used sequentially or simultaneously in an integrated or "layered" behavioral treatment plan. These cyberphysiologic techniques have several common characteristics. Perhaps the most important and generic component of these strategies is the "emphasis on mastery, coping and control achieved by the child or adolescent" (Olness, 1996). Children are often taught several self-regulation techniques, either alone or in combination, and they are encouraged to choose the therapeutic strategies that they find most effective and enjoyable to use in home practice.

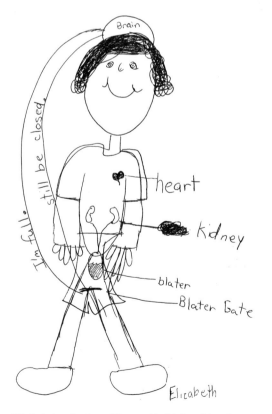

Figure 85–4. A drawing by a 10-year-old girl describing the connections between her brain and her bladder.

except Laura. Additionally, Laura's parents had intermittently restricted her fluids and taken her to the bathroom to urinate in the middle of the night. Laura had become increasingly anxious, because she was afraid that her younger siblings would tell her friends about "her problem" or that they would discover the pull-ups that were hidden in the house. She had more recently felt left out because she could not participate in sleepovers with her friends. It was clear that Laura was motivated to resolve "her problem."

During the initial meeting, Laura was taught the normal anatomy and physiology of the urinary tract system. The discussion emphasized the mind-body connections, specifically how her brain instructs her bladder gate to stay shut except when she sits on the toilet. Laura was encouraged to engage in self-hypnosis (review the discussion of her mind-body connections in relation to the urinary system) for 5 to 10 minutes just before bed each evening. She would pretend in her thinking that it was the middle of the night and her bladder was full. Her bladder gate would send the message to her brain, which would then decide whether to wake her body up to go to the bathroom or to send a message back down to the bladder gate to stay shut for the remainder of the night. The daily practice would enable her to "reprogram" her brain to keep her bladder gate shut at night just as she had it programmed to do during the day. Laura was also encouraged to keep a daily calendar to monitor her dry beds. Laura was responsible for practicing her self-hypnosis each night. After the initial meeting, Laura had all dry beds after 2 weeks of the self-regulation program; after 4 months, she had been on three sleepovers and "her problem" was considered only a part of her past.

SLEEP DISORDER

Children with sleep onset difficulties and parasomnias can benefit greatly from learning self-regulated relaxation strategies. Coaching children to fall asleep with a positive perceptual frame using self-hypnosis and positive self-talk can help them achieve a restful, uninterrupted night of sleep. Diaphragmatic breathing and muscle relaxation strategies can help children cultivate a low level of sympathetic nervous system arousal and assist them in an easier transition from a waking to a sleep state. Relaxation also helps to counteract the potential disruptive impact of stress on sleep–wake cycles. Autogenics training works well with children who describe that their mind is "too busy" and "won't shut off" at bedtime.

EXAMPLE

Jeremy was a bright 5 1/2-year-old boy who was having difficulty falling asleep. He also woke frequently during the night and yelled fearfully out to his parents. The nighttime awakenings were associated with nightmares, and Jeremy had a "dream catcher" to help on such occasions. His parents followed a consistent bedtime routine, and he had stars on his ceiling and a night light in his room. Initially, after a nightmare, Jeremy's parents would go to his room to console him and stay in his room until he fell back asleep. More recently, they had encouraged

Jeremy to put himself back to sleep by having a monitor in his room so that he would feel secure knowing that they could hear him at all times. They used a sticker chart to reward Jeremy for the times that he was able to put himself back to sleep without his parents, which were infrequent. The nightmares seemed to increase, causing great disruption and stress to their otherwise stable family and time lost from work for Jeremy's parents.

On Jeremy's first visit, he appeared comfortable and readily discussed the fearful nightmares that he had involving scary monsters and wolves. He admitted that the nightmares made it difficult for him to go to sleep by himself, and he expressed enthusiasm in learning a way to make it easier for him to get to sleep alone after a bad dream. He was invited to imagine a favorite place in his thinking. He readily engaged in favorite place mental imagery and described seeing "a magic door." He spontaneously explained that he was wearing a "special discovery suit with a blue design" and was playing tag with five friends. He was encouraged to notice how happy and content he was while engaged in mental imagery (self-hypnosis). It was suggested that he practice the self-hypnosis before going to sleep each night, so that if he woke up in the middle of the night, he would be able to help himself get back to sleep. Jeremy was then asked to talk about his "nightmares" and create an ending to those dreams in which he would win, or "take out the bad guy." He easily followed through with this suggestion and left the meeting feeling enabled and confident. Follow-up from his parents weeks later revealed that Jeremy quickly learned to do the self-hypnosis on his own and reportedly used it effectively to help himself fall asleep. Soon after the initial visit, Jeremy no longer had frequent nightmares and had no further problems with sleep.

RECURRENT PAIN

Self-regulation strategies are particularly effective when applied to pediatric pain management. In acute pain associated with trauma and related medical procedures, diaphragmatic breathing and self-hypnosis have been shown to be successful in alleviating discomfort and allowing treatment to proceed easily (Kuttner, 1996). Studies of chronic, recurrent pain (e.g., migraine headaches and recurrent abdominal pain) have clearly documented the effectiveness of self-regulation strategies. One prospective study compared propranolol, placebo, and self-hypnosis in the treatment of pediatric migraine and found that self-hypnosis was most effective in reducing the frequency of migraine headaches (Olness, MacDonald, and Uden, 1987).

EXAMPLE

Kara was a 12 1/2-year-old with chronic stomachaches and sore throats. Since her initial complaints 3 to 4 months ago, she had three negative throat cultures, two courses of antibiotics, a normal complete blood count, a normal urinalysis, and an upper gastrointestinal series that showed nonspecific findings. Kara was given a short course of an H_2 blocker, but her stomachaches continued. She had missed several days of school until arrangements were made for her to spend time as needed with the *school nurse instead of being sent home. Kara made several visits to the nurse's office to lie down each day. Kara was being seen by a psychologist weekly for anxiety that was thought to be related to school. Further history revealed occasional headaches, no weight loss, no vomiting or bowel problems, and a normal physical examination.*

Kara described two types of abdominal pain: a sharp constant, epigastric pain that she believed was "a virus," and a lower abdominal pain that occurred intermittently when she was nervous. On a scale of 0 (no pain) to 12 (worst pain), Kara rated her stomachache as 9 on the initial visit. (The worst that it had been was 11 and the best that it had been was 7.) Further laboratory testing determined no organic cause of the stomachaches. When asked how her life would be different when she no longer had the pain, Kara tearfully replied that she "wouldn't have to go to the school nurse" and that she would "eat and feel better."

Kara was given examples of how she gets signals from her body when she has different feelings, and the specific physiologic changes of the body in response to being nervous or scared versus relaxed. Kara was encouraged to hear that many children with problems like hers improve by learning how to use their mind to help their body. She was given a calendar and asked to monitor her stomachaches. On the second visit Kara was taught diaphragmatic breathing and introduced to biofeedback. Through self-regulation training, she quickly learned to control her breathing pattern and slow its rate. At the end of the first session she had lowered her stomachache to a rating of 4, the lowest that it had ever been. She recognized that her stomachache bothered her less when she slowed her breathing rate and relaxed. She agreed to practice the "belly breathing" at home each night before bed. Kara had five subsequent biofeedback sessions in which she mastered the physiologic self-regulation of her peripheral temperature (an indirect measure of sympathetic nervous system activity), muscle activity, and sweat gland response (EDA) in a video game format.

After 5 weeks, Kara's stomachaches had improved dramatically (down to a rating of 1 to 2), with only one visit to the school nurse each day. At follow-up 8 weeks after the initial visit, Kara no longer had any somatic complaints and only visited the school nurse to say hello.

TIC DISORDER

Self-regulation strategies have been applied successfully to treat repetitive behaviors including habits, tics, obsessive-compulsive disorder, and Tourette syndrome (Kohen, 1995). A significant number of patients with mild to moderate tics who are seen by developmental-behavioral pediatricians improve with self-regulation techniques alone. It is important to discuss with the patient the significant impact that anxiety and stress may have on the repetitive behaviors. During treatment, self-awareness of behavior patterns and an enhanced sense of self-control are emphasized.

EXAMPLE

Nick was a 17-year-old boy with a chronic motor tic disorder who was referred for self-regulation training. Nick

had recently been on a psychotropic medication trial to help with the tics, but he did not respond optimally to the medication and did not want to consider alternative medication options. Nick had had difficulties with motor tics since he was 10 years old. At that time, he developed facial tics, which seemed to come and go over the next several years but did not impair him functionally. However, within the past 18 to 24 months, the tics had worsened considerably and had become widespread (occurring in muscle groups all over his body), more frequent, and quite intense. He had been seen several times by a pediatric neurologist who had established the diagnosis of chronic motor tics and had prescribed the medication trial.

Nick described tics of his wrists and ankles that were so repetitive and severe that his joints would become sore. At the time of referral, he also noticed that his eyeblink and head-throw tics were interfering with his reading. Nick reported that the tics occurred daily and that he thought they were exacerbated by stress.

Despite the severity of the tics, Nick was well adjusted and had a very close and supportive group of friends at school. Nick was a well-rounded and highly successful high school student. Not only was he doing well academically and was on the honor role but he was also a key player on the football team. Additionally, Nick had a part-time job.

Nick's facial tics were evident throughout the first visit. Initially, the potential triggers of the tic flare-ups and the role of stress and anxiety on the tic exacerbations were discussed. Nick was then coached through a progressive muscle relaxation exercise and encouraged to let go of any muscle tension that he felt in his body. His tics stopped abruptly. Nick spontaneously closed his eyes and was encouraged to enjoy his choice of pleasant mental imagery. Particular attention was given to Nick's experience of a sense of warmth, heaviness, and comfort in his facial muscle groups. Nick was excited and surprised at how his tics had stopped so suddenly while using the relaxation technique. The session concluded with teaching Nick the basic diaphragmatic breathing techniques. Nick was encouraged to practice the progressive muscle relaxation and breathing techniques at least twice a day for 5 minutes and when he felt stressed or anxious. He was also encouraged to self-monitor through the use of a symptom diary.

Nick returned as scheduled for a follow-up visit 1 month later. He reportedly used the relaxation techniques regularly every day with great success, and he was excited to share the noticeable decrease in his motor tic activity that he had experienced. He described the use of very vivid and colorful mental imagery as part of his practices. The application of self-hypnosis was discussed in more explicit terms, and the use of progressive muscle relaxation and diaphragmatic breathing strategies was reviewed. A peripheral temperature sensor was attached to Nick's left index finger prior to the practice session. Nick once again demonstrated the ability to quickly and deeply relax soon after the practice began. He did an excellent job and raised his peripheral temperature 12 degrees over the 20-minute relaxation session. Nick stated that he felt quite confident that he had good control over his tics by using the self-regulation strategies that he had learned.

At a final follow-up visit 1 month later, Nick exhibited only mild facial tics at the beginning of the session. Since his last visit, he had been chosen for one of the lead roles in his school play. Self-hypnosis strategies were reviewed, including an imagined "rehearsal" of his performance in the play. Once again, while actively involved in the relaxation techniques, Nick's facial tics completely resolved. He stated that he had been using diaphragmatic breathing and progressive muscle relaxation between scenes in the play when he was performing and had continued excellent symptom control.

Training and Certification

Child health care professionals who would like to acquire and apply these techniques should have appropriate training and experience. Cyberphysiologic techniques are not viewed as a separate discipline or profession, but they are meant to be used in the context of the practice of medicine, nursing, dentistry, psychology, and social work. Therefore, competency and licensure in a defined medical or mental health related discipline is required before training or certification in self-regulation techniques. Hypnosis and biofeedback in particular have strong professional organizations, training opportunities, and formal testing and certification standards.

Child health care professionals who desire training in hypnotherapeutic methods should take a basic workshop sponsored by the Society for Developmental and Behavioral Pediatrics, the American Society of Clinical Hypnosis, or the Society for Clinical and Experimental Hypnosis or through an appropriate academic offering, usually at a university medical center or psychology department. After adequate training, supervision, and clinical experience, individuals seeking formal certification for hypnosis training can contact the American Society of Clinical Hypnosis, the American Board of Medical Hypnosis, the American Board of Psychological Hypnosis, the American Board of Dental Hypnosis, or the American Board of Hypnosis in Clinical Social Work for information.

Training in biofeedback techniques is offered at meetings of the Association for Applied Psychophysiology and Biofeedback and through private training seminars. Board certification in biofeedback is available through the Biofeedback Certification Institute of America. Table 85–3 lists the names and addresses of the organizations referred to in this section.

Conclusion

A growing body of literature and successful clinical experience documenting the utility and cost efficiency of the self-regulation strategies described in this chapter underscore the increasing importance of these techniques in the armamentarium of the developmental-behavioral pediatrician and other pediatric health professionals. It is also clear that parents are increasingly interested in nonpharmacologic treatment modalities for their children with biobehavioral

Table 85–3 • Organization/Resource Guide

Hypnosis certification and training
    American Society of Clinical Hypnosis, 2200 East Devon Ave., Suite 291, Des Plaines, IL 60018
    Society for Clinical and Experimental Hypnosis, 3905 Vincennes Rd., Suite 304, Indianapolis, IN 46268
    Society for Developmental and Behavioral Pediatrics, 19 Station Lane, Philadelphia, PA 19118
    American Board of Medical Hypnosis, c/o Donald Lynch, M.D., Sentara Cancer Institute, 600 Gresham Dr., Norfolk, VA 23510; 757-668-4264
Biofeedback certification and training
    Association for Applied Psychophysiology and Biofeedback, 10200 West 44th Avenue, Suite 304, Wheat Ridge, CO 80033
    Biofeedback Certification Institute of America, 10200 West 44th Avenue, Suite 304, Wheat Ridge, CO 80033

problems. Biofeedback, hypnosis, and the other cyberphysiologic techniques offer children the option of "skills for pills" (Wickramasekera, 1988). Once children learn self-regulation strategies, they commonly apply the techniques to other challenging situations that they encounter and continue to use these techniques throughout their life. It is hoped that these techniques would become part of all child health care providers' curricula, including medical and nursing school programs, Child Life programs, and pediatric residency programs.

Pioneering research in pediatric self-regulation supports the ability of children to voluntarily modulate certain aspects of immune system function (Olness, Culbert, and Uden, 1989). Research in this area, termed *psychoneuroimmunology,* documents children's ability to eradicate warts, change levels of salivary immunoglobulins, and influence the activity of certain white blood cell types (Olness, 1990). Researchers are exploring the role of relaxation, directed mental imagery, and related cyberphysiologic strategies on children with cancer, autoimmune disorders, and infectious processes. The links of mental imagery and emotions to physiologic response patterns are also being clarified.

Practitioners in this field look forward to the day when biofeedback computers, hypnotherapy, and breathing control training are part of the general pediatrician's daily office practice. The idea of proactive stress management, or stress "inoculation," for the pediatric population using training in cyberphysiologic techniques is also timely. The idea that early training in self-regulation techniques may help certain at-risk populations in reducing morbidity from conditions such as asthma, essential hypertension, hemophilia, migraine headache, and Tourette syndrome is promising. A preventive approach to these disorders using training in hypnosis, biofeedback, diaphragmatic breathing, and related skills could result in huge savings in medical costs over time.

With the advance of computer graphics technology, it is likely that children will be able to learn and practice these self-regulation skills in interactive multimedia formats—playing a "video game for your body" in a way that is both therapeutic and enjoyable for pediatric patients. Children's interest and ability in learning about mind-body connections was demonstrated in a special exhibit at the Cleveland Health Science Museum. A program was designed on a computer that teaches children about mind-body connections through the use of friendly animated graphics and touch screen technology. Pilot studies with more than 350 children on the "mind-body" machine determined that only two subjects could not modulate their EDA in the desired direction within the first few minutes (Olness, Kohen, 1996).

It would seem likely, given the studies and clinical experiences to date, that biofeedback, self-hypnosis, and related self-regulation techniques will become the primary "treatments of choice" for a variety of biobehavioral problems of childhood, including headaches, somatization disorders, anxiety spectrum problems, enuresis, sleep disorders, and disorders of autonomic nervous system arousal.

REFERENCES

Attansio V, Andraski F, Burke E, et al: Clinical issues in utilizing biofeedback with children. Clin Biofeedback Health 8:134–141, 1985.

Culbert T, Reaney J, Kohen D: Cyberphysiologic strategies for children: the clinical hypnosis/biofeedback interface. Int J Clin Exp Hypnosis 42:97–117, 1994.

Jacobson E: The origins and development of progressive relaxation. J Behav Ther Exp Psychiatry 8:119–123, 1977.

Kajander R: The Pediatric Self-Regulation Series Monographs: Diaphragmatic Breathing. Minneapolis, Just Imagine, Inc., 1997.

Kendall P: Child and Adolescent Therapy—Cognitive-Behavioral Procedures. New York, Guilford Press, 1991.

Kohen DP: Ericksonian communication and hypnotic strategies in the management of tics and Tourette syndrome in children and adolescents. *In* Zeig I, Lankton S (eds): Difficult Contexts for Therapy. New York, Brunner/Mazel, 1995, pp 116–138.

Kohen DP, Olness K: Hypnosis with children. *In* Rhue JW, Lynn SJ, Kirsch I (eds): Handbook of Clinical Hypnosis. Washington, DC, American Psychological Association, 1993, pp 357–382.

Kohen DP, Olness K, Colwell S, et al: The use of relaxation mental imagery (self-hypnosis) in the management of 505 pediatric behavioral encounters. J Dev Behav Pediatr 1:21–25, 1984.

Kuttner L: A Child in Pain—How to Help, What to Do. Point Roberts, WA, Hartley and Marks, 1996.

Kuttner L: Management of young children's acute pain and anxiety during invasive medical procedures. Pediatrician 16:39–44, 1989.

Lee LH, Olness KN: Effects of self-induced mental imagery on autonomic reactivity in children. J Develop Behav Pediatr 17:323–327, 1996.

Linden W: Autogenic Training: A Clinical Guide. New York, Guilford Press, 1990.

Olness K: Introduction. J Dev Behav Pediatr 17:299, 1996.

Olness K: Cyberphysiologic strategies in pediatric practice. Pediatr Ann 20:115–119, 1991.

Olness K: Pediatric psychoneuroimmunology: hypnosis as a mediator. Potentials and problems. *In* Hypnosis: Current Theory, Research and Practice. Amsterdam, VU University Press, 1990.

Olness K: Unrecognized biologic bases of behavioral symptoms in patients referred for hypnotherapy. Am J Clin Hypn 30:1–8, 1987.

Olness K: The use of self-hypnosis in the treatment of childhood nocturnal enuresis: a report on forty patients. Clin Pediatr 14:273–279, 1975.

Olness K, Culbert T, Uden D: Self-regulation of salivary immunoglobulin A by children. Pediatrics 83:66–71, 1989.

Olness K, Kohen D: Hypnosis and Hypnotherapy with Children, 3rd ed. New York, Guilford Press, 1996.

Olness K, MacDonald J, Uden D: Prospective study comparing propranolol, placebo, and hypnosis in the management of juvenile migraine. Pediatrics 79:593–597, 1987.

Schwartz MS: Biofeedback: A Practitioner's Guide, 2nd ed. New York, Guilford Press, 1995.

Wickramasekera I: Clinical Behavioral Medicine: Some concepts and Procedures. New York, Plenum Press, 1988.

86 Referral Processes

David A. Pangburn

At the end of 1995, more than 60% of Americans belonged to some form of managed care health plan.

The single largest negative finding in managed care systems has consistently been lower patient satisfaction rates, which may have more to do with the form of organization than with the capitation strategy.

Whether care is delivered in a staff-model health-maintenance organization (HMO), group model HMO, physician network, or independent practice association (IPA), there are incentives to reduce specialty referral.

The Tinman found he had what he thought he lacked.
—TRACY CHAPMAN, "REMEMBER THE TINMAN"

The primary care physician is uniquely situated to provide needed services to children and families. The inclusion of the physician in some of the most intimate aspects of a family's life experience—joy accompanying the birth of a child, distress surrounding illness, consolation in recovery, fear of death and disability, and delight in a child's achievements—affords clinicians a unique vantage and responsibility. The care of children with special health care needs and developmental disabilities perhaps epitomizes this special role of the physician. Families beckon, and at times demand, an extra measure of consideration and engagement that may send the primary care physician on the quest for a "wizard," that consultant of amazing skill and accomplishment who can conjure up a solution to the family's needs. In fact, L. Frank Baum's *The Wonderful Wizard of Oz* may be an appropriate allegory for the referral process in the age of managed care: the referral for specialty care ("the Wizard") is complicated by incentives ("opium fields") and disincentives ("flying monkeys").

The Social Context of the Care of Children With Disabilities

The past 30 years of social reform have created the conditions for inclusion of children with disabilities in their communities. From the passage of Public Law 94-142, the Education for All Handicapped Children Act of 1975, and the Education of the Handicapped Act Amendments of 1986, to the Individuals with Disabilities Education Act (IDEA) and the Americans with Disabilities Act of 1990, there has been increasing legislative support for individuals with disabilities to lead full lives at home, in the public schools, in recreational activities, and in access to health care. Fewer and fewer children with developmental disabilities are receiving their primary care in specialty clinics,

hospitals, and residential facilities; rather, they are visiting the primary care physician in their communities.

Managed Care

At the same time that these reforms are occurring, another movement is shaping the future of health care delivery—the emergence and development of "managed care," now the predominant method of organization of the delivery of care and health care financing. At the end of 1995, 161 million Americans—more than 60% of the total population—belonged to some form of managed care health plan. Figure 86–1 shows the growth of enrollment in health maintenance organizations (HMOs) from 1976 to 1995.

A definition of managed care follows:

> Managed care refers to a variety of methods of financing and organizing health care in which attempt is made to control costs by controlling the provision of services. The term encompasses health maintenance organizations (HMOs), preferred provider organizations (PPOs), and point-of-service (POS) financing and delivery systems. (Iglehart, 1994)

In clinical terms, managed care describes a system that determines the most *appropriate* and *efficient* treatment for the individual patient. Eliminating unnecessary testing and procedures, streamlining the processes of care, rationalizing decision making about when and where to refer and admit patients, measuring outcomes, and improving quality are all aspects of well-managed care.

Prospective payment, the method typically used in a managed care setting, is intended to shift services more toward preventive care and primary care and away from costly and unnecessary procedures and tertiary care.

The impetus toward managed care is the upward spiral of health care costs, which, by 1993, absorbed 14% of the gross national product and threatened to bankrupt the government. Health benefits now represent between 7% and 8% of employee compensation and are predicted to rise to 10% by the latter half of this decade.

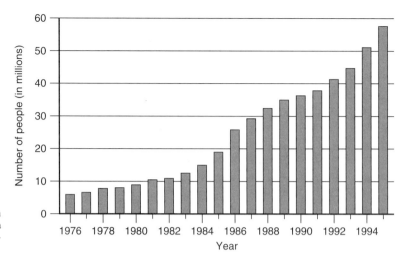

Figure 86–1. Number of HMO enrollees, 1976 through 1995. (From Health Insurance Association of America [HIAA]: Sourcebook of Health Insurance Data. Washington, DC, HIAA, 1996.)

QUALITY CARE OR COST CONTAINMENT?

In general, the literature consistently shows that the care of patients in managed care systems costs less, with quality equal to or better than that in fee-for-service models. Several studies suggest that preventive services, such as immunization and screening tests, have been more reliably delivered in managed care systems than in fee-for-service systems. The single largest negative finding in managed care systems has consistently been lower patient satisfaction rates, which may have more to do with the form of organization than the capitation strategy.

From the earliest models of managed care in the 1960s, the Kaiser Plan and Harvard Community Health Plan HMOs, to today's for-profit plans, managed care has undergone a significant transformation. For-profit HMOs surpassed not-for-profits organizations in total members in 1993 and are continuing to grow at a more brisk pace. "Managed care" has become increasingly synonymous with "cost containment." The trends stimulated by competition for markets, including mergers and affiliations of hospitals, downsizing of specialty departments, and HMO restrictions on referral to preferred providers, are affecting the relationship between primary and specialty care providers. Whether care is delivered in a staff-model HMO, group model HMO, physician network, or independent practice association (IPA), there are incentives to reduce specialty referral.

Payment for care through various forms of capitation may offer financial incentives for limiting specialty referral. Capitation, strictly speaking, refers to the payment of a designated amount of money for the ongoing care of an individual or group for a specified period of time. The sum is set in advance of the actual delivery of services and represents the "best guess" of the amount of money that will be required to provide that care. A 1995 survey found that primary care physicians in 56% of network or IPA-model managed care plans, 34% of physicians in group- and staff-model HMOs, and 7% of physicians in preferred-provider organizations (PPOs) were paid on a capitated basis.

DIAGNOSIS-RELATED GROUPS AND LEVEL OF SERVICE

During the 1980s, the effort to control costs initiated by Medicare, the diagnosis-related group (DRG) approach, began a process to quantify reimbursement based on the severity of illness. The latest system for coding diagnoses is the *International Classification of Diseases, 9th Revision, Clinical Modification (ICD-9-CM)*.

The Health Care Financing Administration (HCFA) has taken the lead in stimulating reform of the systems of health care reimbursement. In collaboration with the Harvard School of Public Health, HCFA developed a new methodology for financing health care services called the *resource-based relative value scale* (RBRVS). The RBRVS attempts to adjust the amount of payment for physician services by the actual amount of work involved in providing a particular service. The aim is to shift compensation to reward primary care and evaluation of patients more and to reward the performance of procedures less. The specifications most widely used for reimbursement are found in the American Medical Association's *Current Procedural Terminology, 4th edition (CPT-4)*.

Reimbursement for services within a managed care system requires the informed and accurate use of *CPT-4* and *ICD-9-CM* coding. This is true for both primary care and specialty encounters. Use of codes that adequately reimburse for time spent doing case management, including reviews of extensive records, telephone consultations, and coordination and planning meetings, can ensure that at least part of the time spent can be billed for.

INTEGRATION OF HEALTH CARE SYSTEMS

Integration of health care systems provides another strategy for ensuring comprehensive and efficient health care delivery. Vertical integration of a health care delivery system creates efficiencies of scale as well as the ability to market a unique business entity. A network of primary care providers, specialists, hospitals, long-term care facilities, pharmacy, laboratory, and radiology departments, linked by a single administration, can plan for and develop programs designed to meet the needs of the communities and populations it serves. The combination of hospital with IPA or PPO exemplifies this form of vertically integrated system.

QUALITY IMPROVEMENT

Quality improvement strategies, supported by the financial goals of reducing the use of specialty referral, emergency room, and inpatient hospital, have demonstrated the ability to improve health outcomes while controlling costs. An example of this is the improved treatment of asthma and decreased hospitalization rates following training of both patients and providers in modern asthma management and providing the patient with effective medications via home nebulizers. The coordinated efforts of primary care physicians, specialists, pharmacists, nurses, educators, vendors of medical equipment, and family members are necessary to accomplish this kind of improvement. Programs such as this can flourish under integrated systems.

MEDICAID-MANAGED CARE

Managed care has so successfully controlled the cost of health care that by 1994 many employer health plans had achieved modest decreases in premiums. This is in sharp contrast to the cost of Medicaid expenditures, which, for fee-for-service care, rose through the 1980s at 10% a year and by 1990 through 1991 rose at an astounding rate of 31%. In 1980 the total state and federal expense for Medicaid was $25 billion, and by 1995 Medicaid spending totaled $159 billion. Individuals with disability are enrolled in Medicaid at higher rates than in the private sector, constituting 15% of all Medicaid recipients, their care accounting for about 37% of all Medicaid expenditures. Confronted with these staggering increases in costs, most states are considering, or have implemented, managed care programs for individuals with Medicaid coverage.

While state Medicaid programs have always had the ability to offer Medicaid recipients the *choice* of managed care plans (as long as the beneficiary had the ability to enroll and disenroll voluntarily), many states are moving toward *mandatory* enrollment in managed care. States are able to do this under special waivers of the Medicaid law (the freedom of beneficiaries to choose health care providers is *waived*). Nearly all states are currently in the process of considering, developing, or implementing such waivers.

Referral to Specialists

Whereas most children require only a single provider for most of their health care and supervision, children with special health care needs or disabilities frequently have multiple providers and multiple treatments. A child with cerebral palsy may have contact with a pediatrician, a neurologist, an orthopedist, an orthotist, a physiatrist, a physical therapist, a speech pathologist, an occupational therapist, a psychologist, and a social worker, among others (see Chapter 61). The task of the primary care physician is to coordinate these referrals and to assist the family in understanding the services that different specialties pro-

vide. The division of labor within the team of primary care and specialty providers must be clearly understood by the family as well as by team members. Most managed care plans require the initial contact to be with the primary care physician.

The referral to specialists must be well planned and requires communication concerning the goals of referral, the sharing of historical, examination, and laboratory data relevant to the referral, and the plan for follow-up with the family subsequent to the specialty consultation. Information may be shared through a variety of media, including electronic, or through automated medical record systems, but no method is perhaps more suitable to building the relationship between primary care physician and specialist than person-to-person contact.

The team of providers involved with the child and family is typically broader than the scope of health care services, including early intervention program personnel, educators, therapists in the community, and extended family members. The recommendations of any one member of this group may vary from those of another, and families must often choose among conflicting advice. In continuing health care, there usually are trade-offs among some choices, such as the optimal time to do a surgical procedure or the choice between seizure control and alertness. In all of these, the primary care physician can help families make informed choices.

EXPECTED OUTCOMES OF REFERRAL

The comparative rarity of most childhood chronic conditions may make families feel isolated. They may wonder why they have been singled out by an unusual condition and feel that no other families share their experiences. Programs in specialty centers (e.g., programs for children with Down syndrome, Williams syndrome, or cerebral palsy) and parent advocacy programs have worked to break this sense of isolation through groups that help parents learn from each other how to raise children with chronic disorders.

Many of these conditions are unpredictable in their implications, longevity, complications, and developmental impact on the individual child. Parents speak frequently of how difficult this unpredictability is for them and how they wish for clear answers to difficult questions, even if the answers may be unfavorable. Many important aspects of chronic disease or disabling conditions are unpredictable, both because of great variability in environmental influences and biological responsiveness to specific conditions and treatments and because little information is available about many rare diseases. Expertise from the fields of genetics and neurology, with access to new knowledge from ongoing research, can best inform these questions of prognosis.

Chronic conditions have a pervasive influence on a child's daily life. Frequent interactions with the medical care system, occasional hospitalizations, and greater dependency on parents and health care providers characterize their experience. A chronic condition may create a sense of "differentness," of being unable to do many things that other children can do.

A chronic condition creates additional stresses and

demands on families and on children that more typically developing children and their families do not face. Perhaps as a result, chronically ill children have about twice the frequency of psychological or behavioral problems than is found in healthy control subjects; children with significant developmental disabilities or sensory deficits have as much as a five times greater risk for these problems. Despite this greater risk of psychological maladjustment, most children with chronic conditions are psychologically healthy. Mental health referrals should be proactive as well as used for crisis intervention. Referral should be made to experienced clinicians cognizant of the needs of a child with special health care needs, especially children with cognitive deficits who may benefit from nonverbal forms of therapy or behavioral approaches.

All of these factors reinforce the importance of thoughtful consideration and planning of specialty referral. The goal is to prevent secondary conditions that may be associated with the underlying chronic condition and to promote the best possible adaptation of the child and family.

BARRIERS TO REFERRAL

There is growing concern, primarily based on the anecdotal reports from developmental specialists in tertiary hospitals, that there has been a marked decline in referral for developmental consultation and management over the past decade. There is also evidence that pediatricians are experiencing difficulty referring patients in managed care systems. A 1992 survey of Fellows of the American Academy of Pediatrics (Cartland and Yudkowsky, 1992) found that pediatricians were less likely to refer patients in managed care systems than patients in traditional, fee-for-service plans. Of these pediatricians, 8.7% reported that they referred their managed-care patients less frequently than their fee-for-service patients. The reported barriers to specialty care referral are listed in Table 86–1. The table compares the types and rates of barriers to referral to specialty care reported by pediatricians (n = 684) caring for patients enrolled in managed-care versus traditional fee-for-service plans. Types of barriers reported included administrative barriers, financial barriers, availability of proper care (or lack thereof), and community barriers. The mean number of barriers reported by each pediatrician increases from 2.3 for traditional fee-for-service patients to 5.7 for managed-care patient referrals.

The most compelling finding from this study, and from other informal reports, is the inaccessibility of specific specialty providers due to panel restrictions of managed care plans. Since children with special health care needs often have rare conditions, only a few subspecialists in any one geographic area may have the experience and expertise necessary to provide quality consultation. Whereas other barriers to referral, including administrative and financial barriers, may be more easily overcome, inaccessibility to specific specialists has potentially far greater implications for quality care.

Models of Managed Care for Children With Disabilities

Managed care has the potential to control the costs of health care as well as to improve quality through coordination of care and incentives for preventive health care. It

Table 86–1 • Pediatrician-Reported Barriers to Referring Patients to Specialized Care

Barrier Categories*	Patient Type	
	Managed Care, % (n)	Traditional Pay, % (n)
Administrative barriers	91.3 (578)	71.6 (373)
Time-consuming verbal (telephone) authorization process	61.1 (391)	24.4 (129)
Burdensome paperwork	58.2 (370)	28.0 (150)
Peer review process	58.8 (365)	42.5 (224)
Complex appeals process for utilizing out-of-plan specialists	49.4 (306)	7.8 (39)
Other administrative procedures	59.1 (369)	36.1 (191)
Past reimbursement denials	49.6 (307)	32.6 (169)
Financial barriers	66.3 (414)	26.4 (135)
Peer pressure to contain costs	52.4 (330)	23.0 (124)
Financial disincentives	40.6 (250)	4.8 (24)
Availability of proper care	53.5 (332)	11.7 (57)
Physician panel restrictions	40.4 (250)	4.7 (24)
Hospital restrictions	28.2 (177)	4.3 (22)
Pressure to refer to adult specialists/subspecialists	20.2 (126)	3.7 (20)
Pressure to refer to adult inpatient care	5.5 (34)	1.3 (7)
Community barriers	—	30.0 (169)
Lack of pediatric specialists in the community	—	27.9 (158)
Lack of availability of pediatric inpatient care	—	6.9 (39)
Mean number of barriers	5.7	2.3
Mean	6.0	2.0
Mode	5.0	0

*Findings presented in this table represent those differences between managed care and traditional pay that reached a statistical significance of p<.01.
Adapted from Cartland DC, Yudkowsky BK: Barriers to pediatric referral in managed care systems. Pediatrics 89(2):183, 1992.

has also been shown to reduce out-of-pocket expenses for families of children with disabilities. Inherent in managed care is the potential to limit the choice of primary care and access to specialty providers. There are, however, examples of "best practices" that have been developed in managed settings that may serve as models for the future of managed care for children with disabilities. These three examples vary greatly in scope and scale but share common themes relevant to the managed care referral process: (1) care coordination services, bringing together community providers and health care providers, which enhance the quality of care, and family and provider satisfaction and may reduce the cost of care; (2) interdisciplinary teamwork that may enhance the quality of referral outcomes; and (3) managed care networks, which, owing to their size, integration, emphasis on preventive services, and communication systems, make programs of this nature possible.

Health Care Services for Children With Special Needs, Inc. An HMO in the District of Columbia for children who are eligible for Supplemental Security Income (SSI) began operation in December 1995. The benefit package includes care management by a full interdisciplinary team and includes coverage for all acute and long-term needs. The HMO is paid $1000 per month on a prospective basis and reimburses primary care providers on a fee-for-service basis for the first 2 years of operation. It is anticipated that, beginning in the third year, this program will begin paying its providers on a capitated basis, essentially sharing risk with its providers at that point. Potential for cost savings is expected to be generated from deinstitutionalization of children currently residing in out-of-home placements. Accordingly, Health Care Services for Children With Special Needs has developed annual targets for the reduction of long-term care utilization.

The Developmental Consultation Services (DCS), Harvard Pilgrim Health Care. A centralized program of the staff model division (formerly known as Harvard Community Health Plan) of this New England HMO, the DCS serves all pediatric members for whom specialized consultation may be of benefit. The DCS provides general developmental consultation as well as a specialized Down syndrome program and diagnostic team for children with pervasive developmental disorders. The administrator of the program also coordinates all Early Intervention Program referrals for this HMO. Referrals come from 65 staff pediatricians as well as from pediatricians in other divisions of this HMO. Referrals are triaged by a team composed of a developmental pediatrician and specialized social workers who begin care coordination at the point of referral. When more thorough consultation is needed, an interdisciplinary team, made up of a developmental pediatrician, social work case manager, and combinations of speech pathologist, physical therapist, psychologist, and child psychiatrist, may meet with the child and family. Often invited to the session, with the involvement of the family, are members of the broader community-based team working with the child, such as Early Intervention Program personnel and representatives from schools or state agencies. The goals of the program are improved care coordination, preventive services, and communication between primary and specialty care providers and the family. Families and primary care providers served by the program have been surveyed and

register high levels of satisfaction. Cost savings are postulated to result from decreased utilization of out-of-plan providers and reduced primary care visit rates.

The Center for School Problems, Department of Pediatrics, Kaiser-Permanente. This program was founded in 1974 to investigate and clarify school problems referred to the Department of Pediatrics. The service is considered a medical benefit. Upon receipt of a written referral, a developmental questionnaire and teacher questionnaire are mailed to the member family and are subsequently reviewed by the program director. Based on the pattern of expressed concerns, the child is seen for any combination of service, including screening triage, school readiness screening, a medical evaluation for attentional difficulties, psychological evaluation of developmental abilities, and neuropsychological evaluation for those with medical conditions that affect adaptive functioning. The child may also be referred for other diagnostic and therapeutic services, such as speech and language therapy. The focus of the program is on diagnosis and advocacy, and treatment is referred to appropriate facilities within the health plan, the public sector, or the school system. Review of use indicated a 30% decline in physician contacts by the family, and an ongoing quality assurance survey indicated very high approval ratings by members.

Conclusion

Providing primary and specialty care in a managed care environment presents unique challenges and opportunities. The era of fiscal constraints on health care is likely to persist into the next century. However, advocates for better health care for individuals with disability, as well as other groups of health care consumers and providers, will provide pressure to ensure that health care spending remains equitable.

The tasks of participation in consultation, communication among multiple providers and with the family, and ongoing surveillance may appear daunting. Primary care physicians must find within themselves or seek out the tools necessary to accomplish these tasks. The tools are the compassion to care for and develop lasting relationships with children and their families; the knowledge of developmental pediatrics and the integration of a developmental framework into day-to-day interactions; and the courage to advocate for the needs of children and their families, including by thoughtful and well-defended referral. There are no "yellow brick roads" to follow.

REFERENCES

Cartland JDC, Yudkowsky BK: Barriers to pediatric referral in managed care systems. Pediatrics 89(2):183, 1992.
Iglehart JK: Physicians and the growth of managed care. New Engl J Med 331:1167, 1994.

SUGGESTED READINGS

Berwick DM: Quality of health care: Part 5. Payment by capitation and the quality of care. N Engl J Med 355:1227, 1996.
Blackman JA, Healy A, Ruppert ES: Participation of pediatricians in early intervention: impetus from public law 99-457. Pediatr 89:98, 1992.

Committee on Children With Disability, American Academy of Pediatrics: Pediatric services for infants and children with special health care needs. Pediatrics 92:163, 1993.

Crocker AC: Improved support for children with disabilities. Pediatrics 88(5):1057, 1991.

Dorwart RA, Epstein SS: Financing of services. *In* Privatization and Mental Health Care: A Fragile Balance. Westport, CT, Auburn House, 1993, pp 37–56.

Edmunds M, Frank R, Hogan M, McCarty D, Robinson-Beale R, Weisner C (eds): Managing Managed Care: Quality Improvements in Behavioral Health. Committee on Quality Assurance and Accreditation Guidelines for Managed Behavioral Health Care, Division of Neuroscience and Behavioral Health [and] Division of Health Care Services, Institute of Medicine. Washington, DC, National Academy Press, 1997, pp 15–33.

Fontanesi JM, Richards JH: A learning disability clinic within the HMO setting. HMO Pract 8(3):141, 1994.

Ireys HT, Grason HA, Guyer B: Assuring quality of care for children with special needs in managed care organizations: roles for pediatricians. Pediatrics 98:178, 1996.

Kassirer JP: Editorial: access to specialty care. N Engl J Med 331:1151, 1994.

Kastner TA, Walsh KK, Criscione T: Overview and implications of Medicaid managed care for people with developmental disabilities. Mental Retardation 35:257, 1997.

Kastner TA, Walsh KK, Criscione T: Technical elements, demonstration projects, and fiscal models in Medicaid managed care for people with developmental disabilities. Mental Retardation 35:270, 1997.

Newacheck PW, Hughes DC, Stoddard JJ, Halfon N: Children with chronic illness and Medicaid managed care. Pediatrics 95:497, 1994.

Perrin JM, Shonkoff JP: Developmental disabilities and chronic illness: an overview. *In* Behrman RE, Kliegman RM, Arvin AM (eds): Nelson Textbook of Pediatrics, 15th ed. Philadelphia, WB Saunders, 1996 pp 123–128.

PART VIII

Legal and Ethical Issues

87 *Legal Issues*

Kathleen Bradley Kapsalis • Walter P. Christian

Legal precedents for the pediatric population are interwoven with ethical and moral considerations.

The right to due process is a basic protection afforded patients when their autonomy is threatened.

Informed consent includes at least three elements: competence, knowledge, and voluntariness.

Documentation is an essential feature of appropriate treatment.

Given the inadequate knowledge of the efficacy of aversive interventions, the potential harm to the pediatric patient, *and* the availability of efficacious positive interventions, it is more wrong than right on moral grounds to use aversive procedures.

The basic legal issues that ensure a pediatric patient's rights to treatment are the doctrine of the least restrictive alternative, due process, informed consent to treatment, privacy, confidentiality, appropriate treatment, and protection against harm. The pediatric practitioner must recognize that the legal rights of patients have a dramatic impact not only on the relationship between the care provider and the patient but also on the diagnostic and treatment services that the practitioner can legally provide. This practitioner, no matter how well intentioned, is not the ultimate authority in treatment decisions. He or she must be knowledgeable of all legal restraints to practice competently.

Quality of Life and the Pediatric Patient

Laws and their ensuing regulations are only one end of the practice continuum. Practice standards and guidelines developed by advocacy groups reflect the values and precepts that arise from public opinion. Basic concern with the quality of life for pediatric patients with disabilities is ultimately reflected in the law. Legal precedents for this population are interwoven with ethical and moral considerations. Although the subject is outside the scope of this chapter, it is important to consider the social framework within which laws have been enacted. The reader is referred to Chapter 88 for further details on the legislative changes affecting children.

Practitioners need to recognize the relationship between values, rights, and laws. All pediatric patients deserve access to legal protections and safeguards to provide the highest quality of life achievable. The continuum of

safety, defined as institutionalization in earlier decades, to full community inclusion has been interrupted by a false freedom. Freedom from institutionalization does equal access to the educational and legal system enjoyed by children without disabilities. What was previously viewed as benevolence is now protected by legal rights. Legal protections for pediatric patients are increasing.

It is important for the practitioner to recognize that measures for the quality of life for children with disabilities are no different from the measures used for typical children. A useful benchmark is to evaluate the child's access to opportunities for education, health care, and social supports. Pediatric practitioners must be knowledgeable about the legal protections extended to their patients, which provide the framework to move from the dead ends of institutions to real ends; patients who reach adulthood with opportunities for health care, education, and subsequently, employment.

Civil Rights

Legal precedents for a patient's civil rights in the United States stem from four sources: the Constitution, legislation and resulting governmental regulation, judicial precedent, and codes of conduct of professional organizations. The Constitution provides for the equal protection of all citizens, regardless of age. These protections include the right to free speech and association; to protection against involuntary servitude; to not be deprived of property; to manage one's own affairs; to make contracts; and to exercise religious beliefs (Mental Health Legal Advisors Committee 1996). In addition, the practitioner must provide services to patients without discriminating on the basis of race, sex, medical condition, or behavioral or physical disability. Federal and state legislation results in specific regulations that govern the care and treatment of children. For example, the practitioner may be governed by state regulations for the implementation of the Individuals with Disabilities Education Act of 1990 (IDEA); Education for All Handicapped Children Act of 1975 (PL 94-142); Section 504 of the Rehabilitation Act of 1973; the Developmentally Disabled Assistance and Bill of Rights Act of 1975; or any of the various entitlements of the Social Security acts. Judicial decisions set precedents that determine rights of patients and standards for services. Courts will typically specify the extent to which a given treatment service deprives a patient of liberty and hence the due process procedures that the practitioner must follow.

A code of conduct, such as the "Principles of Medical Ethics," specifies professional standards for practice. Then, whenever a practitioner provides a professional service to a patient, the courts will find that a common law contract based on this code was established between the practitioner and patient. The professional standards are interpreted by the courts as implicit covenants in the contract, whether they were formally agreed to or understood at the time of service. Published professional reviews or the opinions of expert consultants of what constitutes standard practices (the professional community standard of care) may also be interpreted to form implicit covenants or are used to judge the appropriateness of the service.

The limits of the law tend to expand based on the precedents established in various localities and jurisdictions. A precedent that is clearly interpreted in one fashion in one state may be ignored or interpreted inconsistently in another, however. Therefore, although this chapter includes a review of general principles of law and sample precedents from various states and professional disciplines, practitioners must be careful to review the standards of practice within their own profession and the regulations of their own state prior to applying the information in this chapter to their own practice. In particular, practitioners should be careful to review any concerns about specific practices with a lawyer, rather than rely on these general guidelines.

Autonomy

The right to autonomy is a fundamental concept of constitutional law—the right of individuals to make the decisions about what happens to their mind or body, free from all restraint or interference of others. The courts have consistently maintained that for the state to encroach on this right to be left alone there must be a compelling interest that is directly related to the accomplishment of a permissible policy. The practitioner is reminded that the pediatric patient with special needs holds legal and social status as a community member. His or her individual civil rights and personal autonomy must be viewed in this context (Rowitz, 1992).

Any treatment intervention in a pediatric patient's life represents a potential deprivation of liberty sufficient to raise constitutional issues. Recent court decisions suggest that assignment of a patient to a special treatment

program or even the provision of any type of medical, educational, or psychological treatment may constitute a deprivation of liberty. For example, charging students with misconduct could give them a label that could damage their standing with fellow students and their teachers, thus depriving them of an essential element of liberty. Similarly, PL 94-142 and PL 105-17 (IDEA) specify the rights of students with disabilities in assignment to special programs. When there may be behavioral justification or need for which the treatment service is offered, the decision to provide the service must still follow due process.

The procedural safeguards in IDEA "are essential to ensure parents' rights to be informed about and stay involved in their children's education. IDEA's due process provisions have leveled the playing field by correcting the imbalance of the legal and fiscal resources available to school districts and . . . families" (Herr, 1997).

When a treatment procedure may be particularly effective in terms of a patient's cognitive or physical behavior (controlling the behavior to some extent), the courts are more likely to identify the procedure as posing a threat to the patient's right to autonomy. The more effective the control, the more restriction on the patient's autonomy. Restrictive treatment procedures and special programs that have come under the most scrutiny include segregated treatment and education programs, hospitalization, psychotropic medication, electroconvulsive therapy, surgery, deprivation, restraint, isolation, or aversive stimulation. The courts have shown a particular interest in protecting children from the involuntary administration of these restrictive procedures.

The Law and the Pediatric Patient

Respect for the legal rights of children has evolved only gradually, lagging far behind respect for the rights of adults. Table 87–1 illustrates the need for recognizing the

---

Table 87–1 • Rights for Children With Special Needs

Children with special needs such as mental retardation, autism, brain injury, and other pervasive developmental disabilities are entitled to the same civil and legal protections as all other children.
The following are based on "The Rights of People with Mental Retardation," from the Arc of the United States:
1. Children with mental retardation have the same legal, civil and human rights as all citizens. Fairness and justice dictate the need for additional legal protection to enable children and their families who exercise these basic rights.
2. The rights of children with special needs should never be limited or restricted without compelling state interests and due process.
3. Children with mental retardation who need supports, services, and protection to fully exercise their rights should have these provided to them, or to their guardians.
4. Children with mental retardation have the right, in turn, to be protected from decisions made by parents or guardians when these decisions threaten their health, life, safety or general well-being.
5. Constitutional, legislative, administrative, and judicial means should be vigorously pursued to protect the rights of children with mental retardation.

Arc of the United States, Delegate Body: The Rights of People with Mental Retardation. Arc of the United States Web Page. October 1995a. http://thearc.org/posits/posindx.html

Table 87–2 • Principles of the Least Restrictive Alternative as Applied to Involuntary Commitment by the State

1. The burden of proof is on the state to explore and exhaust all less restrictive alternatives as inadequate.
2. Full-time hospitalization is justified only when less restrictive alternatives have been proven ineffective.
3. The deprivation of liberty should not go beyond what is necessary for the patient's or others' protection.
4. Each patient must have a treatment plan that states the least restrictive treatment conditions necessary to achieve the purposes of commitment.
5. The patient must have a diagnosable mental disorder.
6. The choice of alternative must be based on the patient's assessed needs rather than availability.

rights of children with mental retardation and other special needs. Much of this comes from the child's inherent or assumed incompetence to make legal decisions. For example, the child is not considered to be the holder of privilege with regard to the rights to privacy, confidentiality, and informed consent. In other words, the parent or guardian actually holds these rights when these issues arise in the treatment of the child. The practitioner is obligated to respect the rights of the parent or guardian rather than of the child, with a few qualifications. However, the courts are likely to interpret legal precedents rather broadly, attributing the rights of adults to those of children in many cases. Furthermore, in some cases the child may be judged to be "competent" and therefore entitled to the rights of an adult. In other cases, the child may have rights that are extended beyond those of the adult. For example, children may not sue until they come of age, and, concomitantly, a statute of limitations for an offense against a minor patient will not come into effect until after his or her 18th birthday, thus extending protection to children longer than it is extended to adults.

THE LEAST RESTRICTIVE ALTERNATIVE

The selection of the most appropriate service for the pediatric patient will be the service that represents the least restrictive alternative for meeting the patient's needs. Table 87–2 contains a list of these basic principles. This doctrine may be applied to any treatment procedure or treatment setting contested by any person with a legal interest in the welfare of the patient, regardless of the issue of commitment or confinement. The concept was most notably applied to children in PL 94-142. The courts have held that each child's treatment procedures must consist of the least restrictive alternative available that would not result in deterioration. The child may not be discriminated against in this regard on any basis, including having a medical condition such as carrying hepatitis B or being infected with the human immunodeficiency virus (HIV). The practitioner may expect the courts to refer to professional standards in deciding the issue of restrictiveness.

DUE PROCESS

The right to due process is a basic protection afforded patients when their autonomy is threatened. The threat here is usually in the form of the recommendation of a more restrictive treatment procedure or setting. Table 87–3 contains a list of the due process safeguards that are usually imposed. These rights will be imposed on patients who are voluntarily admitted to treatment programs as well as on those who are involuntarily committed. Within a treatment program, each procedure may also require due process, with the more restrictive procedures, such as those involving deprivation, requiring more safeguards.

In general, the rights of adults to due process have been extended to children whenever contested. Furthermore, when such rights as human rights review or court review apply, they must be protected regardless of the consent of the guardian. In the case of the institutionalization of juvenile delinquents, the youths receive full due process rights. The purpose of juvenile detention is generally considered to be to provide rehabilitation, and therefore the patients have the right to due process review of the specific treatment procedures to be conducted within the setting.

Any proposed "special" treatment of a student, even a disciplinary procedure within a regular school placement, would require at least a notice and a hearing. Due process should be followed in prescribing psychotropic medication or a service that would be provided in a segregated setting. Practitioners cannot simply appeal to their own authority in prescribing special treatments.

Public Law 94-142 (Martin, 1979) and subsequently IDEAct, PL 105-17, further defined the rights to due process of students. In general, all school-aged children are entitled to a public education and to be placed in regular public school classrooms. This has specifically extended to children with the disabilities of traumatic brain injury and autism. In addition, states must actively publicize early intervention programs to both parents and agencies serving children with special needs (Savage, 1995). Children with disabilities can be provided with other educational placements only if the alternative is more suited to their educational needs and only after notice and a hearing to challenge the reassignment is provided. The special placements must be regularly re-evaluated with notice and a hearing. If the school fails to provide timely due process, the affected students may be entitled to compensatory education. If the

Table 87–3 • Components of Due Process

Each patient has the following rights:
1. To notice of the issue or charges
2. To a hearing
3. To counsel at the hearing
4. To be present at proceedings
5. To cross-examine witnesses
6. To call witnesses
7. To receive an independent evaluation (a "second opinion")
8. To challenge the form of treatment offered
9. To human rights review of experimental treatment services
10. To a court review of certain treatment procedures (in some instances for psychotropic medication)
11. To a record or transcript of any hearing
12. To appeal
13. To notification of the patient's specific rights with respect to the treatment service

school intends to expel a student with disabilities, the school must wait until the due administrative review process has been completed.

The courts have held that this process is owed to all children regardless of disability. For example, the practitioner may expect that the right to due process in determining the least restrictive alternative will be extended to the child who is infected with HIV. Furthermore, professional standards and current scientific evidence will be interpreted to support the right of the child with HIV infection to education in the regular classroom.

INFORMED CONSENT

Consent refers to the pediatric patient's right not to be touched or treated without his or her authorization. However, because the patient typically depends on the practitioner for all information concerning the proposed treatment, the practitioner must take great care to ensure that the patient fully understands (is *informed* of) the decision to be made and its implications. The practitioner cannot, in these cases, substitute his or her own "superior" judgment for that of the patient. Patients must give their "express" or "implied" consent. Express consent is that which is spoken or written by the patient, although the patient's written consent should always be secured. Implied consent is that which is reasonably implied by the conduct of the patient, although patients must be aware of what they are implying in a particular context.

Informed consent includes at least three elements: competence, knowledge, and voluntariness (Martin, 1975). The patient must be competent to make a well-reasoned decision, to understand the nature of the choice presented, and to *meaningfully* give consent. The routine use of a standard consent form is inadequate for this purpose, and authorization by such a form might serve as evidence that informed consent was *not* given. The patient must have knowledge of the nature of the treatment, the alternatives available, and the potential benefits and risks involved. The patient must voluntarily agree to participate in treatment. Voluntariness may not be as obvious an element, but it is crucial. For example, after a patient has been involuntarily confined, the use of a procedure that requires consent may not be allowable, given the inherent involuntariness of the patient's placement in the overall program.

As noted previously, the parent is considered to be the client in a professional treatment contract, and this principle is generally based on the child's incompetence in giving informed consent. Therefore, in general, the practitioner is expected to obtain the informed consent of the guardian for any treatment service (Melton, Koocher, and Saks, 1983). Exceptions to this proposition include emergencies in which immediate treatment is required to preserve the life of or prevent the serious impairment of the health of a child. If parents or persons standing in loco parentis cannot be located within the time available in these situations, the courts have usually held that the existence of an emergency obviates the need for informed consent. Courts have also recognized the consent of a minor for simple treatment of a nonemergent nature if the minor can demonstrate the capacity to understand and appreciate the risks and benefits of the treatment. The practitioner may

Table 87–4 • Informed Consent Disclosures

Prior to treatment, the practitioner shall fully disclose and give a fair and reasonable explanation of the following:
1. The patient's condition or problem
2. The nature and purpose of the proposed treatment
3. The risks and benefits of the proposed treatment
4. The probability that the proposed treatment will be successful
5. Possible alternatives to the proposed treatment
6. The prognosis if the proposed treatment is not given
7. The potential for professional breaches of confidentiality
8. Who is responsible for authorizing and providing the treatment service
9. The nature of any research or educational activities that might affect the patient's care or treatment

safely see a child for an initial consultation; however, in most states, practitioners forfeit their right to obtain reimbursement from parents or guardians unless the parents give informed consent for the care and treatment being provided to the child (Table 87–4).

Except for emergency situations, the pediatric patient has the right to decide his or her treatment, particularly to accept or refuse clinical interventions. In Massachusetts, a physician must obtain the patient's informed consent prior to administering any form of treatment, including medication. In spite of having been admitted to or committed to a mental health facility, for example, the pediatric patient over the age of 16 years is presumed competent, unless a court has established incompetence. Minority age, in this case, does not presume incompetence. Furthermore, in this example, written consent of the parent or guardian for treatment must be obtained by the practitioner for all interventions for patients under the age of 16. Consent is waived only in legally defined emergency situations.

PRIVACY

The right to privacy is actually a special case of the constitutional right to autonomy. Privacy refers to the right of persons to refuse to disclose and to keep information about them out of the hands of others, including other persons, agencies, and officials of government. These private facts include identifying characteristics of the individual, test scores, diagnoses of illness and disability, and medical services. This right was advanced by the Buckley Amendment of the Family Educational Rights and Privacy Act of 1974 and was extended to persons with disabilities in PL 94-142 and the Developmentally Disabled Assistance and Bill of Rights Act of 1975.

This right prevents the practitioner from subjecting a patient to a test for the presence of HIV or illicit drugs, for example, without his or her informed consent. Other forms of invasion of privacy include commercial exploitation (as in using the testimony of patients in advertising a service), opening a patient's mail (as in a residential treatment setting), examining private bank accounts, and using electronic recording devices. This right may be limited if through due process there is found to be reasonable cause to suspect that greater benefit may accrue for the invasion, as in searching a patient suspected of harboring a weapon upon return from an authorized leave of absence from an inpatient hospital unit.

The child's right to privacy has been supported in several areas. The identification of the behavior and drug use of specific public school students through a self-report questionnaire has been ruled an invasion of privacy. The invasion of privacy may consist of a public disclosure of private facts, publicly placing a child in a false light, psychological testing without adequate consent, or testing conducted by persons other than well-trained practitioners.

CONFIDENTIALITY

Whereas privacy is concerned in part with the right to guard disclosure of information, the patient's right to confidentiality is concerned with what happens to private or privileged information after it has been disclosed. By statute, confidentiality concerns the practitioner-patient privilege of information in legal proceedings. Confidentiality is also an ethical concept that is primarily based on codes of professional conduct. The difference between *confidentiality* and *privilege* is important. Privilege applies to court or administrative hearings and must be asserted by the pediatric patient or his or her guardian. Confidentiality demands that the practitioner refuse to disclose information about a patient without his or her express, written consent (Mental Health Legal Advisors Committee, 1996).

Privilege of Information

The concept of privilege of information refers to "a legal right existing by statute which protects the patient from having his or her confidences revealed publicly, without permission, during legal proceedings" (Schwitzgebel and Schwitzgebel, 1980). This right of the patient has often been assumed to be a protection for the practitioner as well. However, when a conflict of interest exists, the patient, rather than the practitioner, is the holder of privilege. Furthermore, Schwitzgebel and Schwitzgebel (1980) suggested that "in actual practice so many exceptions to the physician-patient privilege have been found necessary, in order to prevent fraud or to promote the public interest, that the privilege is meaningless. Psychotherapists [however] are protected because, presumably, the matters dealt with are less understandable or more socially sensitive."

Confidentiality as an Ethical Practice

The concept of confidentiality is also an ethical practice that is addressed in the codes of conduct of various professional organizations. These codes are intended to safeguard the patient's confidentiality and to provide sanctions for professional misconduct. As defined by Section 9 of the Principles of Medical Ethics, a physician "may not reveal the confidences entrusted to him [or her] in the course of medical attendance, or the deficiencies he [or she] may observe in the character of patients unless it becomes necessary to protect the welfare of the individual or of the community." Breaches of confidentiality may be disclosed verbally, through film or other recordings, and through written material. For example, a therapist was found liable for publishing a book about a patient that included informa-

tion sufficient to reveal the patient's identity to a number of readers. Computer-generated patient records are also vulnerable to disclosure. The practitioner is responsible for the use of passwords, codes, and other information management protocols to prevent the unauthorized disclosure of patient information.

Although the parent or guardian has generally been considered to be the holder of privilege, the practitioner may safely respect the confidentiality of the child except in cases of potential harm to any person. However, the best professional-patient relationship is usually maintained when the practitioner clearly communicates to both the parent and the child the fact that parents are entitled to have full access to the child's communications. The practitioner should be careful to offer specific examples of the duty to protect being in conflict with the right to confidentiality. The practitioner may also warn the child to withhold any information that the child does not want disclosed (the child's putative right to privacy). In divorce cases, both parents generally retain the right to review the child's records, regardless of custody, unless a specific court order prevents a parent from seeing the record.

The "Tarasoff Warning"

The patient's right to confidentiality may be abridged when there would be greater benefit than injury resulting from such disclosure. In general, the practitioner's duty to protect any person, whether patient or not, is greater than any duty to protect confidentiality. In *Tarasoff v. Regents of the University of California* (1974), the California state supreme court held that "once a therapist does in fact determine, or under applicable professional standards reasonably should have determined, that a patient poses a serious danger of violence to others, she or he bears a duty to exercise reasonable care to protect the foreseeable victims of that danger . . . to warn the intended victim or those who reasonably could be expected to notify the person of the peril. The protective privilege ends where the public peril begins."

In these cases, when a warning appears to most reasonably fulfill the duty to protect, the accepted standard of practice is to obtain informed consent from the patient, obtain professional consultation to ground the action in the community standard of care, and then inform both the threatened party and the authorities by telephone and in writing. The medical record should contain documentation of all activities. Note, however, that the obligation is to *protect* rather that to *warn* the intended victim. Roswell (1988) suggested alternatives to warning the third party. These include making frequent telephone contact with the patient, providing medication to the patient, bringing the third party into therapy, and committing the patient. The practitioner must carefully weigh the disincentives of the managed care environment with the risk of failing to extend additional treatment options to patients at risk. These alternatives may more reasonably fulfill the practitioner's duty to protect the intended victim, given the lack of proven ability of practitioners to predict actual violence. Furthermore, the practitioner may not be able to effectively warn the intended victims.

Other Limits of Confidentiality

Direct information about certain crimes is not protected. All persons who ordinarily come into contact with children in their professional capacity are mandatory reporters of child abuse and neglect (Child Abuse Prevention and Treatment Act of 1974). In general, when they obtain direct evidence or the direct report from a witness of such behavior as defined by state statute, they shall make an immediate oral and written report to the state children's protective service, usually within 48 hours. Civil immunity is typically provided for practitioners from lawsuits by patients alleging harm. Table 87–5 lists a variety of cases in which the right to confidentiality was not upheld.

Medical Records

The issue of confidentiality of medical records is complicated by the increasing emphasis now being placed on the ready accessibility of fiscal and treatment-related information. Whatever the source of a request for records (including insurance companies, subsequent treatment providers, or law enforcement agencies) the patient's rights are violated when the information is disclosed unless the patient grants consent for the release of the information. Typically, if a patient challenges the release of information at a later date, the court will require that the practitioner have the patient's written permission for the release of specified information to the specified receiver for the specified purpose and that the permission has been granted prior to the release (Table 87–6).

The practitioner does not have the right to release written information that was obtained from another source, even with the permission of the patient. This often abused practice deserves special vigilance on the part of the pediatric practitioner, when convenience may outweigh prudence. The patient or his or her guardian must grant that permission only to the original source of the record. Also, the courts have routinely enjoined the secondary collection of records of sensitive information.

Another issue concerns patients' ability to gain ac-

Table 87–5 • Limitations on the Right of Confidentiality

Confidential information may be disclosed when
1. The practitioner determines that the patient poses serious danger of violence to self or others
2. The practitioner reasonably suspects a situation of child abuse or neglect
3. The practitioner reasonably suspects an instance of abuse or neglect of an incompetent person
4. There is a legal dispute between the practitioner and patient
5. The practitioner's services are solicited for illegal activity
6. The patient is involved in workers' compensation litigation
7. The patient is prosecuted for homicide
8. The patient is involved in a legal contest over the validity of a document such as a will
9. The court orders or permits the loss of privilege
10. The patient's mental condition is used as part of a claim or defense in a child-custody case
11. The patient is informed that the communications will not be privileged for the purpose of a court-ordered examination
12. The patient introduces his or her mental condition as an element of his or her claim or defense in a civil proceeding

Table 87–6 • Information to Be Included in Medical Records

The medical record should contain the following:
1. An intake evaluation that contains the rationale for a diagnosis
2. A treatment plan or contract, signed by both the patient and the practitioner if possible
3. The rationale for the intervention and for disregarding more traditional approaches if the treatment was especially innovative or experimental
4. The patient's informed consent, especially regarding risks and potential pain
5. Reassessments and recommendations made with the patient's active participation at regular intervals
6. Any lack of treatment compliance on the part of the patient
7. The patient's statements of dissatisfaction with progress and remedies offered, such as referrals to outside consultation
8. Any releases for transmitting confidential information
9. A record of all services provided
10. A summary of treatment, including the final diagnosis, recommendations for future services, and referral activity

cess to their own medical records. The Freedom of Information Act provides that anyone has the right of access to (and to receive copies of) any record, document, or file in the possession of the federal government. The Buckley Amendment gives students 18 or older and their parents the right to inspect relevant school records. In addition, the student or parent may enter his or her own comments into the written record. However, in the amendment, those records "created or maintained by a physician, psychiatrist, psychologist, or other recognized professional or paraprofessional acting in his or her professional or paraprofessional capacity or assisting in that capacity, [and those records] created, maintained or used only in connection with the provision of treatment to the student [are not to be] disclosed to anyone other than individuals providing the treatment." In addition, state and private organizations may not be required to disclose medical information from a patient's medical record.

The courts have decided that hospital records are typically hospital property but that parties with a legitimate interest could inspect the record, provided it resulted in no danger or harm to the patient. Some professional codes of conduct specify and many professionals would hold that patients should have access to records concerning themselves. Alternatively, the courts have also ruled that the constitutional protection of privacy does not give patients any interest in viewing their own medical records.

In the eventuality of a malpractice suit, however, the practitioner may expect records to be subpoenaed and thus must take care to routinely enter written records of all decisions and practices, the absence of which could result in a negative judgment. It is important that the practitioner realize that activity that is not documented is considered to have not occurred. The practitioner should not enter extraneous information that might be interpreted negatively, however. If the information is not necessary to document a significant professional activity, then there is more risk in its inclusion in the chart. Information that might be defamatory or libelous would not be a concern here, since the record is confidential. To prevent patients' access to specific items in the record under the provision of protecting them from danger or harm, the practitioner is often required to identify such items at the time of entry into the record.

APPROPRIATE TREATMENT

When a patient enters into a professional relationship with a practitioner, the practitioner is obligated to provide an acceptable standard of appropriate treatment. The acceptability of the treatment may be judged in court according to the community standard of care. To meet the community standard, the practitioner must understand and conform to the tenets of the school of treatment that the practitioner professed to follow, the reasonableness of the treatment (as might be decided by a judge or jury or both), the research base for the treatment, the judgments of an ethics committee, the state regulatory and professional organization standards, the professional protocols of the hospital or agency in which the treatment was delivered, and the legal precedent for that treatment (Roswell, 1988). Although these determinations may be made in court, the court often defers to the judgment of a qualified practitioner to determine the reasonableness of the treatment plan. Table 87–7 presents a list of basic legal standards of practice in providing any treatment service.

The temporary intervention with a restrictive program may be used to accomplish goals to which the patient has agreed. Even when the program may be claimed to ultimately free the patient of a debilitating behavior pattern, however, the program must also be warranted according to accepted standards of professional practice and the opinion of the lay public. In particular, the treatment plan must specifically address the remediation of the behaviors that are being used to justify the program. The courts have termed this concept the *right to minimally adequate habilitation*.

Documentation is an essential feature of appropriate treatment. This issue is not a simple issue of proof of provision of services. The courts may interpret a lack of adequate records as *resulting in* inadequate care. Table 87–6 lists the activities that should be documented in the

medical record to demonstrate that the practitioner has provided appropriate treatment.

If the practitioner cannot provide treatment or refuses to provide treatment, due, for example, to the patient's inability to pay, the practitioner's lack of qualifications to treat the particular problem, or the practitioner's bias, the practitioner ethically must refer the patient to an alternative provider. Again, the role of managed care and ready access to alternative treatments by other professionals must be confronted. Under most professional standards, the practitioner has an ethical duty to promote the welfare of all persons, but that duty may be better discharged by making a referral than by providing inadequate treatment because of a bias or lack of experience (American Medical Association, 1987).

When making a referral, the practitioner must be able to document that an appropriate, realistic referral was made, that the alternative provider was contacted by the practitioner, and that the practitioner made a personal and written attempt to contact the patient if the patient broke off treatment prematurely. A referral to more than one alternative practitioner will help to ensure that an appropriate referral was made. If the patient is potentially dangerous, then a special attempt must be made to ensure that an appropriate practitioner contacted the patient in person. It is helpful to follow up on the patient's informed decision to prematurely terminate treatment by sending a written summary of the current status of treatment, any recommendations, and an appropriate referral to the patient.

Minimal standards for the types of educational services to be provided to children with disabilities are articulated in PL 94-142 and PL 105-17. IDEA specifically extends traditional "special education" to other settings and services, which may include rehabilitation counseling, social work services, or therapeutic recreation (Savage, 1995). The courts have found that an educational program must offer a reasonable likelihood that a child will benefit from it. The courts have interpreted state statutes to mean that each child has a right to those educational services that will produce the maximum feasible benefit for the student. In this regard, Kauffman (1981) provides an excellent discussion of the issue of whether all children are educable. When the school has discriminated against a student on the basis of his or her disability, in not providing an appropriate education, the student may be entitled to compensatory education. The courts have also held that the state must provide direct services to a student with a disability when the school district fails to do so.

Segregated Treatment

A number of court cases have found that patients have a right to individualized programs of treatment based on their special needs. This right is most strongly interpreted when the patient has been involuntarily committed to a restrictive treatment program (Simon, 1987). In *Wyatt v. Stickney* (1972), it was held that involuntarily committed patients "unquestionably have a constitutional right to receive such individual treatment as well as give each of them a realistic opportunity to be cured or to improve his or her mental condition." The courts have also held that the patient has a right to treatment or release and that when the justifica-

---

Table 87–7 • Basic Legal Standards
for Appropriate Treatment

The practitioner should be able to demonstrate the following:
1. That the patient has entered into and maintained a contractual treatment plan with the practitioner
2. That the plan objectively identifies the diagnosis of the presenting problem
3. That the diagnosis meets the accepted standards of professional decision making
4. That the plan identifies the objective goals of treatment
5. That the plan identifies the proposed method of treatment
6. That the plan identifies the anticipated course of treatment
7. That any restrictive treatment plan is individualized to meet the patient's unique needs
8. That any restrictive treatment plan specifies a projected timeline for meeting specific, measurable goals
9. That any restrictive treatment plan specifies criteria for movement to less restrictive conditions and discharge
10. That adequate provisions for 24-hour, year-round responses to emergencies are made

tion for confinement is treatment, it violates due process if the treatment is not provided. Similarly, if the justification for confinement is that the patient is dangerous to himself or herself or to others, treatment is the quid pro quo that society must pay as the price of the extra safety it derives from the denial of a person's liberty. Once a patient is committed, the practitioner has the equally weighty responsibility to demonstrate that the released patient is not a danger to himself or herself or to others according to statutory standards.

The courts have held for a variety of standards for segregated treatment. These have included rights to reasonably safe conditions of confinement, freedom from unreasonable bodily restraints, such as minimally adequate training as reasonably may be required, and a humane physical and psychological environment. The courts have held that they could determine whether care was adequate and formulate workable standards for institutional treatment. The courts have also found that basic rights may not be used as earned privileges in purported rehabilitation programs and that work must be part of an individualized treatment plan to meet the patient's needs and that compensation must be provided for that work.

The courts have held that the purpose of juvenile detention was to provide rehabilitation and therefore the patients had the same rights to treatment as have been discussed previously. The courts have found that the simple provision of a structured program (including level and point systems) does not constitute an individualized professional treatment program. They have also suggested that the provision of adequately trained and supervised staff is necessary to avoid subjecting the patients to cruel and unusual punishment. Table 87–8 summarizes some of the requirements that have been needed in advocacy for patients in segregated treatment programs.

Psychotropic Medication

Various states are initiating strict standards for the administration of psychotropic medications. Court rulings have suggested that the administration of a drug without the patient's consent might be considered cruel and unusual

Table 87–8 • Restrictions on Segregated Treatment Services

Clients have a right to the following:
1. Keep and use personal possessions
2. A comfortable bed
3. Personal privacy
4. Access to television and recreational facilities
5. Adequate meals
6. Be free of therapy for the sole purpose of institutional convenience
7. A limit on therapeutic isolation of 1 hour per application
8. Qualified and adequate staff
9. Send and receive sealed mail from anyone
10. Have interactions with persons of the opposite sex
11. Voluntarily participate in institutional maintenance work for the minimum wage
12. Access to medical facilities and nursing services
13. Exercise and to be outdoors on a regular basis
14. Free exercise of religion

punishment or unpermissible tinkering with the mental processes. The courts have ruled that no medication may be administered without a written order of a physician. In addition, the use of medication must be consistent with the patient's program of treatment, may not be administered in excessive quantities, and may not be used as a punishment procedure or as a substitute for other treatment.

Court decisions regarding psychotropic medication have been determined largely on the basis of whether the treatment in question is a recognized medical practice, that is, whether it is experimental, the extent to which it interferes with the patient's thought processes, and whether it is therapeutic or is being used primarily to control the patient's behavior. Pediatric patients with developmental disabilities may require special attention to the impact of psychotropic medication and the stage of their neurologic development. The decisions also depend on the patients' assessed needs and their competency to give informed consent (American Bar Association, 1980). Significant liability has been found for negligent prescription of psychotropic medication. Increased scrutiny is also being given to the issue of monitoring for tardive dyskinesia and other side effects.

Evaluation for Educational and Treatment Services

Assessment and diagnostic evaluation may result in significant consequences for the patient, such as civil commitment, segregation, or eligibility for services. Historically, evaluations have come under scrutiny for discriminating against various groups (eg, when black children were both identified in greater proportions for special education and put on unreasonable waiting lists for services). Indeed, the issue of eligibility for state-funded services continues to be carefully scrutinized.

In most states an evaluation of eligibility for services begins with a determination of a diagnosis and then an assessment of appropriate services. When the child may be entitled to special educational services, the diagnosis must conform to the state's interpretation of the diagnostic categories in PL 94-142 and IDEA. The criteria for eligibility vary widely among states. Guidelines for the appropriate selection and administration of a standardized test are specified in various professional codes (Joint Committee on Testing Practices, 1989). In general, for an assessment to be valid, the test must have been standardized for the population being evaluated, the testing conditions must conform with the recommendations of the manual, and the practitioner who selects and administers the test and interprets the results must have been trained in the use of the test in question.

Evaluation for the Courts

The practitioner may also provide the service of evaluating a patient for the purpose of a legal proceeding. These proceedings may involve civil commitment, juvenile delinquency, custody, or child maltreatment. An essential challenge to the practitioner is to remain within the bounds of competence when receiving the varied requests for assistance from the parties involved.

The results of the evaluation, when presented in court, may not include opinion or inference; rather they must be facts that are based on accepted professional research, standards of practice, or skilled knowledge of the subject matter. The courts then make the legal judgment based on the facts that are presented by the expert witness. Melton and Limber (1989) emphasized that "when a clinician enters the courtroom, he or she should don a scientist's hat. Presentation of greater certainty than is scientifically warranted does not assist the fact finder. Rather it misleads the fact finder and, in doing so, undermines the pursuit of justice and the exercise of legitimate legal authority."

When the practitioner is providing testimony on the most appropriate form of treatment for a patient, the legal issues are less problematic. Here, the practitioner can testify to the extent to which the patient's presenting problems suggest a given treatment modality, given a body of standard practices. Suggesting an innovative treatment procedure requires more extensive rationale, but also is within the practitioner's purview. The practitioner needs to refrain from predicting efficacy, however, since outcome studies are routinely lacking in clear support for any treatment to date. In the area of civil commitment of a child, the Supreme Court has determined that professionals, rather than the courts, are most qualified to assess the child's needs. The court, however, will hear the factual results of the practitioner's assessment and make the actual judgment on commitment.

In the area of juvenile delinquency, the practitioner is most likely to be involved in the determination of whether the child should be tried as a juvenile or as an adult. This is a very serious issue given the marked discrepancy between the potential legal outcomes of the two alternatives. The practitioner may competently provide factual evidence on the mental and physical condition of the child and the child's amenability to rehabilitative treatment. However, the court will also take into account evidence from other sources on the child's age, record, and history, the nature of the offense, and the safety of the public (Whitebread and Heilman, 1988).

In the area of child maltreatment, the practitioner may be expected to provide a psychological evaluation of the patient to help determine whether the patient was the perpetrator or the victim of abuse. Unfortunately, the scientific basis for a practitioner's determination is usually lacking in these proceedings. For example, the relatively straightforward practice of comparing a patient's characteristics to those of a known group of perpetrators or victims and then inferring the likelihood of an episode of abuse is inappropriate, given the leaps of reasoning involved, and is considered unduly prejudicial according to legal standards.

In the area of child custody evaluations, the practitioner may competently present the factual results of an evaluation of the interaction and interrelationship of the child with the parents and others, the child's adjustment to home and community, and the mental and physical health of all parties. The court uses these facts in combination with its knowledge of the wishes of the child and parents and of the demonstration of physical violence of the potential custodians to determine the best interest of the child. The court may not use its knowledge of any conduct by a potential custodian that does not affect the child (Uniform Marriage and Divorce Act of 1971).

PROTECTION AGAINST HARM

Practitioners have a duty to protect the patients in their care from harm. The courts have extended the definition of injury resulting from treatment to a variety of outcomes. A list of common injuries is provided in Table 87–9. Most injuries to patients are not regulated by statute; rather, they are violations of ethical standards of professional organizations.

Suicide

The practitioner should take steps to assess all patients for suicide risk and to document that the assessment was made according to professional standards for predicting such risk. The practitioner is not obligated to inform relatives of the suicide risk, since such action would likely be considered a breach of confidentiality. However, the practitioner should attempt to obtain the patient's informed consent to involve significant others or potential social supports in the management of the risk. In addition, the practitioner should ensure that the patient can always contact the practitioner or a referral source for professional help, establish a more consistent or frequent schedule of visits, engage the patient in a treatment contract in which the patient agrees not to commit suicide, and document all contacts and attempts to contact the patient. If the practitioner's service is part of a restrictive treatment program, the practitioner should provide a safe environment, routinely brief all staff of the risk, and monitor their activities. Finally, if the patient breaks off contact unexpectedly, the practitioner should make persistent, documented attempts to appropriately resolve treatment.

Severely Restrictive Treatment Procedures

Any treatment intervention that exposes the patient in a restrictive service setting to harm or danger may be found

Table 87–9 • Injuries Claimed by Patients

1. Exacerbation of the patient's presenting problem
2. Appearance of new problems
3. Client misuse or abuse of therapy such as accepting a dependent relationship
4. Clients overextending themselves by taking on tasks before they can adequately achieve them, possibly to please the therapist or due to inappropriate directives, leading to failure, guilt, or self-contempt
5. Disillusionment with therapy, leading to feelings of hopelessness in relationships
6. Iatrogenic injuries, including damages due to reliance on a therapist's directives, leading to divorce, job loss, economic loss, emotional harm, injury to reputation, loss of companionship, incarceration, suicide or death of a third party, self- or non-self-inflicted injuries, deprivation of constitutional rights, and/or loss of liberty or privacy
7. Damages due to unethical acts by the practitioner such as sexual contact with a patient or engaging in any dual relationship such as bartering services, employing the patient, or engaging in a social activity with the patient

Adapted from Roswell VA: Professional liability: issues for behavior therapists in the 1980s and 1990s. Behav Ther 11:163, 1988.

to be in violation of the constitutional prohibition against cruel and unusual punishment. According to Schwitzgebel and Schwitzgebel (1980), "a procedure may constitute cruel and unusual punishment if it violates minimal standards of decency, is wholly disproportionate to the alleged offense, or goes beyond what is necessary." In determining what procedures may meet these tests, the courts may hear the testimony of various professional organizations that have issued statements on the use of restrictive procedures.

Severely restrictive treatment procedures such as physical restraint and isolation, which are often employed in restrictive service settings, must conform with strict regulatory guidelines for implementation. Table 87–9 reviews the basic rights for all patients in segregated treatment. Basic safeguards would include "clear written policies, periodic monitoring and review; staff training on appropriate implementation . . . ; periodic external review; and patient consent" (Czyzewski, Sheldon, and Hannah, 1986). Other severely restrictive treatment procedures, such as deprivation, electric shock, psychosurgery, and related aversive procedures, are rarely, if ever, allowable. Relative to the preceding section reviewing the patient's right to autonomy, aversive procedures are strictly regulated. There is inadequate knowledge of the impact of aversive procedures. Therefore, the practitioner should consider the potential harm to the child, access positive interventions instead, and preclude the use of aversive procedures on purely moral grounds.

Physical Restraint

In general, physical restraint by manually holding the patient may be used only when there is an immediate threat of injury to the patient or others or of damage to the environment. It may not be used as a form of punishment or behavior control, for the purpose of staff convenience, or as a substitute for an appropriate treatment program. The courts have stipulated that the mechanically restrained patient be given bathroom privileges every hour and be bathed every 12 hours. The Joint Commission on Accreditation of Healthcare Organizations set a 30-minute limit on the application of restraint.

Staff must also ensure that the patient is not threatened by injury due to unexpected events such as a fire. In addition, the patient must be taught appropriate behaviors as alternatives to those that result in restraint. In *Youngberg v. Romeo* (1982), an individual resident of Pennhurst was held by the courts to have a constitutional right to training and to live in safety and free from undue restraints. In this case the court also recognized that the judgments of a mental retardation professional are due judicial respect if they follow professional standards (Herr, 1997). The courts have also held that the decisions made by the appropriate professionals in the use of such treatment procedures are entitled to a presumption of validity, thus protecting them from civil liability in the absence of negligence.

Isolation

Isolation may include the long-term or brief "time out" seclusion of a patient in a closed room. Long-term isolation of patients has been ruled to be cruel and unusual punish-

ment. The courts have established the right of patients to be free from isolation and specified 1 hour as the time limit for therapeutically justified isolation. It has also been held that the patient in isolation must be checked every 30 minutes or even continuously. The court will usually find that isolation of a child may be psychologically harmful, and at least is an unwarranted interruption in his or her educational programming. For example, courts have held that juveniles could not be placed in isolation for treatment purposes for a period exceeding 1 hour, but that lesser periods do not require due process protection. This isolation cannot serve as a substitute for individualized professional treatment.

The clinical procedure termed *time out from positive reinforcement* will also be considered to consist of isolation whenever the patient is removed to a room or area that obstructs the patient's view of his or her peers. In this case, a room with a closed door with a viewing device may be employed, but the door may not be locked or mechanically barred and a staff person must be in close proximity to continuously view the child. The room must be no smaller than 2 meters square, well lit, carpeted, well ventilated, clean, and empty of all dangerous items. The procedure should last for no longer than 1 hour per application, and typical practice is to require the patient to become calm in the room for up to, but no longer than, 5 minutes in order to terminate each application of the procedure.

Discipline

Cruel and unusual punishment as defined in case law has included deprivation of basic amenities (bed, clothing) as a disciplinary action; the forceful injection of a drug into a juvenile as a disciplinary procedure; and the performance of degrading, unnecessary acts (the use of make-work for children in which nothing is accomplished by the work, e.g., moving rocks from one place to another) as a disciplinary procedure. Furthermore, disciplining a student with disabilities for behavior that is considered part of the disabling condition has been considered discriminatory.

The courts, however, have found that various techniques are appropriate to discipline serious misconduct by students with disabilities. These acceptable techniques include the use of study carrels, time out, detention, restriction of privileges, and suspensions of up to 10 school days. The schools must prove the likelihood of injury to extend suspensions beyond 10 days. The courts have consistently found, however, that expulsion of students for behavior that is a manifestation of their disability is considered a change in placement and, in fact, discrimination in the provision of education against the students on the basis of their disability (Bartlett, 1989).

Corporal Punishment

Corporal punishment is societally unacceptable in any service setting, and state regulations and professional standards are being promulgated to this effect. This may be due to the increased attention given to the issue of child abuse in the 1980s. In any event, the use of corporal punishment with a child who is a patient would be certain to be proscribed. The courts have ruled that corporal punishment, as well as any actions generally described as causing physical pain or discomfort, is unacceptable. Spanking as a disciplinary procedure is not considered a violation of the Constitution but may be proscribed by local civil and criminal laws.

Supervision of Children

When a child is placed under a professional's care, no matter for how long or for what purpose, the professional then has physical custody of the child and is expected to take reasonable steps to protect the child from injury (Sheldon, 1983). The practitioner must provide a certain level of supervision in concordance with the dangerousness of the activity, the likelihood of injury occurring under greater supervision, whether the possibility of an injury is foreseeable without the presence of a supervisor, and whether the child is known to engage in dangerous behavior, even despite the supervisor's instructions. When there is the adequate presence of a supervisor, the supervisor should be reasonably active in interrupting dangerous acts. The practitioner is also expected to be aware of potential dangers in the practitioner's facility and to take effective steps to correct them. If an activity, such as a trip, may include inherent dangers, the requirement of having parents sign a waiver of liability will not protect the practitioner from liability for negligent supervision.

The more disrupted the family situation, the more likely that the practitioner will face unexpected challenges in providing care for the child. A common issue is parents' failing to pick up their child at appointed times. In this case, the practitioner is expected to provide for the care of the child until an appropriate authority discharges them. An appropriate alternative to the parents in these cases is a legally identified police officer or child protection worker. If the practitioner's facility closes for the day, the child is most safe if the practitioner ensures that staff members who have the normally delegated responsibilities of supervising such a child remain in the given setting with the child. The practitioner is then continuing to provide the customary service within applicable regulations.

A second issue is releasing the child to the care of unauthorized persons. At intake, the practitioner should obtain a written list of those persons authorized to pick up the child and to obtain prior written permission to release a child to other persons. Both parents are always assumed to have this permission. If a parent claims that one parent's rights are restricted, the parent making the claim must produce a court order outlining those very restrictions. When an unauthorized person does attempt to remove a child, the practitioner must take all reasonable steps (including safely hiding the child) to prevent this and to call authorities if unsuccessful.

ACCESS TO JUSTICE

The criminal justice system overlooks the impact of having a disability. The pediatric practitioner may be called to evaluate a child or adolescent involved within the system. Due to lack of training or awareness, many justice professionals fail to have a basic understanding of the impact of mental retardation and related disabilities. Few organized

Table 87–10 • Limitation of Rights in the Criminal Justice System

Persons with mental retardation may have cognitive impairments that may limit their ability to fully exercise their rights in the criminal justice system. These include:
1. Failure to be identified as an individual with mental retardation by attempting to hide their mental retardation.
2. Disclosing incriminating information or confessions due to confusion or a desire to please.
3. Incompetence to stand trial due to failure to understand the criminal justice system and procedures.
4. Inability to actively assist in their own defense.
5. Unknowingly waiving rights such as the Miranda warning.

Arc of the United States, Delegate Body: The Rights of People with Mental Retardation. Arc of the United States Web Page. October 1995b. http://thearc.org/posits/posindx.html

resources are available to the child or adolescent with special needs in the criminal justice system. The Arc has adopted a position statement regarding the relationship between the individual with mental retardation and the criminal justice system (Arc, 1995a, 1995b). Table 87–10 illustrates the most frequently cited limitations facing the individual with mental retardation involved in the criminal justice system.

Conclusion

At all levels of our judicial system, litigation on behalf of patients is increasing. The challenge facing the health care practitioner is to provide a high quality of service based on the patient's individual needs, but to do so only within the limits of the patient's rights under the law. This requires the practitioner to understand the law and its implications for health care as well as the various procedures that can be employed to protect the patient's rights. The challenge for the pediatric practitioner is even more demanding, since the rights of pediatric patients are only just emerging and vary greatly from state to state. Continuing education in the areas of patient's rights and children's rights is therefore essential for the present-day pediatric practitioner.

Medical and psychological techniques have the potential to produce dramatic and irreversible changes in a person, and the patient must be protected against their misuse. This is particularly true for the pediatric patient who is not always capable of understanding the risks and benefits of a health care procedure and of reaching an informed decision to cooperate. This incompetence does not confer the authority to make treatment decisions to the practitioner; rather it requires the practitioner to make efforts to ensure that the patient's rights are protected and that the practitioner can demonstrate that the rights were protected. The practitioner must make every effort to include pediatric patients with special needs in decision-making. This not only supports their rights but also reinforces their inclusion in the community. The practitioner must ultimately be guided by the purpose of treatment.

REFERENCES

American Bar Association, Commission on the Mentally Disabled: Summary and analysis. Ment Dis Law Reporter 4:299, 1980.

American Medical Association: Ethical issues involved in the growing AIDS crisis. JAMA 259:1360, 1987.

Arc of the United States, Delegate Body: Access to justice and fair treatment under the criminal law for people with mental retardation. Arc of the United States Web Page. October 1995a.

Arc of the United States, Delegate Body: The rights of people with mental retardation. Arc of the United States Web Page. October 1995b. http://thearc.org/posits/posindx.html

Bartlett L: Disciplining handicapped students: legal issues in light of Honig v. Doe. Except Child 55:357, 1989.

Czyzewski MJ, Sheldon J, Hannah GT: Legal safety in residential treatment environments. *In* Fuoco FJ, Christian WP (eds): Behavior Analysis and Therapy in Residential Programs. New York, Van Nostrand Reinhold, 1986.

Herr S: Reauthorization of the Individuals With Disabilities Education Act. Mental Retardation 35:2, 1997.

Joint Committee on Testing Practices: Code of fair testing practices in education. Am Psychol 44:1065, 1989.

Kauffman JM (ed): Are all children educable? [special issue]. Ann Int Dev Disabil 1:1, 1981.

Martin R: Legal Challenges to Behavior Modification: Trends in Schools, Corrections, and Mental Health. Champaign, IL, Research Press, 1975.

Martin R: Educating Handicapped Children: The Legal Mandate. Champaign, IL, Research Press, 1979.

Melton GB, Koocher GP, Saks MJ: Children's Competence to Consent. New York, Plenum, 1983.

Melton GB, Limber S: Psychologists' involvement in cases of child maltreatment. Am Psychol 44:1225, 1989.

Mental Health Legal Advisors Committee: The Handbook on the Legal Rights of Minors. Boston, Author, 1996.

Roswell VA: Professional liability: issues for behavior therapists in the 1980s and 1990s. Behav Ther 11:163, 1988.

Rowitz L (ed): Mental Retardation in the Year 2000. New York, Springer-Verlag, 1992.

Savage C: Public Law 101-476. (Fact Sheet). The May Center for Behavioral Pediatrics, Norwood, Massachusetts, 1995.

Schwitzgebel RL, Schwitzgebel RK: Law and Psychological Practice. New York, John Wiley & Sons, 1980.

Sheldon JB: Protecting the preschooler and the practitioner: legal issues in early childhood programs. *In* Goetz EM, Allen KE (eds): Early Childhood Education: Special Environmental, Policy, and Legal Considerations. Rockville, MD, Aspen Systems Corporation, 1983.

Simon RI: Clinical Psychiatry and the Law. Washington, DC, American Psychiatric Association Press, 1987. *Tarasoff v. Regents of the University of California*, 17 Cal. 3d 425, 131 Cal. Rptr. 14, 551 P. 2d 334, 83 ALR 3d 1166 (1976).

Whitebread C, Heilman J: An overview of the law of juvenile delinquency. Behav Sci Law 6:285, 1988.

Wyatt v. Stickney, 325 F. Supp. 781, 784, aff'd on rehearing 344 F. Supp. 341 (M.D. Ala. 1971), aff'd on rehearing 344 f. Supp. 373, aff'd in separate decision, 344 F. Supp. 387, 390, 392, 394-407 (M.D. Ala. 1972), aff'd sub nom. *Wyatt v. Aderholt*, 503 F. 2d 1305 (5th Cir. 1974).

Youngberg v. Romeo, 457 U.S. 307 (1982).

88 Legislation for the Education of Children With Disabilities

Judith S. Palfrey • John S. Rodman

The existence of strong legislative underpinnings for special education attests to the power of collaboration between family and professional.

Some chapters of the Individuals with Disabilities Education Act (IDEA) saga delineate successes for children with severe physical disabilities and sensory impairments. Others document tragedies of promises half fulfilled for high school–aged youngsters from minority backgrounds who have learning disabilities. Monitoring, vigilance, and advocacy are warranted to ensure that high-quality services are furnished at every level and that providers have adequate training and support to carry out their assignments.

Family–Professional Partnership

The story of special education legislation is now a quarter-century saga of an evolving relationship between families and professionals. Drawn together by common goals to improve the life chances of children with disabilities, parents and child health care providers have learned that there is increased leverage when the two groups work in concert.

This combined constituency has achieved a number of remarkable legislative victories that have resulted in substantial legal protections and programmatic advances for children with disabilities. No legislation is free from attack and no program is immune from the vagaries of inadequate funding and inept implementation. Nonetheless, the existence of strong legislative underpinnings for special education attests to the power of family–professional collaboration.

In the United States, education is a right, an entitlement. This fact makes the schools fundamentally different from most other institutions. Recognizing that every child has a right to education, advocates, including parents and pediatricians, have pushed for legislative assurance that all children with disabilities will have access to proper school programs. In the late 1960s and early 1970s, parent groups, child-helping professionals, and lawyers joined together in an effective lobby to establish legal precedents clarifying the rights of all children with disabilities. Two landmark cases, *Pennsylvania Association for Retarded Citizens v. Commonwealth of Pennsylvania* and *Mills v. The Board of Education of the District of Columbia,* provided that bulwark. Through these two court cases, the right to a free appropriate public education for children with developmental disabilities was upheld.

Advocacy moved rapidly in the 1970s into policy formation and legislative initiatives. The time was right and the mood of state legislators and the US Congress was receptive to the advocates' message. As a result, one of the most extensive programs affecting children in the United States, namely, the Education for All Handicapped Children Act (PL 94-142), was passed by large majorities in Congress in 1975.

Over the ensuing 20 years, the initial legislation has been added to, modified, and refined based on experience at the state and local levels (Horne, 1991). Currently, the legislation is entitled the Individuals with Disabilities Education Act (IDEA).

Individuals with Disabilities Education Act (PL 105-17)

In 1991, two federal initiatives, PL 99-457, the early intervention legislation, and PL 94-142, the Education for All Handicapped Children Act, were combined into the Individuals with Disabilities Education Act (PL 101-476). This comprehensive act covers children with disabilities from birth to 21 years of age (Table 88–1). IDEA was recently reauthorized as PL 105-17.

EARLY INTERVENTION

Families and professionals have argued persuasively for the value of early intervention services for children with a

Table 88–1 • Individuals with Disabilities Education Act: Key Components

Early Intervention (birth to 3 years)
  Identification of children with disabilities or at risk
  Evaluation
  Individualized Family Service Plan (IFSP)
Special Education (3 to 21 years)
  Identification
  Individualized Education Plan (IEP)
  Least restrictive environment
  Related services
  Parental due process
  Transition services

wide range of physical and developmental disabilities. Early intervention encompasses identification at the time of diagnosis, direct services for the disabling condition, and preventive services to avoid secondary disability. The services should be provided in the community and, whenever possible, at home. Parents should be involved at every level of the planning, including their participation in the the Individualized Family Service Plan (IFSP).

Eligibility for IDEA services is met by children from birth to 3 years of age with developmental delays or diagnosed with a physical or medical condition (e.g., cerebral palsy, Down syndrome), or those who are at risk of having substantial developmental delays if early intervention services are not provided (e.g., low birth weight, mother addicted to cocaine). This particular criterion is at the discretion of each state (IDEA, 1990, Vol. 20 USC§1472[1]).

The *services* covered under early intervention include family training, counseling and home visits, special instruction, speech therapy and audiology, occupational therapy, physical therapy, case management, diagnostic medical services, health services, social work, vision services, assistive technology, transportation, and psychological services (IDEA, 1990, Vol. 20 USC§1472[2]). States vary in whether these are discretionary or mandated services.

The *process* for obtaining early intervention services for a child requires referral to the appropriate state agency. This may be public health, education, the state's department of human services, or another special agency. Each state must have an Interagency Coordinating Council that ensures that multidisciplinary services are available no matter which state agency is in the lead position. If a clinician is unaware of how to make a referral, the best first place to call is the public education authority that can steer the family to the proper agency, if it is not the schools.

Once a child is identified as eligible for early intervention, assessments are carried out to determine the extent of needs, and then all concerned parties (including family members and professionals) prepare an IFSP. The "F" in IFSP acknowledges the central role of the family in the process of early intervention.

SPECIAL EDUCATION FOR CHILDREN AGED 3 TO 21 YEARS

When parents and professionals forged the original bonds to enact special education legislation, it was recognized that the legislation would need to be broad enough to accomplish three major goals. First, uniform standards for appropriate educational services were seriously wanted. Second, a concerted shift toward community and school system responsibility was essential if children with disabilities were to receive the most appropriate services. And, third, the legislation must ensure the entitlement that previously had systematically been withheld for children with disabilities. To attain these goals, the authors of the federal legislation created a program that is comprehensive in scope and specific in detail.

Under the regulations of IDEA, states are required to provide "a full appropriate public education" for all children with disabilities. The law applies to children who are mentally retarded, hard of hearing, deaf, speech impaired,

visually limited, or seriously emotionally impaired and those who have other health impairments or multiple disabilities as well as children with specific learning disabilities. Priority is given to children with the most severe impairment.

The state education agencies are required to identify, locate, and evaluate all children with disabilities and to prepare and implement individualized education plans (IEPs) for these children. They are further required to ensure placement of children in the least restrictive environment possible and to uphold procedural safeguards for children in public schools. "Related services" needed by students to benefit from special education are also to be provided. These include transportation, counseling, physical therapy, occupational therapy, speech and hearing therapy, school health services, and diagnostic health services. Finally, states must provide in-service training for special and regular education teachers.

The *pediatric role* in special education is implied rather than delineated. Because pediatricians care for children with a wide range of disabilities, special educational services are either a resource for families or the bane of everyone's day. To work with school systems in the most effective manner, it is helpful for pediatricians to understand and engage in all aspects of the special education program, especially evaluation, services, and parent advocacy.

Individual diagnostic *evaluation* is the pivotal component of IDEA. Individual evaluations are required for every child receiving special education. The basic planning team consists of the child's teacher, a representative of special education, one or both parents, and other individuals at the discretion of parents or agencies, as well as the child when appropriate.

Although IDEA does not specifically require physician input in regard to the individualized education plan, many states do. There is considerable variation, however, in the extent of the involvement required. In some states, all that is necessary is a statement regarding a recent physical examination. In others, specific questionnaires are used to pinpoint areas of educational relevance. In still others, the physician or the physician's representative is asked to be present at the IEP meeting (Palfrey, 1989).

Because pediatricians are being asked to participate in the evaluation of children with a range of disabilities from severe retardation and physical disability to emotional disorders to sensory problems and learning disabilities, it is important for clinicians to recognize the issues and questions that are foremost in the minds of the educators and parents (Walker, 1984; Porter et al, 1992). When children are referred to pediatricians for the "medical" portion of the IEP, it is likely that the evaluation team wants a number of issues to be addressed. First, there is the lingering hope that somehow the physician can determine the cause of the child's problem and that then the child can be cured. It is thus extremely important that the physician document the efforts that have been made to establish a cause or cure for the disorder and spend some time explaining what is and is not understood about the child's problem, treatment, and prognosis. Second, educators wish to know the behavioral consequences of the child's disorder. Will the child be experiencing seizures in the classroom; is he or she likely or unlikely to interact with other children; are there any safety considerations? Third, the team will probably want as full an exploration of the child's history, current neurodevelopmental status, and attention-activity modulation as possible.

Although assessment of some of these areas will undoubtedly be covered by other specialists, the pediatrician is often in a good position to synthesize many issues, adding the longitudinal perspective derived from history taking or from a long-term relationship with the child. To have a better personal understanding of the developmental, functional, and behavioral issues under team consideration, the physician may wish to obtain some observational data (Levine, Brooks, and Shonkoff, 1980). This process can help the pediatrician to concentrate the medical reports on issues of highest relevance for the evaluation team.

The major *service* to be provided under IDEA and state laws is special education. However, the law also calls for the provision of "related services" needed by the student to benefit from special education.

The "related services" aspect of the law challenges school systems to work with community health and mental health agencies to ensure that no barriers to special education remain unaddressed. A variety of systems have been established by school districts across the United States to meet the related services section of the law. Although many of these have worked well, there have been persistent problems in a number of areas, including counseling, supervision, and the extent to which school systems should be involved in the diagnosis of and therapy for certain mental and physical conditions (Palfrey, 1994).

For pediatricians, one of the most important developments in special education has been the increasing call on schools to provide health-related services and school-based nursing care. Because of advances in medical knowledge and technology availability, more and more severely ill children are living longer lives depending on devices such as tracheostomies, oxygen administrators, respirators, suctioning, gastric feeding lines, central venous lines, ostomies, ureteral or urethral catheterization, and dialysis (Office of Technology Assessment, 1987). Most of these children are well enough to attend school if the necessary nursing support programs are available. In 1984, the Supreme Court heard *Tatro v. the Irving Independent School District*, which involved a young girl with myelomeningocele who required clean intermittent catheterization during school. The court ruled that clean intermittent catheterization should be seen as a "related service" that must be provided to remove the barrier to the child's education.

The Tatro case has extensive ramifications. Schools now must provide any nursing service required by a child in special education. A new manual is now available on the care of children with health technologic needs in the classroom (Porter et al, 1997). Payment remains the ultimate responsibility of the state. Over the past few years, significant clashes and controversies have revolved around this issue. Pediatricians with patients who are assisted by medical technology are advised that the state does, in fact, have the final fiscal responsibility for such services. As a result of the OBRA legislation of 1989 (PL 100-360, Medicare Catastrophic Coverage Act), schools are now reaching out to the Medicaid agency for coverage of such services for children who are Medicaid eligible (Fox Health Policy Consultants, 1991).

Central to the concept of special education is *parent participation*. IDEA is in many ways a "consumer law." The position of parents vis-à-vis the educational system is protected by the due process clauses within the law. Physicians are in a position to help parents share actively in the decision-making process. This is a role to which parents are unaccustomed, and they often want to have a helping professional available for consultation and advice. This is particularly true for parents of low socioeconomic status and ethnic minority background (Palfrey et al, 1989). Pediatricians can play a major advocacy role for families by acquainting them with their rights and coaching them in ways to approach school systems.

Parents also frequently want a second opinion, and IDEA allows them to seek this from their physicians. When this happens, physicians should consider the request as a call for mediation by the parents between themselves and the school. They should therefore obtain as much educational information as possible while maintaining some distance from the school. In addition, physicians should try to avoid preconceived biases toward one or another specialty. They should try to interpret the specialists' reports within the context of the whole child.

As advocates for children, physicians can join with parents to monitor their state education laws to see that these conform to IDEA. This is especially important in times of federal and state funding cutbacks, when compromise of quality and standards may be the consequence.

Future Directions

Legislation provides a foundation upon which people build living, working structures. The outcomes depend on many factors, including the resources allotted, the commitment and support provided, and the presence or absence of competing demands. Some chapters of the IDEA saga delineate successes for children with severe physical disabilities and sensory impairments. Others document tragedies of promises half fulfilled for high school–aged youngsters from minority backgrounds who have learning disabilities. Monitoring, vigilance, and advocacy are warranted to ensure that high-quality services are furnished at every level and that providers have adequate training and support to carry out their assignments.

Such monitoring is best carried out by professionals and families working in concert. Several vehicles for such collaboration exist. One of the most accessible is Family Voices, a membership organization that provides information on a reliable and timely basis to parents and professionals so that, if need be, a combined voice can speak out to protect and advance special education services for children with disabilities.

REFERENCES

Fox Health Policy Consultants, Lewin and Associates: Medicaid Coverage of Health-Related Services for Children Receiving Special Education: An Examination of Federal Policies. Washington, DC, US Government Printing Office, 1991.

Horne RL: The education of children and youth with special needs: what do the laws say? NICHCY News Digest 1:1, 1991.

Individuals with Disabilities Education Act (PL 101-476). Vol. 20 USC, Chapter 33, §1400–1485 (1990).

Levine MD, Brooks R, Shonkoff J: A Pediatric Approach to Learning Disorders. New York, John Wiley & Sons, 1980.

Mills v. Board of Education of the District of Columbia: 348 F. Supp. 866 (DDC 1972).

Office of Technology Assessment: Technology-dependent children: hospital vs. homecare. Washington, DC, US Government Printing Office, 1987.

Palfrey JS: Community Child Health: An Action Plan for Today. Westport, Praeger, 1994.

Palfrey JS: Health care needs of children in special education programs. *In* Rubin L, Crocker A (eds): Developmental Disabilities: Delivery of Medical Care for Children and Adults. Philadelphia, Lea & Febiger, 1989.

Palfrey JS, Walker DK, Butler JA, Singer JD: Patterns of family response to raising a child with chronic disabilities: an assessment in five metropolitan school districts. Am J Orthopsych 59:94, 1989.

Pennsylvania Association for Retarded Citizens v. Commonwealth of Pennsylvania. 334 F Supp 1257 (ED Pa 1971) and 343 F Supp (ED Pa 1972).

Porter S, Burkley J, Bierle T, et al: Working Toward a Balance in Our Lives: A Booklet for Families of Children With Disabilities and Special Health Care Needs. Boston, MA, Project School Care, The Children's Hospital, 1992.

Porter S, Haynie M, Bierle T, et al (eds): Children and Youth Assisted by Medical Technology in Educational Settings: Guidelines for Care. Baltimore, Paul H. Brooks Publishing Co, 1997.

Walker DK: Care of chronically ill children in schools. Pediatr Clin North Am 31:221, 1984.

89 *The Right to Be Different*

Melvin D. Levine • William B. Carey •
Allen C. Crocker

 As the chapters of this book have come together, we have gathered stories from a notable assemblage of children and families amid diverse circumstances and conditions. Spurred by varied messages from the cell nucleus, buffeted sometimes by unsettling environmental forces, or reacting to injury or inner conundrums, these children and their families find themselves differing from most others. Even more commonly, individual children are unusual merely through the chaos of natural variation or the innate range of personal expression found in human beings. In this final chapter, we pause to reflect on the personal meaning and effects of being different.

There is a societal expectation that persons will conform in appearance and style, and often an impatience toward substantial variation. Reduced options and lack of social acceptance may be costs incurred by being different. Respect for pluralism is believed to be an element of our founding resolves; in practice, differentness may invoke isolation. Those most familiar with human dissimilarity, however, ultimately become captivated by the commonality of values and the continuum of contribution.

Human Rights

A gratifying by-product of an American social revolution that began in the 1960s has been a clarification and codification of the fundamental liberties and prerogatives of all humans. A remarkable sequence of liberating and supporting measures has become part of our law and culture, providing an important remedy for many of the earlier penalties imposed on children having different attributes or needs. Much of the campaign has surrounded young persons with serious disability, but the effects have been more broadly applicable. Landmark legislation has secured and stabilized the central elements, with special acclaim appropriate for Public Law 94-142 (now incorporated in PL 105-17; see Chapter 88), Title XIX, the Developmentally Disabled Assistance and Bill of Rights Act, the Section 504 amendment to the Vocational Rehabilitation Act, and the Americans with Disabilities Act. Similar legislation has been enacted in other nations throughout the world.

Most listings of human rights as they pertain to exceptional individuals deal with a common basic inventory (Crocker and Cushna, 1976). They invoke a defense of "normal rights," such as family living, educational opportunities, treatment and rehabilitation services, employment opportunities, establishment of contracts, and confidentiality in personal records. It is then essential to state as well certain "special rights" that acknowledge particular vulnerability, including issues of guardianship, protection in drug or behavioral treatments, consent in experimental procedures, counseling regarding reproduction, and intelligent exposure to life situations involving risk. In recent times an increasing emphasis has been placed as well on securing a setting of specifically "nor-malized" experiences and circumstances and freedom from architectural and environmental barriers.

It is reasonable to state that a good amount of success has been achieved regarding the right to education, treatment, employment, the legalistic aspects of protection, and elimination of architectural barriers, although vigilance is continually needed. A substantial lag pertains in the social realm.

The Very Standard Deviation

What is meant by *different*? This has quantitative and qualitative elements. Not uncommonly an instrument-dependent norm is established (e.g., regarding intelligence or visual acuity) by studies of an accessible population. In the same human group, 1 standard deviation of measurement away from the norm then represents a "borderline" situation, with troubling unusualness but redemption if personal factors are favorable. It is a reality that 2 standard deviations of "downward" variation indicate true exceptionality (e.g., mild mental retardation; see Chapter 56). Four or 5 such standard deviations produce an abnormality so assertive as to be culturally startling, and a sequence of potential exclusion begins. These difficulties are multiplied when behavior or social style is simultaneously aberrant.

The relativity of exceptionality is further demonstrated by consideration of special human circumstances. Groce (1980) has described the responses on the island of Martha's Vineyard in the 18th and 19th centuries to an extraordinary incidence of hereditary deafness, potentiated by environmentally conditioned consanguineous mating. Serious deafness existed in some remote villages at a rate ranging from 4% to 25%, producing a situation in which this usually exceptional disability became a "normal" element of rural life. As a consequence, young persons grew up learning sign language as a natural aid to local relations; church services were automatically conducted in sign and verbal communication simultaneously; and no prejudicial implications existed for deafness.

Other instances of acceptance of pervasive disability are known in certain large pedigrees in which "the disease" in the family has become a fact of life (such as the unusual reticuloendotheliosis described by Omenn [1965]). This is particularly true in X-linked syndromes, in which there can be a quiet tolerance of the fatal involvement of many male children. A special population of persons with Hunter disease exists in the Catskill area of New York State, in which death from this disabling mucopolysaccharidosis occurs typically in the 4th or 5th decade (Beebe and Formel, 1954). The involved males have been well integrated into the rural setting, although they have compelling personal special needs.

It has been appropriately championed that virtually all humans who have some degree of differentness resemble "normals" in many more ways than they differ from them. Moreover, they may differ from each other in more ways than they differ from normalcy. They harbor the same emotional feelings, yearnings for rewarding social relations, potential for growth, and liability to injury, suffering, and disease. Brightman (1975), in a small book for the instruction of children, has warmly expressed this universality across diversity by voicing, "I hope you can see, just how much you're like me. . . ."

The Enabling of Labeling

Issues relating to the effects of assigning diagnostic "labels" to variant children have been vigorously discussed in the past decade, with a predictable ambiguity in the conclusions. In the educational or clinical milieu there is a tempting utility in appropriating an accurate descriptive term linking a child to others with the same or similar characteristics so that specialized services can be mobilized. Furthermore, it is a reality that consumer group achievements in the promotion and defense of programmatic rights have rallied around common convictions solidified by categorical labeling. At the same time, fears of elaborating self-fulfilling prophesies and biased service design are well founded. Mandell and Fiscus (1981) summarized some risks of diagnostic labels in the educational setting as follows:

- Labeling detracts from the development of appropriate individualized programs.
- Labels once assigned are difficult to remove.
- Labeling and subsequent categorical placement limit the opportunities for normal children to become familiar with pupils with disabilities.
- Labeling tends to establish conditions for mistakes in assessment of minority group children.
- Labeling minimizes the significance of societal and environmental factors.

Unquestionably the act of labeling courts the risk of mislabeling. This can occur in a variety of ways. It is perhaps best illustrated in considering children with behav-

ioral and relatively low-severity learning problems. In responding to the compulsion to find a diagnostic tag for a child, a clinician may seek to identify and feature only one aspect of a child's complex plight. There may be endless discussions about whether his or her failure to learn is primarily "emotional" or a "learning disability." In reality it is likely that such students suffer from an amalgam of factors that may include neurologic predispositions, negative educational experiences, unresolved stresses at home, maladaptive coping strategies, difficulties with attention, or inadequate or overly coercive role models. To reduce such factors to one diagnosis may represent a real injustice and, more importantly, may thwart the mobilization of a much-needed multifaceted intervention program.

Diagnostic labels also run the risk of reflecting the training and disciplinary biases of the labeler. A professional who is most comfortable in dealing with family problems may brand a child who is having school problems as "emotionally disturbed." One who is more neurologically biased may relate the same observable phenomena in school to cortical abnormality. Although disciplinary inclinations never can be totally eliminated, it is likely that labels will encourage these propensities.

Diagnostic labels may become as permanent as a tattoo. They may penetrate so deeply as to be nearly impossible to excise from the identity of a person. This may affect how others view the person and also how that person perceives himself or herself. In short, children grow and they change; their labels may grow and not change. Labels may artificially exceed the scientific limits of assessment. In the field of developmental and behavioral pediatrics, for many clinical conditions diagnostic criteria are far from clear-cut. Features of some disorders tend to overlap. For example, many of the traits described as being typical of children with depression also are applicable to those with deficits of attention. In both groups, self-deprecatory comments, problems with sleep, dysphoria, somatic complaints, agitated behavior, and low self-esteem are common. Whether a child is labeled as having an attention deficit, depression, or both may be a fairly arbitrary decision.

Closely related to the issue of labeling is the broader matter that might be called assessment semantics. The selection of words to describe a child's behavior, a perceived delay, or an individual difference can have major implications in terms of the way in which the world views and treats that child. For example, a particular youngster may be called "immature" by his or her teacher. The teacher may be referring to a pattern of behavior that includes impulsivity, emotional lability, overactivity, and an inability to persist at tasks. The entire complex of traits, in fact, may be secondary to some underlying learning problems that are impairing the child's adjustment to school. However, because the word "immaturity" was selected to describe the phenomenon, the implication is that the child will "outgrow it," that no service is needed, and perhaps that the child should be retained in first grade! The more basic decision about whether a child really has a problem can be influenced strongly by choices of words to describe phenomena. A youngster may be described as "highly independent," or, alternatively, the same child may be thought of as "a disciplinary problem" or "a loner." The connotations differ considerably. A child who has unusual interests tending toward noncomformity might be described by some observers as "socially maladjusted," whereas others might commend the child's willingness to "do his or her own thing." It is of interest that the term *eccentric* is seldom used in describing children. This may reflect a tendency to characterize and label unusual behavior in children as pathologic.

Responses to Variation: Public and Private

Bewilderment is a common reaction to the unfamiliar. Social ostracism by peers and adults may be practiced against a child with unusual physical features or behavior, generally as a reflection of observer uncertainty. In earlier times this often led to a lasting residential segregation (Cushna, 1976). Now armed with legislative support of the right to education in the least restrictive environment, the child with special needs also poses a perceived economic threat to the mainline citizenry. Development of individualized educational plans is undertaken in 10% to 20% of school children, varying in proportion to the basic affluence and resources of the school district. The fact is that these support systems (even when they include psychotherapy, other special services, recreational components, and 12-month coverage) are still less costly than the outcomes of neglect (or care under the old institutional system).

Bewilderment is assuredly also shared by the unusual child, who is awash in the phenomena of a world he or she never made. Being out of synchrony with one's peers robs one of needed positive feedback and is destructive of self-image. In recent times, supported by the Association for Retarded Citizens groups, young adults with mental retardation have launched a productive movement of self-advocacy.

Differentness in their children exacts a toll from parents as well. Featherstone (1980) documented eloquently the universal responses of guilt, fear, loneliness, and anger felt by mothers and fathers of children with developmental disabilities. "This type of child should not be in a public place," a mother was told by another shopper when she took her non-acting-out but unusual-appearing daughter with profound retardation to a supermarket (reported in a recent clinic experience). Effects on brothers and sisters are significant, but the outcomes are notably successful (Crocker, 1983).

In recent years there has been a gratifying new awareness of stylistic differences. Variations in styles of being parents present a wide range of workable and interesting modes of nurturance. At the same time, enhanced appreciation of infant and child temperament has promulgated a greater clinical tolerance for behavioral variation and the expression of unique styles during childhood. With this has come a new awareness of "the match," the nearly fortuitous but critical encounter between a child's unique stylistic and cognitive repertoire and the personal needs, expectations, and values of an important adult, such as a parent or a teacher.

Getting Children Changed

Attempts to remedy variation can result from a complex of motivations. Pressing to change a child into a more con-forming presentation, to relieve the stress of unusualness per se, must be thoughtfully reviewed. The use of psychoactive medications, for example, as a quick alleviation of the burden in children with atypical behavior may be a substitute for a more penetrating, child-focused program of primary assistance in behavioral adaptation or, alternatively, tolerance by adults. Another example is the undertaking of cosmetic surgery on the faces of young children with Down syndrome. Revisions of the special phenotypic features of the eyelids, nose, ears, and tongue can be safe but have no clinical defense.

Counseling and guidance also raise significant ethical questions. Is there a danger that the therapist or counselor will superimpose his or her own values on a naive child? To what extent do various forms of therapeutic counseling edge the child toward uniformity and conformity? Should one press the development of social skills for a youngster who prefers to be alone? If a child appears to have gross motor delays and shows little or no interest in sports, is the adult world privileged to insist on physical education for the child? It may be that such a child would prefer not to feature motor pursuits in his or her activities. Children, in fact, may have a right to "specialize." They may need help in resisting the overriding drive of adults to make them good at almost everything. Specialization appears to be a right that is reserved for grown-ups. In certain instances it may need to be afforded to children also. At the very least, one should pause when a youngster about to undergo therapy protests, "You know, I like the way I am." One must modulate one's zeal to promulgate a standard form of adjustment. There may be some youngsters who are not fitting in particularly comfortably during childhood but are destined to be more effective adults than they are children. Altering their childhood conformation, in fact, may worsen their prognosis.

A Final Word

If there is a commitment to the vitality of a pluralistic society, with its enrichment by the contributions of diverse citizens, there is indeed "the right to be different." There are increasing examples of this in our culture:

- The movement for assistance in adoption of "hard to place" children (e.g., those who have developmental disabilities or behavioral disorders) has been strikingly successful. In effect this has transformed the rejected child into the avidly chosen child. Many hundreds of adoptions of children with Down syndrome have now taken place, and in most major cities there is a waiting list of couples for adoption of infants and young children with Down syndrome.
- The reform of "deinstitutionalization," bringing persons with serious disabilities into circumstances of community living, has led to substantial victories. Major functional gains are commonplace when individualized programs are provided.
- In the "new" special education, the excitement of learning has been successfully incorporated into a vastly broader scope. The child who is nonverbal but then speaks with the use of augmentative communi-

cation, the young child with autism who is able to be established in a regular class after home parent training, the atypical youth who receives reimbursement for graded accomplishments in a vocational training program—these are victories of the social revolution.

- When parent–professional communication is thoughtfully developed, the quality of parenthood in unusual circumstances can be enormously reinforced, to the gain of all parties. Self-help groups have been important as well in improving parental understanding of differentness. As one mother reported, "First I realized what she would never be, then I learned what she did not have to be, and finally I think I have come to terms with what she is and can be" (Pueschel, 1978).

- The orientation of young adults to the helping professions developed a momentum in the 1960s and 1970s and has been sustained. "Working with children" remains a major preoccupation of thoughtful youth, and assuredly youthful enthusiasm and insights are needed in developmental and behavioral programs. Acceptances of differences in human style and expression have characterized the recent generation.

The variations in human presentation delineated in this book can be considered the products of phenotypic, genotypic, sociocultural, and individual circumstances that characterize our species. The concept of "normal" or "average" is statistically perceivable but often subject to political inducement, and it is assuredly humanistically irrelevant on many occasions. We have much to learn from a far broader view and much to celebrate.

REFERENCES

Beebe RT, Formel PF: Gargoylism: sex-linked transmission in nine males. Trans Am Clin Climatol Assoc 66:199, 1954.

Brightman AJ: Like Me. Cambridge, MA, Behavioral Education Projects, 1975.

Crocker AC: Sisters and brothers. *In* Mulick JA, Pueschel SM (eds): Parent-Professional Partnerships in Developmental Disabilities Services. Cambridge, MA, The Ware Press, 1983.

Crocker AC, Cushna B: Ethical considerations and attitudes in the field of developmental disorders. *In* Johnston RB, Magrab PR (eds): Developmental Disorders: Evaluation, Treatment, and Education. Baltimore, University Park Press, 1976.

Cushna B: They'll be happier with their own kind. *In* Koocher GP (ed): Children's Rights and the Mental Health Professions. New York, John Wiley & Sons, 1976.

Featherstone H: A Difference in the Family: Living with a Disabled Child. New York, Basic Books, 1980.

Groce N: Everyone here spoke sign language. Nat Hist 89:10, 1980.

Mandell CJ, Fiscus E: Understanding Exceptional People. St. Paul, MN, West Publishing Co, 1981.

Omenn GS: Familial reticuloendotheliosis with eosinophilia. N Engl J Med 273:427, 1965.

Pueschel SM (ed): Down Syndrome: Growing and Learning. Kansas City, Sheed Andrews & McMeel, 1978.

Index

Note: Page numbers in *italics* refer to illustrations; page numbers followed by (t) refer to tables.

PEERAMID (Pediatric Examination of
  Educational Readiness at Middle
  Childhood) *(Continued)*
  attention testing with, 513, *513*
PEEX (Pediatric Early Elementary
  Examination), 701
Pelizaeus-Merzbacher disease, *738*
Pemoline, 812(t)
  as abused drug, 486(t)
Penetrance, genetic principle of, 215
Penis, adolescent sexual development
  affecting, 72, *460*, 461(t)
  pubertal lengthening of, 72
Perception. See also *Attention; Cognitive
  function; Sensory function.*
  haptic, 572–573, 575
  middle childhood level of, 56–57, 62(t)
  newborn level of, 19–20
  spatial. See *Visual-spatial ability.*
Perfectionism, child "hothoused" by,
  163(t), 169
Peripheral nervous system, disorders
  related to, 738, 740
Persistence, temperament categorized by,
  91, 93(t), 97(t)
Personal history theory, 4
Personality. See also *Behavior;
  Individuality; Temperament.*
  giftedness effect on, 654–655
  historic studies related to, 1–12, *2*
  psychological testing of, 729(t), 730
Perspiration, adolescent development
  and, *460*, 461
  axillary, *460*, 461
Pervasive developmental disorder, 594,
  594
  atypical, *594*
  autism in, 589–590, 590(t)
  diagnosis of, 617
  not-otherwise-specified, *594*, 595–596
Petechiae, meningococcemia causing, 286
Petting, sexual development role of,
  463–464
Peyote, 485(t)
Phencyclidine (PCP), 485(t)
  analogues of, 487(t)
Phenobarbital, 281(t), 282(t)
  effects of, 282(t)
  pharamacokinetics of, 281(t)
  seizure therapy using, 280(t)–282(t),
  281
Phenothiazines, 815(t)
Phenotype, 215
  behavioral, 226(t), 226–228
  congenital anomalies associated with,
  252–253
Phenylketonuria, 306(t)–307(t)
  aspartame warning related to, 839
  biochemistry of, 306(t)
  neuropsychological testing affected by,
  734–735
  symptoms of, 307(t)
  treatment of, 307(t)
Phenytoin, 281(t), 282(t)
  effects of, 282(t)
  pharamacokinetics of, 281(t)
  seizure therapy using, 280(t)–282(t),
  281
Phobias, anxiety disorder with, 644–645

Phobias *(Continued)*
  drug therapy and, 826
  school avoidance due to, 542, *544*,
  546(t), 546–549
  simple, 645
  social, 644–645
Phonation, definition of, 621
Phonemes, disabilities related to, 524,
  529
  English language, 524
  motor production of, 625, 626
Phonetics, language dysfunction role of,
  523(t), 523–524
Phonology, consonant production and,
  626
  definition of, 621
  disorder of, 626
Phototherapy, premature infant in, 265
Phylogeny, 1
Physical abuse, 163–169. See also *Child
  abuse.*
  child impacted by, *164*, 164(t),
  164–166, *165*
  contributing factors for, 164, 164(t)
  definition of, 163–164, *164*
  developmental effects of, *164*, 164(t),
  164–166, *165*
  diagnosis or identification of, 166(t),
  166–167, *167*
  family dysfunction accompanied by,
  163, 163(t), 163–169, *164*, 164(t),
  165, *167*
  food related to, 163(t), 167–168
  forms of, 163(t), 163–169, 164(t)
  health care neglect as, *163*, 163(t),
  168–169
  housing inadequacy aspects of, 163(t),
  168
  management approach to, 166–167,
  167
  signs and symptoms of, 166(t),
  166–167, *167*
Physical restraint, legal issues about, 866
Piaget, Jean, beaker experiment of, 58
  pioneer role of, *2*, 2–3, 10–11
  sexual development theory of, 459(t)
  stages of infant cognitive function
  classified by, 32–34, 33(t)
Pica, 396
  lead ingested in, 304
  parental concern about, 396
Picking, 436
  fingernail affected by, *435*
  nose affected by, 436
Pimozide, tic disorder treated with, 438,
  439(t)
Pineal gland, sleep regulation by, 423
Pink disease (acrodynia), mercury
  causing, 318
Pinna, 257, *257*
  congenital anomalies of, *256*, *256*
  minor, 252–253
  normal landmarks of, 257
Pitch, audiometric testing and, 560, *561*
  common sounds possessing, 560, *561*
Pituitary gland, puberty initiation role of,
  460
Placenta, 17, 210
  behavioral development studies related
  to, 210, *212*

Placenta *(Continued)*
  substances crossing, 17
Play, 25(t), 33(t), 34
  cross-cultural variations in, 110, *110*
  disaster reenactment in, 193
  infant development of, 25(t), 33(t), 34
  Piagetian stage related to, 33(t), 34
  sexual aspects of, 458–459
Pleasure-seeking, development theory
  role of, 9–10
Poisoning, 312–319
  aluminum, 318
  arsenic, 318
  carbon monoxide, 318–319
  heavy metal, 315–318
  lead, 180, 303–304, *315*, 315–318, *316*.
  See also *Lead.*
  manganese, 318
  mercury, 318
  neural development affected by, 312,
  316
  solvent, 319, 485(t)
  thallium, 318
Polydactyly, 259
  racial factors in, 253
Polysomnography, indications for, 427(t)
Pompe disease, *738*
Ponderal index, 21
Poorness, economic. See *Poverty.*
Poorness of fit model, 89–90
  behavioral development in, 89–90, *90*,
  93(t)
  individuality development in, 89–90,
  90
Poppers, as abused drug, 485(t)
Popularity, giftedness effect on, 654–655
  middle childhood and, 60
Population density, cross-cultural
  variations and, 108–109
  low vs. high, 108–109
Positive reinforcement, behavior
  management using, 767–769, 768(t)
Positron emission tomography, CNS
  disorder diagnosed with, 741
Possessions, overabundance of, 185–186
Posttraumatic stress disorder, 645–646
  accidental injury causing, 830–831
  course of, 646
  definition of, 645–646
  disasters eliciting, 192–195, 193(t)
  epidemiology of, 646
  treatment of, 646
Posture, low birth weight baby handling
  and, 270–271, *271*, *272*
Potter sequence, 249–250
  oligohydramnios and, 249
Poverty, 177–184
  clinical impact of, 178–181
  child mortality increase in, 178–179
  developmental aspects of, 179–180,
  184
  homelessness associated with,
  180–181
  morbidity increase in, 179–180
  trauma in, 179
  definition of, 177
  formulation of public policy on, 184
  index of, 177
  interventional programs directed at,
  181(t), 181–184